Comprehensive Child
and Family Nursing Skills

# Comprehensive Child and Family Nursing Skills


EDITOR

**DONNA PHILLIPS SMITH, RN, MS**
Pediatric Nurse Consultant
Clinical Nurse I, Pediatrics
Saint Francis Hospital
Formerly Assistant Professor
University of Tulsa School of Nursing
Tulsa, Oklahoma

UNIT EDITORS

**KRISTIE S. NIX, RN, EdD**
Associate Professor
University of Tulsa School of Nursing
Tulsa, Oklahoma

**JOAN YOUNG KEMPER, RN, MS**
Nursing Instructor
University of Wyoming at Casper
Formerly Chief Nurse, Pediatrics/Pediatric ICU
City of Faith Hospital
Tulsa, Oklahoma

**ROSEMARY LIGUORI, RN, MSN, CPNA**
Assistant Professor
Northeastern State University Division of Nursing
Tahlequah, Oklahoma
Maternal-Child Health Consultant
Oklahoma State Health Department
Formerly in association with
Richard Lisciandro, MD, FAAP
Jamestown, New York

**DEBORAH KAY BRANTLY, RN, MS**
Director of Nursing and Quality Assurance
Shadow Mountain Institute
Therapist, Private Practice
Tulsa, Oklahoma

**JUDY HOLT ROLLINS, RN, MS**
Child Health Care Consultant
National Consultant for Very Special Arts
Washington, D.C.

**NANCY VALENTINE STEVENS, RN, MS, CPNP**
Doctoral Candidate
Oklahoma State University
Stillwater, Oklahoma
Formerly Assistant Professor
Northeastern State University, Division of Nursing
Tahlequah, Oklahoma

**LYNN B. CLUTTER, RN, MSN**
Child Health and Parenting Consultant
Tulsa, Oklahoma

CONSULTANT

**DONNA L. WONG, RN, MN, PNP**

With original photography by

**JOHN ROY**
Saint Francis Hospital
Tulsa, Oklahoma


With 364 illustrations


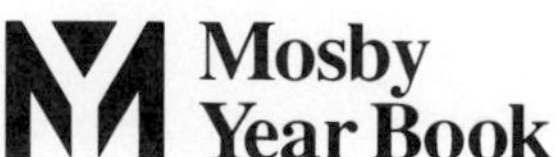


St. Louis Baltimore Boston Chicago London Philadelphia Sydney Toronto

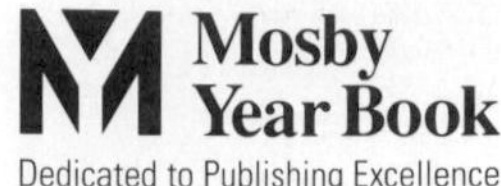


Editor: William Grayson Brottmiller
Developmental editor: Winifred Sullivan
Project manager: Carol Sullivan Wiseman
Production editor: David S. Brown
Cover Design: David Zielinski



Printed in the United States of America

Mosby–Year Book, Inc.
11830 Westline Industrial Drive
St. Louis, Missouri 63146

Comprehensive child and family nursing skills / editor, Donna Phillips Smith; unit editors, Kristie S. Nix ... [et al.]; consultant, Donna L. Wong.
p. cm.
Includes bibliographical references and index.
ISBN 0-8016-5209-X
1. Pediatric nursing. 2. Family nursing. I. Smith, Donna Phillips. II. Wong, Donna L., 1948-
[DNLM: 1. Family--nurses' instruction. 2. Nursing Process. 3. Pediatric Nursing. WY 159 C7365]
RJ245.C626 1990
610.73′62—dc20
DNLM/DLC
for Library of Congress 90-13648
CIP

GW/VH/VH 9 8 7 6 5 4 3 2

# Contributors

***LISA K. ANDERSON, RN, BSN**
Patient Care Supervisor, Pediatrics
Saint Francis Hospital
Tulsa, Oklahoma

**MARY M. ARUDA, RN, MSN, CPNP**
Adolescent Nurse Practitioner
Children's Hospital
Boston, Massachusetts

**CATHERINE C. AYOUB, RN, MN, EdM**
Clinical Nurse Consultant in Private Practice
Clinical Fellow in Psychology
Harvard Medical School
Cambridge, Massachusetts

**MARY C. BARON, RNC, MS**
Clinical Nurse Specialist, Neuroscience
Children's Hospital of Los Angeles
Los Angeles, California

***SHERRY BAZE, RN, MA, CPNP**
Pediatric Nurse Practitioner
Muskogee County Health Department
Muskogee, Oklahoma

**PATRICIA BEACHY, RN, MS**
Clinical Nurse Specialist
University Hospital at the
University of Colorado Health Sciences Center
Denver, Colorado

**DEBBIE R. BERRY, RN, MS**
Pulmonary Clinical Nurse Specialist
Oklahoma Children's Memorial Hospital
Oklahoma City, Oklahoma

**DORA BRADLEY, RN, MS**
Former Nursing Development Program Manager
Oklahoma Children's Memorial Hospital
Oklahoma City, Oklahoma
Doctoral Candidate, University of South Carolina
Columbia, South Carolina

***MARY BREEN, RN, MS**
Craniofacial Clinical Nurse Specialist
Children's Medical Center
Dallas, Texas

**PAMELA A. BROWN, RN, MS, CCRN**
Clinical Nurse Specialist
Pediatric Intensive Care Unit
Children's Hospital of Los Angeles
Los Angeles, California

**PAMELA K. CHRISTENSEN, RN, ADN**
Former Charge Nurse, Pediatrics
City of Faith Hospital
Tulsa, Oklahoma
Cross Country Health Care Personnel
Boca Raton, Florida

**JANE DEACON, RNC, MS, NNP**
Neonatal Nurse Practitioner
The Children's Hospital
Denver, Colorado

***DONNA MARIE DE SIMONE, RN, MS, CNS**
Clinical Nurse Specialist, Pediatrics
Saint John Medical Center
Tulsa, Oklahoma

***BONNIE UTHOFF DOLSON, RN, MS**
Formerly Assistant Professor
BSN Department Nursing
Houston Baptist University
Houston, Texas

**JACQUELINE DOWLING, RN, MS**
Director Nursing Laboratory, School of Nursing
University of Lowell
Lowell, Massachusetts

***PEGGY J. DRAPO, RN, PhD**
Professor, Texas Women's University
Denton, Texas

**MELANIE C. DREHER, RN, PhD**
Dean and Professor
University of Massachusetts at Amherst
School of Nursing
Amherst, Massachusetts

---

*Also reviewed selected skills.

***MIDGE ELLIOT, RN, MA, MS**
Assistant Professor
University of Tulsa School of Nursing
Tulsa, Oklahoma

**KAREN S. FARR, RN, CPNP**
Clinical Nurse II
Pediatric Intensive Care Unit
Saint Francis Hospital
Tulsa, Oklahoma

**SANDRA L. GARDNER, RN, MS, PNP**
Director, Professional Outreach Consultation
Neonatal/Perinatal/Pediatric Consultant
Aurora, Colorado

**SHARON M. GLASS, RNC, MS, CNNP**
Neonatal Nurse Clinician
Eastern Oklahoma Perinatal Center
Saint Francis Hospital
Tulsa, Oklahoma

***KAREN T. GRAVES, RN, MN, CNSN**
Clinical Specialist, Nutrition Support Team
Children's Hospital of Los Angeles
Los Angeles, California

**JANICE S. HAYES, RN, PhD**
Associate Dean
University of Miami School of Nursing
Research Consultant
Miami Children's Hospital
Miami, Florida

**KELLY LANNON HENDERSON, RN, BSN**
Clinical Nurse I, Pediatrics
Saint Francis Hospital
Tulsa, Oklahoma

***CARYN STOERMER HESS, RN, MS**
Nurse Consultant
Englewood, Colorado

**MARGARET P. IRETON, RN, BSN**
Staff Nurse
Children's Medical Center
Tulsa, Oklahoma

**PATRICIA A. JAMERSON, RN, MSN**
Outreach Coordinator, Clinical Nurse Specialist
Eastern Oklahoma Perinatal Center
Saint Francis Hospital
Tulsa, Oklahoma

**LYDIA JOHNSON, RN, BSN**
Diabetes Education
Saint Francis Hospital
Tulsa, Oklahoma

***CHRISTINA ALGIERE KASPRISIN, RN, MS**
Quality Attainment Coordinator,
Saint Francis Hospital
Assistant Clinical Professor
University of Oklahoma College of Nursing
Tulsa, Oklahoma

**SYLVIA KERR, RN, MS**
Associate Professor
University of Tulsa School of Nursing
Tulsa, Oklahoma

**DEBORAH S. LAMMERT, RN, MSN, CCRN**
Pediatric Cardiovascular Clinical Nurse Specialist
Saint Francis Hospital
Tulsa, Oklahoma

**JANET LUDGAR, RN, MSN, CNS**
Clinical Nurse, Pediatric Hematology/Oncology
Loma Linda University Medical Center
Loma Linda, California

***BOBBIE J. MACKAY, RN, MSN, MSW**
Pulmonary Clinical Nurse Specialist
Washington University Medical Center
St. Louis, Missouri

**TERESA MARGAGLIO, RN, MSN, IBCLC**
Certified Lactation Consultant in Private Practice
Instructor in Pediatrics
University of Southwestern Louisiana
Lafayette, Louisiana

**BARBARA L. MARINO, RN, PhD**
Nurse Researcher
Children's Hospital
Boston, Massachusetts

***ELIZABETH A. MARKS, RNC, MS**
Clinical Nurse Specialist, Nutrition Support Team
Children's Hospital of Los Angeles
Los Angeles, California

**BARBARA MARTIN, RN, MS**
Professor
University of Tulsa School of Nursing
Tulsa, Oklahoma

**KELLY McCAMPBELL, RN, MS**
Genetic Counselor/Nursing Education
Children's Hospital of Oklahoma
Oklahoma City, Oklahoma

**FRANCES LYNN McCULLOUGH, RNP, MNSc, ONC**
Orthopedic Clinical Nurse Specialist
Arkansas Spine Center
Little Rock, Arkansas

***NOREEN HEER NICOL, RN, MS, FNC**
Dermatology Clinical Specialist
National Jewish Center for
Immunology and Respiratory Medicine
Denver, Colorado

**MARY C. OBERC, RN, MSN**
Former Instructor of Nursing
Anna Vaughn School of Nursing
Oral Roberts University
Tulsa, Oklahoma

***LYNDA LOWE ODAFFER, RN, MS**
Assistant Professor
University of Tulsa School of Nursing
Tulsa, Oklahoma

***RITA J. PAYTON, RN, MS, DA**
Former Director and Professor
University of Tulsa School of Nursing
Tulsa, Oklahoma

***KATHRYN A. PERRY, RN, MSN**
Pediatric Clinical Nurse Specialist
Saint Francis Hospital
Tulsa, Oklahoma

**BEVERLEE E. REDDING, RN, MS**
Family Therapist, LaFortune Cancer Center
St. John Medical Center
Marriage/Family Therapist in Private Practice
Tulsa, Oklahoma

**JAYNE E. ROGERS, RNC, MSN**
Nurse Manager, Children's Hospital
Boston, Massachusetts

**ANNE SCOTT, RN, PhD**
Instructor, Anna Vaughn School of Nursing
Oral Roberts University
Tulsa, Oklahoma

**CECILIA E. SHAW, RN, MS, OCN**
Clinical Supervisor/Research Coordinator
Cancer Care Associates
Tulsa, Oklahoma

***ANNA L. SUMMERFIELD, RN**
Director, Perinatal Nursing Services
The Women's Hospital of Texas
Houston, Texas

**DONNA J. TAKACS, RNC, MS**
Director, Quality Attainment
Laureate Psychiatric Clinic and Hospital
Tulsa, Oklahoma

**CAROLYN TESTI, RN, MS**
Maternal/Child Speciality Area Instructor
St. Anthony Hospital
Oklahoma City, Oklahoma

**PATTI J. TOMBRIDGE, RN, BSN**
Clinical Nurse II, Pediatrics
Saint Francis Hospital
Tulsa, Oklahoma

***KRENA HUNTER WHITE, RN, MA, MS**
Director of Nursing Education
Associate Degree Nursing Program
Rogers State College
Claremore, Oklahoma

**ROBERTA S. WILSON, RN, BA**
Assistant Head Nurse, Burn Center
Burn Nurse Specialist
Coordinator of In-service Education
Oklahoma Children's Memorial Hospital
Oklahoma City, Oklahoma

***DONNA L. WONG, RN, MN, PNP**
Nurse Consultant
Saint Francis Hospital
Tulsa, Oklahoma

# Additional Reviewers*

**GEORGIA ADAMS, RN, DNSc, CS**
Formerly Director Mental Health-Outpatient
Hillcrest Medical Center
Tulsa, Oklahoma

**ANNE ALLEN, RN, CPAN**
Patient Care Supervisor, Post-Anesthesia Care Unit
Saint Francis Hospital
Contributing Editor for Journal of Post Anesthesia Nursing
Tulsa, Oklahoma

**CONNIE MORAIN BAKER, MS**
Child Life Specialist Consultant
Oklahoma City, Oklahoma

**JANICE ELAINE BROWN, RN, BS, CPNA**
Program Coordinator, Research in Pediatric Neurology
John F. Kennedy Institute
Johns Hopkins University
Baltimore, Maryland

**PAULETTE BURNS, RN, PhD**
Division Director, Assistant Professor
University of Oklahoma, Tulsa Campus
Tulsa, Oklahoma

**CONNIE STEWART CARPENTER, RN, EdD**
Assistant Professor
Boise State University
Boise, Idaho

**MARGUERITE CHAPMAN, JD, LLM**
Associate Professor of Law
University of Tulsa
Tulsa, Oklahoma

**VAN G. CHAUVIN, RNC, MSN, MHS**
Family Nurse Practitioner
Dallas Independent School District
Dallas, Texas

**NOREEN CLARKE-SHEEHAN, RN, MSN**
Clinical Nurse Specialist, Craniofacial Team Coordinator
Children's Hospital of Los Angeles
Los Angeles, California

**ELLEN RUDY CLORE, RN, MSN, FNP**
Assistant Professor, Graduate College of Nursing
University of Florida
Orlando, Florida

**PATRICIA CLUNN, RN, EdD**
Professor
University of Miami School of Nursing
Miami, Florida

**DONALD R. CRAIG, DDS**
General Dentistry
Tulsa, Oklahoma

**CATHERINE CROPLEY, RN, MN**
Neonatal Nurse Educator
Charles R. Drew Medical School
Los Angeles, California

**GAIL DANEK, RN, MSN**
Clinical Nurse Specialist
Shands Hospital at University of Florida
Gainesville, Florida

**PATRICIA DEAN, RN, MSN**
Nurse Coordinator for Comprehensive Epilepsy Center
Miami Children's Hospital
Miami, Florida

**JENNIFER A. DISABATO, RN, MS**
Clinical Nurse Specialist,
Pediatric Neurosurgery
The Children's Hospital
Denver, Colorado

**JUDITH P. DOLL, MS**
Education Specialist, Automotive Safety for Children Program
James Whitcomb Riley Hospital for Children
Indianapolis, Indiana

**DIANNE FOCHTMAN, RN, MN, CPNP**
Clinical Specialist, Pediatric Oncology
Children's Memorial Hospital
Chicago, Illinois

**JACK FOREMAN, MS**
Associate Professor, Communicative Disorders
University of Tulsa
Tulsa, Oklahoma

*Reviewed selected skills.

**MARY KAY GARCIA, RN, MN**
National Consultant, Asthma and Allergy Foundation
Nurse Educator and Consultant
Missouri City, Texas

**DEBRA A. GAYER, RN, MS, CPNP**
Pulmonary Clinical Specialist
University of Missouri Hospital and Clinics
Columbia, Missouri

**MEG GILLESPIE, RN, MS**
The Children's Hospital
Denver, Colorado

**FRANCES H. GOLDMAN, EdD, LPC**
Outpatient Supervisor, Loudoun County Mental Health Center
Leesburg, Virginia

**MOLLIE L. HALL, RN, BSN, CETN**
Enterostomal Therapist
Saint Francis Hospital
Tulsa, Oklahoma

**LORI J. HOWELL, RN, MS**
Clinical Nurse Specialist, Pediatric Surgery
Assistant Clinical Professor
University of California Medical Center
San Francisco, California

**SANDRA JACOBS, RN, BSN**
Apnea Nurse Clinician
Children's Hospital of Columbus
Columbus, Ohio

**JACQUELINE C. JONES**
Automotive Safety for Children Program
James Whitcomb Riley Hospital for Children
Indianapolis, Indiana

**BETTY R. KUPPERSCHMIDT, RN, EdD**
Director of Nursing, Clinical Services
Tulsa Regional Medical Center
Tulsa, Oklahoma

**RENEE LEASURE, RN, PhD, CCRN**
Assistant Professor
College of Nursing
University of Oklahoma
Oklahoma City, Oklahoma

**MARGO McCAFFREY, RN, MS, FAAN**
Consultant in the Nursing Care of People with Pain
Santa Monica, California

**LORI A. McCLURE, RN, BS**
Health Care Consultant
Hillcrest Healthcare Systems
Tulsa, Oklahoma

**MEGAN McKEE, RN, MS**
Adolescent Nursing Coordinator
Springwood Psychiatric Institute
Leesburg, Virginia

**JOANNE B. MICHALEK, RNC, MSN**
Nurse Consultant, Child Protection Program
Children's Hospital
Boston, Massachusetts

**JULIE A. MONTGOMERY, RN, MSN**
National Rehabilitation Hospital
St. Rita's Medical Center
Lima, Ohio

**MARY BETH OGLE, RN, MS**
Education Specialist
Department of Nursing Education
Saint Francis Hospital
Tulsa, Oklahoma

**CATHEY PIELSTICKER, RN, MS, CDE**
Program Manager
Saint Francis Hospital Diabetes Center
Tulsa, Oklahoma

**KATHLEEN SIMONS PIGGOTT, MS, RN**
Pediatric Nursing Consultant
Seattle, Washington

**CAROLE L. PILES, RN, PhD**
Associate Professor
Anna Vaughn School of Nursing
Oral Roberts University
Tulsa, Oklahoma

**MARIE POGGENPOEL, RN, PhD**
Professor
Anna Vaughn School of Nursing
Oral Roberts University
Tulsa, Oklahoma

**LAURA PRATT, RN, MSN**
Health Care Missionary
Matehaula, Mexico

**MAELYNN REECE, RN, CDE**
Territory Sales Representative
Squibb-Novo, Inc.
Princeton, New Jersey

**JENNIFER J. ROARK, RN, BSN, CETN**
Enterostomal Therapist
Saint Francis Hospital
Tulsa, Oklahoma

**MARY LISA ROTH, RN, MN**
Critical Care/ECMO Clinical Nurse Specialist
The Children's Hospital
Denver, Colorado

**CINDY HYLTON RUSHTON, RNC, MSN**
Clinical Educator III, Neonatal/Infant Specialist
Children's Medical Center
Washington, D.C.

**KRISTINE M. SCHUEREN, RN, BSN**
Clinical Nurse II, Pediatric Intensive Care
Saint Francis Hospital
Tulsa, Oklahoma

**JUDITH ALLEN SHELLY, RN, BSN, MAR**
Nurses Christian Fellowship, Resource Development
Author
Frederick, Pennsylvania

**CARMEN SMITH, RN**
Head Nurse, IV Therapy
Hillcrest Medical Center
Tulsa, Oklahoma

**CINDY GREENBERG SMITH, RN, MS, CPNP**
Nurse Manager Pediatrics
Saddleback Hospital and Health Center
Laguna Hills, California

**KATHRYN SMITH, RN, MN**
Public Health Nurse Specialist/Community Care Coordinator
Los Angeles County Children's Services
Los Angeles, California

**MARY SNYDER, RN, MS**
Assistant Professor
University of Tulsa School of Nursing
Tulsa, Oklahoma

**F.L. SOMMER, DDS, MS**
Diplomate, American Academy of Pediatric Dentistry
Fellow, American Academy of Pediatric Dentistry
Tulsa, Oklahoma

**MICHAEL A. STOIKO, MD, FAAP**
Pediatric Intensivist
Director of Pediatric Intensive Care
Saint Francis Hospital
Tulsa, Oklahoma

**RHONDA STORIE, BS, ECE/CHILD LIFE**
Child Life Specialist
Hillcrest Medical Center
Tulsa, Oklahoma

**KAREN BRUNER STROUP, PhD**
Automotive Safety for Children Program
James Whitcomb Riley Hospital for Children
Indianapolis, Indiana

**LINDA A. SUMPTER, RN, BSN**
School Nurse, Tulsa Public Schools
Tulsa, Oklahoma

**LORETTA THOMPSON, RN, MS**
Century Health Care
Tulsa, Oklahoma

**IRIS TORVIK, RN, MS**
Clinical Nurse Specialist, Special Care Nursery
Hillcrest Medical Center
Tulsa, Oklahoma

**JAMES TRIPPLEHORN, BS, RRT**
Respiratory Therapy Clinical Specialist
Eastern Oklahoma Perinatal Center
Saint Francis Hospital
Tulsa, Oklahoma

**JANE TUTTLE, RNC, MS, PNP, FNP**
Assistant Professor, Nurse Practitioner
Yale School of Nursing
New Haven, Connecticut

**GARY VANCE, RN, RRT**
Clinical Nurse II
Pediatric Intensive Care
Saint Francis Hospital
Tulsa, Oklahoma

**CHRISTINE WALDMAN-WAGNER, RN, BSN**
Nurse Educator
Allergy Associates of Houston
Houston, Texas

**KAREN MULLER WHITSON, RN, BSN**
Former Patient Care Supervisor, Pediatrics
Saint Francis Hospital
Tulsa, Oklahoma

**DAVID WILSON, RN, MS**
Clinical Instructor
Eastern Oklahoma Perinatal Center
Saint Francis Hospital
Tulsa, Oklahoma

**LORRAINE T. ZANGHI, RN, AA, SNT**
Lakewood School District (Retired)
Lakewood, New York

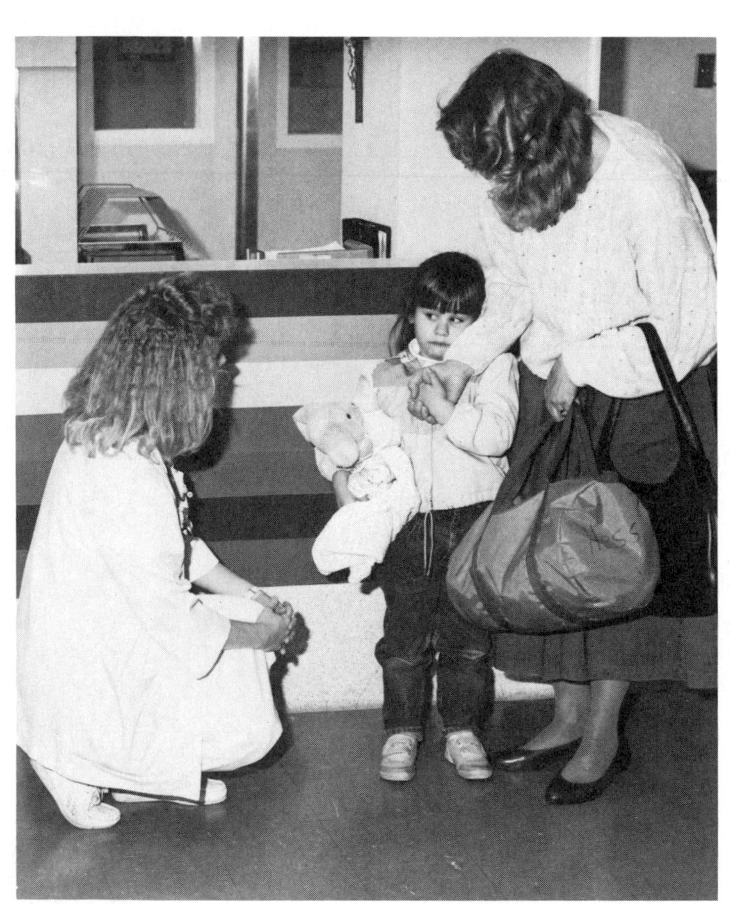

# Preface

## PHILOSOPHY

So often the transition from theory to actual practice is much more difficult than it seems. For example, a significant gap may exist between knowing that a child and family should be appropriately prepared for a procedure and actually being able to do so competently. Knowledge does not necessarily impart skill. *Comprehensive Child and Family Nursing Skills* serves not as a substitute for a theoretical background, but as a guide to implementing theoretical knowledge. It can help bridge the gap between theory and practice so that the full potential of the professional nurse-child-family encounter is realized.

As presented in this book, *skills* are broadly defined to include any technique or intervention in which theory or principles are applied in a practical manner to an interaction with a child or family. Therefore skills are not limited to traditional hands-on procedures, but include physical and developmental assessment, as well as psychosocial and teaching interventions. Although the skills were written assuming that the user possesses fundamental nursing knowledge, many skills are appropriate for nursing students. The entry level nurse needing to develop and refine skills will benefit from the book's more advanced content as will the experienced nurse who wishes to update and expand his or her practice based on current research and technological progress. Thus this book is a unique and valuable resource for students and nurses functioning in a wide variety of settings and roles.

Adopting a broad definition of "skills" made the selection of which skills to include difficult. Several criteria guided the decision. Skills unique to children or that differ significantly from the adult version of the procedure are included. Also, if developmental considerations were a major factor in a skill, it was included. Although a fundamental nursing knowledge is assumed, it is also recognized that some of the more practical aspects of caring for children are not always addressed in nursing programs, and students may not have basic child care experience. Therefore some skills provide practical information to enable the inexperienced student or nurse not only to provide care but to teach families with confidence. At the other end of the spectrum, many complex skills are included, especially those that are increasingly needed on general care units, as well as in intensive care areas. In all, 126 skills are presented offering a comprehensive, yet specific scope of current child and family nursing practice.

Whether simple or complex, all skills reflect current research-based practice when possible. If research is lacking, skills follow theoretical principles and professional standards of care, while considering practicality and convenience. However, the steps in the skills are intended as *guidelines only;* facility policies, regional practices, personal preferences, equipment and supplies availability, and the acuity of the child's clinical status are all factors that vary with actual implementation of a skill. Similarly, although the authors made every effort to provide up-to-date information regarding drugs and pediatric dosages, the reader should recognize how frequently such information changes and is encouraged to seek current data.

Expert reviewers from different geographic regions helped to refine the skills to universal application as much as possible. It is our belief that defining the steps of a skill, even if variations exist, is preferable to the omission of guidelines. Defining steps allows testing and refinement to further professional practice.

As a multicontributed book, skills were written or reviewed by clinical specialists and others with expert clinical backgrounds. Although multiple contributors results in variability among skills, the gain of tapping nursing practice expertise far outweighs the acknowledged disadvantage. The unit editors—each a clinical expert—have sought to diminish that variability and maintain a consistent presentation.

## ORGANIZATION

One hundred and twenty-six skills are presented in logical unit groupings to allow easy access. Unit I contains foundational skills in assisting the child and family to interact with the health care system. Unit II contains skills to provide psychosocial care to the child and family in all settings and across a range of situations. Unit III provides basic physical and developmental assessment skills that can be applied in many settings. Unit IV addresses the influence of the family, environment and culture on the child, and provides skills to assess and intervene appropriate to these influences. Unit V skills focus on health and wellness aspects with teaching concepts to be applied to preventative and well child care. Units VI through XIX contain skills that describe interventions used in a health care facility such as a hospital, clinic, or practitioner/physician's office, although many skills contain modifications for implementation in the home with important teaching points for the child and family. Skills are grouped by concepts or topics rather than by health patterns or systems approaches, so that the user may easily identify the most likely unit under which to find a desired skill. Four appendices contain additional information essential to the provision of thorough nursing care to children and their families.

Each skill contains an introductory statement to present the focus and preliminary information to orient the user. Next, possible *Nursing Diagnoses* which are appropriate for nursing care related to the skill, but not the condition(s) leading to the need for the skill, are listed to help the user develop an individualized plan of care. Nursing diagnoses follow current North American Nursing Diagnosis Association (NANDA) nomenclature. Although part of the nursing process, the nursing diagnoses did not conform easily in the planned skill format, so were placed at the beginning for easy reference.

The body of the skill is presented in a two column, step by step, nursing process format. Adapting the steps of the skill into nursing process provides an organizational framework, mindful of the dynamic, rather than linear quality of assessment, planning and goal setting, implementation, and evaluation. The actual "how-to" steps of the skill are located in the left column, and may be quickly perused for review or in an emergency situation. The right side of the column contains well-developed *Rationales* and *Special Considerations*, which provide a knowledge base for the user. The Special Considerations category encompasses related research, modifications or alternate steps, age-specific or developmental guidelines, additional explanation, helpful tips, and other useful information.

The *Assessment* section outlines needed information to safely and appropriately implement or perform, and evaluate the skill, such as the child's age and developmental level, the history, and baseline assessment. The *Planning and Goal Setting* section generally addresses needed equipment and supplies, and timing considerations. Goals are written as nursing goals or child and family goals as appropriate. Goal setting is presented in general terms, to allow an individualized approach to the clinical or client situation. The *Implementation* section provides detailed step by step actions, with illustrations and photographs as instructional aids. Often one skill actually encompasses several subskills, and when appropriate, the reader is referred to other skills in the book. The *Evaluation Outcomes/Observational Guidelines* section provides not only the expected outcomes in detail, but the observable behaviors and means of evaluating if the outcomes have been achieved. Specific guidelines to *Documentation* are provided with each skill. Appropriate documentation is a key to validation of professional nursing practice, and increasingly important for legal verification. References are generously cited with each skill to validate the strong literature and research base of the content. The most up-to-date sources have been used, along with classic citations when appropriate.

Additional special features with selected skills enhance the book's usefulness. While skills generally contain teaching information, some include a *Child/Family Teaching* section at the end of the skill that provides additional information. Another special feature is the *Home Care Modifications* section accompanying skills that are commonly taught to the family so that the child may be cared for at home. Many skills also provide product manufacturer information, organizations, and books, pamphlets and other literature for the professional and the child and family in the *Product References and Teaching Resources* section at the end of each unit.

Changes in infection control practices prompted the use of a special feature designed to increase the user's awareness of skills in which precautions might apply. Symbols (top right), designed by Walt Lenz for the Body Substance Isolation system, designate precautions that might apply to a particular skill, and are located next to the heading for the Implementation section. The user is advised to use these barrier precautions based on anticipated/actual contact with applicable substances, equipment or situations (see Skill 50 for guidelines on barrier precautions and body substances for which precautions are recommended). The handwashing and gloving symbols apply only to barrier precautions. Sterile gloving is addressed as appropriate to individual skills, and handwashing prior to patient contact is discussed below.

## GENERAL INSTRUCTIONS

Certain steps or precautions should always be applied to any clinical skill. These include:

1. Identify the child prior to any medication administration or procedure. The most reliable method is to check the patient identification bracelet.
2. Check for allergies to medication, diagnostic substances, antiseptic solutions, or food prior to administering, using, or providing the child any of these.
3. Wash hands thoroughly with soap for 10 seconds under running water before the initial patient contact at the beginning of work time, and after toileting and breaks. Also wash hands before preparing food/for-

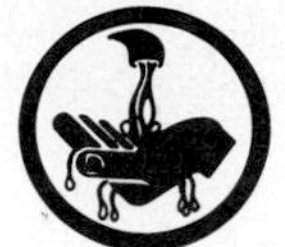

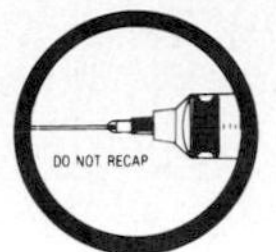


**Wash hands.**

Wear gloves when likely to touch body substances, mucous membranes or nonintact skin.

Wear plastic apron when clothing is likely to be soiled.

Wear mask/eye protection when likely to be splashed.

Place intact needle/syringe units and sharps in designated disposal container. **Do not** break or bend needles.

Courtesy Walt Lenz, San Diego Forms

mula, medications, and assembling supplies for a procedure. For handwashing guidelines between patient contacts, see skill 50.

4. Prepare the child and family for any procedure that will be performed (see Skill 1). Although life-threatening events may preclude adequate preparation, a few well-chosen words may provide needed emotional comfort and facilitate a measure of coping.
5. Consider the child's age and developmental level, and intervene in an accommodating manner.
6. The steps and recommendations in the skills are guidelines only. Refer to facility policy and procedure manual.

## ACKNOWLEDGMENTS

A true collaborative effort, this book represents a nationwide network of health care professionals dedicated to providing the best nursing care possible for children and their families. Fifty-four contributors shared our vision for what this book could be, and demonstrated clinical expertise, dedication, professionalism, and responsiveness despite concurrent demands of career and family. Without their immeasurable efforts, and the sacrifices of countless unnamed people who helped and supported them, this book would not have been possible. We thank these colleagues for their outstanding contributions, not only in this book, but to the profession. Many contributors also served as reviewers of other skills, and we are especially indebted to them for their valuable critiques. We are also grateful for the excellent work by Jackie Dowling, MS, RN, for developing all of the nursing diagnoses for the skills. Many thanks also to the additional reviewers who made significant contributions to the quality of the book, providing refinement through their constructive critiques.

The special talents of Donald O'Connor, medical illustrator, provided clear, instructive and pleasing illustrations to accompany the skills. A special thanks to John Roy, Medical Photographer, Saint Francis Hospital, Tulsa, Oklahoma and his assistants for most of the original photographs, and also to Patti Muller, RN, EdD, Director of Nursing Education at Saint Francis Hospital, for arranging the services. We also appreciate the efforts of others to take or arrange photographs for specific skills: Rosemary Liguori, Maternal-Child Health Consultant Oklahoma State Health Department; Sharon Glass, Neonatal Nurse Clinician and Pat Jamerson, Outreach Coordinator and Clinical Nurse Specialist, Eastern Oklahoma Perinatal Center, Saint Francis Hospital; Lynn McCullough, Orthopedic Clinical Nurse Specialist, Arkansas Spine Center; Pam Brown, Clinical Nurse Specialist, Children's Hospital of Los Angeles; and Lisa Anderson, Patient Care Supervisor for Pediatrics, Saint Francis Hospital; and all the nurses, children and families who agreed to be in the photographs.

We are especially indebted to people at C.V. Mosby with whom we were directly involved, those who provided us with this opportunity, and those who toiled countless hours making it a reality. Linda Duncan, Editor, first believed in our abilities and helped us develop the idea. William Brottmiller, Editor, encouraged us through the seemingly endless writing process with grace and enthusiasm. Winnie Sullivan, Developmental Editor, provided attention to detail, creativity, and objectivity when our capabilities were lagging; she was also patient and unfailingly pleasant. Thanks also to Dave Brown, Production Editor, and Carol Wiseman, Project Manager, for hours of work to ensure a quality presentation.

As part of Pediatric Nurse Consultants, a truly unique collaboration of professionals, we are grateful to those who were not able to serve as unit editors, but helped develop the initial proposal and list of skills to include, especially Krena White, Caryn Hess, Mary Beth Ogle, and Chris Kasprisin. The member to whom we owe the most is Donna L. Wong, RN, MN, PNP. She provided the initial idea and opportunity, and assisted throughout its execution. Although she is designated as book consultant, she has been a mentor, a cheerleader, and a friend, nurturing and challenging us to strive for quality. Through her publications, research, clinical consultation, speeches, and advocacy, she has improved the quality of pediatric nursing care.

The deepest and perhaps most poignant gratitude is expressed to our children and families. In our drive to improve the health care of children and families everywhere, we sacrificed irreplaceable moments in the lives of our own children, and asked incalculable sacrifices of our families. We dedicate this book to our children, husbands, parents, and other loved ones; their love gives spirit to our lives, and our faith gives life meaning.

At the initiation of this project, the fear was expressed that if the stress and pressure might eventually disrupt our relationships, we preferred not to pursue publication. Confident however, we continued, and the personal and collaborative growth experienced has provided serendipitous rewards. Through support, hard work, encouragement, constructive criticism, frustration, crises, exhaustion, humor, and tears, we have developed the deep bonds of having shared an uncommon experience. We salute each other, and are proud to offer this collaborative contribution to further professional nursing practice.

***Donna Phillips Smith***
***Kristie S. Nix***
***Joan Young Kemper***
***Rosemary Liguori***
***Deborah Kay Brantly***
***Judy Holt Rollins***
***Nancy Valentine Stevens***
***Lynn B. Clutter***

### *UNITED NATION'S DECLARATION OF THE RIGHTS OF THE CHILD*

All children need:

- To be free from discrimination
- To develop physically and mentally in freedom and dignity
- To have a name and nationality
- To have adequate nutrition, housing, recreation and medical services
- To receive special treatment if handicapped
- To receive love, understanding, and material security
- To receive an education and develop his/her abilities
- To be the first to receive protection in disaster
- To be protected from neglect, cruelty and exploitation
- To be brought up in a spirit of friendship among people

# Contents

# UNIT I Children and Families in the Health Care System

# SKILL 1 Preparing the Child for Procedures

*Judy Holt Rollins and Deborah Kay Brantly*

Children are prepared for procedures to increase cooperation, to help them cope, and to promote a sense of self-esteem and mastery. Although the purpose of preparation is not "education," knowledge may improve coping skills for the school-age or older child.

## NURSING DIAGNOSES

Anxiety related to unmet informational need about procedure; Ineffective coping related to unrealistic procedural expectations or inadequate coping method; Situational low self-esteem related to impending procedure; Powerlessness related to illness-related regimen.

| Steps | Rationale |
|---|---|
| **Assessment** | |
| 1. Review information before the procedure.<br>a. What the procedure entails.<br>b. Time it will occur.<br>c. Sensations the child may experience (Table 1-1).<br>d. Age and developmental level.<br>e. Motivation to accomplish new skills. | Reviewing information prior to preparation allows more confidence, facilitates planning, and helps assure the most complete preparation possible. Knowledge of age and developmental level provides predictive clues to fears and anticipated reaction to the procedure (Table 1-2).<br>***Special Considerations:*** *In an emergency situation, preparation may consist of a few words of explanation and assurance of emotional support given almost concurrently with the procedure.* |
| 2. Communicate with the family.<br>a. What the child has been told.<br>b. Prior experiences.<br>c. The child's usual coping style.<br>d. The family's decision regarding participation in the preparation and/or procedure. | Parents are the best resource for information about the child's past experiences and behaviors. Communication also facilitates parental participation, cooperation, and shows recognition that parents are essential members of their child's treatment team. Parents' wishes regarding participation are respected. |

**TABLE 1-1** Sensations Associated with Commonly Performed Procedures

| | Emotions | Smells | Sights | Sounds | Taste | Touch |
|---|---|---|---|---|---|---|
| Fingerstick; injection; venipuncture | Fear<br>Anxiety<br>Guilt (being punished)<br>Powerlessness<br>Curious | Alcohol | Perhaps a stranger wearing a white coat or other uniform<br>Band-Aid<br>Gloves<br>Alcohol pad<br>Bubble of blood<br>Glass pipettes/slides<br>Lancet<br>Syringe with needle<br>Syringe may be clear or colored<br>Tubes may be colored and have different colored top (stoppers)<br>"Big rubber band" (tourniquet) | Tearing of paper to open Band-Aid and lancet<br>"Smacking" of gloving<br>"Pop" of needle cap | None | Cool and wet (alcohol)<br>Rubbery feeling of gloves<br>Squeezing of finger<br>"Pressure," "sting," or "prick" of needle<br>"Some children say it feels like a chicken pecking or kitty scratching. I wonder how it will feel for you?"<br>Perhaps a squeeze or a tight feeling at site<br>"Someone may help you hold still<br>Same as injection<br>Tightness of tourniquet<br>Tapping on skin by fingers |
| IV insertion | Same as fingerstick | Same as fingerstick | Same as venipuncture<br>Plastic tubing<br>Glass bottle or plastic bag (may be colored)<br>Tape<br>Board<br>Machine on a pole (pump) | Same as venipuncture<br>Buzzer (alarm of the pump) | None | Same as venipuncture<br>Skin pulled tight from tape<br>Heavy or stiff from board |
| Bone marrow; lumbar puncture | Same as fingerstick<br>Restricted | Same as fingerstick<br>Alcohol | Same as IV insertion<br>Different room with a hard bed<br>People in gloves, aprons, and masks<br>Sleep (from anesthesia) | Same as IV insertion<br>"Pop" of needle cap | None | Same as IV insertion<br>Feel yourself falling asleep (bone marrow)<br>Prick from xylocaine<br>Numbness<br>"Someone may help you hold still." |
| Heart catheterization | Same as lumbar puncture<br>Hunger<br>Embarrassment (from exposure) | Special soap (bath the night before)<br>Alcohol<br>Soap at time of procedure | Same as injection<br>Large machine<br>Long table<br>Large camera<br>Machines that look like TV sets<br>Tiny tube<br>Lights sometimes dimmed, sometimes brighter<br>Clear plastic hood over head to breathe in for a few moments<br>BP cuff<br>Stethoscope | Stomach growling (from hunger)<br>Humming<br>Clicking<br>People talking to each other | None | Cool<br>Pressure on thigh<br>Band-Aid being applied<br>Camera will come close but will not touch you<br>"Sticky Band-Aids" (electrodes)<br>Snug feeling on arm from BP cuff<br>Soap warm and wet in groin<br>May feel table move slightly<br>Warm when fluid goes in |

***TABLE 1-1*** **Sensations Associated with Commonly Performed Procedures—cont'd**

| | Emotions | Smells | Sights | Sounds | Taste | Touch |
|---|---|---|---|---|---|---|
| X-ray; CT scan | Same as fingerstick<br>Motion of x-ray machine may seem "funny" | None | "Big machines" or "Cameras" (X-ray machines) over you<br>Lead shield or apron on self, x-ray technician, and/or parent | Noises of machine "buzzing," sliding of x-ray plates | None | Cold room and table<br>Weight of lead shield |
| NG tube | Same as fingerstick | Plastic | Plastic tube in paper<br>Gloves<br>Masks<br>Apron | Opening paper | Water to help tube go down<br>Plastic tubing | Gag when tube goes down<br>Irritating and want to get it out<br>Tube follows throat |
| Magnetic resonance imaging (MRI) | Same as fingerstick plus feeling trapped, feeling alone, fear of not being seen or heard, fear that machine can see inside head and "see" thoughts, sleepy (if medicated), bored or tired | None | Big machine<br>Skinny table going into a tunnel<br>Lights inside tunnel<br>When inside can see above but may not be able to see beginning and end of tunnel | Thumping sounds<br>Rat-a-tat—like a drumbeat that starts and stops<br>Voice from "nowhere" that tells when noise is coming and asks if you are OK<br>Sliding sound when table goes into tunnel | None | Gown, own underwear (unless metal snaps)<br>Blanket or sheet and belt over body<br>Helmet<br>Metal jewelry removed |

| Steps | Rationale |
|---|---|
| | Parents are a major source of support to children and their presence minimizes the stress imposed by separation. Young children tend to be more attentive and better able to concentrate if a parent is present.<br>***Special Considerations:*** *The most complete care for the child demands a family-centered focus. Although controversy exists among health care professionals about parental presence during a procedure, most agree that there are more advantages than disadvantages. In one study of 250 parents, the majority (78%) expressed a preference to be present during lab work or IV starts (Bauchner, Vinci, and Waring, 1989). The older child or adolescent may gain a greater sense of independence and mastery if parents are not present. Another option is to allow parents to be close by, if they are not directly participating. If child's wishes conflict with parents, the choice should always be made by the child.* |

## Planning and Goal Setting

| | |
|---|---|
| 1. Choose the time for preparation.<br>a. Younger children are generally best prepared closer to the time of the procedure.<br>b. Older children may be prepared farther in advance of the procedure.<br>c. For less complicated procedures (e.g. injections, finger sticks, temperature), children of all ages may be prepared just before the procedure. | Choosing the most appropriate time for preparation better facilitates coping and cooperation. In addition to decreasing anxiety level, the ability to exhibit mastery of skill is maximized.<br>***Special Considerations:*** *For some procedures, school-age children and adolescents may be prepared in a group setting, preferably 2 to 3 at a time.* |

**TABLE 1-2** Guidelines for Preparing Children for Procedures

| Developmental Characteristics | Responsibilities |
|---|---|
| **INFANCY: DEVELOPING TRUST** | |
| Attachment to parent | Involve parent in procedure if desired<br>Keep parent in infant's line of vision<br>If parent is unable to be with infant, place familiar object with infant, such as stuffed toy |
| Stranger anxiety | Have usual caregivers perform or assist with procedure<br>Make advances slowly and in nonthreatening manner<br>Limit number of strangers from entering room during procedure |
| Sensorimotor phase of learning | During procedure use sensory soothing measures (e.g., stroking skin, talking softly, giving pacifier)<br>Use analgesics (e.g., local anesthetic, sedation) to control discomfort<br>Cuddle and hug child after procedure; encourage parent to comfort child |
| Increased muscle control | Expect older infants to resist<br>Restrain adequately<br>Keep harmful objects out of reach |
| Memory for past experiences | Realize that older infants associate objects or persons with prior painful experiences<br>Keep in mind that older infants will cry and resist at sight of objects or persons that inflict pain<br>Keep frightening objects out of view<br>Perform painful procedures in a separate room, not in crib |
| Imitation of gestures | Model desired behavior (e.g., opening mouth) |
| **TODDLER: DEVELOPING AUTONOMY** | |
| | Use same approaches as above in addition to following: |
| Egocentric | Explain procedure in relation to what child will see, hear, taste, smell, and feel<br>Emphasize those aspects of procedure that require cooperation, such as lying still<br>Tell child it is OK to cry, yell, or use other means to verbally express discomfort |
| Negative behavior | Expect treatments to be resisted; child may try to run away<br>Use firm, direct approach<br>Ignore temper tantrums<br>Use distraction techniques<br>Restrain adequately |
| Limited language skills | Communicate using behaviors<br>Use few and simple terms that are familiar to child<br>Give one direction at a time, such as "Lie down" and then "Hold my hand"<br>Use small replicas of equipment; allow child to handle equipment<br>Use play; demonstrate on doll but avoid child's favorite doll as child may think doll is really "feeling" procedure<br>Prepare parents separately to avoid child's misinterpreting words |
| Limited concept of time | Prepare child shortly or immediately before procedure<br>Keep teaching sessions short (about 5 to 10 minutes)<br>Have preparations completed before involving child in procedure<br>Have extra equipment nearby (e.g., alcohol swabs, new needle, or Band-Aids) to avoid delays<br>Tell child when procedure is completed |
| Striving for independence | Allow choices whenever possible but realize that child may still be resistant and negative<br>Allow child to participate in care and to help whenever possible (e.g., drink medicine from a cup, hold a dressing) |
| **PRESCHOOLER: DEVELOPING INITIATIVE** | |
| Preoperational thought; egocentric | Explain procedure in simple terms and in relation to how it affects child (as with toddler, stress sensory aspects)<br>Demonstrate use of equipment<br>Allow child to play with miniature or actual equipment<br>Encourage "playing out" experience on a doll both before and after procedure to clarify misconceptions<br>Use neutral words to describe the procedure |
| Increased language skills | Use verbal explanation but avoid overestimating child's comprehension of words<br>Encourage child to verbalize ideas and feelings |

From Whaley LF and Wong DL: Nursing care of infants and children, ed 4, St Louis, 1991, The CV Mosby Co.

**TABLE 1-2** Guidelines for Preparing Children for Procedures—cont'd

| Developmental Characteristics | Responsibilities |
|---|---|
| Concept of time and frustration tolerance still limited | Implement same approaches as for toddler but may plan longer teaching session (10 to 15 minutes); may divide information into more than one session |
| Illness and hospitalization often viewed as punishment | Clarify why all procedures are performed, such as "This medicine will make you feel better"<br>Ask child his or her thoughts regarding why a procedure is performed<br>State directly that procedures are never a form of punishment |
| Fears of bodily harm, intrusion, and castration | Point on drawing, doll, or child where procedure will be performed<br>Emphasize that no other body part will be involved<br>Use nonintrusive procedures whenever possible (e.g., axillary temperatures, oral medication)<br>Apply a Band-Aid over puncture site<br>Realize that procedures involving genitals provoke anxiety<br>Allow child to wear underpants with gown<br>Explain unfamiliar situations, especially noises or lights |
| Striving for initiative | Involve child in care whenever possible (e.g., hold equipment, remove dressing)<br>Give choices whenever possible but avoid excessive delays<br>Praise child for helping and cooperating; never shame child for lack of cooperation |
| **SCHOOL-AGE: DEVELOPING INDUSTRY** | |
| Increased language skills; interest in acquiring knowledge | Explain procedures using correct scientific/medical terminology<br>Explain reason for procedure using simple diagrams of anatomy and physiology<br>Explain functioning and mechanism of equipment in concrete terms<br>Allow child to manipulate equipment; use doll or another person as model to practice using equipment whenever possible (doll play may be considered "childish" by older school-age child)<br>Allow time before and after procedure for questions and discussion |
| Improved concept of time | Plan for longer teaching sessions (about 20 minutes)<br>Prepare in advance of procedure |
| Increased self-control | Gain child's cooperation<br>Tell child what is expected<br>Suggest ways of maintaining control (e.g., deep breathing, relaxation, counting) |
| Striving for industry | Allow responsibility for simple tasks, such as collecting specimens<br>Include in decision making, such as time of day to perform procedure, preferred site<br>Encourage active participation, such as removing dressings, handling equipment, opening packages |
| Developing relationships with peers | May prepare two or more children for same procedure or encourage one to help prepare another peer<br>Provide privacy from peers during procedure to maintain self-esteem |
| **ADOLESCENTS: DEVELOPING IDENTITY** | |
| Increasingly capable of abstract thought and reasoning | Supplement explanations with reasons why procedure is necessary or beneficial<br>Explain long-term consequences of procedures<br>Realize that adolescent may fear death, disability, or other potential risks<br>Encourage questioning regarding fears, options, and alternatives |
| Conscious of appearance | Provide privacy<br>Discuss how procedure may affect appearance, such as scar, and what can be done to minimize it<br>Emphasize any physical benefits of procedure |
| Concerned more with present than future | Realize that immediate effects of procedure are more significant than future benefits |
| Striving for independence | Involve in decision making and planning, for example, choice of time, place, individuals present during procedure (such as parents), clothing to wear<br>Impose as few restrictions as possible<br>Suggest methods of maintaining control<br>Accept regression to more childish methods of coping<br>Realize that adolescent may have difficulty in accepting new authority figures and may resist complying with procedures |
| Developing peer relationships and group identity | Same as for school-age child but assumes even greater significance |

| Steps | Rationale |
| --- | --- |
| 2. Inform child and family of feelings other children have experienced or behavior anticipated postprocedure | Misbehavior or other displays of anger, disturbed sleep, or regression are commonly experienced, particularly following painful procedures or those in which a child has perceived little control. The child may also want to reenact the experience through play to gain mastery after the procedure.<br>***Special Considerations:*** *When talking to the child, it is helpful to use the third person (see Skill 12). Aggression toys such as pounding benches and other expressive means to aid children in coping with feelings of anger and loss of control are often needed (see Skill 16). Reenacting the procedure with a doll may also prove helpful, avoiding use of the child's favorite toy. Security and comfort items should be available to the child during the procedure, or if contraindicated, immediately after.* |
| 3. Obtain informed consent, if necessary (see Skill 8). | |
| 4. Select developmentally appropriate preparation aids. | Understanding is greatest when appropriate aids are used.<br>***Special Considerations:*** *Use as much of the actual equipment as possible. Medical toys, dolls, picture books, simple tapes, and videos are ideal for the younger child. Pamphlets, books to read, anatomically correct charts, or drawings may be added to the list of resources for the older child and adolescent. Since fantasy stories, e.g., doctors shrinking and going down into the throat to remove tonsils, are often confusing and misleading, their use is generally contraindicated.* |
| 5. Create an environment conducive to preparation. | Coping and cooperation are best facilitated in an environment that is pleasant, nonthreatening, and free of distractions.<br>***Special Considerations:*** *A lounge, playroom, or patient room is preferable to treatment room or place where procedure will be performed.* |
| a. Approach in a calm, friendly, and confident manner. | ***Special Considerations:*** *The ideal person to prepare the child is someone with whom trust is established. It is helpful if this person has played with the child and they have shared a good experience together. If the nurse is a stranger, a familiar staff person may provide an introduction.* |
| b. Inform the child of the pending preparation. | ***Special Considerations:*** *Provide a general overview of the time and equipment involved in the preparation.* |
| c. Arrange the area considering privacy, comfort, sights, sounds, and safety. | ***Special Considerations:*** *Privacy considerations are a major concern for older children and adolescents.* |
| d. If time permits, leave the room and return after a few minutes. | Allowing the child time to process information provides time to adjust. |
| 6. Develop individualized client and family goals:<br>▪ Will have knowledge of procedure.<br>▪ Will have coping skills to use.<br>▪ Will identify family role.<br>▪ Will develop realistic postprocedure expectations. | |

## Implementation

| Steps | Rationale |
| --- | --- |
| 1. Prepare the child for the procedure using developmentally appropriate teaching aids and communication techniques (see Table 1-2 and box on Procedural Guidelines on p. 7). | Preparing children for a procedure using developmentally appropriate tools and techniques increases the likelihood that children will be capable of cooperating and coping with the experience.<br>***Special Considerations:*** *If the preparation is done immediately before the procedure, assemble all needed equipment before this step. Watch the child for interest and attention span. If the child is losing interest, cover only the basic steps.* |
| a. Inform the child of time, place, and purpose of the procedure, including who will be present. | Giving some of the essential facts in the beginning may aid in comprehension of the details. Knowing "when" allows the child to set a time frame for absorbing information. |
| b. Address the child's previous knowledge and experiences of similar procedures, e.g., ask, "How was it when you had this done before?" "What did you or someone else do to make it easier for you?" | Children have a tendency to generalize situations and events. Discussing previous knowledge is helpful to children for the assimilation of information.<br>***Special Considerations:*** *If the child has had a negative experience, allow the opportunity to ventilate feelings and discuss that this time can be different.* |

| Steps | Rationale |
|---|---|
| c. Give permission to interrupt with questions at any time and answer questions honestly. | Often a misunderstood word or phrase will result in confusion for the child. Anxiety may be elevated to the level where the child is no longer listening. **Special Considerations:** *Assess bewilderment in the child by observing facial expressions.* |
| d. Inform the child of the procedure in a step-by-step manner. | Dividing large segments of information into smaller parts aids in mastery as well as understanding. **Special Considerations:** *Choose words carefully, avoiding those with dual meaning (see box below right). Clarify unfamiliar words. Save anxiety-laden information for last. Explanations to adolescents may be as detailed as the adolescent requests. Suggestions for how the child may assist elicits cooperation and often offers much needed sense of control.* |
| e. Using visual aid(s), describe what body part is involved, emphasizing that no other part is involved. | Children tend to absorb information more readily when it is visualized. Emphasizing noninvolvement of other body parts addresses unspoken fears. **Special Considerations:** *Stress whether or not there will be a change in ability or function of a part, even if the change is only temporary, such as "soreness for a few days."* |
| f. Describe what sensations may be experienced. See Table 1-1. | Describing sensations presents a more accurate explanation. In addition to being more honest, it also is helpful in building trusting relationships (Johnson et al, 1976.) |
| g. Explain what is expected of child and offer choices when they exist. | Offering choices provides some sense of control. **Special Considerations:** *Positive comments such as "you can help by holding still," are more helpful than, "you must not move."* |
| h. Help the child find an appropriate and comfortable coping technique. For example, "Does It help you to see what is going on, or do you like to keep your eyes closed?" See box on p. 8 for list of coping techniques. | When a child feels some control over a situation, feelings of helplessness are lessened. |
| i. Practice the coping technique. | Practice allows for further explanation, correction, or individual adjustment to a technique. It also provides an opportunity to judge probable effectiveness. **Special Considerations:** *It is helpful to practice the coping technique one final time immediately before the procedure.* |

### *PROCEDURAL GUIDELINES*

**DURING THE PROCEDURE**

1. Maintain a running dialog throughout the procedure, reinforcing what is being done and will be done, how it will feel, smell, and so on.
2. Comment on child's behavior, e.g., "You are doing a good job holding your arm still."
3. For some children it is helpful to let them know where they are in the procedure (e.g., "We are halfway through," "We are just about finished,") or what is specifically happening.
4. Mark the point at which the child no longer need worry: "Now, it's over."

**AFTER THE PROCEDURE**

1. Focus on the positive aspects of the child's coping, no matter how trivial.
2. Praise specifically for accomplishing expected behavior, e.g., "You really held your arm still," Comments such as "you were a good boy," are not particularly helpful.
3. Provide opportunities for therapeutic play (see Skill 16).

### *GUIDELINES FOR SELECTING NONTHREATENING WORDS OR PHRASES*

| WORDS/PHRASES TO AVOID | SUGGESTED SUBSTITUTIONS |
|---|---|
| Shot | Medicine under the skin |
| Organ or tissue | Special place in the body |
| Test | See how ____ is working |
| Incision | Special opening |
| Edema | Puffiness |
| Stretcher | Rolling bed |
| Stool | Child's usual term for stool |
| Dye | Special medicine (for dye) |
| Pain | Hurt, discomfort, "owie," prick |
| Deaden | Numb, make sleepy |
| Cut, fix | Make better |
| Take (i.e., "take your temperature") | "I want to see how warm you are" |
| Put to sleep | Special sleep |

From Whaley L and Wong D: Nursing care of infants and children, ed 4, St Louis, 1991, The CV Mosby Co.

| Steps | Rationale |
|---|---|
| j. Summarize and rehearse the procedure. | Rehearsal provides an opportunity to gain mastery of skills (e.g., effective coughing) and provides feedback for the child's understanding of the explanation. ***Special Considerations:*** *Preschoolers and school-age children can return a demonstration of the procedure through use of therapeutic play or a drawing. Older children and adolescents may simply verbally repeat the steps.* |
| k. Tell what will happen after the test or procedure. | Children are curious about what happens to the specimen, what will happen to them after the procedure is over, how they will feel, and when normal activities may be resumed. ***Special Considerations:*** *Emphasize the end of the procedure and highlight realistic pleasant outcomes. For example, "After I put the medication under your skin, you may go to the playroom."* |
| l. Give the child and family an opportunity to ask additional questions. | This time offers an opportunity to provide additional information and clarify misunderstandings. ***Special Considerations:*** *Paper and pencil may be left with the child or family to list other questions or concerns. These may be answered presently or at an arranged follow-up session before the actual procedure.* |
| m. Provide a follow-up session, often immediately before the procedure. | Questions or concerns may surface after child and family have had time to process information. Additionally, they may want to review the procedure one final time. |

## Evaluation Outcomes

1. The child and family are able to demonstrate knowledge of the procedure.
2. The child can demonstrate an effective coping skill.
3. The family can identify their role during the procedure.
4. The child and family are able to verbalize knowledge of postprocedure expectations.

## Observational Guidelines

Observe the family's and child's ability to demonstrate the procedure.
Ask the child to demonstrate one coping skill that was taught.
Ask the family to identify their role during the procedure.
Interview the child and family regarding their expectations postprocedure.

## Documentation

On the child's chart, document the name of the procedure, the place and time when preparation occurred, and the type of preparation/education aids used. List people (family members or staff) who were present. Comment on the child's behavior, the parent(s) reaction and anticipated role, the coping skill identified, and the child's success in demonstration. Identify positive points, as well as problem areas, and add suggestions for future preparation/teaching. Because the patient chart is a legal document, this information supports and validates the signed informed consent form.

### *COPING TECHNIQUES*

Count to 10, count backwards from 10 or 100
Cry
Sing a song
Tell a story
Relax and exhale
Take a deep breath
Hold or squeeze a hand
Pretend you are somewhere else doing something you enjoy
Close your eyes
Teach the child to memorize the steps of the procedure, then he or she may recall the steps during the procedure
May help to be told progress of procedure: "half finished," "finishing up"
Distraction
Say "ouch"

# SKILL 2 Preparing for Hospitalization

*Deborah Kay Brantly*

Hospitalization is a stressful experience for the child. The experience can be growth producing (Dixon and Stein, 1987) or cause emotional harm. Although some form of preparation may initially increase anxiety and fear during the hospitalization experience, it "has been shown to lessen fears, fantasies, and behavioral symptoms" during the year following hospitalization (Dixon and Stein, 1987). Orientation to the hospital best occurs before the child is admitted (Zweig, 1986), but the intervention may still be effective with the child for whom advanced preparation was not possible.

## NURSING DIAGNOSES

Anxiety related to unmet informational needs about hospital experience; Fear related to separation from support system during hospitalization; Altered family processes related to hospitalization transition.

| Steps | Rationale |
|---|---|
| **Assessment** | |
| 1. Determine the child's age and developmental level. | The child's support, coping needs and ability to comprehend differ according to maturation levels (Zurlinden, 1985). |
| 2. Assess the child/family's previous experiences with hospitals and health-related contacts.<br>a. Relatives that have been hospitalized or ill.<br>b. Personal illnesses, procedures or hospitalizations.<br>c. "Open house" or other tour program when the child was healthy. | Each child and family member reacts uniquely to health care contact and each may have differing knowledge about illness/hospitalization, including information that is inaccurate. The child's perception of present events can be influenced by those personal experiences, e.g., past painful procedures. Family anxiety over past experiences can be also transmitted to the child. |
| 3. Identify the reason for hospitalization: tests, surgery, illness, trauma, etc. | Planned admissions allow time for proper preparation. For example, admissions for elective surgery can allow for needed additional preparation (see Skill 112).<br>***Special Considerations:*** *Urgent or emergency admissions will usually require immediate medical attention, delaying or permitting only minimal preparation.* |
| 4. Explore the fears of the child. Common fears include:<br>a. Harm or injury.<br>b. Separation from significant others and usual routine.<br>c. Unknown environment and personnel.<br>d. Unclear limits and role expectations.<br>e. Loss of control and abilities (Zurlinden, 1985). | These five fears, identified by Visintainer and Wolfer, are "common to all hospital experiences" (Zurlinden, 1985). However, each age group would experience the fear with a different focus, e.g., the 4- to 7-year-old would fear separation from parents, whereas the adolescent would be more concerned with separation from peers (Zurlinden, 1985). |
| 5. Determine the child's usual responses to identified fears (Zurlinden, 1985).<br>a. Desired presence of significant others.<br>b. Use of blankets, pacifiers, or other security items.<br>c. Maintaining phone contact with peers and extended family members. | Continuity of usual responses facilitates coping with hospitalization, e.g., if a child clings closer to one particular parent when in an unfamiliar surrounding, that parent's presence in an unfamiliar x-ray room may reduce fears. |
| 6. Assess the child's social supports. | Children need to maintain usual social supports during stressful situations such as hospitalization.<br>***Special Considerations:*** *Young children tend to rely more on parents, grandparents, and siblings for support. Adolescents rely heavily on peer support.* |
| **Planning and Goal Setting** | |
| 1. Determine types of preparation needed. | Focusing on specific preparation needed provides individualized care and guides implementation. |
| 2. Collaboratively plan with the family members who will be responsible for preparation. The task may be shared or be the sole responsibility of the family or the professional. | Collaborative planning provides the basis for a future working relationship with the family, gives them a sense of control in the health care setting, and gives more of an opportunity for planning of individualized care. |

| Steps | Rationale |
|---|---|
| | ***Special Considerations:*** *Some sources suggest that parents alone are the best preparers of their children (Azarnoff, 1985; Gross, 1986).* |
| 3. Gather needed materials (e.g., booklets, pamphlets, videos, story books) to provide information on: the hospital (for the child), general hospital information (for parents), and/or the child's specific illness, procedure or type of surgery (see box on Guidelines for a Hospital Orientation booklet on p. 12). | Information is best given in written form for future reference. Audiovisuals enhance the learning process. |
| 4. Develop individualized client and family goals:<br>▪ Will be adequately prepared for hospitalization.<br>▪ Will demonstrate decreased anxiety. | |

## Implementation

| Steps | Rationale |
|---|---|
| 1. Provide the family with information by giving materials to them directly, sending through the mail, or distributing during a physician's office visit. | Distributing information ahead of time allows the parents the opportunity to look over materials themselves before they share it with the child and provides time for the parents to prepare the child in the nonthreatening environment of the home.<br>***Special Considerations:*** *Phone follow-up is desirable after the parents have had time to review materials.* |
| 2. Prepare the family for the hospitalization, especially if the child is younger. Include information on:<br>a. The child's developmental perception of the illness.<br>b. Descriptions of helpful parent-child interactions to prepare the child.<br>c. A review of pediatric hospital policies.<br>d. Potential alterations in the parent-child relationship during hospitalization (Pass and Pass, 1987). | Pass and Pass (1987) suggest that sessions to prepare the parents are important to facilitate an interactive relationship between the parents and health care team, as well as preparing parents to be a valuable source of information and comfort for their child.<br>***Special Considerations:*** *If the admission is not planned, preparation can occur during or just after admission (see Skill 3).* |
| 3. Invite the child to visit the hospital unit. Include as part of the orientation (Table 2-1):<br>a. Play in the playroom or recreation room (for the adolescent).<br>b. Demonstrations of simple procedures, e.g., vital signs.<br>c. Needle and equipment play/exploration (see Skill 16).<br>d. Tour of the unit.<br>e. Tour of x-ray.<br>f. Tour of the lab.<br>g. Discussion of what hospitalization will be like.<br>h. Answer questions. | Visitation before admission familiarizes the child with the hospital unit, simple procedures, equipment, and rooms. The visit allows for fears to be discussed and a trusting relationship to begin. |
| 4. Provide preadmission teaching in a group or individually as appropriate to the reason for admission, e.g., surgery (see Skill 112 for guidelines for presurgical teaching). | Many hospitals offer preadmission teaching to ease transition to hospitalization. This can be done in a group to conserve time. |
| 5. Discuss rooming-in decisions with the parents. | Parents who room in with their child may feel more at ease about the hospitalization. Advance knowledge about rooming in allows parents to plan and manage other responsibilities |
| 6. Facilitate discussion of hospital unit policies and services, e.g., visitation or availability of special groups or programs. | Parents and children usually have many questions about the unfamiliar structure of the hospital and are unaware of some services or programs. |
| 7. Schedule a time for the child's admission with the parents and physician. | When admission time can be arranged, it allows for optimal staff planning, e.g., allowing staff who are familiar with the child to be free to greet the child and to communicate with other unit members regarding the child's arrival and needs. |

| Evaluation Outcomes | Observational Guidelines |
|---|---|
| 1. The child and parents are knowledgeable and prepared for hospitalization. | The child and parents ask questions relevant to hospitalization, participate in preadmission preparation, and readily interact with the professional during prehospital visit. The parent/child correctly identifies information covered during preparation. |
| 2. The child/family will exhibit a greater sense of mastery over the hospitalization experience. | The child/family appear to have a low level of anxiety, are able to express fears or concerns to the professional, and plan for the hospitalization experience. |

**TABLE 2-1** Developmental Guidelines to Preparation for Hospitalization

| Age Group | Guidelines |
|---|---|
| Infant to Toddler | Preparation is done to enhance the needs of the parents with their infant. Encourage parents to tour hospital without child(ren) to become familiar with the setting, admission process, and other routines to allay their own fears and more successfully support their infant. |
| Toddler to 5 years | Suggest parents encourage medical play in the child's play routine before hospitalization is discussed. Encourage parents to tour the hospital; 4 to 5 year olds may attend also.<br>Allow only about 2 days advanced preparation.<br>Preparation should be brief and simple.<br>Educate the child about what will happen to him or her and the feelings he or she may have.<br>Play out scenes in the hospital and allow time for questions (to reinforce this, suggest parents act out events while still at home).<br>Verbalize common fears and psychosocial concerns, e.g., separation (abandonment), mutilation (or death), physical pain, guilt, or beliefs that hospitalization is a punishment for "being bad."<br>Address misconceptions about illness (e.g., when the outside of the body looks all right, the person is healthy; confusion about functions of organ systems; if bleeding occurs, all blood will be released; diseases are always contagious, or procedures that hurt can't be helpful).<br>Use aids, e.g., puppets, simply designed coloring books, simple storybooks, medical play equipment, dolls, and doctor and nurse kits. |
| 6 to 12 years old | Preparation can be done more than 2 days before admission so the child can discuss the event with friends and decide what to take to the hospital (e.g., clothing, personal hygiene items, and favorite toys and stuffed animals). Provide a suggested list of items to bring.<br>Give a more detailed description of the need for hospitalization.<br>Emphasize feelings the child may have and stimulate his or her imagination of what it might be like to be in the hospital.<br>Identify resources for the child to appropriately express feelings, e.g., through play or art activities.<br>Explore the child's concerns, e.g., about physical harm, death, disability, or feelings of inferiority.<br>Encourage the child to take pictures of the hospitalization or write a story (or keep a diary) about his or her experiences while in the hospital, using parents as secretaries, if necessary.<br>Use aids, e.g., booklets, simple diagrams of the body or diseased part, coloring books, videos, films, self-instruction material, puppets, medical play equipment, dolls, stories designed for the older child, and doctor and nurse kits. |
| Adolescents | Incorporate adolescent needs in the plan of care from the beginning, e.g., if hospitalization is for planned surgery, allow the patient to help decide the admission date.<br>Present information as far in advance as possible and reasonable to allow the adolescent time to tell his or her peers of the hospitalization and solicit their support, as well as gather personal belongings. Provide a list of appropriate items to bring.<br>Inform the adolescent of special programs designed to meet the needs of an adolescent.<br>Include details of the illness or surgical procedure.<br>Encourage time for questions; however, if no questions are asked, communicate availability to answer questions later if any should arise.<br>Present aspects of preparation in a group format, when possible, to initiate contacts with peers who are being hospitalized.<br>Encourage the adolescent to keep a diary of daily events and feelings.<br>Include aids, e.g., pamphlets, booklets, diagrams of illness/body, videotapes, films, age-appropriate self-instruction materials, games, or art media. |

Adapted from Steele S: Nursing care of the child with long-term illness, New York, 1977, Appleton-Century-Crofts.

## Documentation

Document previous hospital experiences of the child and family. Identify fears and child's response, with supports needed to alleviate fears on the child's plan of care. Delineate type of preparation given and persons responsible. Document any booklets, pamphlets, or other materials that are given to the parents and any prehospital visits.

Note questions asked by the parents and child. Document child's response to preadmission preparation and the tour of facilities. Note child's affectual response when admitted to the hospital and any other notable information. Document child's response to play and observations that indicate unidentified fears or questions the child may have.

### GUIDELINES FOR A HOSPITAL ORIENTATION BOOKLET

GOAL: To aid parents in the preparation of their child for hospitalization.

1. Include a picture of the hospital.
2. Show pictures or illustrations of common hospital rooms, equipment, and procedures. Include:
   - Patient room
   - Playroom
   - X-ray rooms and machines
   - Blood pressure cuffs
   - Thermometers
   - Needles, IVs, and pumps
   - People in various uniforms, masks, gowns, and gloves
3. Orient the child to some of the sights and sounds of the hospital, as well as a typical schedule. Stimulate the child's imagination about what it might be like, e.g., "What do you think it might be like to eat in your bed from a tray?"
4. Throughout the booklet, emphasize the role of the parent in the child's hospitalization to alleviate fears of abandonment.

Adapted from Zweig, C: Reducing stress when a child is admitted to the hospital, MCN 11:25-27, 1986.

# SKILL 3 Admitting a Child to the Health Care System

*Donna Marie De Simone*

The environment of a health care agency can be confusing and frightening, creating a number of real, imagined, or potential threats for the child and family. The process of being admitted to a health care agency generates the threat of the strange, the unknown, and the possibility of surprise. Therefore the admission process for the child and family should be made as comfortable as possible.

## NURSING DIAGNOSES

Health-seeking behaviors (admission) related to child's need for health care; Anxiety related to unmet informational need about health care facility, policies, and admission procedures; Fear related to unfamiliarity with admission process.

| Steps | Rationale |
|---|---|
| **Assessment** | |
| 1. Determine the child's age. | The age of the child guides planning for almost all aspects of care in a health care system. |
| 2. Review admitting diagnosis. | The reason for admission determines assessments indicated, priority of interventions, and preparation needs, as well as room assignments. |
| 3. Review admitting orders, if available. | A review of admitting orders assists in setting intervention priorities. |
| **Planning and Goal Setting** | |
| 1. Select appropriate room (and roommate if necessary); prepare room for admission. | A prepared room makes the family feel expected and welcome. A child is usually placed in a room with a child of similar age, sex, and diagnosis. Infectious disease precautions and anticipated length of stay also guide roommate selection.<br>***Special Considerations:*** *Psychosocial and developmental needs are more adequately met when children are grouped according to age. However, this is not always possible, especially on small or speciality units.* |
| a. Obtain appropriate size crib/bed; place bed in lowest position. | For the child's safety and easy accessibility, the bed should be in the low position.<br>***Special Considerations:*** *Admission kit contents vary by institution but may include: water pitcher, soap and soap dish, lotion, measuring tape, and bath basin.* |

| Steps | Rationale |
|---|---|
| b. Have an admission kit opened and assembled. | |
| c. Have admission equipment available for easy access. Common items needed include:<br>▪ Height/weight equipment<br>▪ Stethoscope<br>▪ Sphygmomanometer<br>▪ Admission forms<br>▪ Identification bracelet | |
| d. Inform roommates of impending admission. | A child/family who already occupies a room will appreciate being informed about an incoming roommate. |
| 2. Organize and prioritize admission activities, based on available information on child's condition and admitting orders. | To reduce anxiety inherent in any admission, care must be taken to organize the child's experience. An organized, smooth admission process calms the child and family and increases their confidence in the health care team (Zweig, 1986). |
| 3. Develop individualized goals of nursing care:<br>▪ Adequate and developmentally appropriate introduction to health care facility will be given to child and family.<br>▪ Child and family experience admission process in an orderly and professional manner.<br>▪ Child and family anxiety over admission procedure will be minimized.<br>▪ Family receives appropriate information concerning their child. | |

## Implementation

| Steps | Rationale |
|---|---|
| 1. Greet family and child. Introduction should include name and position (see Skill 10). | Introduction permits the family to address the caregiver by name and facilitates the beginning of a trusting relationship and positive initial impression.<br>***Special Considerations:*** *If the child and family receive prehospitalization preparation by a staff member, provide for that staff member to greet child and family. A familiar face may put the family at ease. Be aware that the order of this and the following interventions may change in priority based on the assessment and needs of the child (e.g., a seriously ill child will need attention to physical needs first).* |
| 2. Determine developmental and cognitive ability. | Tailoring explanations of illness and orientation to the health care facility to a child's level of cognitive development enhances comprehension, reduces anxiety, and increases cooperation (Robinson, 1987).<br>***Special Considerations:*** *This process should occur throughout hospitalization.* |
| 3. Apply identification band to child's wrist, ankle, or both. | Band provides method for positive identification of child. |
| 4. Orient the family and child to the hospital room. | Impressions developed through the admission process can affect the entire stay. A confusing introduction to the health care agency may add tension to a situation that already is very stressful for the child and family. Orientation to the health care agency and its equipment helps to reduce the fear of the strange and unknown for the child and parents (Gohsman and Yunck, 1979). |
| a. The hospital bed should be in a low position, near the floor. | A hospital bed in a high position frightens younger children (Zweig, 1986) and may pose a safety threat.<br>***Special Considerations:*** *Reinforce that the bed should remain in lowered position for safety reasons.* |
| b. Point out similarities of hospital room to child's room. | Noting similarities assists in demystifying the unfamiliar environment. |
| c. Suggest parents/child unpack and place special objects where the child desires. | Allowing for individuality of surroundings encourages self-esteem and provides a sense of control. Adolescents especially feel this loss of control when they are faced with hospitalization. |
| d. Demonstrate how to work call light and other equipment. If appropriate, allow child hands-on experience to operate equipment (Siaw, 1986). | Orientation to equipment provides basic knowledge of the immediate environment and communicates that the child/parent's needs are important. |
| e. Show child/family location of the bathroom. | |
| 5. Orient to unit: physical layout, services provided, policies, and visiting hours. Provide written material, if available. | Knowledge facilitates adjustment to and comfort with surroundings.<br>***Special Considerations:*** *When one member of the family is hospitalized, all family members are affected and will have needs related to the admission. Therefore it is important that family members be allowed to visit the child (Miller, 1979).* |

| Steps | Rationale |
|---|---|
| 6. Introduce or identify unit personnel: manager, other nurses, nurse's aides, housekeepers, lab technicians. Explain roles and, if appropriate, corresponding uniforms. | The child/family's anxiety decreases as they become familiar and comfortable with hospital staff and environment. Understanding roles and uniforms of personnel helps the child and family identify who may be entering the child's room. |
| 7. Encourage parental presence during child's hospital stay. Describe meal services, sleeping arrangements, and other services for family members. | Fear of separation is paramount when the child is being admitted and may continue through hospitalization. Provision of services demonstrates belief in the importance of family presence. |
| 8. Encourage child/family to ask questions. | New or unfamiliar situations frequently generate questions. Providing time to answer questions eases adjustment to the hospital. |
| 9. Complete nursing admission history (see box) and facilitate resolution of other admission paperwork. Provide a play area for the child. | Admission procedures and paperwork can be confusing and time consuming for parents. ***Special Considerations:*** *The child will probably want parents to be within sight to allay separation fears. For the child who has encountered a significant loss (e.g., death of a parent, divorce, or adoption), fear of separation can intensify to fear of abandonment. It is also helpful to have the older child nearby as a source for his or her own history.* |
| 10. Encourage parental participation during admission and hospitalization. Let the parent know how they can help, e.g., holding child during vital signs and maintaining close proximity during examination. | Parental presence and participation reduces both parental and child anxiety. Parents are able to learn, improve, or maintain parenting skills, and the parent-child dyad maintains attachment and bonding. |
| 11. Prepare child for any admission procedure using age-appropriate methods (see Skill 1). | Play is the natural medium the child uses to work through conflicts. |
| 12. Measure vital signs and assess physical growth measurements (e.g., height, weight, head circumference)(see Skill 28). | These data provide baseline information that may be used throughout hospitalization. |
| 13. Perform physical and developmental assessment (see Skills 25 and 27). | Physical and developmental assessments contribute to optimal care planning and delivery and provide important baseline information. |
| 14. Communicate with family on all aspects of child's care, including lab work, special tests, x-rays, planned procedures (e.g., IVs), and diet. Discuss physicians' visits, meal trays, or other events of significance. | Informing parents helps decrease anxiety. Parental anxiety can have implications for the ill child. Anxious parents are often hampered in their ability to provide emotional support for their child and may communicate that anxiety to the child (Alexander, White, and Powell, 1986). Informing parents may enable them to realize that their input is valued and that they are considered essential members of the health care team. ***Special Considerations:*** *A child's ability to understand, accept, and master illness may coincide with parent's ability to cope successfully.* |
| 15. Encourage the family to bring a few of the child's significant things from home, e.g., favorite toys, blanket, or picture of family. | Child maintains ties with home while making the hospital environment similar to home (Gohsman and Yunck, 1979). |

| Evaluation Outcomes | Observational Guidelines |
|---|---|
| 1. Child is oriented to health care facility according to developmental and cognitive age. | Child demonstrates developmentally appropriate understanding of the surroundings. Child displays behavior appropriate to development and knows that he or she is in the hospital. |
| 2. Child retains usual home routines. | Child participates in usual home routines: similar feeding times, playtimes, and usual bedtime routines. |
| 3. Family demonstrates adequate knowledge concerning care of child, procedures, and policies. | Family asks pertinent questions about child's care and procedures and adheres to policies. |
| 4. Family takes an active role in care of child. | Family participates in as much care of child as desired (feeding, bathing, etc.). |
| 5. Family exhibits minimal anxiety. | Family demonstrates minimal signs of anxiety: minimal tension, restlessness, and apprehension. Parents feel comfortable to take breaks from hospital. |

## Documentation

Note date and time of arrival of child, admitting physician, room to which admitted, and persons who accompany child and their relationship to child. Note admitting procedures completed: ID band applied, growth measurements, vital signs, nursing history and assessment (in nursing notes, refer reader to other forms that have been completed). Document orientation to room, unit, and hospital, highlighting written materials given. Record information shared with family about lab work, special tests or x-rays, diet, and planned procedures. Note child's and family's response to orientation information and admitting procedures.

## *NURSING ADMISSION HISTORY ACCORDING TO FUNCTIONAL HEALTH PATTERNS*

### HEALTH PERCEPTION-HEALTH MANAGEMENT

1. Why has your child been admitted?
2. How has your child's general health been?
3. What does your child know about this hospitalization?
   a. Ask the child why he or she came to the hospital.
   b. If answer is "For an operation or for tests," ask the child to tell you about what will happen before, during, and after the operation or tests.
4. Has your child ever been in the hospital before?
   a. How was that hospital experience?
   b. What things were important to you and your child during that hospitalization? How can we be most helpful now?
5. What medications does your child take at home?
   a. Why are they given?
   b. When are they given?
   c. How are they given (if a liquid, with a spoon; if a tablet, swallowed with water, or other)?
   d. Does your child have any trouble taking medication? If so, what helps?
   e. Is your child allergic to any medications?

### NUTRITIONAL-METABOLIC

1. What are the family's usual mealtimes?
2. Do family members eat together or at separate times?
3. What are your child's favorite foods, beverages, and snacks?
   a. Average amounts consumed or usual size portions.
   b. Special cultural practices, such as family eats only ethnic food.
4. What foods and beverages does your child dislike?
5. What are your child's feeding habits (bottle, cup, spoon, eats by self, needs assistance, any special devices)?
6. How does the child like food served (warmed, cold, one item at a time)?
7. How would you describe your child's usual appetite (hearty eater, picky eater)?
   a. Has being sick affected your child's appetite?
8. Are there any known or suspected food allergies; is your child on a special diet?
9. Are there any feeding problems (excessive fussiness, spitting up, colic); any dental or gum problems that affect feeding?
10. What do you do for these problems?

### ELIMINATION

1. What are your child's toilet habits (diaper, toilet trained—day only or day and night, use of word to communicate urination or defecation, potty chair, regular toilet, other routines)?
2. What is your child's usual pattern of elimination (bowel movements)?
3. Do you have any concerns about elimination (bedwetting, constipation, diarrhea)?
4. What do you do for these problems?
5. Have you ever noticed that your child sweats a lot?

### SLEEP-REST

1. What is your child's usual hour of sleep and awakening?
2. What is your child's schedule for naps; length of naps?
3. Is there a special routine before sleeping (bottle, drink of water, bedtime story, nightlight, favorite blanket or toy, prayers)?
4. Is there a special routine during sleep time, such as waking to go to the bathroom?
5. What type of bed does your child sleep in?
6. Does your child have his or her own room or share a room; if shares, with whom?
7. What are the home sleeping arrangements (alone or with others, such as sibling, parent, or other person)?
8. What is your child's favorite sleeping position?
9. Are there any sleeping problems (falling asleep, waking during night, nightmares, sleep walking)?
10. Are there any problems awakening and getting ready in the morning?
11. What do you do for these problems?

### ACTIVITY-EXERCISE

1. What is your child's schedule during the day (nursery school, daycare center, regular school, extracurricular activities)?
2. What are your child's favorite activities or toys (both active and quiet interests)?
3. What is your child's usual television viewing schedule at home?
   a. What are your child's favorite programs?
   b. Are there any TV restrictions?
4. Does your child have any illness or disabilities that limit activity? If so, how?
5. What are your child's habits and schedule for bathing (bath in tub or shower, sponge bath, shampoo)?
6. What are your child's dental habits (brushing, flossing, fluoride supplements or rinses, favorite toothpaste); schedule of daily dental care?
7. Does your child need help with dressing or grooming, such as hair combing?
8. Are there any problems with the above (dislike of or refusal to bathe, shampoo hair, or brush teeth)?
9. What do you do for these problems?
10. Are there special devices that your child requires help in managing (eyeglasses, contact lenses, hearing aid, orthodontic appliances, artificial elimination appliances, orthopedic devices)?

NOTE: Use the following code to assess functional self-care level for feeding, bathing/hygiene, dressing/grooming, toileting:

O: Full self-care
I: Requires use of equipment or device
II: Requires assistance or supervision from another person
III: Requires assistance or supervision from another person and equipment or device
IV: Is dependent and does not participate

*Continued.*

## *NURSING ADMISSION HISTORY ACCORDING TO FUNCTIONAL HEALTH PATTERNS—cont'd*

### COGNITIVE-PERCEPTUAL

1. Does your child have any hearing difficulty?
   a. Does the child use a hearing aid?
   b. Have "tubes" been placed in your child's ears?
2. Does your child have any vision problems?
   a. Does the child wear glasses or contact lenses?
3. Does your child have any learning difficulties?
   a. What is the child's grade in school?

### SELF-PERCEPTION—SELF-CONCEPT

1. Describe your child (e.g., takes time to adjust, settles in easily, shy, friendly, quiet, talkative, serious, playful, stubborn, easygoing)?
2. What kinds of things make your child angry, annoyed, anxious, or sad? What helps?
3. How does your child act when annoyed or upset?
4. What have been your child's experiences with and reactions to temporary separation from you (parent)?
5. Does your child have any fears (places, objects, animals, people, situations)? How do you handle them?
6. Has your child's illness changed his or her self-perception (e.g., more shy, embarrassed about appearance, less competitive with friends, stays at home more)?

### ROLE-RELATIONSHIP

1. Does your child have a favorite nickname?
2. What are the names of other family members or others who live in the home (relatives, friends, pets)?
3. Who usually takes care of your child during the day/night (especially if other than parent, such as babysitter, relative)?
4. What are the parents' occupations and work schedules?
5. Are there any special family considerations (adoption, foster child, stepparent, divorce, single parent)?
6. Have any major changes in the family occurred lately (death, divorce, separation, birth of a sibling, loss of a job, financial strain, mother beginning a career, other)? Describe child's reaction.
7. Who are your child's play companions or social group (peers, younger or older children, adults, prefers to be alone)?
8. Do things generally go well for your child in school or with friends?
9. Does your child have "security" objects at home (pacifier, thumb, bottle, blanket, stuffed animal, or doll)? Did you bring any of these to the hospital?
10. How do you handle discipline problems at home? Are these methods always effective?
11. Does your child have any speech or hearing problems? If so, what are your suggestions for communicating with him or her?
12. Will your child's hospitalization affect the family's financial support or care of other family members, such as other children?
13. What concerns do you have about your child's illness and hospitalization?
14. Who will be staying with your child while he or she is in the hospital?
15. How can we contact you or another close family member outside of the hospital?

### SEXUALITY-REPRODUCTIVE

(Answer questions that apply to your child's age-group.)

1. Has your child begun puberty (developing physical sexual characteristics, menstruation)? Have you or your child had any concerns?
2. Does your daughter know how to do breast self-examination?
3. Does your son know how to do testicular self-examination?
4. How have you approached topics of sexuality with your child? Do you feel you need help with some topics?
5. Has your child's illness affected the way he or she feels about being a boy or a girl? If so, how?
6. Do you have any concerns with behaviors in your child, such as masturbation, asking many questions or talking about sex, not respecting others' privacy or wanting too much privacy?
7. Initiate a conversation about adolescent's sexual concerns with open-ended to more direct questions and using the terms "friends" or "partners" rather than "girlfriend" or "boyfriend":
   a. Tell me about your social life.
   b. Who are your closest friends? (If one friend is identified, could ask more about that relationship, such as how much time they spend together, how serious they are about each other, if the relationship is going the way the teenager hoped it would).
   c. Might ask about dating and sexual issues, such as the teenager's views on sex education, "going steady," "living together," or premarital sex.
   d. Which friends would you like to have visit in the hospital?

### COPING-STRESS TOLERANCE

(Answer questions that apply to your child's age-group.)

1. What does your child do when tired or upset?
   a. If upset, does your child want a special person or object? If so, explain.
2. If your child has temper tantrums, what causes them and how do you handle them?
3. Whom does your child talk to when worried?
4. How does your child usually handle problems or disappointments?
5. Have there been any big changes or problems in your family recently? How did you handle them?
6. Has your child ever had a problem with drugs or alcohol or tried suicide?
7. Is your child "accident prone?" If so, explain.

### VALUE-BELIEF

1. What is your religion?
2. How is religion or faith important in your child's life?
3. What religious practices would you like continued in the hospital, such as prayers before meals/bedtime; visit by minister, priest, rabbi, or prayer group?

From Whaley LF and Wong DL: Essentials of pediatric nursing, ed 3, St Louis, 1989, The CV Mosby Co.

# SKILL 4 Facilitating a Multidisciplinary Health Care Team

*Donna J. Takacs*

A multidisciplinary approach to health care is a planned, coordinated system for delivering services to a child and family. Collaborative efforts by the child, family, and members of health care disciplines are focused on identifying and implementing treatment goals. The manner of implementation may vary with the setting; however, a leader, often a nurse, is designated to coordinate the function of the team and be an advocate for the child and family. Each discipline intervenes in its own way; however, assessment, planning, and evaluation occur in conjunction with members of other disciplines to assure consistent, integrated, quality care (Koerner, Cohen, and Armstrong, 1986).

## NURSING DIAGNOSES

Ineffective family coping (compromised or disabling) related to the lack of information or misinformation, inadequate support systems, ineffective coping methods, or chronicity of child's illness; Impaired home maintenance management related to child's illness or injury, insufficient finances, or inadequate community resources; Powerlessness related to illness-related regimen.

| Steps | Rationale |
|---|---|
| **Assessment** | |
| 1. Review the child's chart and care plan to identify problem areas or needs, including physical (e.g., nutritional, respiratory, infectious disease, mobility); psychological (e.g., crisis, grief, self-esteem); social (e.g., peer relationships); or spiritual. | The identification of problems delineates which disciplines are appropriate to include in a multidisciplinary team meeting (Boatwright and Crummette, 1987). |
| 2. Ask family members to identify and prioritize needs; assess family strengths, resources, and ability to meet these needs. | Each family is unique and may perceive needs or problems differently from the nurse or other professionals. |
| 3. Identify specific health care professionals who have been assigned responsibility for working with the child. | Composition of the team will vary depending on needs of the individual child and family. In some settings, all health professionals may be asked to attend. In other settings, a smaller, identified core group may consult with other professionals as indicated. |
| 4. Discuss with the child/family their desire to be present at the planning conference. | Collaboration with the family is vital, since their ability to contribute information can lead to more comprehensive and appropriate care plans. Family participation also enhances parental competence. ***Special Considerations:*** *The age and physical condition of the child and ability and desire of the family to attend must be considered (Shelton, Jeppson, and Johnson, 1987).* |
| 5. Determine willingness and availability of identified health care professionals to participate in a multidisciplinary planning conference. | Commitment to the process increases the likelihood of its success. Geographic assignment of professionals also affects their ability to attend multidisciplinary conferences (Koerner, Cohen, and Armstrong, 1986; Zimbelman, 1988). |
| **Planning and Goal Setting** | |
| 1. Establish objectives for the planning conference. Objectives generally focus on identifying or meeting treatment needs or discharge planning. | Clearly defined objectives will assist the group to be more focused and enhance effectiveness of the team conference (Boatwright and Crummette, 1987). |
| 2. In collaboration with identified team members, establish a convenient date, time, and place for conference. | Available time is limited and will not be convenient to all. Attempt should be made to include as many team members as possible (Boatwright and Crummette, 1987). ***Special Considerations:*** *Interdisciplinary collaboration may occur in the absence of a formal meeting. A regular weekly meeting time could be established if the same group of professionals work with many of the same patients.* |

| Steps | Rationale |
|---|---|
| 3. Send a reminder of the meeting to team members. Provide written objectives or an agenda with the notice. | Knowledge of the objectives allows team members to come to the meeting prepared. |
| 4. Develop a nursing goal of care:<br>▪ To organize a multidisciplinary health care team to collaboratively develop and maintain a comprehensive treatment plan for the child and family. | |

## Implementation

| Steps | Rationale |
|---|---|
| 1. To begin the meeting, briefly review objectives for multidisciplinary team meeting and child's history, if necessary. | Sharing the planned objectives with the team will help keep the group on task (Boatwright and Crummette, 1987). |
| 2. Request each team member to summarize professional involvement with the family. Ask each team member to state planned interventions based on assessed needs. If the family or child is present, ask them to share their perspective. | Collaboration results in greater communication and understanding of each team member's role, facilitating a holistic plan that benefits the child (Bersky, Keys, and Dickens, 1987). The family viewpoint increases comprehensiveness and understanding (Shelton, Jeppson, and Johnson, 1987). |
| 3. Using input from the child and family, formulate and discuss each care objective, including the intervention strategies of each discipline. Discuss and reach consensus on strategies that may be conflicting. For each intervention, identify responsibility for implementation and target date for completion. | Each professional's input enriches the process and contributes to delivery of comprehensive care (Bersky, Keys, and Dickens, 1987; Warden et al, 1988). Identifying responsible persons and target dates promotes accountability.<br>***Special Considerations:*** *The approach of each discipline is similar in format; however, priorities for care differ. There is a body of knowledge shared by many disciplines, as well as a body of knowledge unique to each. Issues of role definition and need for negotiation emerge when territorial concerns arise and must be addressed (Bersky, Keys, and Dickens, 1987; Cumberledge et al, 1987).* |
| 4. As a group, plan successive meeting(s) to determine progress or goal achievement. | Successive meeting(s) can be used for evaluation and alteration of the treatment plan, if indicated (Boatwright and Crummette, 1987). |
| 5. If family was not included in the team meeting, share and discuss the results of the team conference with them. | Participation of the child and family increases satisfaction with care and promotes compliance (Boatwright and Crummette, 1987). |
| 6. Incorporate decisions into the nursing care plan. | It is important that the nursing care plan be in concert with the multidisciplinary plan to help ensure consistent care (Boatwright and Crummette, 1987). |
| 7. Discuss plan with nursing professionals who will implement it. | Communicating the plan with other nursing professionals will enhance its implementation. |
| 8. As previously planned with the team, organize and call follow-up meeting(s). Discuss the treatment objectives and interventions set at the planning conference to determine progress and response of the child/family to the plan. | Team members may see similar or differing responses of the child/family. Pooling information provides more data with which to evaluate interventions and revise care plan. |
| 9. Based on the response of the child/family, determine if alterations in the plan are indicated. Make changes accordingly. | |

| Evaluation Outcomes | Observational Guidelines |
|---|---|
| 1. A multidisciplinary health care team is formed according to the child/family's needs. | Written documentation includes the child/family's problem areas or needs, and a list of identified health professionals who agree to work collaboratively. |
| 2. A comprehensive treatment plan, including objectives and intervention strategies, is developed by the multidisciplinary health care team. | Minutes from the care conferences include objectives and intervention strategies, with identified target dates and responsible person(s). |
| 3. The treatment plan is implemented by the target date and evaluated for goal achievement and revision. | Minutes from successive care conferences include documentation of goal achievement, suggested revisions or alternative strategies, and new target dates. |

## Documentation

Record the date(s) of the team meeting, disciplines represented, family participation, and decisions and plans made by the team. Following discussion with the child/family concerning treatment goals and plans, document their responses to the plans in the patient record. As interventions occur, child/family responses should also be recorded in the patient record.

# SKILL 5 Planning Discharge

*Donna J. Takacs*

Discharge planning is an organized process whereby the nurse evaluates, in collaboration with the child and family, readiness for discharge from the acute setting, care needed after hospitalization, and necessary resources for continuation of care. Discharge planning also encompasses investigating and securing resources to provide a smooth transition to another facility or home. The nature and degree of discharge planning varies according to needs of the child/family. It may range from simple teaching, e.g., care at home following a tonsillectomy to involved care, e.g., suctioning a tracheostomy.

## NURSING DIAGNOSES

Altered family process related to transition of child from hospital to another facility, home, or school; Altered health maintenance related to insufficient information about medical condition, medications, diet, activity, and/or special procedures; Potential for impaired home maintenance management related to child's illness or injury, unfamiliarity with resources, or inadequate support systems.

| Steps | Rationale |
|---|---|
| **Assessment** | |
| 1. Review nursing care plan goals and outcomes desired at time of discharge. | The use of outcome criteria assists in determining readiness for discharge (Feetham, 1986; Mezzanotte, 1987). |
| 2. Collect pertinent information about the child/family, including physiological, psychological, and social needs. | The collection of relevant data serves as a baseline for evaluation of discharge planning. It allows comparison of current patient status with desired status at discharge, assisting to identify gaps and coordinate discharge planning efforts. |
| 3. In collaboration with the family, assess factors that play a part in determining readiness for discharge (see Skill 38). | The family plays a vital role in decision-making for future care of the child (Feetham, 1986; Shelton, Jeppson, and Johnson, 1987).<br>***Special Considerations:*** *Including older children and adolescents in discussions is helpful and consistent with their increased need for autonomy.* |
| 4. Identify potential barriers to smooth and timely transition from the hospital. Barriers may include:<br>a. Psychosocial factors (e.g., family support or integrity, cultural values or beliefs).<br>b. Financial resources (e.g., lack of insurance to cover needed services).<br>c. Transportation needs.<br>d. Educational needs (e.g., need for information about disease process, medications, treatments).<br>e. Health condition/functional status of child and possible need for emergency medical support. | Early identification of potential barriers provides an opportunity to include additional intervention strategies in the care plan when formulating a discharge plan (Feetham, 1986; Seigel, 1988).<br>***Special Considerations:*** *It is vital that health professionals see continuity of care as their responsibility.* |
| 5. In collaboration with the family and team, assess appropriate placement options for the child, if home discharge is not feasible. | Should barriers to home discharge be prohibitive, alternative care settings, such as long-term care, foster care, or respite care may be important choices to consider (Feetham, 1986; Larkin, 1987; Slevin and Roberts, 1987). |
| 6. Determine if a discharge date has been targeted. | A target date provides parameters for the timely implementation of interventions. |
| **Planning and Goal Setting** | |
| 1. Using assessment data, determine knowledge and skills needed by family. | Teaching should be tailored to meet the assessed needs of the family. |
| 2. Plan schedule for teaching knowledge and skills. If possible, arrange for family to stay at hospital for 24 to 48 hours to provide care if complex skills are involved (e.g., apnea monitoring). | Provision of care under guidance promotes confidence of family members. |

| Steps | Rationale |
|---|---|
| 3. Collaborate with multidisciplinary team members to coordinate plans for discharge (see Skill 4). | Collaboration yields coordinated, comprehensive care.<br>***Special Considerations:*** *In some settings, a discharge planning specialist may be available to assist with specific tasks of discharge planning and is included in the team.* |
| 4. Based on assessments, identify available resources needed to meet health needs that continue after discharge, e.g., support groups, home health care, alternative care settings, and resources for medical supplies and equipment. | The provision of information and services to the family facilitates continuity of care.<br>***Special Considerations:*** *If the child's family has familiar and dependable resources, this information should be incorporated into the process of planning.* |
| 5. Develop individualized goals of nursing care.<br>▪ Formulate a discharge plan based on assessed child/family needs. | |

## Implementation

| Steps | Rationale |
|---|---|
| 1. Discuss child's illness and anticipated changes of daily living with the child and family. | Knowledge of condition and possible forthcoming events related to the illness assist the family to cope. The child and family will be faced with explaining the illness to others (e.g., extended family, school officials, friends). Depending on the illness and the child's stage of development, he or she may feel different from others and socially isolated.<br>***Special Considerations:*** *The need for explaining the illness to others will vary depending on whether the illness is short-term or long-term or the extent of effect on others.* |
| 2. Provide child/family education of needed skills: demonstration, return demonstration by child/family, reinforcement, and written materials for reinforcement of teaching, if appropriate. Focus areas may include assessment skills, equipment maintenance and operation, potential complications, and guidelines for seeking professional care (see Skill 43 and Home Care Modifications for individual skills). | At home, the family independently implements prescribed therapy. Feedback about the performance of procedures builds confidence of the caregivers (Shelton, Jeppson, and Johnson, 1987).<br>***Special Considerations:*** *Should the child be discharged to an environment other than the family home, other appropriate caretakers should be included in the education process.* |
| 3. Provide family with written names and phone numbers of health professionals and support groups in addition to dates and times of scheduled appointments. | The impending discharge is a time of increased anxiety for family members. Specific, written information is helpful in providing a smooth transition (Cagan and Meier, 1979; Kruger and Rawlins, 1984). |
| 4. Provide family with a list of supplies needed at home. If appropriate, provide list of special equipment suppliers. | Advanced knowledge of items needed allows family time to acquire them before discharge.<br>***Special Considerations:*** *Consulting with social service agencies may be important if family requires financial assistance to obtain needed items.* |
| 5. Encourage family to identify and schedule backup assistance—additional people or agencies (friends, church members, extended family, respite care) who can provide emotional or physical relief to the primary caregiver(s). | Caring for a family member is a stressful activity that normally elicits mixed emotional responses. Addressing the need for parents to take breaks from caregiving to reduce stress and maintain marital relationship may prevent a crisis in the family (Feetham, 1986; Feuer, 1987).<br>***Special Considerations:*** *Relief caregivers may be encouraged and/or required to attend family education sessions.* |
| 6. If the child is school-age, collaborate with school personnel regarding home-bound education or return of the child to the classroom as indicated by child's health status. | School is a child's major "work" and success in that environment is important for growth and development (Weitzman, 1984). |
| 7. If child is to return to the classroom, contact or assist family in contacting school nurse, counselor, teachers, or principal. Obtain written parental consent to discuss information about child's illness and collaborate on child's reentry into school. Information important to share includes:<br>a. Description of child's illness.<br>b. Day-to-day effects of the illness.<br>c. Realistic expectations of the child's abilities.<br>d. Physical limitations caused by illness.<br>e. Long-term projected needs of child (see also Skill 18). | Without accurate information, school personnel are forced to make their own interpretations. Information assists school personnel to understand the uniqueness of the child. Appropriate expectations from teachers are important to provide opportunity for the child's achievement (Goodell, 1984; Weitzman, 1984). Written consent prevents violation of confidentiality.<br>***Special Considerations:*** *Considering possible limitations as a result of illness, efforts can be directed at encouraging the child to develop an interest area through which feelings of success and achievement can be realized (Goodell, 1984; Weitzman, 1984). The school or hospital-based nurse may provide age-appropriate information to classroom peers to promote acceptance of the ill child and increase the likelihood for normal growth and development (Goodell, 1984).* |

| Steps | Rationale |
|---|---|
| 8. Before the discharge date, communicate with family and receiving providers concerning needs of the child and family (e.g., procedures, medications, psychosocial needs). | Knowledge of the needs of the child and family by receiving providers allows them an opportunity to be prepared to provide appropriate and needed services without delay (Dumas, 1987). |
| 9. On a regular basis, review with the family the care plan goals and outcomes. | Comparison of current condition to preestablished outcome criteria measures progress toward discharge (Feetham, 1986; Mezzanotte, 1987). |
| 10. Arrange for transportation from hospital, if needed. | In some cases, the family may not have transportation or a child may have special needs that prevent transporting in the family vehicle. |
| 11. Provide follow-up care after discharge by:<br>a. Telephoning the family to inquire about status after discharge.<br>b. Telephoning care providers regarding status of child and family.<br>c. Making a home visit (see Skill 6). | Follow-up provides evaluation of discharge planning effectiveness. Also, information received from the family and community professionals provides feedback and permits adjustment of hospital procedures for enhanced effectiveness of other discharges (Slevin and Roberts, 1987).<br>***Special Considerations:*** *In some settings, a home care department is designated to provide follow-up for discharged patients.* |

| Evaluation Outcomes | Observational Guidelines |
|---|---|
| 1. A discharge plan is developed in collaboration with child and family as a part of the nursing care plan. | Review written documentation of objectives and intervention strategies with target dates and identified responsible persons. |
| 2. Care plan goals are achieved, and the family (or alternate provider) is prepared to assume full responsibility for child's care by the discharge date. | Review minutes from care conferences and documentation of goal achievement in the patient record. Interview family as to comfort level regarding care of the child. |
| 3. Follow-up review of the child and family indicates satisfactory adjustment following discharge. | The record includes documentation of responses from the family and receiving professionals regarding outcome of discharge and adjustment of child and family to new environment. |

## Documentation

Document in the child's record the discharge plan, action taken, and response of the child and family. Note information such as issues addressed during hospitalization, referrals to various providers, and the result of follow-up contacts.

# *SKILL* 6 Conducting a Home Visit for Follow-up Care

*Donna Marie De Simone*

Home visits for follow-up care are becoming more frequent as early discharge is promoted for economic reasons. Before discharge from a health care agency, discharge planning initiates the preparation for home visits. It is important that nurses who are making home visits become skilled in adapting the plan of care to fit the family's environment.

### NURSING DIAGNOSES

Altered family processes related to transition of child/family from hospital to home; Altered health maintenance related to insufficient information about medical condition, medications, diet, activity, physician instructions, and/or special procedures; Impaired health maintenance management related to child's illness, insufficient finances, or inadequate support systems.

| Steps | Rationale |
|---|---|
| **Assessment** | |
| 1. Identify indications for home visit, generally one or more of the following:<br>a. Perform procedure.<br>b. Physical assessment.<br>c. Reinforce teaching.<br>d. Observe/evaluate technique.<br>e. Check equipment.<br>f. Assess transition of child/family from hospital to home. | Identifying purpose of visit helps direct planning and assists in selection of materials and equipment needed for the visit. |
| 2. Review agency record for history, plan of care, and discharge plan. | Information supplies important background data in addition to providing an opportunity to review child's discharge plan or current plan of care (Rusch, 1986). |
| 3. Review child's age and family characteristics (see Skills 38 and 41). | The child's age affects other aspects of planning. Assessing family structure and culture also assists in planning (Rushing, 1987). |
| **Planning and Goal Setting** | |
| 1. Contact family to make/confirm appointment. Ask if there are any special needs or concerns or if there are special items that could be brought, such as supplies, equipment, or educational materials. | Responses to these questions help guide planning and referrals.<br>***Special Considerations:*** *Initially, many parents prefer face-to-face contact with a health care professional as compared to a phone conversation (Brandon and Huber, 1987).* |
| 2. Gather equipment, information, and teaching material. | Nature of the visit will dictate needed items. |
| 3. Develop a nursing goal of care:<br>▪ To organize and conduct home visit to meet identified child/family needs. | |
| **Implementation** | |
| 1. Arrive on time and introduce self, if needed. Take a few moments to exchange social pleasantries. | A pleasant interchange helps put family at ease and facilitates communication. |
| 2. Review discharge plan or current plan of care with family. Determine child/family's knowledge base regarding:<br>a. Medical condition.<br>b. Medications.<br>c. Diet.<br>d. Activity.<br>e. Physician's instructions.<br>f. Plan of care.<br>g. Special procedures.<br>h. Handling emergencies. | Poor comprehension is a major cause of noncompliance and failure to achieve desired results. In addition, family may have had difficulty attending to instructions that were provided at discharge because of a high anxiety level (Kruger and Rawlins, 1984). |
| 3. Identify any new concerns/problems.<br>a. Ask child/family to describe a typical day.<br>b. Discuss new problems or concerns.<br>c. Identify necessity for referrals for physical needs (e.g., physical therapist or dietician), psychosocial problems, financial concerns, or other needs. | New concerns arise when the child/family is back in their own environment. When a typical day is reviewed, family may be reminded of concerns that might otherwise be forgotten.<br>Physician, social worker, clinical nurse specialist, or other referrals may be appropriate and initiation of referrals should be made as needs arise. Because of the nature of home health care delivery, coordination is more complex to facilitate than institutional care (Bock, 1985). |
| 4. Identify problems child is experiencing in transition from hospital to home.<br>a. Attending school.<br>b. Playing with friends.<br>c. Eating.<br>d. Sleeping.<br>e. Behavior changes.<br>f. Disciplinary problems. | Unanticipated problems may have arisen for the child in resuming daily activities. A child's psychosocial development is facilitated when he or she is able to participate in family, community, and school life (Perrin, 1985)<br>***Special Considerations:*** *Parents may express relief in having a health care professional's advice regarding their child (Noga, 1982).* |
| 5. Identify problems family is experiencing in transition.<br>a. Redefining or reorganizing roles.<br>b. Work schedules.<br>c. Participation in family, community, and school life. | All family members are affected when the health of one is disrupted (Terry, 1987).<br>***Special Considerations:*** *Role changes may occur in the family unit. A parent may become a case manager for the child, interacting with health care providers continuously. An at-home mother may begin to work to pay medical expenses, or an employed parent may have to quit to provide unavailable or unaffordable care for a child with special needs. A single parent's role becomes more burdened. Siblings often redefine parent-child relationships as self-reliance develops and may participate in the home care of the affected child (Feinberg, 1985).* |

| Steps | Rationale |
|---|---|
| 6. Have the family identify some transitional changes that were successfully managed. | Having family members identify their strengths and ability to solve problems successfully increases self-confidence for future problem solving. |
| 7. Explore family's knowledge of community resources.<br>a. Professional organizations.<br>b. Support groups.<br>c. Respite care.<br>d. Day care. | The family may not be aware of resources available to them or may not be aware that they are eligible for assistance. |
| 8. As needed, perform assessments of the following:<br>a. Physical and developmental (see Skills 25 and 27). | Ongoing assessment provides evaluative information for previous assessments and a baseline for future comparison.<br>***Special Considerations:*** *Document successful approaches to the child during assessments.* |
| b. Family (see Skill 38). | A family assessment provides information as to the interaction, functioning, and needs of the family in adapting to a disruption in a family member's health. |
| 9. Reinforce teaching to family, providing written instructions. | Greater compliance with instruction occurs when parents receive instruction sheets written at their level of comprehension (Streiff, 1986), compared to receiving verbal instructions (Kruger and Rawlins, 1984). In addition, it is legally prudent to have documented instructions (Cushing, 1984). |
| 10. Prepare child for procedures according to cognitive and developmental age (see Skill 1). | Preparation helps the child know what to expect, how he or she can cooperate, and gives the child a measure of control. |
| 11. Perform specialized procedures or observe family perform.<br>a. Evaluate technique.<br>b. Provide feedback and reinforcement. | Observing family member performing a procedure ensures that the procedure is being performed effectively and provides encouragement to the caregiver. In some situations, family may prefer not to perform skills.<br>***Special Considerations:*** *On a home visit a health care professional must adapt to the family's environment, which may vary significantly in cleanliness, space, and availability of resources (Creighton, 1987).* |
| 12. Inspect any medical equipment used for the care of the child. Observe for correct operating and maintenance techniques. | Medical equipment already in the home should be checked and adjusted to assure proper functioning (O'Malley and Ness, 1987).<br>***Special Considerations:*** *Mechanical problems should be managed by appropriate servicing centers.* |
| 13. Update/revise plan of care to fit child/family needs. | Adjustments may need to be made in child's plan of care to fit current needs (Rushing, 1987).<br>***Special Considerations:*** *Strive for a workable plan of care that regards the family as team leader (Bock, 1986).* |
| 14. Close home visit by reviewing care, reinforcing teaching, and confirming next visit date and time (if another visit is planned). | These elements provide appropriate closure and ensure continuity for next visit. |

| Evaluation Outcomes | Observational Guidelines |
|---|---|
| 1. Child/family progress toward goals is assessed. | Documentation includes description of problems and progress. Plan of care reflects any updates or revisions. |
| 2. Family shows adaptation to readjustment of roles and routine. | Family reports maintenance or adjustments of daily activities (e.g., child attending school, playing with peers, adhering to bedtime). Family shows progress in returning to previous roles or adjusting to new ones. |
| 3. Nurse or family performs assessments or specialized procedures. | Charting reflects assessments. Observe family performing procedures, identifying problems or proper techniques. Charting reflects procedures done and equipment or supplies used. |
| 4. Appropriate referrals are made for family. | Family states decision regarding use of referrals such as professionals, community organizations, and support groups. Note documentation of referrals. |

## Documentation

Include the following in the child's record: date and time, including reason for the home visit; assessments performed, as well as procedures done; new teaching or reinforcement of previously learned information, including any written materials given to family; a revised or updated plan of care that includes nursing diagnosis, goals, interventions, and outcomes; child/family's adaptation to home environment and any role changes that have occurred; strengths and weaknesses; support systems that are being used; level of family participation in care of child; equipment checked and supplies used; questions verbalized by family and answers given; and referrals identified and made.

# SKILL 7 Protecting the Child with Alleged Maltreatment

*Catherine C. Ayoub*

In 1986 more than 1.5 million children nationwide experienced abuse or neglect (National Center on Child Abuse and Neglect [NCCAN], 1988). Identification and intervention of child maltreatment prevents or ameliorates significant short-term and long-term physical and emotional/developmental risks to the child's health and well-being. All 50 states in the United States have reporting statutes that include nurses as professionals mandated to report suspected maltreatment.

## NURSING DIAGNOSES

Altered growth and development related to inadequate or inappropriate caretaking; Ineffective family coping, disabling, related to unrealistic expectations or unmet psychosocial needs of the child by parent; Altered parenting related to physical and psychosocial abuse of nurturing figure; Powerlessness related to physical, emotional, or sexual abuse.

| Steps | Rationale |
|---|---|
| **Assessment** | |
| 1. Review presenting situation with consideration to complaint, age of child, and presence and state of mind of parent or accompanying adult. | Child abuse presents in a wide variety of ways. Direct admission of the problem by the perpetrator is rare. Cues are often subtle and require careful assessment of the child and family.<br>***Special Considerations:*** *Urgency is not based on the severity of the injury itself but on the etiology of the insult and the presentation of the family. Younger children (0 to 5 years) have a limited ability to communicate their situation, are less able to meet their own needs, and are more vulnerable to severe or fatal injury than older children (NCCAN, 1988). Classic presentation is of a child in distress brought in by a parent describing a vague or unknown complaint. Abuse is seldom given as primary reason for concern. For example, a very young child with linear bruises around the neck who is in no physical distress should raise concerns beyond the immediate impact of the present injury. Child abuse should be considered a potentially life-threatening health emergency.* |
| 2. Review possible signs and symptoms of abuse/neglect (see boxes on Types of Abuse and Emotional Maltreatment) and behavioral/environmental signs that may signal maltreatment (see box on Alerts to Maltreatment on p. 28) and compare findings to this situation. | Child maltreatment takes on many forms that require individualized approaches (Kempe and Helfer, 1980). |
| 3. Review age-appropriate developmental expectations of involved child (see Skill 25). | Discrepancy between developmentally possible or appropriate tasks is helpful in assessing the nature of the condition/injury to the child (Gallmeier and Bonner, 1988; Kempe and Helfer, 1980). |
| 4. Obtain information about available institutional supports (child abuse consultation team), mandated agency (usually local child welfare department), and juvenile legal system. | Child abuse requires a multidisciplinary, multiagency approach and mandatory reporting of suspicion of abuse or neglect. |
| **Planning and Goal Setting** | |
| 1. Tend to the details of the evaluation immediately on presentation. Rearrange personal schedule to allow abuse/neglect evaluation to take top priority. | Regardless of the extent of the injury, the potential for further abuse/neglect is always present and presents an immediate threat to the child. |
| 2. Consider time and process needed for each evaluation. | |
| a. Determine order of assessment events based on preliminary information about severity and etiology of injury/condition and socioemotional presentation of child and accompanying adult. | Nature and severity of the problem (acute vs. subacute injury) should be considered to order the assessment process. The child's physical needs or safety should not be jeopardized. The accompanying adult's emotional needs of stress, shame, or fear should be addressed supportively. |

| **Steps** | **Rationale** |
|---|---|
| b. Allow enough time for history taking and psychosocial interview of parent/accompanying adult and child, physical examination, and needed laboratory tests. | A thorough, paced assessment may take an hour or more. A calm, unhurried, supportive attitude is central to productive information gathering and stress reduction in the child and family. |
| c. Plan and implement immediate referral to special team or group for evaluation if time and present role do not allow for further evaluation. | Immediate evaluation is imperative for the protection of the child when abuse is suspected. ***Special Considerations:*** *Consultation with special teams or individuals with cultural expertise may be indicated if families from different ethnic or cultural backgrounds are involved. This practice serves as a check for personal bias.* |
| 3. Coordinate with other professionals who will share in the assessment. | Nurses are often part of a special evaluation group. Careful planning of each professional's role reduces miscommunication in a situation where coping mechanisms are frequently stressed. |
| 4. Create an environment conducive to discussion. a. Approach all involved in a calm, nonjudgmental manner. b. Arrange area for maximum privacy for all parties. | Cooperation is built with trust and concern. Assessment is the first step to change and sets the tone for future intervention. |
| 5. If serious, immediate danger to the child is present or guardian refuses to allow or continue examination, alert mandated agency or police. | Protection of the child should supersede attempts to engage parents in complete assessment. Legal intervention should be requested if immediate threat or harm to child is present. ***Special Considerations:*** *Parents who appear to be out of touch with reality, intoxicated, or intensely anxious or hostile should be approached with extreme caution. Interview may be deferred or done with two professionals present, if necessary.* |
| 6. Develop individualized goals for nursing care: ▪ Assess nature and extent of injuries. ▪ Determine possible etiologies and implications for health and safety of the child. ▪ Act on suspicious findings of maltreatment by notifying appropriate authorities. ▪ Provide safe environment for the child until authorities intervene. ▪ Provide emotional support for child. ▪ Provide emotional support for family. | |

## Implementation

| | |
|---|---|
| 1. Obtain detailed history from parent to include: a. Psychosocial history to include family environment information (see Skill 38). | A sense of the family environment and the individual interrelationships of those people close to the child are central to understanding the situation. ***Special Considerations:*** *Include an assessment of child care arrangement(s), a potential source of maltreatment.* |
| b. Developmental history of child (see Skill 25). | The child's developmental history provides a framework in which to consider compatibility of the described events surrounding the injury/condition with the child's developmental skills. |
| c. Health history (see Skill 23). | Health history contains clues to the child's general well-being and specific issues that may be related to the child's injury/condition. |
| d. History of events surrounding injury or condition including: ▪ When the injury/condition occurred. ▪ Who was present. | The clarity and congruity of the events are indications of the truthfulness and attentiveness of the child's caretakers. |
| ▪ Sequence of events from the time of the injury/event to present. | Parents who do not know the time or circumstances surrounding injury/condition raise concern. |
| ▪ Reasons for which the parent sought medical attention for the child. | Histories that are not compatible with the physical findings are suspicious. ***Special Considerations:*** *Delay in seeking medical attention and children with multiple injuries in different stages of healing are suspicious, and explanations for each should be requested.* |
| 2. Obtain separate history from the child privately if he or she is old enough to communicate. Child should be placed at ease in an environment that is safe and comfortable. Age-appropriate toys or games are helpful. | Child may confirm the parent's story or arouse suspicion about its accuracy. Children need time to feel at ease and may need to be reassured that they are safe. Children use toys to relax, as well as to communicate feelings and situations. |

## *EMOTIONAL MALTREATMENT*

**I. IGNORING**

The parent is psychologically unavailable to the child, i.e., the parent is preoccupied with self and unable to respond to the child's behaviors. Ignoring includes lack of sustained attention, prolonged periods of unavailability, limited emotional access, lack of responsiveness to the child's cries or requests, a pattern of coolness and lack of affect, failure to engage the child in activities, failing to protect the child from others, and demonstrating no interest in the child's activities or interests.

**II. ISOLATING**

The parent prevents the child from taking advantage of normal opportunities for social relationships or withdrawal or avoidance of interactional opportunities. Isolating includes leaving young children unattended for long periods in cribs or closed areas, punishing social overtures, removal of the child from interaction with peers, and punishment for engaging in normal social interactions.

**III. REJECTING**

The parent engages in behaviors that communicate or constitute abandonment. Rejecting may be occasional or continuous, generalized or categorical. Rejecting includes refusal to return smile and respond to social gestures, exclusion of the child from family activities, communication of a negative definition of self to the child, name calling, scapegoating, failure to acknowledge changing social roles (i.e., infantilizing), and subjecting child to humiliation and excessive criticism.

**IV. TERRORIZING**

The parent threatens the child with extreme or vague but sinister punishment, intentionally stimulating intense fear, creating a climate of unpredictable threat, or setting unmeetable expectations and punishing child for not meeting them. Terrorizing includes the use of scare tactics in discipline, direct threats to the child's security, deliberate violation of the child's tolerance for change, extreme gestures to intimidate, punish, verbal threats of extreme harm, frequent raging at the child, placing the child in intolerable double binds, forcing the child to choose between competing parents, frequently changing the rules, constantly criticizing, exposing the child to public humiliation, and ridiculing the child in public.

**V. CORRUPTING**

The parent reinforces antisocial or deviant patterns of behavior, particularly in the areas of substance abuse, aggression, and sexuality. Corrupting includes behaviors that encourage the child's unsuitable behavior in these areas either by conveying approval, reinforcing such delinquent behavior, or creating and sustaining patterns of behavior that risk permanent social dysfunction, including addiction, illegal activity, compulsive sexual acting out, or repetitive acts of violence.

Adapted from Garbarino J, Guttmann E, and Seeley J: The psychologically battered child, San Francisco, 1986, Jossey-Bass Publishers.

## *TYPES OF ABUSE*

**I. PHYSICAL ABUSE**

a. Soft tissue injury
   - Multiple bruises, particularly on the face, head, arms, or buttocks (not bony prominences such as knees, elbows)
   - Bruises with identifiable shape—lamp cord, belt buckle, hand, etc.
   - Human bites
   - Burns—scald, immersion, splash, contact, cigarette, chemical/ignitable substance

b. Head and central nervous system injury
   - Cerebral contusions, intracranial hemorrhage
   - Shaking injury-subdural hematoma, retinal hemorrhage, hidden fractures
   - Asphyxia—suffocation, strangulation

c. Chest and abdominal organ injury
   - Chest compression—Putscher's syndrome
   - Bruising or rupture of abdominal organs—kidney, spleen, pancreas, stomach, intestine

d. Skeletal injury
   - Fractured ribs with or without perforation
   - Skull fracture
   - Twist fracture of long bones, particularly femur
   - Epiphyseal-metaphyseal fracture
   - Any fracture with fractured rib

**II. SEXUAL ABUSE**

a. Intrusion—genital contact with penetration
b. Molestation—genital contact without penetration
c. Other sexually stimulating acts—fondling, voyeurism, exhibitionism.

| Steps | Rationale |
|---|---|
| | ***Special Considerations:*** *Special disclosure interviews for sexual abuse should be arranged with psychological experts in the field, as should any other special form of questioning to the child because the legal standard of proof needed in such situations may involve the criminal justice system.* |
| a. Child should be interviewed by one person (a second may be present) rather than by a series of individuals. | Repeated questioning is not only stressful, but may create a situation in which the child refuses to respond at all. ***Special Considerations:*** *Children can be interviewed in front of two-way mirrors or may be videotaped to reduce the number of interviews as long as the child and legal guardian have knowledge of and approve the procedure. These procedures remain controversial and policies differ among agencies.* |
| b. Child should be interviewed alone if possible; however, if a relative or adult friend provides support for child to proceed with process he or she can be included. Child should not be interviewed in the presence of the alleged perpetrator or anyone who sympathizes with that person. | The stress of subjecting a child to disclose abuse in the presence of the perpetrator is enormous. The child victim should not be further victimized in this way. |
| c. Questions should be:<br>▪ Tailored to the child's developmental level of understanding (see Skill 12).<br>▪ Open and nonleading (e.g., "Tell me about that boo-boo?" rather than "Did your mommy hit you?"). | Nonleading questions allow the child to tell the story without superimposing adult ideas. |
| d. Child should not be pressured to respond if he or she initially refuses to do so. | Pressuring may lead to further resistance and fear. ***Special Considerations:*** *Child may need to be interviewed by one special evaluator over time if found to be resistant.* |
| 3. Prepare child for physical examination and other procedures (see Skill 1). | Maltreated children may be particularly fearful of examination because of their abuse experiences. Preparation enhances trust and reduces fear and anxiety. |
| 4. Perform or assist with physical examination of child (see Skill 27). | Children with suspected abuse or neglect require complete physical exams to determine the presence of other injuries or conditions. ***Special Considerations:*** *Colposcopy is used with increasing frequency in sexual abuse examination (Gallmeier and Bonner, 1988).* |
| 5. Perform or assist with laboratory collections. | Children with suspected physical abuse may have hidden injuries that are only identified through laboratory investigation. Laboratory procedures should be ordered on a case-by-case basis after careful consideration of the medical findings and history of presenting problem. |
| a. Skeletal survey (long bones and/or bone scan). | Exploratory x-ray studies are indicated, since healing fractures are often identified only by x-ray. |
| b. Bleeding screen (PT, PTT, platelet count). | Rule out bleeding disorders in children with bruises since they may have thrombocytopenia purpura or other unusual bleeding problems. ***Special Considerations:*** *Careful physical examination and laboratory analysis can avoid false allegations.* |
| c. Sexual abuse lab protocol (acid phosphotase, gram stain, and cultures of any genital or anal discharge, *Neisseria gonorrhoeae* from the mouth, vagina, penis and anus; *Chlamydia trachomatis,* and serologic tests for syphilis; wet preparations for trichomonads and clue cells, Whiff test, vaginal culture for *Trichomonas vaginalis* and *Gardnerelia vaginalis*). | Sexual abuse requires specific laboratory specimens depending on the time of assault and the specific findings. Special protocols are frequently used in gathering of physical evidence for legal purposes (Ellerstein, 1981; Gallmeier and Bonner, 1988). |
| d. Other specialized laboratory tests may be required depending on the child's specific injury or condition. | ***Special Considerations:*** *See Ellerstein, 1981; Gallmeier and Bonner, 1988; Eman et al, 1987, for further details regarding specific protocols.* |
| 6. Review findings with other team members. | All information gathered should be discussed and integrated before presenting to parents or mandated authorities. This should be done with expediency while the child and family are still available. Child may require hospitalization for injuries, further assessment, or safety/protection precautions. |
| 7. Present findings to parents unless such informing presents a risk to child. If a report of suspected abuse is to be filed, explain the procedure to parents. Parents can be told "Your child's unexplained/confusing injuries/condition is of concern, and this requires us by law to report to the (mandated agency)." Aid in filing report as necessary. | The development of trust demands honesty and clarity (Racusin and Felsman, 1986). It is important to continue to treat suspected offenders in a nonaccusatory style. Support and a nonjudgmental attitude are required toward all parties present. |

### BEHAVIORAL/ENVIRONMENTAL ALERTS TO POSSIBLE MALTREATMENT

1. Contradictory or vague history
2. Delay in seeking treatment
3. Inappropriate food, clothing, shelter
4. Poor hygiene
5. Erratic or absent health care
6. Unsanitary environment
7. Child seen as "bad"
8. Parentification or pseudomaturity (child routinely takes care of parent)
9. Danger-oriented, hyperalert child
10. Depressed or socially withdrawn child
11. Emotional difficulties, especially nightmares, somatic complaints, sleep disorders, substance abuse, running away
12. Delayed development in a normal child
13. Premature erotization (specific to sexual abuse)
    a. Preoccupation with genitals
    b. Repetitive seeking to engage others in sexualized behavior
    c. Excessive and indiscriminate masturbation or masturbation with objects
    d. Precocious seductive behavior
    e. Depiction of differentiated sexual acts in doll play or during play therapy (specific reenactment of intercourse or other adult sexual acts)
14. Inappropriate/absent supervision/safety

| Steps | Rationale |
|---|---|
| 8. Provide further support with the process as needed. | Individual aid for parents or children is often required. Accompany for admission, serve as facilitator in contacts with mandated agency professionals, or provide individual support to child or family. |
| 9. Document all aspects of the process carefully, including conversations with child, significant others, process of interviews, exams, laboratory collections, consultation with inhouse personnel and involved outside agencies. | The chart is a legal document often subjected to scrutiny throughout any legal proceedings resulting from findings of assessment. **Special Considerations:** *Student nurses should leave charting to professional staff in cases of child maltreatment.* |

| Evaluation Outcomes | Observational Guidelines |
|---|---|
| 1. The etiology of the child's condition/injury has been carefully evaluated, considering the physical findings, presenting situation, and psychosocial dynamics of individuals. | Observe for physical and emotional signs of maltreatment, obtain and review detailed information that relates to injury, and assure that complete physical evaluation is conducted and evaluated in light of all known information from child, family, and others. |
| 2. An interdisciplinary team has coordinated efforts to maximize the integration of information and clarification of interventions on behalf of the child. | Adequate consultation has been obtained. Child has been referred to a safe place (hospitalization, emergency foster care if situation cannot be fully evaluated). |
| 3. Action (based on 1 and 2) has been taken to improve the child's safety. | Oral and written reports of "suspicion" of abuse have been filed with mandated agency if needed. Referrals for other supportive services made as needed. |
| 4. The proper mandated agency has been contacted and additional information shared (if indicated). | Contacts are documented. (Examples of multidisciplinary team records can be found in Schmitt, 1989.) |
| 5. The process has been completed with respect and concern for reducing distress for the child and family. | Both child and family have received explanation of events and have had offers to discuss feelings and concerns. |
| 6. Continued contact with any one of the parties is negotiated if appropriate. | Parents desire to discuss or refrain from doing so should be respected. The effectiveness of reporting is evaluated through follow-up with the mandated agency, or with the primary caregiver (with parental permission) to assure implementation of discharge plan. |
| 7. Assessment and interventions have been carefully documented for the medical record. | Review documented information and interventions for completeness, objectivity, and detail. |

## Documentation

Document the following: date and time of contact with child and family; identifying information on all parties involved; description of general appearance of child and parent(s) or accompanying adult; medical and psychosocial history provided by each party; developmental and psychosocial impression of child; physical examination including description of injury/condition to include identification of each finding in terms of location, appearance, age, and possible etiology; description of circumstances surrounding injury/condition as conveyed by all persons providing history; results of all laboratory and x-ray findings; parental responses to the process noted and intervention initiated; team assumptions and conclusions; phone call documented in medical record followed by written referral to mandated agency if indicated; follow-up plans delineated.

# *SKILL 8* Obtaining Informed Consent for Minors

*Kristie S. Nix*

The nurse, as the child's advocate, has a duty to ensure that a child and the parents are properly informed regarding treatments, procedures, and research. Informed consent is defined as a process of shared decision-making based upon mutual respect and participation; it is necessary and important because families have the responsibility and right to make decisions on issues affecting their lives. Nurses often share the responsibility with other health team members to ensure that families give informed consent.

## NURSING DIAGNOSES

Health-seeking behaviors (informed consent) related to medical/nursing procedure; Anxiety related to unmet informational needs about consent for medical/nursing procedure; Decisional conflict related to alternatives, benefits, and risks for medical/nursing procedure.

| Steps | Rationale |
|---|---|
| **Assessment** | |
| 1. Determine legal guardian of child, whether parent or court-appointed guardian. | A legal guardian is necessary to provide consent for a minor child.<br>***Special Considerations:*** *Court orders for legal guardianship should be a part of the child's record. A child in foster care usually has a court-appointed guardian with legal authority to give consent. With divorced parents, either parent can give consent (Hogue, 1988).* |
| a. Determine if child qualifies as an emancipated or mature minor. | Emancipated minors are legally capable of giving consent without parental permission. A minor may become emancipated by military service; judicial decree; marriage; graduation from high school; self-employment; consent of parents; or failure of parents to meet legal responsibilities (Silva, 1984; Selbst, 1985).<br>***Special Considerations:*** *State laws vary regarding child's age or conditions that qualify a child as an emancipated minor. Some states have a "mature minor" doctrine, which allows minors to consent to medical/surgical therapy if they are capable of understanding the nature of the procedure and its consequences. Many states have statutes that allow minors to be treated without parental consent for sexually transmitted diseases, examination following rape, substance abuse, birth control, pregnancy, or abortion (Silva, 1984).* |
| 2. Assess competency (Silva, 1984) of the child and family based on the following: | Competency relates to decision-making ability; requirements of the decision to be made (e.g., conceptual difficulty or gravity of the decision); consideration of possible adverse effects of decision; consistency in choices that are tied to a set of values and goals; communication skills; and ability to reason and deliberate (Taylor and Hobaugh, 1986).<br>***Special Considerations:*** *The child's participation is variable and depends on emotional maturity, family dynamics, physician philosophy regarding child's involvement, and gravity of decisions to be made (Erickson and Hopkins, 1987).* |
| a. Goals and values; use the following to assess:<br>▪ Chronological age.<br>▪ Mental age.<br>▪ Legal status.<br>▪ Developmental status. | |

| Steps | Rationale |
|---|---|
| ▪ Family situation and arrangement.<br>▪ Family's goals and values.<br>▪ Minor's goals and values.<br>▪ Minor's ability to verbalize relationship between values and choices. | ***Special Considerations:*** *Child's or family's goals and values are best assessed over time as a relationship is established. Assessment of goals and values may be difficult. Listen for congruency in statements. Clarify meaning (e.g., ask, "Did I hear you say . . .").* |
| b. Comprehension and communication abilities; use the following to assess:<br>▪ Presence of psychological or motor impairment.<br>▪ Presence of memory impairment.<br>▪ Degree of orientation.<br>▪ Overall capacity to understand information.<br>▪ Present capacity to understand information.<br>▪ Ability to summarize information related to an informed consent. | The family must have the capacity to understand information provided during the process of informed consent (Hogue, 1988).<br>Ability to understand information may be affected by inner forces (e.g., anxiety, pain, medication) or external factors (e.g., culture, terminology, or speed of presentation) (Taylor and Hobaugh, 1986).<br>***Special Considerations:*** *Pay attention to questions asked, facial expressions, and other body language to determine comprehension. Use open-ended questions to elicit family's perceptions. For example, ask "In your own words, can you explain to me what you understand about what we've just discussed?"* |
| c. Reasoning capability and ability to make choices; use the following to assess:<br>▪ Health status.<br>▪ Perception of reality.<br>▪ Past history of decision-making.<br>▪ Typical thought processes involving decisions.<br>▪ Ability to verbalize relationship between condition and proposed treatment. | Ability to reason and make choices influences capacity to give consent.<br>***Special Considerations:*** *Ask questions that provide insight into decision-making (e.g., "In the past when you've had to make a difficult decision, what did you do?"). Assess for congruency of statements over time. The need to use assessment parameters in each category (a, b, and c) will vary based on the nature of decisions to be made.* |
| 3. Determine primary language and competency in English, if spoken. | ***Special Considerations:*** *It may be necessary to provide a translator who is competent in medical terminology to ensure that informed consent is properly obtained.* |
| 4. Cultural/religious background. | Cultural and religious traditions influence a family's decisions about care. Beliefs may prohibit parents from consenting to certain medical or nursing treatments.<br>***Special Considerations:*** *Sometimes it is necessary for health professionals to strike a balance between the presumed best interests of the child (e.g., a life-saving blood transfusion) and the rights of the parents to refuse treatment (Erickson and Hopkins, 1987). If the views of the parents and best interests of the child conflict, the judicial system may be invoked to protect the best interests of the child. All states have legal procedures to authorize needed medical treatment for children when parents refuse to permit it; they also have provisions for expediting the issuance of a court order when time is of the essence for medical action. Refer to agency protocol for requesting the hospital or county attorney to obtain court authorization for needed treatment (Rhodes, 1987). Parents may be limited by law in consenting for a child to donate organs or bone marrow, be sterilized, or terminate pregnancy. These cases may also require deliberation and consent of the court. In difficult cases, ethics committees may be a resource to assist health professionals or families in decisions related to informed consent (see also Skill 9).* |

## Planning and Goal Setting

| | |
|---|---|
| 1. Determine nursing responsibilities pertaining to informed consent process for: | Informed consent is active, shared decision-making between the provider and the recipient of care (Silva and Zeccolo, 1986). The person who will perform the procedure (whether physician or nurse) holds legal responsibility for assuring that the family clearly and completely understands the treatment to be performed and all the risks, consequences, or results that may or may not occur from the treatment (Whaley and Wong, 1991). |
| a. Medical procedures. | The legal duty to obtain informed consent resides with the physician who is going to perform the medical/surgical intervention (see box). |

### *INFORMED CONSENT DOCUMENTATION*

Separate informed permissions must be obtained for each surgical or diagnostic procedure, including:

1. Major surgery.*
2. Minor surgery, e.g., cutdown, biopsy, dental extraction, suturing a laceration (especially one that may have a cosmetic effect), removal of a cyst, and closed reduction of a fracture.*
3. Diagnostic tests with an element of risk, e.g., bronchoscopy, needle biopsy, angiography, electroencephalogram, lumbar puncture, cardiac catheterization, ventriculography, and bone marrow aspiration.*
4. Medical treatments with an element of risk, e.g., blood tranfusion, thoracentesis or paracentesis, radiation therapy, and shock therapy.*
5. Research.*†

Other situations that are not directly related to medical treatment but require consent:

1. Taking photographs for medical, educational, or other public use.*†
2. Removal of the child from the hospital against the advice of the physician.*†
3. Postmortem examination except in unexplained deaths, e.g., sudden infant death, violent death, or suspected suicide or abuse.*
4. Willingness to donate dying child's organs and tissue (bone, skin).*†
5. Examination of medical records by unauthorized persons, e.g., attorneys or insurance representatives (family members have the legal right to medical records).*†‡

Situations in which a parent cannot consent independently and may also require consent of the courts:

1. Organ or bone marrow donation from a healthy child.*
2. Sterilization of a minor.*
3. Termination of a minor's pregnancy.*

Adapted from Whaley LF and Wong DL: Nursing care of infants and children, ed 4, St Louis, 1991, The CV Mosby Co.
*Physician responsibility.
†Registered nurse responsibility.
‡Responsibility of others, e.g., attorneys.

| Steps | Rationale |
|---|---|
| | ***Special Considerations:*** *The nurse's role is to communicate with the child and family to ensure that they are not confused or that they have not changed their minds about proposed medical testing or therapy. Notify physician and document when the parents appear to have additional questions about procedures or have decided to withdraw consent.* |
| b. Nursing procedures. | Although a general consent for nursing and medical procedures provided by a hospital is usually obtained on admission and is a part of the patient record, obtain informed consent before beginning for general nursing procedures (e.g., vital signs) when explaining the procedure to the child or parent. Consent may be verbalized or manifested by the conduct of the child or family, such as when the parent assists with obtaining vital signs (Brent, 1987). In some cases, e.g., nursing research, responsibility for obtaining informed consent resides with the nurse (see box). In these cases, disclosure of information requirements (see next step) applies equally to a nurse or physician. |
| 2. If responsible for obtaining consent, prepare information related to: | These elements are considered essential to the process of providing informed consent. |
| a. Condition or problem.<br>b. Nature and purpose of proposed treatment.<br>c. Risks and consequences of proposed treatment.<br>d. Feasible alternatives.<br>e. Consequences of nontreatment.<br>f. Prognosis. | Although it is unnecessary to divulge all potential risks, statistically significant risks should be discussed. Risks that are not statistically significant should be discussed if the child has unique characteristics that make risk more probable or if risk could be meaningful to child or family. The doctrine of informed refusal provides that information should be given to the family regarding probable injury/harm to health for refusing rec- |

| Steps | Rationale |
|---|---|
| | ommended treatment (Creighton, 1986). |
| 3. Prepare appropriate documents for signatures. | The consent form serves as evidence that the process of informed consent occurred. ***Special Considerations:*** *Legally, it is not necessary to sign a consent, but a signed document serves as evidence that the obligation to provide necessary information was met and serves to protect nurses, physicians, and hospitals or other agencies. However, the fact that consent is written does not mean that it is either valid or informed (Working Group, 1986). Alternative methods to written consent include tape recordings, a witness, or providing written information about the treatment. Nevertheless, most agency policies require written signatures on specific forms (Hogue, 1986).* |
| a. Ensure that documents are legible and comprehensible. | Language that is too technical or detailed to understand may contribute to *uninformed* consent. ***Special Considerations:*** *Whereas a nonprofessional may transcribe information from a physician's order to consent document, responsibility often rests with the nurse to check for correct spelling of the procedure or treatment and names of persons authorized to participate.* |
| b. Determine if the child is cognitively capable of and should be included in signing consent forms (see Skill 25). | The child's participation is variable and depends on emotional maturity, family dynamics, physician philosophy regarding child's involvement, and gravity of decisions to be made (Erickson and Hopkins, 1987). |
| 4. Select an optimal time and place for obtaining informed consent. | Time and setting for explaining and discussing proposed diagnostic tests, treatments, procedures, or research should reinforce the voluntary nature of the process. Setting should be as quiet and free of distractions as possible. |
| 5. Develop individualized client and family goals:<br>▪ Participates in shared planning and decision-making regarding medical and nursing care. | |

## Implementation

| Steps | Rationale |
|---|---|
| 1. When informing a family about a nursing treatment, include the following elements (Taylor and Hobaugh, 1986): | In court cases, these elements are considered to determine if consent is based on adequate information. |
| a. Current status, including likely course if no treatment is provided. | One option a family may choose is to take no action or refuse treatment. The informed consent process requires that possible consequences of the option be divulged. |
| b. An objective discussion of treatment alternatives, including a description of the procedures involved and the probable related risks and benefits. | The family may experience difficulty making a choice. Working through options with the family (see Skill 9) may help. |
| c. An explanation of the role uncertainty plays in any course of action, i.e., there are no guarantees in health care. | |
| d. On request, a professional opinion as to the best alternative. | The family may ask "What would you do in this situation?" It is reasonable to give a professional opinion or offer referral sources (clergy, social worker, psychologist, etc.) to help the family. |
| 2. Before any medical/surgical procedure, ensure that the parents understand what has been explained to them by the physician. | Language that is too technical for the parents to understand may lead to uninformed consent. ***Special Considerations:*** *Inform the physician when parents indicate confusion. Avoid explaining procedures for which the physician is responsible (Bernzweig, 1984; Silva and Zecollo, 1986).* |
| a. Encourage questions about proposed diagnostic or treatment procedures. | |
| b. If no questions are forthcoming, use an open-ended question to verify understanding, e.g., "Can you tell me in your own words what is going to happen?" | The child/family may be hesitant or unable to ask questions because of variables such as anxiety, fear of appearing uninformed, or feeling intimidated. |
| 3. Allow the family adequate time to make decisions. | Time should be allowed for the family to consider options, ask questions, and weigh risks and benefits. |
| 4. Ensure voluntary nature of the decision-making process. | Freedom to make a decision may be compromised by saying things like, "The care of your child will improve if you participate" (De Leon Siantz, 1988). Ultimatums, e.g., "This is your only choice," may later be held to constitute duress, coercion, or undue influence. |

| Steps | Rationale |
|---|---|
| 5. Witness signatures on informed consent forms. | In most cases, the physician will be responsible for explaining proposed treatments, but the nurse is often required to obtain signatures on consent forms. **_Special Considerations:_** *When required to witness signatures for medical procedures, document "witnessing consent only" with signature to signify nonprovision of information related to the medical treatment or procedure (Northrup, 1985).* |
| a. Provide family with a copy of consent form. | A copy of the form communicates to the family that they are full partners in the decision and nothing has been withheld. |
| 6. If necessary, obtain consent by telephone. | In cases when a parent/guardian cannot be present to sign a consent form, consent may be verbal. |
| a. Have a second nurse listen to the conversation on an extension or speaker phone.<br>b. Both nurses should cosign documentation that includes:<br>1) Name of person giving permission and legal relationship to child.<br>2) Date and time.<br>3) Telephone consent. | **_Special Considerations:_** *A tape recording of the conversation would be useful; however, all parties should be aware of the recording and give permission.* |
| 7. Inform family that they can withdraw consent at any time, even after authorized treatment has begun (Bernzweig, 1984). | Parents may fear that their child will not receive adequate treatment if unwilling to comply with proposed treatment. **_Special Considerations:_** *Guard against labeling a family as "difficult" when choices are made that conflict with personal opinions and values. Such action may be interpreted as manipulation, infringing on the voluntary nature of informed consent.* |

| Evaluation Outcomes | Observational Guidelines |
|---|---|
| 1. The child/family have received adequate information with which to make a decision. | Information has been shared regarding current medical status and course of treatment, risks and benefits of various treatment alternatives, and prognosis. |
| 2. The child/family comprehend alternatives for health care. | Ask the family to list or explain alternatives as they understand them. Compare with actual identified alternatives. |
| 3. The child/family demonstrate competence to make a decision regarding health care. | Child/family demonstrate capacity to reason and deliberate and make consistent choices; ask appropriate questions or verbalize understanding in own words. |
| 4. The child/family understand the voluntary nature of informed consent. | Freedom to withdraw consent or refuse treatment are presented as options, including potential injury/risks related to such choices. |

## Documentation

Documentation should include: assessments; family members present or contacted; place and time when consent occurred; family reaction or statements; notification of physician when family is hesitant or confused regarding medical information; whether patient was capable of refusing/withdrawing consent; refusal of diagnostic tests or treatment; acceptance of treatment regardless of risks; declining or withdrawal of consent; all attempts to contact parents who are not present to give consent; use of translator and translator's name; "witnessing signature only" when not giving information.

## Home Care Modifications

Teach parents to provide caretakers with emergency authorization forms. Authorization to seek medical treatment should be granted to responsible parties (relatives, babysitters, and day care, school, or camp personnel) in writing by parents. Inform parents that even with such written authorization, health care providers have a duty to contact parents.

# SKILL 9 Assisting the Family in Making Ethical Decisions

*Rita J. Payton*

Families and health care professionals are faced with choices during the delivery of health care. Available choices often reflect conflicting values about health, illness, quality of life, and individual versus societal rights. Conflict and resultant tension about what they "ought" to do may exist within the family unit. Ethical decision-making often involves not only the family, but also health care professionals, the community, and society in general. This skill, however, focuses on the nurse's role in assisting the family with a decision-making process when an ethical decision must be made.

## NURSING DIAGNOSES

Decisional conflict related to lack of relevant information about choices and consequences or lack of experience with decision making; Ineffective family coping (compromised or disabling) related to situational crises, inadequate information, or family disorganization.

| Steps | Rationale |
|---|---|
| **Assessment** | |
| 1. Communicate with family to assess:<br>a. Past experiences with the health care system. | Past personal experiences and those of others may affect perceptions that families have of certain treatment options. Misconceptions about the health care system may be present. |
| b. Family's desired level of involvement in health care decision-making. | Families may desire variable levels of involvement in decision-making. Many families are aware of their right to make informed decisions that affect their health and well-being and desire to be more actively involved in health care decisions than has been true historically. However, a family may express an autonomous desire to defer to authority rather than participate in decision-making, e.g., "We trust the staff here to decide." A family that makes autonomous decisions may do what is suggested to them by persons on the health care team because they agree with what has been suggested and not because they have been told to do it.<br>***Special Considerations:*** *No matter what the family's level of involvement, support and value the uniqueness of the family unit and their desire to participate in decision-making.* |
| c. Knowledge base for decision-making. Ask the family the following: "Do you have the information needed to make a decision? What is unknown? What can be clarified or explained for you?" | An adequate knowledge base is essential for good decision-making. |
| d. Coping strategies used in the past and present. Ask the family: "How have you handled previous decisions? What has worked for you in the past?" | Some coping methods such as intellectualization directly affect the extent to which families wish to engage in ethical decision-making. Other methods such as denial impede decision-making. |
| e. Ability to freely ask questions and express conflict about what to do. | An adequate knowledge base is facilitated by open communication and an opportunity to express feelings and concerns. A collaborative relationship with the family is desirable for optimal decision-making. |
| f. Cultural factors affecting decision-making ability, e.g., religion and family roles (see Skill 41). | Cultural attitudes and beliefs affect family's relationship toward authority, level of involvement in health care, perceptions of life and death, and relationships within the family. |
| 2. Communicate with the child to determine:<br>a. Chronological and developmental age; grade in school (if appropriate). | These factors are indicators of child's ability to engage in problem-solving and decision-making. |

| Steps | Rationale |
|---|---|
| b. Ability and interest to engage in problem-solving. | A positive therapeutic benefit is derived when a child participates in decision-making. The consenting child plays an active role as a partner and participant in treatment and is not simply a subject submitting to distasteful therapies.<br>***Special Considerations:*** *Consent implies a complete and voluntary commitment to the intervention, whereas assent indicates that the child poses no objection.* |
| c. Role of this child in decision-making within the family. | The role the child holds in decision-making offers clues to his or her experience with expressing opinions. Families vary widely in decision-making patterns (e.g., parents share equally or one person has ultimate authority). These patterns are often well established and become even more pronounced when the family unit is stressed.<br>***Special Considerations:*** *Tension may exist between the child's right of self-determination and the more traditional rights of parents as decision-makers for the child.* |
| 3. Determine whether an ethical conflict confronts the family and whether they believe a dilemma exists. | An ethical dilemma exists when there is conflict between choices about what to do. The family may have strong beliefs about the choices and their consequences. Conflict may exist between family members, family and health care team members, or family and institution or society.<br>***Special Considerations:*** *Differentiate between problems with communication, administrative issues, or personality conflicts.* |

## Planning and Goal Setting

| Steps | Rationale |
|---|---|
| 1. Clearly define the nature of the dilemma and the participants (e.g., staff, physician, child, family). | At times dilemmas arise that do not directly involve the nurse. However, the nurse may advocate for the family and provide support during the decision-making process. |
| 2. Identify supports for the family during decision-making (e.g., clergy or a close friend). | Resolving ethical dilemmas often involves the active participation of several health care team members and external support systems identified by the family. |
| 3. Identify strategies to facilitate family understanding and knowledge base. | The family is provided with opportunities for obtaining information/knowledge necessary for decision-making.<br>***Special Considerations:*** *One method to equip the family is through a multidisciplinary meeting involving the family and support personnel. Another strategy is to give the family verbal and written information related to the nature of the dilemma (e.g., diagnosis, treatment options).* |
| 4. Identify an ethical decision-making process that may be useful in helping this family resolve the dilemma if a defined process is needed. | Whereas some families exhibit well-developed problem-solving skills, others are immobilized when confronted with an ethical dilemma. There are several ethical decision-making models available (Payton, 1979; Fowler and Levine-Ariff, 1987; Thompson and Thompson, 1985). The most success in helping the family work through the dilemma will occur if a familiar decision-making process is used. |
| 5. Prepare any written material that might be helpful for understanding the decision-making process. | A sketch of the decision-making process and a list of possible choices can be helpful for the family. |
| 6. Decide who to work with:<br>a. Both parents and child.<br>b. Parents only.<br>c. Child and parents separately. | Legal requirements mandate that the professional work with the parents or the legally responsible party. Ethical requirements mandate that the professional work with the child as well. This may require initially meeting with the parents and the child separately, especially if there is reason to believe there may be a conflict between the decisions made by the parents and child.<br>***Special Considerations:*** *If there is conflict, determine strategies for mediating the conflict. This may place the nurse in a difficult situation between the child and family. Situations beyond one's expertise should be referred.* |
| 7. Personally work through the dilemma using the selected process. | Working through the dilemma personally will help determine if all necessary data has been collected. This step is not done to help the family "see" the "right" decision, but to assist problem-solving. |
| a. Identify all possible action choices. | ***Special Considerations:*** *At this point be exhaustive. Do not be limited by legal parameters or personal value set. Remember that to choose to take no action is in itself a powerful action choice. Also, consider that the human mind prefers "either/or" thinking; do not quit after identifying two action choices.* |

| Steps | Rationale |
|---|---|
| b. Rule out action choices in conflict with personal values. | All persons value some actions more than others. Some actions violate a deeply held personal value, e.g., taking a patient's life by ceasing ventilator function. |
| c. Develop an ethical statement for the action choice that appears most desirable. | An ethical statement declares *who* is going to do *what* under *which* circumstances. It includes the power verb *ought* as its verb, e.g., "Nurse practitioners ought to provide contraceptives to sexually active minors regardless of whether or not parental consent is given." An ethical statement implies by its "ought" that in theory the statement applies to all people in similar circumstances. |
| d. Determine the consequences of the chosen action. | By defining both immediate and long-term consequences, one can hypothesize outcomes if everyone took the action proposed in moral statement.<br>***Special Considerations:*** *People frequently tend to be more concerned with immediate short-term consequences than with long-term global consequences.* |
| e. Compare the consequences identified with personal value set. | As nursing is inherently a human-to-human interaction, the consequences are generally congruent with the nurse's personal values. |
| ▪ Action choice ethically valid if consequences are in agreement with value set. | ***Special Considerations:*** *Values clarification exercises may be applied to increase awareness of own value set (see Uustal, 1987).* |
| ▪ Inconsistency between values and consequences requires either making another action choice or modifying the conditions under which the action would be taken. | ***Special Considerations:*** *When a different action choice is made or the moral statement conditions are modified, the new action choice or moral statement must be analyzed through steps of the decision-making model.* |
| 8. Select an optimal time and place for helping the family work through the dilemma. | Avoidance of distractions eases communication and facilitates decision-making (see Skill 43). |
| 9. Develop individualized client and family goals:<br>▪ The family engages in ethical decision-making.<br>▪ The family reaches consensus about a desired action. | |

## Implementation

| Steps | Rationale |
|---|---|
| 1. Use the identified decision-making process with the family. Review the steps slowly and thoroughly. | Families may be unfamiliar with this type of decision-making and need time to process and reflect on a new way of approaching a decision. |
| 2. Have other members of the health care team available as resource persons as needed. | Some decisions, e.g., treatment options involving both medical and nursing interventions, require that several health care team members be present or at least available for clarification. |
| 3. Serving as a resource person, have the family problem-solve the dilemma. | Clarifying information and providing additional data increases the family's knowledge base.<br>***Special Considerations:*** *This process may occur rapidly in terms of actual arrival at the decision or may occur very slowly over a period of days or even months, e.g., with a decision about termination of care. Discussions regarding potential ethical conflicts should occur at the earliest possible time.* |
| 4. Verify the decision with the family both verbally and in writing, stated in their own words. | Having the family state their decision in their own words minimizes the possibility of misinterpretation.<br>***Special Considerations:*** *Advocate for the family by adapting nursing interventions to coincide with decisions made by the family.* |

| Evaluation Outcomes | Observational Guidelines |
|---|---|
| 1. Family recognizes options related to health care issues. | Assessment information is documented. Family asks questions and seeks clarification. |
| 2. Family understands choices and their consequences. | Written options are given to family and documented. Decision-making model is used to facilitate selection of choice. |
| 3. Family reaches a consensus about a desired course of action. | Ask family about desired action that was selected. Review chart for documentation of family's decision. Review care plan for interventions appropriate to choices made by the family. |
| 4. Child assents or consents to decision. | Child is able to express preferences. |

## Documentation

Document questions raised by the child/family. Note attempts to involve or actual involvement of other health care team members in decision-making. Note action choices considered by the family and choice(s) they have made. Document treatment plan to meet mutual goals of care.

## UNIT I

### PRODUCT REFERENCES AND TEACHING RESOURCES
### Patient Education Materials

Braznick D: Becky's story, Washington, DC, 1981, Association for the Care of Children's Health.

"Going to the Hospital", Association for the Care of Children's Health, 1986, Washington, DC.

Hill E: Spot Visits the Hospital, New York, 1987, GP Putnam's Sons.

Howe J: The Hospital Book, New York, 1981, Crown Publishers, Inc. (Also available through the Association for the Care of Children's Health.)

Ped Pals
P.O. Box 4089
380 Victoria Road
Youngstown, Ohio 44515
(216) 797-0277

This comprehensive pediatric patient education program offers informational pamphlets to prepare children for procedures.

Reit S: Some busy hospital, Racine, Wis., 1985, Western Publishing Co Inc.

Rogers F: Going to the Hospital, Pittsburgh, 1977, Family Communications.

Wong DL and Whaley LF: Clinical manual of pediatric nursing, ed 3, St Louis, 1990, The CV Mosby Co.

You're Gonna Do What?
Arkansas Children's Hospital
800 Marshall Street
Little Rock, AR 72202-3591

This series of pediatric preparation pamphlets covers 72 commonly performed procedures.

### Organizations

National emergency child abuse hotline number is 1-800-422-4453 (1-800-4-A-CHILD).

Telephone numbers of local Child Welfare Departments are usually listed under "Child Abuse" in the business white pages of local telephone directories.

Association for the Care of Children's Health
7910 Woodmont Ave.
Bethesda, Md 20814
(301) 654-6549

This organization is dedicated to children's health and has numerous books and brochures available to help children and their families cope with experiences with health care.

Clearinghouse on Child Abuse and Neglect Information
P.O. Box 1182
Washington, DC 20013
(703) 821-2086

Pediatric Projects
P.O. Box 1880
Santa Monica, CA 90406-1880
(213) 828-8963
Hearing or speech impaired callers - 1-800-342-5966 (CA only)

This nonprofit organization offers medically oriented materials (toys, books, games, etc.) to help children and their families understand experiences in health care. A catalog of materials and a quarterly newsletter are available.

## REFERENCES


Alexander D, White M, and Powell G: Anxiety of nonrooming-in parents of hospitalized children, Children's Health Care 15(1): 14-20. 1986.

Arkansas Children's Hospital: You're gonna do what? Little Rock, Ark, 1984, Arkansas Children's Hospital.

Azarnoff P, editor: Preparation of young healthy children for possible hospitalization: the issues, Santa Monica, Calif, 1983, Pediatric Projects, Inc.

Azarnoff P: Preparing well children for possible hospitalization, Pediatr Nurs 11(1): 53-56, 1985.

Bartholomew WG: The child-patient: do parents have the right to decide? In Spicker SF, Healey JM, and Engelhardt HT, editors: The law-medicine relation: a philosophical exploration, Boston, 1981, D Reidel.

Bauchner H, Vinci R, and Waring C: Pediatric procedures: do parents want to watch? Pediatrics 84(5): 907-909, 1989.

Berksy AK, Keys EJ, and Dickens RN: Learning interdisciplinary and assessment skills through videotaped client interviews and collaborative planning, J Nurs Educ 26(5): 202-204, 1987.

Bernzweig EP: Don't cut corners on informed consent, RN 47(11): 15-16, 1981.

Boatwright D and Crummette BD: How to plan and conduct a patient care conference, Nursing 17(2): 64, 1987.

Bock RH: State of the art, Caring 4(5): 26-28, 1985.

Brandon DH and Huber CJ: Evaluating cost-effectiveness of preevaluation client visits, Nurs Econ 5(2): 65-76, 1987.

Brent NJ: How informed are you about consents? Nursing Life 7(6): 37-39, 1987.

Brody H: Ethical decisions in medicine, Boston, 1976, Little, Brown & Co.

Broome ME: The relationship between children's fears and behavior during a painful event, Children's Health Care 14(3): 142-145, 1986.

Cagan J and Meier P: A discharge planning tool for use with families of high-risk infants, JOGN 8(3): 146-148, 1979.

Cerne F: Collaborative practice benefits nurses, patients, Hospitals 62(3):78, 1988.

Creighton H: Informed consent, Nurs Man 17(10): 11-13, 1986.

Creighton H: Legal implications of home health care, Nurs Man 18(2): 14-17, 1987.

Cumberlege J et al: Whose patient is it, anyway? Nurs Times 83:22, 1987.

Cushing M: Legal lessons on patient teaching, AJN 84(6): 721-722, 1984.

De Leon Siantz ML: Defining informed consent, MCN 13(2): 94, 1988.

Dixon S and Stein M: Encounters with children: pediatric behavior and development, Chicago, 1987, Year Book Medical Publishers.

Droske S and Francis S: Pediatric diagnostic procedures, New York, 1981, John Wiley & Sons.

Dumas L: How to tie up the discharge plan, RN 50(4): 81-82, 1987.

Ellerstein N, editor: Child abuse and neglect: a medical reference, New York, 1981, John Wiley & Sons.

Eman S et al: Genital findings in sexually abused symptomatic and asymptomatic girls, Pediatrics 79(5): 778-785, 1987.

Erickson S and Hopkins MA: Gray areas: informed consent in pediatric and comatose adult patients, Heart and Lung 16(3): 323-325, 1987.

Erlen J: The child's choice: an essential component in treatment decisions, Children's Health Care 15(3): 156-160, 1987.

Feetham S: Hospitals and home care: inseparable in the '80s, Pediatr Nurs, 12(5): 383-386, 1986.

Feinberg FA: Family stress in pediatric care, Caring 4(5): 38-41, 1985.

Feuer L: Discharge planning: home caregivers need your support, too, Nurs Man 18(4): 58-59, 1987.

Fowler MD and Levine-Ariff J: Ethics at the bedside, Philadelphia, 1987. JB Lippincott Co.

Gallmeier T and Bonner B, editors: For kids sake: an advanced curriculum in child sexual abuse for health care professionals, Oklahoma City, 1988, University of Oklahoma Health Science Center.

Garbarino J, Guttmann E, and Seeley J: The psychologically battered child, San Francisco, 1986, Jossey-Bass Publishers.

Gaylin W: The competence of children: no longer all or none, The Hastings Center Report 12(2): 33-38, 1982.

Gill KM: Parent participation with a family health focus: nurses' attitudes, Pediatr Nurs 13(2): 94-96, 1987.

Gohsman B and Yunck M: Dealing with the threats of hospitalization, Pediatr Nurs 5(5): 32-35, 1979.

Goodell A: Peer education in schools for children with cancer, Issue Compr Pediatr Nurs 7:101-106, 1984.

Gross S: Pediatric tours of hospitals - positive or negative? MCN 11: 336-338, 1986.

Hansen B and Evans M: Preparing a child for procedures, MCN 6(6): 392-397, 1981.

Harvey S: Parents are the best preparers of young children. In P. Azarnoff, editor: Preparation of young healthy children for possible hospitalization: the issues, Santa Monica, Calif, 1983, Pediatric Projects, Inc.

Healey JM: Patient rights and nursing. In Murphy CP and Hunter H, editors: Ethical problems in the nurse-patient relationship, Boston, 1983, Allyn and Bacon.

Hogue EE: Informed consent: implications for critical care nurses, Pediatr Nurs 14(4): 315-316, 1988.

Hogue EE: What you should know about informed consent, Nursing 16(6): 47-48, 1986.

Johnson JE, Kerchhoff KR, and Endress MP: Easing children's fright during health care procedures, MCN 1(4): 206-210, 1976.

Kempe H and Helfer R, editors: The battered child, ed 3, Chicago, 1980, The University of Chicago Press.

Knafl KA: How families manage a pediatric hospitalization, WJ Nurs Research, 7(2): 151-176, 1985.

Koerner BL, Cohen JR, and Armstrong DM: Professional behavior in collaborative practice, J Nurs Adm 16(10): 39-43, 1986.

Kruger S and Rawlins P: Pediatric dismissal protocol to aid the transition from hospital care to home care. Image 16(4): 120-125, 1984.

Larkin J: Factors influencing one's ability to adapt to chronic illness, Nurs Clin North Am 22(3): 535-542, 1987.

Lynn MR: Children have rights, too, J Pediatr Nurs 1(10): 345-349, 1986.

MacFarlane K et al: Sexual abuse of young children, New York, ed 3, Chicago, 1986, The Guildford Press.

McClowry SG: Research and treatment: ethical distinctions related to the care of children, J Pediatr Nurs 2(1): 23-27, 1987.

Mezzanotte J: A checklist for better discharge planning, Nursing 17(10): 55, 1987.

Miller S: Children's fears: a review of the literature with implications for nursing research and practice. Nurs Res 28(4): 217-223, 1979.

National Center on Child Abuse and Neglect, U.S. Department of Health and Human Services: Study finding: study of national incidence and prevalence of child abuse and neglect: 1988, Washington, DC, 1988, National Center on Child Abuse and Neglect.

Noga KM: High-risk infants—the need for follow-up nursing care. JOGN 11(2): 112-115, 1982.

Northrup CE: The ins and outs of informed consent, Nursing 15(1): 9, 1985.

O'Malley ST and Ness PL: Intensive care at home: establishing a program in Washington state, Home HealthC Nurse 5(1): 8-11, 1987.

Pass M and Pass C: Anticipatory guidance for parents of hospitalized children, J Pediatr Nurs 2(4): 250-258, 1987.

Payton RJ: Pluralistic ethical decision making, In Clinical and scientific sessions, 1979, Kansas City, Mo, 1979, American Nurses' Association.

Perrin E and Gerrity P: Development of child with a chronic illness, Pediatr Clin North Am 31(1): 19-31, 1984.

Perrin JM: Chronically ill children in America, Caring 4(5): 16-22, 1985.

Perry S: Teaching tools made by peers: A novel approach to medical preparation, Children's Health Care 15(1): 21-25, 1986.

Pridham KF et al: Helping children deal with procedures in a clinic setting: a developmental approach - competence and self-esteem, J Pediatr Nurs, 2(1): 13-22, 1987.

Prugh DG et al: A study of emotional reactions of children and families to hospitalization and illness, Am J Orthopsychiatry 23: 70-106, 1953.

Racusin R and Felsman K: Reporting child abuse: the ethical obligation to inform parents, J Am Acad Child Adolesc Psych 25(4): 485-489, 1986.

Rhodes AM: Obtaining consent to treat minors, MCN 12(3): 209, 1987.

Rhodes AM: When parents refuse to consent, MCN 12(4): 289, 1987.

Robertson J: The fallacy of "preparing" young healthy children for possible hospitalization. In P Azarnoff, editor: Preparation of young healthy children for possible hospitalization: the issues, Santa Monica, Calif, 1983, Pediatric Projects, Inc.

Robinson CA: Double bind: a dilemma for parents of chronically ill children, Pediatr Nurs 11(2): 112-115, 1985.

Robinson CA: Preschool children's conceptualizations of health and illness, Children's Health Care 16(2): 89-95, 1987.

Rusch SC: Continuity of care: from hospital unit to home, Nurs Man 17(12): 38-41, 1986.

Rushing P: The challenge of caring for a patient at home, RN 50(1): 61-62, 1987.

Rushton CH: Ethical decision making in critical care part 1: the role of the pediatric nurse, Pediatr Nurs 14(5): 411-412, 1988.

Rushton CH: Ethical decision making in critical care part 2: strategies for nurse preparation, Pediatr Nurs 14(6): 497-502, 1988.

Schmitt B: The child protection handbook, ed 2, New York, 1989, Garland STPM Press.

Seigel H: Nurses improve hospital efficiency through a risk assessment model at admission, Nurs Man 19(10): 38-46, 1988.

Selbst SM: Treating minors without their parents, Pediatr Emerg Care 1(3): 168-173, 1985.

Sgroi S: Handbook of clinical intervention in child sexual abuse, Lexington, Mass, 1982, Lexington Books.

Shelton TL, Jeppson ES, and Johnson BH: Family-centered care for children with special health care needs, ed 2, Washington DC, 1987, Association for the Care of Children's Health.

Silva MC: Assessing competency for informed consent with mentally retarded minors, Pediatr Nurs 10(4): 261-265, 306, 1984.

Silva MC and Zeccolo PL: Informed consent: the right to know and the right to choose, Nurs Man 17(6): 18-19, 1986.

Siaw SN: Knowledge about medical instruments and reported anxiety in pediatric surgery patients, Children's Health Care 14(3): 134-141, 1986.

Slevin A and Roberts A: Discharge planning: a tool for decision making, Nurs Man, 18: 47-50, 1987.

Stanford G: Beyond honesty. Presentation at the twenty-fifth annual conference of the Association for the Care of Children's Health, Boston, Mass, 1985.

Steele S, editor: Nursing care of the child with long-term illness, New York, 1977, Appleton-Century-Crofts.

Streiff LD: Can clients understand our instructions, Image 18(2): 48-52, 1986.

Taylor SC and Hobaugh R: The role of the critical care nurse in developing informed consent, Dimen Crit Care Nurs 5(2): 98-106, 1986.

Terry DG: The needs of parents of hospitalized children, Children's Health Care 16(1): 18-20, 1987.

Thompson JE and Thompson HO: Bioethical decision making for nurses, Norwalk, Conn, 1985, Appleton-Century-Crofts.

Uustal DB: Values: The cornerstone of nursing's moral art. In Fowler MD and Levine-Ariff J, editors, Ethics at the bedside, Philadelphia, 1987, JB Lippincott Co.

Waidley, P: Preparing children for invasive procedures, Am J Nurs 85: 811-812, 1985.

Warden GD et al: Multidisciplinary team approach to the pediatric burn patient, QRB 14(7): 219-226, 1988.

Waters H: All for one and one for all, Nurs Times 83(18): 61-62, 1987.

Weitzman M: School and peer relations, Pediatr Clin North Am 31(1): 59-69, 1984.

Whaley LF and Wong DL: Nursing care of infants and children, ed 4, St Louis, 1991, The CV Mosby Co.

Working Group of the Northern Health Region in current Medical/Ethical Problems: Consent to treatment by parents and children, Child Care Health Dev 12(1): 5-12, 1986.

Zimbelman LK: A team approach: considerations in developing diabetes care teams, The Diabetes Educator 14(2): 113-116, 1988.

Zurlinden J: Minimizing the impact of hospitalization for children and their families, MCN 10: 178-182, 1985.

Zweig CD: Reducing stress when a child is admitted to the hospital, MCN 11(1): 24-27, 1986.

# UNIT II Psychosocial Support of Children and Families

## SKILL 10 Conducting an Interview

Deborah Kay Brantly

Interviewing the child/family effectively requires specialized skills and empathy. Trust must be established quickly, and interviewing questions must be focused, yet comprehensive. Interviewing is used during initial hospital admissions, clinic visits, or follow-up visits to gain assessment and evaluative data. Many times interviewing is a formal process, but it can also be an informal process to obtain information while other tasks are performed. This skill will focus on the formal process of interviewing.

**NURSING DIAGNOSES**

Health-seeking behaviors (admission/follow-up) related to infant/child health promotion/maintenance; Decisional conflict related to lack of experience with priority setting.

| Steps | Rationale |
|---|---|
| **Assessment** | |
| 1. Determine the child's age and developmental level. | The child is able to assume more active participation in the interviewing process as he or she grows developmentally. |
| 2. Review the purpose of the interview; general areas to be discussed, specific information needed, and stage of the nurse-patient relationship. | General areas to be covered and methods of gathering information differ depending on the purpose of the interview. |
| 3. Determine who is to be interviewed. | Defining who is to be interviewed aids in preparation. Infants and younger children will most effectively be interviewed with at least one parent (or guardian) present. Adolescents may wish to be interviewed privately. ***Special Considerations:*** *With society's multiple changes in family structure, check the relationship of adults to the child (e.g., parents, guardians, grandparents, stepparent, adoptive parents). In some situations the child will need to be interviewed separately (e.g., if child abuse is suspected).* |
| 4. Assess the physical environment for the interview. a. Quiet b. Private c. Comfortable | A quiet, private, and comfortable environment makes the process more pleasant and sends the message that those interviewed are important enough to be a priority during the interview—an important consideration for establishing and maintaining trust. |
| **Planning and Goal Setting** | |
| 1. Determine the time of the interview. | Determining the interview time allows for scheduling of a sufficiently long and uninterrupted period. |

| Steps | Rationale |
|---|---|
| 2. Prepare the environment.<br>a. Adequate space and enough seating with all adults at eye level. | Adequate seating that does not invade personal space provides an atmosphere of comfort. Maintaining parents at eye level communicates equality (Stein, 1987).<br>***Special Considerations:*** *The infant or young child may wish to be held or sit very close to the parent. A rocking chair, larger comfortable chair, or couch may be considered. A desk between the parent and nurse can set up a barrier, especially on an initial interview (Stein, 1987).* |
| b. Soft lighting. | Soft lighting is more relaxing than bright examination lights. |
| c. Comfort, quiet, and privacy. | When comfort and privacy are maintained, the child/family feels valued, facilitating trust in the relationship.<br>***Special Considerations:*** *It may be necessary to place a "Do Not Disturb" sign on the door to ensure privacy.* |
| d. Place for play. | Selecting toys and other play materials that are age-appropriate enables the child to begin playing and to feel comfortable soon after entering the room. |
| 3. Prepare the materials needed.<br>a. Toys and art supplies.<br>b. Interview guide (appropriate to purpose).<br>c. Writing materials. | Gathering the needed assessment guide and writing materials before the interview is an efficient use of time. |
| 4. Develop individualized goals of nursing care:<br>▪ Establish trust with the child/family.<br>▪ Gather assessment data.<br>▪ Establish priority needs. | |

## Implementation

| Steps | Rationale |
|---|---|
| 1. Introduce yourself to the child/family. Communicate: | Introducing yourself follows socially acceptable norms, provides a transaction for interview communication, and informs the child/family.<br>***Special Considerations:*** *If a relationship has already developed, greet the child/family in a friendly manner. It would be appropriate to make reference to the last meeting.* |
| a. At eye level to the child/family member. | Communicating at eye level sends the message that the child/family member is valued and important.<br>***Special Considerations:*** *The younger child may desire more distance until he or she has developed a relationship with the clinician (Stein, 1987).* |
| b. By smiling. | A smile communicates warmth and caring and can help to ease tension. |
| c. By setting aside articles that are being held. | Carrying objects creates physical distance and communicates a nonapproachable professional air. |
| d. Name, title, and role. | Children/families can be confused by the different types of health care professionals. Informing them of the nurse's role eases their confusion and educates them about nursing (Whaley and Wong, 1991). |
| e. By using child/family member's name (preferably the name he or she is normally called). | Using the child/family member's familiar name implies a recognition of individuality. |
| f. By using touch (e.g., shaking hands, touching on the back, shoulder, arm or hand, or holding, patting, stroking, or rocking infants). | Touching communicates caring and is especially effective in calming infants and younger children when coupled with verbal comfort.<br>***Special Considerations:*** *Touching has not been shown to be as effective with older children (Willison and Masson, 1986). Touching is never to be used in a manipulative manner or when the child/family indicate that they do not like to be touched (Older, 1982).* |
| 2. Facilitate comfortable seating arrangements.<br>a. Keep personal space limits. | Comfortable seating, about 1½ feet apart, maintains personal space limits and decreases anxiety.<br>***Special Considerations:*** *When in the working phase of the nurse-patient relationship, more spontaneous interviewing can occur (e.g., walking down a hall or during a bath) without offending the child/family member. Do not, however, get so involved in tasks to forget to notice nonverbal responses and establish closeness.* |

| **Steps** | **Rationale** |
|---|---|
| b. Direct the child to specific toys, the toy area, or an art project, e.g., drawing a picture of the family (Stein, 1987). | Play is an effective medium to use while interviewing the child or as a diversion while interviewing the parent. ***Special Considerations:*** *If the child is to participate in the interview and play is not used, inform the child that he or she may play with toys after the interview.* |
| 3. Make social conversation. a. Comment on things seen (e.g., "I noticed you're wearing a baseball cap. Are you a baseball fan or player?"). b. Ask the child his or her age, things he or she enjoys, hobbies, or if the family has a pet. | Beginning the interview with comments on the child/family communicates interest in them as people and can ease some tension. |
| 4. Obtain verbal consent for the interview by: a. Discussing the purpose. b. Describing the length of time the interview will take. c. Explaining the purpose of taking notes. d. Validating permission to proceed. | Obtaining consent for the interview involves the child/family from the beginning and establishes the family's sense of control in the health care setting. ***Special Considerations:*** *Some professionals take notes during the interview, some do not. If doing so, explanations are important, as well as keeping notes within view and offering to show what is written.* |
| e. Answering questions. | The child/family may have questions that have emotional impact or are not brought out by interview questions. Addressing the child/family's concerns sends the message they are valued and is helpful in establishing priorities. |
| 5. Determine the child/family's past encounters with health care professionals and use information to direct interactions, e.g., ask "Have you been satisfied with health care services in the past?" If not, ask "What is important to you when you are in the hospital or come in to the clinic?" | The child/family may have had prior experiences with health care professionals that influence the interview (both positively and negatively). ***Special Considerations:*** *When in the working phases of the nurse-patient relationship, this step is usually unnecessary.* |
| 6. Obtain interview data (see Skills 12 and 13 for further examples of communication techniques). | |
| a. Squarely face the child/family member with direct eye contact. | Directly facing the child/family member creates greater immediacy and communicates interest in what is being said. It has been associated with higher information retention levels by the client (Larsen and Smith, 1981). ***Special Considerations:*** *When interviewing a family, sit in sight of all family members.* |
| b. Maintain an open and relaxed body posture. | Open and relaxed body posture communicates a willingness to listen and assists the child/family in feeling comfortable. |
| c. Lean forward. | Leaning forward communicates interest and a willingness to listen. This can result in the client paying greater attention to what is being said and an increase in understanding (Larsen and Smith, 1981). |
| d. Focus attention on what the speaker is saying (active listening). | When distracted, valuable information can be missed and disinterest communicated. ***Special Considerations:*** *Most often distraction occurs when thinking of what needs to be said next or while taking notes. If this occurs, apologize and ask for the information to be repeated.* |
| e. Use open-ended questions to explore information and closed-ended questions to obtain specifics; direct questions to most appropriate person in the family. | Open-ended questions "generate more spontaneous, less structured responses" (Stein, 1987), which provide an opportunity for concerns to be expressed. ***Special Considerations:*** *Closed questions can be effective when the child/family member is noncommunicative or embarrassed about the topic of discussion. Asking a closed question can open up the topic for discussion.* |
| f. Use easily understandable language. | Using clinical words or abbreviations the child/family does not understand can lead to fear, confusion, or anxiety (Petrillo, 1976). ***Special Considerations:*** *The child/family member may give verbal or nonverbal communication that indicates he or she does not understand what was said (e.g., puzzled look, inappropriate response, or a question indicating misunderstanding). If this occurs, repeat the message in simpler terms or clarify what was said (Petrillo, 1976).* |
| g. Pause and use silence effectively. | Pausing allows the child/family member time for thought and verbal expression. It also communicates an air of concern (Stein, 1987) and patience. |

| Steps | Rationale |
|---|---|
| h. Note responses between family members (see Skill 38). | Observing communication patterns can give clues to the structure of the family (e.g., degree of closeness between family members, parenting styles, or emotional climate). |
| i. Pay attention to the child/family and acknowledge their perceptions of illness and etiologies (Korsch, Freemon, and Negrete, 1971). | Families have closely held ideas about the nature of the illness and its etiology. When these assumptions are accurate, they can provide valuable data when analyzing problems. When assumptions are incorrect, they become vital teaching needs.<br>***Special Considerations:*** *Consider the child/family's culture when discussing etiology of disease or treatment of symptoms.* |
| j. Communicate empathy, genuineness, and honesty (e.g., through voice tone, willingness to listen, admitting when a mistake is made, or saying "I don't know" and offering to obtain an answer). | Empathy, genuineness, and honesty facilitate trust. |
| k. Determine essence of what is being said by using reflection techniques. | Many feeling states are not communicated directly, but through a general sense of what is meant. If the essence of the dialog is not grasped, vital feelings can be missed. |
| l. Identify themes by listening to content and feelings (e.g., fear, sadness, dependency, misunderstanding, lack of information, or recurring ineffective coping strategies). | Identifying themes can reveal coping patterns, problem areas, and feeling states (especially fears). |
| m. Summarize and clarify content and feelings (e.g., "What I hear you saying is you are fearful of managing the medical regime at home. Is that correct?"). | Summary and clarification verify the information given and analysis of feeling states.<br>***Special Considerations:*** *When interviewing the child directly, clarify information with the parent for accuracy.* |
| 7. Speak to parent(s) in private when necessary. | Parents sometimes hint when desiring a private discussion without the child. The parent may be seeking guidance about something concerning the child of which the child is not aware (Whaley and Wong, 1991).<br>***Special Considerations:*** *It is important not to perpetuate secrecy or cause the child to feel left out during private discussions. These could impede maintaining trust with the child.* |
| 8. Note and respond to nonverbal communication.<br>a. Note:<br>▪ Body posturing and spacing, which indicate degree of closeness desired.<br>▪ Facial expressions.<br>▪ Degree of relaxation, tension, or excessive movements of hands, arms, face, or neck.<br>▪ Spontaneous, open responses, or hesitant, restricted, or guarded ones.<br>▪ Responsiveness to interviewer's nonverbal communication, e.g., touch.<br>b. Respond by:<br>▪ Maintaining spatial needs.<br>▪ Emulating nonverbal cues.<br>▪ Giving feedback, e.g., "I noticed you are clenching your teeth . . ."<br>▪ Providing an opportunity for expression of feelings, e.g., "Something seems to be bothering you." | Nonverbal communication "is used to communicate feelings, attitudes, and preferences, and tends to reinforce or contradict feelings that are conveyed verbally" (Larsen and Smith, 1981). Responding to the child/family member's nonverbal communication can be comforting.<br>***Special Considerations:*** *Even though parents of smaller children answer interviewing questions, the child may provide important nonverbal cues.* |
| 9. Establish priority needs with the child/family. | Involving the child/family in nursing care from the beginning opens the door to a collaborative relationship. |

| Evaluation Outcomes | Observational Guidelines |
|---|---|
| 1. Trust is established. | The child/family seems relaxed and comfortable. They share information, fears, and feelings with a minimum of difficulty. |
| 2. Interview information is obtained. | The child/family provides assessment data and elaborates on information as necessary. |
| 3. Priorities are established. | The child/family identifies and agrees with priorities. |

## Documentation

Document the purpose of the interview and the persons present. Describe avenues of interviewing (e.g., play, discussion). Describe the initial response of the child/family to the interviewer and the general trust level established during and after the interview process. Refer to assessment data collected. Describe themes noted during the interview and general relationships between family members. List mutually defined priority needs of the child/family.

# *SKILL* 11 Conducting a Psychosocial Assessment of the Child

*Deborah Kay Brantly*

In recent years, the acuity level of hospitalized children and those cared for at home following discharge has risen dramatically. Attention to psychosocial needs may be overlooked in the urgency of providing physiologic care. Psychosocial assessment, however, is an important aspect of the total care of the child. It encompasses many areas of the child's psychologic/emotional state, including affect, temperament, self-concept, coping ability, use of defense mechanisms, attachment, and spirituality.

## NURSING DIAGNOSES

Ineffective coping related to situational crisis, ineffective coping methods, or inadequate support systems; Self-esteem disturbance (chronic or situational) related to developmental conditions, changes in relationships, or unrealistic expectations; Impaired adjustment related to inadequate situational support.

| Steps | Rationale |
|---|---|
| **Assessment** | |
| 1. Determine the child's age and developmental level. | Knowing the child's developmental level assists in planning methods of data collection and interpretation of findings. **_Special Considerations:_** *The child's ability for verbal expression improves with developmental growth.* |
| 2. Determine the need for assessment, e.g., routine assessment, determine psychosocial functioning, use psychosocial information in plan of care. | The reason for the assessment will determine the depth of assessment needed. |
| **Planning and Goal Setting** | |
| 1. Arrange time to gather assessment data. | When a specific time for assessment can be arranged, attention is focused on analysis of psychosocial information. **_Special Considerations:_** *It is important to remember, however, that psychosocial assessment is an ongoing process that can occur on a formal or informal level.* |
| 2. Gather needed materials (e.g., assessment tools, paper and pencil, puppets or other toys). | Gathering materials before the assessment is an efficient use of time. |
| 3. Develop a nursing goal of care:<br>▪ To obtain accurate psychosocial information about the child.<br>▪ To integrate psychosocial data into the plan of care. | |
| **Implementation** | |
| 1. Determine the child's affect.<br>a. Happy (e.g., smiling).<br>b. Flat (e.g., little expression on face, "blank" look).<br>c. Sad (e.g., looking downward, mouth downturned).<br>d. Depressed.<br>e. Lability or pervasiveness of affect (affect changes rapidly or remains constant). | Affect nonverbally expresses the child's inner state. **_Special Considerations:_** *Sometimes the child's words and affect will not express the same message (incongruent); this is called an inappropriate affect.* |
| 2. Assess the child's temperament (Table 11-1). | Temperament is the basic mood or behavioral style of the individual (Thomas and Chess, 1977); assessment provides guidance for development of specific nursing interventions to meet the child's needs. For example, "children with high activity levels, intense reactions, and negative moods can be helped to deal with their aggressive feelings and given appropriate outlets through play therapy. By the same token, children with low activity levels might prefer television and board games" (Ruddy-Wallace, 1987). |

**TABLE 11-1** Dimensions of Temperament

| Dimension Label | Range | Definition | Behavioral Examples |
|---|---|---|---|
| Activity level | High to low | Amount of movement displayed; proportion of time spent in motor activity | Active movement; running and jumping; quiet play |
| Rhythmicity | Arrhythmic to very rhythmic | Predictability of bodily functions | Takes a long time to fall asleep; eats similar amounts each day |
| Approach | Withdrawn to approachable | Initial response to new stimuli | Holds back in new situations; outgoing with visitors |
| Adaptability | Slowly adapts to very adaptable | Ease in which initial reactions can be altered | Changes in plans bother the child; adjusts quickly to changes in household rules |
| Threshold | Low to high | Strength of stimulation needed to elicit an overt response | Cries over a minor fall; able to fall asleep in a noisy room |
| Intensity | Intense to mild | Indicates the energy level of responsiveness | Outwardly expressive of emotions; complains briefly when unable to watch TV |
| Mood | Negative to positive | Proportion of happy/unhappy behavior | Frequent periods of crankiness; laughs and smiles while playing |
| Distractibility | Distractible to nondistractible | Effect of environmental stimuli in altering activity | Stops playing when telephone rings; does not "hear" parent when involved in favorite game |
| Persistence | Nonpersistent to high persistence | Includes attention span and the length of time an activity continues | Spends less than 15 minutes with a new toy; not willing to leave before a puzzle/game is completed |

From Ruddy-Wallace M: Temperament: assessing individual differences in hospitalized children, J Pediatr Nurs 2(1):30-36, 1987.

| Steps | Rationale |
|---|---|
| 3. Determine the child's ability to communicate and interact with peers, adults, and family (see Skill 12; see Skill 13 if communication is impaired). | Young children communicate psychosocial needs primarily nonverbally through actions and interactions. Older children and adolescents generally have verbal skills needed to discuss psychosocial needs.<br>***Special Considerations:*** *Even though ability to express feelings generally increases with age, some children are able to verbalize feelings at a very young age, e.g., at 5 years; others may still have difficulty past adolescence.* |
| 4. Determine recent family/personal stressors the child is facing (e.g., divorce, birth of a sibling, hospitalization of a close relative, death in the family or the death of a pet, move or change in school or teacher). Signs the child may be experiencing stress are: an increase in physical illness or injury (e.g., stomach aches, headaches, colds, flu, or accidents), a change in daily activities, a change in grades at school, or a change or disinterest in friends. | Children have multiple life stressors that affect them differently according to their developmental stage and that may impede coping ability. Hospitalization and illness distinctly increase the child's stress factor.<br>***Special Considerations:*** *Gifted children are especially vulnerable to stress at school (Johnson, 1981). Children who are heavily engaged in sports activities at a young age can show a decrease in athletic performance when under stress.* |
| 5. Assess the child's ability to cope.<br>a. Usual coping style: Ask how the child usually reacts to a new environment (e.g., cries, approaches with caution, approaches with fearlessness, clings to parent, requests help from adults, becomes sullen, whines, becomes aggressive, uses breathing or relaxation techniques, screams, reads, listens to music, counts to 10).<br>b. Current methods of coping. Ask if child has learned any new coping techniques, uses methods formerly dropped, or stopped using former methods of coping.<br>c. Coping style of the parents.<br>d. Support to try new coping techniques and function independently.<br>e. Energy level. | Coping involves efforts at dealing with new and stressful situations and, in this way, is related to problem-solving (Vipperman and Rager, 1980). When children are under a great deal of stress, they typically use coping methods consistent with their coping style and may regress to an earlier developmental level. Vipperman and Rager (1980) also describe five factors that contribute to differences in coping capacities: (1) the environment and its support systems, (2) past coping experiences, (3) temperament and developmental level, (4) range of positive coping resources (gratification, positive attitude toward life, range and flexibility of coping devices and defenses), and (5) intervening variables (present state of health and energy level, information received before a new experience, usual level of parental coping and opportunities for independence/autonomy).<br>***Special Considerations:*** *Questions can be addressed to the child or parents. Adolescents can be asked directly.* |
| 6. Assess the amount and type of defense mechanisms the child uses (e.g., denial, repression, or projection). | Determining the extent of defense mechanisms used can assist in developing strategies to help the child cope more effectively. |

| Steps | Rationale |
|---|---|
| | ***Special Considerations:*** *It is important to allow the child to use defenses until he or she is ready to give them up (Vipperman and Rager, 1980).* |
| 7. Determine the child's self-concept and level of self-esteem. Notice:<br>a. Statements the child makes about himself or herself.<br>b. Ability to be goal oriented.<br>c. Readiness with which the child takes risks.<br>d. Need for approval from adults.<br>e. Ability to delineate strengths and weaknesses.<br>f. Ability to make independent choices based on likes and dislikes.<br>Self-esteem can also be measured by paper and pencil self-report scales, such as the Tennessee Self-Concept Scale, the Coopersmith Self-Esteem Inventory, or the Piers–Harris Self-Concept Scale. | The child's level of self-esteem will influence the ability to master tasks and seek solutions to problems. Children may have fluctuations in self-esteem because of developmental considerations (e.g., struggling with task mastery), however, this is only a temporary modification in the child with a healthy sense of self (Whaley and Wong, 1991).<br>***Special Considerations:*** *Parent-child interactions strongly influence the child's self-esteem, as do stressful situations (e.g., hospitalization and chronic conditions). The early school-age child's self-esteem is influenced by daily school routine (peer and teacher relationships and achievement); older children are more influenced by extraneous events that may affect achievement of developmental tasks (e.g., school progress and competition) (Riffee, 1981). Riffee (1981) found that older children who were hospitalized for surgery had a lower self-esteem than children hospitalized for a nonsurgical reason. Gifted children often feel isolated from peers, lack self-confidence, and have a lowered self-esteem (Betts, 1986).* |
| 8. Determine attachment level of the child by noticing bonding behaviors (see Skill 40). | Cassidy (1988) reported attachment influences self-esteem and behavior. |
| 9. Assess the child's spirituality (see Skill 42). | Meeting spiritual needs may provide support and comfort the child. |
| 10. Incorporate psychosocial assessment into the plan of care by identifying and diagnosing psychosocial strengths and problems and integrating appropriate strategies (Table 11-2). | Effective use of psychosocial data individualizes care of the child and family. |

***TABLE 11-2*** Psychosocial Interventions for the Hospitalized Child

| Age | Intervention |
|---|---|
| **ENHANCING SELF-CONCEPT/SELF-ESTEEM** | |
| Infancy | Encourage positive, parent-child interaction (e.g., encourage parent to smile directly at child and play games such as peek-a-boo).<br>Encourage touching and talking to the infant.<br>Encourage play according to child's developmental level.<br>Support parents (e.g., by enhancing their sense of competency with their ill child, being an empathetic listener, and assisting them in building a support network with other parents). |
| Preschool | Encourage developmentally appropriate play and medical play.<br>Incorporate parents in the plan of care, encouraging rooming in or suggesting appropriate parental substitutes when parents cannot be with the child.<br>Allow child to make age-appropriate decisions about care and activities.<br>Provide positive reinforcement when the child is appropriately cooperative. |
| School-age | Encourage daily contact with child's teacher.<br>Assist child to complete school work.<br>Encourage school-age friends to visit, call, and write.<br>Assign to a room with a same-aged peer.<br>Encourage alternative forms of play.<br>Plan for speedy return to school after discharge, beginning with half-day involvement. |
| Adolescent | Self-disclosure in a group or 1 : 1 setting (see Olds, 1987).<br>Encourage visits by family and friends (including peers), phone calls, letters, cards, and gifts.<br>Emphasize the attention adolescent is receiving by these significant others.<br>Reassure confidentiality of information shared.<br>Emphasize privacy and avoid situations that may be embarrassing. If the latter must occur, acknowledge feelings of embarrassment.<br>Maintain limits of behavior.<br>Limit number of caregivers.<br>Include adolescent in planning care and give choices when possible.<br>Provide self-monitoring activities (e.g., charts, checklists, calendars, diary). |

*Continued.*

**TABLE 11-2** Psychosocial Interventions for the Hospitalized Child—cont'd

| Age | Intervention |
|---|---|
| Adolescent—cont'd | Encourage questions about health status and air concerns; clarify misconceptions.<br>Provide explanations/preparation of procedures and routines.<br>Avoid negative criticism and use positive reinforcement.<br>Provide short passes from hospital, if possible.<br>Provide unit activities with other adolescents.<br>Encourage identification of support systems.<br>Emphasize adolescent's abilities and strengths.<br>Role play situations in which the adolescent may feel uncomfortable (e.g., questions from friends about his or her illness or appearance).<br>Provide education to adolescent's class about the illness, with his or her permission. |
| **ENHANCING COPING ABILITIES** | |
| Infant | Stroke, massage, cuddle, rock, talk to, and touch the infant.<br>Provide ample time for sleep and rest.<br>Provide mobiles and colorful infant toys for stimulation.<br>Play tapes of music or parental voice.<br>Encourage maximal parental involvement in nurturing and care activities. |
| Preschool | Accept defense strategies (regression, denial, repression, projection, withdrawal, aggression, and temper tantrums) within defined limits, while providing opportunities for use of more appropriate defenses when the child is ready.<br>Provide expressive play activities, e.g., use of puppet play, role reversal, drawing, water play, and aggressive play (see Skill 16).<br>Provide stories about children in similar situations.<br>Encourage parental contact through rooming-in, tape of parents' voices during absences, and family photos. If rooming-in is not possible, encourage frequent parental visits and visits from others the child is close to.<br>Talk to child about home activities.<br>Encourage child to bring familiar objects from home (e.g., toys, stuffed animals, blanket or other security items).<br>Accept use of fantasy and use it to gain an understanding of child's fears.<br>Hold and cuddle the child.<br>Provide for playroom time after stressful events.<br>Give simple choices when possible. |
| School-age | Encourage contact with parents, other family members, teachers, and schoolmates. Ask them to keep child filled in on events; send cards, letters, and gifts.<br>Provide familiar objects/games from child's home environment.<br>Accept defense strategies within defined limits, while providing for more effective coping when child is ready.<br>Use guided imagery (see Skill 17).<br>Encourage questions about hospitalization/illness; clarify misconceptions.<br>Encourage verbal expression of feelings.<br>Encourage use of what has helped the child cope in the past.<br>Provide activities for self-expression using play role reversal situations.<br>Provide opportunities for child to control the situation by making a hospital scrap (or memento) book, taking pictures, making drawings or games about the hospital, and manipulating equipment.<br>Allow the child to read books about hospitalization and children who have a similar illness.<br>Encourage fantasy play, e.g., "Let's pretend we're riding on a bicycle."<br>Allow child to carry out aspects of care (e.g., recording I & O or assisting in a dressing change). When possible, allow the child to direct what care is being given (e.g., "You tell me what to do and I will change your dressing").<br>Ask child to explain a procedure to another child.<br>Use humor (ask child to tell jokes and riddles and share cartoons). Play humorous videos, (e.g., The Three Stooges, cartoons).<br>Provide for adequate gross motor activities and aggression activities. |

**TABLE 11-2** Psychosocial Interventions for the Hospitalized Child—cont'd

| Age | Intervention |
|---|---|
| **ENHANCING COPING ABILITIES—cont'd** | |
| Adolescent | Accept use of defense strategies within appropriate boundaries and supply opportunities for more effective coping.<br>Ask adolescent what his or her perception of the illness is and why the adolescent thinks he or she has the illness; clarify misconceptions.<br>Assist in discrimination of normal versus abnormal body changes; assist in anticipation of future body changes, if appropriate.<br>Identify feelings seen in the adolescent and encourage him or her to talk about them; encourage self-expression through music, arts and crafts, drawing, and writing.<br>Emphasize strengths.<br>Encourage peer interaction with letters, cards, phone calls, and unit group attendance.<br>Encourage adolescent to wear his or her own clothes and bring personal belongings from home.<br>Facilitate planning of and participation in self-care/treatment; allow him or her to make as many choices as possible.<br>Encourage creative thinking and problem-solving.<br>Use imagery and imaginative thinking to promote stress release.<br>Allow for diversity of hospital routine, when possible.<br>Promote activities that provide optimal motor functioning when appropriate.<br>Use adolescent to orient new adolescent to unit or a procedure. |

## Evaluation Outcomes

1. Psychosocial assessment is completed.
2. Collected psychosocial information is incorporated in the plan of care.

## Observational Guidelines

Psychosocial information is recorded on the child's chart (e.g., temperament, coping style, communication style, self-esteem and behaviors indicating stress).

Review child's care plan, noting presence of psychosocial diagnoses, interventions, and goals (e.g., play activities are used that are consistent with the child's temperament; coping methods that are most comforting to the child are encouraged). Care documentation records, e.g., nurses' notes, reflect implementation of planned interventions.

## Documentation

Describe the child's temperament type, level of self-esteem, general stress level and specific identified stressors, coping style, and current coping mechanisms. Document the child's psychosocial needs and use of psychosocial factors in the plan of care.

# SKILL 12 Communicating with Children: Age-Related Techniques

*Deborah Kay Brantly*

Communicating with the child is essential to promote effective coping and facilitate nursing care. Special sensitivity to the child's developmental needs and cognitive ability is necessary. Children are highly sensitive to both verbal and nonverbal means of communication and internalize their personal interpretations of communicated messages. They are normally not as likely to share their interpretations unless prompted by an adult, thus placing the bulk of the responsibility for effective communication on the nurse.

## NURSING DIAGNOSES

Impaired verbal communication related to developmental level, language, physiologic or cultural barriers; Fear or anxiety related to unmet informational needs about or changes in health status, or threat to self-concept.

| Steps | Rationale |
|---|---|
| **Assessment** | |
| 1. Identify nature of the child's diagnosis and prognosis. | This information provides a basis for predicting feelings the child may be experiencing and the type of information that needs to be communicated. |
| 2. Determine the child's age and developmental level (Table 12-1). | Age and developmental level influence factors such as word selection, complexity, and approach. Younger children are more concrete in their communication, whereas adolescents can think abstractly. |
| 3. Determine presence of developmental or perceptual disorders (e.g., developmental delay, deafness) (see Skill 13). | Developmental or perceptual disorders may influence or alter the communication process. |
| 4. Assess family's basic value system and other culturally prescribed determinants of communication (see Skill 41). | The more understanding of the family's value orientation, the greater probability communication will be appropriate and responsive to the family's and child's needs (Selig and Selig, 1983). Culture can affect communication patterns and word meanings. For example, in the Indian and Oriental cultures, direct eye-to-eye contact is considered disrespectful. |
| 5. Consider readiness for communication, e.g., the ability to focus thoughts. | In a crisis situation or when in a state of fear or denial, the child may not be able to listen. |
| 6. Determine past medical events and experiences with professionals. | Children's past experiences with medical professionals may have an effect (either positively or negatively) on communication. |
| 7. Determine purpose of communication (e.g., to elicit information, to provide information, to offer psychosocial support, to prepare the child for an event, or to build rapport). | Communication with the child is an on-going process. Determining the purpose of each communicative encounter guides selection of techniques and choice of communication setting. |
| 8. Assess personal feelings and attitudes about the child. | Feelings and attitudes are easily communicated to the child nonverbally. The appropriate person to interact with the child is someone who is capable of communicating positive feelings and attitudes. If this is not possible, reassignment should be strongly considered. |
| **Planning and Goal Setting** | |
| 1. Choose where communication will occur. | Much communication is effected during the routine course of the day. However, if the purpose of the communication demands privacy, a quiet room may be more appropriate.<br>***Special Considerations:*** *If play materials are to be used, the playroom may be the most appropriate setting.* |

***TABLE 12-1*** Age-related Communication Needs

| Developmental Stage | Developmental Communication Guidelines |
|---|---|
| **INFANTS** | ▪ Infants communicate primarily nonverbally and by vocalizations, e.g., crying.<br>▪ Parents are best able to discriminate differences in meaning of their infant's cry.<br>▪ Sounds that were familiar in utero tend to calm the infant, e.g., music or singing.<br>▪ Gentle touching, cuddling, patting, and light bouncing are comforting to the infant, as well as a soft, low calm voice.<br>▪ Smile at the infant and respond to his or her cues.<br>▪ Approach the infant slowly, as sudden movements may be frightening.<br>▪ Play pat-a-cake, peek-a-boo, or "this little piggy" with the child.<br>▪ Duplicate the parental style of holding the child. If unknown, hold the child in an upright manner.<br>▪ Keep the mother in the infant's view. |
| **TODDLER TO 5 YEARS** | ▪ Preschoolers have limited verbal communication, therefore they continue to rely heavily on nonverbal communication.<br>▪ Kneel to look at the child at eye level when speaking.<br>▪ Touch the child gently on the shoulder to gain attention.<br>▪ Introduce yourself in terms the child can understand.<br>▪ Show interest in the child, e.g., ask about a toy in the child's hand or comment on his or her appearance.<br>▪ Speak to the child in familiar terms, e.g., use the family term for urination.<br>▪ Provide positive reinforcement through words and tangible objects, e.g., say, "I like the way you are sitting in that chair," or "Your mommy and I are talking right now. If you continue to play quietly until we are finished, you can play with my favorite puppet."<br>▪ Use short, concrete descriptions and terms.<br>▪ If it is essential to communicate more than one statement at a time, pause briefly between sentences or at the end of phrases to allow time for the child to grasp the information.<br>▪ Avoid words/phrases with literal and figurative meaning, e.g., "coughing your head off" or "a little stick in the arm."<br>▪ Respect the child's ability to animate inanimate objects, taking care not to dehumanize toys. Use play to project feelings and gain information (see Skill 16).<br>▪ Use communication techniques of third person, therapeutic responding, storytelling, bibliotherapy, "what if" questions, and three wishes.<br>▪ Allow the child to sit on the lap of the parent or nurse or beside him or her, if the child desires.<br>▪ Repeat explanations several times if the child has not grasped the content. When possible, couple explanations of objects with a child-sized replica of the object or with simple fantasy play.<br>▪ Answer persistent "why" questions with pleasant but short answers.<br>▪ Explain how things might feel in simple terms. Give the child a name for what he or she seems to be feeling, e.g., "You look upset right now."<br>▪ Use humor. Laugh when the child sees humor in a situation; make funny faces, imitate, or tickle the child in an appropriate manner.<br>▪ Set limits firmly, but gently, in a nonaccusatory manner. Reward acceptable behavior, e.g., "The toys are not to be thrown. Sit here beside me right now. When you are calm you may play with the toys again." |
| **6 TO 12 YEARS** | ▪ Younger school-age children desire explanations. They are better able to grasp the information they seek. When providing answers to questions, give the how, when, where, and why as the child requests.<br>▪ Use humor by laughing at things the child finds humorous, telling simple jokes and riddles, making funny faces, and using dramatizations.<br>▪ Use simple role play, therapeutic play (see Skill 16), three wishes, "what if" questions, bibliotherapy, and storytelling.<br>▪ Allow fearful children to sit with parents.<br>▪ If the parents desire, ask them to perform the activity/explanation. Allow the child to participate at his or her own pace. |

Adapted from Wong D and Whaley L: Clinical manual of pediatric nursing, ed 3, St. Louis, 1990, The CV Mosby Co.

*Continued.*

**TABLE 12-1** Age-related Communication Needs—cont'd

| Developmental Stage | Developmental Communication Guidelines |
|---|---|
| **ADOLESCENTS** | ▪ Adolescents communicate most often in verbal form and develop a "language" that is shared by their peers; ask for clarification of terms, if needed. Use adolescent terms in moderation.<br>▪ Because of the adolescent's fluctuating emotions and behavior, communication may be adultlike one moment and childlike the next. Anticipate shifts in communication by using a variety of techniques: third person technique, bibliotherapy, storytelling, "what if" questions, three wishes, rating game, word association game, sentence completion, pros and cons, writing, and drawing.<br>▪ Use humor by taking advantage of funny events that happen, telling jokes and riddles, listening to the adolescent's jokes, or watching a funny video.<br>▪ Play a board game or card game with an adolescent to facilitate discussion.<br>▪ Express a nonjudgmental attitude by not reacting to issues that differ with personal values.<br>▪ Adolescents may at one time reveal feelings and at another be silent.<br>▪ Attend to conversations without interruption and avoid comments that are value-laden.<br>▪ Remain aware of developmental issues that the adolescent may wish to talk about, (e.g., peer relationships, sexuality, parental relationships, and identity concerns).<br>▪ Decide whether to talk with the adolescent and parents together or separately; when possible, communicate directly with the adolescent and retain confidentiality.<br>▪ Inform the adolescent of limits to confidentiality, e.g., if the adolescent would have suicidal or homicidal ideations.<br>▪ Assist with resolution of conflicts with parents by role playing assertive communication, arbitrating a family meeting, or brainstorming solutions. |

| Steps | Rationale |
|---|---|
| 2. Select an appropriate time, considering factors such as timing, readiness, and the child's schedule. | A consideration of these types of factors offers the greatest possibility for successful communication. |
| 3. Develop a nursing goal of care:<br>▪ To engage in an accurate and communicative exchange.<br>▪ To establish open communication.<br>▪ To establish a therapeutic relationship. | |

## Implementation

| Steps | Rationale |
|---|---|
| 1. Communicate a caring attitude to the child.<br>a. When speaking to the child, use his or her name.<br>b. Speak directly to the child at eye level.<br>c. Touch the child (e.g., pat the child on the arm or hand, touch his or her shoulder, or hold the infant).<br>d. Handle the child and speak in a gentle and loving manner.<br>e. Attend to responses of the child, especially when performing procedures. Allow enough time for the child to complete a statement or ask a question.<br>f. Convey the recognition of the uniqueness and individuality of the child, e.g., refer to a special endearing characteristic of the child. | Providing communication with a caring attitude establishes a safe emotional environment in which trust can develop. Nonverbally, a statement is made that this child is lovable and that all children are worthy of being loved regardless of appearance, behavior, or life situation. If there is a conflict between verbal and nonverbal communication, the nonverbal communication will commonly be believed above the verbal.<br>***Special Considerations:*** *Avoid extended eye contact, which can be uncomfortable to some children. Also a child may be distrustful of a new face with too broad of a smile, or of an overly friendly manner.* |
| 2. Be an empathetic listener.<br>a. Active listening (e.g., "It's sounds like you are concerned you won't be able to use your hand after the surgery").<br>b. Reflective listening (e.g., "Are you saying you think your blood might all come out if you have an IV?"). | Empathetic listening facilitates establishment of a trusting relationship. An active listener demonstrates interest and concern about what the listener perceives is important to the person. A reflective listener rephrases what was said for clarification. |
| 3. Provide opportunity for ventilation of feelings. Acknowledge feelings expressed. If the child is unable to express feelings verbally, use play to encourage self-expression (see Skill 16). | When the child ventilates feelings, he or she is able to cope more effectively. Young children especially have difficulty expressing feelings and need an adult to help name their feelings. A child learns it is acceptable to feel/express emotions when an adult acknowledges the feelings. |
| 4. Use silence when appropriate. | A quiet presence can communicate caring and concern. A common misconception is that something needs to be said to be therapeutic. |
| 5. Communicate as honestly and as accurately as possible.<br>a. Give accurate information. Tell the child if the information is a guess. | Honest, accurate communication facilitates trust and establishes safe parameters in which concerns and questions can be aired. |

***TABLE 12-2*** Communication Techniques for Children

| Technique | Description |
|---|---|
| **THIRD PERSON** | Express a feeling using the third person, then be silent to allow the child to respond. For example, "Sometimes when other children get medicine from a needle a lot, they tell me they feel angry about being hurt so much." If the child fails to respond, ask, "Have you ever felt that way?" The child may open up and express feelings. If he or she denies feeling angry, ask, "It sounds like you feel another way." If the child responds with silence or further denial, he or she may not be ready to express feelings yet. Allow the use of denial while encouraging opening up by saying, "If you ever feel that way, just let me know." |
| **FACILITATIVE RESPONDING** | Listen for underlying feelings and expression of major themes. Then clarify these to the child with the statement "You feel ________ because __________." For example, a child wakes up from a nap and discovers his mother is gone. He states, "Where's my mommy? She said she'd stay here." A facilitative response would be to say, "You are feeling scared because you are afraid your mom isn't going to return." |
| **STORYTELLING** | Children often make up stories (using fantasy) to reflect what they are thinking and feeling. Storytelling takes advantage of this typical activity. Ask the child to tell a story about a theme or event (e.g., "going to surgery" or showing a picture of the idea). If the child has difficulty giving details about the story, ask specific questions, e.g., "What did the little boy feel when he was lying on the table?" If the child has difficulty beginning the story, suggest using "Once upon a time . . . ." Developing comic strip words is an effective method of storytelling for children who can write. Older children can also write a story or draw a picture about a story, then talk about it. Children with verbal skills can tell their story into a tape recorder, if they desire. A variation on the technique, mutual storytelling, allows for direct intervention. The child begins by telling a story, then the nurse tells a similar story with a more realistic but positive outcome. For example, a child was asked to tell a story about having an x-ray. In the story he told, his pregnant mother was allowed to stay in the room because the child was afraid of the dark. The nurse, using different names, told a similar story about a child whose pregnant mother accompanied the child to the x-ray department and waited right outside the door so the x-ray would be finished more quickly and they could be together again. |
| **BIBLIOTHERAPY** | Using books about experiences common to the hospitalized child/family can be a therapeutic means of communication. This technique helps the child face feelings and concerns, whether being read to or reading the books himself or herself. Many available books are educational, providing information about procedures or hospitalization, or providing the child with an opportunity to become familiar with an anticipated experience. Verify that the book is appropriate to the child's age and developmental level. Allow the child to express what was learned from reading the book by retelling the story, rereading parts of the book, telling what the book means, or drawing a picture about the theme of the book. |
| **FAIRY TALES** | Tell the child a familiar fairy tale that brings out a conflict the child seems to be experiencing. Through the story, the child may find meaning in his or her experience. |
| **DREAMS** | When the child/family member brings up a particularly disturbing dream, it is helpful to discuss the dream with them. Often, underlying conflicts will emerge as the dream is revealed. If not readily divulged, ask questions about particular figures in the dream. Also, ask "What does the dream mean to you?" Occasionally, the dream can be used to provide further direct intervention. Use disturbing parts of the dream and allow the child/family member to respond to what was disturbing; suggest the child rewrite (or refantasize) the disturbing part to be the way they would like it to be. |
| **"WHAT IF" QUESTIONS** | In considering potential situations, ask the child to respond to a "What if" question, e.g., "What if you had to have surgery on your stomach?" The answer will probably reveal the child's knowledge level and feelings. |
| **THREE WISHES** | Ask the child what he or she would wish for with three wishes. This may reveal the things that are the most important or disturbing to the child. Acting on a child's wish, e.g., a short visit from a family pet, powerfully communicates a sense of caring. |
| **RATING GAME** | The child is asked to rate something on a scale from 1 to 10. For example, "Rate your day today on a scale from 1 to 10, with 1 being the worst day possible, and 10 being the best." After the child's rating, discuss the results. |

Adapted from Wong D and Whaley L: Clinical manual of pediatric nursing, ed 3, St. Louis, 1990, The CV Mosby Co.

*Continued.*

**TABLE 12-2** Communication Techniques for Children—cont'd

| Technique | Description |
|---|---|
| **WORD ASSOCIATION GAME** | Using a list of key words, ask the child to say the first word that comes to mind. This is best used when desiring information about a particular area. Begin with nonthreatening or neutral words, then proceed to possible anxiety-producing words, e.g., needles. |
| **SENTENCE COMPLETION** | Using sentence completion encourages the child to communicate areas of concern. Present the sentence stems and ask the child to fill in the ending. Allow the younger child to verbally complete them, or have the older child or adolescent read the sentences and complete them in writing. Sample questions are:<br>The thing I like to do best (least) is ________.<br>What I like (dislike) about school is ________.<br>What I like (dislike) most about mom/dad is ________.<br>The happiest (saddest) moment in my life was ________.<br>What I like best (least) about being in the hospital is ________.<br>Generally, ask questions with potentially less strong emotions attached at the beginning, proceeding to those that evoke stronger feelings. |
| **PROS AND CONS** | Select a topic and have the child list five good things and five bad things about it. Topics can concern experiences (e.g., being in the hospital) or things they like or don't like about themselves (to elicit information about self-esteem) or family members. |
| **WRITING** | Writing can be used in a variety of ways, by itself or in conjunction with other techniques, as previously noted. Suggest the child keep a diary (e.g., of the hospitalization experience), write about his or her feelings in a journal, write letters to someone that are never mailed (to express strong emotion, to a make-believe pen pal, or to say good-bye to someone who has died.) Frequently, the child may need to discuss what is written. Offer to read the writing if the child would like; if he or she doesn't wish to share, respect the child's privacy. Suggest the child go back at a later time to read what was written. |
| **TAPE OR VIDEO RECORDING** | Tape or video recording can be used for the same purposes as writing. However, it is frequently used to share information with someone or as a gift of remembrance before death. For example, one girl used a tape recording to tell a "fantasy" story about a girl who had been sexually abused. She gave it to her therapist to reveal those secret, fearful memories she could not discuss in person. |
| **DRAWING** | A child's drawings are projections of his or her personality, relationships with others, and experience. Drawing is an active medium of communication that provides the child an active mode of self-expression. Drawings can be spontaneous or directed. Spontaneous drawings can be elicited by giving the child a variety of art supplies and asking him or her to draw a picture. Directed drawings are elicited by suggesting the child draw something specific, e.g., "Draw a person for me." Through this task, the child can reveal basic knowledge about developmental level and feelings. Interpretation of the drawings should be developmentally based and validated with the child and the child's experience. The Kinetic Family Drawing (see Skill 39) is used to elicit the child's or family member's feelings about the family relationships. Another such technique is the sociogram. |

| Steps | Rationale |
|---|---|
| b. Offer to get answers; locate information when necessary. | |
| c. Use terms the child understands; explain medical terms when used. | |
| d. Use visual aids, e.g., charts, drawings, or models to promote accuracy. | |
| 6. Allow time for questions, both at the time and later. Provide paper and pen or pencil. | Absorbing information is a process. Additional questions may surface after the passage of time and the opportunity for reflection. With paper and pen or pencil, questions can be written to remember to ask at a later time. |

| Steps | Rationale |
|---|---|
| 7. Convey sincerity. | |
| a. When choosing phrases of comfort or support. | Phrases such as "I understand" are of no value unless the person saying it has truly been in that situation. Furthermore, most situations are viewed as unique, and such a statement may provoke well-deserved anger. ***Special Considerations:*** *The use of the third person could be more effective, e.g., "Other children in your situation have told me they felt very helpless. Is that how you're feeling right now?"* |
| b. When sharing private information about self. | Traditionally, personal disclosure was discouraged. A more open approach is advocated today. However, relating private information should have a purpose. Validation of feelings through personal experience can prove very supportive to the child. |
| 8. Use humor when appropriate. | Sharing humor invites those present to come a little closer. Humor provides a common ground to soften cultural and economic barriers. |
| 9. Use a variety of communication methods (Table 12-2). | Using a variety of communication techniques may elicit a more effective response. |

| Evaluation Outcomes | Observational Guidelines |
|---|---|
| 1. Communication is effective. | Techniques of therapeutic communication are employed. The child communicates and interacts in a comfortable manner. Needed information is exchanged. |
| 2. The child communicates needs and fears. | The child asks questions and expresses fears in a developmentally appropriate manner. |

### Documentation

Document significant conversations with the child on his or her chart. Use direct quotes as much as possible. Describe the child's response to the use of specific techniques.

# *SKILL* 13 Communicating in Special Situations

*Deborah Kay Brantly*

Nurses frequently find themselves in situations where the usual avenues of communication are impaired, causing frustration for the nurse, child, and family. Communicating in special situations due to a hearing impairment, speech impairment, intellectual/learning impairment, or gown and mask isolation necessitates the use of special communication techniques.

### NURSING DIAGNOSES

Impaired verbal communication related to auditory/speech impediment; Impaired social interaction related to communication barriers, therapeutic isolation, or sociocultural dissonance.

| Steps | Rationale |
|---|---|
| **Assessment** | |
| 1. Determine the child's age and developmental level. | Age and developmental level provide a basis for communication, teaching, and intervention selection. ***Special Considerations:*** *It is often incorrectly assumed that the child with communication difficulties is developmentally delayed.* |
| 2. Assess nature of communication problem. | Early attention to the problem spares misunderstandings and further difficulties and facilitates a therapeutic alliance. |
| a. Length of time impairment has existed. | The child who has had an impairment longer may have more communicative resources than the child whose impairment has recently surfaced. |
| b. Ability to hear: assess for prelingual or postlingual deafness. | The child with postlingual deafness is more familiar with spoken language (DiPietro and Knight, 1986). |
| c. Ability to speak: assess enunciation and cause of speech impairment (e.g., deafness, tracheostomy, intubation, or physiologic impediment). | If the child is able to enunciate so that he or she is understood, he or she will have less difficulty communicating. |
| d. Ability to comprehend others: assess cultural language differences or intellectual and learning difficulties. | When comprehension is impaired, communication may need to be more concrete—using symbols, signs, and simple words. |
| e. Ability to read and write. | The child can use written communication to the extent he or she can read and write. |
| 3. Assess alternative communication channels available. | Using existing communication channels is comforting to the child. |
| a. Ability to use sign language: determine type used. | Sign language is a typical mode of communication for the hearing impaired and is an appropriate alternate mode of communication for the young ventilator-dependent child (Hall and Weatherly, 1989). ***Special Considerations:*** *American Sign Language (ASL) is commonly used in the United States, although other systems exist that follow the English syntax and can be easily learned. Some children are learning cued speech along with ASL, however, this has had limited acceptance in the United States.* |
| b. Ability to read lips. | Lipreading (or speechreading) is another form of communication used with the hearing impaired. |
| c. Electronic devices, (e.g., hearing aids, assistive listening devices, or amplification systems). | A disabled child may use electronic writing devices to facilitate communication; these may or may not have voice feedback. |
| 4. Determine cultural influences on communication. | The child's cultural values may influence communication patterns (see Skill 41). |
| 5. Determine availability of someone to facilitate communication, unless personally qualified.<br>a. Family members.<br>b. Friends.<br>c. Interpreters, including those for sign language or nondominant language. | The child will be more able to communicate with someone to help bridge the gap. ***Special Considerations:*** *Direct communication to the child, unless the facilitator is a family member who would normally supply the needed information.* |
| 6. Determine psychosocial factors, e.g., fear, that may affect communication. | Fear and anxiety adversely affect communication. ***Special Considerations:*** *The child who is under total isolation precautions may be fearful of persons in isolation dress.* |
| **Planning and Goal Setting** | |
| 1. Facilitate other health care providers' understanding of the communication problem.<br>a. Plan a patient care conference.<br>b. Provide a written care plan. | Increased communication among health care members decreases frustration of interacting with the child and gives a basis for quality care. |
| 2. Gain consensus of child/family and other nurses about which interventions to select.<br>a. Appropriate to the communication problem.<br>b. Realistic to implement. | When the child and family and other nurses collaborate on the plan of care, a more quality product emerges, contributors are more likely to follow through on planned interventions, and a sense of camaraderie is established between staff members and with the child/family. |
| 3. Develop individualized child/family goals:<br>▪ Communicates pain, needs, wants, or fears to health professionals.<br>▪ Communicates and plays with other children.<br>▪ Acknowledges messages are understood.<br>▪ Exhibits diminished fear. | |

**Steps** | **Rationale**

## Implementation

### *Nonverbal communication techniques*

Nonverbal skills are learned before verbal skills (Mundy et al, 1988), thus providing a basis for communication.

***Special Considerations:*** *Nonverbal communication exists at all times through body spacing, body positioning, gesturing, smiling, frowning, nodding, etc. These all send messages to the child, which, if in conflict with verbal communication, could give the stronger message.*

1. Body language.
   a. Use pointing and gesturing.

Acting out an idea or pointing to an object is understood universally by those who can see.

***Special Considerations:*** *Although inappropriate for those without sight, it is useful to others, especially as an initial intervention. Establish signals for common requests or responses.*

   b. Use sign language (Figs. 13-1 and 13-2).

If the hearing impaired child normally communicates by sign language, the facility has a duty to provide communication by that means, including obtaining a qualified interpreter if necessary. For aphonic infants and children, especially those that have been ventilator dependent since birth, early introduction of sign language can increase their communication potential and foster cognitive development (Hall and Weatherly, 1989). Some agencies in some states provide interpreters free of charge. To avoid legal complications, always use a certified interpreter.

   c. Approach child in a slow, calming manner.

A child is more likely to be calm when around an adult who is calm.

2. Touch.
   a. Cuddling.
   b. Stroking.
   c. Patting.
   d. Gentle touching of arm, shoulder, etc.

Used effectively with or without verbal communication, touch can provide assurance, comfort, and direction.

***Special Considerations:*** *Extra effort to touch the child who is in isolation or who is blind assists in diminishing alienation. Gentle, but firm, touch on the shoulder of the child with intellectual difficulties can direct his or her attention, limit the amount of sensory stimulation, and increase information processing.*

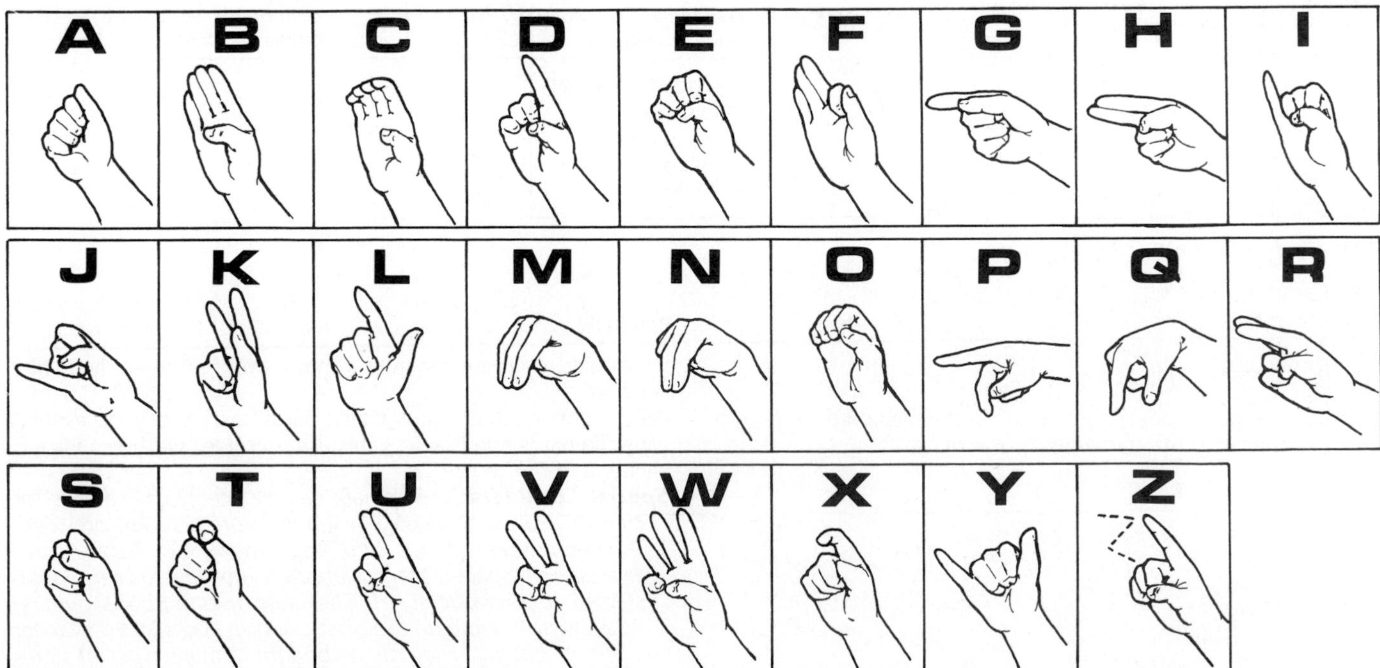


***FIG. 13-1*** The American Sign Language alphabet.

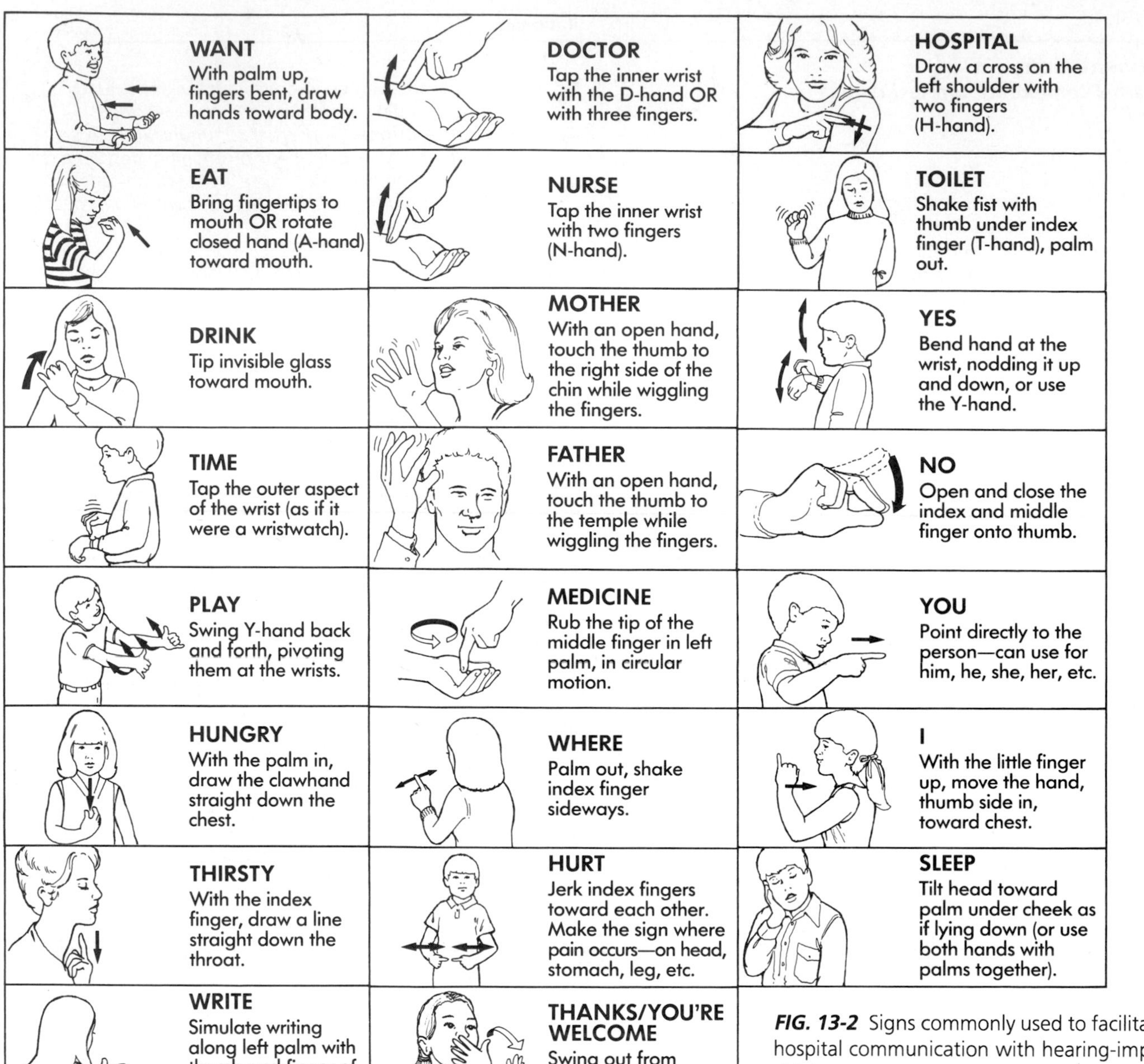


***FIG. 13-2*** Signs commonly used to facilitate in-hospital communication with hearing-impaired children.

| Steps | Rationale |
|---|---|
| 3. Visual aids. | Visual aids are more concrete in nature and more easily understood. |
| a. Use pencil and paper, chalk and chalkboard, or Magic Slate to write messages or ask questions. | Pencil, paper, chalk, and chalkboards are readily accessible. Chalkboards and Magic Slates are reusable. All three aids are easy and fun to use.<br>***Special Considerations:*** *Chalk can be messy, but allows for creative expression, especially when colored chalk is provided. Colored pencils, crayons, and magic markers provide creative expression on paper. Magic Slates are wax-covered cardboard, stapled to a plastic sheet. The child uses a special writing instrument to write on the plastic, which sticks to the wax for words or designs. They can be bought at many types of stores and are inexpensive. Magic Slates are especially useful when messages do not have to be saved.* |

| Steps | Rationale |
|---|---|
| b. Provide an alphabet board for the child with poor handwriting or diminished strength. | With alphabet boards, the child only needs to point to spell out a word.<br>***Special Considerations:*** *Make an alphabet board by taking cardboard and writing the letters of the alphabet or signs on it with a marker. The child can point to the letters or signs to spell words. (Gallaudet Press makes a pocket-sized plastic card with alphabet and signs that can be used for pointing.) Magnetic letters on a metal board can be used the same way. This can be purchased at a toy store.* |
| c. Use word cards written in the child's primary language. | Using prepared word cards saves the child time and energy. Writing the words in the child's primary language is comforting to him or her.<br>***Special Considerations:*** *To make word cards, write common requests, phrases, or words on a 4 × 6 inch flip chart. Use pictures for children who are younger, have a language barrier, or are intellectually impaired. If using sign language symbols or different language, seek help from an interpreter. Include the English meanings of those words chosen.* |
| d. Provide lap board. | The lap board combines the advantages of an alphabet board with word cards.<br>***Special Considerations:*** *Make a lap board with a piece of cardboard. On one side write the alphabet and on the other side write frequently used phrases or words (McGinnis, 1986). Laminate the cardboard with clear contact paper for durability.* |
| e. Use pictures and simple drawings to represent complex ideas/concepts. | Pictures or graphic representations sometimes present an idea easier than words.<br>***Special Considerations:*** *Select pictures that are developmentally appropriate.* |
| 4. Electronic devices.<br>a. Use direct selection devices for the child who cannot use handwriting but has some motor control.<br>b. Use a scanning communication system for the child who is unable to use selection devices. | Electronic devices are used to improve communication of the disabled child.<br>***Special Considerations:*** *A direct selection device has a keyboard and may or may not have voice capabilities. A scanning device is similar to a direct selection device, but easier to use (see Product Resources for a listing of companies that supply these devices; telephone devices are also available for the deaf through A.G. Bell Association; see Product Resources).* |
| ***Verbal communication techniques*** | Verbal communication is the most commonly used form of communication.<br>***Special Considerations:*** *Some deaf children can speak, although the quality of speech is different. Listen carefully, then repeat the message as necessary to make sure it was understood. When entering a room of a child on total isolation, always speak to the child before and during care.* |
| 1. Use a soothing tone of voice and mood. Make nonverbal messages consistent with verbal messages. | The meaning of a message can be altered by tone of voice. A soothing voice quality can allay fears even though the child does not understand the words.<br>***Special Considerations:*** *Many people unconsciously raise their voice when speaking to a child who has difficulty with or does not understand the language. This is frightening for the child and does not enhance comprehension. Also, always speak when entering the room of a child who is blind or with eye dressings to prevent anxiety and feelings of isolation.* |
| 2. Use lipreading when appropriate. Consider lighting and visibility. Speak clearly and only slightly slower but do not exaggerate or shout. | The child who lipreads may understand spoken messages.<br>***Special Considerations:*** *Lipreading can be difficult to understand, especially for young children. It may be more effective to use a more concrete method of communication, e.g., sign language or alphabet board.* |
| 3. Provide an interpreter when needed. | Using someone who speaks the child's language can provide him or her with a sense of familiarity and increase the ability to communicate.<br>***Special Considerations:*** *The facility has a duty to provide a certified interpreter if necessary to provide adequate standards of nursing care.* |

| Steps | Rationale |
|---|---|

### Evaluation Outcomes

1. The child comprehends messages given by health professionals.
2. The child is able to communicate with other children.
3. The child communicates needs, wants, and desires to health professionals.
4. The child has a decrease in fear.

### Observational Guidelines

Clarify messages by asking for verbal or nonverbal restatement of message.
Observe for improved interaction among peers.
Child does not repeat message and seems satisfied when provided with item, information, or assistance.
Notice nonverbal cues indicating the child is less fearful (e.g., smiling, communicating more often, or showing increased creativity).

### Documentation

Detail descriptions about communication strengths and deficits: type of problem; length of time it has existed; ability to hear, speak, and comprehend others; ability to read and write; and alternative communication channels available. Define cultural influences on communication. Describe availability of others to facilitate communication. Document amount of fear the child is exhibiting. Detail how interventions were planned (e.g., patient care conference) and which interventions were chosen. Describe the child's response to the intervention. Document future need for assessment and intervention. Describe need for an interpreter and plans to obtain devices needed to facilitate communication. Indicate other community resources and referrals given.

# *SKILL 14* Intervening in a Crisis

*Deborah Kay Brantly*

Crisis occurs when an individual perceives a problem as unsolvable and experiences increased inner tension, anxiety, and inability to function (Caplan, 1961). Crisis can be viewed as a pivotal point. If coping attempts are unsuccessful, the crisis can be overwhelming. The subjective distress can lead to depression, disrupted interpersonal relationships or other psychosocial problems, and psychosomatic disease. Conversely, the crisis can be an opportunity for growth. New coping strategies are defined and old ones rekindled to reestablish homeostasis. At the minimum, a return to the precrisis level of coping is desired. At the maximum, the child/family establishes a higher level of functioning. During a crisis, people are more susceptible to outside influence, therefore intervention is more readily received (Moore, 1989). Because nurses often see children and their families during crisis situations, such as with a critically ill or injured child, mastering crisis intervention techniques is of utmost importance (Moore, 1989).

## NURSING DIAGNOSES

Anxiety related to situational/maturational crisis; Ineffective family coping, compromised, related to situational/developmental crisis, ineffective coping methods, or inadequate support systems; Potential for violence, self-directed, related to suicidal behaviors.

| Steps | Rationale |
|---|---|
| **Assessment** | |
| 1. Determine the child/family's perception of the crisis: precipitating event, meaning of the crisis. | Perception influences the child/family's ability to return to equilibrium (Aguilera and Messick, 1986). |
| a. Precipitating event: what led the child/family to seek help, when it occurred, individuals involved, circumstances that led to the crisis. For example, begin by asking "What has happened that you feel the need for help?" or "What has happened recently that disturbs you the most?" | The more specifically the problem can be defined, the more likely the best answer can be found (Aguilera and Messick, 1986). Precipitating events usually occur within the previous day, normally at least within the previous 14 days (Aguilera and Messick, 1986). Time can distort events or give a different perspective of the event, which can influence accuracy of data and interventions needed. Precipitating events are not always the main source of the crisis. Discussing circumstances can bring other stressors into focus. |

| Steps | Rationale |
|---|---|
| | ***Special Considerations:*** *Younger children are more likely to act out behaviorally when they feel tension. Data gathered from them can be obtained through play, storytelling about "someone else" who feels similar to the child's perceived feelings, or the family can supply information. Older children or teenagers are more likely to discuss events. If the entire family is involved, be sure every family member is invited to express his or her personal perception of events.* |
| b. Perception of event realistic or distorted. | Perception gives information about reality testing and directs intervention to clarify distorted perceptions. |
| c. Effect of the event on the present and future, e.g., ask, "What has been the most difficult thing for you to handle?" or "What is important about that?" | Getting a perspective of the crisis' future meaning can indicate what basic needs are being threatened. |
| d. Type of crisis:<br>▪ Maturational—predictable; a result of growth and development (e.g. separation anxiety).<br>▪ Situational—unexpected life situations (e.g. sudden illness, a move, being fired from a job).<br>▪ Adventitious—unexpected but less common and more catastrophic events (e.g., rape, flood, fire, murder). | The type of crisis directs teaching and intervention needs.<br>***Special Considerations:*** *Some crises fall into more than one category. In this case, decide which seems most appropriate.* |
| e. Seriousness of the crisis. | The severity indicates the immediacy and type of intervention, e.g., a threat to human life would take highest priority.<br>***Special Considerations:*** *If the child is verbally aggressive, it is essential to calm the child before proceeding with assessment. If the child's behavior is threatening to self, property, or others, intervention is immediately needed. Assessment and further intervention can occur later. (Specific interventions for the suicidal, homicidal, or aggressive child are given later in this skill.)* |
| 2. Assess other psychosocial stressors contributing to the child/family problems. | The effects of stress are cumulative. It is more difficult to cope with several major stressors at once than it is to cope with each individually over a period of time.<br>***Special Considerations:*** *Holmes and Rahe (1967) have designed stress rating scales to determine the degree of stress in children and adolescents.* |
| 3. Discuss which factors are preventing the child/family from solving problems. | Children/families tend to view situations congruently with their perceptions of the world. Unless they discover what is preventing them from solving the problem, they will continue to function using the same coping mechanisms (White, 1987). |
| 4. Determine the strategies the child/family has used to cope with stressors and outcomes of the strategies. | Coping mechanisms are highly individualized and what may be effective for one person may not be as effective for another. |
| a. Usual methods of coping.<br>b. Coping used in similar events.<br>c. Coping used in this situation.<br>d. Previous coping methods that have worked in the past but have been dropped. | When under stress, more familiar methods of coping are used; some effective methods of coping may have been inadvertently dropped. |
| 5. Observe the child/family's emotional responses during the interview.<br>a. Expressive movements.<br>b. Emotional tone.<br>c. Verbal responses.<br>d. Attitudinal changes.<br>e. Defense mechanisms used. | Emotionally charged responses may represent unresolved feelings. The overuse of defense mechanisms indicates coping is ineffective. |
| 6. Determine the level of anxiety present in the child/family. | Anxiety interferes with the cognitive problem-solving process and must be decreased to a moderate level before effective problem-solving can occur.<br>***Special Considerations:*** *The Child Anxiety Scale (CAS) is a 20-item instrument designed to measure anxiety in children in kindergarten through fifth grade (Gillis, 1980).* |
| 7. Determine the child/family's available supports.<br>a. Family members.<br>b. Other individuals.<br>c. Institutions, e.g., churches, government agencies, or other community agencies. | Support systems affect the child/family's ability to return to equilibrium (Aguilera and Messick, 1986). |

| Steps | Rationale |
|---|---|
| 8. Discuss the child/family's ability to carry on with usual activities and responsibilities. | Inability to function in expected roles (e.g., get along reasonably well with peers, maintain grades at school, or participate in expected family functions) gives an indication of severity of crisis.<br>***Special Considerations:*** *If roles are compromised, consider a referral to a child and family therapist or hospitalization.* |
| 9. Determine each family member's ideas concerning what needs to be done about the problem. | Considering all members' suggestions provides more options from which to choose, allows everyone to express an opinion, and can foster a sense of family. |
| 10. Determine suicidal risk.<br>a. History of suicidal ideations or attempts, e.g., ask, "Have you ever thought about suicide?", "Have you ever thought about harming yourself?", or "Have you attempted suicide before?"<br>b. Specific plan, e.g., ask, "Do you have a plan in mind?" "What are the details of your plan?"<br>c. Means to carry through with the plan, e.g., ask, "How would you carry through with your plan?"<br>d. Desire to carry out the plan, e.g., ask, "Do you want to go through with it?" or "Do you think you would carry the plan through?" | Susceptible individuals (those who have a previous attempt, have a family history of suicide, or have had suicidal thoughts) are more prone to suicide during a crisis event. The more specific the plan, the more serious the risk.<br>***Special Considerations:*** *If the crisis was precipitated by an injury to a child, a family member who feels responsible should be assessed for suicidal thoughts (Moore, 1989).* |
| 11. Determine homicidal risk.<br>a. Name of the person to be harmed.<br>b. Specific plan. | Extreme emotions and a decrease in cognitive awareness are experienced during a crisis, which may lead to homicidal feelings. |

## Planning and Goal Setting

| Steps | Rationale |
|---|---|
| 1. Determine type of intervention needed.<br>a. Individual therapy.<br>b. Family therapy.<br>c. Group therapy.<br>d. Social services.<br>e. Hospitalization. | Determining needed interventions facilitates planning referrals and nursing interventions. |
| 2. Determine the type of professional needed.<br>a. Staff nurse.<br>b. Psychiatric nurse therapist.<br>c. Other health professional. | Determining the type of professional needed further guides the referral-making process.<br>***Special Considerations:*** *It is important to recognize one's own personal strengths and limitations and the definitions of one's role. When those boundaries are exceeded, referral is essential.* |
| 3. Determine the community resources available. | Familiarity with community resources provides the opportunity for an appropriate and timely referral linkage. |
| 4. Determine the expected length of time that services will be needed. | Crisis intervention is a short-term, problem-solving therapy, generally considered to be under 12 sessions in length. If further intervention is needed, a referral is in order.<br>***Special Considerations:*** *The number of sessions needed is sometimes difficult to identify during initial presentation. This is determined in joint effort by child/family and therapist.* |
| 5. Develop individualized child and family goals:<br>▪ Increased ability to cope.<br>▪ Resolution of the crisis. | |

## Implementation

| Steps | Rationale |
|---|---|
| 1. Remain calm; approach the child in a warm, unhurried manner. | A calm approach communicates a sense of calm to the child/family. |
| 2. Use clear, simple language. | Hearing is the first sense to be affected during a crisis. |
| 3. Allow for venting of emotions. | Intense emotions interfere with cognitive skills. After emotions are decreased, the child/family is better able to provide information and problem-solve.<br>***Special Considerations:*** *When the child/family is experiencing intense emotions during the assessment process, use this intervention before continuing with data collection.* |
| 4. Assist the child/family to gain an intellectual understanding of the crisis. | Often the child does not see the connection between the crisis event and the extreme discomfort that is experienced (Morley, Messick, and Aguilera, 1967). |

| Steps | Rationale |
|---|---|
| a. Connect events of the crisis to the emotional discomfort that is felt.<br>b. Connect related events. | ***Special Considerations:*** *With younger children, use play therapy to make this connection. Ask questions to allow the child to think and project personal feelings, e.g., "Do you think Janey is sad?" "What is Janey sad about?" or "When Janey is sad, what does she do?"* |
| 5. Assist in bringing suppressed emotional reactions to the surface. | The child may have emotions that have been denied, but are affecting coping ability. |
| 6. Support the child/family's ability to cope with the problem thus far. | Children/families can forget they have had some success dealing with the problem, even though the situation has become overwhelming. Positive support encourages the child/family and increases coping.<br>***Special Considerations:*** *When the child/family sees nothing positive and focuses on the negative, praise the child/family's ability to talk about the problem.* |
| 7. Assist the child/family in problem-solving. | Assisting with problem-solving models the process and mobilizes the child/family to an action orientation. |
| a. Identify the problem clearly and realistically, considering all aspects of the situation. | A clear, concise definition of the problem will provide a firm basis for problem-solving. |
| b. Support the child/family's ability to come up with solutions to the problems. | Supporting the child/family's problem-solving abilities raises esteem and promotes independence. |
| c. Assist the child/family in identifying all alternatives. Consider all possibilities at this point and encourage creative suggestions. | Identifying all alternatives stimulates the child/family's creativity.<br>***Special Considerations:*** *When working with a family, all members (except infants) can participate. Even the younger child can be involved by coming up with ideas while the adult acts as "secretary." Write down suggestions in a notebook (Faber and Mazlish, 1982).* |
| d. Suggest trying old coping mechanisms that have worked in the past but have not been tried in this situation. | If methods have worked in the past, they may succeed in helping the child/family cope with the current crisis. |
| e. Suggest alternate ways of coping not yet proposed. | Suggesting coping mechanisms the child/family has not thought of may empower them to try other methods. |
| f. Identify pros and cons of each coping method or alternative. | Identifying pros and cons provides strengths and limitations of each alternative. The situation and alternatives are viewed realistically, increasing coping ability and establishing a foundation for selecting the best choice. |
| g. Select the coping methods or alternatives that are feasible. | The child/family exercises the right of choice, facilitating a sense of accomplishment and increased self-esteem.<br>***Special Considerations:*** *If a family is involved, find solutions that are acceptable to all members. Do not let personal or cultural values interfere with what the family feels is feasible and what is realistic in the situation.* |
| h. Discuss how the plan will be implemented and who will be involved in implementation. | Detailing the plan clarifies implementation and reinforces commitment. |
| 8. Assist the child/family in identifying potential support persons. | When others are involved, they can continue to give support after professional intervention is terminated.<br>***Special Considerations:*** *Determine and encourage use of the existing intrafamilial system of support.* |
| 9. Refer the child to more intensive therapy if needed. Make the referral by writing down the name and telephone number of the referral for the family or call for an appointment in their presence.<br>a. Individual therapy.<br>b. Family therapy.<br>c. Hospitalization.<br>d. Crisis intervention group therapy. | Referral is needed when problem-solving is ineffective, the family requests it, or the skills of the interviewer are inadequate to meet the needs of the client.<br>***Special Considerations:*** *Individual or family therapy may be provided by a nurse clinical specialist, nurse therapist or other psychiatric-mental health professional. Some mental health centers have a crisis intervention therapy group. When hospitalization is indicated, refer to a physician or directly to the hospital.* |
| 10. Refer for further situational support and socialization.<br>a. Support group.<br>b. Church group.<br>c. Governmental agencies, e.g., human services.<br>d. Community agencies.<br>e. Social services.<br>f. Interest groups. | Referring the child/family to groups, agencies, and institutions broadens the support base, which increases potential for coping. |

| Steps | Rationale |
|---|---|
| 11. Write the local crisis hotline telephone number for the family. | The crisis hotline is a quick means to intervention. |
| 12. Teach about the nature of stress and the necessity to promote a stress-reducing lifestyle. | When the individual leads a lifestyle that promotes stress reduction, energy is mobilized for coping when a crisis occurs. |
| ***Intervening with the suicidal or homicidal child*** | |
| 1. Indicate concern for the suicidal child's safety and make a commitment to keep him or her safe, e.g., say, "I care about your safety and I will keep you safe to the best of my ability." | The child feels safer when with an adult who cares about his or her safety. |
| 2. Establish a no suicide contract written and signed by the child. | Even a child recognizes the seriousness of signing a contract and will only on rare occasions break his or her word. |
| 3. Maintain close observation of the child. | Close supervision maintains safety of the child and others.<br>***Special Considerations:*** *In the community or in an outpatient setting, it may be difficult to keep a suicidal adolescent near. In this case, immediately notify the family (see Step 5). When the child is in a psychiatric unit, keep the child under strict observation. Document the child's behaviors at least every 15 minutes.* |
| 4. Secure dangerous objects (e.g., glass objects, knives, scissors, razors, guns, OTC medications, and toxics). | When dangerous objects are secured, the options for carrying through the plan are diminished.<br>***Special Considerations:*** *Some adolescents view this as a challenge. They may then come up with a new plan and not divulge it.* |
| 5. Inform the family of the child's suicidal or homicidal intentions. | The parents are the legal guardians of the child and must be informed of these intentions. |
| 6. Discuss treatment options with the family. | Providing options gives the parents information to make a decision about treatment.<br>***Special Considerations:*** *If parents choose outpatient therapy even though hospitalization is indicated, it may be necessary to consult with a mental health professional to discuss submission of a petition to determine need for treatment. (Check with local mental health council for details of this procedure.) When the homicidal child is in the community and deemed dangerous, the person who is the object of potential harm has a legal right of notification by the health professional.* |
| ***Intervening with the aggressive child*** | |
| 1. Remain calm and confident. | When a child senses others feel calm and confident, he or she feels more calm and secure. |
| 2. Maintain adequate space between self and child. | The child may feel his or her body space is being invaded and therefore feel threatened.<br>***Special Considerations:*** *Adolescents especially resent body space invasions during crises and generally require others to be at least an arm's length away.* |
| 3. Place self between the child and the door. | Positioning of this nature defines boundaries for the child and provides a means of escape from aggressive acts initiated by the child. |
| 4. Maintain eye contact and face the child at all times. | Facing the child and establishing eye contact focuses the child's attention, facilitates rapport, and provides awareness of aggressive acts. |
| 5. Make movements and gestures slowly. | Sudden movements encourage aggression in the child, whereas slow movements promote calming. |
| 6. Use short, concrete sentences. | Auditory perception is the first sense to be impaired in a crisis. Short, concrete sentences are more easily understood by children of all ages. |
| 7. Give the child specific instructions on what behavior is expected. | The child is more likely to fulfill the request when it is specific. |
| 8. Use grounding techniques. | Grounding techniques bring the child's emotions and perceptions into focus, producing a calming effect. |
| a. Instruct the child to look you straight in the eye. | When the child focuses on another person, he or she focuses his or her attention and is under more control. |
| b. Lightly, but firmly, touch the child's shoulder at arm's length. | This helps establish a therapeutic alliance and the child senses the adult has control of the situation. |

| Steps | Rationale |
|---|---|
| | ***Special Considerations:*** *Make sure the child is ready for an invasion of his or her body space. Approach the child slowly and touch the child first at arm's length. Adolescent males sometimes are not responsive to this intervention, therefore, use more verbal directives and eye contact.* |
| c. Move with the child to remain in his or her view. | This technique establishes rapport and maintains safe boundaries. |
| 9. Reaffirm the child's ability to get under control, e.g., say, "I'm certain you can calm yourself." | Reaffirming the child's ability to control himself or herself reinforces self-control and gives the child permission to do so. |
| 10. Make sure other persons are available for support if necessary. | In case of further escalation, additional help may be required to protect the child and others. |
| 11. With further escalation, use restraint or holding techniques. | Holding and restraining prevents the child from harming self, others, or the surroundings when he or she is out of control. ***Special Considerations:*** *Holding techniques must be learned through trained personnel. Restraint with cloth or leather restraints requires a physician's order. (Check facility policy statements and procedures.)* |

| Evaluation Outcomes | Observational Guidelines |
|---|---|
| 1. The child/family experiences relief from the crisis. | The child/family state they feel relief from the crisis. |
| 2. The child is free from physiologic manifestations of the crisis. | Interview the child/family to determine presence of physiologic manifestations of stress (eating disturbance, sleep disturbance, intestinal disturbance, headaches, muscle tension or pain). |
| 3. Anxiety has diminished or is absent. | Interview and observe the child for a lower level of anxiety. |
| 4. New and preexisting support systems are used and considered effective. | Interview the child/family to determine support systems being used and effectiveness. |
| 5. Problems are being resolved using the problem-solving method. | Interview the child/family to determine what problems have arisen and how they were resolved. |
| 6. Coping mechanisms are used and considered effective. | Interview the child/family to determine the use of coping methods and their effectiveness. |
| 7. Current affective responses are more positive than those previously noted. | Observe for more positive affective responses (e.g., smiling, language indicating optimism, absence of crying). |
| 8. Changes have been made in lifestyle to reduce stress. | Interview to determine changes in nutrition, rest, exercise, and leisure time activities. |

## Documentation

Clearly and concisely describe the precipitating event and problem as viewed by all those involved. Describe the child/family's affective responses, usual coping mechanisms, and coping mechanisms tried during this crisis. Describe support systems identified and the nature of the support given. Document physiologic symptoms associated with the crisis and stress. Identify any teaching done, interventions used, and those strategies the child/family decides to try. Document the child's response to all interventions, as well as referrals and plans for follow-up visits.

# SKILL 15 Meeting the Child's Developmental Needs through Play

*Judy Holt Rollins*

Play is a natural and essential activity for every child that provides many opportunities to learn and grow—physically, mentally, and socially. Supervised play allows nurses to optimize normal development in children and enrich the family's involvement with their child. Observing a child at play provides information about cognitive, intellectual, social, and emotional development. Play and playthings challenge children, and with mastery comes satisfaction and the desire to master problems in general.

While many hospitals are fortunate enough to have child life specialists who develop and supervise play activities for hospitalized (and often outpatient) children, it is important that play remains a part of nursing care. If play is viewed as solely the responsibility of the child life specialist, and the rest of the staff performs only medical procedure duties, it creates a system in which some staff may be viewed by the child as "nice," while others will be viewed as "mean" (Jolly, 1968). Play should be incorporated into care of children by all staff, including nurses and physicians.

## NURSING DIAGNOSES

Health-seeking behaviors (play) related to infant/child's ability to master developmental tasks; Altered growth and development related to environmental and stimulation deficiencies; Diversional activity deficit related to long-term hospitalization or confinement at home, immobility, or sensory-peceptual alteration.

| Steps | Rationale |
|---|---|
| **Assessment** | |
| 1. Review information about the child: | |
| a. Age.<br>b. Developmental level.<br>c. Interests. | Chronologic age provides guidelines for selecting play materials and experiences (Table 15-1). Play that is developmentally appropriate is likely to be more enjoyable and worthwhile for the child. For example, a 4-year-old child would probably be very frustrated and unable to complete a puzzle with a large number of pieces.<br>***Special Considerations:*** *It is common for children to regress when hospitalized or experiencing other potentially traumatic events, possibly affecting the child's play abilities.* |
| d. Physical limitations, restrictions, and abilities. | Choice of play activities or materials is often determined by factors such as the child's limitations, restrictions, or abilities. |
| e. Temperament. | Some children enjoy details and instructions; others prefer gross motor activity. |
| 2. Consider the availability of family members. | Knowledge of the availability of family members aids in planning some activities around playtimes when family members can be included. |
| 3. Determine the need for: | |
| a. Group vs. individual play. | Individual play allows for a more intense intervention with a focus on the child's unique needs. Children, particularly school-age and above, find group play with others sharing similar conditions to be very valuable.<br>***Special Considerations:*** *For the young hospitalized child experiencing separation anxiety, developing a relationship with an adult is of primary importance and usually necessary before group play is enjoyed. Children who have had emotional difficulties before hospitalization, are expected to be in the hospital for a long period of time, or have a chronic, terminal, or progressive illness may also benefit initially from individual play (Clatworthy, 1981).* |

| Steps | Rationale |
|---|---|
| b. Structured vs. nonstructured play. | A structured play session may be necessary to evaluate a child's development or to work on a particular task. Nonstructured play usually offers a greater opportunity to discover what the child is thinking, fearing, anticipating, misunderstanding, and so on. Nonstructured play takes much more constraint on the part of the adult who has little control over the ultimate outcome.<br>***Special Considerations:*** *Children with high anxiety levels are often unable to engage in nonstructured play.* |
| 4. Assess personal attitude. | Play may be enhanced by a flexible and accepting attitude. It is not only permissible to play with a child, but it is an essential part of total care for the child. |

***TABLE 15-1*** **Guidelines for Toy Selection and Play Activities**

| Guidelines | Suggested Toys & Activities |
|---|---|
| **BIRTH TO 6 MONTHS** | |
| Toys for this age are primarily for looking, listening, sucking, or fingering. Infants 0 to 2 months enjoy seeing and hearing interesting things. Infants 2 to 6 months show growing interest in touching, holding, batting, turning, shaking, kicking, mouthing, and tasting objects. Infants like to see bright primary colors, high contrast, simple design, clear lines and features, human face features (especially eyes), and bull's eye patterns. They enjoy watching hanging objects or "mobiles" that move by wind, wind-up action, or infant's own activity. Toys for watching should be suspended 8 to 14 inches from the infant's eyes at first and angled toward the eyes, then moved up out of reach when the infant can touch them. Toys for watching are more appealing if they move and make noise (but movement should be slow and noise should not be too loud or sudden). Infants enjoy variety and producing effects on toys by their own activity. Toys for holding should be light, easily graspable, and mouthable. | ▪ Hang brightly colored objects, e.g., mobiles, or black and white bull's eye patterned objects within 8 to 14 inches of infant's face.<br>▪ Place a nonbreakable mirror where the infant can see himself or herself.<br>▪ Talk soft and gently to infant.<br>▪ Play soft, soothing music from music boxes, radio, record player, television. Move away and toward infant to change loudness and attract attention.<br>▪ Hold, cuddle, rock, and touch infant.<br>▪ Take infant on excursions, holding head erect for visual inspection.<br>▪ Rub soft cuddly toys against infant's skin.<br>▪ Place infant on tummy and give colorful objects to look at.<br>▪ Provide toys such as rubber animals and teething rings. Older infants can use rattles.<br>▪ String brightly colored beads within reach across crib.<br>▪ Play water games—splash water gently, have baby float on back with firm support, blow bubbles.<br>▪ Touch, tickle, and stroke older infant.<br>▪ Prop up in infant seat to scan environment.<br>▪ Attach "busy box" to crib. |
| **6 TO 12 MONTHS** | |
| Infants 6 to 9 months are interested in longer and more extensive exploration of toys. They like to bang, insert, poke, shake, bite, throw, open and shut, empty and fill. Infants 10 to 12 months show beginning interest in object mastery and like many objects to explore. They like stacking, putting in and taking out, pouring out, fitting one object into another, opening and closing, pressing levers, turning things, pushing balls and cars. Generally, infants in this age range are interested in operating simple mechanisms, containers, and the container/contained relationship, appearing and disappearing objects. As at earlier ages, infants enjoy producing effects by their own actions. Toys for infants should:<br>1. Be nontoxic materials.<br>2. Have no sharp points or edges.<br>3. Be safe for mouthing.<br>4. Be nonbreakable; no glass or brittle plastic.<br>5. Have no small parts to be lodged in throat, ears, or nose.<br>6. Have no parts to entrap fingers, toes, or hand. | ▪ Talk to and mimic sounds infant makes.<br>▪ Provide safe, clear area for crawling.<br>▪ Provide walker, Johnny-jump-up, swing.<br>▪ Ride in stroller or wagon.<br>▪ Retrieve objects they throw down over and over to give sense of control over environment.<br>▪ Play pat-a-cake, bye-bye, peek-a-boo, finger and toe games, e.g., "This little piggy."<br>▪ Read and tell child simple nursery rhymes.<br>▪ Give push-pull toys.<br>▪ Help child with walking by holding hands. |

*Continued.*

**TABLE 15-1** Guidelines for Toy Selection and Play Activities—cont'd

| Guidelines | Suggested Toys & Activities |
|---|---|
| **1 YEAR** | |
| This age group prefers action toys that produce movement or sounds by child's efforts. Toys need not be highly detailed but should be realistic looking, lightweight, and preferably in bright colors. This child is always on the move—large muscle activities, e.g., running and climbing, dominate over small muscle activites, e.g., exploring objects, construction. The child begins to combine, put together objects, and also begins imitative play.<br><br>**2 YEARS**<br>Beginning of cooperative, social play with an increasing interest in pretend play. Child loves physical, active play and prefers action toys and toys that produce movement or sounds by child's own efforts. More realism is preferred and child begins to pay attention to qualities of objects. Prefers toys with working parts. Toys should be lightweight for easy lifting and carrying. Bright colors are preferred. Toys should meet safety regulations for age:<br>1. Sturdy, unbreakable; not likely to break into small pieces and strong enough for child to stand on or in.<br>2. Nontoxic materials.<br>3. No sharp points or edges.<br>4. Too large to be lodged in windpipe, ears, or nostrils.<br>5. No detachable small parts.<br>6. No parts that could pinch or entrap fingers, toes, or hair.<br>7. Not put together with easily exposed straight pins, sharp wires, or nails.<br>8. No electrical parts, unless supervised by adult. | ▪ Provide wide variety of objects to play with and touch, e.g., shoes, boxes, cans, toys.<br>▪ Provide fill and dump containers, large cardboard blocks, dolls, stuffed toys, pedal-propelled toys, low rocking horse, transportation toys.<br>▪ Play "Simon says" in identifying body parts.<br>▪ Play with puppet, with adult as the performer.<br>▪ Play "pretend" with animals, phone calls.<br>▪ Provide large picture books, books of rhymes, puzzles with squares and pegs.<br>▪ Talk about pictures in books, e.g., "Look at the three blue birds."<br>▪ Provide large crawl-into boxes.<br>▪ Offer crayons and paper for scribbling. |
| **3 TO 5 YEARS** | |
| Preschoolers prefer toys with realistic detail and working parts. There is an increasing interest in dramatic and pretend play by age 5 (the peak period for dramatic play) with all sorts of props. This is also the period of peak interest in puppet play. The preschooler enjoys increasing construction activity, often with a plan or goal. Interest peaks at this age in play scenes, small figures, and cars. Toys for this age should:<br>1. Be sturdy and not likely to break easily into small pieces or leave jagged edges.<br>2. Have no sharp points or edges.<br>3. Not be made of glass or brittle plastic.<br>4. Be made of nontoxic materials.<br>5. Have no electrical parts unless supervised by adult. | ▪ Provide tricycle.<br>▪ Play show and tell games, dance activities.<br>▪ Offer toys such as jigsaw puzzles with large pieces, pounding bench, balls of varying sizes, dolls and stuffed animals, set of farm toys, tea sets, play telephone, housekeeping and carpentry toys, rocking horse, wooden train sets, materials for safe cutting, finger paints, dress-up clothes.<br>▪ Provide low stable objects for supervised climbing.<br>▪ Use story or sound effects tapes and records.<br>▪ Storytelling by child.<br>▪ Guessing games. |
| **6 TO 8 YEARS** | |
| Child is primarily interested in goal rather than means or process. Experimentation becomes increasingly "scientific." Child is less dependent on concrete object for concept. Child can sort and classify using more than one criterion; increasingly makes use of reading, writing, and simple arithmetic in games and toys; does simple sewing, weaving, braiding, ceramics, jewelry kits; uses simple mechanical toys (cars, trains); and has greatly increased fine motor control. Child is interested in time and seasons and in toys marking time, collections of things, line between fantasy and reality (likes magic tricks and disguise kits), producing arts, crafts, woodworking, etc., kits (science, craft, models). Child can follow simple directions, adult roles, and likes realistic costumes and props for character play, and rudiments of sports and skill development. Children show increasing variation in interest and abilities. Reading interests vary, but child is beginning to be able to use dictionary. Beginning interest in giving "shows." Great interest in fairness, but hates to lose and will cheat to win in games. | ▪ Offer skates, scooter, bicycles, doll houses or other miniature sets.<br>▪ Provide child-sized furniture.<br>▪ Play group games, jump rope, hopscotch, rough and tumble games.<br>▪ Provide opportunities for organized play.<br>▪ Play board games or card games with child.<br>▪ Provide older school-age child with materials for more solitary activities, e.g., reading, crafts, collections (e.g., dolls or stamps), and other special interest activities (e.g., magic).<br>▪ Provide more complex board games for older child.<br>▪ Provide multipiece puzzles for the older child.<br>▪ Support children's productions (shows, plays, exhibits) at whatever level children desire (e.g., helping to locate props and other materials, publicizing the event).<br>▪ Encourage attendance at events of special interest to individual children (athletic events, musicals, plays, movies, art shows, model or collector's shows).<br>▪ Provide opportunities for children with special interests to meet other children and adults with similar interests. |

**TABLE 15-1** Guidelines for Toy Selection and Play Activities—cont'd

| Guidelines | Suggested Toys & Activities |
|---|---|
| **9 TO 12 YEARS** | |
| At this age there is a great increase in individual differences in abilities and interest—may be interested in reading (and in specific kinds of books), science (with some specific interest like chemistry or astronomy), computers (some like to make their own programs), hobbies, crafts (skill approaches adult level by age 12), building models, collections (some become serious collectors and many enjoy small collections), formal training in arts (music, drama, drawing) or specific crafts (pottery, weaving, carpentry, sewing, etc.), producing shows or plays (live actors, animals, puppets, etc.). Both sexes enjoy athletics or competitive sports, but specific interests vary—child may be interested in formal training in some athletic skill. Fine motor abilities begin to approach that of an adult—may enjoy dexterity games, complex constructions, or puzzles. Interested in more complex table games and enjoys strategy and competition—can now stick to the rules and lose gracefully. | |
| **ADOLESCENCE** | |
| Teenagers are interested in adult forms of play. The young adolescent is not content with toy versions of anything. Competitive sports are enjoyed and community recognition for sports and hobbies are important to this age group. They tend to be very self-critical, and activities that they are unable to excel in (e.g., drawing realistically) are usually dropped. They enjoy dancing, parties, reading, movies, rock concerts, part-time employment, watching television, experimenting with their appearance, and talking to or being with peers. | ▪ Provide opportunities for competitive sports and games, watching movies and television, talking on telephone, attending parties and dances, experimenting with cosmetics, hairstyles, and dress.<br>▪ Provide electronic games, books, construction, and craft sets.<br>▪ Play card and board games with adolescent, help with craft activities.<br>▪ Provide opportunities for interested adolescent to help younger children with special activities, e.g., face painting or crafts. |

| Steps | Rationale |
|---|---|
| **Planning and Goal Setting** | |
| 1. Consider the play environment:<br>a. Safety.<br>b. Light.<br>c. Comfort.<br>d. Color.<br>e. Scale. | Although children will engage in play in almost any environment, one conducive to play is desirable. In the hospital, the play environment, whether it be the child's room or a playroom, should attempt to recreate the home environment as closely as possible. Homelike furniture and a playroom with familiar toys lend an air of permission to play that helps a child attain a sense of well-being.<br>***Special Considerations:*** *A child who is immobilized in bed (e.g., a child in traction) may be brought to the playroom in the bed with physician permission. A toy cart can be wheeled to the child who is unable to leave the room (e.g., a child in isolation). Outpatient waiting areas often have a corner devoted to play.* |
| 2. Develop individualized nursing goals of care:<br>▪ To promote and maintain physical, intellectual, social, and emotional development.<br>▪ To provide a means of ongoing psychosocial and developmental assessment. | |
| **Implementation** | |
| 1. Restrict playroom use to "safe" activities. | Restricting certain unpleasant, embarrassing, or painful activities keeps the playroom a safe place for children. Many hospitals have a rule that no procedures, painful or unpainful, embarrassing or not, are allowed in the playroom. Some hospitals have also extended this rule to the patient room. |

| Steps | Rationale |
|---|---|
| | ***Special Considerations:*** *Often children become upset when their play is interrupted. Therefore, at times procedures such as vital signs, oral or IV medications are performed in the playroom, but only with the permission of the child and the other children present. Care must be taken to assure that other children in the playroom understand and are not confused or fearful about the event.* |
| 2. Define limits for child. | |
| a. Time available for play. | Children dislike being interrupted in the middle of mastering a task. It is often helpful before starting an activity to know how much time is available. ***Special Considerations:*** *Once play is underway, it is useful to remind the child, "You have about 5 more minutes before clean-up," or for younger children, "You have until the big hand on the clock reaches the top."* |
| b. Behavior to be limited. | Children need to know that they may not hurt others, themselves, or destroy property. ***Special Considerations:*** *Therapeutic play is used for dealing with aggressive behavior (see Skill 16). Note: What looks like destructive play may only be a search for new effects in manipulating objects.* |
| 3. Choose or help child select a play activity. | Choosing or helping the child select a play activity invites a child to play and helps familiarize the child with available materials and activities. ***Special Considerations:*** *More than one activity or toy can serve the same developmental purpose. Children sometimes want a demonstration of a particular plaything to understand how to use it, taking care not to stifle the child's creativity. Children also often use toys in creative ways never envisioned by the manufacturer. Playthings need not be expensive; common objects are suitable and even preferable for many play activities (see Table 15-1). For the child in isolation, consider using playthings that are disposable or can be washed in a washing machine or dishwasher.* |
| 4. Adapt plaything or activity for the child with physical limitations, disabilities, or restrictions. | Generic toys and common play activities can frequently be adapted for a child with special needs (see Product References and Teaching Resources). ***Special Considerations:*** *Switches to control battery-operated toys provide a way for even severely disabled children to play independently with toys (see Product References and Teaching Resources). The growth of computer technology has greatly expanded play opportunities for disabled children.* |
| 5. If a child is very weak or immobile, "play" for him or her, e.g., move playthings, game or puzzle pieces, and so on, following child's instructions. | The child can still benefit from the problem-solving and decision-making aspects of play. |
| 6. Be flexible, creative, and willing to do the unconventional. | Flexibility creates an atmosphere of fun and adventure. The child is offered the message that he or she is limited only by his or her imagination. |
| 7. Remain available for the child, letting the child indicate desired level of adult involvement in play activity. | The play environment consists not only of playthings, but also of people. Children observe how other people react, and it either encourages or discourages a child's imaginative play. Children often like to play near adults. Young children, in particular, feel safer when an adult is in view. ***Special Considerations:*** *Remaining available also provides an excellent opportunity for the child and nurse to get to know each other on a different, nonthreatening level.* |
| 8. Offer encouragement by expressing interest and praise in the child's activity (e.g., asking questions such as "What happens next?" "Please tell me more" or "That's a fine, sturdy house you built"). | Encouraging children to be creative provides positive reinforcement, leading to greater self-esteem. Children who are encouraged to tell their own stories, paint their own pictures, act out their own fantasies, and construct their own worlds are better able to hold onto their own hopes and dreams (Stapleton and Yahraes, 1978). |

| Steps | Rationale |
|---|---|
| 9. Challenge the child each time a new skill is learned. Provide new levels of difficulty by having available a balanced variety of toys encompassing numerous areas of development. | Children who try more challenging tasks gain security and confidence from knowing that they can return to what they have already mastered if they chose to do so. |
| 10. Encourage family members to play with child. | The availability of play materials and parental involvement correlates positively with subsequent developmental outcomes (Gottfried, 1985). Play offers the opportunity to reinforce family supporting and nurturing in a healthy and desirable manner (Goldberger, 1988). Observing the child in a normal activity often provides family with hope for recovery. ***Special Considerations:*** *Serve as a role model for parents who may think their child is too sick or fragile to play.* |
| 11. Facilitate play by incorporating it into as many aspects of care or interactions as possible (see Table 15-1). | Play is an essential part of a child's development. Using play not only helps restore normal aspects of living by allowing children to be in control, it also provides an enjoyable experience for participants. |

## Evaluation Outcomes

1. Child will demonstrate developmental maintenance or growth.
2. The child's environment will approximate a normal home environment.
3. The child and family will have enjoyable interactions.
4. Child's play behavior will provide information regarding cognitive, emotional, and social development.

## Observational Guidelines

Observe child's ability to perform a new task. Reassess developmental level; compare to previous assessment.

Observe the presence of toys and child's willingness to participate in play.

Observe quality and quantity of family interaction.

Observe child's behavior and ability to master developmental tasks. Observe child's interactions with other people.

## Documentation

Document the child's approach and response to play, behavior, interests and abilities, interaction with other people, any parent teaching, and plans for future interventions.

## Home Care Modifications

For the child confined to bed at home, the Toy Manufacturers of America offers the following suggestions for families:

1. Use a bed tray, ironing board lowered to the correct height, or a leaf from a table covered with an old sheet or plastic tablecloth as an activity center (also, lap boards are commercially available).
2. Use a large carton cut out to fit over the legs to serve as a playspace and to protect bedcoverings from messy spills.
3. Provide a play area large enough to allow space for coloring books, paint sets, craft and model kits, construction sets, building blocks, puzzles, and small chalkboards and slates.
4. Use extra pillows to provide back support and be sure that there is adequate light.
5. Introduce new experiences, e.g., a musical instrument.
6. Bring faraway places to the child through slide viewers.

# SKILL 16 Assisting With Therapeutic Play

*Judy Holt Rollins*

Often children, particularly hospitalized children, require more than recreational play. Therapeutic play, structured by an adult for a specific purpose, combines play with communication. It provides children with the opportunity to express themselves while giving them appropriate feedback (Meer, 1985). The use of play in health care settings not only reduces anxiety but also improves coping abilities, mastery, and feelings of control (Bolig, 1988). Medical play is a form of therapeutic play that includes medical themes or use of medical equipment. Play therapy may be used to assist children in understanding their own behavior and in changing those behaviors that are inappropriate (Gibbons and Boren, 1985).

## NURSING DIAGNOSES

Anxiety related to unmet informational needs about upcoming events/procedures; Ineffective individual coping related to unrealistic perceptions, unpleasant experiences, and/or inadequate support systems; Altered role performance related to lack of information about expected role behaviors/responsibilities; Anticipating/dysfunctional grieving related to perceived/actual loss of well-being, significant other, or personal possession.

| Steps | Rationale |
|---|---|
| **Assessment** | |
| 1. Determine the child's age and developmental level. | The child's cognitive ability helps determine his or her understanding of the hospital experience. The child's behavior, in turn, is influenced by this understanding. A basic knowledge of age-appropriate concerns is helpful in planning therapeutic interventions. |
| a. Children 2 to 4 years old are most susceptible to separation anxiety as a result of hospitalization. | Children of this age lack the cognitive sophistication to understand their illness and resultant hospitalization, as well as the social maturity required for separation (Golden, 1987). They may regress to the degree that they are unable to play until a transitional attachment to another adult is established.<br>***Special Considerations:*** *It is estimated that over 50% of pediatric hospital beds are filled by children under 3 years of age (American Academy of Pediatrics, 1986).* |
| b. Children 4 to 7 years old worry primarily about mutilation to their bodies. | Cognitive development may still be insufficient for adequate understanding of condition and resultant procedures. Because they are no longer burdened with the overwhelming anxiety of separation, they may experience a great deal of anger at perceived injustices and the assaults against their bodies (Golden, 1987). |
| c. Children 8 years old to puberty are concerned primarily with mastery in peer relationships. | Cognitively, they are able to grasp the reasons for their hospitalizations and often require detailed explanations of their condition and procedures. Comprehensive plans of care will consider the importance of peer relationships.<br>***Special Considerations:*** *This age group often benefits from group interactions with peers sharing similar experiences.* |
| 2. Review history and present condition for physical limitations, restrictions, and abilities. | Therapeutic play can be adapted to meet the unique needs of the child, regardless of limitations. |
| 3. Review behaviors for areas that commonly cause concern. | Therapeutic play provides the child with an opportunity to communicate and learn in the medium children understand best—play. |
| a. Separation. | Therapeutic play allows the establishment of a nurturing relationship with an adult other than parent (Golden, 1987). |

| Steps | Rationale |
|---|---|

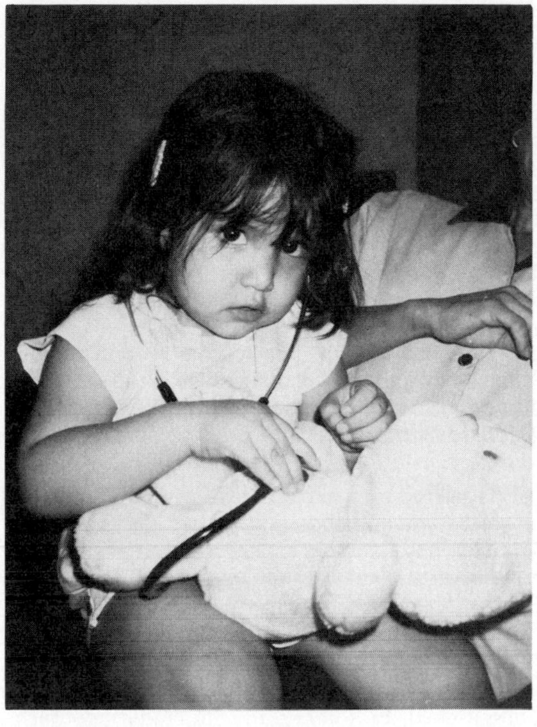

***FIG. 16-1*** Therapeutic play helps identify misconceptions and provides the child an opportunity to communicate.

| Steps | Rationale |
|---|---|
| b. Autonomy and mastery. | Hospitalization places the child in the role of passive recipient of an active treatment often provided by strangers. Play therapy, particularly medical play, helps the child become involved in the treatment (even if only in a very small way) and retain a sense of competence (Fig. 16-1). |
| c. Medical information and procedures. | Children's fears and anxieties are based on their perceptions, which sometimes differ from reality. Medical play therapy helps identify misconceptions and can be used to dispel myths and establish trust. |
| d. Surgery. | Research has determined that preoperative play interventions are effective in reducing or preventing an increase in presurgical and postsurgical anxiety (Chan, 1980). |
| e. Injections. | Along with the sometimes painful event of receiving an injection, children are often confused about the purpose. Play therapy provides an opportunity for desensitizing and clarifying. |
| f. Disability or a chronic condition. | Therapeutic play is especially helpful for the child dealing with altered body image and low self-esteem. |
| g. Grief. | Children typically find the difficult and frequently unfamiliar feelings of grief easier to express through play. |
| 4. Assess behavior for severe reactions to hospitalization (e.g., severe withdrawal, infantile regression, loss of cognitive skills, excessive somatization, and emotional lability). | While some difficulties are expected, observe for severe reactions that may require more vigorous and immediate intervention. |
| 5. Determine degree of expected family involvement in child's hospitalization. | Differing from simple visitation, the need for family involvement in the hospitalization of young children has been acknowledged for many years. Involvement often helps ease anxiety in children of all ages and in the parents themselves (Golden, 1987). In addition to providing an excellent opportunity for parents to expand their knowledge and develop skills, play may reinforce family support and nurturing in a healthy and desirable manner (Goldberger, 1988). **Special Considerations:** *In the relaxed and nonthreatening play environment, parents can practice new skills that can be used with their children at home. This is also a good opportunity to model positive interactions and play for the parents who are having difficulty relating to their child. Furthermore, seeing their children play gives parents hope.* |

| Steps | Rationale |
|---|---|

## Planning and Goal Setting

1. Determine the type of therapeutic play intervention based on the specific issue to be addressed.
   a. Preparatory play (see Skill 1).

Preparatory play helps to explain upcoming events and prepare children for procedures. Children who are prepared are more cooperative and less emotionally traumatized than those who are left to cope without assistance (Gibbons and Boren, 1985).

   b. Need for cathartic play following stressful events.

Cathartic play is a means for children to act out unpleasant experiences and minimize the negative psychologic impact that results. Fantasy and imagination meet reality, fears and conflicts are confronted and conquered, and children achieve a sense of control and mastery.

   c. Play to promote intervention compliance.

Using play to encourage children to comply with a procedure, e.g., bubble blowing to encourage deep breathing, makes the procedure fun for the child and helps achieve a goal.

***Special Considerations:*** *Pediatric nursing offers a challenge to incorporate play in the child's care plan at every opportunity.*

2. Decide whether a group or an individual play intervention is appropriate (see Skill 15).

Individual play allows for a more intense intervention with a focus on the child's unique needs.

3. Consider the play environment (see Skill 15).

Although children will engage in play in almost any environment, one conducive to play is desirable.

***Special Considerations:*** *For privacy when working with an individual child, some playrooms are closed to the other children for a period of time.*

4. Determine whether a structured or nonstructured session is appropriate, depending on therapeutic goals.

When very specific information is to be conveyed, e.g., when preparing a child for surgery, the structured approach is favored. After surgery, with goals of allowing the child an opportunity to ventilate and regain a sense of mastery, the nonstructured approach may be most helpful (Golden, 1987).

5. Assemble materials for the play session. Tip: Compile a play therapy box to have therapeutic play equipment readily available (see box on p. 73 and Product References and Teaching Resources).

Children can communicate a wide range of feelings and messages with a limited number of toys and materials. While it is good to have a variety of things available for the child, a child usually responds to whatever is provided.

6. Develop nursing goals of care:
   - To provide a means of expression through play.
   - To offer a sense of control and mastery.
   - To encourage compliance with procedures.

## Implementation

1. Define limits for child.
   a. Time available for play.

Children dislike being interrupted in the middle of mastering a task. It is often helpful before starting an activity to know how much time is available.

***Special Considerations:*** *Therapeutic play takes a tremendous amount of energy and some children, especially younger ones, need to have other outlets for play when the work becomes too intense.*

   b. Behavior to be limited.

Children need to know that they may not hurt others or themselves, or destroy property.

***Special Considerations:*** *In therapeutic play, destruction of certain predetermined items, e.g., the smashing of old egg cartons, is permitted.*

   c. Gently redirect aggressive behavior. For example, a child who has experienced several invasive procedures might begin needle play with giving the doll injections in the eyes or some other particularly sensitive area. After several injections, the nurse might say, "It looks like you are enjoying giving the patient a shot in the eye. Where do you get stuck with needles? Will you show me how it is done?"

Medical play, particularly needle play, is often very aggressive at first. By gently redirecting unrealistic play, children will not feel their play is being criticized.

### *SUGGESTED MATERIALS FOR THERAPEUTIC PLAY*

Alcohol swabs
Anesthesia mask
Armboards for an IV
Band-Aids and bandages
Blood pressure cuff
Blue CHUX pads
Clipboard and paper
Cotton and cotton swabs
Doctor bags
Dolls
Flashlight
Gauze
IV supplies: empty bottles or bags, tubing, cassette for IV infusion pumps
Needles (IV, syringe, and butterfly)
NG tubes
Otoscope
Oxygen masks
Plaster for casting
Reflex hammer
Stethoscope
Suction catheter
Surgical gloves, hats, gowns, sponges, drapes, masks
Syringes—all types
Tape, adhesive, and paper
Thermometer-empty IVAC cases
Tongue depressors
Tourniquet

Adapted from Gustafson M: Ideas for activities with hospitalized children, Washington DC, 1982, Association for the Care of Children's Health.

| **Steps** | **Rationale** |
|---|---|
| 2. Use issue specific therapeutic techniques. | |
| a. Separation.<br>Develop a nurturing relationship.<br>▪ Use cuddling, rubbing, and reinforcing.<br>▪ Avoid trying to get the child to "do something."<br>▪ Communicate caring through physical contact, eye contact, proximity, laughter, and soft tones.<br>▪ Use following, describing, and imitating sounds and actions.<br>▪ For more active relationships include wrestling (thumb, arm, leg, full body), lifting the child, rolling, and playing together in finger paints or water.<br>▪ Give and receive messages, (e.g., smiles, coos). | The development of the nurturing relationship helps the child in the transition between the parents' departure and their return. Additionally, it helps keep the child from repressing and denying feelings of attachment (Golden, 1987).<br>***Special Considerations:*** *It is helpful to have the parents involved during the formation of the relationship for the child who might have loyalty issues, feeling he or she is betraying parents by bonding with the nurse.* |
| b. Autonomy and mastery.<br>Provide opportunities for the child to be an active agent in his or her own care.<br>▪ Allow child to make choices, e.g., type of food, toy selection, location for injection.<br>▪ Encourage child to demonstrate creative skills through drawing, paintings, modeling with clay, paper folding or cutting, or writing.<br>▪ Activities such as stacking blocks, building houses or forts, pounding wood, stringing beads, assembling puzzles, and pasting can help the child demonstrate construction skills.<br>▪ Encourage play activities of almost any type that will allow the child to experience his or her strengths.<br>▪ Encourage child to do things on his or her own whenever possible. | Involving children in their treatment helps restore a sense of autonomy and mastery. Play can be used to help children feel competent. Activity alone can help children achieve autonomy and mastery while hospitalized.<br>***Special Considerations:*** *Children who are unable to play can achieve autonomy and mastery by supervising the nurse playing "for" the child. For example, the child can instruct where to move game pieces, e.g., checkers.* |
| c. Medical information and procedures (Table 16-1; see Skill 1 and box on p. 75).<br>Provide children with opportunities to play.<br>▪ Bring medical equipment into the playroom whenever possible and allow child to handle.<br>▪ Demonstrate on a doll, stuffed animal, or puppet. (Do not use the child's love object for painful or traumatic procedures unless it is the child's choice).<br>▪ Encourage the child to reenact the procedure (Fig. 16-1).<br>▪ Anticipate and dispel fears by clearly showing and explaining the limits of commonly feared procedures (e.g., what body parts are involved).<br>▪ Observe and listen to the child for his or her perception of the procedure and clarify misconceptions. | Most children, regardless of age, benefit from some type of exposure to medical equipment before it is used on them.<br>***Special Considerations:*** *Restrict playroom use to "safe" activities (see Skill 15, Implementation step 1).* |

**TABLE 16-1** Medical Play

| Type | Comments | Equipment | Example |
|---|---|---|---|
| Role rehearsal/role reversal | Children take on the roles of health care professionals and reenact medical events on models, e.g., dolls, puppets, or stuffed animals. May be structured or unstructured. | Medical (see box on suggested materials for therapeutic play). | Children reenact actual events they have experienced, especially those that are ongoing or were intrusive or traumatic. |
| Medical fantasy play | Role playing and fantasy with medical themes.<br>Allows child to avoid contact with feared objects, yet can still play out topics of concern. | Building blocks, doll houses, cars, trucks, play animals, etc. | If a child is playing an active game with cars and trucks and causes a car to crash, the adult might inquire whether the car was hurt. If the child affirms that the car was injured, the adult might then ask what would happen to the injured car. Children will often decide to take it to a doctor or to a car hospital. |
| Indirect medical play | Provides opportunity for familiarization, exploration, and education related to medical experiences. No role play or fantasy.<br>For the child who is passive, very fearful, noncommunicative, or simply too sick to engage in unstructured play, this indirect play offers important potential for providing information and establishing relationships. | Puzzles, games, and songs with a medical theme; the use of medical equipment in nonmedical ways. | Syringe squirt guns. |

Adapted from McCue K: Medical play: an expanded perspective, Children's Health Care 16(3):157-161, 1988.

| Steps | Rationale |
|---|---|
| d. Surgery. | Impending surgery can raise a great many questions and conflicts for the child. Children may never be fully "prepared" (Chan, 1980). (See Table 16-1 and Skill 112).<br>***Special Considerations:*** *Many hospitals allow the child to take a favorite doll or stuffed animal to the operating room. This decision should be the child's. The doll is bandaged identically to the child, and as the child progresses, so does the doll.* |
| Provide the opportunities for play listed under step C while considering some additional concerns that may be demonstrated through play.<br>▪ Allow child to act out a surgical event spontaneously with a puppet or doll, clarifying misconceptions and redirecting child to a better understanding of the reality. | Clarifying children's misconceptions about surgery gives them the message that a surgical insult to the body is done for a good reason (Linn, 1978). |

## *PLAY ACTIVITIES FOR SPECIFIC PROCEDURES*

### FLUID INTAKE

Make freezer pops using child's favorite juice
Cut Jell-O into fun shapes
Make game of taking sip when turning page of book or in games like "Simon Says"
Use small medicine cups; decorate the cups
Color water with food coloring or Kool Aid
Have tea party; pour at small table
Let child fill a syringe and squirt it into his mouth or use it to fill small decorated cups
Cut straws in half and place in small container (much easier for child to suck liquid)
Decorate straw—cut out small design with two holes and pass straw through; place small sticker on straw
Use a "crazy" straw
Make a "progress poster"; give rewards for drinking a predetermined quantity

### DEEP BREATHING

Blow bubbles with bubble blower
Blow bubbles with straw (no soap)
Blow on pinwheel, feathers, whistle, harmonica, balloons, toy horns
Practice band instruments
Draw face on rubber glove to expand when blown up
Have blowing contest using balloons, boats, cotton balls, feathers, marbles, Ping-Pong balls, pieces of paper
Blow such objects on a table top without falling over a goal line, over water, through an obstacle course, up in the air, against an opponent, or up and down a string
Suck paper or cloth from one container to another using a straw
Use blow bottles with colored water to transfer water from one side to the other
Dramatize stories, e.g., "I'll huff and puff and blow your house down" from the Three Little Pigs
Do straw blowing painting
Take a deep breath and "blow out the candles" on a birthday cake

### RANGE OF MOTION AND USE OF EXTREMITIES

Throw bean bags at fixed or movable target, wadded paper into wastebasket
Touch or kick balloons held or hung in different positions (if child is in traction, hang balloon from trapeze)
Play "tickle toes"; wiggle them on request
Play Twister game or "Simon Says"
Play pretend and guessing games, e.g., imitate a bird, butterfly, horse
Have tricycle or wheelchair races in safe area
Play kick or throw ball with soft foam ball in safe area
Position bed so that child must turn to view television or doorway
Climb wall like a "spider"
Pretend to teach "aerobic" dancing or exercises; encourage parents to participate
Encourage swimming, if feasible
Play video games or pinball (fine motor movement)
Play "hide and seek" game—hide toy somewhere in bed (or room, if ambulatory) and have child find using specified hand or foot
Provide clay to mold with fingers
Paint or draw on large sheets of paper placed on floor or wall
Encourage combing own hair; play "beauty shop" with "customer" in different positions

### SOAKS

Play with small toys or objects (cups, syringes, soap dishes) in water
Wash dolls or toys
Bubbles may be added to bath water if permissible; move bubbles to create shapes or "monsters"
Pick up marbles, pennies from bottom of bath container
Make designs with coins on bottom of container
Pretend to make a boat a submarine by keeping it immersed
Have "Instant Products" for child (a capsule filled with a design that when immersed in warm water dissolves and foam rubber animals or other surprises appear)*
Read to child during soaks, sing with child, or play game, e.g., cards, checkers, or other board game (if both hands are immersed, move the board pieces for the child)
Sitz bath—give child something to listen to (music, stories) or look at (Viewmaster, book, etc.)

### INJECTIONS

Let child handle syringe, vial, alcohol swab and give a "shot" to doll or stuffed animal
Use syringes to decorate cookies with frosting, squirt paint, or target shoot into a container
Draw a "magic circle" on area before injection
Allow child to have a "collection" of syringes (without needles); make "wild" creative objects with syringes
If multiple injections or venipunctures, make a "progress poster"; give rewards for predetermined number of injections.

### AMBULATION

Give child something to push
  Toddler—push-pull toy
  School-age—wagon or decorated IV pole
  Teenager—a baby in a stroller or wheelchair
Have a parade—make hats, drums, etc.

### EXTENDING ENVIRONMENT (PATIENTS IN TRACTION, ETC.)

Make bed into a pirate ship or airplane with decorations
Put up mirrors so patient can see around room
Move patient's bed frequently, especially to playroom, hallway, or outside

*Instant Products, Inc., P.O. Box 33068, Louisville, KY 40232.
From Whaley LF and Wong DL: Nursing care of infants and children, ed 4, St. Louis, 1991, The CV Mosby Co.

| Steps | Rationale |
|---|---|
| ▪ Use a doll, drawing, or other means of expression to discover and address child's fears and concerns, e.g., fear of loss of a body part, fear of mutilation of the body, or concern that the surgeon will remove something the child needs.<br>▪ If a child will be disabled either temporarily or permanently, demonstrate this change on doll or puppet before surgery.<br>▪ Have child practice play activities before surgery, e.g., bubble blowing to encourage deep breathing (see box on p. 75). | |
| e. Injections.<br>Provide opportunities for needle play that address the fear surrounding any type of needle puncture—from a finger stick to a bone marrow aspiration (Gibbons and Boren, 1985).<br>▪ Choose equipment based on the type of needle procedure the child is preoccupied with at the time.<br>▪ If close supervision is available, actual needles should be used (see box on opposite page).<br>▪ Begin with an explanation that the child is going to be able to start an IV (or do a lumbar puncture or other procedure) on a doll.<br>▪ When preparing a child for a new experience, give a demonstration of the procedure and a verbal explanation of what the doll is feeling. In the reenactment of a procedure, talk the child through the experience, letting him or her demonstrate how it was done.<br>▪ The child may imitate the procedure. | Needles are often frightening to a child and the reason for receiving one may not be understood. Needle play provides the opportunity for desensitization for the child who must receive multiple injections, leading to a reduction in stress and fear.<br>***Special Considerations:*** *Some children need to begin with syringes without needles. Others direct the nurse with needle placement, and then begin to use the needles themselves. It is especially helpful to let the child start the IV so that the child (and parents) can see that the needle comes out leaving only a pliable sheath of tubing in the vein (Morain-Baker, 1988).* |
| ▪ Assume the role of the doll and respond to the doll's expressions. | Responding in a realistic manner helps dispel fears and conveys empathy. |
| ▪ Continue to play for children who are too anxious or are physically unable to participate. | Some children are extremely anxious at the sight of needles and cannot play. By playing for the child and then later pretending to require assistance with the task, children will sometimes join in the activity.<br>***Special Considerations:*** *Needle play with a small group allows children the opportunity to encourage each other. Older children may require a less structured session.* |
| f. Disability or a chronic condition.<br>During play intervention:<br>▪ Encourage the child to be active and involved.<br>▪ Place emphasis on the whole child to avoid preoccupation with his or her medical problems.<br>▪ Encourage participation in regular playroom and recreational activities whenever possible.<br>▪ Help the child identify his or her competencies by providing a variety of activities and encouraging demonstration of his or her skills. | Play therapy is an effective intervention for disabled children or those with chronic conditions who may suffer feelings of inferiority, insecurity, and exclusion, and who lack motivation (Golden, 1987).<br>***Special Considerations:*** *Group play therapy is often the treatment of choice after the age of 4 or 5 years. This promotes learning social skills at an early age.* |
| ▪ Provide opportunities for cathartic play by offering aggression toys, e.g., pounding benches, or materials that can be pounded or crushed, e.g., empty egg cartons. | Limitations inherent in many disabilities and chronic conditions often lead to frustration and anger. |
| ▪ Encourage imaginative play, e.g., in the management of pain, encourage the child to imagine pleasant, positive situations or distract the child through play from the painful sensations (Donnelly, 1988).<br>▪ Assist child in obtaining special play equipment, e.g., a hand-operated tricycle for the child unable to pedal. | Imaginative processes and language can assist children with disabilities to achieve a measure of control over difficult situations and, at least symbolically, remove themselves from the situational constraints of their disabilities. |
| g. Grief (see Skill 21). | Therapeutic play is useful for children dealing with a variety of grief issues: death, chronic illness, divorce, anticipatory grief.<br>***Special Considerations:*** *Play and other expressive modalities often work very well in a group setting, whether the group is a family, children on the unit, etc.* |

| Steps | Rationale |
|---|---|
| ▪ Observe the child in unstructured play, noting concerns, misconceptions, and expression of feelings, e.g., anger. | An unstructured play session is helpful in learning where the child is in the grief process. ***Special Considerations:*** *Avoid overinterpretation and combine information from play session with other information about the child.* |
| ▪ Accept the child where he or she is in the process at that particular moment by providing activities to encourage expression (e.g., provide pounding activities for the child dealing with anger). | Acknowledgment of the child's feelings demonstrates understanding and helps build trust. ***Special Considerations:*** *Clay is good for pounding, squeezing, smashing, rolling. After anger has passed, these activities may become more playful.* |
| ▪ Include family members whenever appropriate. It may be helpful to include siblings in a session that deals with divorce, the entire family when working through a death, and so on. | Because the family is a system, when one member is going through a stressful period, other members will be affected in some way. Additionally, family members may find the nonthreatening atmosphere of play an easy arena to provide support for the child and each other. ***Special Considerations:*** *It is helpful to assemble affected children on a unit when a child dies to process feelings together.* |
| ▪ Group or individual sessions could include an activity such as "A Book about Daddy Dying" (Junge, 1985). Have family members compile a book. A variety of means of expressing feelings—pictures, drawings, comments, poetry—may be included in the book. | Through this activity there is a sense of commemoration, and at the end of the book, closure. The child may look back on the book as often as he or she likes, further facilitating grieving. |
| ▪ Observe for behaviors such as withdrawal or extremely aggressive behavior that indicate that the child may need more intensive intervention. | Play and expressive therapy usually work very well for the grieving child. ***Special Considerations:*** *The grieving process is often lengthy.* |
| 3. Through words and activities, offer encouragement to the child that he or she will feel better, gain mastery, and so on. Ask the child to keep a diary or draw pictures of how he or she is feeling at a particular moment. At a later date have the child look back at the evidence of progress. | Children who are encouraged to tell their own stories, paint their own pictures, act out their own fantasies, and construct their own worlds, are better able to hold onto their own hopes and dreams (Stapleton and Yahraes, 1978). ***Special Considerations:*** *Even a child who is too young to understand words will hear encouragement in a positive tone.* |

| Evaluation Outcomes | Observational Guidelines |
|---|---|
| 1. Therapeutic play session facilitates child's adjustment to his or her condition or situation. | Note that child's behavior and mood are appropriate. |
| 2. Therapeutic play session facilitates child's expressions of feelings. | Child freely expresses a variety of feelings (verbally and nonverbally). |
| 3. Therapeutic play activities provide child with a sense of control and mastery. | Child makes choices, is able to reenact a demonstration, and displays competence in an activity. |
| 4. Therapeutic play activities increase child's compliance with procedures. | Child follows directions, uses coping strategies, and minimizes distress. |
| 5. Therapeutic play activities facilitate ongoing assessment of child. | Observe child's play activity, noting feelings expressed and misconceptions. |

## Documentation

Note on child's chart his or her approach to play session, length of time session lasted, behavior, competence in reenacting a demonstration, mastery, feelings expressed, misconceptions corrected, family involvement, and planned follow-up activity or recommendations.

# SKILL 17 Teaching Relaxation as a Coping Technique

*Deborah Kay Brantly*

Jacobson (1938) proposed that anxiety and relaxation cannot coexist. When a child uses relaxation techniques, he or she gains a sense of mastery by participating in the treatment and experiencing a sense of control over threatening events (Cotanch, Hockenberry, and Herman, 1988) and his or her body. The child with a chronic condition can use relaxation techniques in long-term pain management, in learning self-help skills, or in coping with the psychosocial effects of a disability. Other indications for relaxation include reducing anxiety and stress, controlling (or diminishing) nausea and vomiting because of chemotherapy, preparing for and coping with procedures, decreasing effects of migraine headaches, and promoting sleep. A variety of techniques that produce relaxation include distraction, rhythmic breathing, letting-go, progressive muscle relaxation, imagery, color exchange, visualization, systematic desensitization, autogenic training, sensory pacing, and using background music or environmental sounds. These can be used alone or in combination.

## NURSING DIAGNOSES

Ineffective individual coping related to inadequate relaxation, situational crisis, or ineffective coping methods; Anxiety related to perceived threat to health status; Sleep pattern disturbance related to anxiety response.

| Steps | Rationale |
|---|---|
| **Assessment** | |
| 1. Determine child's age and developmental level. | The child's age and developmental level have implications as to the appropriate type(s) of relaxation technique(s) (see Appendix B on p. 814). |
| 2. Determine level of anxiety. | Jacobson (1938) proposed that anxiety causes muscle tension, which contributes to mental and physical illness. By reducing muscle tension, anxiety and its effects upon mental and physical illness can be reduced (Titlebaum, 1988).<br>***Special Considerations:*** *If the child's anxiety level is in the panic stage, relaxation training is contraindicated until anxiety level is decreased.* |
| 3. Assess current mental status and history of mental illness to determine appropriateness of relaxation. | Relaxation is not to be used with persons with psychosis, schizophrenia, hysterical tendencies, or a poor sense of reality testing (Griffin, Ling, and Staley, 1985). |
| 4. Identify relaxation techniques the child may have used previously and the response to the techniques. | Assessing previous experience with relaxation will give further direction for planning.<br>***Special Considerations:*** *If the child has successfully used relaxation in the past, determine whether the child would like to continue with that technique or try new techniques. If experiences were negative, assess the circumstances that contributed to the negative experience. Facilitate resolution of the event, if possible. Discuss with the child his or her desire to use that technique again.* |
| 5. Ascertain when relaxation is needed.<br>a. Ask which events cause the anxiety and stress.<br>b. Ask if certain times of the day or days of the week are more difficult.<br>c. Ask the child if he or she can tell when feeling anxiety, tension, and stress.<br>d. Ask the parent what behaviors the child manifests when under stress. | Individuals experience anxiety and tension at different times.<br>***Special Considerations:*** *Bedtime is the most common time children experience anxiety and tension. It may take the form of demanding behavior, not remaining in bed, hesitation in or objections to performing bedtime routine, crying or whining, or disturbing siblings. Adolescents may identify specific situations, e.g., before a test, that would require relaxation. More often this occurs after adolescents have used relaxation techniques regularly.* |

| **Steps** | **Rationale** |
|---|---|
| 6. Determine if the child prefers a support person to assist in relaxation or to relax on his or her own. If the child prefers a support person, identify who can assist him or her and the extent of the person's role. | Identifying support persons in the child's environment can provide accountability and security for the child.<br>***Special Considerations:*** *Adolescents may want to relax on their own without adult intervention.* |
| 7. Judge the child's readiness to learn.<br>a. Ask the child if he or she knows what relaxation is. If not, provide information.<br>b. Ask if the child would like to learn to relax.<br>c. Ask if the child has any fears about relaxation, e.g., say, "Does any of this scare you?" If yes, ask, "What scares you about that?" or "What are you afraid might happen?" | If the child is not ready to learn, teaching efforts will be futile.<br>***Special Considerations:*** *If the child is fearful and desires the parents' presence, allow parents to be present. Assure child of your presence. Give the child permission to stop or continue with the exercise at will. If, during implementation, the child appears reluctant to relax, reassess learning readiness.* |
| 8. Determine amount and location of tension in the child's body.<br>a. Note facial or neck tension.<br>b. Note clenched fists or rigid legs. | This gives baseline data for intervention and evaluative purposes.<br>***Special Considerations:*** *If overt tension in muscles is not obvious on inspection, observe a general sense of the child's level of calmness or anxiety, e.g., by observing for nervous movements (e.g., tapping pencil, swinging legs, twisting or biting hair strands, or biting nails).* |

## Planning and Goal Setting

| | |
|---|---|
| 1. Prepare the environment. | Environmental stimuli influence the child's ability to concentrate and relax. |
| a. Quiet room without distractions. | A quiet environment allows the child to concentrate. |
| b. Comfortable seating. | Comfortable seating allows for initial release of muscle tension. |
| c. Adequate space. | Adequate space prevents interruptions if repositioning is needed (especially when relaxation is in a group setting) and promotes concentration and release of tension.<br>***Special Considerations:*** *Relaxation can be taught individually or in a group. If a group setting is chosen, ideally place 3 to 5 children in a group, considering spatial and developmental needs.* |
| d. Soft lighting without obvious shadows; lights off. | Soft lighting decreases stimulation in the room and decreases inhibitions.<br>***Special Considerations:*** *Some children, particularly younger children, may be frightened with the lights completely off.* |
| e. Serene background sounds, e.g., white noise, tapes of music or environmental sounds. | Background noise blocks out other noises and creates a focus for the mind.<br>***Special Considerations:*** *Not all children may wish to have background noise, although it is particularly beneficial for children with attention deficit disorder.* |
| f. Nonstimulating room, e.g., walls painted blue, green, or beige. | These colors are more conducive to relaxation. |
| 2. Determine the method most useful to the child (see Appendix B on p. 814).<br>a. Type of technique.<br>b. Individual or group instruction. | Choosing techniques that best suit the child tends to increase the child's use of the technique. |
| 3. Gather needed aids, e.g., tape recorder, appropriate tape, exercise pad, or neck support. | Preparing aids decreases distractions when instruction begins. |
| 4. Develop individualized client and family goals:<br>▪ To learn and use relaxation techniques effectively. | |

## Implementation

| | |
|---|---|
| 1. Discuss the purpose of relaxation training. | Clarifying when to use relaxation gives the child information for choosing coping techniques in stressful situations. Consider known specific stressors during which the child may decide to use relaxation (e.g., during a procedure, while in pain, before bedtime, or before and during chemotherapy). |
| 2. Describe what will happen during the first relaxation session.<br>a. What the support persons will be doing.<br>b. What the nurse will be doing.<br>c. What the child will be doing. | Providing a description of events prepares the child for what is to come and can decrease anxiety. |

| Steps | Rationale |
|---|---|
| 3. When the child is ready, describe the proper positions (see Appendix B on p. 814), and allow him or her to choose which one to use. | Allowing the child to choose the position increases his or her sense of control and mastery, facilitates a mutual relationship, increases cooperation, and facilitates an optimal comfort level to begin relaxation.<br>***Special Considerations:*** *If the child has physical limitations that do not permit certain positions, help the child find a comfortable position.* |
| 4. Instruct the child to close his or her eyes and get as comfortable as possible. | This initial position prepares the child for further relaxation.<br>***Special Considerations:*** *If the child is afraid of closing the eyes, has a hard time keeping them shut, or just prefers to keep them open, he or she can focus upon an object in the room.* |
| 5. Read the relaxation script to the child (see Appendix B on p. 814).<br>a. Slowly.<br>b. Calmly.<br>c. Soothingly; low tonalities with some voice fluctuation.<br>d. Pausing according to technique need. | Research suggests that live instructions during teaching sessions are generally more effective than those taped or written (Hillenberg and Collins, 1982), and reading the script for the child the first two or three times models the techniques for use during self-instruction. |
| 6. Contract with the child and family to practice relaxation on his or her own and return for future sessions. | Relaxation training seems to be most effective when the program lasts at least 6 weeks (Lamontagne, 1985), most commonly with teaching sessions once a week and daily practice. |
| 7. Assist the child in making a relaxation tape or assist in finding a premade tape.<br>a. Choose the script the child likes best.<br>b. Have the child practice the script until comfortable with it.<br>c. Assist the child during taping, stopping the tape if needed.<br>d. Review the tape with the child and, if he or she desires, assist in remaking it. | Relaxation is thought to be a learned skill that improves with practice (Griffin, Ling, and Staley, 1985). Making the child's own relaxation tape creates a sense of pride and mastery and encourages responsibility for treatment.<br>***Special Considerations:*** *Younger children will need adult help when practicing and will not be able to make a tape. Suggest the parent make a tape for the younger child.* |
| 8. Encourage the child to change the technique to meet his or her needs as time progresses. | As time progresses the child may prefer to use or try alternative techniques. Encouraging a change in technique better individualizes care. |

| Evaluation Outcomes | Observational Guidelines |
|---|---|
| 1. The child learns the relaxation technique. | Note completion of a session; child is able to repeat technique without assistance. The child states or demonstrates the ability to relax on internal command. |
| 2. The child experiences decreased muscle tension. | During a session, the child's leg or arm can be easily lifted, and, when released, readily drops to the supporting surface. After the session, observe for tension behaviors noted in the assessment. |
| 3. The child's anxiety is eliminated or diminished. | The child expresses feelings of calm, relaxation, peacefulness, serenity, unwillingness to move, or similar statements indicating relaxation. |
| 4. The child uses relaxation during stressful times or as per contract. | The child reports practicing relaxation as per contract. Observe the child's use of the technique during a stressful event. |
| 5. The child copes more effectively. | The child reports or demonstrates decreased tension, anxiety, and stress when facing stressful situations. The child expresses more positive feelings about other aspects of treatment. |
| 6. Behavioral manifestations of stress are diminished. | Ask parents if they have noted a change in behaviors identified as stress-related. Observe for a decrease in these behaviors. |

## Documentation

Note the child's initial level of anxiety and any notable changes after relaxation. Document assessment data of previous techniques used, manifestations of stress, use of support persons, learning readiness and tension in the child's body. Describe the technique used and the child's positioning. List the child's subjective descriptions of feelings after the procedure and apparent degree of relaxation. Document the contract for teaching, use, and practice of relaxation. During future sessions, begin by documenting the child's own practices and the results of using relaxation during identified stressful situations. Describe any changes the child wishes to make in the technique. Then document above information about the current session.

# *SKILL* **18** Supporting the Child

*Judy Holt Rollins*

Pediatric nurses are becoming increasingly concerned with meeting the psychosocial needs of children. The best possible physical care and cure does not always prevent deep emotional scars. Children have needs for nurturing, security, love, safety, privacy, and freedom from pain and fear, as well as the normal physiologic and developmental needs of a growing child, including nutrition, rest and sleep, warmth, activity, and freedom to move and explore (Association for the Care of Children's Health, 1980). Highly sophisticated physiologic care should be matched with a high level of developmentally appropriate emotional support for the child. A model of care that includes psychosocial support can improve pediatric care at all phases of the health care spectrum for children with acute illness and those with chronic conditions.

## NURSING DIAGNOSES

Ineffective situational coping related to situational crisis, ineffective coping methods, or inadequate support systems; Anxiety related to unmet informational needs about health condition and treatment; Self-esteem disturbance related to life-threatening, acute, or chronic illness.

| Steps | Rationale |
|---|---|
| **Assessment** | |
| 1. Review information about child.<br>a. Age and developmental level. | Age and developmental level influence children's perception and understanding of experiences such as illness and, therefore, their ability to cope. Children are continually developing, by and large in an orderly, sequential, and cumulative manner. They remain vulnerable at each stage of development to external stress (Magrab, 1985).<br>***Special Considerations:*** *Children, particularly very young ones, can change physically and developmentally very rapidly, requiring continual reassessment to modify nursing care plans to reflect these changes. Children 1 to 4 years old are most vulnerable to negative effects of hospitalization (Adams and Fras, 1988).* |
| ▪ Infancy. | The infant's concept of illness is a generalized perception of discomfort and pain. |
| ▪ Preschool. | Preschoolers conceive illness as a punishment for bad behavior. They operate from a magical point of view: adults could magically cure the illness if they so wished. |
| ▪ School-age. | For the school-age child, self-causation of illness from disobedient or imprudent behavior still occurs but may take longer to express. The child can have an accurate awareness of the location of body parts and begin to understand body processes and functions. |
| ▪ Adolescence. | For the adolescent the focus is on discrete symptoms rather than overall impact of illness. The adolescent has the ability to intellectually question and deal with information about illness. He or she may use denial of illness or overcompensation in areas not affected (Magrab, 1985). |
| b. Nature and severity of illness or injury. | Bodily injury or disease stress the child. Chronic conditions inherently cause more anxiety than acute episodes of illness or injury. The child who is chronically ill continually endures various physical symptoms, including pain, shortness of breath, and lethargy, that cannot be completely prevented and must be managed in ways compatible with normal living. A chronic illness or injury may change physical appearance in ways that are potentially stigmatizing, restrict mobility, or result in physical isolation. |

| Steps | Rationale |
|---|---|
| ▪ Age of onset and etiology. | Children with a chronic illness diagnosed early in infancy do not have to cope with the implications of the emerging awareness of their disease until their preschool or early elementary school years. For the previously physically healthy child, diagnosis presents a multifaceted crisis in which the child must adapt to the loss of normal functioning, tolerate and comply with new medical procedures, and struggle with feelings about the meaning of the disease and its treatment. Illnesses with a hereditary component entail a sense of parental responsibility for the disease with implications also for the child's interpretation that differs from illness of undetermined cause (Drotar and Bush, 1985). |
| ▪ Prognosis. | Life-threatening or potentially fatal illnesses pose special psychologic threats, e.g., facing the issue of possible or inevitable early death (see Skill 21). |
| ▪ Needs created by the condition that threaten health, life, and comfort. | Needs that arise in response to symptoms such as pain are of the first priority and require optimal physical, physiologic, and pharmacologic support (Association for the Care of Children's Health, 1980). |
| c. Psychosocial assessment (see Skill 11). | An individualized plan of care considers characteristics unique to the child (e.g., coping style, temperament). |
| d. Assessment of family (see Skills 38 and 41). | Knowledge of a family's strengths and needs assists in planning a realistic, family-centered, culturally sensitive approach to support. |
| 2. Identify needs and concerns of child through interview and assessment of child and family. Issues to consider often include the following: | There are many predictable needs and concerns, but a truly individualized plan of care results only when a child/family's unique needs and concerns are considered in planning a realistic, family-centered approach to support.<br>***Special Considerations:*** *Child and family input also allows for prioritizing of needs.* |
| a. Information or clarification about condition, treatment, or prognosis. | While it is important to know what the child has been told about the condition, it is essential to remember that his or her perception is far more important. This knowledge allows the opportunity to clarify misconceptions that are barriers to the child's coping and ultimate adjustment. |
| b. Hospitalization (Table 18-1). | Hospitalization has long been recognized as a stressful event for children. A hospital is an unfamiliar environment and disrupts the child's routine and often development. Conversely, with appropriate support for the child, hospitalization provides an opportunity for growth.<br>***Special Considerations:*** *Children who are more active and perhaps more strong-willed seem to fare better. Those with preexisting anxiety will usually do worse (Adams and Fras, 1988).* |
| c. School. | Children may be concerned about getting behind in their work. Additionally, children worry about school reentry and their teacher's and classmates' reactions. Older children may be concerned about scholarship opportunities and colleges with resources available to meet their needs. |
| d. Recreation. | Children sometimes question what limitations their condition will place on activities and if restrictions are temporary or permanent. Previously active children are often very concerned about renewing participation in recreational activities and sports. |
| e. Peer relationships. | Feeling different becomes increasingly important as children enter adolescence. Isolation may cause children to withdraw. Teenagers may be concerned with the possible negative effect their condition may have on their sexuality. |
| f. Concerns about the future. | Children, particularly adolescents, sometimes have very valid concerns about employment, marriage, reproduction, and the ability to obtain or maintain health care insurance coverage. |
| g. Spirituality (see Skill 42). | Children and adults, in an attempt to find meaning for their condition, are sometimes confused over spiritual issues. |
| h. Cultural variables (see Skill 41). | Children have the right to support from health care professionals that preserves the integrity, values, and customs of their culture. |

**TABLE 18-1** Age-related Concerns and Needs of Hospitalized Children

| | Concerns | Possible Responses | Positive Parent/Nurse Responses |
|---|---|---|---|
| Infancy | The infant needs to have parents close by; parents are seen as powerful. Parents' presence and reactions provide best support in handling fear, pain, and separation. | Inappropriate bonding; development of distrust; anxiety due to separation and new environment; delayed skills development. | Close proximity to child (rooming in); frequent contact with child; stroking, cuddling, rocking, talking and singing, reading; communicating love for child. |
| Toddler | Separation from parents is a major issue. Loss of control is viewed in terms of physical restriction, loss of routine and rituals, and dependency. The toddler fears bodily injury and pain. | Regression to infantile behavior; lack of cooperative behavior; not eating; no interaction with others; protest (e.g., verbal cries for parent; verbal attack on others; kicking, biting, hitting, pinching; may try to escape to find parent; clings to parent); depair (e.g., passive, depressed, disinterested in environment; uncommunicative; loss of newly learned skills); negativism; temper tantrums; resistance. | Praise for appropriate behavior (e.g., putting on slippers without help); restate reasons for hospitalization; rooming-in; continue with usual home routine (e.g., read a bedtime story); communicate love for child. |
| Preschool | The presence of parents continues to be of primary importance. Hospitalization is perceived as rejection or punishment. There may be fears of mutilation. Treatment may be seen as hostile or punishment. Child is concerned with bodily penetration by surgery or injections. | Anger toward primary caretaker (parent); acting out (e.g., throwing toys, inappropriate verbalizations); refusal to listen to or look at or speak to parent; refusal to participate in hygiene and play activities; protest (e.g., less direct and aggressive than toddler, may displace feelings on others); despair and detachment similar to toddler; physical and verbal aggression; dependency; withdrawal; feelings of fear, anxiety, guilt, shame; physiologic responses; immature behavior. | Accept and provide outlets for child's anger; communicate love for child; maintain behavior limits (appropriate discipline); restate reasons for hospitalization; use play conversation to continue hospital experience explanation. Reassure child that hospitalization is not a punishment. |
| School-age | The school-age child is primarily concerned with lack of body control and mastery. There may be feelings of inadequacy. The child may become demanding and rebellious to maintain semblance of control. Knowledge about illness is effective in handling anxiety. | Regression to previous developmental level behaviors; inability to complete some tasks; anger related to confinement, inability to be mobile, lack of contact with friends; refusal to ambulate; loneliness; boredom; isolation; withdrawal; depression; displaced anger; hostility; frustration; excessive sleeping or TV watching; seek information. | Establish consistent visiting pattern; implement plan for continued education and teacher visit; set limits for self-care tasks that are attainable; praise for appropriate behavior (e.g., completing homework); arrange peer visit. |
| Adolescence | Hospitalization to the adolescent may be viewed as a threat to independence. Conflicts over control issues become a focal concern. Separation from family and peers may interfere with developmental task mastery and can be interpreted as abandonment and substantiate a sense of worthlessness. There is concern about status in peer group after hospitalization. | Rejection; uncooperativeness; withdrawal; self-assertion; self-control; cooperativeness; fear; anxiety; overconfidence; may capitalize on gains from pain; depression; loneliness; withdrawal; boredom. | Support the adolescent's need for independence, confidentiality, and decision-making. Encourage opportunities to meet normal developmental tasks while in the hospital (e.g., schoolwork, visits with peers). |

Adapted from Association for the Care of Children's Health: Guidelines for adolescent units, Washington, DC, 1980, Association for the Care of Children's Health; Magrab P: Psychosocial development of chronically ill children. In Hobbs N and Perrin JM, editors: Issues in the care of children with chronic illness, San Francisco, 1985, Jossey-Bass; Pass M and Pass C: Anticipatory guidance for parents of hospitalized children, J Pediatr Nurs 2(4):250-258, 1987; Whaley L and Wong D: Nursing care of infants and children, ed 4, St Louis, 1991, The CV Mosby Co.

| Steps | Rationale |
|---|---|
| 3. Ask child what information, assistance, action, or resources he or she believes would be helpful. | Recognizing the uniqueness of the individual shows respect and increases the possibility that a thorough assessment will be performed.<br>***Special Considerations:*** *While promoting the growth of a supportive relationship, encouraging input from the child sends the message that, as a health care consumer, he or she is a valuable member of the team planning the care. This message is especially important for the chronically ill child who will gradually be assuming more responsibility for his or her care.* |
| 4. Looking to the family, extended family, and community, examine what support, both emotional and practical, is available to the child. Determine how well it meets the child's current needs. | Parents are typically the most meaningful resource for emotional support. Meeting the needs of a child with a chronic condition usually requires multidisciplinary collaboration. |
| **Planning and Goal Setting** | |
| 1. Meet with the family (and child, if appropriate) to discuss the child's needs and to plan together how they might best be met. | Parents are the best resource for support for their child and are the constant in the life of the child. It is fitting that they be given the opportunity to be included in all phases of their child's care.<br>***Special Considerations:*** *Incorporate what the child believes would be most helpful from Assessment step 3. Serve as an advocate for the child's wishes with other family members.* |
| 2. Plan interventions based on identified needs and concerns. | Needs and concerns identified in assessment serve as a framework for a plan of care. |
| a. Gather age-related resource materials and information. | Establishing a good network of resources provides an excellent base for offering support. A growing number of booklets, videos, programs, and support groups are available.<br>***Special Considerations:*** *Play materials are especially useful for younger children (see Skills 15 and 16).* |
| b. Consider age-related needs of the child and availability and wishes of the family when planning support for the child in the hospital (Table 18-1). | An understanding of age-related concerns and needs provides a focus for appropriate support. The availability and wishes of family to be involved will help determine schedules for care and procedures, or the need to identify extended family members, friends, volunteers, or staff to substitute. |
| 3. Plan to reassess support needs on a formal and regular basis. | Children are growing and developing rapidly and needs and priorities change often, especially during illness. |
| 4. Develop nursing goals of care:<br>▪ To provide the child with information about his or her condition.<br>▪ To provide emotional support for the child.<br>▪ To allow for the expression and management of the child's feelings. | |
| **Implementation** | |
| 1. Provide information concerning the child's condition and treatment, considering age and desire to know. Indicate that whenever the child is ready, information will eagerly be shared. When parents are resistant to the child receiving information, stress that children, in the absence of accurate information, will make up their own versions of what is occurring and why. These misconceptions may produce more stress for the child. | Age-appropriate communication techniques ensure the most accurate understanding.<br>***Special Considerations:*** *Although the child may be reluctant to ask questions in the beginning, using the third person technique is often helpful (e.g., "Children often tell me that they are curious about how they got sick"). Some children may not be ready to learn about their condition. Frequently children need to express their feelings before they are prepared to receive information (see Skill 12).* |
| a. Ask what the child thinks caused the condition, what a particular treatment is for, etc., and clarify as needed. | Children often hold two views of the cause: one from the medical information they may have heard from the doctor or parents and a "private version" (Sourkes, 1987). There are often misconceptions concerning reasons for treatment and procedures (see Skill 1).<br>***Special Considerations:*** *Using a doll and asking what the child thinks caused the doll to get sick will often uncover the "private version."* |

| **Steps** | **Rationale** |
|---|---|
| b. Tell the child that any topic he or she wishes to discuss is acceptable (e.g., "Some kids tell me that having cancer is hard, but that other things in their lives are difficult, too. We can talk about any of those other kinds of things, too"). | Giving the child permission to discuss whatever may be troubling provides the opportunity to address concerns that may be unrelated to the condition (e.g., an alcoholic parent, a pending divorce for parents, a parent's announcement of remarriage). Many issues could be more stressful than those directly related to the condition. (For more on communication, see Skill 12). |
| 2. Provide the following when the child is hospitalized: | |
| a. Normalize the environment as much as possible. | Humanizing or normalizing the environment to seem more like home will make the strange setting less stressful and minimize interference with the child's normal development.<br>***Special Considerations:*** *Some suggestions may require policy changes in hospitals. Advocating for the best interests of the child and family is a traditional role for the pediatric nurse.* |
| ▪ Welcome parents at all times. | Parents are not "visitors" and should be treated as valued members of the health care team. They are the most valuable source of support, particularly for the young child. Reasonably comfortable sleeping accommodations should be available at the child's bedside.<br>***Special Considerations:*** *When parents are not able to be present, encourage photographs of family members (including the family pet) and tape recordings of family members' voices.* |
| ▪ Provide parents with information about ways they can be helpful. | Developmentally appropriate parental responses offer the best opportunity for adequate support (Table 18-1). |
| ▪ Encourage parents to participate in the child's care at their level of comfort. | Parents may be afraid they will harm a fragile child or sophisticated equipment. Offer to help parents become familiar with care and role model for them.<br>***Special Considerations:*** *With experienced parents of a chronically ill child, it is useful to solicit advice from them on preferred techniques, child's preferences, etc.* |
| ▪ Provide for sibling visitation. | Liberal visitation for siblings (even in critical care units) is typically supportive for both the child in the hospital and the siblings. |
| ▪ Provide for friends to visit. | Friends are an excellent resource for support, particularly for the adolescent. |
| ▪ Plan procedures and treatments around the child's routines and rituals as much as possible. | The less disruption to the child's normal routine, the less stress is experienced. Such scheduling also provides maximum periods of rest instead of continual interruptions. |
| ▪ Help the child and family establish a comfortable routine that reflects the child's preillness patterns of discipline. | In the hospital, the child often loses a former set of checks and balances or controls. Without the security that children receive from having limits at home, they begin to construct their own limit system (Hall, Hardin, and Conatser, 1982). A system that may be without limits and expectations can be confusing and stressful for the child. |
| ▪ Provide opportunities for play. | Play is a very important activity in a child's development (see Skills 15 and 16). |
| ▪ Encourage toys or transitional objects from home. | Familiar objects are a source of comfort and often essential to a child's self-comfort routine.<br>***Special Considerations:*** *A transitional object is a stuffed toy, blanket, etc., that the child cuddles to feel secure and comforted.* |
| b. Prepare child for all procedures and offer opportunities to work through experiences after they occur. | Preparing the child for procedures reduces anxiety and provides experiences to develop mastery (see Skill 1).<br>***Special Considerations:*** *A child may work through an experience after it occurs verbally, in play, or in other appropriate ways.* |
| c. Help child develop coping techniques to manage stressful or painful events (see Skill 17). | Although many stressful events cannot be avoided, age-appropriate coping strategies can reduce stress. |
| d. Offer choices whenever possible. | Even seemingly trivial choices provide the child with a sense of control in an environment where very little is in the child's control. |
| e. Protect children, whenever possible and appropriate, from frightening and unfamiliar sights, sounds, and equipment. Help them prepare for and understand those experiences that are unavoidable. | Strange sights and sounds can be frightening and confusing for the child.<br>***Special Considerations:*** *Try to evaluate the sights and sounds in the environment from the child's point of view. Sometimes simple and harmless stimuli are taken for granted by those who work in the environment (see Table 1-1 on p. 2).* |

| Steps | Rationale |
|---|---|
| f. Find ways to "soften" equipment, e.g., clipping a bear to a stethoscope or decorating an IV pump with paper, fabric, or stickers to resemble a friendly animal. | Combining familiar or comforting sights with the unfamiliar relieves much of the harshness of equipment. |
| g. Encourage primary care. | Having the same nurses care for the child promotes continuity of care and the development of supportive relationships. |
| h. Provide opportunities for expression of feelings (see Skill 16). | Children in the hospital often experience many new and sometimes painful or frightening emotions. Knowing that this is normal and that it is okay to express them appropriately is supportive.<br>***Special Considerations:*** *Young children in particular use play to express emotions.* |
| 3. Discuss current education options with child and parents. Ask if child and family would like someone to speak to the child's class in preparation for reentry. Gather information about educational opportunities and scholarships for the older child (see Product References and Teaching Resources). | Most school districts have a provision for home study. A tutor may be needed for the child who has missed a significant amount of schoolwork. Most states require hospitals to offer school for children who are hospitalized over a certain number of days.<br>***Special Considerations:*** *For the child with special needs, provide parents with information about P.L. 94-142 (Education for All Handicapped Children's Act) and P.L. 99-457 (Education of the Handicapped Act).* |
| 4. Provide information about recreational opportunities for the child with a chronic or disabling condition (see Product References and Teaching Resources). A referral to a recreation therapist may be helpful. | Children may be able to resume previously enjoyed activities. Sometimes adaptive equipment is necessary. Other times new activities and interests should be explored. |
| 5. Share information about support groups, peer support, or support programs for the child (see the box below). For the adolescent with a chronic condition, encourage relationships with groups. The experience will smooth the transition to a meaningful relationship with one person. | Support from those who have shared similar experiences provides an inexpensive and effective means of support.<br>***Special Considerations:*** *When contacting resources, respect confidentiality and do not use the child's or family's name without permission.* |
| 6. Provide material, contact appropriate resources, or provide referral for information relating to future concerns. | As an increasing number of children with chronic illness live through childhood and adolescence, adult issues surface (e.g., employment and financial considerations) that may best be served by adult care practitioners.<br>***Special Considerations:*** *Model programs are developing to smooth the transition from adolescence to adulthood for children with chronic illnesses. Adult practitioners are learning to care for young adults with childhood diseases such as cystic fibrosis where the average life expectancy is presently 27 to 28 years of age (Cystic Fibrosis Foundation, 1988). Whereas some young adults may choose to remain in pediatric care, as more programs develop, young adults should be offered a medically sound and appropriate option.* |
| 7. Explore with child and family the identification of a person, e.g., the family pastor, who would be an appropriate resource for spiritual concerns. | While written information is helpful and should be obtained, it is often valuable to have the opportunity to discuss these concerns with someone.<br>***Special Considerations:*** *For the child in the hospital, most hospitals have either a chaplain or a pastor in the community on call.* |

### *LOCATING SUPPORT GROUPS*

Resources such as the local telephone directory or a community services telephone directory provide an excellent starting point in the search for local self-help groups. Although usually only a small number of groups are listed, local chapters of organizations serving children with a specific disease or disability often list self-help groups in the area. The Encyclopedia of Associations, which is available in most public libraries, includes the names of national organizations. These organizations usually have information about local groups. Appendices of books relating to children with chronic illness or disability will sometimes offer sources of self-help.

Before recommending a group, try to visit a meeting and assess for (1) purpose(s), (2) group members, (3) group leader(s), (4) benefits, (5) people for whom the group would not be suitable, and (6) problems. Attempt to answer the question: "Is the group preventing further emotional distress?" (Newton, 1984).

Write information about groups on index cards and store in a file box. This system will allow the addition of new groups and the updating of old ones. Keep the cards in alphabetical order for easy access.

| Steps | Rationale |
|---|---|
| **Evaluation Outcomes** | **Observational Guidelines** |
| 1. Child is knowledgeable concerning condition, treatment, and resources appropriate to age. | Ask child to explain condition and treatment. Have child list possible resources specific to the condition. Child assists in treatment and rehabilitation regimen. |
| 2. Child effectively uses coping techniques. | Ask child how using coping techniques has worked. Ask child to demonstrate an effective coping technique. |
| 3. Child expresses and manages feelings appropriately. | Listen to child express feelings and cope with them. Observe for feelings of anger and sadness, as well as confidence and optimism when outlook is better. Observe child express feelings to family members, or ask them if child is discussing feelings with them. |
| 4. Child achieves or maintains a positive self-image. | Observe for child's verbal and nonverbal expressions of pride in completing a task or doing a good job. Note the child taking pride in personal appearance. Listen for child expressing desire to improve ability or identifying with a role model. |

### Documentation

Document psychosocial, developmentally supportive care with the same importance and frequency as physical aspects of care. Chart intervention and response of child and family members. Note resource materials given to child or family. Any follow-up plans should be noted, as well as future areas of concern.

# *SKILL* 19 Providing Support for Parents

*Judy Holt Rollins*

When a child experiences a serious illness, accident, or disability, the event presents a crisis for the entire family. Even a less severe or temporary disruption in a child's health will, because of the nature of the family system, cause a change in the everyday life of all members. An important role for the nurse is assisting all family members in coping with the situation. Because the family environment is probably the greatest influence on the child's health, it seems reasonable that the proper approach should be a family-centered one. Parents need adequate support in order to provide support to their children, including the healthy siblings.

## NURSING DIAGNOSES

Ineffective family (parental) coping related to situational crisis, ineffective coping methods, or inadequate support systems; Anxiety related to unmet informational need about child's health condition or treatment; Parental role conflict related to interruptions of family life due to health care regimen.

| Steps | Rationale |
|---|---|

## Assessment

1. Assess emotional response of family members through observation and conversation. Common responses are
   a. Powerlessness.
   b. Loss of control.
   c. Fear.
   d. Guilt.

The most useful support begins by acknowledging the family member's emotional response at the present time (see Skill 14).

***Special Considerations:*** *In the case of chronic illness or disability, parents often grieve the loss of the "perfect child" or, in the case of birth defects, the loss of "a dream" (Moses, 1984). All of the emotions of the grieving process—denial, anger, bargaining, depression, and finally acknowledgment or acceptance—may, at one time or another, be present. Parents may experience feelings of powerlessness, lack of control, and fear about prognosis or ability to care for child. Guilt may be felt when parents wonder if their child's condition is due to something they did (or didn't do), and is frequently experienced with genetic disorders. In the case of a preventable accident, the responsible family member may experience extreme feelings of guilt and shame. Adoptive parents may be spared the feelings of guilt associated with genetic disorders, but otherwise are vulnerable to the same emotions.*

2. Determine if child's condition challenges the family's view of the world. Common beliefs include:
   a. Only the very sick are hospitalized.
   b. Only elderly people are sick.
   c. With the increase in technology, surely there is a cure for everything.
   d. Children should not suffer.
   e. Being born in America guarantees a happy, healthy life.
   f. In the case of cancer, most malignancies are fatal.
   g. Diseases are punishment for previous sins or shortcomings.

Faulty notions in the existential environment may affect the family's perception of the child's condition and treatment (Hall, Hardin, and Conatser, 1982).

***Special Considerations:*** *An evaluation of one's own feelings and attitudes regarding these notions must be done before attempting to support families.*

3. Determine the family structure and the present and anticipated changes within the structure (see Skill 38).

Initially, the family structure is disorganized. There may be role changes and changes in the family's daily routine.

***Special Considerations:*** *In a single-parent family, parental figures may be a mother with maternal grandmother, or father with oldest sibling (Hall, Hardin, and Conatser, 1982).*

4. Determine the family's usual coping patterns and family communication (see Skill 38).

Knowledge of family's usual coping and communication patterns gives more direction for interventions and support.

***Special Considerations:*** *Research indicates that families are happier and marital satisfaction greater when communication between spouses is easy, when disagreements are less frequent and not always resolved in favor of the same spouse, and when more decisions are made together rather than by one spouse alone (Stuifbergen, 1987).*

5. Determine stage of the family life cycle by reviewing number and ages of children.
   a. Beginning-married, no children.
   b. Expecting-pregnant until birth of first child.
   c. Childbearing-oldest child: birth to 30 months.
   d. Preschool-oldest child: 2½ to 6 years.
   e. School-age-oldest child: 6 years to 13 years.
   f. Teenage-oldest child: 13 years to 20 years.
   g. Launching Center-first child gone to last child gone.
   h. Middle Years-empty nest to retirement.
   i. Aging-retirement to death of both spouses.

The family changes constantly with the maturation of its members (Duvall, 1977). Because some stages of the family life cycle are predictably more stressful, degree of stress is often related to the stage of the family life cycle.

***Special Considerations:*** *One of the most stressful times in the family life cycle is when children are in their adolescent years.*

6. Assess nature of the affected child's condition.

The nature of the condition is particularly significant in the case of chronic illness, where the stress of the illness continues over an extended period of time and may be somewhat unpredictable and uncontrollable.

7. Identify needs and concerns. There are many predictable needs and concerns that parents share:
   a. Information about their child's condition.
   b. Financial concerns.
   c. What to tell siblings.

An approach built on the unique needs and concerns of the family helps assure that the most valuable support is provided.

| Steps | Rationale |
|---|---|
| d. How to interact with other family members, including grandparents and friends. | ***Special Considerations:*** *Often family and friends will avoid parents because they do not know what to say. Others will press parents for information or question the child's care. In many cases the parents usual support system of family and friends is either unavailable or adding more stress.* |
| e. Educational disruption.<br>f. Discipline.<br>g. Parental role in the care of the child.<br>h. Concerns about the future.<br>i. Home or work responsibilities neglected due to time spent with hospitalized child.<br>j. Lack of time and energy to devote to other children in family. | ***Special Considerations:*** *Parents of disabled children are particularly concerned about meeting educational needs, care of the child should something happen to them, and the future employability of their child.* |
| 8. Ask family what assistance they believe would be helpful. | Families have unique needs and are in the best position to prioritize them (e.g., a parent of an ill or disabled child might consider occasional help with meals a most important form of support). Also, giving parents the message that they are recognized as important members of the health care team helps to build the therapeutic relationship. |
| 9. Examine what support, both emotional and practical, is available to the family and how well it meets their current needs.<br>a. Emotional.<br>b. Practical, e.g., financial, medical management, household management, child care, and respite care. | Identifying the current support system reduces duplication of services.<br>***Special Considerations:*** *Families may be surrounded by many supportive people through their extended family, neighbors, friends, church, and other organizations. A particularly desperate situation is the growing number of homeless families with little or no support (Wood, 1989).* |

## Planning and Goal Setting

| Steps | Rationale |
|---|---|
| 1. Gather information about resources available to meet parents' particular needs. Consider:<br>a. Family resource libraries.<br>b. Organizations, associations, churches.<br>c. Support groups.<br>d. Other parents.<br>e. Social services.<br>f. Legislators.<br>g. Helplines. | Establishing a good network of resources provides an excellent base for offering support.<br>***Special Considerations:*** *Obtain permission from parents before giving their name to any resource.* |
| 2. Develop nursing goals of care:<br>▪ To provide parents with information about the ill or disabled child's condition, developmental functioning, treatment, and prognosis.<br>▪ To help parents define their role in child's care.<br>▪ To reduce the dysfunctional effects of stress in the family system. | |

## Implementation

| Steps | Rationale |
|---|---|
| 1. Communicate a caring attitude to the family by treating their child in a caring manner. | Treating their child with tenderness and care communicates a caring attitude to family members.<br>***Special Considerations:*** *Actions such as these provide good opportunities to serve as a role model for family/members, particularly for those who are having difficulty bonding with their child.* |
| 2. Be an empathic listener. | The importance of listening cannot be overemphasized. Assuming the roles of active and reflective listener is truly helpful and provides the basis for the type of trust and support necessary in a family professional partnership (Dunst, Trivette, and Deal, 1988).<br>***Special Considerations:*** *A family member is not likely to take advice from a care provider without feeling that their needs and thoughts have been carefully heard and considered (Selig and Selig, 1983).* |

| Steps | Rationale |
|---|---|
| a. Active listening. | An active listener demonstrates interest and concern about what is important to a family, and how different members feel or perceive family circumstances. For example, "You seem very concerned about your child's future. What are the things that worry you?" (Dunst, Trivette, and Deal, 1988). |
| b. Reflective listening. | In reflective listening, what a family member says is rephrased to help clarify exactly what is being said. For example, "Am I understanding you to say that you have doubts about your child's future, and that this is causing you to feel down and depressed?" (Dunst, Trivette, and Deal, 1988). |
| 3. Allow family members the opportunity to vent feelings and show emotion (e.g. guilt), "I really feel that it is my fault that Joey was born with one arm." | Encouraging family members to express feelings may relieve tension, provide information for intervention, and set the tone that in open communication, anything can be discussed. |
| 4. Acknowledge their feelings. For the example in Step 3, it would be helpful to reply, "If you really believe that you are responsible, then no wonder you feel so bad" (Moses, 1984). | Acknowledgment of feelings conveys understanding without agreeing on accuracy of facts. The facts can be discussed later. ***Special Considerations:*** *Avoid tendency to make statements such as "You shouldn't worry about that; it's not your fault" as it belittles their feelings.* |
| 5. Use silence when appropriate. | A quiet presence can communicate caring and concern. ***Special Considerations:*** *This is sometimes difficult for nurses who feel they have to "say something" to be therapeutic.* |
| 6. Provide information for the family according to their needs, including medical information, community resources, support groups, and pros and cons of treatment choices (Shelton, Jeppson, and Johnson, 1987).<br>a. Offer information in understandable terms and provide corresponding medical terminology.<br>b. Write specific information relating to child's management.<br>c. Share information in manageable doses.<br>d. Allow adequate time for questions and follow-up conversation.<br>e. Provide booklets, videos, handouts, etc., when available. | Knowledge reduces anxiety and brings a sense of power and control. It is also a critical factor in enabling parents to participate fully in the decision-making process—not only ongoing and daily decisions about the child's care, but more basic decisions regarding the provision of medical treatment. ***Special Considerations:*** *Information also helps to minimize the development of a dependent relationship between parents and professionals that can undermine the competence of parents. Information should also be shared with siblings (Skill 20), grandparents, and other family members, and with the child at the discretion of the parents. Remember that information sharing is an ongoing process, not a one time intervention (Shelton, Jeppson, and Johnson, 1987).* |
| f. Vary the method of teaching, if possible. | Some people learn best by reading, others by listening, observing, or doing. |
| g. Clarify information provided by other health professionals.<br>h. Provide parents with paper and pencil or pen. | |
| i. Offer to explain and clarify information to family members who are not present. | Expecting family members to relate a large number of details to others may be a burden when they are trying to process the information themselves. Additionally, other family members may have different questions than the ones asked by those present. |
| 7. Help parents define their role in the care of their child, remembering that some parents desire or are able to assume a more active role than others. | Parents often are confused and insecure about their role in the care of their child. Helping them to define their role provides security and benefits the child. ***Special Considerations:*** *The family is the constant in the child's world. Parents of children with special needs must be prepared to assume the role of providing the overall management to coordinate the efforts of many specialists and the needs of the child within the context of the family (Anderson, 1985).* |
| a. Encourage input from parents. | Because parents know their child better than anyone, their contributions are unique and invaluable. |
| b. Regard families as capable. | Every family has strengths. In stressful situations, families may need help identifying theirs. |
| c. Remind parents that professionals are always available for them—this is a family/professional partnership. | Giving permission to ask for help allows parents to do so without feeling like failures. |
| 8. Be sincere:<br>a. When choosing phrases of comfort or support. | Phrases such as "I understand" are of no value unless the person saying it has truly been in that situation. Furthermore, most situations are viewed as unique, and such a statement may provoke well-deserved anger. ***Special Considerations:*** *The use of the third person could be more effective: "Other mothers in somewhat similar situations have told me they felt very helpless. Is that maybe some of what you're feeling now?"* |

| Steps | Rationale |
|---|---|
| b. When sharing private information about self. | Traditionally, personal disclosure was discouraged. A more open approach is advocated today. However, relating private information should have a purpose, e.g., it may be very supportive to a single mother to know that the nurse truly understands the problems of being a single parent because she is one also. |
| 9. Encourage honest and open communication within the family. | Accurate information allows the child and family members the opportunity to define the problem and develop means of coping. Much time and energy is expended in an effort to "spare" someone from the painful truth. These efforts are usually not successful and cause mistrust. Information deficits can establish a pattern of diminished communication that may spread to other aspects of family life, producing a generalized "web of silence" (Turk, 1964). |
| 10. Use a variety of methods to convey to the family an awareness of their feelings and be available for parents to talk about them. | Setting aside time to meet the needs of the family can be as important as any other element on the child's care plan. Reduced anxiety in parents generally leads to a better outcome for the child. |
| 11. Encourage parental presence and participation when the child is hospitalized. | Creating an environment with family members in familiar roles is supportive for parents and the hospitalized child. |
| a. Support liberal visiting policies for parents and other family members, and rooming-in provisions. | Liberal visiting policies and comfortable accommodations indicate a respect for maintaining the integrity of the family unit. Flexible visiting hours respect unique needs of parents with jobs or other responsibilities.<br>***Special Considerations:*** *Hospitals can make a statement of the importance of parental presence by eliminating the word "visitors" when referring to parents.* |
| b. Communicate that parents are welcome through written material, including signs, and choice of words. | Parent handbooks discuss rooming-in and encourage parents to provide some of their child's care. This notifies parents that the staff recognizes this as a difficult period and helps parents feel welcome.<br>***Special Considerations:*** *A sign stating "Parents* welcome *at all times" delivers a more supportive message than "Parents* allowed *at all times."* |
| c. Provide guidelines and other assistance to help parents and other family members learn to care for the child (e.g., how to bathe a child who has an NG tube). | Guidance helps reduce anxiety of the unknown and fear of harming child. Providing daily care for child maintains normal parental role and routine, offering a source of comfort and security for parent and child. |
| d. Encourage parents to play with their child, helping them to adapt favorite play to present restrictions (e.g., IV) (see Skill 15). | Play can be a pleasant activity, one that is not new to the parent and offers an opportunity for a successful intervention and resulting praise.<br>***Special Considerations:*** *Parents often mistakenly believe an ill child is uninterested or unable to play.* |
| e. Orient parents to the facility environment. Show them where to go for coffee, food, bathroom, playroom, showers, chapel. | Familiarity with the facility is comforting for families. |
| f. Encourage parents to take a break by offering to watch child in parent's absence, by bringing child to nurses station, or arranging for volunteer to stay with child. | Constant attendance to a hospitalized child can be physically and emotionally draining to a parent. Refreshed parents are better able to care for and support their child. Parents may be reluctant to leave child, often feeling that the child's needs may go unmet. Knowing a trusted person will be with the child offers a sense of security.<br>***Special Considerations:*** *Parents are also often reluctant to leave because they do not want to miss the visit from the physician. Hospitals can equip parents with beepers and notify them when the doctor is on the unit.* |
| g. Inform parents of their right to be kept apprised of their child's condition and their right to ask for clarification when needed. | Parents are sometimes passive, not wanting to "bother" the busy physician or afraid their child's care will be jeopardized if they question treatment methods, policies, and other issues. |
| 12. Encourage parental involvement with other parents.<br>a. Provide information about parent groups (see box on p. 86).<br>b. Introduce parents to other parents. | Parents indicate that they have a need to feel that someone truly understands (Lynam, 1987). Creating opportunities for parents to meet others in similar situations increases the likelihood that this will occur. |
| c. Maintain an environment conducive to informal gathering of parents. | Comfortable seating in cluster arrangements encourages conversation. |

## GRANDPARENTS

While much has been documented about the effects of disabled or chronically ill children on their parents, only recently has there been concern about the impact on grandparents. For many families, grandparents are an important and active part of the family network. The grandparent-grandchild relationship is often a very important one—for both the child and the grandparent.

When the grandchild is diagnosed with a disability or chronic condition, this important relationship is jeopardized. Initially, grandparents may experience the same reactions as the child's parent. When grandparents have difficulty adapting, their attitude may affect other family members' reactions and adaptation.

Grandparents of special needs children are frequently unable to offer child care advice. They have many unanswered questions of their own. They may feel powerless and sad when unable to fulfill their function as role models for the younger generation.

Grandchildren represent the family's promise for the future and the extension of family through its descendants. This is comforting for grandparents. The disabled child upsets this certainty. The future is now unpredictable, not only for the grandchild, but for the parents as well. Grandparents often experience a double grief, for both their grandchild and their child.

Grandparents instinctively want to help when they hear the diagnosis, but when faced with a problem about which they are poorly informed, they really don't know how. Information is provided for parents, but grandparents typically have to seek out the answers themselves.

Additionally, parents are frequently supported through the expected grief and depression, whereas these emotions are not acknowledged in grandparents. Grandparents are left to adapt on their own (Vadasy, 1987).

There is a true need to include grandparents in the full spectrum of family-centered care. In addition to meeting their needs, with appropriate support grandparents prove to be excellent resources to the child with special needs, the child's siblings, and parents.

Grandparents, like parents, benefit from peer support. Workshops, self-help groups, and even reading about the experiences of other grandparents through a newsletter are all helpful in meeting this need.

| Steps | Rationale |
|---|---|
| d. Invite the parent who has been successful in overcoming a particular aspect of hospitalization or illness experience to talk about it with another parent struggling to resolve a similar issue (Lynam, 1987). | Acknowledging successful management of problem increases parents' self-esteem and reinforces their ability to solve future problems. In addition, their solution is likely to prove useful to other parents in similar situations. |
| e. Help interested parents start a self-help group if none are available (See Product References and Teaching Resources). | ***Special Considerations:*** *Although one out of every three self-help groups is started with the help of a professional, success seems to be greatest in those groups where parents assume leadership (Rollins, 1987).* |
| 13. Help parents maintain existing support systems. | The existing support system serves as a foundation for additional support. |
| a. Identify overloaded and underused sources of support. | |
| b. Facilitate less involved family member's understanding of condition, treatment, and so on. | Frequently, one parent is involved in the child's care—hospitalizations, clinic appointments, etc. It is not entirely reasonable to expect one parent to effectively and consistently "orient" the other to the child's care. They may also be at different stages in dealing with the situation and have difficulty relating to one another's needs (Lynam, 1987).<br>***Special Considerations:*** *There is also a growing recognition of the importance of considering grandparents (see box above).* |
| 14. Encourage parent participation in activities where it is important that the parent voice be heard.<br>a. Parent advisory boards.<br>b. Membership on policy making committees.<br>c. Multidisciplinary organizations (see Product References and Teaching Resources).<br>d. Legislative and lobbying. | Support is most likely to be favorably received if it can be reciprocated and the possibility of "repaying" is sanctioned and approved but not expected (Fisher, Nadler, and Whitcher-Alagna, 1983). Repaying need not be material in nature and in fact is often informational (Dunst, 1988).<br>***Special Considerations:*** *Parents' perspective is not available from any other source than a parent.* |
| 15. Advise parents to make an effort to provide for their own and other family members' needs. | Meeting the needs of all family members helps assure that the family system will function in a healthy manner.<br>***Special Considerations:*** *Parent and sibling needs are often overlooked when family is absorbed with concerns of ill or disabled child.* |
| a. Encourage scheduling time for normal family activities. | Continued participation in normal activities provides a sense of stability to the family unit. |
| b. Help identify child care and respite services. | Constant care for a child with special needs can deplete physical and emotional resources of family members. Respite services provide opportunities for participation in normal family activities. |

| Steps | Rationale |
|---|---|
| | ***Special Considerations:*** *Maintain a network of resources in the community offering respite care. An increasing number of states offer a data base of community resources, including agencies providing respite services.* |
| c. Emphasize the importance of the marital relationship in times of stress. | The marital relationship is the axis around which all other relationships are formed. The couple relationship is particularly vulnerable during times of stress. ***Special Considerations:*** *Continuing activities previously enjoyed as a couple (e.g., dinner at a favorite restaurant or going to the movies with friends) provides opportunities to maintain the couple relationship.* |
| 16. Help parents explore and evaluate individual's and family's present methods of coping and communicating, suggesting new ones when appropriate (see Skill 17). | Communication techniques and coping strategies proven effective in the past are likely to be successful in the present situation. ***Special Considerations:*** *Families may need professional counseling if methods of communicating and coping are ineffective or dysfunctional to the family system.* |
| 17. Reassess needs of parents at regular intervals. | Needs may be different as children and families develop or child's condition changes. Providing resources is an ongoing service. ***Special Considerations:*** *The use of the term "resource" may be more acceptable to some families than "support."* |

| Evaluation Outcomes | Observational Guidelines |
|---|---|
| 1. Parents and other family members are able to cope effectively. | Parents and other family members state they feel supported/understood and model effective and appropriate coping behaviors. |
| 2. Parents are knowledgeable about child's condition. | Parents are able to discuss child's condition, treatment, prognosis, ask appropriate questions, and use some medical terminology. |
| 3. Parents have defined their role in their child's care. | Parents adequately perform child care tasks at the present level of parental comfort. |
| 4. Parents are able to identify needs and use resources. | Equipment and other medical resources are obtained. Nonmedical resources, e.g., support group membership, are used effectively. |

## Documentation

Document on the child's chart an assessment of the family's needs, their strengths, available support, and any contacts, literature, or other information given to family. Note family interaction and coping ability of individual members, using examples of behaviors. Update with reassessments and future interventions.

# SKILL 20 Providing Support for Siblings

*Judy Holt Rollins*

A family member's state of health will have an effect on everyone within the family system. While focusing on the ill or disabled child and the parents, nurses and other health care professionals often overlook siblings. Studies indicate that siblings of children who are ill, hospitalized, or have a disabling or chronic condition may at some point experience more stress than parents or even the ill or disabled child (Spinetta, 1981). Siblings assist in the socialization process, aid in identity formation, and serve in a variety of roles. Perhaps the most unique of all features of the sibling relationship is its duration. The sibling relationship lasts through a lifetime, often 50 to 80 years in duration, likely the longest relationship one will share with another human being (Bank and Kahn, 1975).

## NURSING DIAGNOSES

Ineffective family (sibling) coping related to situational crisis, ineffective coping methods, or inadequate support systems; Anxiety related to unmet informational need about sibling's health condition or treatment.

| Steps | Rationale |
|---|---|
| **Assessment** | |
| 1. Review:<br>a. Age and birth order of sibling(s).<br>b. Age and birth order of child with special needs and other siblings.<br>c. Sex of sibling(s). | The age, birth order, sex, and many additional factors often influence the sibling reaction.<br>***Special Considerations:*** *Because of the need for attention, the child just younger than the child with special needs is often at greatest risk. Older siblings often feel very protective. The oldest sibling, particularly if female, may be responsible for providing care for the child with special needs or for the other siblings. Preschoolers are concerned about time and attention devoted by family members and professionals to child with special needs; parental distress and preoccupation with the disabled child; etiology of condition; and worry that they will be affected as well. This is often reflected in acting out behavior. Child may act out concerns about bodily injury and death in dramatic play. Without realistic information, the child uses magical thinking to supply his or her own explanations. School-age healthy siblings are concerned with changing roles within family as they possibly gain skills faster than disabled brother or sister, additional responsibilities, how to tell peers, talking to parents about their role, and uncertainty as to the exact nature of their brother or sister's disability or condition. Adolescents are concerned about need for more sophisticated information about the condition, its cause, treatment, and prognosis; they also worry about the future.* |
| d. Brother's or sister's condition, limitations, and prognosis.<br>e. Location of brother or sister at present.<br>f. Type of family, degree of support, cultural heritage, and socioeconomic status. | Research findings differ; some report more adjustment problems among siblings of severely disabled children, whereas other studies report the opposite (McKeever, 1983). Visibility of the condition may be a factor (Lavigne and Ryan, 1979). Siblings typically have more difficulty if the disability is ambiguous or undefined (McHale, Simeonsson, and Sloan, 1984), the prognosis for the child's recovery is not good, the family lives far from the hospital, they are living in a single-parent family with little money, and they have limited family or friends for support (Laker, 1988). Siblings in larger families tend to cope more easily than those from smaller ones (Powell and Ogle, 1985). |

| **Steps** | **Rationale** |
|---|---|
| | ***Special Considerations:*** *With some conditions, e.g., cancer, remissions are possible. Even remissions may be difficult times for siblings. They see that their parents are no longer spending time in the hospital or clinic and feel that it is finally their turn for attention. Exhausted physically and emotionally, parents often use the time to relax. The sibling's unfulfilled expectations lead to disappointment (Spinetta, 1981).* |
| g. Parental style. | If parental style is dysfunctional (e.g., overprotective and overpermissive with special needs child), then the sibling subsystem is equally vulnerable to dysfunction (Minuchin et al, 1975). |
| 2. Assess behavior and adjustment of sibling by observation and/or interview of sibling/parents, noting presence of:<br>a. Negative self-image.<br>b. High level of anxiety.<br>c. Increased guilt.<br>d. Jealousy.<br>e. Resentment.<br>f. Feelings of rejection.<br>g. Severe separation anxiety.<br>h. Stammering.<br>i. Nightmares.<br>j. Poor peer relationships. | A healthy child's response to being a sibling of a child with special needs is often reflected in behavior or adjustment difficulties.<br>***Special Considerations:*** *Healthy siblings are more likely to experience adjustment or behavior problems than are their peers without brothers and sisters with special needs (Gallo, 1988). Siblings can often provide significant insight to understanding the strengths and needs of the entire family (Steiner, 1984; Roche, 1987). Preschoolers tend to become withdrawn and irritable. Older children act out socially. Female school-age siblings tend to have more problems than school-age males. In adolescence, it reverses and seems to be easiest on females, except for female who is placed in caregiver role for special needs child (Powell and Ogle, 1985).* |
| k. Poor school performance. | ***Special Considerations:*** *Occasionally siblings will overachieve and get good grades with the hope of being noticed.* |
| l. Enuresis.<br>m. Appetite problems.<br>n. Headache.<br>o. Recurring abdominal pain.<br>p. Preoccupation with own health. | ***Special Considerations:*** *Symptoms should be taken seriously and evaluated by a thorough physical examination. If no physical basis is found, then underlying emotional stress should be recognized. The examination reassures sibling that he or she is healthy (Cairns et al, 1979).* |
| 3. Determine sibling's usual style of coping with stress. | Methods of coping that have worked in the past are likely to be helpful in dealing with subsequent stressful situations.<br>***Special Considerations:*** *An effective coping style may be minimizing the dysfunctional effects of the stress sibling is experiencing.* |
| 4. Determine through interview, observation of sibling, or family members or friend if sibling's basic needs are adequately met. | Financial and emotional resources may be limited as more of these resources are primarily channeled to the ill child. |
| 5. Assess sibling's knowledge of brother's or sister's condition, developmental functioning, prognosis, and treatment. | Siblings typically have less information than anyone in the family. Parents often feel insecure about providing information, sometimes evading answering questions accurately or completely. Siblings are hesitant to approach parents who are perceived as being overburdened, anxious, and unwilling to discuss the problem (Gallo, 1988).<br>***Special Considerations:*** *Although siblings are usually the least informed, they are often treated by friends and neighbors as the family informant. Not knowing what to say may lead to further distress.* |
| 6. Determine parents' ability or willingness to support sibling. | Parents may be overwhelmed with the child with special needs and not have the ability or willingness to devote time to the sibling.<br>***Special Considerations:*** *Support is often available outside and inside the family through extended family, church, friends, neighbors, and others.* |
| 7. Determine additional stressors in the sibling's life. | A recent divorce or remarriage of a parent, a move, a new baby, a new school, a bully, or an alcoholic parent may add to the sibling's stress level, sometimes causing more concern than having a brother or sister with special needs. |

| Steps | Rationale |
|---|---|
| **Planning and Goal Setting** | |
| 1. Meet with parents to discuss concept of family-centered care and sibling issues. | Parents need to know that illness in the family affects every member of the system. ***Special Considerations:*** *Occasionally families desire that siblings not receive information about their brother's or sister's condition. Family wishes are to be respected, but continued communication with the family, encouragement from the nurse, and physician support may change their minds over time.* |
| 2. Gather age-related resource materials and information to provide to sibling or parents. | Establishing a good network of resources provides an excellent base for offering support. Booklets, videos, programs, and support groups for siblings of special needs children are available (see Product References and Teaching Resources). ***Special Considerations:*** *When contacting resources, respect confidentiality and do not use the family's name without permission.* |
| 3. Select a convenient time to meet with sibling. | Considering the sibling's needs and wishes offers the best possibility for successful support. ***Special Considerations:*** *For very young siblings, plan to meet with the parents (with child present, if appropriate) to provide information on sibling support.* |
| 4. Develop nursing goals of care:<br>▪ To provide information to the sibling about the brother's or sister's condition, developmental functioning, prognosis, and treatment.<br>▪ To provide sibling support.<br>▪ To allow for the expression and management of sibling's feelings. | |
| **Implementation** | |
| 1. Provide information concerning the condition of the ill or disabled child. | Knowledge reduces anxiety and allows a sense of power and control. Furthermore, siblings are accustomed to everyone focusing on the child with special needs. The offering of information helps siblings realize that their needs are important, too. ***Special Considerations:*** *Frequently siblings need to express their feelings before they are able to receive information. Information may be provided through discussion with an individual child, in a group, as part of a sibling day, through literature or videos, or by parents.* |
| a. Ask sibling what he or she thinks caused the condition. Although siblings may be reluctant to speak or ask questions in the beginning, use the third person technique (see Skill 12). For example, say, "Children often tell me that they wonder how their brother or sister got sick. Have you ever thought about that?" to get the conversation started. | Children often hold two views of the cause of illness: one from the medical information that they may have heard from parents or a doctor, and a "private version" based on their cognitive ability of understanding (Sourkes, 1987). ***Special Considerations:*** *Young children often view illness as punishment; ages 7 to 11 as contagion. Children 12 and older are able to use logic. Siblings, particularly young ones, often think that they caused their brother's or sister's condition and feel guilty.* |
| b. Repeat the actual cause of the brother's or sister's condition. | Reaffirming the medical view clarifies misunderstandings. ***Special Considerations:*** *With young children, encourage parents to use everyday situations to show the child that simultaneity or sequence does not necessarily imply cause. Ask parents to note if sibling is avoiding an activity out of fear that it will cause the condition.* |
| c. Discuss the visibility of the condition and reinforce that the child is the same person. When the child's condition is not visible, stress that even though he or she looks the same, an inner change is making the child sick. | Because children rely so much on their senses to understand their world, it is sometimes difficult for them to understand that someone is the same person when he or she looks, sounds, etc., so different. On the other hand, when the condition is not visible, the sibling may question whether the brother or sister is really sick. ***Special Considerations:*** *It is often helpful to ask the sibling to draw a picture of the ill brother or sister to provide insight on his or her understanding.* |

| Steps | Rationale |
|---|---|

d. Discuss treatment.
   - Ask sibling about treatment aspects, duration, side effects, etc.

     An awareness of the sibling's knowledge provides a starting point for learning and allows an opportunity for the discovery of misconceptions.

   - Provide the sibling with a tour of the facility where treatment is given, the special school the child will be attending, etc.
   - Introduce the sibling to professionals who are involved in their brother's or sister's treatment and allow them to explain what they do.

     Siblings frequently see the treatment facility as a threatening place, or envy their brother's or sister's treatment times as time spent with parents and missed from school. Observation of the experience clarifies understanding.

   - Allow hands-on exposure to equipment when possible.

     Children learn more easily when several senses are stimulated.
     ***Special Considerations:*** *Medical play can be very helpful for sibling understanding (see Skill 16).*

e. With parental consent, honest and accurate information should be given about prognosis in amounts sibling can tolerate and process at the time. Siblings are particularly concerned with how the prognosis will affect them; as much as possible, this information should be provided.

   Open communication provides a forum for expressing feelings and sharing support. Additionally, it allows the opportunity to role model communication with siblings, both in technique and content.
   ***Special Considerations:*** *Parents should be present for support if potentially upsetting news is given. Upsetting news is usually more appropriate if initiated by parents with explanation and clarification by professionals then or at a later time.*

2. Offer resources for support.

   a. Have child and parent identify a relative or friend the child likes who is available to spend time with the sibling.

      Having someone provide extra attention when parents are unavailable conveys that the sibling has not been forgotten.
      ***Special Considerations:*** *It is especially valuable if the sibling is comfortable sharing feelings with the person.*

   b. Sponsor a Sibling Day—a special time for siblings that usually includes a tour of the treatment site, films, discussion, and other activities.

      A sibling day provides an opportunity to support several children and allows siblings to meet peers in similar situations.

   c. Encourage participation in a sibling support group.

      Groups help siblings overcome the social isolation and communication difficulties they may experience in their families or communities.
      ***Special Considerations:*** *Although it is optimal to have siblings with brothers or sisters with the same conditions, because sibling concerns are so similar, a mixed group can provide a great deal of support.*

   d. Offer to speak to the sibling's class, church group, scout group, or other groups about the brother's or sister's condition.

      Misinformation among peers, e.g., fear of contagion, can cause much pain for the sibling.

   e. Offer information about subscriptions to publications focusing on sibling issues (see Product References and Teaching Resources).

      Newsletters and other literature provide information and decrease loneliness, particularly for those unable to attend support meetings.

   f. Provide parents with information for helping their healthy children (see box on next page).

      Parents are often very much aware that their healthy children are experiencing the impact of a special needs brother or sister, yet are uncertain of what to do.
      ***Special Considerations:*** *When interacting with the child with special needs, model acceptance of the child's condition. Parents may in turn model behavior for siblings.*

   g. Offer information about scholarships, camps, and other benefits that are available to siblings of children with special needs.

      Agencies are becoming increasingly aware of the stress experienced by siblings. Organizations for children with special needs are excellent resources for information concerning providers of services for siblings.

3. Give child permission to choose whether or not to act as family informant. If sibling decides not to, offer something to say to questions, e.g., "I'd rather not talk about it." If the child does decide to answer questions, help him or her anticipate them.

   The child may believe that withholding information from someone, especially an adult, is rude or disobedient.
   ***Special Considerations:*** *Although many siblings enjoy the role of family informant, some do not. Many times siblings feel uncomfortable in the role because they lack information about their brother's or sister's condition. Reassure siblings that should they choose to share information, they may feel embarrassed at first, but the feeling will go away as they get used to it.*

### PARENTAL STRATEGIES FOR SUPPORTING SIBLINGS

1. Value each child individually and avoid comparisons. As often as possible, remind each child of his or her positive qualities and contribution to other family members.
2. Limit caregiving responsibilities and give recognition when siblings perform them.
3. Use respite care and other supportive services.
4. Seek to be fair in terms of discipline, attention, and resources.
5. Develop a library of children's books on special needs.
6. Schedule special time with the sibling and use a friend or family member to help out during tough times.
7. Let siblings settle their own differences. (Naturally, parents should never let siblings hurt one another.)
8. Welcome other children and friends into the home. This provides a powerful model of accepting a child's condition and reasserts the family's willingness to fully participate in community life.
9. Praise siblings when they have been patient, have sacrificed, or been particularly helpful. Don't expect siblings to always act in this manner.
10. Help sibling recognize the uniqueness of the family and avoid making comparisons with other families. Although perhaps hidden, other families usually have a whole range of problems, too.
11. Listen to siblings. Asking the sibling to talk or in other ways prompting communication between family members will let siblings know that their thoughts and suggestions are valued.
12. Involve the siblings by:
    a. Inviting them to attend school meeting to develop educational plan for child with special needs.
    b. Discussing future plans with them.
    c. Soliciting their ideas on treatment and service needs.
    d. Having them visit with professionals working with the special needs child.
    e. Helping them develop competencies to teach the disabled child new skills.
    f. Providing opportunities to advocate for the disabled child.
13. Require the disabled child to do as much for himself or herself as possible.
14. Encourage sibling to join or help establish sibling support group.
15. Recognize special stress times for siblings and plan to minimize negative effects.
    a. Birth of a new sibling.
    b. Disabled child goes to school.
    c. Sibling starts to date.
    d. Friends reject the disabled child.
    e. Disabled child becomes critically ill or dies.
    f. Problems related to the child are handled in secrecy.
    g. Parent dies.
    h. For conditions with remission, when the child is off treatment or in remission.
16. Use the services of professionals when needed. If parent feels that such a service is necessary, it should be provided in as vigorous a manner as a service for the disabled child.
17. Teach the sibling to interact. Many need help in learning how to socially interact with a child with a disability or chronic condition.
18. Provide opportunities for a normal family life and normal family activities, which is often difficult when a family's energy and resources are focused on providing care to the special needs child. Encourage siblings to participate in community activities with as much parental participation as possible.

Adapted from Powell TH and Ogle PA: Brothers and sisters: a special part of exceptional families, Baltimore, 1985, Paul H. Brookes.

| Steps | Rationale |
|---|---|
| 4. Encourage communication between sibling and child with special needs through sibling visitation, participation in treatment, phone calls, and letters. | Often the sibling feels guilt about being the healthy one. Additionally, the special needs child may feel angry at the healthy sibling for escaping the condition. Communication may be uneasy until feelings are acknowledged and explored. |
| 5. Provide opportunities for expression of feelings. | |
| a. Use active listening communication technique. | By acknowledging the sibling's feelings, a safe environment is created for further expression. Information may be clarified. |
| b. Use nonverbal methods to encourage expression of feelings and concerns (see Skills 12, 16, and 39). | Nonverbal means are much easier to use for younger siblings and for siblings of all ages who are struggling with difficult feelings. |
| c. With sibling, develop appropriate coping techniques to deal with troublesome feelings, behavior, and family situations. For example, going for a walk when an autistic sibling is screaming. | Mastery of effective coping techniques should reduce dysfunctional effects of stress.<br>***Special Considerations:*** *Literature for siblings of children with special needs often includes coping techniques (see Product References and Teaching Resources).* |
| 6. Identify need for further professional intervention by routinely reassessing behavior and adjustment (refer to Assessment step 2). | Some siblings may need professional counseling. Keep in mind that family situations change, special needs child's condition may change, and all family members are undergoing developmental changes. |

| Steps | Rationale |
|---|---|
| **Evaluation Outcomes** | **Observational Guidelines** |
| 1. Sibling is knowledgeable about brother's or sister's condition. | Observe sibling's ability to relate information concerning brother's or sister's condition, developmental functioning, treatment, and prognosis. |
| 2. Sibling copes with stress in an effective, appropriate manner. | Sibling demonstrates an effective coping technique. |
| 3. Sibling expresses and manages feelings. | Observe sibling's behavior and ability to communicate feelings, verbally or nonverbally, in an appropriate manner. Older siblings may verbally express feelings of support. Observe relationships with parents, child with special needs, and other siblings. |

### Documentation

Record sibling assessment and intervention on the child's chart. Note techniques and materials used, the sibling reaction to the intervention, and any future plans (e.g., the sibling's intent to attend a sibling day). Note sibling's level of comprehension, coping, or expression/management of feelings. Record strengths, identified problems needing further assessment, and plans of action.

# *SKILL* 21 Facilitating Grieving

*Beverlee E. Redding*

A child's death and the dying process is one of the most traumatic events a child and family can experience. Unresolved grief is cumulative and can have detrimental physical and psychologic side effects because the immune system is greatly compromised in the grieving person. Interventions and responses of health care professionals can significantly affect the child's and family members' immediate and subsequent adjustment. While it is difficult and perhaps undesirable to prescribe specific procedures for helping families cope with an experience as personal and traumatic as death, certain guidelines can be suggested (Jost and Haase, 1989). When grieving is facilitated, significant spiritual and emotional growth can result for the dying child, for the family, and for health care professionals involved in the care. Although the primary focus of this skill is the dying child, many of the principles are applicable in situations of unexpected death, e.g., an accident.

### NURSING DIAGNOSES

Anxiety related to unmet informational needs about dying process or perceived threat of death; Grieving (anticipatory or dysfunctional) related to perceived or actual loss of life; Altered family process related to dying child; Parental powerlessness related to inability to prevent child's death; Spiritual distress related to crisis of death.

| Steps | Rationale |
|---|---|
| **Assessment** | |
| 1. Examine attitude and comfort level in functioning in a role that will require caring for a dying child. | Health professionals' feelings and attitudes help determine whether their actions are perceived as helpful or unhelpful by the child and family. Helpful actions are related to a helpful attitude, which includes some aspect of caring and involvement (Jost and Haase, 1989). The child and family will need a quiet, caring person who can be available to them. |
| 2. Assess the child for the presence of pain (see Skill 52) and other physical complications. | If the child is in pain or physical discomfort, any attempts at psychosocial intervention with the child or family will be ineffective. |
| 3. Explore the child's understanding of the condition. | Knowledge of the child's understanding facilitates appropriate and effective intervention. |

### *CHILDRENS' PERCEPTION OF DEATH*

**INFANTS AND TODDLERS**

Sleep-wake patterns and "peek-a-boo" games reflect infant awareness of existence and nonexistence. Infants become very dependent and bonded to primary caregiver (usually mother) and cry or fuss when she moves out of their line of vision; loss is the absence of this security, her person. The parent's grief will key the infant to sad circumstances.

**3- TO 5-YEAR-OLDS**

Experience death as a departure or sleep, but it is not irreversible; some bodily processes go on in death, e.g., eating, breathing, hearing (Nagy, 1948). The child knows himself or herself as living and therefore views the world in a state of livingness, which includes lifeless objects and dead people.

**5- TO 8-YEAR-OLDS**

Personify death—often viewed as a frightening clown, angel, or someone who has already died, but "if you run fast enough and lock the door you may be able to beat it" (Nagy, 1948). The child's impression of death in this stage is a composite of contradictory paradoxes surrounded by the unknown (Miya, 1972).

**9-YEAR-OLDS**

By this age a child understands that death is a final, inevitable, irreversible fact (Nagy, 1948).

**ADOLESCENTS**

This is the most difficult of *all* age groups to face death. Adolescents waver between experiencing a sense of total invulnerability to having a catastrophic sense of doom. It is also a time when concern about body image is at its height.

| **Steps** | **Rationale** |
|---|---|
| a. Determine the child's age and developmental level. | Knowledge of age and developmental level provides a starting point for predicting the child's perception and understanding of death (see box above) (McCown, 1988). |
| b. Determine what the child has been told about the condition.<br>▪ Check chart for documentation of verbal or written communication with child or family about child's condition and prognosis.<br>▪ Ask parents what they have told child. | In trying to protect the child from additional emotional distress, parents and health care providers may withhold information, which results in the child filling in the gaps with fantasy thinking. When unrealistic assurances of physical healing and wellness are expressed to the dying child by the family or health professionals, the child becomes isolated from those who normally are the source of emotional support and comfort.<br>***Special Considerations:*** *Many children are altruistic enough to participate in this game of deception to protect loved ones from further pain. The child quickly learns that it is not okay to express real feelings. The bond of trust is thus broken; the high cost for the dying child is emotional isolation.* |
| c. Be alert for verbal and nonverbal clues of the child's understanding of the condition, which may range from themes of life returning to normal to death and dying. | Children will frequently make comments about death or use the theme in play. Comments of play may also reflect unrealistic expectations. |
| d. Look for magical thinking in the child's explanations of what is happening. | Children engage in magical thinking and believe their thoughts influence the external world. This thinking pattern makes them vulnerable to guilt and fears regarding their part in the death (McCown, 1988).<br>***Special Considerations:*** *The child's behavior, e.g., angry outbursts, may also be an indicator of his or her understanding.* |
| 4. Assess the effect of the child's condition on other members of the family. | A child's death or dying constitutes a crisis for all members of the family. "Survivor guilt" (feeling somehow responsible for the death of another) is common on some level to each family member. |
| a. Marital dyad. Consider the following questions for parents:<br>▪ "How has your child's illness affected your relationship?" | The marital relationship is frequently dysfunctional with the dying of a child. Feelings of guilt, shock, blame, anger, and sadness may be projected onto the spouse. |

| Steps | Rationale |
|---|---|
| ▪ "When was the last happy time you spent together as a couple?"<br>▪ "How does your wife/husband handle stress?"<br>▪ "Who usually gets the most upset?"<br>▪ "Where do you find the greatest source of comfort and support?" | ***Special Considerations:*** *The child represents a love object that unifies the parents and makes them feel a part of each other through the child. The loss of a child reactivates earlier disappointments or losses in the parents' lives, which affects the relationship to each other and to other key people (Sanders, 1989). The mother may experience guilt over not having protected the child enough or for having erred in some way during her pregnancy. Both parents may feel robbed of their future, angry at the forces that did this, and extremely impotent (powerless) to protect their child. Fathers, particularly, will often try to regain a sense of control by spending more time at their jobs, which is frequently interpreted as insensitivity to the child's condition.* |
| b. Siblings (see Skill 20). | Siblings of a dying child have been described as having behavior problems, e.g., school difficulties, somatic complaints, enuresis, nightmares, loneliness, depression, clinging, crying, confusion, antisocial behavior, and jealousy (McCown, 1988). With the child's death, siblings may feel their own guilt for having survived when their dead sibling did not. If a long illness has preceded the death, they probably have resented the attention their sick sibling received. If the atmosphere remains tense and hostile, it will be difficult for surviving siblings to sort out their involvement in the situation (Sanders, 1989). |
| c. Grandparents. | Grandparents may experience a double grief reaction: the loss of their grandchild and perhaps the loss of their own child who is immersed in grief. Grandparents also grieve for their own child's pain. The grandparents' own grief may render them unavailable as a resource to support the child and parents. |
| 5. Examine child's and family's previous experiences with death and dying. | Negative experiences may be generalized by the child and family. For example, a dying uncle may have experienced a great deal of pain, and the child and family anticipate the same circumstances for the child. |
| 6. Assess for any cultural or religious implications for the meaning and treatment of the dying (see Skill 41). | Cultural and ethnic heritage are significant factors in shaping the child's and family's view of death and dying. Certain religions have practices necessary at the time of death or after the death has occurred. |
| 7. Assess the family's ability to discern the need for inclusion or exclusion of those outside the immediate family. Check with the family to see who has been significant in the child's life. If the parents are resistant to having these individuals visit, stress the need for facilitating their grieving process by having some closure with the child. | In situations of impending death, parents may be unaware of the needs of others and their grief. Grandparents, relatives, significant friends, teachers, and others who need to say "goodbye" may be isolated from the child by the parents' need to "protect" the child from further stress. The child, too, may have a need to see these significant others. Conversely, parents may be unable to discern or may exclude less significant persons, further stressing themselves and the child. |
| 8. Assess process of faith development in the child (see Skill 42). | Faith is a source of strength for many children. An awareness of the child's developmental conception of faith assists in providing appropriate and effective support. |
| 9. Assess the spiritual needs of child and family (see Skill 42). | The experience of grief and loss frequently gives rise to existential thought and questions of faith and belief.<br>***Special Considerations:*** *If the clergy is not a part of the family support, the availability of appropriate resources may need to be offered. This can include a referral for a clergyperson.* |

## Planning and Goal Setting

| Steps | Rationale |
|---|---|
| 1. Establish a relationship with child and parents. | Health care professionals who have established a relationship with the family are best suited for relaying information concerning any change in the child's status (Hall, Hardin, and Conaster, 1982). |
| 2. Develop nursing goals of care:<br>▪ To provide physical and emotional support for the child.<br>▪ To provide emotional support for the family, including attention to siblings. | |

**Steps** | **Rationale**

- To educate the family regarding the dying process when death is expected.
- To educate the family and facilitate their grieving process.
- To provide the opportunity for emotional and spiritual growth for the entire family and the health care professional.

## Implementation

### *The child*

1. Meet the child's need for physical comfort.
   a. Provide pain relief.
   b. Address other physical symptoms, nausea, vomiting, constipation, diarrhea, mouth care.
   c. Provide a clean, dry environment free of noxious odors.

   Physical comfort facilitates a less stressful period of time in which grieving can be a priority.

   d. Encourage parents and siblings to provide physical care for the child at their level of comfort.

   Feelings of helplessness and powerlessness are often lessened when parents assume their natural nurturing and caregiving role. Such ministrations help fill the parents' and siblings' need to "do something," and are comforting to the child. Caring for a loved one is a great facilitator for productive grief work.

2. Truthfully disclose facts when asked: gear communication and interventions to child's cognitive level; answer only what is asked, adhering strictly to the belief system of the child's family in matters of faith.

   Being truthful with the child establishes a trusting relationship and provides the information needed for the child's adaptation to dying.

   ***Special Considerations:*** *Withholding information often gives rise to magical thinking as the child tries to fill in the informational gaps. Truthful explanation of what is happening will help eliminate the need for magical thinking.*

3. Allow the child to grieve: provide the security needed for the process to occur; do not deny the child's feelings or disallow grief; be present to the emotional pain; make appropriate statements such as "You must feel very sad" or "I'll sit here with you" (see Skill 12).

   Permitting the grieving process validates the child's feelings and further strengthens the therapeutic relationship.

4. Model appropriate grieving behavior; do not be afraid to show sadness.

   Modeling appropriate grieving behavior gives child permission to express feelings.

   ***Special Considerations:*** *Tears are appropriate when sad; do not be afraid to let the child witness tears; a hug at this time can often open communication with the child, enabling the child to share emotional pain.*

5. Use humor or lighthearted play appropriately.

   The appropriate use of humor or play is not disrespectful, but rather can allow the child a temporary escape from the burden of facing death. It can allow the child to feel normal, if only for a few moments (Hinds, Martin, and Vogel, 1987; and Carosella, 1986).

6. Recognize that the grief of children may be evidenced only intermittently.

   Lack of observable grieving behavior does not indicate that grieving is failing to occur; children's inner feelings are not always conveyed by external behavior (Rando, 1984).

7. Use play and art therapy whenever possible (see Skill 16). Frequently, even the very sick, young child will want to draw a picture with pencil or crayons.

   Much of the young child's grief will be expressed through play, acting out behaviors, or artistic creation.

   ***Special Considerations:*** *Attempt to understand the symbolic messages that are conveyed through these mediums (Rando, 1984).*

8. Help the child feel secure by assisting in identifying feelings and avoiding excessive changes in the routine or environment.

   Identification of feelings is the first step in dealing with them. Consistency is critical for the child whose world is diminishing.

   a. Maintain the same health professionals in the child's routine care.
   b. Maintain the same schedule for treatments, baths, etc.
   c. Be alert for signs of restlessness or agitation in the child.

   The child will often become restless or agitated if equilibrium is disturbed.

   ***Special Considerations:*** *Note if there have been new or different visitors or if there is a disturbance between family members. Stress to the family that the child who appears to be sleeping may yet be aware of tension and discord.*

| Steps | Rationale |
|---|---|
| 9. Work with the parents to arrange visits from significant people in the child's life (grandparents, school friends, teacher, neighbors). | Children suffer from separation from people to whom they have been connected (Rando, 1984).<br>***Special Considerations:*** *It may be desirable to talk with visitors before seeing the child to prepare them for any physical changes in the child and to offer suggestions on how they might relate best to the child.* |
| 10. Be creative, imaginative, and flexible in regard to the child's hospitalization; encourage the family to bring in favorite objects or foods from home, or pets. For example, Carosella (1986) reported immeasurable benefit to a dying child when a visit was arranged from "Ronald McDonald," the boy's favorite character (see Skill 18). | It is important to create as comfortable and homelike an atmosphere as possible. Normalizing the environment provides the child and family with comfort and a much needed sense of control. |
| 11. Encourage the continuation of schoolwork and craft activities as long as possible. | The potential for human growth continues up until the time of death; these activities also provide a sense of accomplishment. |
| ***The parents*** | |
| 1. Support the natural nurturing role of parents by involving them in the child's physical care as much as possible. Teach them bedside nursing functions as appropriate. | Maintaining their natural caregiving role offers parents a much needed sense of control in a situation where little control exists. Parents need to feel that they are doing everything possible for their child. Their physical involvement is also beneficial for the child.<br>***Special Considerations:*** *Be sensitive not to "compete" with the parents for the child's attention and affection. Most parents are grateful for the loving attention to their child, but some may feel threatened.* |
| 2. Support the parents by facilitating their closeness with the child (see box on following page). | Parents begin the grieving process before the actual death of their child.<br>***Special Considerations:*** *In a crisis such as awaiting inevitable death, grief stricken parents often feel extremely helpless and become immobilized.* |
| 3. Keep parents informed of their child's condition and treatments. | Insufficient information can interfere with grieving (Jost and Haase, 1989). Information regarding the child's condition and treatments offers parents the opportunity to make informed decisions and to feel that everything possible is being done for their child.<br>***Special Considerations:*** *It is often argued that parents of seriously ill or injured children are too anxious to participate in the decision-making process. Most parents can actively participate with adequate information and support (Thompson, 1989).* |
| ***Siblings*** | |
| 1. Encourage the siblings to ask questions and express feelings (see Skill 20). | Siblings, like the dying child, may have incomplete or inaccurate information regarding their brother's or sister's condition. Discussion provides an opportunity to dispel misconceptions and deal with feelings. |
| 2. Encourage the parents to include siblings in their activities and ministrations with the dying child. | Parents are often hesitant or forget to include the other children in the family at the time of death. |
| 3. Arrange or assist parents to arrange for a warm, empathetic person to help care for each sibling. Possible resources include a favorite relative, family friend, or neighbor. | Consistency is a very important part of the sibling's feeling nurtured and secure while parents are preoccupied with the dying child. |
| 4. Assist family in informing significant others in the sibling's life of what is happening (teachers, coaches, friends) (McCown, 1988). | As important support resources for siblings, significant others need an explanation for likely behavioral changes in siblings, e.g., somatic complaints, difficulties with concentration, daydreaming, and changes in eating habits.<br>***Special Considerations:*** *Behavioral changes are a concomitant mechanism of a child's grief but may seem inappropriate to adults. It is one of the ways their grief is experienced and expressed (Fox, 1985).* |

## *STRATEGIES FOR SUPPORTING THE PARENTS OF THE DYING CHILD*

**DO**

1. Give them permission to cry with the child and siblings.
   Rationale: This behavior provides good modeling with the other children for appropriate expression of feelings of grief. It also enables the child to express feelings more openly as many children, even young ones, will try to protect their parents from emotional pain, particularly if they (the parents) always maintain a false sense of cheerfulness around the child, telling the child he or she is getting better; this behavior only further isolates the child.
2. Be a quiet listening presence in the room.
   Rationale: Being present but unobtrusive is a source of strength to the parents at this time; nonverbal communication can be a powerful tool. Careful listening and observation will enable the formulation of appropriate interventions with the family after death has occurred.
3. Use physical touch: a hand on the arm, holding a hand, arm around the shoulder, or a hug.
   Rationale: Touching can convey caring, compassion, concern, acceptance, and understanding far more poignantly than words in this situation.
4. Encourage the parents to touch or hold their child; provide a rocking chair or comfortable chair if they would like to do this; if the child cannot be moved from the bed because of equipment, remove side rails and place chairs close to the child, or a parent may want to lie beside the child.
   Rationale: This enables them to have better closure with their child: they who brought this child into the world can see him or her out; this also facilitates grief.
5. Offer the parents the opportunity to bathe their child.
   Rationale: This can provide a ritual of closure for the parents with their child; this permits them to do something physical, providing comfort while touching and tending to the child.
6. Encourage them to talk to the child even if he or she appears comatose.
   Rationale: It is thought that hearing is the last sense to go. Their verbal reassurance to their child will also reinforce their feelings of being able to help in some way.
7. Validate humor; give the parents permission to laugh.
   Rationale: Humor can be a very therapeutic coping mechanism for all at this time.
8. Encourage the parents to take an active part in the decision making regarding their child's treatment at this time.
   Rationale: Assist them in processing the value of routine treatments when the child is clearly dying, e.g., the drawing of blood specimens, nebulizer treatments, physiotherapy.
9. Encourage the parents to make the necessary funeral plans and arrangements in advance. Plan a service that can be a legacy from the child to the living. Reassure parents that planning the service will not make death occur.
   Rationale: The numbness after the death occurs can be debilitating to the parents.
10. Encourage the parents to consider talking with a professional counselor or their clergy at some point after the death.
    Rationale: Husbands and wives frequently have very different ways of expressing their grief after the death of a child; this may lead to a breakdown in communication, feelings of alienation, or a rupture in the family.
11. Allow for spiritual exploration and growth; ask if a chaplain or other clergy would be helpful at this time.
    Rationale: Death raises many existential and spiritual questions.
12. Encourage the parents to attend support groups, e.g., Compassionate Friends or Candlelighters.
    Rationale: There is comfort in being in the company of parents who have shared the same experience and are still able to go on with their lives.

**DO NOT**

1. Try to cheer up the parents or the child.
   Rationale: They have a legitimate right to be sad and depressed.
2. Expect the parents to be logical or objective.
   Rationale: Emotions and feelings are at an all-time high; feedback gently given will often enable them to process enough to make the necessary decisions sensibly.
3. Impose personal spiritual or philosophical beliefs that are contrary to those of the family at this time of extreme vulnerability.
   Rationale: It is important to support their basic belief system and to encourage them to draw whatever strength they can from it at this time of life crisis.
4. Offer platitudes such as "God only gives his crosses to those he loves." "It's for the best, he was suffering so." "You're lucky to have other children."
   Rationale: All of these sayings are empty words to the grieving parent and only engender feelings of rage. If they ask "Why?" they really aren't looking for a response. They are just reacting to their feelings of hopelessness and helplessness.

| **Steps** | **Rationale** |
|---|---|
| 5. Encourage sibling inclusion in the grieving process, e.g., share knowledge about the illness and death and facilitate the sharing of feelings. | Parents need to keep siblings apprised of the child's changing status so they may prepare themselves; to withhold information regarding the child's condition often gives rise to feelings of jealousy and anger towards the excessive attention and gifts received from parents, other family members, and friends. When death is acknowledged as a possible outcome, the family can share their grief, thus providing siblings the opportunity to acquire coping skills, which will enhance their ability to manage future grief experiences (Miya, 1972). When death is acknowledged, spiritual resources may be mobilized for comfort, strength, and peace. |
| ***Grandparents*** | |
| 1. Keep grandparents apprised of any changes in the child's condition. Do not assume that they have access to this information through their children. Empathy can be conveyed through a hug, a touch, or just attentive physical presence. | Acknowledging the grandparents' feelings for the child and recognizing their place in the family can facilitate their grieving process.<br>***Special Considerations:*** *These same guidelines apply for other close family members and friends.* |
| **Facilitating Grieving After Death** | |
| 1. Review circumstances of death. | |
| a. Expected or unexpected. | When a child dies suddenly, parents may experience more guilt, a prolonged period of numbness and shock, intense loneliness and emptiness, anxious fear that someone else will die, and intense anger at those responsible for the injury (Miles and Perry, 1985). When the death is expected over a long period of time, the opportunity exists to complete all "unfinished business," e.g., helping the child and siblings understand and cope with a fatal prognosis. Unexpected death, e.g., an accident or suicide, deprives survivors of time to prepare and begin the grief process. Under these circumstances, families often experience intense guilt and remorse for not having done something additional or different with the child (Whaley and Wong, 1991). |
| b. Whether or not family members were present at time of death and their understanding of the event. | Notification of death is an event that is remembered vividly. If family members were not present, they will likely know less about the circumstances surrounding the death than when they are present. To facilitate grieving, parents need adequate information, including the cause of death, an explanation of treatments or tests performed in an effort to save the child, and information about the child's mental state at the time of death (Jost and Haase, 1989). Parents should also be informed of any measures used to relieve discomfort or pain. |
| 2. Clean the child and the room (see box on following page). | It is important for their future grieving process that the family remember their last moments with the child as ones in which the child appears comfortable and peaceful. |
| 3. Sit quietly with the family and allow them to express their feelings. | The death of a child elicits strong emotions. Providing the opportunity to ventilate feelings facilitates the grieving process. |
| a. Allow them the safety of expressing any frustration or anger at deities, medical person, etc., but do not assume that all anger is displaced. | Anger and rage are normal expressions of grief in the face of what appears to be injustice. Although much anger may be displaced, sometimes it may be justified regarding errors in the management of the child or with attitudes of caregivers. |
| b. Do not try to answer the "Why's?". | This is a natural expression of grief and just deserves to be heard. |
| c. Do not offer platitudes or praise at this time. | It is impossible to ventilate pain and rage when being told one is handling things well or doing a wonderful job. |
| d. Do not be afraid to weep with the parents. | It is often very comforting for family to know caregivers deeply cared for their child and how much their pain and loss is felt. |
| e. Do not suggest they should be grateful if they have other children. | Human beings are individuals with a unique personality, characteristics, and qualities that are not interchangeable. Death ends a life, not a relationship. |
| f. Reassure the parents that they made the best decisions possible for their child's care. | "What if's?" only result in feelings of frustration and guilt. |

## *SENSITIVE AFTERCARE*

The final moments family members spend with the child after death will be remembered most vividly in the weeks and months to follow. It is important to make this time as peaceful as possible. Sensitive aftercare can be a very therapeutic process for the family.

1. Offer parents the opportunity to bathe their child with warm water. This procedure can be an effective ritual for the facilitation of grief. Symbolically, parents were given the washed child as he entered the world and now they are bathing and returning their charge.
2. If they decline, provide the care as they wait outside the room.
3. Place the child in a fresh gown, comb the hair, freshen the bed, using colored sheets and spread if available.
4. Check before removing medical lines and equipment. In some instances, e.g., if there is to be an autopsy or the case is to be reviewed by the medical examiner, lines and medical equipment must remain in place to comply with local laws. If that is the case, change soiled tapes, clamp tubes, and conceal equipment with sheets.
5. Raise the head of the bed slightly, side rails down, place hands outside the covers alongside the body; close the eyes if necessary with gentle pressure for several seconds.
6. If the mouth gapes, place the body in a semi-sitting position. Place a tightly rolled face cloth, a roll of tape, or a pill bottle under the chin to keep the mouth closed. Conceal with a small towel across the neck and shoulders.
7. Use subdued lighting rather than harsh ceiling lights.
8. Place chairs by the bed so the family may sit by the child's body.
9. Suggest holding the child, perhaps in a rocking chair, or lying on the bed next to the child.
10. Stay with the family until they feel more comfortable with the body, then allow privacy.
11. Do not rush this "leave-taking" experience. The family should have unlimited time alone with the child.

| **Steps** | **Rationale** |
|---|---|
| 4. Offer specific information, suggestions, and choices to the family. | Parents frequently feel numb and immobilized at the time of death and are unable to ask for what they need (Jost and Haase, 1989). |
| a. Assist the family in identifying and contacting a friend, relative, or other support person. | The death of one's child is probably the most devastating life experience any parent will ever have. Never assume any parent will be able to manage his or her grief alone. Because of their own intense grief and need for support, couples may not be able to support each other at the time of death (Jost and Haase, 1989). |
| b. Suggest inviting clergy to assist the family, if desired. If clergy has not been present during the dying process, ask if the family would like one called. | Spiritual support is vital to many families' sense of peace regarding death. |
| c. Encourage family to view their child's body, clearly explaining the procedure and what to expect. | Viewing the body provides a sense of closure. Parents who choose not to view the body frequently express regret at a later time (Jost and Haase, 1989).<br>***Special Considerations:*** *Offer the choice again later if the parents initially refuse. Their feelings may change after some time for introspection.* |
| d. Clearly explain requests for autopsy or organ donation, the procedures, and any papers requiring signatures. Use words such as "options" or "choices" to reiterate that the decision is theirs and no pressure will be applied. | Parents need adequate information to make informed decisions that may provide answers to pressing questions (e.g., the cause of death) or offer comfort in the knowledge that their child has helped another child. Health professionals often avoid discussing these options with families out of fear of upsetting them. |
| e. Explain that there will probably be a period of time that they will feel extremely empty and devoid of feelings and that this experience is often protracted in mothers (Wong, 1980). Feelings eventually do return, but it may be many months and it is important that they be patient with themselves and with one another. Stress that grief is a process that must be addressed. It can be postponed, but not put off indefinitely. | After the death of a child the grieving process is slow and long; it is often a year or more before the parents can begin to experience more normal living without such intense pain.<br>***Special Considerations:*** *Fish (1986) found that grief of mothers was more intense after 2 years than it was in the beginning and it did not taper off until after 5 years. For fathers, the same rise in intensity was present up to 2 years, but with a steady tapering after that. Rando (1983) reported that bereaved parents whose children died of cancer actually had intensified grief during the third year. There is often a vast underestimation of the length of time it takes to survive the death of a child (Sanders, 1989).* |

| Steps | Rationale |
|---|---|
| f. Suggest seeking marriage or family counseling with a mental health professional or clergy in a month or two. | The death of a child places a great deal of stress on most marriages. |
| g. Make parents aware that the siblings of the deceased child will need some special attention. Offer to talk to the siblings or to be present when parents talk to them. | In addition to their grief, siblings may have feelings of guilt over their imagined contribution to the death, or anguish over their feelings of jealousy towards the child and the attention he or she received. |
| h. Ask parents' permission to contact Compassionate Friends, a support group for parents who have lost a child (see Product References and Teaching Resources). | Parent-to-parent support from someone who has shared a similar experience, e.g., the death of a child has been identified as a significant and inexpensive resource to supplement or even prevent the need for professional mental health services (Madara, 1986). |
| i. Give family the names of recommended books and other literature for coping with grief (see Product References and Teaching Resources). | Information about the grieving process provides families with guidelines on what to expect, which helps validate feelings and dispel fears. |
| 5. Let the family spend as much time with child's body as they need, then assist them with packing and personally escort them to their car. | This is a very traumatic time for the family; they will be experiencing many mixed emotions as they leave the hospital. At this juncture, the health care professional is the caring link between the world of medicine and their child's death and the empty world in which they must now live. |

| Evaluation Outcomes | Observational Guidelines |
|---|---|
| 1. Child is free of pain and comfortable. | Facial expressions and body appear relaxed. Child states he or she is comfortable. Vital signs are consistent with pain-free state. |
| 2. Child expresses feelings freely and appropriately. | Child can speak at times of pending death; expresses sadness and joy. The small child can give and receive affection. |
| 3. Family members express feelings freely and appropriately. | Family members can speak at times of the child's pending death; express sadness and joy. Family members, including siblings, speak and interact freely with each other and give and receive affection with the child and other family members. |
| 4. Family members understand the expected course of dying for their child. | Parents recognize and relate signs and symptoms of changes in the child's condition. Parents use this information to guide their actions with the child, other family members, and significant others, e.g., inviting the child's teacher to visit to say goodbye. |
| 5. Child and family have a basic understanding of the grieving process. | Child and family can identify and relate feelings such as anger or guilt as part of the grieving process and cope with these feelings appropriately, e.g., crying when sad. |
| 6. Survivors (family members and health professionals) grow emotionally or spiritually. | Healthy methods, e.g., talking about feelings, are chosen to cope with stresses in life. Unhealthy methods, e.g., alcohol abuse, are abandoned. Survivors reach out to help others, e.g., start support groups. |

## Documentation

Document all information, verbal or written, given to the child or family on the patient's chart. Interventions and the child's or family members' reaction should be documented. Feedback from child and family regarding referrals to self-help groups should also be noted.

## Home Care Modifications

Some families choose to care for their dying child at home. With appropriate systems and support in place, the child and family can be comfortable with the decision. Parents need answers to the following questions (Jones, 1985):

1. How will the child die?
2. Whom should they contact if help is needed during the day, at night, or on weekends?
3. Can they manage alone or will help be needed from any health care professionals?
4. Is there a local hospice organization that can help them make arrangements and offer support?
5. How can their family best provide the necessary nursing care?
6. How can they best provide for the child's daily nurturing care?
   Consider:
   - Equipment
   - Bedding
   - Toileting
   - Bathing
   - Hair care
   - Mouth care
   - Eye care
   - Massage
   - Food and liquid
7. What medical care does the child need?

# *SKILL* 22 Facilitating Adjustment to Divorce

*Deborah Kay Brantly*

It is projected that one third to one half of marriages in the United States that began in the 70s will end in divorce. Divorce creates the need to adjust to new family roles (with new and perhaps different individual responsibilities), new living arrangements for some (or all) family members, and the entry of parental dating or stepparents. It is estimated that 6.5 million children live in stepfamilies (Skeen, Covi, and Robinson, 1985), which necessitates an alteration in societal norms.

Adjustment to divorce and loss of family as the child knows it is a grieving process, and, as such, precipitates feelings of denial, guilt, anxiety, anger, and depression. Children typically must redefine love, marriage, and the family. Psychosomatic problems may develop as a result of anxiety and stress, e.g., stomachaches, headaches, dizziness, muscle aches and pains, as well as an increased occurrence of accidents, susceptibility to infectious disease (Ludder-Jackson and Runyon, 1983), school problems, and social problems.

## NURSING DIAGNOSES

Altered family processes related to loss of family member due to divorce; Ineffective individual coping related to perceived loss of parent, unrealistic reconciliation expectations, or inadequate coping method; Anxiety related to change in family role functioning or interaction patterns; Grieving related to loss of noncustodial parent.

| Steps | Rationale |
|---|---|
| **Assessment** | |
| 1. Determine age, gender, cultural background, and developmental level of the child. | These factors influence the child's response to the divorce and help guide planning and implementation. For example, preschool-age children most often experience a heightened fear of abandonment (Rossiter, 1988). Younger school-age children have a tendency to act out behaviorally as a response to parental divorce; adolescents tend to become depressed (Siemon, 1978) (Table 22-1). Differences in the effects of divorce according to gender have also been noted. Although studies are controversial, Zaslow (1988) finds that while males tend to show immediate effects of the divorce, females may be more adversely affected in the long run, especially when the custodial mother remarries. |
| 2. Assess the child's current level of stress and previous experience with crises and coping abilities. | Children who have successfully coped with crises in the past can use that experience to enhance present coping, although coping may be less effective if the child has multiple stressors. ***Special Considerations:*** *The child who has experienced or is experiencing a divorce may be afraid of situations that would lead to a loss of a parent (Frischman, 1989).* |
| 3. Assess the child and family's support resources and use of these resources. | Support systems may diminish with divorce as family members and friends "may have difficulty maintaining relationships with both partners" (Ludder-Jackson and Runyon, 1983) or new support systems may be gained. |
| 4. Construct a family genogram (see Skill 38). | Genograms graphically identify when divorce (and other related problems) become a multigenerational family pattern. |
| a. Family constellation (including extended family). | Determining family constellation defines the family. |
| b. Previous divorces in the family. | Multiple family divorces may lead to increased family stress. |
| c. Physical or mental illness since the separation or divorce. | Families that have experienced divorce are more susceptible to physical and mental illness, e.g., physical complaints, infections, and accidental injuries (Ludder-Jackson and Runyon, 1983). ***Special Considerations:*** *Children with chronic conditions may have exacerbation of the illness from the stress and anxiety of a divorce (Ludder-Jackson and Runyon, 1983).* |

***TABLE 22-1*** Potential Developmental Responses to Divorce

| Age | Responses |
|---|---|
| Infant/Toddler | ▪ Increased irritability, whining, tantrums<br>▪ Difficulty separating<br>▪ Fear of abandonment<br>▪ Frightened and confused |
| Preschool (3-5 years of age) | ▪ Low self-esteem<br>▪ Sadness<br>▪ Denial of divorce (e.g., indicates both parents are in the home)<br>▪ Clinging to parent (especially remaining parent) and excessively tearful departures<br>▪ Developmental regression (e.g., loss of feeding skills or bowel and bladder control)<br>▪ Aggression toward peers, siblings<br>▪ Nightmares and other sleeping disorders (e.g., fear of the dark and sleeping alone)<br>▪ Temper tantrums and other misbehavior<br>▪ Fighting with siblings for attention<br>▪ Blaming self for loss of noncustodial parent<br>▪ Idealization of noncustodial parent<br>▪ Intense reunion fantasies<br>▪ Complaints of stomachache, headache<br>▪ Increase in accidental injuries |
| School-age (6-11 years of age) | ▪ Profound depression, fear, and insecurities<br>▪ Feelings of deprivation—loss of parent, attention, money, security<br>▪ Loss of appetite<br>▪ Increase in psychosomatic complaints, frequent illnesses, greater risk of accidental injury<br>▪ Preoccupation with parental health/activities (fear of abandonment)<br>▪ Placing blame on custodial parent for loss of noncustodial parent<br>▪ Divided loyalties<br>▪ Ashamed of parental behavior<br>▪ Intense desire for reconciliation<br>▪ Decreased interest in play activities<br>▪ School phobia, diminished school performance, or difficulty concentrating in school (day-dreaming)<br>▪ Domination of younger children<br>▪ Aggression and fighting<br>▪ Altered peer relationships—become bossy, demanding, manipulative |
| Adolescent | ▪ Withdraw from family and friends<br>▪ Intense anger at one or both parents<br>▪ Worry over finances<br>▪ Regression to childhood activities<br>▪ Profound sense of loss<br>▪ Inconsistent attendance at school<br>▪ Increased time spent with peers, or increase in conflicts with peers, or a change in peer group<br>▪ Substance abuse<br>▪ Aberrant behavior, e.g., lying, stealing<br>▪ Initiation of or increase in sexual activity<br>▪ Feelings of anxiety concerning family members |

| Steps | Rationale |
|---|---|
| 5. Determine when divorce is to occur or length of time since divorce. | The more recent or impending the divorce, the more it may be experienced as a crisis. Less recent divorces with lingering problems require a more in-depth assessment. |
| 6. Assess the manner in which the divorce is proceeding or has occurred.<br>a. Planned or impulsive.<br>b. Presence or absence of expressions of anger, guilt and blame.<br>c. Pursued through litigation or mediation.<br>d. Child to testify. | Divorce is more stressful for the child when it is impulsive or characterized by guilt, anger, or blame. Divorces pursued through prolonged litigation have been identified as more potentially damaging (Koopman and Hunt, 1988), especially when the child has been involved in the litigation.<br>***Special Considerations:*** *If the child has yet to be involved in court proceedings, it would be important tp assist the parents in preparing the child for the court experience or obtaining a child advocate.* |

| Steps | Rationale |
|---|---|
| 7. Assess the child's feelings and perceptions of the divorce.<br>a. What the child has been told.<br>b. Feelings the child has expressed.<br>c. Verbal or nonverbal indicators of difficulties and misperceptions, e.g., the child may think the noncustodial parent no longer loves him or her.<br>d. Feelings of responsibility.<br>e. Feelings of anger, fear, depression, grief or abandonment (e.g., ask "How do you feel about your parents' divorce?" or "Other children have said they feel angry or sad when their parents got a divorce. Have you felt that way?").<br>f. Hopes for reconciliation (reconstruction fantasy) (e.g., ask "Have you ever wished mom and dad would get married again?"). | Many parents feel inadequate to discuss the divorce with their child and may only tell the child the divorce is occurring, without discussing the reason for the divorce and how it will affect the child's life. The distress that the parents feel can prevent them from effectively coping and facilitating resolution of their child's anger or grief.<br>***Special Considerations:*** *Interview the parent(s) and child separately and together, if possible. This allows them to identify real feelings and provides information about their interactions. Ask the parents what emotions the child has revealed to them, and then assess the child's current feelings.* |
| 8. Determine custody and visitation rights/desires of the noncustodial parent, stepparents, grandparents, and other members of the noncustodial parent's family.<br>a. Custody rights.<br>b. Restraining orders.<br>c. Previous involvement with the child.<br>d. Wishes of the custodial parent.<br>e. Wishes of the child. | Custody and visitation rights may limit the noncustodial parent's interaction with the child. Stepparents, although usually not under legal constraints, may or may not desire visitation. All states have some provisions for grandparent visitation.<br>***Special Considerations:*** *In the case of joint custody, the parents share legal custody and make decisions jointly. Visitation can be especially complicated when the child is hospitalized. It is important to know the custody laws of the state. When parental arguing occurs in the hospital, it can cause undue stress on the child and affect progress. Some solutions to this problem have been: monitoring visits; setting limits on the parents, e.g., parents agree to not argue in front of the child and restrict negative comments about the absent partner; and scheduling visits to avoid parental conflictual interaction (Coucouvanis and Solomons, 1983).* |
| 9. Discuss actual involvement of the noncustodial parent (visitation).<br>a. Frequency of visits, phone calls, participation in school events and extracurricular activities.<br>b. Where visits occur.<br>c. Relationship of the child with noncustodial parent.<br>d. Feelings that visits elicit, e.g., greater feelings of loss, sadness, confusion, satisfaction, or joy. | Furstenberg et al (1983) noted that in divorced families in which the mother was the custodial parent only one out of three children saw their (noncustodial) father at least once each month. Frequent contact with the noncustodial father seems especially beneficial to sons (Zaslow, 1988).<br>***Special Considerations:*** *Since the noncustodial parent sees the child less often, it is tempting to make the outings fun and special. In this artificial environment, the relationship may become viewed one-dimensionally and the child may perceive one parent as fun (and good) and the other parent as demanding and no fun (and bad).* |
| 10. Determine the effect the divorce has had on daily living tasks and roles.<br>a. Parental roles and responsibilities.<br>b. Child's and sibling's roles and responsibilities.<br>c. Living and sleeping arrangements.<br>d. Financial status.<br>e. School attendance. | Changing from a two-parent to a one-parent family usually increases the custodial parent's responsibilities, increasing parental loneliness and altering family roles. The child may have additional household responsibilities and changes in interactional patterns to decrease parental loneliness. Frequently, children are allowed to sleep with the custodial parent. |
| 11. Determine the effects of the parent's reentry into dating or remarriage on the child.<br>a. What child has been told.<br>b. Child's relationship with dating partner or stepparent.<br>c. Child's feelings/perceptions regarding parent's sexuality.<br>d. Role and responsibilities of stepparent. | Children often maintain the reconstruction fantasy in which they envision their parents reuniting. When dating begins or stepparents enter the picture, this fantasy is threatened. Children who continue to cling to this fantasy, remain fearful of being abandoned by the custodial parent, or who have a strong identification with the absent parent are more likely to have problems when one or both parents remarry (Skeen, Covi, and Robinson, 1985).<br>***Special Considerations:*** *Older children and adolescents are less prone to accept a stepparent than are younger aged children (Skeen, Covi, and Robinson, 1985).* |
| 12. Assess the family's economic resources.<br>a. Custodial parent income.<br>b. Child support payments awarded/received.<br>c. Other sources (e.g., Social Security). | Economic difficulties are common for the custodial parent because of a decrease in overall income and a decrease in spendable income (because of an increase in financial responsibilities), while the noncustodial parent's spendable income may increase. Collection of child support payments may be unpredictable and difficult to obtain. |

| Steps | Rationale |
|---|---|

## Planning and Goal Setting

1. Gather needed materials for intervention, e.g., play materials, pamphlets, resource information, book lists (see Product References and Teaching Resources), handouts or telephone numbers of assisting agencies, paper and pen for recording of information.

Gathering play materials before intervention decreases interruptions.

***Special Considerations:*** *Younger children may respond best to play therapy.*

2. Develop individualized client and family goals:
   - To effectively cope with divorce.
   - To facilitate the process of grieving the loss of the family as an intact unit.

## Implementation

1. Further explore the child's feelings and perceptions of the divorce.
   a. Meaning of love, divorce, or other ideas the child may be hearing (e.g., ask, "Some children tell me they don't understand how someone can stop loving another person. Have you felt like this?").
   b. Cause of the divorce (e.g., ask, "Have you ever thought it was your fault your parents divorced?" or "Many children tell me they think the divorce was their fault. How do you feel?").
   c. Finality of the divorce (see also Step 6).
   d. Feelings such as anger, hurt, or grief.

Allowing the child the opportunity to discuss feelings and questions about foundational issues, e.g., love and marriage, offers ventilation of feelings and identifies where perception and reality are incongruent.

***Special Considerations:*** *Younger children will best respond to play and storytelling, e.g., use a doll family to reenact aspects of the divorce and ask the child how different dolls feel.*

2. Encourage the child to identify his or her feelings about the divorce as normal (e.g., say, "Many children whose parents are divorced feel sad and angry at their parents" or "Your feelings are important and OK to talk about").

Defining common feelings as normal relieves the child's fears and helps to decrease feelings of isolation.

3. Supply the older child with reading materials written by children of their age who have been through a divorce (see Product References and Teaching Resources).

Reading materials further reassure the child that his or her feelings and perceptions are normal and felt by others. If reading materials express situations that are coped with effectively, it provides the child with hope of doing the same.

***Special Considerations:*** *Younger children or children with developmental delay need resources appropriate to their level of comprehension.*

4. Assure the child the divorce was not his or her fault.

Preschoolers especially feel they caused the divorce and may feel guilty or attempt to make up for past wrongs in hope that the noncustodial parent will return.

***Special Considerations:*** *The younger child needs simple explanations of the divorce, coupled with frequent reassurance that both parents will continue loving him or her. The school-age child and adolescent will require more explanation, with references to events or problems the child may remember, e.g., specific arguments the parents may have had (Ludder-Jackson and Runyon, 1983).*

5. If not already done, encourage each parent to talk separately with the child to:
   a. Discuss the reason for the divorce with the child.
   b. Allow for expression of the child's feelings.
   c. Reassure the child of continued love and care.
   d. Discuss the impact of the divorce on the family, e.g., living and custody arrangements.

The child has limited understanding of marriage, love, and divorce. The child frequently will feel that if the parents could divorce one another, they might abandon him or her.

6. Discuss any reconstruction fantasies with the child.
   a. Contents of the fantasy.
   b. Actions the child may have already taken.
   c. Reality of parents' reuniting.

Reconciliation (also called reunion or reconstruction) of the marriage is a universal fantasy as the child wishes for the former sense of perceived security and stability. Sometimes this fantasy is acted out and the child spends energy trying to reunite the parents, either on a conscious level, e.g., by sending gifts to one parent from the other (Ludder-Jackson and Runyon, 1983), or on an unconscious level, e.g., by developing an illness.

7. Validate that the child and family are experiencing a loss and are grieving.

Understanding assures the child that his or her feelings and experiences are a natural part of the grieving process.

***Special Considerations:*** *For the family who sustained abuse by the noncustodial parent, the family may express relief.*

| Steps | Rationale |
|---|---|
| 8. Encourage the child to cry, if needed, and express feelings to a support person. | Crying and expressing feelings facilitate resolution of grief. Expressing feelings freely to a support person outside the family provides an important emotional outlet. |
| 9. Discuss the child's part in litigation disputes.<br>a. Feelings about the litigation and being (or having been) a witness.<br>b. If proceedings are pending, teaching or observation of court proceedings or meeting the judge before the trial may help. | Children may be involved in the litigation dispute, causing feelings of fear and confusion. Testifying against a parent or being asked to choose between parents may produce an internal conflict of feeling disloyal to the other parent. |
| 10. Discuss multigenerational patterns with the parent(s) and perceived causes (e.g., ask, "Have you noticed there are several divorces in your family?"). | Frequently, multigenerational patterns are maintained subconsciously. Bringing this to the attention of the parent gives them the option of seeking solutions to stop destructive patterns. |
| 11. Assist the parent in defining the child's roles and responsibilities developmentally (e.g., performing chores the child can master, while maintaining time for age-appropriate play, school activities or homework; avoiding treating the child as a peer). | Defining new roles of the child in an age-appropriate manner maintains the child's developmental integrity and prevents the child from being expected to take on adult roles left vacant by the noncustodial parent (e.g., confidante, supplying emotional support, financial advisor, or doing housework or yardwork). |
| 12. Encourage the custodial parent to find mature emotional support primarily from other adults. | When the custodial parent finds emotional support from other adults, generational boundaries and satisfactory emotional resolution are maintained. |
| 13. Encourage redefinition or strengthening of the child's relationships with the noncustodial parent, relatives, grandparents, and stepparents.<br>a. Encourage visits, special outings, and overnight stays.<br>b. Encourage shared mutual interests/hobbies.<br>c. Encourage letter writing and telephone conversations. | Continuation and modification of relationships reassure the child that abandonment will not occur.<br>***Special Considerations:*** *If the noncustodial parent or other relatives are not available for visitation, do not respond to the child's requests, or do not follow through on committments over a period of time, suggest seeking alternative role substitutes. Consider the need to refer to counseling for resolution of feelings of abandonment. It may be necessary to encourage other relationships, e.g., aunts, uncles, or cousins.* |
| 14. Encourage stepfamilies to clearly define realistic family roles and responsibilities as well as allow time for bonding to occur. Educate the stepfamily on the six stages stepfamilies typically go through (Frischman, 1989).<br>a. Friendship—a time for getting acquainted.<br>b. Honeymoon—few problems exist and there is excitement over the new family.<br>c. Disillusionment—flaws are exposed and family members have unmet expectations.<br>d. Crisis—explosions of feelings occur; children may run away.<br>e. Decision-making—time to reevaluate relationships, roles, etc.<br>f. Equilibrium—new relationships are established and harmony/balance exists in the home. | A strong bond usually develops between the child and custodial parent while in the single parent stage. Although normal, this bond may be resistant to the integration of a stepparent (Reutter and Strang, 1986). Stepfamilies immediately are faced with "dual-family membership, lack of common history, instant multiple relationships, and lack of norms and societal support" (Reutter and Strang, 1986). Issues of loyalty, degree of involvement of ex-spouse, stepsibling relationships, and parenting responsibilities of stepparent to stepchildren are common sources of difficulties when families unite. Integration of stepfamilies often takes about 4 years (Frischman, 1989). |
| 15. Refer the child/family to divorce groups and resources for support (see Product References and Teaching Resources). | Support groups offer an inexpensive and effective means of help for the child and family. |
| 16. Encourage parents to identify needs to outside agencies, e.g., schools to send records or invitations to both sets of parents or include stepparents and noncustodial parents when making Father's Day or Mother's Day cards. | Society's inability to respond to the needs of the child whose parents have divorced may contribute to his or her feeling different (Skeen, Covi, and Robinson, 1985). Parents then have the responsibility to inform those persons/systems that affect the child about his or her needs if the child is to optimally cope with the divorce. |

| Evaluation Outcomes | Observational Guidelines |
|---|---|
| 1. The child's perceptions about the divorce are identified. | The child expresses feelings, fantasies, and misunderstandings about the divorce. |
| 2. The child and significant family members have redefined and established new role relationships or maintained established relationships. | The child discusses contact with noncustodial parent, grandparents, and stepparents and expresses satisfaction with the visits. Plans are discussed to redefine relationships, when needed. |
| 3. The child's roles and responsibilities are developmentally appropriate. | Interview the child/family as to home responsibilities and allowances for play time. Observe the parent-child interaction for behaviors appropriate to parenting rather than a peer relationship. |

| Steps | Rationale |
|---|---|
| 4. Child progresses to the stage of acceptance in the grieving of the intact family. | The child reports acceptance of the divorce or play behaviors about family suggest greater comfort with the divorce. Ask the child whether reconciliation fantasies continue to occur. |

## Documentation

Document age, gender, developmental level, and culture of the child. Document information obtained on the family genogram. Describe when the divorce occurred or is to occur, the child's knowledge and response to the divorce, the manner in which the proceedings are occurring/occurred, and the child's participation in the divorce proceedings. Describe the feelings the child has about the divorce, misunderstandings and questions he or she may have, and reconstruction fantasies. Describe involvement of the noncustodial parent, grandparents, and stepparent. Document the child's response to changing roles. Describe the parent's response to the child's questions/need for information. Document reading material given or referred to the child/family. Describe plans to redefine and enhance relationships.

Unit II

**PRODUCT REFERENCES AND TEACHING RESOURCES**

**Books**

Baznik D: Becky's story, Washington, DC, 1981, Association for the Care of Children's Health.
A book that encourages young siblings of hospitalized children to explore and understand their own reactions, needs, and emotions.

Boegehold B: Daddy doesn't live here anymore, New York, 1985, Golden Book.

Bozarth-Campbell A: Life is goodbye life is hello; grieving well through all kinds of loss. Minneapolis, 1982, CompCare Publications.

Brogan J and Maiden U: The kid's guide to divorce, New York, 1986, Ballantine Books.

Burkhart, Linda I
R.D. 1, Box 124
Millvilla, PA 17846
Homemade battery powered toys & educational devices for severely handicapped children
More homemade battery devices for severely handicapped children with suggested ideas

Derrick S, Bachman K, and Parder S: Hospitalized children play and play activities. Lake Mills, Iowa, 1982, Graphic Publishing Company, Inc.

Disabled Guests Guide Book
Guest Letters Department
Walt Disney World
P.O. Box 40
Lake Buena Vista, FL 32830
(305) 824-8009
Gives information about wheelchair access and answers questions concerning accommodations for the sight and hearing impaired and disabled guests who are planning to visit the theme park in Florida.

Eberle B and Stanish R: CPS for kids: A resource book for teaching creative problem-solving to children. Buffalo, 1980, DOK Publishers.

Especially Grandparents
2230 Eighth Avenue
Seattle, WA 98121
A unique quarterly newsletter written for and by grandparents of children with special needs. Each eight-page issue is full of articles, ideas, resources, and stories to help grandparents better understand their grandchild's special needs and enrich relationships with grandchild and his or her parents.

Fassler D, Lash M, and Blakeslee I: Changing families: A guide for kids and grown-ups. Burlington, Vt, 1988, Waterfront Books.

Featherstone H: A difference in the family life with a disabled child. New York, 1980, Penguin.

Gardner R: The boys and girls book about divorce. New York, 1985, Bantam Books.

Goodson B and Bronson M: Which toy for which child, Washington, DC, 1985, U.S. Consumer Product Safety Commission.

Hazel R et al: A community approach to an integrated service system for children with special needs, Baltimore, 1988, Paul H Brookes.

Hendricks S and Willis R: The centering book: awareness activities for children, parents and teachers. Englewood Cliffs, NJ, 1975, Prentice-Hall.

Kushner H: When bad things happen to good people, New York, 1981, Avon Books.

Madera E: How to ideas for developing groups. In Madera E, and Meese A editors: The self-help sourcebook: finding and forming mutual self-help groups. Danville, NJ, 1986, New Jersey Self-help Clearinghouse.

Meyer DJ and Vadasy PF: Grandparent Workshops, Seattle, 1987, University of Washington Press.
For information on this handbook, contact University of Washington Press-Seattle at 1-800-441-4115.

Meyer D, Vadasy P, and Fewell R: A handbook for implementing workshops for siblings of children with special needs, Seattle, 1985, University of Washington Press.

Nathanson M: Organizing and maintaining support groups for parents of children with chronic illness and handicapping conditions, Washington, DC, 1986, The Association for the Care of Children's Health.

Parents Guide to Accredited Camps
The American Camping Association
Bradford Woods
5000 State Road 67 North
Martinsville, IN 46151
1-800-428-CAMP

In addition to noting traditional camps that have facilities for children with special needs, the guide has a listing of "special clientele" camps under the following headings: Blind, Communicably Limited, Deaf, Diabetic, Emotionally Disturbed, Epileptic, General Physical Disabilities, Hemophilia, Learning Disabled, Mentally Retarded, Mobility Restricted, Overweight, and Wheelchair Bound. The book is available at most libraries, many bookstores, or may be purchased from the American Camping Association.

For information about other camps, contact local or national organizations serving children with specific diseases or disabilities.

Rappaport L: Recipes for fun, Washington, DC, 1986, Let's Play to Grow.

Rogers F and O'Brien C: How to break the news: Mister Rogers talks about kids and divorce, Working Mother, 9(3):95-99, 1986.

Schiff HS: The bereaved parent. New York, 1977, Penguin Books.

Simon R: After the tears. New York, 1985, Harcourt Brace Jovanovich.

*The Ultimate Rejection*
Survivors of Suicide
Suicide Prevention Center, Inc.
184 Salem Avenue
Dayton, OH 45406

**Products**

Direct Selection or Scanning Communication Devices
Canon Corporation
One Canon Plaza
Lake Success, NY 11042
(516) 488-6700

Prentke Romich Co
1022 Heyl Road
Wooster, OH 44691
1-800-642-8255

ZYGO Industries Inc
PO Box 1008
Portland, OR 97207-1008
(503) 684-6006

**Organizations**

Alinda Press
PO Box 553
Eureka, CA 95501
(707) 443-2510

Alinda Press produces a Code Book that illustrates many signs that are needed during a hospital stay.

Compassionate Friends, Inc.
PO Box 3696
Oak Brook, IL 60522
(312) 990-0010

Family Friends Project
Box 1214, Cardinal Station
620 Michigan Ave, NE
Washington, DC 20064
(202) 635-5949

A unique intergenerational project that uses senior citizen volunteers to work one-on-one with children with chronic illnesses and disabling conditions and their families.

Federation for Children with Special Needs
95 Berkeley Street
Boston, MA 02116
(617) 482-2915

The Federation is involved in the Collaboration Among Parents and (Health) Professionals (CAPP) project, which is designed to increase and encourage parent involvement in the health care of their children who have a chronic illness or disability while promoting parent/professional partnerships.

National Easter Seal Society
70 E. Lake St
Chicago, IL 60601
(312) 726-6200

General information provided about camps and recreational activities for children with special needs.

National Information System & Clearinghouse
Center for Developmental Disabilities
1244 Blossom Street, 5th Floor
Columbia, SC 29208
(803) 777-4435

National Information System is a computerized data base of information about specialized services available to children with developmental disabilities and special health care needs. National Information Clearinghouse provides information about services available to families and medically fragile infants with disabilities. For either service call 1-800-922-9234 or in South Carolina call 1-800-922-1107.

Sibling Information Network
Connecticut's University Affiliated Program on Developmental Disabilities
991 Main Street
East Hartford, CT 06108
(203) 282-7050

The Sibling Information Network is an organization for those interested in the welfare of persons with disabilities and their families, including siblings, parents, special education teachers, social workers, psychologists, physicians, nurses, journalists, program administrators, and counselors. The Network publishes a quarterly newsletter that often includes a special fun page for siblings. The group is a clearinghouse of information, ideas, projects, literature, and research regarding siblings and other issues related to the needs of families with disabled members.

For additional information, audiovisual material and program information about a particular group of siblings, contact an association that serves the needs of the sibling's brother or sister.

Special Olympics
1350 New York Avenue, NW
Suite 500
Washington, DC 20005
(202) 628-3630

The Alexander Graham Bell Association for the Deaf
3417 Volta Place, NW
Washington, DC 20007
(202) 337-5220

The Association for the Care of Children's Health
7910 Woodmont Ave
Bethesda, MD 20814
(301) 654-6549

Offers literature, videos, and consultative services.

Provides *Ideas for activities with hospitalized children.* 1982. Suggestions for games, activities, hospital play, cooking, and outpatient projects. For use in hospitals, schools, and at home.

Also offers *Activities for children with special needs.* 1986. Activities for children, including children with limited use of extremities, restricted trunk movement, traction, limited sight and hearing, and respiratory problems.

The Candlelighters Foundation
1312 18th Street NW
Suite 200
Washington, DC 20036

The Candlelighters Foundation offers a list of camp programs serving children with cancer and/or their siblings.

The National Association of the Deaf
814 Thayer Avenue
Silver Spring, MD 20910
(301) 587-1788

The National Resource Library on Youth with Disabilities
1-800-333-NCYD or (612) 626-2825.

Brings together comprehensive sources of information related to adolescents, disability, and transition.

Very Special Arts (Formerly National Committee/Arts for the Handicapped)
Education Office
The John F. Kennedy Center for the Performing Arts
Washington, DC 20566
(202) 662-8899

## REFERENCES


Adams P and Fras I: Beginning child psychiatry, New York, 1988, Brunner/Mazel.

Aguilera D and Messick J: Crisis intervention: theory and methodology ed 5, St Louis, 1986, The CV Mosby Co.

American Academy of Pediatrics: Hospital care of children and youth, Elk Grove Village, Ill, 1986, American Academy of Pediatrics.

Anderson B: Parents of children with disabilities as collaborators in health care, part one. Coalition Quarterly 4(2):3-4, 1985.

Anderson B: Parents of children with disabilities as collaborators in health care, part two, Coalition Quarterly 4(3):15-18, 1985.

Association for the Care of Children's Health: Position statement on critical care of children, Washington, DC, 1980, Association for the Care of Children's Health.

Association for the Care of Children's Health: Guidelines for adolescent units, Washington, DC, 1981, Association for the Care of Children's Health.

Bahrick I: Intermodal learning in infancy: learning on the basis of two kinds of invariant relations in audible and visible events, Child Dev 59:197-209, 1988.

Bank S and Kahn M: Sisterhood-brotherhood is powerful: sibling subsystems and family therapy, Family Process 14(3):311-317, 1975.

Bellack J and Fore C: The young child in the critical care unit. In Fore C and Poster EC, editors: Meeting psychosocial needs of children and families in health care, Washington, DC, 1985, Association for the Care of Children's Health.

Betts G: Development of the emotional and social needs of gifted individuals, J Counsel Dev 64:587-589, 1986.

Betz C: The pediatric patient: strategies for improving interactions . . . community nurse practitioners, Home Health Nurse 3(4):11-17, 1985.

Betz C and Poster E: Incorporating play into the care of the hospitalized child, Issues Comp Pediatr Nurs 7:343-355, 1984.

Blackburn A: Support for the caregiver (workshop), Brookhaven Hospital, Tulsa, Okla, March, 1988.

Bolig R: The diversity and complexity of play in health care settings, Children's Health Care 16(3):132-133, 1988.

Bonitatibus G: Comprehension monitoring and apprehension of literal meaning, Child Dev 59:60-70, 1988.

Bullock D and Thompson B: Guidelines for family interviewing and brief therapy by the family physician, J Fam Pract 9(5):837-841, 1979.

Cairns N et al: Adaptation of siblings to childhood malignancy, J Pediatr 95(3):484-487, 1979.

Camps for children with disabilities: making the right choice for your child, Chicago, 1990, National Easter Seal Society.

Caplan G: An approach to community mental health, New York, 1961, Grune & Stratton Inc.

Carosella L: Send in the clown: a reminder, MCN 11(3):148-149, 1986.

Cassidy J: Child-mother attachment and the self in six-year-olds, Child Dev 59:121-134, 1988.

Caty S, Ritchie JA, and Ellerton ML: Helping hospitalized preschoolers manage stressful situations: the mother's role, Children's Health Care 18(4):202-209, 1989.

Chan JM: Preparation for procedures and surgery through play, Paediatrician 9:210-219, 1980.

Clatworthy S: Therapeutic play: effects on hospitalized children, Children's Health Care 9(4):10-13, 1981.

Coburn J and Manderino M: Stress inoculation: an illustration of coping skills training, Rehab Nurs 11(1): 14-17, 1986.

Cotanch P, Hockenberry M, and Herman S: Self-hypnosis as antiemetic therapy in children receiving chemotherapy, Oncol Nurs Forum 12(4):41-46, 1985.

Coucouvanis J and Solomons H: Handling complicated visitation problems of hospitalized children, MCN 8:131-134, 1983.

Curran B: Divorce in clinical practice, J Fam Pract 12(3):471-476, 1981.

Derrick S, Bachman K, and Parder S: Hospitalized children play and play activities, Lake Mills, Iowa, 1982, Graphic Publishing Company, Inc.

DiMotto JW: Relax, Am J Nurs 84(6):754-758, 1984.

DiPietro L and Knight C: When your patient is deaf, Prof Med Assist 19(1):6-16, 1986.

Dixon J: Effect of nursing interventions on nutritional and performance status in cancer patients . . . nutritional supplementation and relaxation training, Nurs Res 33(6):330-335, 1984.

Donnelly G: Imaginative play and the physically disabled child, Hol Nurs Prac 2(2):81-88, 1988.

Drotar D and Bush M: Mental health issues and services. In Hobbs N and Perrin JM, editors: Meeting psychosocial needs of children with chronic illness, San Francisco, 1985, Jossey-Bass Inc, Publishers.

Dunst C, Trivette D, and Deal A: Enabling and empowering families, Cambridge, Mass, 1988, Brookline Books.

Duvall E: Marriage and family development, ed 5, New York, 1977, JB Lippincott Co.

Faber A and Mazlish E: How to talk so kids will listen and listen so kids will talk, New York, 1982, Avon Books.

Field M: Teaching interviewing skills: a three function model, Dimens Crit Care Nurs 6(5):304-312, 1987.

Fish WG: Difference in grief intensity in bereaved parents. In Rando TA, editor: Parental loss of a child, Champaign, Ill, 1986, Research Press.

Fisher J, Nadler A, and Whitcher-Alagna S: Four theoretical approaches for conceptualizing reactions to aid. In Fisher JD, Nadler A, and DePaule BM, editors: New directions in helping: recipient reactions to aid, vol 1, New York, 1983, Academic Press.

Fox SS: Good grief: helping groups of children when a friend dies, Boston, 1985, New England Association for the Education of Young Children.

Frischman D: Talk on stepfamilies. Presented at NAPNAP Conference, Orlando, Fla, March 1989.

Furstenberg F et al: The life course of children of divorce: marital disruption and parental contact, American Sociological Review 48:656-668, 1983.

Gabel S: The draw a story game: an aid in understanding and working with children, The Arts in Psychotherapy 11:187-196, 1984.

Gallo A: The special sibling relationship in chronic illness and disability: parental communication with well siblings, Hol Nurs Pract 2(2):28-37, 1988.

Gibbons M and Boren H: Stress reduction: a spectrum of strategies in pediatric oncology nursing, Nurs Clin North Am 20(1):83-103, 1985.

Gibbons MD: When the dying patient is a child: the challenge for living. In Hockenberry MD and Coody DK, editors: Pediatric oncology and hematology, St Louis, 1986, The CV Mosby Co.

Gillis J: Child anxiety scale manual, Champaign, Ill, 1980, Institute for Personality and Ability Testing.

Goldberger J: Issue-specific play with infants and toddlers in hospitals: rationale and intervention, Children's Health Care 16(3):134-141, 1988.

Golden D: Play therapy for hospitalized children. In Schaefer C and O'Conner K, editors: Handbook of play therapy, New York, 1987, John Wiley & Sons.

Goodson B and Bronson M: Which toy for which child, Washington, DC, 1985, US Consumer Product Safety Commission.

Gottfried A: Intrinsic motivation for play. In Brown C and Gottfried AW, editors: Pediatric round table 13: infant stimulation, Skillman, NY, 1985, Johnson & Johnson Baby Products.

Griffin M: In the mind's eye . . . value of imagery, Am J Nurs 86(7):804-806, 1986.

Griffin W, Ling I, and Staley D: Stress management groups . . . relaxation training in a psychiatric outpatient setting, J Psychosoc Ment Health Nurs 23(10):31-35, 1985.

Gustafson M: Ideas for activities with hospitalized children. Washington, DC, 1982, Association for the Care of Children's Health.

Haber J et al: Comprehensive psychiatric nursing, ed 3, New York, 1987, McGraw-Hill Book Co.

Hahn K: Therapeutic storytelling: Helping children learn and cope, Pediatr Nurs 13(3):175-178, 1987.

Hall M: Using relaxation imagery with children with malignancies: a developmental perspective, Am J Clin Hypn 25(2-3):143-149, 1982-1983.

Hall M, Hardin K, and Conatser C: The challenges of psychosocial care. In Fochtman D and Foley GV, editors: Nursing care of the child with cancer, Boston, 1982, Little, Brown and Company.

Hall SS and Weatherly KS: Using sign language with tracheotomized infants and children, Pediatr Nurs 15(4):362-367, 1989.

Heineken J and Roberts F: Confirming, not disconfirming: communicating in a more positive manner, MCN 8:78-80, 1983.

Hillenberg J and Collins F: A procedural analysis and review of relaxation training research, Behav Res Ther 20:251-260, 1982.

Hinds PS, Martin J, and Vogel RJ: Nursing strategies to influence adolescent hopefulness during oncologic illness, J Assoc Pediatr Oncol Nurs 4(1-2):14-22, 1987.

Hines J: Only five minutes! nurse-patient communications, MCN 5: 271-274, 1980.

Hobbie C: Relaxation techniques for children and young people, J Pediatr Health Care 3(2):83-87, 1989.

Hockenberry M and Bologna-Vaughan S: Preparation for intrusive procedures using noninvasive techniques in children with cancer: state of the art vs. new trends, Cancer Nurs 8(2):97-102, 1985.

Holmes T and Rahe R: The social readjustment rating scale, J Psychosom Res, 11:213-218, 1967.

Honsigner M, Yorkston K, and Dowden P: Communication options for intubated patients, Resp Man 17(3):45-52, 1989.

Jacobson E: Progressive relaxation, Chicago, 1938, University of Chicago Press.

Jolly H: Play and the sick child, Lancet 2:1286-1287, 1968.

Jones M: Home care for the chronically ill or disabled child, New York, 1985, Harper & Row Publishers, Inc.

Jost K and Haase J: At the time of death: help for the child's parents, Children's Health Care 18(3):146-152, 1989.

Junge M: The book about daddy dying: a preventive art therapy technique to help families deal with the death of a family member, Art Therapy 2(1):4-10, 1985.

Klein D: I.C.U.: It's also the intensive communication unit, Nursing Life, 6(1):46-47, 1986.

Koeppen A: Relaxation training for children, Elementary school guidance and counseling 9(1):14-21, 1974.

Koopman E and Hunt E: Child custody mediation: an interdisciplinary synthesis. Am J Orthopsychiatry, 58(3):379-386, 1988.

Korsch B, Freeman B, and Negrete V: Practical implications of doctor-patient interactions and analysis for pediatric practice, AM J Dis Child 12:110, 1971.

Laker B: Scared siblings, Childtimes, 2(4):16-18, 1988.

Lamontagne L: Effects of relaxation on anxiety in children: implications for coping with stress, Nurs Res 34(5):289-292, 1985.

Larkin D and Zabourek R: Therapeutic storytelling and metaphors, Hol Nurs Pract 2(3):45-53, 1988.

Larsen K and Smith C: Assessment of nonverbal communication in the patient-physician interview, J Fam Pract 12(3):481-488, 1981.

Lavigne J and Ryan M: Psychologic adjustments of siblings of children with chronic illness, Pediatrics 63:616, 1979.

Ledbetter B: Needle play must reflect current public health issues, Children's Health Care 16(3):216-217, 1988.

Lee J and Fowler M: Merely child's play? Developmental work and playthings, J Pediatr Nurs 1(4):260-270, 1986.

Levenstein A: Updating your communication skills, Nurs Man 17(5):20-21, 1986.

Linn S: Puppet therapy in hospitals: helping children cope, J Am Med Wom Assoc, 33(2):61-65, 1978.

Ludder-Jackson P and Runyon N: Caring for children from divorced families, MCN 8:126-131, 1983.

Lynam J and Tenn L: Adolescent communication: understanding its dynamics and fostering its development, Nurs Pap 18(1):67-77, 1986.

Lynam M: The parent network in pediatric oncology, Cancer Nurs 10(4):207-216, 1987.

Lynn M: Pediatric nurs practitioner-patient interactions: a study of the process, J Pediatr Nurs 2(4):268-271, 1987.

Madara E: How-to ideas for developing groups. In Madara E and Meese A, editors: The self-help sourcebook: finding and forming mutual aid self-help groups, Danville, NJ, 1986, New Jersey Self-help Clearinghouse.

Magrab P: Psychosocial development of chronically ill children. In Hobbs N and Perrin JM, editors: Issues in the care of children with chronic illness, San Francisco, 1985, Jossey-Bass Inc, Publishers.

McCown DE: When children face death in a family, J Pediatr Health Care 2:14-19, 1988.

McCue K: Medical play: an expanded perspective, Children's Health Care 16(3):157-161, 1988.

McGinnis J: A communication lapboard, Resp Therapy 16(2):37, 1986.

McHale SM, Simeonsson RJ, and Sloan JL: Children with handicapped brothers and sisters. In Schopler E, and Mesibov B, editors: The effects of autism on the family, New York, 1984, Plenum.

McKeever PL: Siblings of chronically ill children: a literature review with implications for research and practice, Am J Orthopsychiatry, 53:109-218, 1983.

Meer P: Using play therapy in outpatient settings, MCN 10(6):378-380, 1985.

Miles M and Perry K: Parental responses to sudden accidental death of a child, Crit Care Quarterly 8(1):73, 1985.

Miller S: Promoting self-esteem in the hospitalized adolescent: clinical interventions, Issues Comp Pediatr Nurs 10:187-194, 1987.

Miller T and Jay L: Cognitive-behavioral and pharmaceutical approaches to sensory pain management, Top Clin Nurs 6(4):34-43, 1985.

Minuchin S et al: A conceptual model of psychosomatic illness in children, Arch Gen Psychiatry 32:1031-1038, 1975.

Miya TM: The child's perception of death, Nurs Forum 11(2):214-220, 1972.

Moore AC: Crisis intervention: a care plan for families of hospitalized children, Pediatr Nurs 15(3):234-236, 1989.

Morain-Baker C: Personal communication, Oklahoma City, Okla, Nov 1, 1988.

Morley W, Messick J, and Aguilera D: Crisis: paradigms of intervention, J Psych Nurs 5:537, 1967.

Moses K: Keynote address. The 19th annual conference of the Association for the Care of Children's Health, Houston, May 1984.

Mundy P et al: Nonverbal communication skills in Down syndrome children, Child Dev 59:235-249, 1988.

Nagy M: Child's theories concerning death, J Genet Psychol 73:3-27, 1948.

Nickerson E: Art as a play therapeutic medium. In Schaefer C and O'Connor K editors, Handbook of play therapy, New York, 1987, John Wiley & Sons.

Norris J: Teaching communication skills: effects of two methods of instruction and selected learner characteristics, J Nurs Ed 25(3):102-106, 1986.

Older J: Touching is healing, New York, 1982, Stein and Day.

Olds R: Enhancing self-esteem through mutual self-disclosure, J School Health, 57(4):160-161, 1987.

Parish L: Communicating with hospitalized children, Can Nurse, 82(1):21-24, 1986.

Pass M and Pass C: Anticipatory guidance for parents of hospitalized children, J Pediatr Nurs 2(4):250-258, 1987.

Pendleton R and Leishman T: Techniques for improving communication, Prof Med Assist, 19(1):17-20, 1986.

Peppers G and Knapp R: How to go on living after the death of a baby, Atlanta, 1985, Peachtree Publishers, Ltd.

Perrin E and Gerrity S: There's a demon in your belly: children's understanding of illness, Pediatrics 67(6):841-849, 1981.

Petix M: Explaining death to school age children, Pediatr Nurs 13(6):394-396, 1987.

Petrillo J: Your patients hear you but do they understand? RN 39:37-39, 1976.

Petrillo M and Sanger S: Emotional care of hospitalized children: an environmental approach, ed 2, Philadelphia, 1980, JB Lippincott Co.

Powell TH and Ogle PA: Brothers and sisters: a special part of exceptional families, Baltimore, 1985, Paul H Brookes.

Pratt A et al: Psychological parameters of chemotherapy-induced conditioned nausea and vomiting: a review, Cancer Nurs 7(6):483-490, 1984.

Rando TA: Investigation of grief and adaptation in parents whose children have died from cancer, J Pediatr Psychol 8:3-20, 1983.

Rando TA: Grief, dying and death: clinical interventions for caregivers, Champaign, Ill, 1984, Research Press.

Raynor C and Maderino M: Color your life: an assessment and treatment strategy for children, J Child Adolesc Psych Ment Health Nurs 2(2):48-51, 1989.

Reutter L and Strang V: Yours, mine and ours: stepparents and their children, MCN, 11:265-266, 1986.

Riffee D: Self-esteem changes in hospitalized school-age children, Nurs Res 30(2):94-97, 1981.

Roche M: A very special status, Sibling Information Network Newsletter 5(4):1-3, 1987.

Romanezuk A: Helping the stepparent parent, MCN 12:106-110, 1987.

Rossiter A: A model for group intervention with preschool children experiencing separation and divorce, Am J Orthopsychiatry, 58(3):387-396, 1988.

Rothery S: Understanding and supporting special siblings, J Pediatr Health Care, 1(1):21-25, 1987.

Ruddy-Wallace M: Temperament: assessing individual differences in hospitalized children, J Pediatr Nurs 2(1):30-36, 1987.

Rutter M: Stress, coping, and development: some issues and some questions. In Garmezy N and Rutter M, editors: Stress, coping and development in children, New York, 1983, McGraw Hill Book Company.

Sanders CM: Grief: The mourning after, New York, 1989, John Wiley & Sons, Inc.

Scott D, et al: Comparative trial of clinical relaxation and an antiemetic drug regiment in reducing chemotherapy-related nausea and vomiting, Cancer Nurs 9(4):178-187, 1986.

Selig A and Selig E: The need for a family orientation. In Thorton S and Frankenburg W, editors: Child health care communications, Skillman, NJ, 1983, Johnson & Johnson.

Shelton T, Jeppson E, and Johnson B: Family-centered care for children with special health care needs, Washington, DC, 1987, Association for the Care of Children's Health.

Siemon M: Mental Health and school-age children, MCN 3(4):211-213, 1978.

Skeen P, Covi R, and Robinson B: Stepfamilies: a review of the literature with suggestions for practitioners, J Counsel Dev 64:121-125, 1985.

Sourkes B: Siblings of the child with a life threatening illness, Feelings and their Medical Significance 28(5):19-24, 1986.

Spinetta J: The sibling of the child with cancer. In Spinetta JJ and Deasy-Spinetta P, editors: Living with childhood cancer, St Louis, 1981, The CV Mosby Co.

Stanford T: Breaking the silence, Emergency 18(8):38-41, 1986.

Stapleton C and Yahraes H: The importance of play. In Caring about kids, Washington, DC, 1978, US Department of Health and Human Services.

Stein M: Interviewing in a pediatric setting. In Dixon S and Stein M, editors: Encounters with children: pediatric behavior and development, Chicago, 1987, Year Book Medical Publishers, Inc.

Stein REK: Home care: a challenging opportunity, Children's Health Care 14(2):90-95, 1985.

Steiner P: The well child and the hospitalized disabled sibling, J Psychosoc Nurs Ment Health Serv 22(3):23-26, 1984.

Stuifbergen A: The impact of chronic illness on families, Fam Comm Health 9(4):43-51, 1987.

Tesler M et al: Coping strategies of children in pain, Issues Comp Pediatr Nurs 5:351-359, 1981.

Thomas A and Chess S: Temperament and development, New York, 1977, Brunner/Mazel, Inc.

Thompson J: Guiding parent and professionals through the maze of ethical decisions. Paper presented at Pediatric nursing conference: Focus for the 90's, Philadelphia, Sept 23, 1989.

Thuma-Rew S, Cigrand K, and Corwin D: Switched on fun for the recuperating child. Presented at the 24th annual conference of the Association for the Care of Children's Health, Houston, May 1984.

Titlebaum H: Relaxation, Hol Nurs Pract 2(3):17-25, 1988.

Trahd G: Siblings of chronically ill children: helping them cope, Pediatr Nurs 12(3):191-193, 1986.

Vadasy P: Grandparents of children with special needs: supports especially for grandparents, Children's Health Care 16(1):21-23, 1987.

Vessey J, Care of the hospitalized child with a cognitive developmental delay, Hol Nurs Pract 2(2):48-54, 1988.

Vipperman J and Rager P: Childhood coping: how nurses can help, Pediatr Nurs 6(2):11-18, 1980.

Wallerstein J and Kelly J: Surviving the breakup: how children and parents cope with divorce, New York, 1980, Basic Books.

Wells N and Anderson B; Collaboration among parents and health professionals (CAPP) project, Boston, 1988, Federation for Children with Special Needs.

Whaley L and Wong D: Effective communication strategies for pediatric practice, Pediatr Nurs 11(6):429-432, 1985.

Whaley LF and Wong DL: Nursing care of infants and children, ed 4, St Louis, 1991, The CV Mosby Co.

Willison B and Masson R: The role of touch in therapy: an adjunct to communication, J Counsel Dev 64:497-500, 1986.

Wong D: Bereavement: the empty mother syndrome, MCN 5(6):385-389, 1980.

Wong D and Whaley L: Clinical manual of pediatric nursing, ed 3, St Louis, 1990, The CV Mosby Co.

Wood D: Homeless children: their evaluation and treatment, J Pediatr Health Care 3(4):194-199, 1989.

Wyka G and Caraula A: Stopping push before it comes to shove, Nursing 16(11):44-45, 1986.

Zaslow M: Sex differences in children's response to parental divorce, Am J Orthopsychiatry 58(3):355-377, 1988.

Zinberg N: Elements of the private therapeutic interview, Am J Psych 144 (12):1527-1533, 1987.

# UNIT III Physical and Developmental Assessment

# SKILL 23 Obtaining a Health History

*Nancy Valentine Stevens*

Obtaining a health history is one of the most important aspects of the total health assessment. It provides subjective identification of the presenting problem and gives direction to the physical assessment. The health history delineates possible causes or patterns in health behaviors with information from birth, details of the present event, and pertinent data about family and social history. "Most clinicians feel that about 80% of the information the nurse will use in the assessment process will be discovered during the history taking" with 15% from the physical examination and 5% from the laboratory test results (Alexander and Brown, 1979).

A health history should be obtained on initial visits or encounters with the child, e.g., on admission to an acute care facility, clinic, and on home health visits. On subsequent visits, data may need to be updated, especially if an extended period of time has elapsed. In a crisis or emergency, a complete health history may need to be postponed until a more appropriate time.

## NURSING DIAGNOSES

Health-seeking behaviors (admission/home visit) related to infant/child health promotion/maintenance.

| Steps | Rationale |
|---|---|
| ***Assessment*** | |
| 1. Determine the child's age and cognitive and developmental level, as well as the child's knowledge of health history. | Knowledge of the child's age and functioning level provides a reference point for obtaining the complete history. If the child is not developmentally able, other family members will need to provide or assist with data collection. Even adolescents may need support during the health history taking. |
| 2. Assess child's and family's readiness to discuss history. | If verbal responses are evasive or behaviors indicate unreadiness, the child/family may not give accurate or reliable information. If the child/family is experiencing extreme stress or fatigue, they may be unable to provide necessary information. |
| 3. Assess urgency of the event or of present circumstances. | In an emergency situation, the health history may be delayed until a more opportune time. Although a health history is essential to a thorough nursing assessment and the planning of individualized care, life-threatening situations take priority. |
| 4. Determine existence of any cultural, language, or perceptual barriers (e.g., deafness) (see Skills 13 and 41). | If barriers exist, additional measures will be needed to successfully obtain the health history.<br>***Special Considerations:*** *Barriers can be subtle, especially with cultural factors. For example, evasiveness can be misconstrued as unwillingness to participate, when in actuality the family, because of their cultural background, feels their privacy is being invaded.* |

| Steps | Rationale |
|---|---|
| **Planning and Goal Setting** | |
| 1. Gather needed equipment: writing instruments, paper, and required forms, if any. | Ready availability of needed supplies facilitates efficient data gathering. |
| 2. Provide a setting conducive to interview (see Skill 10). | The proper setting facilitates the child's and family's concentration on the task of providing health data. |
| 3. Identify family members to participate before beginning procedure. | Identification of participants facilitates flow of data collection and direction of interviewing/questioning. |
| 4. If possible, ask participants to obtain or gather documentation, e.g., immunization records, letters or health care records from other professionals. | The availability of health information can facilitate flow and accuracy and save time for the family and nurse. |
| 5. Develop a goal of nursing care:<br>▪ Obtain an accurate and complete health history. | |
| **Implementation** | |
| 1. Explain procedure and purpose to child and family. Assure them that every question asked has some purpose of the child's present and future care (Alexander and Brown, 1979). | Child/family understanding enhances cooperation with the procedure. |
| 2. Obtain identifying information.<br>a. Name.<br>b. Address.<br>c. Telephone number or number where family can be reached.<br>d. Age and birthdate.<br>e. Birthplace.<br>f. Race.<br>g. Sex.<br>h. Religion.<br>i. Nationality.<br>j. Date of interview. | Information provides characteristics and demographic data. Some diseases or disorders are more common in certain geographic areas and among specific races and sexes.<br>***Special Considerations:*** *Additional information may include temporary and permanent address, occupation, and marital status, especially if adolescent.* |
| k. Informant and relation to child (if child is not informant). | The name of the principal person providing information may be needed for clarification in the future. |
| 3. Determine chief complaint (CC).<br>a. Record in the child's or parent's own words. | Identification of the chief complaint establishes the primary or main reason for seeking health care intervention at this time. For example, a routine physical examination, immunizations, or an illness may be the reason for the visit. |
| b. If they have difficulty isolating *one* problem or symptom, ask to state why seeking health care now. | Clarifying the question may help the child/family to focus their thoughts to provide pertinent information.<br>***Special Considerations:*** *Be aware that the stated complaint may be an excuse; an unstated problem may be the real reason for seeking health care.* |
| 4. Review present illness (PI). | A review obtains details related to chief complaint or reason for visit. |
| a. Onset:<br>▪ Date of onset or last day well.<br>▪ Manner of onset: gradual or sudden. | Concentrating on the reason for seeking help this particular day, especially if symptoms have existed for a length of time or multiple problems exist, keeps interview focused. |
| ▪ Related precipitating or predisposing factors, e.g., injury, fatigue, infection, allergens, etc., recorded in chronological order. | Discussion of related factors aids in clarification of the development of problem. |
| b. Characteristics of present illness.<br>▪ Quality, quantity, intensity, and severity of symptoms.<br>▪ Location and radiation of pain, rash, discomfort, disability, etc.<br>▪ Timing—duration, continuous or intermittent, relationship to other events and activities.<br>▪ Factors—related, aggravating, intensifying, relief providing, anything that occurs with problem. | In-depth and specific description of present illness can clarify the problem. Patterns of symptoms and timing in relation to activities and events may aid in differential diagnosis. In addition to providing diagnostic data, this information can guide appropriate intervention. |
| c. Course of problem since onset.<br>▪ Incidence—if single attack, recurrent, occurrence daily, many times a day, continuous, etc.<br>▪ Progress—if better, worse or same.<br>▪ Effects of treatments/medications (prescribed, OTC, and home remedies). | An outline description of pattern and progress of present illness helps identify characteristics. |

| Steps | Rationale |
|---|---|
| 5. Discuss past history (PH). | Historical information will provide a profile of previous health status to correlate with present problems. |
| a. Maternal pregnancies, including date and length, maternal health, medications taken, family response to pregnancy. | Many problems of childhood, especially infancy, can be explained or clarified in the maternal pregnancy. ***Special Considerations:*** *Include prescription and OTC medications, and illicit drugs, including alcohol and tobacco.* |
| b. Labor and delivery data, e.g., duration of labor, type of delivery, place of delivery, medications, anesthesia used. c. Birth information, e.g., Apgar scores, weight, length, time needed to regain birth weight, presence of congenital anomalies, length of nursery stay; if problems, explain nature of and treatment. | The birth history may clarify developmental lags since a child who had problems in the neonatal period, e.g., prematurity or birth asphyxia, may be slower to return to birth weight and to develop in all realms (Steele, 1988). ***Special Considerations:*** *Parents may state that a baby was "normal" at birth but remained in the hospital nursery for 10 days. Such statements require clarification for a full understanding of presenting problems.* |
| d. Feeding in infancy and childhood, including type of feeding, schedule, problems, introduction of solid foods (see Skill 29). | A nutritional history, especially if significant changes are noted, may reveal potential or actual problems. |
| e. Previous illnesses, injuries, or surgeries, including date, course of treatment, complications, as well as emotional/psychological response and circumstances of injury. Include transfusion of blood or blood products, gamma globulin, and serum, e.g., horse serum. | Present illness may be directly or indirectly related to past occurrences, e.g., a limp related to a past fracture or sprain. This information may also identify areas of need for health care/safety teaching (Alexander and Brown, 1979). Identification as a transfusion or serum recipient may explain certain responses at present, e.g., +Coombs, unusual blood factors, or difficulty with typing and crossmatching. |
| f. Allergic responses, including adverse reactions to foods, drugs, etc.; hay fever, asthma, eczema. | Past allergy history may explain present illness, direct treatment, and identify food, medications, or agents that must be avoided. |
| g. Current medications—name, dose, duration, and reason for usage. | The use of medications may affect present treatment and symptoms either beneficially or adversely. For example, OTC cortisone creams may mask a skin infection by suppressing inflammation. |
| h. Immunizations—name, number of doses, ages when given, adverse reaction, if any and treatment. Include tuberculin test and reaction (see Appendix A). | Immunization history identifies role of preventive and necessary health care in family, as well as the level of protection from certain communicable diseases. Tuberculosis is endemic in certain areas of the world and testing is necessary for early identification. |
| i. Growth and development (see Skills 25, 27, and 28). ▪ Weight—at birth, 6 months, 12 months, and present—correlate with height. ▪ Dentition. | This basic information identifies rate of growth and development to allow comparison with established norms. |
| ▪ Age when obtained head control, sat without support, crawled, walked, and spoke first words. | Developmental history may clarify objective tests, e.g., DDST (see Skill 26). |
| ▪ School performance—past, present, and future goals. | School is the child's "work" along with play. This is where much self-worth is established and groundwork for the future is laid. |
| ▪ Interpersonal relationships with family, peers, and adults. | Children are normally social beings; problems identified here may be indicative of severe maladjustment. |
| j. Habits—Include activities of daily living, e.g., sleep patterns, toilet training, and exercise; nail biting; thumb sucking; pica; rituals; temper tantrums; unusual movements or noises, e.g., tics, head banging, rocking; emotional stability; disposition; response to frustration; and use/abuse of caffeine, cigarettes, alcohol, or other drugs. | A description of both healthy and less adaptive habits can reveal a child's activities at home and away, identifying patterns, syndromes, or disease processes, and areas of needed health-care/safety teaching. ***Special Considerations:*** *Although the primary purpose of the interview is to obtain a health history, teachable moments may occur, and the opportunity to provide education and counseling should be taken.* |
| 6. Review of system (ROS)—Explain relevance to present illness. Make statement about each system, e.g., "Mother denies child has had any vomiting or diarrhea since birth." | A review of each body system provides a framework to elicit information concerning present or potential health problems. |
| a. General. May state, "Please, tell me about Johnny's overall health since birth." Include any recent, recurring or unexplained changes in rest, weight, activity, moods, behavior, or infections. | Responses to questions concerning overall general health may be indicative of child's ability to perform activities of daily living and identify possible problems. ***Special Considerations:*** *If sufficient information has been provided in response to earlier questions, this question may be repetitive and could be omitted.* |

| Steps | Rationale |
|---|---|
| b. Integument. Ask if child has had any rashes, itching, acne, tendency to bruise, and what the growth rate of the hair and nails is. | This information assists in identifying the general condition of skin and hair, in addition to changes or problems such as poor nutritional intake. |
| c. Head. Ask if there have been any head injuries (treated or untreated), or headaches. | This line of questioning will assist in eliciting specific information regarding headaches or head injuries. |
| d. Eyes. "Where does Johnny sit to watch TV and in school? Does he seem to rub his eyes a lot?" Ask about specific problems with the eyes; ask whether child reads or writes with head close to material, squints, or holds head in awkward position. Ask date and results of last optic examination. | Responses may identify visual problems, including myopia, blurred vision, crossed eyes, excessive tearing, and availability and use of corrective devices. |
| e. Ears. Discuss earaches and hearing ability. For example, ask "Does the child talk extremely loud, do you need to repeat information, does the child seem to pay attention when someone is talking to him?" Inquire about date and results of auditory tests. | Assessment may identify actual or potential hearing problems. ***Special Considerations:*** *Hearing problems may manifest in speech disorders or delayed speech because of inability to hear correct enunciation or pronunciation, or obtain verbal feedback.* |
| f. Nose. Discuss frequency of the child having runny or stuffy nose, any difficulty breathing through nose, any injuries or nose-bleeds, if the sense of smell seems appropriate, and color, consistency, and frequency of nasal discharge. | Clarification assists in identifying potential, actual, or recurring problems with nasal passages, sinuses, frequent upper respiratory illnesses, or the ability to smell. |
| g. Mouth. Inquire about condition of lips, gums, teeth, mouth odor, and if child is a mouth breather. | Responses elicit information about daily care, eruption history of teeth, frequency and response to dental visits, and toothaches. |
| h. Throat. Discuss usual color, pain, or discomfort when speaking or swallowing, and describe any lesions. | Assessment will help to correlate frequency of sore throats, especially strep throat (which may be related to heart or kidney problems), hoarseness, choking, difficulty swallowing or voice problems. |
| i. Neck. Discuss any pain or limitation in movement and length of time of symptoms. | This information will identify pain or stiffness, ability to hold head straight, limitation in movement, thyroid or node enlargement, possible meningitis or birth problems involving neck, e.g., torticollis or nerve injury during delivery. |
| j. Chest. Ask about enlarged nodes or masses. Inquire about breast development, if adolescent, and date of last breast examination (male and female). | Responses may identify problems with the lymph system in chest area and breasts, e.g., abnormal growth, unexplained discomfort, or developmental concerns. ***Special Considerations:*** *Both sexes may have breast development concerns and need to be taught breast self-examination. Breast cancer does occur in males, even though it is much more common in females.* |
| k. Respiratory. Discuss any difficulty breathing, shortness of breath at rest or on exertion, frequency of colds or other infections, any wheezing or other sounds when breathing, and date of last chest x-ray. | Assessment will elicit information related to respiratory status, both acute and chronic (e.g., pertussis, asthma, or cystic fibrosis) and identify environmental factors (e.g., air pollution and cigarette smoke) that can compromise oxygenation. |
| l. Cardiovascular. Ask if there is a history of a heart murmur, rheumatic fever, anemia, fatigue on exertion, cyanosis, pain in chest, arms, or calves, or hypertension. Include date of last blood count and any blood transfusions. If adolescent girl, ask if taking or has taken birth control pills. | Responses may identify any existing or potential problem with the heart or circulation, e.g., congenital anomalies or thrombus. ***Special Considerations:*** *Assess cardiac status and correlate findings with other systems, especially the respiratory system, since the symptoms frequently overlap.* |
| m. Gastrointestinal. Include past and present appetite, patterns and frequency of meals, food tolerances, elimination patterns (include recent changes), nausea, vomiting, pain, frequent burping, and excessive flatus. Ask about vitamin intake, especially fat-soluble A and D. If an adolescent, inquire about alcohol consumption. | This information will assist in isolating problems with the digestive system, including dumping syndrome, food allergies, and eating disorders that can alter nutritional, acid-base, and fluid and electrolyte status, and vitamin absorption. |

| Steps | Rationale |
|---|---|
| n. Genitourinary. Discuss characteristics of urine, e.g., frequency, amount, odor, color, force of stream, meatal discharge, placement of urethral opening (if male), redness or swelling around urethra or scrotum, date of last urinalysis, and history of urinary tract infections. If adolescent, ask if has had venereal disease. If male, ask if testicular self-examination is regularly performed. | Responses will help obtain data regarding the urinary tract and identify potential or actual problems, e.g., recurring urinary tract infections, sexually transmitted diseases, and testicular masses. ***Special Considerations:*** *Correlate genitourinary findings with blood pressure readings since the renal system helps regulate fluid balance and blood pressure.* |
| o. Reproductive. Female—Discuss date of first and last menstrual period, regularity, problems, pain, discharge, or pruritis. If sexually active, ask date and results of last Pap test and type of contraceptive using. Obtain obstetric history, if applicable. Male—Elicit information regarding concerns, development of penis and testes, any history of hernias, masses, pain, discharge, or redness or other color change in skin on penis and scrotum. Question regarding sexual activity, including erection, wet dreams, intercourse, and use of contraceptives. If uncircumcised, discuss retractibility of foreskin and hygiene practices. | Responses to these questions may indicate problem areas and potential teaching opportunities related to the reproductive system, especially developmental and sexuality concerns (Muscari, 1987). |
| p. Musculoskeletal. Elicit information regarding gait, stature, sports activities, body symmetry, joint and muscle range of motion, stiffness, weakness, clumsiness, lack of coordination, deformities, abnormalities, and injuries with or without fractures. Discuss x-rays, removal of fluid, and history of skeletal or muscular problems in family. Clarify vague terms, e.g., "a little stiffness" or "occasionally my ankle swells." Question effects of any limitations on self, body image, and relationships. | Assessment obtains information concerning problems that may interfere with activities of daily living, including walking, standing, sitting, dressing, and lifting, since the musculoskeletal system provides the frame and support for the body. |
| q. Neurologic system. Identify general affect, speech problems, coordination, dizziness, memory loss, tremors, seizures, fears, comprehension problems, numbness, tingling, or weakness, nightmares and unusual habits. Discuss past injuries and infections to central nervous system, including head and spinal cord (e.g., sports injuries or meningitis). | Responses help provide data about the nervous system and correlate to overall health and general body functions, since the neurologic system affects many body functions and can alter the child's ability to participate in daily activities. ***Special Considerations:*** *The child with neurologic problems may have difficulty with recall and processing and may need a family member to assist with health history and verify data. Also, they may tire easily, so the interview may need to consist of several short sessions. Encouraging participation is helpful to the child's self-esteem.* |
| r. Endocrine. Question timing of pubertal changes, any excessive thirst or hunger, sweating, unusual taste or smell of skin, fatigue, headaches, nervousness, weight changes, mental status changes, and tolerance to weather changes. Question medication, usage, and its intended actions. | Responses may elicit data about the endocrine system and its interrelationships with other body functions. Endocrine alterations may be a result of hyperfunction or hypofunction. |
| 7. Review family history. a. Family pedigree (see Skill 24). b. Familial or communicable diseases, e.g., heart disease, hypertension, cancer, diabetes mellitus, allergies, asthma, tuberculosis, sickle cell disease, mental retardation, or emotional disorders. Include symptoms, treatment, and sequelae. | Family history identifies genetic traits or diseases with familial tendencies and helps identify exposure to communicable diseases. ***Special Considerations:*** *When discussing child's parentage, use the terminology of "child's father/mother" instead of "your husband/wife" to avoid inaccurate information or erroneous assumptions.* |
| c. Family relationships and interactions—social activities, problem solving, communications, support systems, sharing of space and time, allotment of monies, and respect of individual religious practices. | This information assists in identifying overall family functioning. ***Special Considerations:*** *A screening questionnaire, e.g., the FAMILY APGAR may be useful. For additional information, see Skill 38.* |
| 8. Discuss personal/social history. a. Home and community environment. | This information helps develop an understanding of the child/family and identify factors that may affect the child's physical and emotional health. ***Special Considerations:*** *Rapport may improve and the family may be more likely to discuss confidential matters openly if the personal/social history is performed toward the end of the history-taking session. Maintain awareness that this information is highly subjective and may differ with each family member's individual perception.* |

| Steps | Rationale |
|---|---|
| b. Recent crisis or changes in home or family structure and family response. Discuss deaths of family members, close friends, or pets. Address divorce/separations, siblings moving away to school or living independently, addition of grandparents in home, etc. | Assessing life events helps identify family structure and stability, and the child's reaction to significant changes. |
| c. Occupation and education of family, types and places of employment, division of family responsibilities, child care, adequacy of income, work satisfaction, attitude toward work and education, exposure to hazards. If mother is employed, determine level of coping with work, home, and family responsibilities. | Socioeconomic information regarding sources and adequacy of family income and response of family to roles and labor division in home assists in problem identification and planning care. |
| d. Cultural and religious traditions (see Skills 41 and 42).<br>▪ Adherence to traditions.<br>▪ Language spoken in home. | Assessing cultural and religious influences on the family's attitudes toward health care and health maintenance assists in planning care and identifying potential or actual health problems. |
| e. Recent travel or exposure to foreign visitors. | This assessment helps identify potential endemic diseases. |
| 9. Write a summary of patient profile (P/P).<br>a. Health status.<br>b. Psychologic status.<br>c. Socioeconomic status. | Written documentation provides a comprehensive review summary of individual and family background. It allows completion of the nursing process and development of nursing diagnoses based on both subjective and objective data. Strengths and weaknesses are delineated providing the basis for nursing care. |

| Evaluation Outcomes | Observational Guidelines |
|---|---|
| 1. An accurate and complete health history is obtained. | Review written documentation for completeness and accuracy in each area. Child and family participated in data collection willingly. |

### Documentation

Note date and time(s) of data collection. Include names and relationship of those present along with child and family responses during history taking session. Record data from all sources in organized manner with statement about each area of health history. If information is deleted, state why. Formulate nursing diagnoses that reflect health history.

# *SKILL* 24 Constructing a Family Pedigree

*Deborah Kay Brantly*

"A pedigree is essentially a pictorial representation or diagram of the (genetic) family history," (Cohen, 1984). The nurse can use a pedigree as a data gathering tool to determine if a genetic referral is indicated. If a need for a referral is identified, the nurse must refer the family to a board-certified genetics counselor or medical/genetics clinic, since the pedigree is only the first step of a complete diagnostic evaluation. Such an evaluation would include a physical examination by a medical geneticist, and appropriate laboratory studies, e.g., chromosome analysis. The family would then be counseled about the diagnosed condition (if determined), the risks involved to other family members and future offspring, and would be provided support in decision making.

The pedigree has been expanded and modified to denote psychosocial relationships. This form is called "genogram," which delineates family relationships over a period of time. It is a form of genealogy with information on birth, death, marriage, and other factors that shed light on family behavior patterns and problems (see Skill 38).

## NURSING DIAGNOSES

Health-seeking behaviors (genetic counseling) related to prevention or identification of genetic diseases; Alteration in family processes related to birth of a child with a genetic defect; Potential altered parenting related to lack of knowledge about inheritable diseases/disorders.

**Steps** | **Rationale**

## Assessment

1. Determine reason for gathering pedigree information: information only, birth of a child with a defect, planning to conceive a child, need to identify other members of the family who may unknowingly be affected (e.g., scoliosis or hemophilia), or unusual or delayed growth and development patterns.

The purpose of the pedigree will direct depth and extent of the diagram. In cases of a clear need for genetic counseling, e.g., the birth of a child with Down syndrome, it may be preferable to initiate a referral without obtaining a pedigree.

2. Determine who will provide the history.
   a. Persons available and interested.
   b. The most reliable person(s) possible with thorough knowledge of the family history.

Genetic information may not be known to all persons in the family; the person(s) with the greatest family history knowledge and greatest interest in diagramming the information usually supplies the most complete information for the pedigree.

3. Determine the proband. The proband is the person who has brought about the need for the pedigree. In child health care, it is usually the child with a disease or birth defect.

Identifying the proband provides a starting point for the pedigree.
***Special Considerations:*** *The proband is often called the propositus.*

## Planning and Goal Setting

1. Ask the family to bring photos, and birth, death, and marriage certificates and records.

Records can supplement or substantiate more accurate information than recall alone. Photos may help reveal some genetic conditions, e.g., achondroplasia, and acromegaly.

2. With the family, determine the time and place of the interview.
   a. Allow 15 minutes to 1 hour to gather pedigree data.
   b. Locate space with adequate work surface (especially if using paper and pencil) and room for all persons to be seated comfortably.

Comfortable spacing and convenience of time allows for a more efficient interview.
***Special Considerations:*** *If there are younger children in the family, it may be best to exclude them from the pedigree meeting or provide them with diversional activities. Older children and adolescents generally participate without difficulties and may enjoy hearing family history.*

3. Select and gather diagramming materials: paper and pencil/pen, chalkboard and chalk, erasable marking board and markers, or tabloid and markers.

Gathering materials before the interview is an efficient use of time.
***Special Considerations:*** *Select diagramming materials large enough for all participants to see. The pedigree can later be duplicated in the client's record. Some standardized forms are available (Fig. 24-1).*

4. Review pedigree construction.
   a. Diagrammatic form.
   b. Symbols (Fig. 24-2).

Reviewing symbols and form improves ease of use and speed during the actual diagramming interview.
***Special Considerations:*** *It is helpful to take a chart of symbols for reference during the procedure or include a symbol key directly on the pedigree chart, especially if symbols are not commonly known.*

5. Develop nursing goals of care:
   - To obtain an accurate pedigree of the family.
   - To identify possible/actual familial disease conditions.
   - To initiate a referral to a qualified genetics counselor/counseling center when indicated.

## Implementation

1. Prepare the family for the task.
   a. Assure seating in which all family members can see the pedigree chart and participate in the process.
   b. Describe the task and review its purpose.
   c. Answer questions and acknowledge concerns.

Describing the purpose and answering questions assists in decreasing anxiety about the procedure and facilitates a more successful encounter.

2. Date the pedigree chart and list participants.

Dating distinguishes pedigree from past and future diagrams.

3. Begin pedigree construction by identifying the proband on the chart (Fig. 24-3).

The proband is the focus of the diagram, therefore is the easiest point at which to begin.

   a. Begin in the center, bottom third of the page.

Centering at the bottom allows for room to expand.

   b. Signify a male by a square, a female by a circle.

These symbols are universally used in pedigrees.

   c. Indicate name and date of birth near symbol.

This identifies the person to whom the symbol belongs and age.

   d. Signify proband by an arrow.

This is a commonly used symbol delineating the primary person around whom pedigree is diagrammed.

   e. Shade in symbol if proband is affected by the condition.

Shading distinctly indicates those affected by the condition.
***Special Considerations:*** *If more than one condition is present, it is possible to distinguish between them by using special shading/signs inside the person's symbol and creating a key of each type (see Fig. 24-2).*

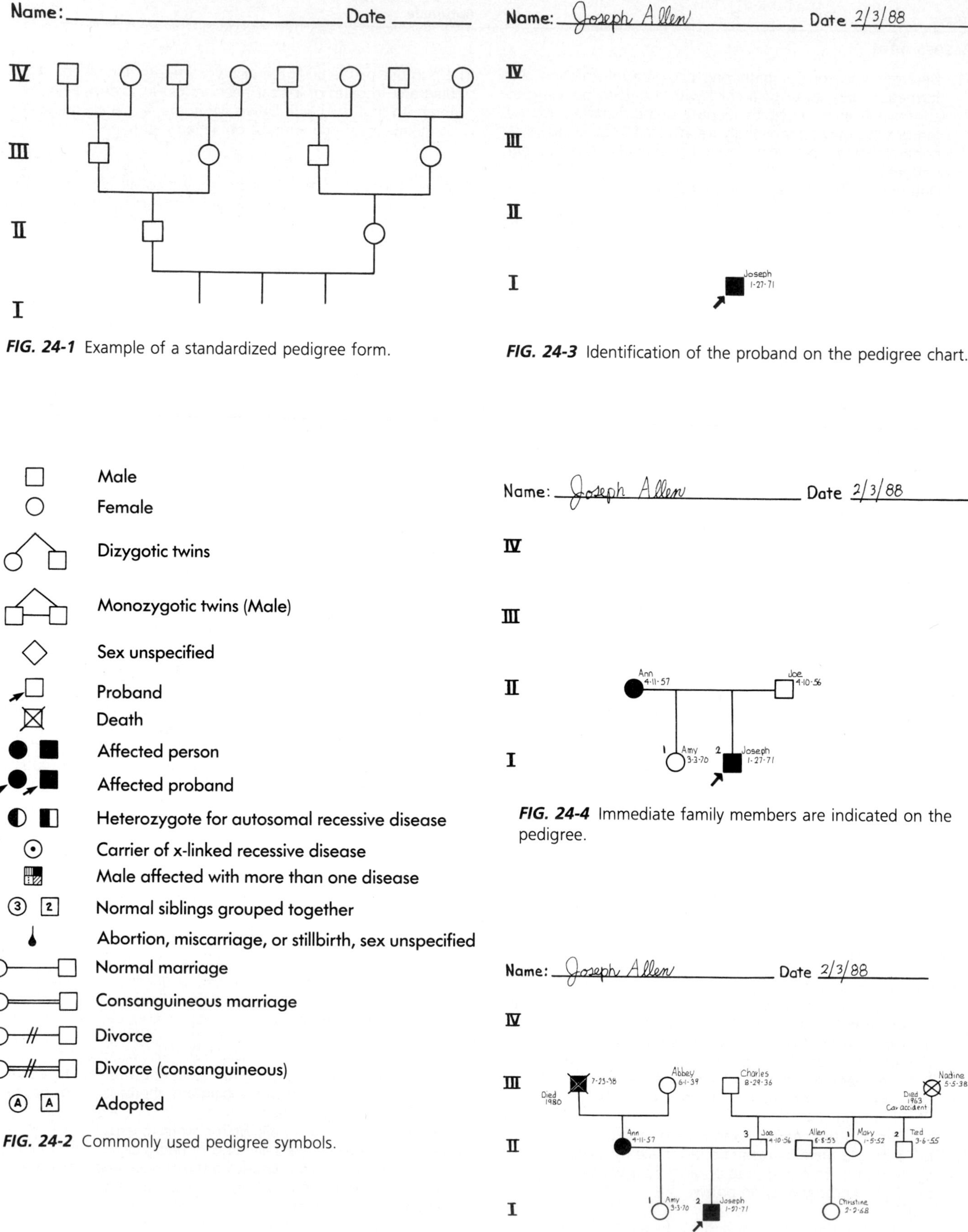


*FIG. 24-1* Example of a standardized pedigree form.

*FIG. 24-3* Identification of the proband on the pedigree chart.

*FIG. 24-2* Commonly used pedigree symbols.

*FIG. 24-4* Immediate family members are indicated on the pedigree.

*FIG. 24-5* Symbols show members of the extended family.

| Steps | Rationale |
|---|---|
| f. Note name of condition(s) and date(s) of onset. | Labeling the disease provides detailed information about those conditions that are inheritable. Notation of the date of onset provides information significant to differential diagnosis in some cases. |
| 4. Identify immediate family members of the proband, including parents and siblings. Write names and dates of birth near the corresponding diagrammatic symbol (Fig. 24-4). | Immediate family members are logically the next people to identify on the pedigree. |
| a. Draw a horizontal line between mates (marital or cohabitant), indicating males on the left. | The male of a union is traditionally diagrammed on the left. **Special Considerations:** *Mates identified with the immediate family of the proband may be the parents or spouse of a sibling.* |
| b. Suspend a line from the union line to include offspring; draw in birth order if possible, indicating birth order with arabic numbers, if desired. | Offspring are commonly represented underneath the parents. **Special Considerations:** *Arabic numbers are sometimes not necessary if offspring are drawn in birth order, but may be helpful. Offspring who are not affected and of the same gender can be combined in one diagrammatic symbol to save time and space (see Fig. 24-2). Special relationships of the offspring can also be noted by symbols, e.g., adopted, twins, or step-siblings (see Fig. 24-2).* |
| c. Note affected members by darkened symbols and note disease(s) with date(s) of onset. | Delineating affected members provides clues to the pattern of the disease history. |
| d. Designate identifiable carriers. Those carrying an X-linked recessive condition are indicated by a dot in the center of the symbol. An autosomal recessive trait is indicated by shading half of the symbol (see Fig. 24-2). | Labeling carriers identifies those at risk for passing the defective gene to offspring. |
| e. Note deaths by drawing a diagonal line or an X through the symbol, and indicate date and cause of death. | Noting deaths and cause of death gives a more comprehensive picture of the possible effects or patterns of inheritable disease in the family. |
| f. Indicate stillbirths, abortions, or miscarriages with the appropriate symbol (see Fig. 24-2). | Stillbirths and spontaneous abortions are sometimes overlooked in the interview, but may have been a result of an inheritable disease. **Special Considerations:** *If reason for spontaneous abortion or stillbirth is known, list or explain it.* |
| 5. Using the same format, identify other family members (Fig. 24-5). Include as a minimum of those diagrammed: parents, siblings, and offspring (if not already identified and appropriate), aunts, uncles, grandparents, and first cousins of the proband (Cohen, 1984). Indicate generations by Roman numerals on the left side of the chart. | A minimum of three generations is needed to establish genetic inheritability. **Special Considerations:** *Depending on the disease and its inheritable pattern, additional generations may be needed.* |
| 6. Identify multiple patterns and encourage discussion of these within the family. "Do you see any patterns evolving?" "It looks like there are several members of your family who died of ________. Was that something you were aware of?" or "Are you aware this particular disease has been found to follow family lines?" | Exploring patterns with the family assists them in becoming aware of their own genetic makeup so they perceive a need for referral. In addition, it provides the health care professionals with valuable information about others who may be affected, facilitating detection and prevention. |
| 7. Ask the family if they have any questions. | Families often have questions after the pedigree information has been collected and will share these if asked. **Special Considerations:** *Since teaching is most effective when interest in learning is high, providing information about a disease, prevention, etc., when it is requested is especially important.* |
| 8. Refer the family to a board-certified genetics counselor or a medical genetics clinic if a need is identified. These might include diagnosed inheritable disease, distinct familial inheritance pattern or high frequency occurrence, birth of a child with a defect, planning to conceive, family concerns, other members possibly unknowingly affected, unusual or delayed growth and development, or advanced maternal age. | Referral is the appropriate action for an identified need because a pedigree is usually not sufficient for an accurate diagnostic evaluation. Additionally, a specialized education in genetics is required to knowledgeably counsel families as to genetic risk factors. Genetic evaluation and counseling will provide the information families need to make informed decisions. **Special Considerations:** *Often nurses become board-certified genetics counselors by completing the necessary specialized education. However, genetics counselors may also be drawn from other disciplines (e.g., social work or science). The additional specialized education is necessary because crucial reproductive decisions within the family may be made using the genetic counseling its members receive. Referral sources for counseling or support can be located by contacting the local chapter of the March of Dimes or the health department.* |

| Steps | Rationale |
|---|---|
| **Evaluation Outcomes** | **Observational Guidelines** |
| 1. A genetic pedigree of the family is obtained. Possible patterns of inheritance are identified. | Review completed pedigree. Pedigree indicates patterns of affected persons and carriers. |
| 2. A referral is made, if appropriate. | Review documentation of referral and delivery of pertinent family records. Verify that family made and kept an appointment. Contact genetics counselor or clinic for results of evaluation and counseling. |

## Documentation

Document time and place of assessment, persons present, and individual responses to the information and procedure. Include a copy of the pedigree in the proband's record. Describe referral sources or genetic counseling provided.

# *SKILL* 25 Assessing Development

*Barbara L. Marino, Jayne E. Rogers, and Mary M. Aruda*

Assessing development is an integral part of nursing care of children in all settings. Assessment of the child's developmental level is indicated not only to identify potential or existing problems but to guide planning, intervention, and evaluation for all aspects of nursing care. Although formal screening and diagnostic tools are available and appropriate in certain situations, often simple guidelines to assess development in a concise, systematic way is a more efficient use of time and all that is needed. The purpose of this skill is to present such guidelines, whether the intent of the developmental assessment is to identify a possible delay during a well-child visit or to prepare a child for a procedure during hospitalization. (Refer to developmental texts for a more in-depth discussion of developmental concepts and processes.)

The infant makes enormous developmental strides in the first 3 years of life at a pace that will never again be equaled. All spheres (motor, social, language, and cognition) progress from rudimentary skills to functional ability, following predictable sequences. Early identification of developmental delay permits intervention to begin at a time when the greatest benefits can be attained. The preschool child is in a period of vast exploration and discovery; a time when imagination is fertile and initiative is strongly developed. The school-age period is one of extensive gains in a child's individual, industrious abilities and need for success. Adolescence is the time of tremendous change where a child matures into a young adult. Coinciding with the dramatic physical changes of puberty, adolescents are distancing from the family and striving for independence and their own identity. Understanding the underlying issues for this period can help to ease the day-to-day conflicts that often arise with teens.

### NURSING DIAGNOSES

Health-seeking behaviors (developmental assessment) related to infant/child health promotion/maintenance; Altered parenting: actual or potential related to unrealistic expectations of infant/child development; Altered growth and development related to parental knowledge deficit, parent-child conflict, school-related stressors, or stimulation deficiencies.

| Steps | Rationale |
|---|---|
| **Assessment** | |
| 1. Determine chronologic age (CA). Correct for prematurity until child is 2 years old by using the formula: CA – (40 – number of weeks of gestation) = adjusted age. For example, a baby born at 32 weeks gestation is 8 weeks early. Obtain corrected age by subtracting 8 from chronologic age in weeks. | Developmental milestones to be assessed are selected at child's corrected age level because prematurity can delay achievement of those milestones. |

| **Steps** | **Rationale** |
|---|---|
| 2. Determine physical growth—measurements of height, weight, and head circumference (up to 2 years of age). Plot measures throughout childhood (see Skill 28). | Serial measurements identify each child's growth curve, and any persistent deviation that could be a subtle indication of early pathology. For example, suppression of the endocrine system will delay puberty, or early triggering will cause precocious puberty. Also, failure to thrive (weight below 5th percentile) will limit developmental progress. |
| 3. Obtain health history (see Skill 23).<br>a. Assess for birth trauma, gestational age at birth, low Apgar scores, extended neonatal hospitalization. | Children at "biological risk" for developmental problems are those who experienced unfavorable perinatal events (Casey et al, 1986). Extended neonatal hospitalization, e.g., for prematurity, can seriously impair infant social skills because of the noncontingent environment (Lawhon, 1986). |
| b. Assess if previously hospitalized and nature of experience. | A previous hospitalization can have significant consequences on development, both physically and psychologically (e.g., motor delay or abnormal tone may follow acute or chronic illness in infancy). Other developmental domains can be unaffected or become impaired secondary to motor delay. Psychologically, the fantasy and magical thinking of preschoolers makes them highly prone to thoughts that they may have caused their illness or hospitalization. They may fear that they are being punished and may experience guilt. They think of their "powers" as magical and dangerous, therefore needing to be repressed and denied. These fantasies may persist into adolescence, often remaining hidden. |
| c. If child has a chronic illness or disability, assess for effect on development. | In both preschool and school-age children chronic illness may result in behaviors more often associated with the next age group as they become sophisticated by their interaction with adults and the medical system. Often their school and peer behavior, however, may be delayed. |
| d. For adolescents, determine growth disorders, congenital abnormalities, radiation exposure, chemotherapy, or drug use. | Existence of these factors may predispose to pubertal delay. |
| 4. Assess current health status:<br>a. Present state on illness-wellness continuum.<br>b. Presence of influencing factors such as pain, fatigue, immobility, isolation from peers, physical disability, severity of illness. | Current illness or disability (acute or chronic) may directly or indirectly inhibit or cause regression of developmental achievement and alter observed behaviors (e.g., an adolescent in pain who is normally striving for independence may plead with a parent to remain at his or her side). |
| c. Medication or other drugs currently taking (including OTC drugs) and dosages. | Drug interactions can often mask behavior problems and depression, especially in the adolescent.<br>***Special Considerations:*** *Question adolescents for smoking, alcohol, and illicit drug use in a confidential manner.* |
| 5. Assess environment.<br>a. Current members of the household; number of siblings, ages, and adoptive status; recent changes in the family unit (e.g., birth, divorce, remarriage, death); and other stressors, e.g., moves, unemployment, emotional disturbance, or substance abuse. | Environmental factors such as family constellation influence development. An environment that provides inadequate care or support places the child at risk for developmental problems (Casey et al, 1986). Recent stress within the home may trigger illness symptoms. Adoption may increase the difficult task of identity formation for the adolescent (Whaley and Wong, 1989). |
| b. For the infant and toddler, ask about a normal day: sleep and feeding schedule, people, favorite toys/objects/games, usual events. If not volunteered, ask about specific sources of stimulation for the child (people, objects, events). | Infants and toddlers develop best in an environment that allows for adequate rest, nutrition, and stimulation from people and objects.<br>***Special Considerations:*** *Appropriate level of stimulation is determined by the tolerance of the individual child.* |
| c. For the preschooler, ask about preschool attendance, play interactions, and usual routines at home. | Preschoolers develop best in an environment that allows for exploration in an emotionally safe setting. |
| d. For the older child and adolescent ask about school performance, sports, and hobbies. Also determine employment and number of hours worked per week. It is often helpful to ask adolescents to do a 24-hour recall of their day. | The opportunity to engage in tasks and activities and complete them provides a sense of achievement for the school-age child. School is also a primary task for adolescents. Sports are a healthy channel for many teens in the emotional upheavals during adolescence. Employment can have beneficial and/or detrimental effects, e.g., increase self-esteem or interfere with school work. |

| Steps | Rationale |
|---|---|
| 6. Assess family expectations regarding development. Elicit parental concerns or expectations about child's development, e.g., ask, "Do you have any concerns about your child's development?" Determine the source of information parents use regarding development. | Parents may have or receive misinformation about normal development and ways to enhance it, which can conflict with information from professionals. However, parents often suspect developmental delay before it is identified by professionals.<br>***Special Considerations:*** *Examples of problematic family expectations are encouraging early attainment of toileting, reading or language before child is ready; looking to schools or health care to try to set limits that they are unable to set at home, e.g., smoking, school attendance; and placing a high value on virginity such that for the teenager to admit to sexual exploration would force exclusion from the home.* |
| 7. Perform physical assessment (see Skill 27). | Physical development and maturation is an essential component of the developmental assessment. Performing a physical assessment also allows identification of neurologic abnormalities and sensory deficits that may hamper task achievement. |

## Planning and Goal Setting

| Steps | Rationale |
|---|---|
| 1. Select an appropriate environment and time for testing/observation. | |
| a. Infants under 3 months: Use a warm, quiet place with indirect lighting. | Reducing stimulation optimizes interactive responses and limits responses to extraneous stimuli. Infants who are overstimulated can exhibit avoidance behaviors so aggressively that they appear blind and deaf. Reducing competing external and internal stimuli allows assessment of true ability. |
| b. Older infants and toddlers: Are most cooperative with parent present (perhaps holding child) and in a nonclinical place (e.g., hospital playroom or in a clinic room without examination equipment in it). | The security derived from parent's presence and from a nonthreatening room optimizes performance. |
| c. Preschool child: An environment that is quiet and without distraction is preferable. Allow children to set their own proximity to parents. Observe the child while interviewing the parents. | Excess stimulation will alter findings. The security secondary to parents' presence will maximize baseline performance. |
| d. School-age child: Use a nonthreatening, nonjudgmental manner. Observe the child when asking questions directly to them and to the parent. | School-age children are very influenced by others' perceptions. |
| e. Adolescent: Separate from the parents and question them in a private place assuring confidentiality. It is helpful to get the past history from the parent and the teen and then compare the versions. | ***Special Considerations:*** *Nurses should be familiar with the laws in their state that govern the "Mature Minor" concept and allow for confidential care to teens related to pregnancy and sexually transmitted diseases (Emans, 1989).* |
| 2. Gather items and tools. | |
| a. For infants: Select toys that are visually appealing (red or black and white contrasting, faces); small; lightweight and safe for grasping; some that make noise and some that do not. | Visual tracking, grasping, and oral exploration can be tested with this variety of toys. |
| b. For toddlers: Choose toys like busy boxes, shape sorters, doll, truck, toy animal, blanket, toy telephone. | These can be used to elicit cause and effect, pretend, and eye-hand coordination behaviors. |
| c. For preschoolers: Provide open space with room to explore, paper and crayons, books, tricycle, dolls, puppets, and dressup clothes. | Imitative, dramatic, imaginative, and cooperative play are most characteristic of the preschooler. Through play they work out life experiences. Preschoolers enjoy playing "school," "house," and "dress-up." |
| d. For school-age child: Provide age-appropriate games, cards, or books. | These items will provide activities to allow observation of them at play/work. |
| e. For more formal tools to assess development, refer to Skill 26 and Product References and Teaching Resources section. | |
| 3. Review expected milestones (Table 25-1). | Knowledge of developmental norms for the age of the child guides screening. |
| 4. Develop individualized goals of nursing care:<br>▪ To identify a delay as early as possible to optimize the effects of intervention.<br>▪ To assure that parental expectations and management are developmentally appropriate for the child.<br>▪ To individualize the nursing care plan according to the child's developmental level. | |

**TABLE 25-1** Selected Milestones in Development

| Age | Expected Behaviors | | | |
|---|---|---|---|---|
| | **MOTOR** | **SOCIAL** | **LANGUAGE** | **COGNITION** |
| 1 to 3 months | Exhibits smooth movements.<br>Has strong grasp reflex (1 month).<br>Grasp reflex disappears; will actually hold rattle but not reach for it (3 months).<br>When prone, pelvis is high and knees flexed (1 month).<br>When prone, pelvis is low and legs extended (2 months).<br>Can lift head momentarily and turn from side to side when prone (1 month) (Fig. 25-1).<br>Has slight head lag when pulled to sitting, head bobs forward when sitting (2 months) (Figs. 25-2 and 25-3). | Is visually responsive (1 month).<br>Smiles responsively (2 months).<br>Follows object to side (3 months).<br>Recognizes caregiver (3 months).<br>Can ignore unpleasant stimulation. | Cries become differentiated (2 months).<br>Turns to sound (hearing development).<br>Coos, chuckles (3 months). | Uses visual skills to learn.<br>Recognizes daily routines. |

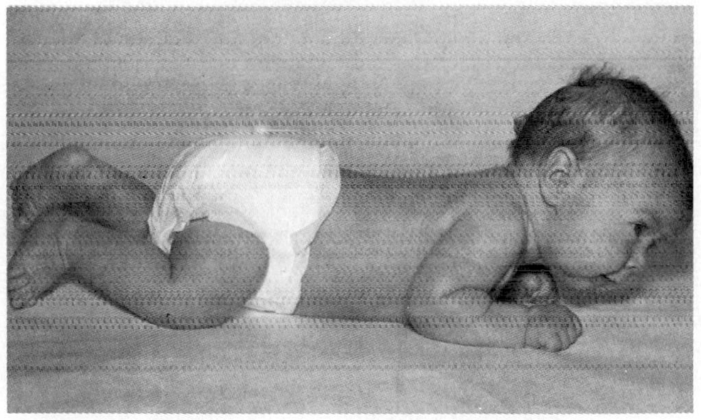

***FIG. 25-1*** Infant momentarily lifts head at 1 month.
From Whaley LF and Wong DL: Essentials of pediatric nursing, ed 3, St Louis, 1989, The CV Mosby Co.

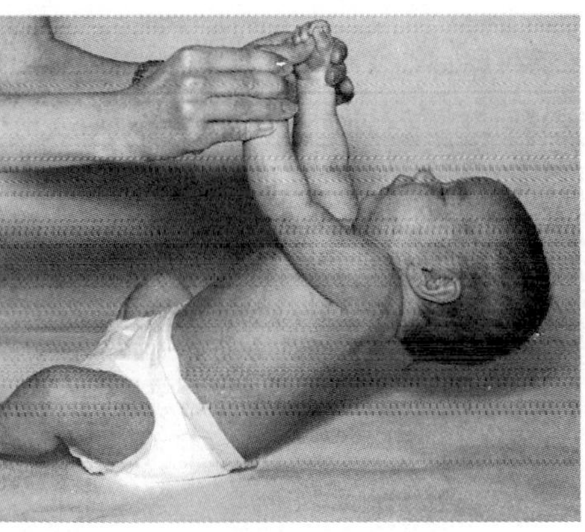

***FIG. 25-2*** Infant shows partial head lag at 2 months.
From Whaley LF and Wong DL: Essentials of pediatric nursing, ed 3, St Louis, 1989, The CV Mosby Co.

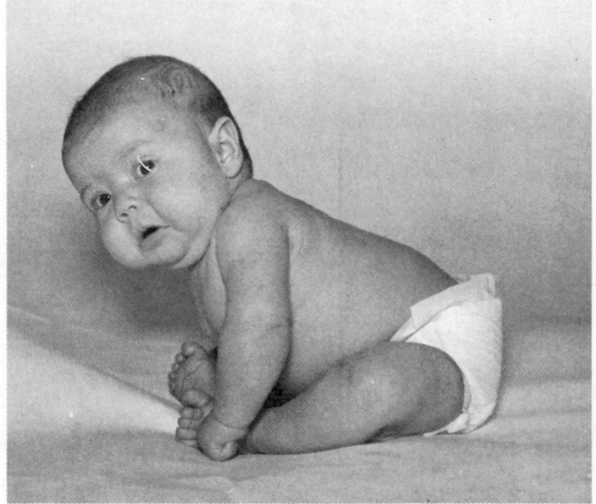

***FIG. 25-3*** Back is still rounded, but infant can sit up momentarily with some head control at 2 months.
From Whaley LF and Wong DL: Essentials of pediatric nursing, ed 3, St Louis, 1989, The CV Mosby Co.

*Continued.*

**TABLE 25-1** Selected Milestones in Development—cont'd

| Age | Expected Behaviors | | | |
|---|---|---|---|---|
| | **MOTOR** | **SOCIAL** | **LANGUAGE** | **COGNITION** |
| 4 to 6 months | Has no head lag when pulled to sitting (4 months).<br>When prone, can raise head and chest up 90 degrees and support with arms (4 months) (Fig. 25-4).<br>Can hold head erect and sit with support (4-5 months).<br>Rolls front to back (6 months).<br>Swipes at dangling toys (4 months).<br>Brings hands to midline; inspects and plays with them (4 months).<br>Brings hands and toys to mouth (5 months). | Trust vs. mistrust.<br>Exhibits attention-getting cues.<br>Smiles at mirror image (5 months).<br>Holds arms out to be picked up (6 months). | Babbles, squeals (4 months).<br>Laughs aloud.<br>Responds to familiar voice (hearing development).<br>Begins to imitate sounds; one syllable utterances, e.g., ma, mu, da, di, hi (6 months). | Learns through touch/mouthing.<br>Anticipates feeding.<br>Shows interest in strange stimuli. |
| 7 to 9 months | Sits leaning on hands (7 months).<br>Sits without support (8 months).<br>Lifts head when supine (7 months).<br>Bears weight on feet (7 months).<br>Pulls to stand (9 months).<br>Begins to crawl (9 months).<br>Transfers objects from one hand to another (7 months).<br>Begins developing pincer grasp (9 months).<br>Chewing replaces sucking. | Develops stranger anxiety.<br>Begins to test limits.<br>Plays peek-a-boo.<br>Demonstrates likes and dislikes.<br>Resists being restrained for diapering and dressing. | Imitates speech sounds.<br>Vocalizes chained syllables e.g., ba ba, da da, ka ka.<br>Understands and responds to inflection and gestures from caregiver's command. | Imitates noises, actions.<br>Searches for hidden objects (beginning object permanence).<br>Recognition of cause and effect, e.g., drops toy, someone will retrieve. |
| 10 to 12 months | Sits from a stand by falling (10 months).<br>Sits down deliberately from a stand (12 months).<br>Cruises holding on (10 months).<br>Stands alone momentarily.<br>Has neat pincer grasp (Fig. 26-4,C).<br>Holds cup to drink, may spill. | Waves bye-bye (10 months).<br>Repeats actions that attract attention.<br>Plays interactive games, e.g., pat-a-cake.<br>Hands toy on request (11 months).<br>Clings to caregiver in strange situations.<br>Exhibits frustration when restricted.<br>Explores away from caregiver in familiar surroundings. | Uses dada, mama deliberately, may use one other word.<br>Uses jargon.<br>Recognizes some objects by name (12 months).<br>Imitates animal sounds. | Learns what objects do, e.g., a ball.<br>Learns differences between objects, e.g., a cow or a dog.<br>Looks at pictures in a book.<br>Searches for object where last seen. |

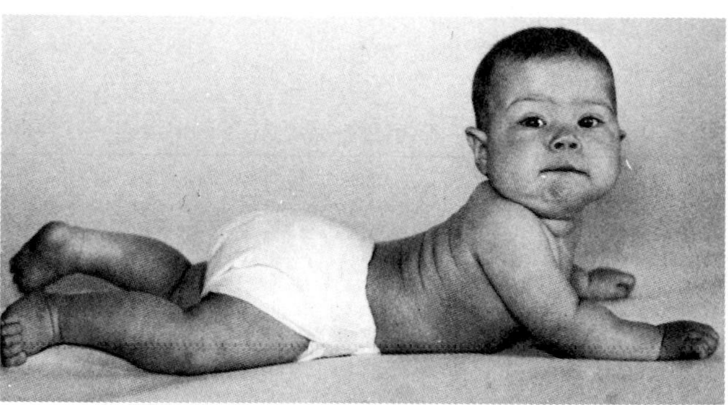

***FIG. 25-4*** Child lifts head and chest 90 degrees and bears weight on forearms at 4 months.

From Whaley LF and Wong DL: Essentials of pediatric nursing, ed 3, St Louis, 1989, The CV Mosby Co.

**TABLE 25-1** Selected Milestones in Development—cont'd

| Age | Expected Behaviors | | | |
|---|---|---|---|---|
| | **MOTOR** | **SOCIAL** | **LANGUAGE** | **COGNITION** |
| 13 to 15 months | Walks without help.<br>Crawls up and down stairs.<br>Can stack 2 blocks.<br>Holds crayon and scribbles (15 months).<br>Puts ball in box. | Shows perseverance in practicing motor skills.<br>Exhibits lessened stranger anxiety.<br>Gives "kisses."<br>Tolerates short separation from caregiver. | Vocabulary increases to 4-6 words.<br>Responds to simple commands, e.g., "bring me the book."<br>Responds with "no" even if agreeing. | Able to match simple geometric objects to appropriate opening.<br>Nesting—fits successively smaller objects together.<br>Opens cabinet doors and drawers to see contents.<br>Learns through imitation. |
| 18 to 24 months | Runs awkwardly (18 months).<br>Removes clothing, socks, and shoes.<br>Pushes and pulls toys.<br>Walks up stairs with help (18 months).<br>Improves balance in stooping, throwing, and kicking (24 months).<br>Runs smoothly (24 months).<br>Jumps (24 months).<br>Kicks a ball (24 months).<br>Uses spoon well. | Begins to feel empathy.<br>Explores from safe base of caregiver.<br>Has a sense of time, able to wait momentarily.<br>Plays in parallel with other children.<br>Tests limits more strongly, temper tantrums.<br>Recognizes ownership: "mine."<br>Attempts to dress self (24 months). | Uses 10 or more words (18 months).<br>Uses 300 words (24 months).<br>Forms 2 to 3 word phrases (24 months).<br>Will repeat new words with encouragement. | Early pretend play (18 months).<br>Looks actively in several places for missing object.<br>Attention span lengthens.<br>Names pictures.<br>Learns through pretend, includes more schemes, actors. |
| 24 to 36 months | Walks up and down stairs with feet together.<br>Jumps with both feet (24 months).<br>Stands on one foot for a few seconds.<br>Pedals tricycle (36 months).<br>Strings beads.<br>Can copy a circle or cross lines.<br>Feeds self well. | Autonomy vs. shame.<br>Dresses self with minimal help.<br>Begins to share (36 months).<br>Begins collaborative play.<br>Explores farther away from safe base.<br>Can put toys away. | Acquires new words from speech of others without encouragement.<br>Understands more complex commands.<br>Uses multiword sentences.<br>Speech is understandable to a stranger about 75% of the time. | Pretend less dependent on realistic toys.<br>Complicated pretend schemes.<br>Knows first and last name. |
| 3 years | Dances, although awkwardly.<br>Broad jumps.<br>Draws a circle with facial features.<br>Walks up steps with alternating feet. | Exhibits a sense of self control.<br>Helps with simple household chores, e.g., setting table and putting away silverware.<br>May exhibit fear of the dark.<br>Knows own sex and sense of sex-role functions. | Has a vocabulary of approximately 900 words.<br>Understands and uses some simple verbs, pronouns, prepositions, and adjectives, e.g., go, me, in, and big.<br>Speaks in complete sentences.<br>Asks frequent questions, e.g., "Why?"<br>Names one or more colors.<br>May stutter. | Preconceptual thinking.<br>Exhibits beginning concept of time through time-oriented expressions.<br>Has egocentric, concrete thought that does not allow movement from the general to the specific.<br>Has a beginning ability to follow commands using spatial direction. |

*Continued.*

**TABLE 25-1** Selected Milestones in Development—cont'd

| Age | Expected Behaviors | | | |
|---|---|---|---|---|
| | **MOTOR** | **SOCIAL** | **LANGUAGE** | **COGNITION** |
| 4 years | Hops and skips on one foot.<br>Walks down stairs using alternate feet.<br>Throws ball overhand.<br>Is able to use scissors successfully.<br>Draws a 3-part stick figure. | Is independent and often rebellious.<br>Tells openly of family "secrets."<br>Is very dramatic.<br>Identifies strongly with parent of the opposite sex.<br>Still has many fears.<br>Cooperates in play.<br>Creates imaginative and dramatic scenarios.<br>Brushes teeth.<br>Obeys limits but does not comprehend right or wrong. | Vocabulary of approximately 1600 words.<br>Makes sentences consisting of 4 to 5 connected words.<br>Understands simple analogies.<br>Knows verses to simple songs.<br>Exaggerates stories or information.<br>Knows several colors. | Intuitive thought.<br>Unable to conserve matter.<br>Can choose longer of 2 lines or heavier object.<br>May count, but little mathematical concepts.<br>Is able to give a connected account of some recent experience.<br>Able to carry out sequence of two simple directions. |
| 5 years | Hops and skips on alternate feet.<br>Good sense of balance.<br>Throws and catches ball.<br>Completely dresses self, including tying shoes.<br>Draws an 8-part stick figure. | Has a sense of clothes that match.<br>Is eager to please and live by the rules, but may cheat if losing at a game.<br>Acts "like a girl" or "like a boy."<br>Begins to demonstrate manners.<br>May identify strongly with parent of the same sex.<br>Cooperative at play.<br>Is able to do complete self care.<br>Often complains over minor hurts, but tries to be brave if major pain anticipated. | Has a vocabulary of approximately 2100 words.<br>Speech is 100% intelligible, although some sounds may be mispronounced.<br>Uses some pronouns correctly.<br>Can carry on a conversation if the vocabulary is within their experience.<br>Matches grammar to the patterns of parents.<br>Uses all parts of speech correctly, except for deviations from the rule.<br>Knows colors.<br>Knows most seasons. | May notice bias or prejudice.<br>Tolerates but does not understand another's perspective.<br>Increases use of time oriented words.<br>Is very curious. |
| 6 years | Has boundless energy and is unable to sit still for long periods.<br>Is clumsy and awkward.<br>Is frustrated by imprecise dexterity, but gradually improves.<br>Likes to draw, color, and do crafts.<br>Is clumsy with pencil but can print uppercase letters. | Can share and cooperate easily.<br>Desires peer interaction.<br>Imitates parental activity.<br>Often engages in rough play.<br>Is unable to admit wrongdoing.<br>Giggles a lot. | Reads from memory.<br>Uses all forms of sentence structure.<br>Ready to learn to read.<br>Recognizes simple words and phrases and sounds out words to pronounce them.<br>Knows days of week.<br>Describes object according to composition, e.g., "a chair is made of wood." | Attends 1st grade.<br>Defines common objects in terms of their use, e.g., "a fork is something to eat with."<br>Understands number concepts.<br>Imitations of reality more exact.<br>Symbolic functioning. |

**TABLE 25-1** Selected Milestones in Development—cont'd

| Age | Expected Behaviors | | | |
|---|---|---|---|---|
| | **MOTOR** | **SOCIAL** | **LANGUAGE** | **COGNITION** |
| 7 to 9 years | Participates more in athletic activities because of muscular development.<br>Practices skills such as gymnastics to master.<br>Can swim and ride bike.<br>Is reasonably cautious with gross motor activities.<br>Begins cursive writing.<br>Has increased smoothness and speed in fine motor control.<br>Moves with more grace and fluidity (8-9 years).<br>Is always on the go.<br>Has fully developed eye-hand coordination.<br>Has quite skillful control of motor activities (9 years). | Helps with routine household tasks.<br>Likes to spend some time alone.<br>Prefers same sex friends.<br>Pleasant attitude at home.<br>Likes to compete and play games.<br>May be interested in opposite sex but reluctant to admit (9 years).<br>Becomes more critical of self (9 years). | Can list months of year, knows date.<br>Speech is sociocentric.<br>Has increased vocabulary and can give a more precise definition.<br>Exhibits mechanical reading—reads in monotone and often skips modifier words. | Attends 2nd grade (7 years).<br>Attends 3rd grade (8 years).<br>Attends 4th grade (9 years).<br>Mental reasoning processes assume logical approaches to concrete problems.<br>Organizes objects and events into hierarchies of classes or along a continuum of increasing values.<br>Attains reversibility, transitivity, and conservation skills. |
| 10 to 12 years | Begin to see noticeable difference in muscular mass development and strength, boys greater than girls (10 years).<br>Has greater stamina (10 years).<br>Appears clumsy, movements more bouncy and jerky (11 years).<br>Exhibits refinement of motor activities (12 years). | Enjoys school and related activities, games, team plays, arts and crafts, and collections.<br>Still considers family important.<br>Shows affection easily.<br>Chooses selectively.<br>Places importance on having a "best friend."<br>Values privacy.<br>Begins to express interest in opposite sex. | Enjoys reading.<br>Likes to memorize.<br>Loves to talk. | Attends 5th grade (10 years).<br>Attends 6th grade (11 years).<br>Attends 7th grade (12 years).<br>True logical thought and manipulation of abstract concepts emerge (12 years).<br>Hypothetical deductive thought begins (12 years). |
| 13 to 15 years | Exhibits improved coordination; as size increases, long-leggedness may make appear awkward and clumsy.<br>Gains mastery and control over increased strength. | Conforms to peer group in dress, activity, and attitudes, including drug/alcohol use.<br>Measures attractiveness by reaction of peers.<br>Daydreams intensely.<br>Develops close, idealized friendship with member of same sex.<br>Experiences cycles of separation from parents.<br>Tests independence and dependence boundaries.<br>Spends considerable time in sports and group activities.<br>Is narcissistic.<br>Has wide mood swings.<br>Experiments with dating and intimacy in a self-centered manner. | Tries out various roles.<br>Effectively uses humor to criticize family and friends.<br>Talks on telephone at length with friends.<br>Expresses anger verbally with outbursts, insults and name calling. | Attends 8th grade (13 years).<br>Attends 9th grade (14 years).<br>Attends 10th grade (15 years).<br>Explores with new ability to think abstractly, though not fully developed.<br>Questions values. |

*Continued.*

**TABLE 25-1** Selected Milestones in Development—cont'd

| Age | Expected Behaviors | | | |
|---|---|---|---|---|
| | **MOTOR** | **SOCIAL** | **LANGUAGE** | **COGNITION** |
| 15 to 18 years | Physically mature (some males later). | Has increased self-centeredness and narcissism (16 years).<br>Is idealistic.<br>Has major conflicts over independence and control with parents: low point in relationship.<br>Continues to allow peer group to set behavioral standards.<br>May experiment with drugs, alcohol.<br>Explores ability to attract opposite sex.<br>Is concerned with dating behavior.<br>Establishes sexual preference decisively (heterosexual or homosexual).<br>Experiences feelings of "being in love", though more romanticism and exploration than actual commitment.<br>Experiments sexually to varying degrees (heterosexual and homosexual). | Has ability to debate effectively. | Attends 11th grade (16 years).<br>Attends 12th grade (17 years).<br>Develops abstract thought.<br>Is able to reason deductively.<br>Worries about school work.<br>Is concerned with philosophic, political, and social problems.<br>Uses intellectualism as defense.<br>Is able to perceive future implications of present behavior and decisions.<br>Exhibits creativity. |

Adapted from Whaley LF and Wong DL: Essentials of pediatric nursing, ed 3, St Louis, 1989, The CV Mosby Co.

| Steps | Rationale |
|---|---|

## Implementation

1. Screen each of the developmental domains: motor, social, language, and cognition (using Table 25-1) and ask the following supplemental questions to elicit/observe for behaviors specific to each age group.

These four domains should be consistently explored for each age group.

***Special Considerations:*** *All domains are interactive, so screening can be done in the order most effective for the particular child.*

### *Infant/toddler*

a. Attempt to elicit/observe behaviors that correspond to child's current age (see Table 25-1). If unattained, move to the next lower level of skills on the chart until behavior is achieved.

Children should demonstrate developmentally appropriate skills for their chronologic age. However, if there are delays, skills normally achieved at an earlier age will be evident, offering an estimate of the child's current developmental age. For example, a 2-year-old child who is mastering skills normally achieved at 18 months of age has a developmental age of 1½ years.

b. Ask parent about any behaviors that appear to be delayed. For example, if language cannot be elicited, ask, "Mrs. Haley, how does Beth tell you she wants something?" Do *not* ask, "Mrs. Haley, can Beth point to something she wants to ask you to get for her?"

Parental information is usually needed to screen early language. For any domain, parental report is useful since it is based on more observations than can be achieved during a screening. Asking a question that can be answered yes or no elicits little substantive information about the child's ability.

***Special Considerations:*** *If the child is hospitalized, primary nurses offer a good substitute for parental input, if parents are not available.*

| Steps | Rationale |
|---|---|
| ***Preschool child*** | |
| *Social domain:* | |
| a. Inquire about child's independence. For example, ask, "What is your child able to do for himself or herself (e.g., dress, feed, brush teeth)?" | Children in this age group are beginning to take initiative for self-care activities and the beginnings of independence. |
| b. Ask about the child's play activities, e.g., ask, "What activities does your child enjoy? Does he or she prefer to play alone or with others? Does he or she pretend often or have an imaginary playmate?" | Fantasy and magical thinking are typical of this age group. The invention of imaginary playmates is normal. |
| c. Gather information about rewards and disciplines used at home. | This gives a baseline understanding of how the family sets limits in the home to maintain desired behavior. |
| d. Ask the parent how the child copes with separation, e.g., ask, "How does your child respond to new or unfamiliar situations, illness, hospitalization (if previously hospitalized)?" | Reaction to separation from the parent and the normal routine at home is seen in the preschooler. |
| e. Ask if the child has any fears. | Fears are typical of this age group and include separation, the dark, being alone, large machines (e.g., C.A.T. scan). |
| f. Observe the child and parent interaction. Ask if the child tends to associate with one parent more than the other. | Parent-child interaction is essential baseline information. It is typical for preschoolers to go through periods of identification with parents of the same or opposite sex. |
| *Cognitive domain:* | |
| a. Ask about the child's understanding of right and wrong, e.g., ask, "Does your child show remorse after doing something wrong?" | Preschoolers have a beginning understanding of moral responsibility. This question may also elicit a sense of parental expectations. |
| b. Assess the child's ability to see things from another's perspective. | Because of concrete thought and egocentricity, preschoolers have a limited ability to see or understand events from another's perspective. |
| c. Ask about the child's concept of time, e.g., ask, "Does your child ask time-related questions using words like when, now, later?" | Time is best explained in relationship to an event. Concrete thought does not allow the preschooler to move from the general to the specific. |
| *Motor domain:* | |
| a. Assess the child's sleep patterns, e.g., ask, "What kind of a sleeper is your child? How many hours at night? Does he or she nap? Does he or she use a security object, toys, or a night light?" | This baseline information allows recreation of a sleep/rest schedule and may identify a pattern indicating an underlying neurologic disorder. More commonly it identifies a sleep problem, e.g., refusal to go to bed or night wakings. |
| b. Ask about the child's ability to dress, feed, and brush teeth independently. | Ability to provide self-care gives baseline information about motor and social function. |
| *Language domain:* | |
| a. Ask how the child expresses himself verbally, e.g., ask, "Approximately how many words does your child use? How many words in a sentence?" | The preschooler has an increased ability to express ideas verbally. |
| ***School-age child*** | |
| The child or parent may be the source of information. | |
| *Social domain:* | |
| a. Assess the child's enjoyment of and functioning in school, e.g., say, "Tell me about school." | School is an integral aspect of the child's life in this age group. |
| b. Inquire about involvement in school-related activities, e.g., ask, "What school-related activities,such as clubs or sports, are you involved in?" | School-age children typically exhibit involvement in school activities and hobbies to derive a sense of accomplishment. |
| c. Ask about peer relationships, e.g., ask, "Do you have a best friend?" | This age group has the ability to get along with others and see friends as a reflection of themselves. |
| d. Ask how the child demonstrates independence, productivity, and achievement. Ask about parental praise for the above, e.g., ask "Does your child enjoy achieving? How do you praise your child?" | The school-age child is striving for independence and productivity. They enjoy doing and achieving, which gives them satisfaction and recognition from others. Self-esteem is gained through achievement and praise, imparting a sense of success. |
| e. Ask how the parent sets limits on behavior. | Children in this age group need parameters of acceptable behavior. The parents' response also gives a sense of their idea of behavioral norms for this age group. |
| f. Ask if there are any fears. | Common fears in this age group are loss of control, bodily injury, pain, and large machines. |

| Steps | Rationale |
|---|---|
| *Cognitive domain:* | |
| a. Ask about the child's grade level and school performance, e.g., ask, "What grade are you in? What subjects do you like/dislike? What kind of grades/scores do you get in these subjects?" | Age-appropriate grade level and performance in school are reliable indicators of a child's developmental age. |
| b. Ask about the child's expression of creativity, e.g., say, "How do you/your child express creativity, e.g., dancing, building things, drawing, etc.?" | Creativity is an expression of intellectual inventiveness and demonstrates cognitive development and flexibility. ***Special Considerations:*** *Indicators of reaction to separation and loss of control include displaced anger, depression, withdrawal, frustration, and hostility.* |
| *Motor domain:* | |
| a. Inquire into child's involvement in sports, interests, and hobbies. | Increased complex muscle use allows the school-age child to participate in sports. Arts and crafts, books, and collections are favorites of this age group. |
| ***Early adolescent (10 to 14 years old)*** | |
| Interview adolescents and parents separately. | |
| *Social domain:* | |
| a. Ask parents about the amount of "mirror time" or time needed to get ready for school. | Body image is the important issue for this age group. Adolescents are especially attuned to body changes as they enter puberty and experience breast development, wet dreams, and voice changes. They need reassurance of the normalcy of these changes with facts to dispel folklore or secret fears. ***Special Considerations:*** *Obese, underweight, or disabled adolescents often have difficulty forming the important peer bonds of this age.* |
| b. Ask parents about the adolescent's activities, e.g., sports, hobbies, summer plans. | At this age there should be beginning separation from the family, with more emphasis on same-sex peer activities. Parental support, e.g., money and transportation, is needed to help young teens participate. |
| c. Give parents an opportunity to voice concerns about behavior, specifically, smoking, alcohol, drug use, dating, or sexual activities. | Although young, this group has the highest increase in pregnancy rates in recent years. Parents often have the first inkling of smoking or drug/alcohol use, but need the opportunity to voice their suspicions to focus their concerns. ***Special Considerations:*** *Smoking is often considered a "gateway" to drug use.* |
| d. Ask the adolescent about peer friendships. | Having a best friend is very important at this stage. Poor impulse control of young adolescents makes it very important to assess peer activity. |
| e. Assuring privacy and confidentiality, ask the adolescent about smoking, alcohol or drug use, and dating or sexual activities. (See also middle adolescent social domain assessment.) | Adolescents must be given the opportunity to be assessed as individuals in a private area. They need to be questioned directly regarding sexual activity and drug or alcohol use. ***Special Considerations:*** *Peer activity is a strong motivator for this age group and it is often helpful to ease into the assessment by asking about the activities of their friends.* |
| *Cognitive domain:* | |
| a. Ask parents about school performance. Request specific information about grades, repeating years, summer school, changing schools. | During junior high, a decrease in grades may occur. This may be related to an increase in peer activities, but may also occur because more abstract concepts are being introduced, and the slower maturing child may not have advanced beyond concrete operations. |
| b. Note whether child's conceptual ability is advancing to an abstract level or is still primarily concrete, e.g., ask, "What are you planning to do after school?" A person whose thought patterns are concrete might answer watch TV, homework, or dinner. If the level of formal operations has been achieved, the child may respond go to law school or be a dancer. | Adult interviewers, who tend to reason more abstractly, may have difficulty communicating with a child who functions at the level of concrete operations. |
| ***Middle adolescent (15 to 18 years old)*** | |
| *Social domain:* | |
| a. Ask parents about current and prior school performance. | Changes in school performance is often one of the first signs of drug or alcohol problems. ***Special Considerations:*** *Educators report a correlation between repeating grades and an increased risk of dropping out. Changing schools is often a parent's attempt to remedy school problems, but may delay identification of drug/alcohol problems.* |

| Steps | Rationale |
|---|---|
| b. Ask parents about rapid mood changes, withdrawn behavior. | Impulse control remains poor for children in this age group. ***Special Considerations:*** *Signs of suicidal behavior include difficulties eating and sleeping. The adolescent often tells a friend of suicide plans.* |
| c. Ask adolescent about participation in sports activities and athletics. | Physical activity can be a healthy outlet for the sexual drive. |
| d. Ask about current job, past work experience, and numbers of hours worked per week. | Teens often test their worth in the world by taking a paying job. Many teens need support and encouragement if their work experience has been a rapid turnover in low-paying jobs. |
| e. Assuring confidentiality, ask adolescent about dating/sexual activity, e.g., ask, "Do you have a special relationship with someone? Does this relationship include sex or might it lead to sex?" Avoid using words such as boyfriend or girlfriend that assume a heterosexual relationship. | A nonjudgmental attitude in eliciting this information will facilitate appropriate counseling regarding contraceptives and information about sexually transmitted diseases. Homosexuality versus heterosexuality is one of the major identity tasks of this age. Use of neutral wording, e.g., partner, conveys a nonjudgmental attitude. ***Special Considerations:*** *Denial is frequently used by teens as a defense mechanism. For example, even when a best friend gets pregnant, the adolescent may deny that she might become pregnant during unprotected intercourse. In denial, multiple somatic complaints may cover real issues. Abdominal pain can often be fear of pregnancy.* |
| f. If sexually active, question regarding contraception, use of barrier contraceptives to prevent sexually transmitted diseases, previous pregnancies or children fathered, abortions, number of partners, and prior sexually transmitted disease. | Because of a general lack of information and use of denial, adolescents are at high risk for pregnancy and sexually transmitted diseases, including HIV. ***Special Considerations:*** *Increased rates of sexually transmitted disease, including gonorrhea, chlamydia, syphilis, condyloma, and herpes lead to early cervical dysplasia.* |
| *Cognitive domain:* | |
| a. Determine the ability to think abstractly. Ask about the courses the adolescent is taking in school and performance. An additional brief cognitive assessment may be conducted by providing a common proverbial expression (e.g., people who live in glass houses should not throw stones) and asking the adolescent to interpret it. | Teens should be capable of formal operational thought patterns. Some coursework, e.g., math, requires abstract thinking. |
| 2. Compare findings to chart or measure being used. Perform a more complete assessment or refer to an appropriate resource if a delay is suspected. | |
| 3. Adapt all nursing interventions to the child's developmental level, e.g., patient teaching, preparation for procedures, and therapeutic play. | Use of appropriate developmental level provides more effective and individualized nursing care than use of chronologic age. |
| 4. Discuss child's development with family. Provide teaching, counseling, or referral to promote development or to address identified needs and concerns. | Improving parental understanding of normal child development and developmental expectations is a significant goal of primary intervention. Additionally, assisting them to understand their child's individual developmental characteristics, promoting sensitivity and responsiveness, and improving parental feelings of confidence and competence to foster the child's development are also important themes (Casey et al, 1986). ***Special Considerations:*** *Ensure that confidentiality is maintained. For age-appropriate activities to promote development, see Skill 15.* |

| Evaluation Outcomes | Observational Guidelines |
|---|---|
| 1. Development is accurately assessed at each well child visit and during any hospitalization. | Documentation reflects milestones achieved to date in all domains and compares them to expected behaviors. |
| 2. Formal developmental testing is arranged for any child with suspected delay. | When milestones achieved are not at expected levels, referrals are made. Reports of formal testing are available. |
| 3. Necessary referrals for services are made. | Name of agency(ies) and case managers are in child's record. |
| 4. Parents demonstrate expectations and management of their child that are appropriate to child's development. | Interview of parents shows a balance between child's abilities and parental actions to discipline, educate, or guide child. |
| 5. The nursing care plan and implemented interventions are appropriate to child's assessed developmental level. | Review care plan and written documentation of intervention for appropriate developmental considerations. |

### Documentation

Document significant information obtained regarding health history, current health status, environmental factors, and the family's expectations related to growth and development. Record and graph, if appropriate, all physical growth measures. Also note developmentally significant findings from the physical assessment.

For developmental screening, note person(s) present, especially if a caregiver is responding to most or all of the questions. For adolescents, note if information was obtained in a private interview. Record at what developmental age level a child is tested, especially if prematurity is a consideration. Record observed/elicited behaviors specific to chronologic age (or previous developmental level), noting failures and areas of advanced behavior. If a child is unable to attain behavioral expectations associated with chronologic age, note the developmental level at which he or she is able to perform.

Document any specific concerns that arose during screening and teaching provided. Document referrals made for any reason, e.g., further developmental testing or drug abuse treatment.

# SKILL 26 Performing a Denver Developmental Screening Test

*Teresa Margaglio*

The Denver Developmental Screening Test (DDST) is a widely used and recognized screening tool that is simple to administer, easy to score and interpret, and useful for repeat evaluations of the same child from 2 weeks to 6 years of age. Screening is beneficial in identifying potential problems of development in the gross motor, language, fine motor-adaptive, and personal-social functions. The DDST is not a diagnostic tool but identifies those children who have a high probability of being developmentally delayed. Identification of problems can result in referral and intervention that can minimize delays. Reassurance and anticipatory guidance from the examiner can further parenting skills and promote an integrated self-concept in the child. This information can be useful when planning care for children in acute or chronic care settings.

Some alternate developmental screening tests are available from the authors of the DDST (see box). For efficiency in screening, use one of the shorter tests; administer a complete DDST only if indicated. The examiner should read and become familiar with the DDST manual before administering the test.

### NURSING DIAGNOSES

Altered growth and development related to physical disabilities and environmental or stimulation deficiencies; Altered parenting, actual or potential related to developmental delays or unrealistic expectations of child; Self-care deficit: bathing, feeding, dressing, toileting related to neuromusculoskeletal impairment; Impaired social interaction related to delayed social skills; Impaired verbal communication related to delayed language skills; Sensory-perceptual alterations related to delays in fine motor-adaptive skills.

## ADDITIONAL DENVER SCREENING TESTS

**REVISED PARENT DEVELOPMENTAL QUESTIONNAIRE (R-PDQ)**

The Revised Parent Developmental Questionnaire (R-PDQ)(Fig. 26-1) is a parent-answered developmental questionnaire that is cost effective, taking about 1 to 3 minutes of staff time to administer. The R-PDQ has been revised to (1) screen children from birth to 6 years of age, (2) make the test items more challenging for the child, (3) provide more information regarding the child's progression for the parent, and (4) provide an easy comparison with the DDST for professionals (Frankenburg, Fandal, and Thornton, 1987). The disadvantage of the R-PDQ is that parent-answered responses may not be correct. The R-PDQ may be used in lower socioeconomic groups, since Frankenburg et al (1987) found a high correlation between the R-PDQ and the DDST in this population. The American Academy of Pediatrics has recommended a two-step process in assessing the development of a child—parent report and an examination of the child (Frankenburg et al, 1988). The R-PDQ meets the parent report recommendation.

If the child has one delay on the R-PDQ, give the family age-appropriate developmental activities and rescreen the child with the R-PDQ in 1 month. If the child fails the rescreen, do a DDST. If the child has two or more delays on the initial R-PDQ, do the DDST as soon as possible.

The R-PDQ forms are only available in English. Four versions based on age range from 0 to 9 months, 9 to 24 months, 2 to 4 years, and 4 to 6 years.

**0-9 MONTHS (R-PDQ)**

## REVISED DENVER PRESCREENING DEVELOPMENTAL QUESTIONNAIRE

Child's Name ____________

Person Completing R-PDQ: ____________

Relation to Child: ____________

For Office Use

Today's Date: ____ yr ____ mo ____ day

Child's Birthdate: ____ yr ____ mo ____ day

Subtract to get Child's Exact Age: ____ yr ____ mo ____ day

R-PDQ Age: (____ yr ____ mo ____ completed wks)

CONTINUE ANSWERING UNTIL **3 "NOs"** ARE CIRCLED — **For Office Use**

**1. Equal Movements**
When your baby is lying on his/her back, can (s)he move each of his/her arms as easily as the other and each of the legs as easily as the other? Answer **No** if your child makes jerky or uncoordinated movements with one or both of his/her arms or legs.
**Yes** **No** (0) FMA

**2. Stomach Lifts Head**
When your baby is on his/her stomach on a flat surface, can (s)he lift his/her head off the surface?
**Yes** **No** (0-3) GM

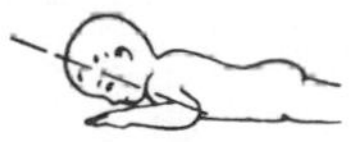

**3. Regards Face**
When your baby is lying on his/her back, can (s)he look at you and watch your face?
**Yes** **No** (1) PS

**4. Follows To Midline**
When your child is on his/her back, can (s)he follow your movement by turning his/her head from one side to facing directly forward?
**Yes** **No** (1-1) FMA

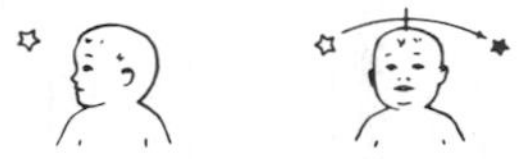

**5. Responds To Bell**
Does your child respond with eye movements, change in breathing or other change in activity to a bell or rattle sounded outside his/her line of vision?
**Yes** **No** (1-2) L

**6. Vocalizes Not Crying**
Does your child make sounds other than crying, such as gurgling, cooing, or babbling?
**Yes** **No** (1-3) L

**7. Smiles Responsively**
When you smile and talk to your baby, does (s)he smile back at you?
**Yes** **No** (1-3) PS

**8. Follows Past Midline**
When your child is on his/her back, does (s)he follow your movement by turning his/her head from one side ***almost all the way to the other side?***
**Yes** **No** (2-2) FMA

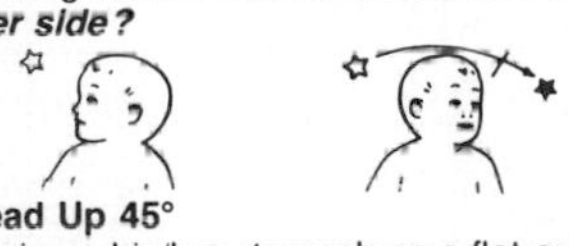

**9. Stomach, Head Up 45°**
When your baby is on his/her stomach on a flat surface, can (s)he lift his/her head 45°?
**Yes** **No** (2-2) GM

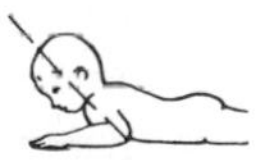

**10. Stomach, Head Up 90°**
When your baby is on his/her stomach on a flat surface, can (s)he lift his/her head 90°?
**Yes** **No** (3) GM

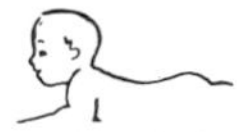

**11. Laughs**
Does your baby laugh out loud without being tickled or touched?
**Yes** **No** (3-1) L

**12. Hands Together**
Does your baby play with his/her hands by touching them together?
**Yes** **No** (3-3) FMA

**13. Follows 180°**
When your child is on his/her back, does (s)he follow your movement from one side ***all the way*** to the other side?
**Yes** **No** (4) FMA

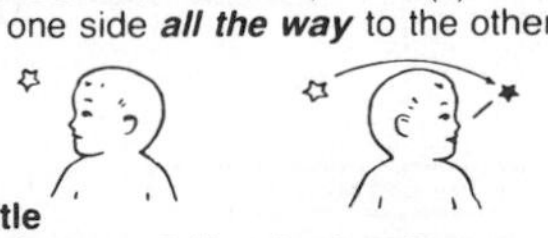

**14. Grasps Rattle**
***It is important that you follow instructions carefully.*** Do ***not*** place the pencil in the palm of your child's hand. When you touch the pencil to the back or tips of your baby's fingers, does your baby grasp the pencil for a few seconds?
**Yes** **No** (4) FMA

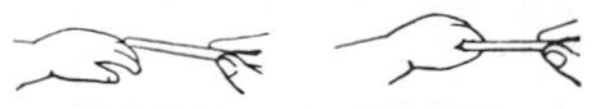

TRY THIS — **NOT** THIS

(Please turn page)



***FIG. 26-1*** Revised Prescreening Developmental Questionnaire.

The first page is reprinted with permission of William K. Frankenburg, MD. Copyright 1975, 1986, WK Frankenburg, MD.

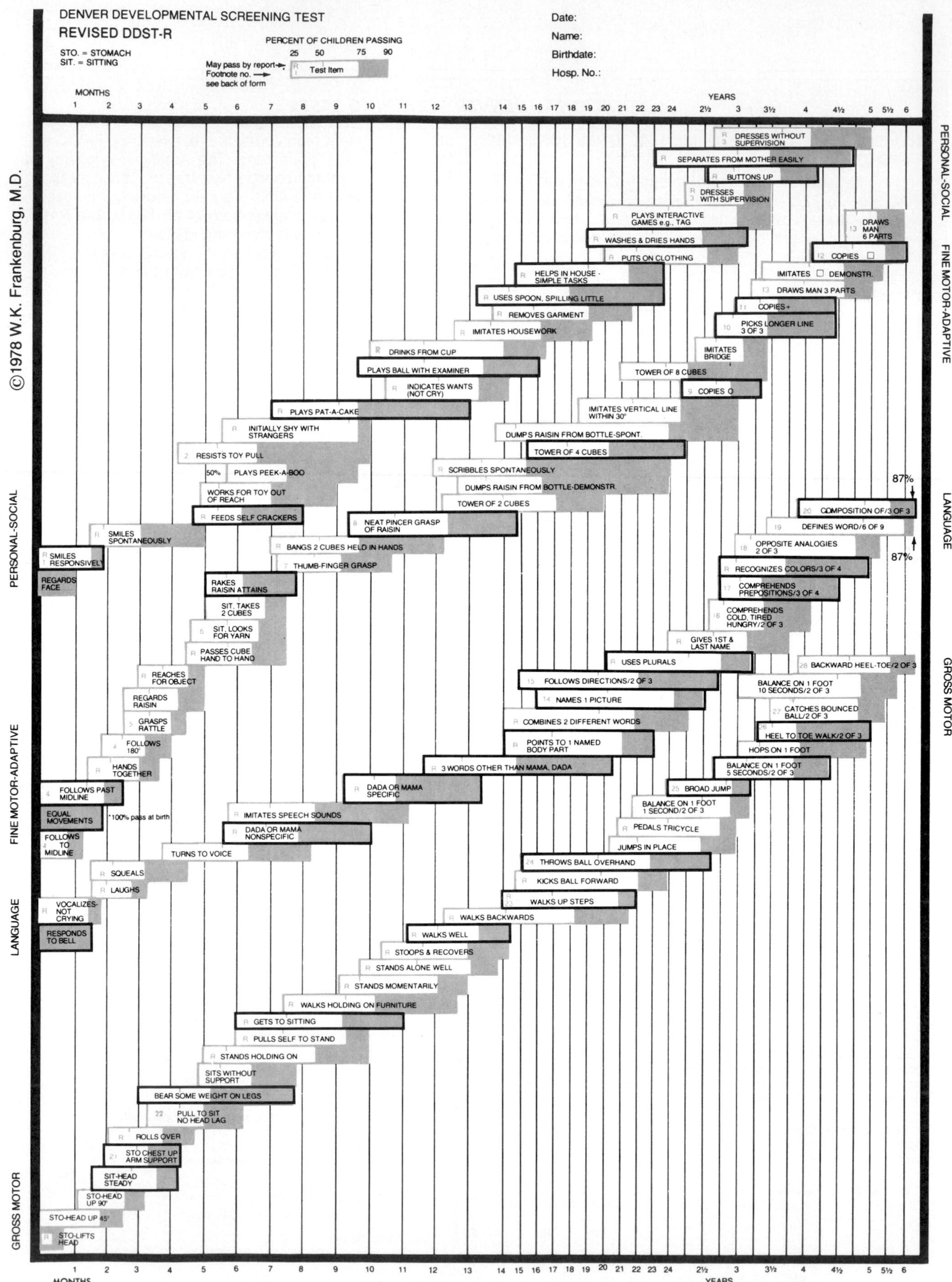


***FIG. 26-2*** The Revised Denver Developmental Screening Test. Resembling a growth curve, this form places items at lowest age level starting at bottom left and progresses upward to right with increasing age. (Refer to actual test for instructions.)

From Frankenburg WK, Sciarillo W, and Burgess D: The newly abbreviated and revised Denver Developmental Screening Test, J Pediatr 99(6):995-999, 1981.

### ADDITIONAL DENVER SCREENING TESTS—cont'd

**SHORT FORM DDST**

The Key Denver Items (KDI) was developed to replace the Short Form DDST. However, it is occasionally used when a R-DDST is not available. Test only the items falling immediately to the left but not touching the age line; there will be 3 in each sector for a total of 12 items. If the child fails or refuses any one or more of the items, administer a complete DDST.

**REVISED DENVER DEVELOPMENTAL SCREENING TEST**

Similar to the original DDST, the items in the Revised Denver Developmental Screening Test (R-DDST)(Fig. 26-2) are arranged in a vertical format, allowing easier administration and interpretation. Either form is acceptable when the complete DDST is administered. The use of the DDST or R-DDST after a child fails the other screening tests (KDI and/or R-PDQ) is to reduce the number of false positives (children with a falsely abnormal score).

## DIRECTIONS

1. Try to get child to smile by smiling, talking or waving. Do not touch him/her.
2. Child must stare at hand several seconds.
3. Parent may help guide tooth brush and put toothpaste on brush.
4. Child does not have to be able to tie shoes or button/zip in the back.
5. Move yarn slowly in an arc from one side to the other, about 8" above child's face.
6. Pass if child grasps rattle when it is touched to the backs or tips of fingers.
7. Pass if child tries to see where yarn went. Yarn should be dropped quickly from sight from tester's hand without arm movement.
8. Child must transfer cube from hand to hand without help of body or table.
9. Pass if child picks up raisin with any part of thumb and finger.
10. Line can vary only 30 degrees or less from tester's line.
11. Make a fist with thumb pointing upward and wiggle only the thumb. Pass if child imitates and does not move any fingers other than the thumb.

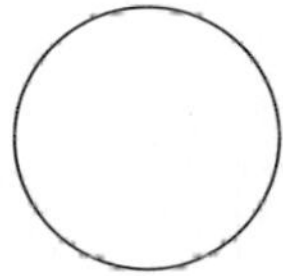

12. Pass any enclosed form. Fail continuous round motions.

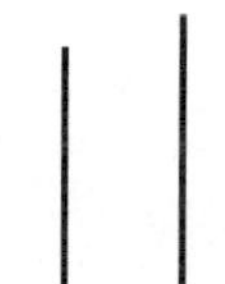

13. Which line is longer? (Not bigger.) Turn paper upside down and repeat. (pass 3 of 3 or 5 of 6)

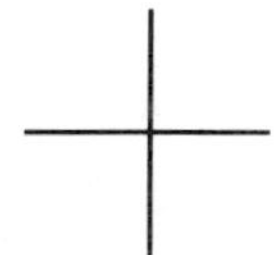

14. Pass any lines crossing near midpoint.

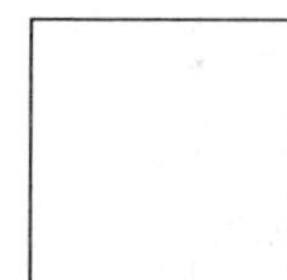

15. Have child copy first. If failed, demonstrate.

When giving items 12, 14, and 15, do not name the forms. Do not demonstrate 12 and 14.

16. When scoring, each pair (2 arms, 2 legs, etc.) counts as one part.
17. Place one cube in cup and shake gently near child's ear, but out of sight. Repeat for other ear.
18. Point to picture and have child name it. (No credit is given for sounds only.) If less than 4 pictures are named correctly, have child point to picture as each is named by tester.

**A**

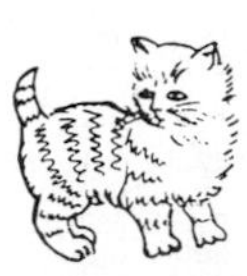
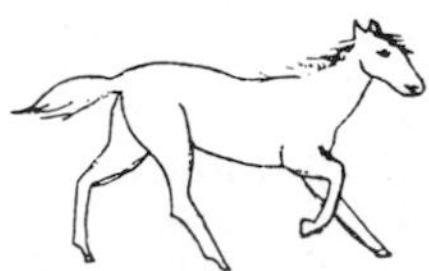
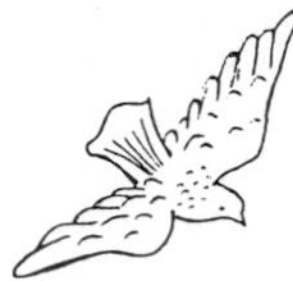
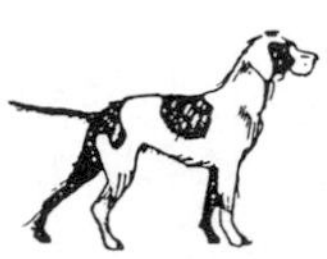
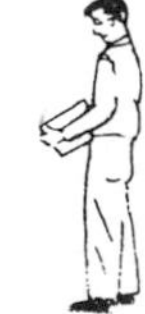

19. Using doll, tell child: Show me the nose, eyes, ears, mouth, hands, feet, tummy, hair. Pass 6 of 8.
20. Using pictures, ask child: Which one flies?... says meow?... talks?... barks?... gallops? Pass 2 of 5, 4 of 5.
21. Ask child: What do you do when you are cold?... tired?... hungry? Pass 2 of 3, 3 of 3.
22. Ask child: What do you do with a cup? What is a chair used for? What is a pencil used for? Action words must be included in answers.
23. Pass if child correctly places and then counts blocks on paper (1, 5).
24. Tell child: Put block **on** table; **under** table; **in front of** me, **behind** me. Pass 4 of 4. (Do not help child by pointing, moving head or eyes.)
25. Ask child: What is a ball?... lake?... desk?... house?... banana?... curtain?... fence?... ceiling? Pass if defined in terms of use, shape, what it is made of, or general category (such as banana is fruit, not just yellow). Pass 5 of 8, 7 of 8.
26. Ask child: If a horse is big, a mouse is __? If fire is hot, ice is __? If the sun shines during the day, the moon shines during the __? Pass 2 of 3.
27. Child may use wall or rail only, not person. May not crawl.
28. Child must throw ball overhand 3 feet to within arm's reach of tester.
29. Child must perform standing broad jump over width of test sheet (8 1/2 inches).
30. Tell child to walk forward, → heel within 1 inch of toe. Tester may demonstrate. Child must walk 4 consecutive steps.
31. In the second year, half of normal children are non-compliant.

* The age of 90% pass for these items varied significantly according to racial/ethnic group, mother's education, and/or residence. The diagnostician is urged to consult the manual (Appendix B) for Colorado data.

***FIG. 26-3 A,*** Instructions and scoring criteria for Denver II.

*Continued*

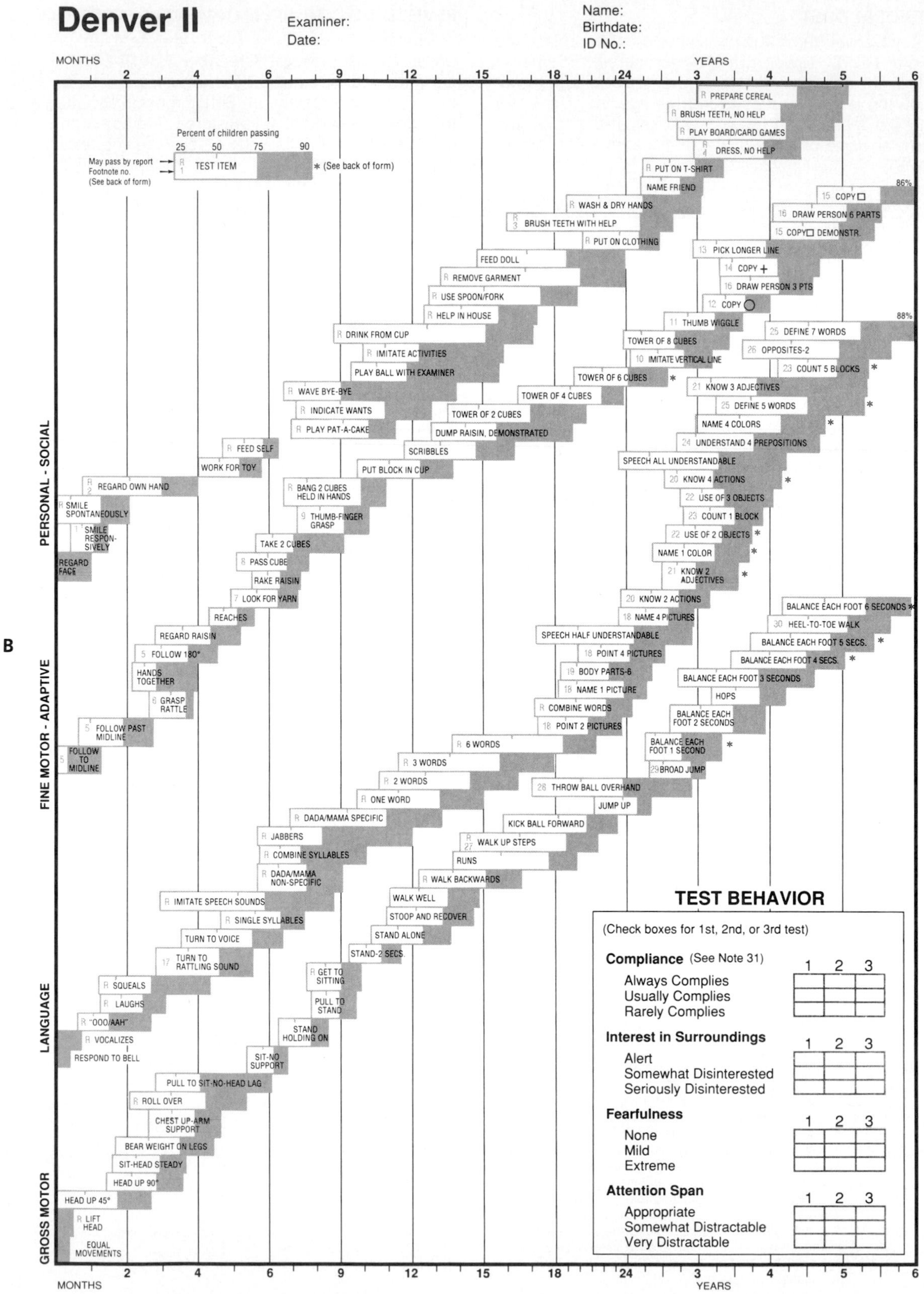


***FIG. 26-3*** cont'd **B,** The Denver II.

## *ADDITIONAL DENVER SCREENING TESTS—cont'd*

**DENVER II**

The DDST has undergone a major revision and restandardization and is now available as the Denver II (Fig. 26-3). The DDST will gradually be replaced by the Denver II but may still be administered while forms are available.

Standardization testing for the Denver II included evaluating each item to determine if significant differences existed between subpopulations. These subpopulations included gender, ethnic group (black, white, or Hispanic), maternal education (less than 12 grades completed or more than 12 grades completed) and place of residence (rural, semirural, or urban).

The Denver II differs from the DDST in the selected items, test form, and interpretation. The total number of items has been increased from 105 to 125; most of the new items are in the language section. Items that were judged as difficult to administer or interpret have been modified or eliminated. The technical manual should be consulted if a delay is identified, since it may be caused by sociocultural differences.

The test form for the Denver II resembles the R-DDST in the vertical placement of items. Key Denver items have been eliminated. The age scale coincides with the American Academy of Pediatrics suggested schedule for health maintenance exams, to facilitate the Denver II's use during these visits. The norms for the distribution bars have been revised to reflect the new standardization data. An addition to the front of the form is a checklist to document the child's behavior during testing.

Scoring and interpretation differences are also present. If a child is able to perform an item to the right of the age line, it is scored as an "advance." If the child passes or fails an item between the 25th and 75th lines, it is an "O.K." If the child fails an item from the 75th to the 90th lines, it is a "caution." If the child is unable to pass an item to the left of the age line, it is a "delay.". Sufficient items should be administered to establish basal and ceiling levels in each sector. To screen only for developmental delays, administer the items located totally to the left of the child's age line. Retesting is recommended in 1 to 3 months for a caution. Retesting for one or more delays, as well as refusals, is done within 1 to 2 weeks.

The Denver II is recommended only as an evaluation of the child's current developmental level and is not a predictor for future development. Abnormalities in more complex functioning may not be recognizable until a later age. Also, changes in the child's biologic or environmental status may affect developmental status.

| Steps | Rationale |
|---|---|
| **Assessment** | |
| 1. Assess child/family's understanding of Denver Developmental Screening Test. | Anxiety and confusion can interfere with performance and reporting of normal results. It is important for the family to realize it is not an IQ test but a screening tool. The child is not expected to perform each item requested on the tool. |
| 2. Obtain health history data. | Risk factors (prenatal, perinatal, and postnatal) can be associated with developmental delays (Table 26-1). |
| a. Maternal health before and during pregnancy. | |
| b. Birth and newborn history. | |
| c. Previous or existing health problems, e.g., hearing or vision loss or neurologic impairment. | Preexisting conditions can influence performance during screening. |
| d. Present health factors: fatigue, illness, hunger, fear. | Present health factors may produce problems in DDST administration and warrant postponement of screening. |
| 3. Assess family's knowledge of growth and development norms. | Parents' perception of expected growth and development may influence child's performance or willingness to succeed as he or she gets older. Parents can have many misconceptions about normal development and expectations of their child. |
| 4. Assess social history: family makeup, adverse economic circumstances, culture, and prior education experiences. | Adverse circumstances may cause the child to not pass certain aspects of the DDST and be scored as abnormal or questionable. Various cultural idiosyncrasies may be misinterpreted, e.g., Puerto Rican children may not establish eye contact (O'Pray, 1980). |
| 5. Assess chronologic age. | Age determines which items are tested.<br>***Special Considerations:*** *Allowances are made for infants born prematurely (see Planning and Goal Setting step 2).* |

***TABLE 26-1*** **Risk Factors**

| Prenatal | Perinatal | Postnatal | Environmental | Family Heritage | Organic Problems |
|---|---|---|---|---|---|
| Inadequate prenatal care | Before or after maturity | Low birth weight <2000 gm | Poverty | History of developmental delays | Seizures |
| Nutritional deficits | Abnormal presentation | Low Apgar score | Interference with maternal-infant interaction | Genetic abnormalities | Congenital malformations |
| Substance abuse | Prolonged labor | Presence of congenital anomalies | Poorly educated mother | History of congenital malformations | Microcephaly, hydranencephaly, hydrocephaly |
| Medication | Precipitous delivery | Respiratory distress | Crowded housing | Inborn errors in metabolism | Sensory losses such as deafness, blindness |
| Maternal age <16 yr or >35 yr | Hypoglycemia | Hyperbilirubinemia | Large family size | | |
| Multiple pregnancy | Hypoxia | Trauma | Poor nutrition and inadequate weight gain | | |
| Maternal diabetes or maternal phenylketonuria | Intracranial hemorrhage | Feeding problems | Lead ingestion | | |
| Infection | | Ingestion of noxious agents | | | |
| Premature rupture of membranes | | Lack of oxygen (near drowning, strangulation) | | | |
| Rh incompatibility | | Head circumference 3 SD above or below the mean | | | |
| Maternal irradiation | | Need for nasogastric feedings | | | |
| Consanguinity | | Thermal instability | | | |
| | | Hypertonia or hypotonia | | | |

From Steele S: Assessing developmental delays in preschool children, J Pediatr Health Care 2(3):141-145, 1988.

| Steps | Rationale |
|---|---|

## Planning and Goal Setting

1. Plan to perform screening in an organized manner; gather equipment and forms (see Figs. 26-2 and 26-3).

Organization promotes complete use of tool and identification of delays or problem.

2. Determine age for testing and draw a vertical line (called the age line) through the four sectors. Place the date of testing at top of the age line.

***Special Considerations:*** *Calculate child's age by subtracting birthdate from test date in years, months, and days. Correct for prematurity until one year old by subtracting the number of weeks born early from the chronological age.*

3. Review the Denver Developmental Screening Test questions and skills for this age child. Items to be administered are:
   a. Items that fall immediately to the left but not touching the age line.
   b. Items crossing the age line.
   c. Items falling immediately to the right of the age line.

Familiarity with the questions will decrease the chances of introducing nonverbal tester bias or missing important parts. Each item is represented on the test form by a bar that is placed between the age scales (Frankenburg and Dodds, 1975).

***Special Considerations:*** *The child will only be tested until receiving 3 failures in each sector, so not all possible items may be tested. The back of the test form provides instruction for items numbered in the left side of the bar. If the item has an "R" on the left side of the bar, it may be passed by report of the caregiver, e.g., "pedals tricycle." It is more reliable, however, if the task is directly observed, e.g., "kicks a ball" or "walks well." For more detailed information, use manual. See Product References and Teaching Resources for test forms and manual availability.*

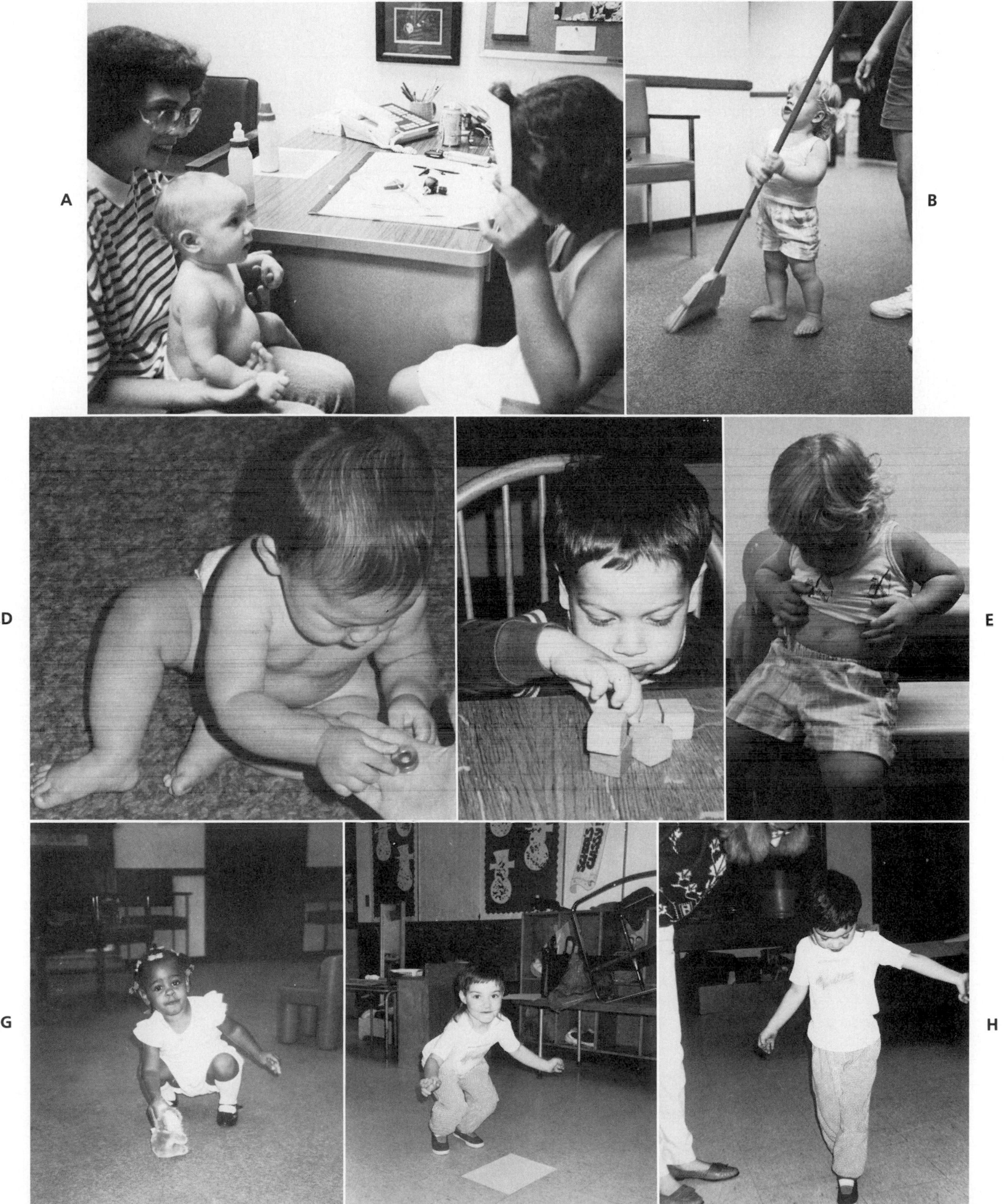

*FIG. 26-4* Developmental screening using the DDST. **A,** Child plays Peek-A-Boo. **B,** Child imitates housework. **C,** Child using the pincer grasp. **D,** Child builds a block tower. **E,** Child points to body part. **F,** Child stoops and recovers. **G,** Child demonstrates broad jump. **H,** Child demonstrates heel-to-toe walk.

(**C** from Whaley LF and Wong DL: Essentials of pediatric nursing, ed 3, St Louis, 1989, The CV Mosby Co.)

| Steps | Rationale |
|---|---|
| 4. Plan for sufficient time to perform DDST (about 15 to 20 minutes). | Adequate time for testing prevents the child from feeling pressured or rushed and allows time afterward for questions. |
| 5. Plan test for time when child is well rested and not hungry or in pain, etc. | Adverse conditions will prevent child from performing his or her best on the DDST. |
| 6. Develop individualized child and family goals:<br>▪ The child is appropriately tested using the DDST.<br>▪ The family demonstrates an understanding of the results.<br>▪ The family is able to promote development specific to the child's needs.<br>▪ The child is referred for further evaluation if appropriate. | |

## Implementation

| Steps | Rationale |
|---|---|
| 1. Explain the DDST to the family. Include that it is a screening tool to observe what the child can do at a particular age. It may help identify possible problems, but not diagnose specific problems. Tell the parent that the child will not be able to do some of the items. | The family has a right to know the purpose and intent of a procedure. Explanations help decrease anxiety over IQ tests, failure, or mental retardation. |
| 2. Inform the family that the results of child's performance will be explained after the test is concluded. | Anxiety may cause the family to interrupt and delay testing. |
| 3. Explain what the child and the family will need to do. | Specific directions on expected roles during testing minimize anxiety. |
| 4. Emphasize and explain that the child is not expected to perform each item on the tool. | Knowing that the child will mostly likely not be able to perform every item will minimize anxiety when the situation does occur. |
| 5. Present the DDST as a game. | Introducing the DDST as a game is nonthreatening, and setting an atmosphere of play increases cooperation. |
| 6. Perform test quickly and present only one toy from the kit at a time in an orderly manner. | Children become easily distracted, which may interrupt performance. |
| 7. Test the child for three items falling immediately to the left but not touching the age line in the first sector. Proceed with items intersected by the age line and those items to the right but not touching the age line until the child fails three items. Test the four sectors in this manner. The child has three opportunities on each item (Fig. 26-4). | Testing the items to the left assures success to provide reassurance to the child and parent, while identifying delays in those not passing.<br>***Special Considerations:*** *If the child refuses to perform an item, allow the parent to make the request.* |
| 8. Scoring—Mark each item on the bar, with "P" for passing, "F" for failing, "R" for refusal and "N.O." for no opportunity.<br>If the child completely fails an item to the left of the age line, it is considered a delay, and should be marked with a dark line on the right side of the bar for easy visibility (see Fig. 26-3). | Scoring the DDST is standard and may be easily interpreted. Failure to perform an item passed by 90% of children of a younger age is considered a delay.<br>***Special Considerations:*** *Interpreting the percentage marks on the bar: left end of the bar indicates that 25% of children perform the item; the hatch mark in the bar indicates that 50% of children perform the item; the left end of the shaded area indicates 75% of children perform the item, and the right end of the bar indicates 90% may perform the item (Frankenburg and Dodds, 1975).* |
| 9. Accept child's reaction to and participation in the screening. | Acceptance helps deal with the participation level and the stress created in an unfamiliar situation.<br>***Special Considerations:*** *Possible reactions include refusal, crying, and easy distractibility.* |
| 10. Praise child's participation in the DDST. | Positive reinforcement encourages cooperation and participation. |
| 11. On completion, ask parents if child's performance is typical. Schedule rescreening if necessary. | Typical performance gives more accurate indications of development. If performance is atypical, retesting may be needed. |
| 12. Review results for interpretation.<br>*Abnormal:*<br>a. Two or more sectors with 2 or more delays.<br>b. One sector with 2 or more delays plus one or more sectors with 1 delay and in that same sector the age line does not intersect a passed item.<br>*Questionable:*<br>a. One sector has 2 or more delays.<br>b. One or more sectors have 1 delay and the age line does not intersect a passed item.<br>*Normal:*<br>a. Any score that does not meet the above criteria. | |

| Steps | Rationale |
|---|---|
| 13. Explain results starting with successful items first, those failed but not expected to pass, and finally those that were delayed. Use the percentage guidelines to reinforce the results. For example, "Mrs. Snow, Jimmy at the age of 4 was able to perform all the items in the personal-social and language sectors. In the fine motor sector he performed the majority of items according to his age. He was unable to draw a 3-part man, which is within normal limits because only 50% of the children his age are able to do this. At 5 years 2 months, 90% of children are able to draw a 3-part man. In the large motor sector, there are some delays present, as Jimmy has difficulty in jumping and balancing for 1 second. Here are some large motor activities to do with Jimmy and we will retest him in 2 to 3 weeks. Remember this is a screening test and not diagnostic of any problems." | Starting with successful items relieves anxiety, allowing more understanding by parent. ***Special Considerations:*** *Frankenburg (1975) states that it is not necessary to share the results or show the test to the parents. If they ask, the examiner should state (if the results are normal) that on this test, the child's development appears normal. If the results are questionable or abnormal, state that there are delays, but remind them that this is a screening and the child needs to be rescreened first and then referred for further evaluation if necessary.* |
| 14. Focus on how well the child performed and reinforce parents' efforts. | Self-concept is affirmed and parental efforts are recognized. |
| 15. Children with abnormal or questionable results should be retested in 2 or 3 weeks. Refer to the child's physician or a child development specialist for a full evaluation if abnormal results are obtained at retesting. | Early referral and intervention minimize delays. |
| 16. Discuss with family ways to foster child's development both in items failed and to achieve next developmental milestones (see Skill 25). | Parenting skills are enhanced and intervention to minimize delays is begun. Developmental screening must be repeated periodically for each child because development is a dynamic process that may be retarded at various ages. (Frankenburg et al, 1976). |
| 17. Support family in following through with any referral for evaluation. | Families will have established a rapport with the original health care provider and need continued support and clarification of the child's progress. |

| Evaluation Outcomes | Observational Guidelines |
|---|---|
| 1. Child participates to the best of his or her ability. | Family reports performance is typical of behavior at other times. |
| 2. Family verbalizes understanding of results and scoring. | Ask family to repeat results of test, naming the areas in which the child passed and areas of delay. |
| 3. Family demonstrates understanding of activities to foster child's development. | Ask family to name some strategies they plan to use to foster development until retesting. |
| 4. The child is retested and/or referred, if appropriate. | A retest is scheduled if performance was atypical, child refuses or otherwise does not complete test, or results are questionable or abnormal. Note documentation of referral, if appropriate. Question family as to follow-up. |

## Documentation

Chart age of child, apparent health status, risk factors that may be influencing delays, score received, teaching, and follow-up recommended (e.g., rescreening in 1 or 2 weeks or if referral is appropriate). Note behavioral observation on back of score sheet.

# SKILL 27 Performing a Physical Assessment

Sherry Baze

Physical assessment is an integral component of nursing assessment. Through inspection, auscultation, percussion, and palpation, important information is added to the data base, which is then used to formulate nursing diagnoses and a plan of care. All nurses should be proficient in these skills. The assessment skills described here are appropriate for registered nurses working with children; pediatric nurse practitioners should be qualified to perform more in-depth assessments. References are provided at the end of this unit if physical assessment study is desired.

## NURSING DIAGNOSES

Health seeking behaviors (physical exam) related to infant/child health promotion/maintenance; Anxiety related to lack of knowledge about physical assessment procedures.

| Steps | Rationale |
|---|---|
| **Assessment** | |
| 1. Review history (see Skill 23). | The history provides important clues to possible findings during physical assessment. |
| 2. Assess age, developmental level, ethnic background, and coping style of child and family (see Skills 11, 25, and 38). | This information will guide preparation and determine approach to be used, as well as being essential to valid interpretation of findings. |
| 3. Identify purpose for physical assessment. | The intended use of the data will determine whether complete assessment is needed or only certain body systems related to specific complaint need to be examined. ***Special Considerations:*** *The child presenting for a well visit will need complete assessment. However, for an acutely ill child, assessment may focus on the specific complaint with complete assessment deferred until child is in less distress. If the child has recently had a complete assessment and presents with a specific complaint, the assessment may be limited to body systems relevant to complaint. Rechecks of positive findings are also generally limited to affected body systems.* |
| **Planning and Goal Setting** | |
| 1. Assemble equipment: stethoscope, ophthalmoscope, otoscope, tongue blades, reflex hammer, penlight, paper, pen. | Although much of physical assessment is done using the senses of sight, hearing, touch, and smell, certain instruments will enhance assessment of specific body systems. Assembling equipment before examination promotes good organization. |
| 2. Plan sequence of assessment based on age, developmental level, and coping style.<br>a. For infants, begin with auscultation of heart and lungs, if quiet. Proceed in head-to-toe sequence, completing invasive procedures (e.g., ear and throat examination) last.<br>b. For toddlers, use minimal physical contact initially and introduce equipment slowly. Auscultate chest and palpate abdomen whenever quiet. Complete invasive procedures last.<br>c. For preschoolers, use head-to-toe sequence if child is cooperative. If child is uncooperative, proceed as with toddler.<br>d. For school-age children and adolescents, use head-to-toe sequence. Genitalia may be examined last. If child is having pain, it is preferable to examine affected areas last. | Adapting approach and sequence to individual child will help decrease child's and family's anxiety and facilitate assessment. A planned, organized approach promotes completeness of assessment. |

| Steps | Rationale |
|---|---|
| 3. Plan diversional activities to be used during examination based on child's age and developmental level. Gather toys and other distractors. | Having toys available helps to put child at ease and avoid restlessness. Hand or finger puppets provide a means of communication with young children, as well as providing distraction. ***Special Considerations:*** *Crayons and paper may also be useful. Rattles, mirrors at eye level, mobiles over examination table, and bright objects are good distractors for infants.* |
| 4. Select location for assessment, taking into consideration lighting, temperature, and privacy. | A well-lighted room with natural or nonglare lighting and neutral coloring assists with accurate assessment. An uncomfortably hot or cold room will affect physical comfort and may alter certain findings. Privacy is a major concern for school-age children and adolescents. |
| 5. Develop individualized goals of nursing care: ▪ Approach and procedures will be adapted to child's developmental level and coping style. ▪ Assessment will be performed using a systematic, organized approach. ▪ Variations from normal physical findings will be identified. | |

## Implementation

### *Approach and preparation*

| Steps | Rationale |
|---|---|
| 1. Approach child, observing readiness to cooperate. Smiling, talking, making eye contact, and allowing nurse to touch him or her are all positive clues to readiness. | ***Special Considerations:*** *If child appears frightened and apprehensive, additional measures may be taken to help adjustment to situation. For example, games such as "Simon Says" may be helpful.* |
| a. Have toys available and allow child to play while interviewing family. | This allows child time to adjust to environment. |
| b. Use personalized approach, greeting by name and complimenting on appearance. Talk to child about toys or dolls; ask child questions about toys. | A personal approach and conversation promotes relaxation. |
| c. Allow choices, when possible, e.g., "Would you like to sit on the table or mom's lap?" Do not, however, give options that do not exist, e.g., "Can you open your mouth?" Instead, say, "Now open your mouth," using a positive manner and tone of voice that suggests that cooperation is expected. | Choices allow child to maintain some control over situation. |
| d. Dolls, hand puppets, or finger puppets may be used to talk with young children (see Skill 12). | Using third-person techniques with a doll or puppet provides an excellent means of communication with young children. |
| e. Begin with activities that may be presented as games, e.g., developmental screening or testing of cranial nerves. | These types of activities tend to minimize anxiety and provide additional time for child to adjust to situation. |
| 2. Prepare child and family for assessment. Give brief overview of what will be done. Proceed to have child appropriately undressed and positioned for the examination. | By alleviating fear of the unknown, involving family, and maintaining comfort, anxiety will be reduced and cooperation improved. Promoting parent's relaxation is essential, since child readily senses parental anxiety. |
| a. Suggest that parent undress infant down to diaper if room temperature permits. Elicit cooperation through use of distractors. The infant may be held on parent's lap or placed on examination table. After 6 months of age, it is preferable to use parent's lap. Approach infant using soft, gentle sing-song voice and smiling; avoid abrupt, jerky movements. | |
| b. Suggest that parent remove toddler's outer clothing; underwear may be removed as body parts are examined. Allow child to inspect and touch equipment. If cooperative, talk about procedure using short, simple phrases. Praise child for cooperative behavior. If uncooperative, perform procedures quickly, but avoid abrupt movements. Toddlers are best examined on parent's lap or standing beside parent. They may be placed lying down across parent's and examiner's laps to complete examination. | |

| Steps | Rationale |
|---|---|
| c. Suggest that preschooler remove clothing down to underpants; if room is cool or child is reluctant, clothing may be removed as examination progresses. Allow child to inspect equipment and briefly demonstrate use. Explain procedures simply. Make up "stories" about procedures, e.g., "I'm going to look to see if Kermit the Frog is in your ear." Always clarify that these are "pretend stories." Give choices, when possible. Preschoolers may be given choice of parent's lap or examination table. If table is used, parent should be in child's view. | |
| d. For school-age children and adolescents, allow child to undress in private and provide gown. Expose only area being examined. Explain procedures, purpose of equipment, and findings as examination progresses. Teach about body function and care as each body system is examined. Emphasize normalcy. School-age children and adolescents are generally cooperative and may be positioned on an examination table. Older children and adolescents may prefer that the family not be present and should be offered that option. | |
| ***General appearance*** | |
| 1. Observe physical appearance, noting whether child appears well, ill, in acute distress, or chronically ill. | General appearance reveals much about health status and provides clues to underlying problems related to malnutrition, poor hygiene, and child abuse or neglect. |
| 2. Observe facies (facial expression and appearance). | Facies provide clues to pain, respiratory distress, acute illness, and emotional status. Diagnostic facies are common in certain chromosomal abnormalities, endocrine diseases, social diseases, and chronic illness. |
| 3. Observe posture, position, and body movements. | Abnormal posturing or movements may indicate musculoskeletal or neurologic disorders. Tilting head to one side may be compensation for vision or hearing loss. A specific body part may be favored because of pain. "Body language" gives important clues to self-esteem and emotional status. |
| 4. Observe level of consciousness, behavior, and activity. Note whether child is alert, lethargic, withdrawn, dull, delirious, or comatose. | An active, chattering, smiling child is usually not acutely ill. |
| 5. Observe interactions between child and family. | Family interactions provide important clues to child's personality, self-esteem, psychosocial status, possible child abuse or neglect, and childrearing practices. |
| 6. Observe hygiene, noting state of cleanliness, any unusual body odors, condition of hair, nails, teeth, and feet, and condition of clothing. | Poor hygiene may be a sign of neglect, inadequate financial resources, inadequate housing, or lack of knowledge of child's needs by the caregiver or of hygiene practices by the child. |
| ***Integument*** | |
| 1. Inspect skin, preferably using natural light or in well-illuminated room with nonglare lighting. Room should be neutral in color. Room temperature should be comfortably warm. | The skin provides clues to problems such as poor hygiene, child abuse, inadequate nutrition, infections, and physical disorders affecting other systems, as well as localized skin disorders. Room colors such as pink, blue, yellow, or orange cast deceiving hues on skin, making accurate assessment difficult. Cold may cause cyanosis or mottling of skin; excessive heat may produce flushing. |
| 2. Observe skin color, noting pigmentation, pallor, jaundice, cyanosis, or erythema. Pay particular attention to sclera, conjunctiva, nail beds, mucous membranes, palms, and soles when assessing skin color. Pressing a glass slide against cheek may assist in evaluating jaundice by producing a blanched background for contrast. | Generalized pallor may indicate anoxia or anemia; edema may produce false pallor by masking skin color. Jaundice, depending on age, may raise suspicions of hemolytic disease, biliary obstruction, or infection. Cyanosis is a late sign of poor oxygenation of blood. Erythema may indicate local inflammation or infection.<br>***Special Considerations:*** *Jaundice is best seen by looking at sclera, skin, and mucous membranes. Carotenemia, a yellow-orange cast to the skin caused by excess carotene ingestion, is most prominent over palms and soles and does not cause yellow sclera. Mongolian spots (large flat blue-black areas) are frequently found over sacrum and buttocks of black and other dark-skinned children. They have no significance and must not be confused with bruising. Black children commonly have a normal bluish pigmentation of gums, buccal mucosa, tongue edges, and nail beds that should not be interpreted as cyanosis. Cyanosis presents as ashen gray lips and tongue in dark-* |

| Steps | Rationale |
|---|---|
| | *skinned children. Erythema, ecchymosis, and petechiae are difficult to visualize in dark-skinned children except in mouth and conjunctiva.* |
| 3. Inspect skin integrity and palpate skin texture for moisture, roughness, rashes, lesions, and birthmarks. Skin is normally smooth and dry to touch. | The skin is a primary defense mechanism against infection; breaks in skin integrity may provide a source of entry for infection. Skin texture provides clues to hydration, nutritional status, hygiene, and presence of infectious disease or allergic responses. Multiple bruises and lesions, particularly over soft tissue areas in varying stages of healing may be a sign of child abuse. Multiple bruises over bony prominences, e.g., shins, knees, and elbows, are common in children. Excessively moist clammy skin may indicate heart disease or other serious illness. |
| 4. Use back of hand to feel skin temperature, comparing different body parts. Compare left and right sides and upper and lower extremities. | Obvious differences in temperature between different body parts may indicate localized exposure to heat or impaired circulation. A key sign for coarctation of the aorta is marked coolness of lower extremities in comparison to upper extremities. |
| 5. Observe skin turgor, elasticity of skin. Pull up 1 to 2 inches of skin on abdomen between thumb and index finger, then quickly release; crease should disappear immediately, without evidence of fingertips. | Skin that remains tented (temporarily suspended and creased) indicates dehydration. |
| 6. Examine nails for color, shape, texture, quality, and hygiene. Nails are normally pink, convex, smooth, hard, and flexible, but not brittle. | Uncut nails with dirt accumulation indicates poor hygiene. Short, ragged nails occur with habitual biting. Abnormalities of nails provide clues to nutritional deficiencies and circulatory and cardiac problems. Fungal infections cause nails to become white with pitted surfaces. Burnished nail surfaces indicate habitual scratching or rubbing of pruritic skin. |
| 7. Observe hair color, texture, amount, and distribution. Note bald or thinning areas. A child's hair is normally lustrous, silky, strong, and elastic. | Stringy, dull, dry, depigmented hair may indicate poor nutrition. Patches of hair loss in infants often indicate trauma or lying in same position for long periods, and may raise suspicions of neglect. Bald or thinning spots may be sign of skin disorder, e.g., tinea capitis. Unusual hair distribution, e.g., low on the neck or forehead, or more than one hair whorl, may indicate genetic disorders (Drapo, 1989).<br>***Special Considerations:*** *Newborns vary in amount of hair, ranging from bald to large amounts of fine, silky hair; however, this hair is normally shed by 2 to 3 months of age and replaced by permanent hair with new texture and often different color. Black children's hair is normally coarse and curly. Braiding or plaiting is common and may lead to hair loss or folliculitis. Grooming with greases and oils is also common and may lead to seborrhea and seborrheic dermatitis (Joyner, 1988).* |
| 8. Examine scalp for cleanliness, lice, ticks, lesions, or signs of trauma. | Any trauma should raise suspicion of possible child abuse.<br>***Special Considerations:*** *Infestations need to be treated (see Skill 82).* |
| ***Lymph nodes*** | |
| 1. Palpate lymph nodes, pressing gently but firmly in circular motion with distal portion of fingers. Generally, lymph nodes are assessed along with that part of body in which they are located (see Fig. 27-1). Note location, size, color, consistency, mobility, temperature, and any tenderness.<br>a. For palpation of cervical nodes, tilt child's head slightly upward.<br>b. For axillary nodes, have arms relaxed at sides but slightly abducted.<br>c. For inguinal nodes, have child supine. | Nodes that are enlarged over 3 mm (1 cm for cervical and inguinal nodes) or are fixed and immobile, warm, red, and/or tender indicate infection, inflammation, or disease proximal to their location.<br>***Special Considerations:*** *Small, nontender, movable nodes, often described as "shotty," are common in children.* |
| ***Head*** | |
| 1. Inspect head for symmetry and shape. Measure head circumference on infants. | Flattening may occur when an infant lies constantly in one position, a possible clue to inadequate knowledge of infant's needs or actual neglect. Asymmetry may be caused by localized swelling, or premature closure of sutures. A prominent forehead (bossing) is found in some genetic conditions, e.g., Hurler syndrome and fragile X syndrome (Drapo, 1989). In neonates, asymmetry may have been caused by position in utero. Unusual shape may be a familial trait. |
| 2. Observe head control and posture. For infant, pull to sitting to observe head control. | Poor head control after 6 months of age indicates slow motor development. Head tilt may be a clue to vision or hearing problems, or brain tumor. |

| Steps | Rationale |
|---|---|

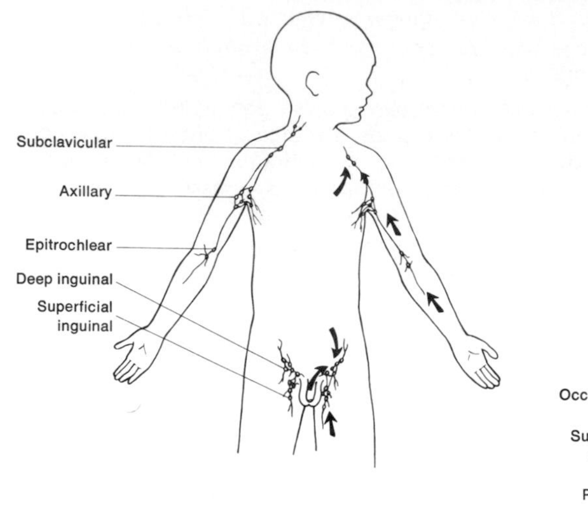


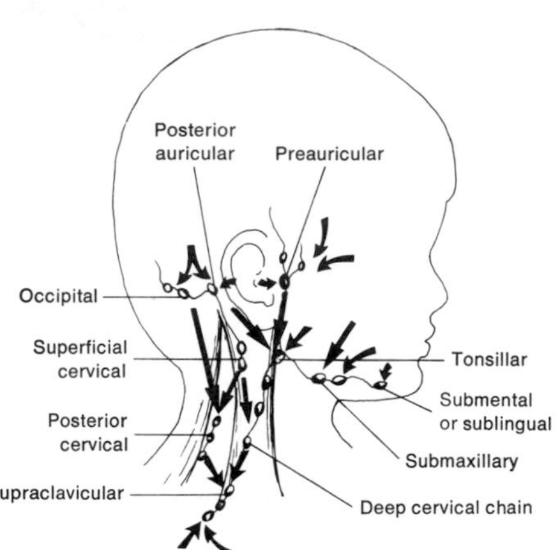


***FIG. 27-1*** Location of superficial lymph nodes. Arrows indicate directional flow of lymph.

From Wong DL and Whaley LF: Clinical manual of pediatric nursing, ed 3, St Louis, 1990, The CV Mosby Co.

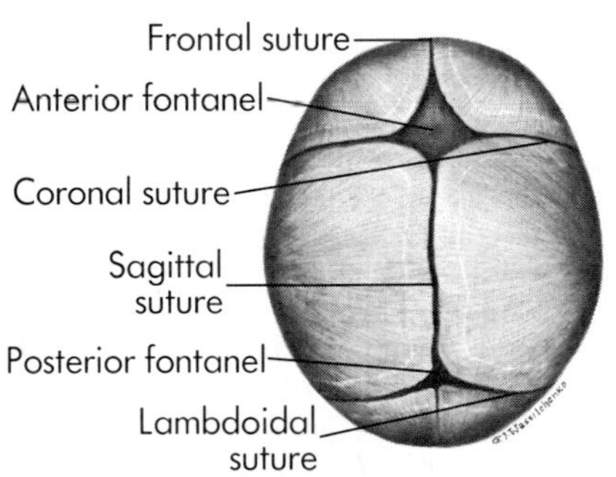


***FIG. 27-2*** Fontanels and sutures.

From Wong DL and Whaley LF: Clinical manual of pediatric nursing, ed 3, St Louis, 1990, The CV Mosby Co.

3. Palpate skull for fontanels, cranial suture lines, masses, or obvious swelling (Fig. 27-2). The anterior fontanel is best palpated while infant is being held in sitting or upright position. It should normally be flat. If open, note size of fontanels, measuring from bone to bone rather than suture to suture.

A tense, bulging fontanel may indicate increased intracranial pressure. A depressed fontanel is a sign of dehydration. Premature or late closure of fontanels may indicate a pathologic condition.

***Special Considerations:*** *In newborns, the posterior fontanel is triangular and measures from 0.5 to 1 cm at widest part; it normally closes from birth to 2 months. The anterior fontanel is diamond shaped and measures from 1.5 to 6 cm in newborns; it gradually closes from 9 to 18 months. A full, bulging fontanel is a normal occurrence with crying, coughing, or while vomiting.*

### *Neck*

1. Inspect neck for size and symmetry, webbing, extra folds and vein distension. Also note excessively small lower jaw (micrognathia) or large lower jaw (macrognathia).

Short or webbed neck may be associated with chromosomal anomalies, e.g., Turner syndrome. Distended veins may indicate cardiac or respiratory problems. Micrognathia can indicate juvenile rheumatoid arthritis or chromosomal abnormalities (Drapo, 1989).

2. Evaluate range of motion (ROM) by having older child look up, down, and to both sides or by passively moving younger child through each position.

Asymmetry and restricted ROM may indicate torticollis, resulting from injury to sternocleidomastoid muscle.

***Special Considerations:*** *Resistance or pain on movement of neck is characteristic of meningeal irritation and requires immediate medical evaluation.*

3. Palpate neck structures (Fig. 27-3). Gently place thumb and finger on each side of trachea and slide fingers up and down, noting any deviations, masses, or nodules. Normally the trachea is in midline or slightly to right of midline.

Deviation of the trachea can indicate a lung disorder, e.g., a tumor or foreign body.

***Special Considerations:*** *Any masses in the neck should be referred to a practitioner for further evaluation.*

4. Palpate carotid arteries, one side at a time to avoid possible carotid occlusion, and observe for protruding veins.

Unequal pulses or protruding veins may indicate cardiac disease or may be a sign of difficult expiration, e.g., asthma or cystic fibrosis.

**Steps** | **Rationale**

***FIG. 27-3*** Anterior view of structures in the neck.

From Whaley LF and Wong DL: Nursing care of infants and children, ed 4, St Louis, 1991, The CV Mosby Co.

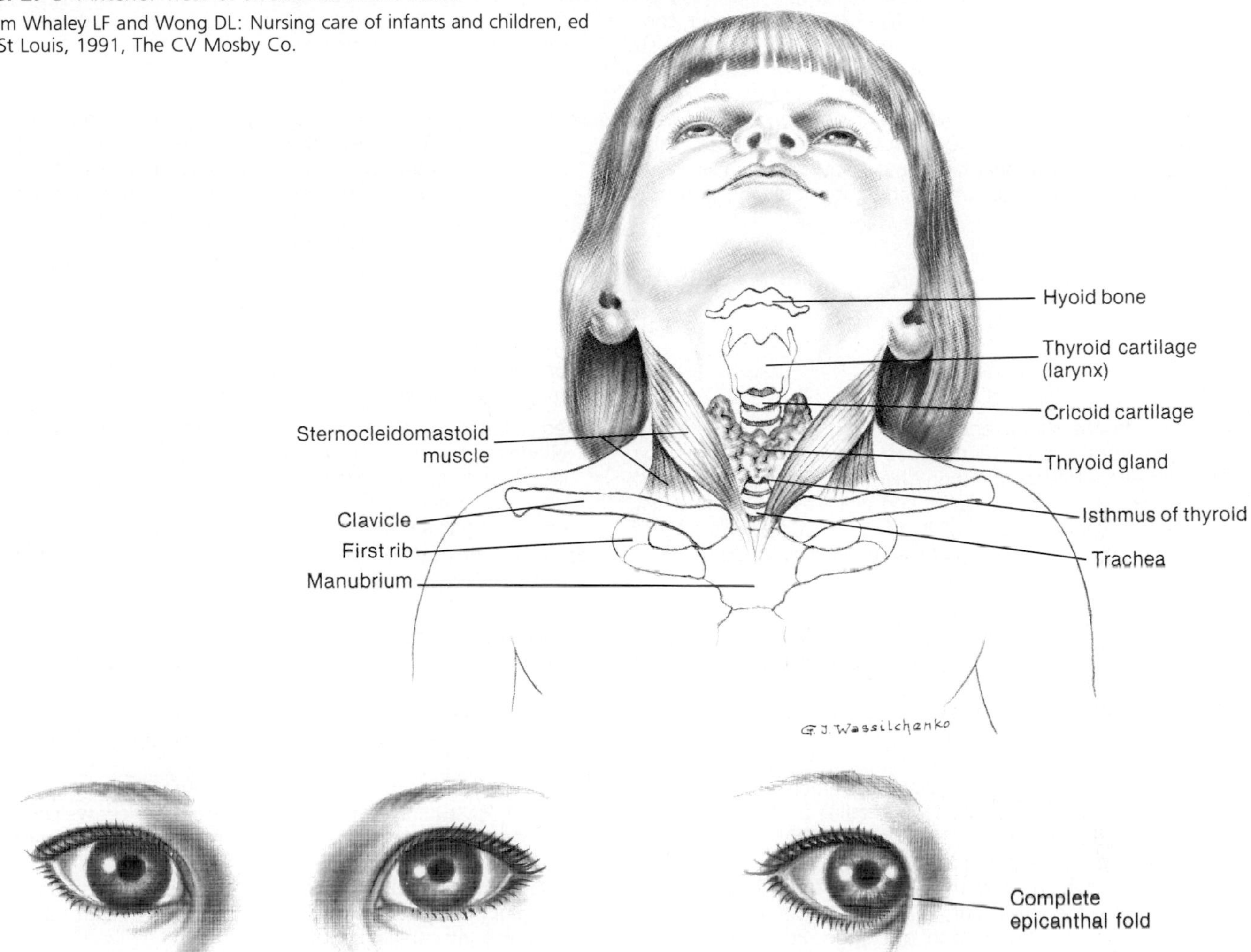


***FIG. 27-4*** Upward palpebral slant.

From Whaley LF and Wong DL: Nursing care of infants and children, ed 4, St Louis, 1991, The CV Mosby Co.

***FIG. 27-5*** Epicanthal folds.

From Whaley LF and Wong DL: Nursing care of infants and children, ed 4, St Louis, 1991, The CV Mosby Co.

### *Eyes*

1. Assess eyes.
   a. Inspect eyes for position, spacing, alignment, and symmetry.
   b. Inspect palpebral slant by drawing imaginary line through two points of medial canthus and across outer orbits, aligning each eye on line. Normally palpebral fissures lie horizontally; in Orientals, slant is normally upward (Fig. 27-4).
   c. Observe lids for placement, movement, and color, noting any ptosis (drooping) of lids, inability to completely close, asymmetry, excessive or infrequent blinking, swelling, or inflammation.
   d. Observe lashes and brows for growth and symmetry.

The eyes may provide clues to chromosomal abnormalities, endocrine disorders, and neurologic status, as well as visual disorders. Hypertelorism, wide spacing between eyes, may be a normal variant; however, when accompanied by other facial anomalies, it may suggest a genetic disorder. For example, hypertelorism, epicanthal folds, and upward palpebral slant are characteristic of Down syndrome. Sunken eyeballs are common with dehydration or chronic malnutrition. Inability to completely close lid over sclera and cornea may lead to chronic eye irritation and infection. Excessive blinking may indicate eyestrain or may be a nervous habit. Long curly eyelashes may indicate Hurler syndrome (Drapo, 1989).

***Special Considerations:*** *Epicanthal folds, an excess fold of skin that overlaps the inner canthus, are common in Asiatic children. They may also be present in other infants, but generally disappear as child grows older (Fig. 27-5). Epicanthal folds may give false appearance of strabismus (see Skill 36).*

| Steps | Rationale |
|---|---|
| 2. Observe conjunctiva. Lower conjunctiva are examined by pulling lower lid down while child looks up. Upper conjunctiva are observed by everting upper lid; gently push down on lid with cotton tipped applicator while pulling upward. Conjunctiva normally appear pink and glossy. | Pallor may indicate anemia. Redness and inflammation may be signs of infection, environmental irritants, fatigue, or eyestrain. Discharge indicates infection. |
| 3. Observe sclera, which should appear white and clear. Check cornea by shining light into eye toward cornea at an oblique angle; it should appear clear and transparent. Observe iris for shape, color, size, and clarity; it should be perfectly round. | Yellow sclera indicate jaundice. Blue sclera may suggest osteogenesis imperfecta. Dilation of blood vessels may indicate irritation, eyestrain, or fatigue. Opacities of cornea may be a sign of scarring or ulceration. Coloboma, a cleft or notching of iris, may indicate a visual field defect. Brushfield spots (black and white speckling of iris) are seen in Down syndrome.<br>***Special Considerations:*** *Scleral hemorrhages are common in newborns and in children who have been violently coughing or vomiting. They are usually of no significance and disappear spontaneously within a few weeks. Tiny black marks in sclera of dark-skinned children are normal and should not be confused with petechiae or foreign body.* |
| 4. Compare size, shape, and movement of pupils; they should appear round, clear, and equal. Test reaction to light by shining light toward and then away from pupil; pupils should constrict as light approaches and dilate as light fades. Test accommodation by having child focus on distant object and then bring object close to face; pupils should constrict as object nears eyes. | Fixed, dilated pupils indicate sympathetic nerve stimulation, blindness, or poisoning. Anoxia, coma, and acidosis cause dilated pupils. Constricted pupils indicate parasympathetic stimulation. White or gray spots observed while looking into pupil indicate opacities or cataracts of lens.<br>***Special Considerations:*** *Normal findings on examination of pupils are commonly recorded as PERRLA, meaning "pupil equal, round, reacts to light, and accommodates."* |
| 5. Check for red reflex by shining light or ophthalmoscope set at "0" directly into pupil; a brilliant, uniform red reflex should be observed. | Visualization of the red reflex rules out most serious defects of the cornea, lens, and aqueous and vitreous chambers. |
| 6. For screening vision, see Skill 35. | |
| ***Ears*** | |
| 1. Inspect pinna for placement and alignment. Normally ears join scalp on or above extension of a line drawn across inner and outer canthi of eye. Note presence of any abnormal openings, skin tags, or sinuses. | Low set ears are common with renal anomalies or mental retardation. Protruding pinna may indicate masses or swelling. Flattened ears in infants may indicate infrequent change of position from side-lying. |
| 2. Inspect for hygiene and any discharge from ear canal. Note color and odor, if present; differentiate between cerumen (wax), which is normal, and discharge. Pull gently on ear lobe to assess for pain. | Purulent discharge or pain indicates infection. Bloody discharge is usually caused by injury of ear canal or foreign body, but may also indicate skull fracture. |
| 3. The ear canal and middle ear structures are examined with an otoscope. The otoscope is held like a pencil with head down and handle resting between thumb and finger.<br>a. Brace examining hand securely against child's head.<br>b. In child under 2 or 3 years of age, ear canal curves upward; the pinna is pulled down and back with free hand in order to straighten canal. In older children ear canal curves down and forward; the pinna is pulled upward and back to straighten canal.<br>c. If child is sitting, tilt the head slightly away from examiner, bringing tympanic membrane into upright position.<br>d. Insert speculum ¼ to ½ inch, using widest speculum that easily accomodates diameter of ear canal.<br>Note any irritation, foreign bodies, or signs of infection. The external canal normally appears pink with minute hairs in outermost portion. The tympanic membrane is normally translucent, pearly-gray with a cone-shaped reflection, with the light reflex at the 5 to 7 o'clock position. Bony landmarks may be visualized behind tympanic membrane: the umbo appears as a small, round, opaque spot near center; the manubrium or handle of malleus (long process) appears as a white line extending from the umbo upward to margin of membrane; the short process of the malleus appears as a short, knoblike protuberance at upper end of long process (Fig. 27-7). | Marked erythema of tympanic membrane and bulging indicated by absence of light reflex and bony landmarks suggest acute otitis media. A dull gray or yellow tinge and retraction of membrane with abnormal prominence of bony landmarks suggest serous otitis media. A small black spot suggests perforation of tympanic membrane. Foreign bodies may be present, a common finding in young children.<br>***Special Considerations:*** *For infants and toddlers, ear examination is best done at end of assessment; for older children, it may be done early using head-to-toe approach. If restraint is necessary, either parent's lap or examination table may be used. On parent's lap, have child sit sideways. Parent restrains arms and chest with one hand and holds head firmly against chest with other hand. Child's legs may be restrained between parent's knees if necessary. On table, place child supine with head turned to side and arms extended along side of head. Parent or assistant holds child's arms at elbows to maintain position. Use upper portion of body to lean over child, restraining the child's body and legs (Fig. 27-6). Slight redness of tympanic membrane is normal in neonates, infants, and young children when crying. Native Americans and children with Down syndrome are at increased risk for otitis media because of a shorter, straighter configuration of eustachian tubes. Next to upper respiratory infections, ear infections are the second most common illness among young children, with peak prevalence from 6 months through 3 years.* |

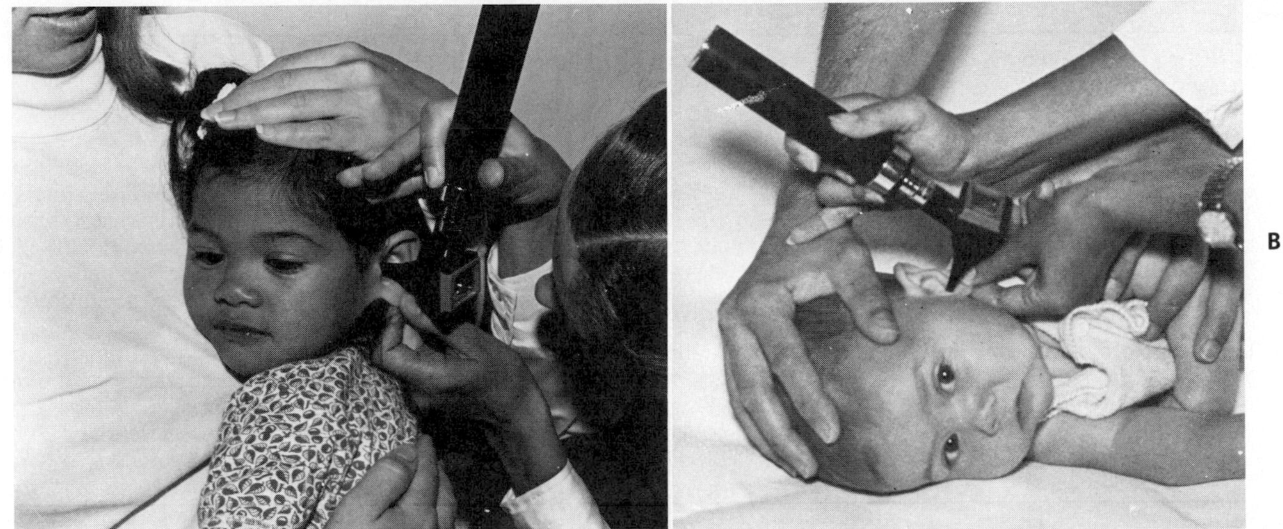


***FIG. 27-6*** Positions for restraint during otoscopic exam. **A,** Child. **B,** Infant.

From Whaley LF and Wong DL: Nursing care of infants and children, ed 4, St Louis, 1991, The CV Mosby Co.

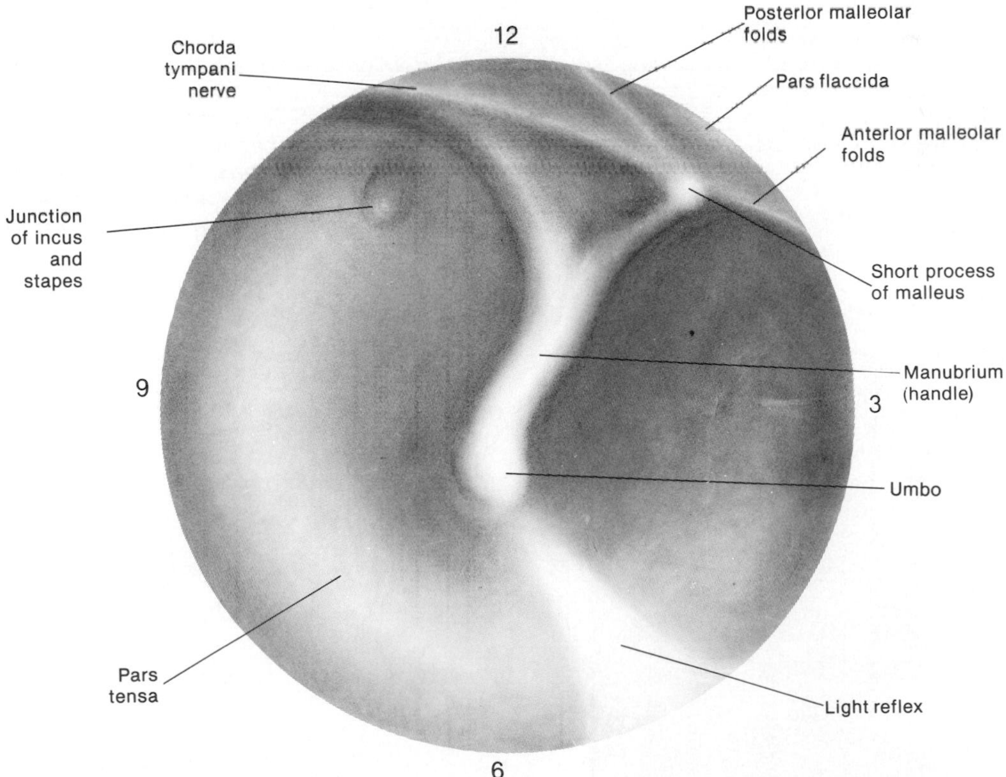


***FIG. 27-7*** Usual landmarks of right tympanic membrane with "clock" superimposed.

From Whaley LF and Wong DL: Nursing care of infants and children, ed 4, St Louis, 1991, The CV Mosby Co.

**Steps** | **Rationale**

4. To screen for air and bone conduction hearing loss the Weber and Rinne tests may be used. Air conduction sound is transferred to the brain via the external, middle, and inner ear. In bone conduction the sound is transferred to the brain via the mastoid bone to the inner ear and auditory nerve.

   a. Assess factors that may affect air conduction: history of upper respiratory infections; otitis media (acute or serous); foreign body in the ear; excessive cerumen; ruptured typmanic membrane.

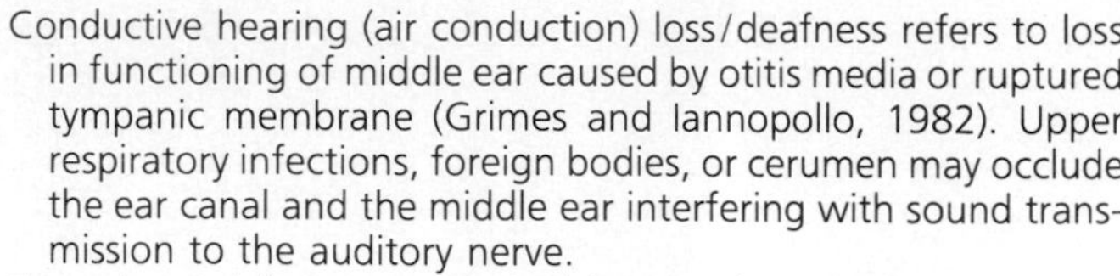

Conductive hearing (air conduction) loss/deafness refers to loss in functioning of middle ear caused by otitis media or ruptured tympanic membrane (Grimes and Iannopollo, 1982). Upper respiratory infections, foreign bodies, or cerumen may occlude the ear canal and the middle ear interfering with sound transmission to the auditory nerve.

   b. Assess factors that may affect bone conduction: trauma from exposure to loud noises, e.g., gunfire or dynamite explosion; chronic middle ear infection that has spread to inner ear; disease such as congenital rubella; cordless telephones; listening to amplified music or attending rock concerts.

Sensorineural (bone conduction) hearing loss/deafness may occur from trauma or disease along the path from the organ of Corti to the brain (Grimes and Iannopollo, 1982).

***Special Considerations:*** *Orchik et al (1985) studied unmodified cordless telephones and hearing loss in young children. The sound levels in the ring of these phones were well above the 115 dB levels and produced hearing loss in the 500 to 2000 Hz range. Listening to loud music may cause hearing loss from nerve damage (Grimes and Iannopollo, 1982).*

   c. Obtain a tuning fork (C octave—512 Hz).

This frequency is within the range of normal speech (300 to 3000 Hz). Lower pitch tuning forks may be felt as vibrations instead of sound, and bone conduction may be overestimated (Bates, 1987).

   d. Explain the procedure to the child. Describe it as a listening game with vibrations or music.
   e. Demonstrate the test by gently striking the tuning fork prongs on own palms, then placing the handle end on own head or forehead.
   f. Again strike tuning fork on own palms, place near the child's ears, and ask if the vibrations can be heard.
   g. Perform the Weber test.
      - Strike the fork against own hand.
      - Touching only the handle, place fork in the center of the child's head or forehead in the midline (Fig. 27-8).

***Special Considerations:*** *Do not handle or touch the prongs as it slows down the vibrations.*

      - Ask if the child hears the sound the same in both ears or louder in one ear.

Hearing the sound better in one ear indicates pathology.

***Special Considerations:*** *To verify that the child understands, have him or her place a finger in one ear. The sound should be louder in that ear, simulating a conductive hearing loss.*

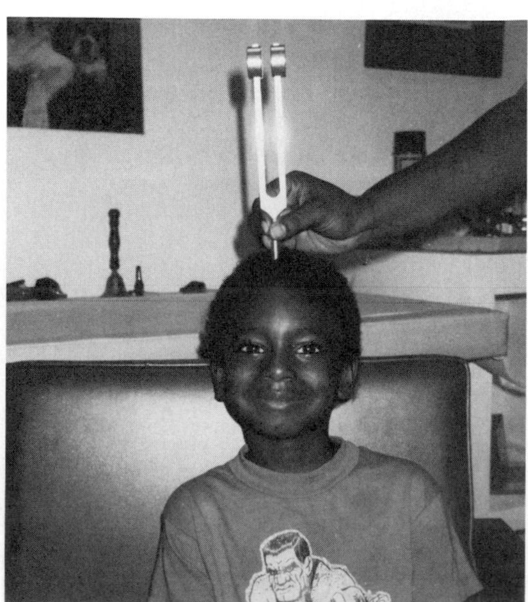

***FIG. 27-8*** Tuning fork is placed in the center of the child's head.

| Steps | Rationale |
|---|---|
| ▪ Repeat testing if the child is confused or hears it louder in either ear. | |
| ▪ Record the results: | |
| (1) If the sound is heard the same or equally in both ears, record: Weber Test—no lateralization. | The normal results would be that child hears the sound equally in both ears. |
| (2) If the child hears the sound better in one ear, write, e.g., Weber Test lateralization to rt (or lt) ear. | Hearing the sound better in one ear indicates either a conductive or sensorineural loss. In a conductive loss, the sound lateralizes to the poorer ear. This occurs because the noise in the room tends to block hearing in the normal ear. The ear with the conductive loss will not be able to hear the noise in the room and will hear the bone conductive sound (Grimes and Iannopollo, 1982). In a sensorineural loss the sound will be heard better in the normal ear because the sound cannot be transmitted to the brain via a damaged nerve. |
| h. Perform the Rinne Test: | |
| ▪ Strike tuning fork against own hand. | |
| ▪ Place the handle of the fork on the child's right mastoid bone directly behind the right ear (Fig. 27-9). | Sound will be transmitted to brain via the mastoid bone. |
| ▪ Ask the child to indicate when the sound is no longer heard or felt. Note the elapsed time. | ***Special Considerations:*** *This requires concentration and cooperation on the part of the child.* |
| ▪ Move the vibrating tuning fork to 1 to 2 inches in front of the auditory meatus, but not touching the ear. Face the "U" of the fork forward to maximize the sound (Fig. 27-10). Do not restrike the fork. | The sound travels to the brain via air conduction. ***Special Considerations:*** *Do not touch the vibrating prongs because it will stop the sound from being produced.* |
| ▪ Ask the child if he or she can hear the vibrations. If it can be heard, have child indicate when sound can no longer be heard. | Since air conduction is about twice as long as bone, the sound should be heard when fork is placed in front of the ear. |
| ▪ Repeat the test with the other ear. | |
| ▪ Record the results: | |
| (1) Positive Rinne is if the child hears the sound longer via air conduction and it is written "AC > BC." | This is the normal response, as air conduction should be twice as long as bone (Bower, 1980). |
| (2) Negative Rinne is if the child does not hear the sound when the fork is placed in front of the ear. It is written "BC > AC." | This is an abnormal response that may mean that there is a conductive hearing loss. The child would not hear vibrations when the fork is placed in front of the ear. ***Special Considerations:*** *With a conductive hearing loss, bone-conducted sound lasts longer than air-conducted sound in the affected ear because the normal pathway through the external and middle ear is blocked (Bower, 1980).* |
| i. Perform audiometric screening (see Skill 34) or refer for audiometric evaluation if lateralization is noted on the Weber Test or if a negative Rinne is obtained. | Further evaluation is necessary for abnormal results on either test. Audiometric testing will screen the hearing range of the child. |

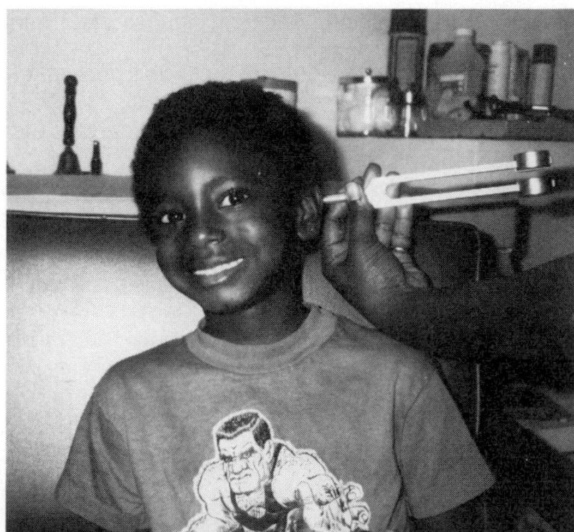

***FIG. 27-9*** Handle of tuning fork is placed on child's right mastoid bone directly behind the ear.

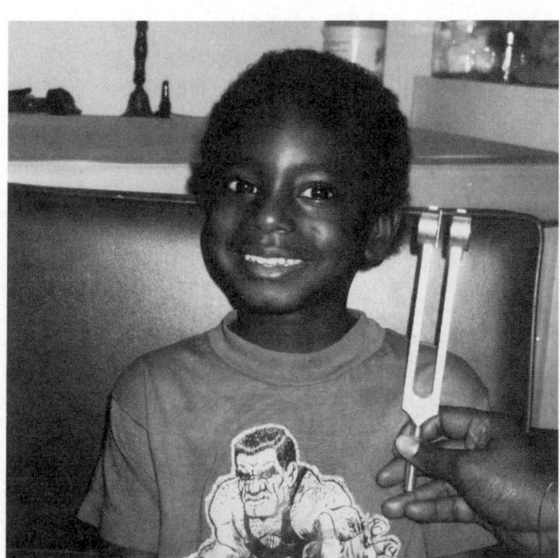

***FIG. 27-10*** Vibrating fork is placed in front of the auditory meatus.

| Steps | Rationale |
|---|---|
| ***Nose*** | |
| 1. Observe nose for size, shape, placement, and symmetry. Observe external nares for patency, flaring, and/or excoriation. | Lack of patency may indicate presence of foreign body. Flaring of nares indicates respiratory distress. |
| 2. Observe nasal membranes and septum by tilting head back, pushing tip of nose up, and illuminating with light. Note color, integrity, swelling, discharge, foreign bodies, or deviated septum. Normally nasal membranes are firm, pink, and slightly darker than oral membranes. Septum should equally divide vestibules. | Pale, swollen, boggy membranes with clear discharge are characteristic of allergies. Red swollen membranes with purulent discharge indicate upper respiratory infection. Discharge from only one nostril suggests foreign body. Deviation of septum may interfere with air passage. |
| 3. For assessment of sense of smell, see cranial nerves. | |
| ***Mouth, throat, and teeth*** | |
| 1. Observe lips, noting color, texture, integrity, and any lesions or excessive salivation. Drooling is normal up to 2 years of age. | Cheilitis (painful, or inflamed, cracked lips) may be caused by harsh environmental conditions, habitual biting or licking, mouth breathing, or dehydration. Fissures at corners of lips may indicate nutritional deficiencies. Excessive salivation may be seen with mouth or salivary gland infections and mental retardation.<br>***Special Considerations:*** *A young child with croupy cough, hoarseness, drooling caused by difficulty swallowing, and respiratory distress with a preference for sitting position may have epiglottitis. Do not proceed to examination of internal mouth structures because of risk of complete airway obstruction. Refer immediately for medical evaluation.* |
| 2. Inspect internal mouth structures by instructing child to open mouth wide, stick out tongue and say "Ah," or by demonstrating for younger child. A tongue blade is usually not necessary with a cooperative child. For younger child who clenches teeth shut, tongue blade is passed through lips to side of mouth, then between molars toward throat, forcing mouth open. Blade is inserted with slightly downward motion, pushing tongue forward and base of tongue downward. Light is needed for illumination (Fig. 27-11). | The mouth provides clues to nutritional status, hydration, infections, and congenital anomalies.<br>***Special Considerations:*** *As with the ear, throat examination is best done at end of assessment up to about 3 years of age. If restraint is necessary, same basic approaches as those described with ear examination may be used.* |

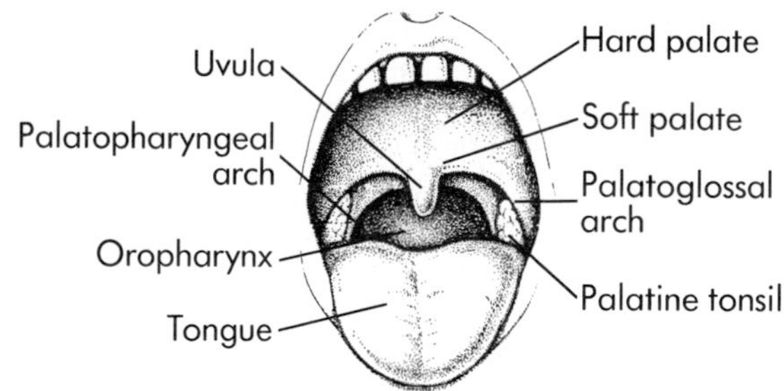


***FIG. 27-11*** Internal structures of the mouth.

From Wong DL and Whaley LF: Clinical manual of pediatric nursing, ed 3, St Louis, 1990, The CV Mosby Co.

| Steps | Rationale |
|---|---|
| a. Observe mucous membranes, gums, and tongue, noting color, moistness, texture, and any lesions or masses. Membranes normally appear pink, smooth, and moist. Gums are normally coral pink with stippled surface texture. | Inflammation or lesions may indicate local or systemic infection, disease, nutritional deficiencies, or poor oral hygiene. White plaques that bleed when scraped are characteristic of thrush. Dryness may indicate dehydration and fever.<br>***Special Considerations:*** *In dark-skinned children, gums are more deeply colored with brown or blue tinge along gum line.* |
| b. Observe size and range of motion of tongue. Tongue movement is observed as child cries or speaks. Tip of tongue should extend at least to gum line. | Restricted movement may interfere with speech development. A large, protruding tongue is seen in some children with mental retardation. |
| c. Observe hard and soft palates. Assess shape and movement of uvula. | Clefts may interfere with nutrition and speech. A bifid uvula is a possible indication of incomplete soft palate. |
| d. Inspect throat and tonsils, noting color and any lesions, postnasal drainage, exudate, or enlargement of tonsils. Tonsils are normally same color as surrounding mucosa with a glandular appearance. | Enlargement of tonsils, erythema, lesions, and exudate indicate infection.<br>***Special Considerations:*** *Tonsils are small in infancy, appear largest during preschool years, then diminish in size as child approaches puberty.* |
| 3. Note any unusual odors from mouth. | Sweet odor of acetone occurs with diabetic acidosis, dehydration, and malnutrition. Odor of ammonia occurs with uremia. Halitosis may indicate tooth decay, poor oral hygiene, mouth breathing, or infection. |

| Steps | Rationale |
|---|---|
| 4. Listen to voice and cry, observing for pitch, hoarseness, shrillness, whining, or weakness. Also note any grunting or stridor. | Voice and cry can provide clues to respiratory and neurologic status. |
| 5. Inspect teeth, noting number, color, any staining, obvious caries, chips in enamel, oral hygiene, and occlusion of upper and lower jaw (Fig. 27-12). | Discoloration of enamel with obvious plaque is sign of poor oral hygiene. Caries appearing as brown spots may indicate inadequate nutrition or poor oral hygiene. Poor tooth formation or decayed appearance may occur with some metabolic diseases, nutritional disturbances, or severe infections. Abnormalities of teeth and malocclusion may lead to pain and poor nutrition. Staining of teeth may result from jaundice, iron or tetracycline therapy, or excess fluoride ingestion. Black lines along gingival margins arouse suspicion of heavy metal ingestion, e.g., lead. |

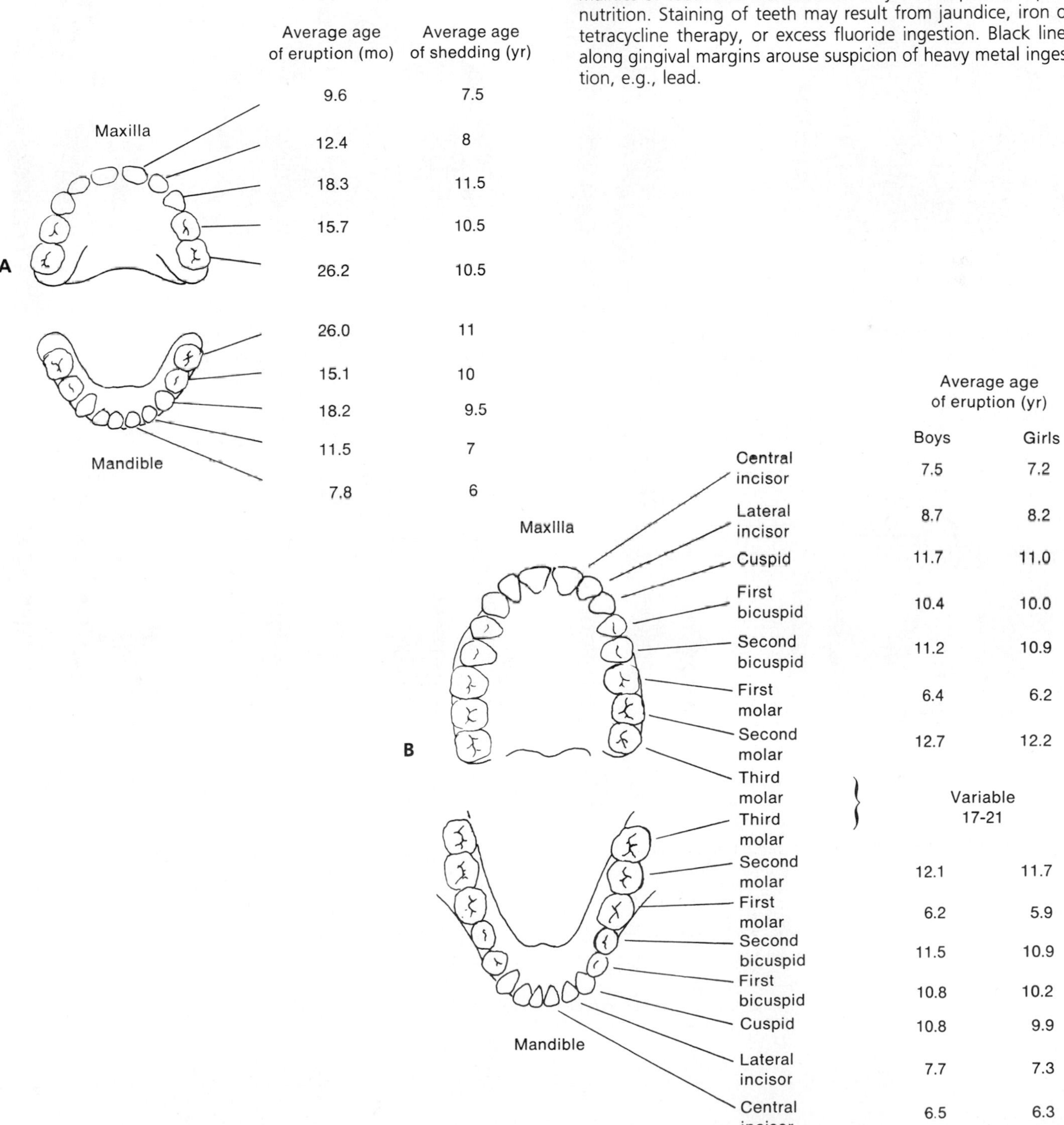


***FIG. 27-12*** Sequence of tooth eruption and shedding. **A,** Primary teeth. **B,** Secondary teeth.

From Wong DL and Whaley LF: Clinical manual of pediatric nursing, ed 3, St Louis, 1990, The CV Mosby Co.

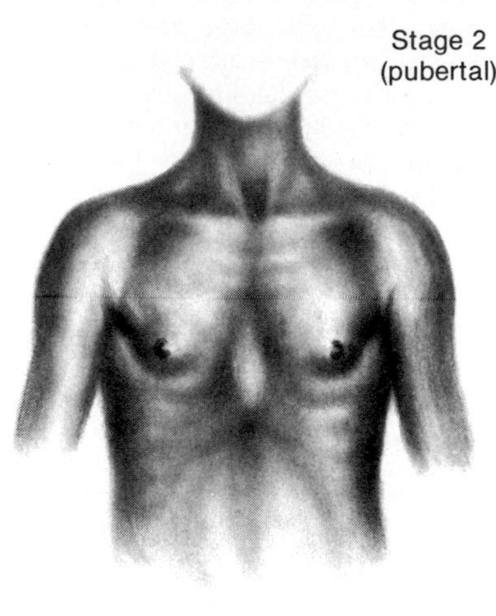


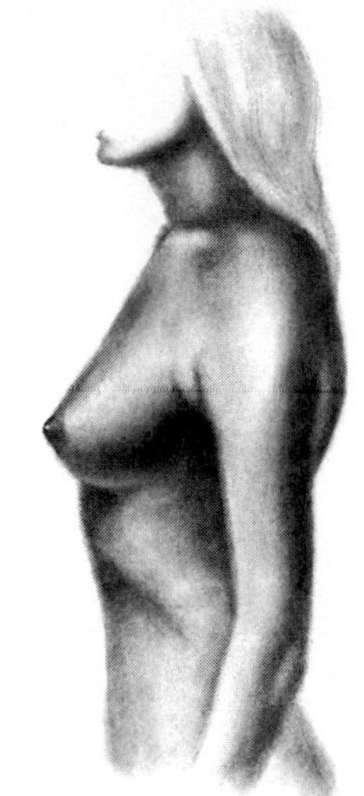


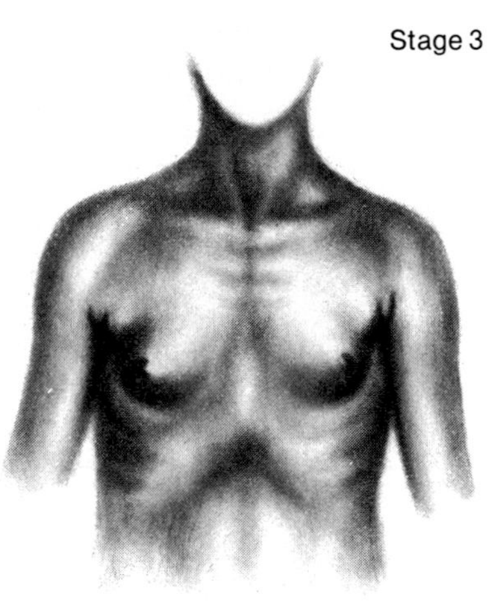
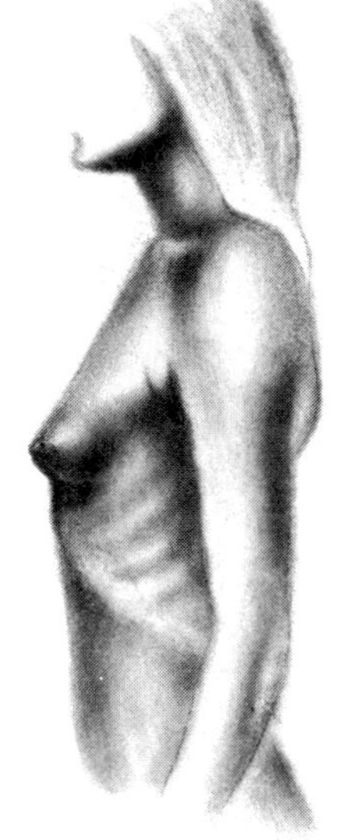


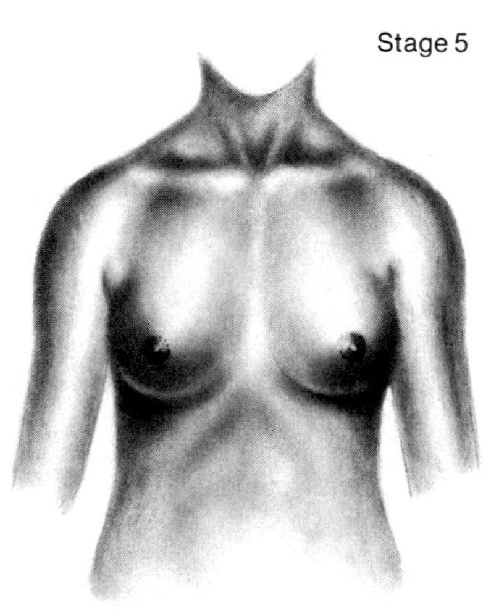
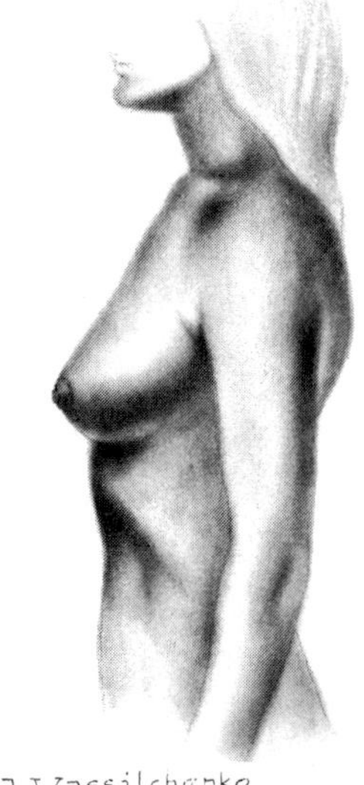


***FIG. 27-13*** Development of the breast in girls. Average age span is 11 to 13 years. Stage 1 (prepubertal—elevation of papilla only) is not shown.

Modified from Marshall WA and Tanner JM: Arch Dis Child 44:291, 1969 and Daniel WA and Paulshock BZ: Patient Care, May 13, 1979, pp 122-124.

| Steps | Rationale |
|---|---|
| ***Chest*** | |
| 1. Inspect chest, noting size, shape, symmetry, and respiratory movement. Chest circumference is measured at nipple line. | Appearance of chest can arouse suspicion of many disease states such as chronic pulmonary disease, rickets, osteoporosis, or congenital anomalies. Abnormal or asymmetrical movements indicate pulmonary dysfunction. ***Special Considerations:*** *Poor posture may lead to poor air exchange.* |
| 2. Inspect breasts, nipples, and areola for shape, size, color, symmetry, and discharge. Palpate adolescent's breasts for masses or hard nodules. Tanner stages are used in assessing female breast development, which usually begins between 10 to 14 years of age (Fig. 27-13). | ***Special Considerations:*** *Precocious or delayed development needs referral for medical evaluation. While the majority of breast masses in adolescents are benign fibroadenomas, prompt referral for medical evaluation is indicated any time a mass or nodule is palpated. Breasts of newborns may normally be enlarged and engorged with secretion of white substance for 1 to 2 weeks because of effect of maternal estrogen. Gynecomastia (enlargement of breast tissue) in male teens is commonly due to adipose tissue from obesity or transitory body change during early puberty, although it may be caused by hormonal or systemic disorders. All adolescents should be taught breast self-examination.* |
| ***Lungs*** | |
| 1. Observe respiratory movements for rate, rhythm, depth, quality, and character during inspiration and expiration. Note type of breathing, e.g., abdominal or thoracic, and presence of retractions. | Tachypnea occurs with lower airway obstruction, early cardiac failure, infection, fever, poisoning, acidosis, and shock. Slow respiratory rate occurs with increased intracranial pressure, depressant drugs, alkalosis, and poisoning. Retractions suggest pulmonary or airway problem. Depth of respirations indicates degree of anoxia, status of respiratory center, and presence of acidosis or alkalosis. Abdominal breathing in child over 6 to 7 years of age may indicate respiratory disorder or fractured rib. ***Special Considerations:*** *In infants and children up to 6 or 7 years of age, respirations are normally abdominal or diaphragmatic; in older children respiratory movement becomes predominantly thoracic. Respirations are less rhythmic in infancy and short periods of apnea may be normal in newborns.* |
| 2. Observe any coughing, stridor, wheezing, hoarseness, grunting, or snoring. Note whether cough is productive or nonproductive, loose or tight. Note appearance of sputum. | Cough may result from infection, pulmonary anomalies, chronic pulmonary disease, foreign body, cardiac failure, allergy, emotion, or habit. Stridor, hoarseness, and barking cough are signs of croup. Grunting and stridor may indicate respiratory distress. |
| 3. Palpate chest for symmetrical movements by placing each hand flat against chest or back with thumbs in midline; assess excursion and expansion. Note any masses or areas of tenderness on chest. | Asymmetrical movements suggest pulmonary dysfunction. |
| 4. Percuss each side of chest in sequence from apex to base. For anterior chest, have child sitting or supine; for posterior chest, have child sitting (Fig. 27-14). | Percussion may assist in identification of liver or heart enlargement, lung collapse, pulmonary edema, lung consolidation, accumulation of fluid in pleural space, emphysema, tumors, and obstructive foreign body. |

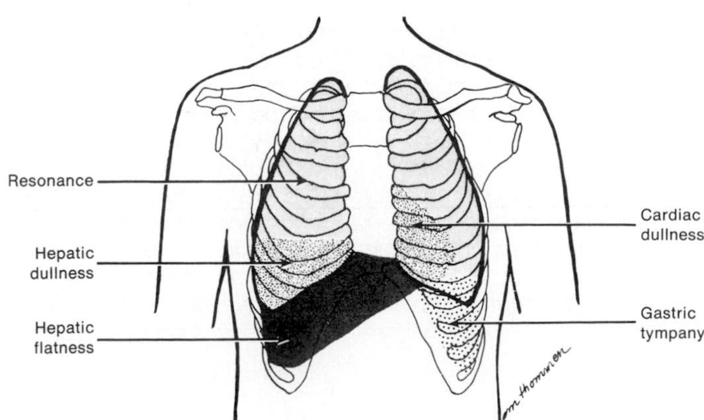


***FIG. 27-14*** Percussion sounds in the thorax.

From Wong DL and Whaley LF: Clinical manual of pediatric nursing, ed 3, St Louis, 1990, The CV Mosby Co.

**Steps**

a. Place finger of one hand on chest wall; use index or middle finger of other hand as percussing hammer; no other fingers should touch chest wall.
b. The percussing finger should move like a piano hammer with very loose hinge-joint action at wrist.

Resonance (a long, low-pitched hollow sound) is expected except for dullness (a soft, high-pitched, thudlike sound) over liver, heart, diaphragm, and scapula, and tympany (a loud, high-pitched, musical note) is expected over stomach.

5. Auscultate breath sounds for intensity, pitch, quality, and relative duration of inspiration and expiration. Note any adventitious sounds, e.g., crackles, wheezes, or pleural friction rub.
   a. The entire chest, including anterior, posterior, and axillary areas, is auscultated, moving side to side for comparison.
   b. Bell or small diaphragm of stethoscope must be placed firmly against chest wall. In infants and young children, it is usually easier to get a tight fit if bell is placed in interspaces rather than over ribs.
   c. Breath sounds are heard best with deep inspiration. The older child can be encouraged to take deep breaths by demonstration. Younger children can be asked to make a pinwheel spin, "blow out" light on otoscope, or blow up balloon.

### *Heart*

1. Observe chest wall from front and at angle for symmetry. Note any bulging, visible pulsations or heaving.
2. Using fingertips, palpate anterior chest wall for point of maximum impulse (PMI). For infant, PMI is normally at fourth to fifth intercostal space (space immediately below corresponding rib) and lateral to left sternal border. For a child over 7 years of age, PMI is normally at fifth intercostal space and near left nipple line. With ball of palm, palpate for thrills or rubs.
3. Auscultate heart sounds: $S_1$ is "lub" heard at beginning of systole as mitral and tricuspid valve close; $S_2$ is "dub" heard at beginning of diastole as aortic and pulmonic valves close. Listen with child in both sitting and supine positions, using both bell and diaphragm of stethoscope.
   a. Evaluate sounds for quality, which should be clear and distinct; rate, which should be same as radial pulse; and rhythm, which should be regular and even.
   b. Note any murmurs, clicks, or pericardial friction rub. Murmurs are distinct, swishing sounds; note location on chest wall where best heard, timing in $S_1$ $S_2$ cycle, intensity or loudness, and quality. Pericardial friction rubs are high-pitched grating sounds that are not affected by breathing; pleural friction rubs stop when child holds breath.
   c. Auscultate systematically (Fig. 27-15):
      - Aortic area at second right intercostal space close to sternum—here $S_1$ is louder than $S_2$ and aortic valve closure is heard best.
      - Pulmonic area at second left intercostal space close to sternum—here splitting of $S_2$ is heard best, with normal widening on inspiration, and pulmonic valve closure.
      - Erb point at second and third left intercostal space close to sternum—this is a frequent site for both innocent murmurs and those of aortic or pulmonic origin.
      - Tricuspid area at fifth right and left intercostal spaces close to sternum—here $S_1$ is heard as a louder sound preceding $S_2$. $S_1$ is synchronous with carotid pulse.

**Rationale**

***Special Considerations:*** *A thin chest wall and small muscles make chest seem more resonant in young children.*

Absent or diminished breath sounds are always abnormal and indicate pulmonary disease or presence of foreign body. Adventitious sounds indicate abnormality of lower respiratory tract and potential for interference with ventilation.

***Special Considerations:*** *Breath sounds in infants and young children seem louder and harsher than in adults because of thinness of chest wall. They are almost all bronchovesicular with medium pitch and expiration equal to inspiration, or even bronchial with high pitch and long, loud expiration.*

Chest bulging is a sign of right-sided heart enlargement.

***Special Considerations:*** *Visible pulsations may be normal in thin child.*

PMI gives indication of heart size because it is usually located at apex; with cardiac enlargement, apex is displaced downward and laterally.

***Special Considerations:*** *PMI may be difficult to feel in children under 2 years of age or in children with pericardial effusion, or heart failure. A forceful apical beat is common after exercise, with excitement, and in a child with a thin chest wall, impending heart failure, fever, hyperthyroidism, anemia, or anxiety.*

Dysrhythmia (failure of heart to beat at regular intervals) interferes with the heart's ability to pump effectively. Extra heart sounds may indicate impaired heart or vascular function. Murmurs are characteristic of changes in blood flow through heart or abnormalities in valve closure.

***Special Considerations:*** *Heart sounds in children may seem louder and higher pitched because of thin chest wall. $S_3$, an additional heart sound, results from vibrations produced during ventricular filling and is normal in some children. Murmurs may be asymptomatic and are common in children; differentiation must be made by physician between innocent (functional) and organic murmurs. Innocent murmurs are usually heard loudest in pulmonic area, and are systolic (occurring with or after $S_1$), of short duration and low intensity, and with low-pitched musical quality; they may disappear with change in position, are not associated with physical signs of cardiac disease, and do not affect growth. Sinus dysrhythmia, in which heart rate increases with inspiration and decreases with expiration, occurs normally in many children; it may be differentiated from abnormal arrhythmias by having child hold breath momentarily, which will cause heart rate to remain steady.*

| **Steps** | **Rationale** |
|---|---|

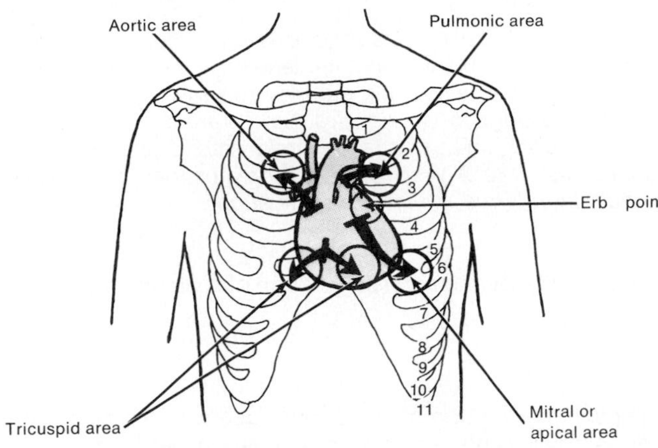


***FIG. 27-15*** Direction of heart sounds from anatomic valve sites.

From Wong DL and Whaley LF: Clinical manual of pediatric nursing, ed 3, St Louis, 1990, The CV Mosby Co.

- Mitral or apical area at fifth intercostal space at left nipple line or, for infants, at fourth to fifth intercostal space lateral to left sternal border—here $S_1$ is best heard.

### *Abdomen*

1. Inspect contour, size, muscle tone, and movement of abdomen, at eye level and from above. Note condition and color of skin, scars, discolorations (e.g., ecchymoses or cafe-au-lait spots), and distension.

These are good indicators of nutritional status and muscular development. Visible peristalsis may be sign of obstruction.
***Special Considerations:*** *"Potbelly" is generally considered normal until child reaches puberty. Abdominal respirations are normal up to 6 or 7 years of age; even in older children, abdomen usually moves with respirations when supine.*

2. Auscultate bowel sounds before palpation or percussion by pressing stethoscope firmly against abdominal wall. Sounds may be stimulated, if necessary, by stroking each quadrant of abdominal wall lightly with fingertip. Peristaltic sounds are a metallic, short tinkling, gurgling, or growling, normally heard every 10 to 30 seconds.

Percussion and palpation may distort bowel sounds. High-pitched, frequent sounds occur with diarrhea, early peritonitis, intestinal obstruction, and gastroenteritis. Decreased or absent sounds may indicate paralytic ileus or peritonitis.

3. Percuss abdomen. Tympany (a high-pitched, hollow, musical note) is normal over stomach and most of abdomen; dullness occurs over liver just below right costal margin.

Lack of tympany suggests fluid or solid masses. Above symphysis pubis, lack of tympany may indicate full bladder.

4. Palpate abdominal organs, beginning in left lower quadrant and proceeding to left upper quadrant, right upper quadrant, and right lower quadrant (Fig. 27-16).
   a. Palpate first superficially and then repeat deeply.
   b. The abdominal muscles must be relaxed; relaxation is promoted by having child take deep breaths and flex knees. Tickling sensation may be lessened by placing child's hand on top of examiner's palpating hand; distraction with talking or toys is also useful.
   c. Warm hands before palpation of abdomen. Note any tenseness, tenderness, or masses. Note pupils while palpating; when tender area is touched, pupils constrict.

Tense abdomen with marked rigidity or resistance to pressure is indicative of surgical condition needing immediate evaluation. Any masses require medical evaluation.
***Special Considerations:*** *For infants and young children, it may be useful to examine abdomen early in assessment if child is quiet; or it may be necessary to return to abdomen later if child becomes tense, is crying on palpation, or complains of pain in abdomen. Young children almost always point to umbilical area when asked where abdomen hurts. Pointing to any other part of abdomen may be significant. In infants and young children, the liver may normally extend 1 to 2 cm below right costal margin and should feel firm and smooth. The spleen may extend 1 to 2 cm below left costal margin and is felt as a soft, slightly curved organ.*

***FIG. 27-16*** Location of organs in the abdomen.

From Wong DL and Whaley LF: Clinical manual of pediatric nursing, ed 3, St Louis, 1990, The CV Mosby Co.

| Steps | Rationale |
|---|---|
| 5. Assess for hernias.<br>a. Inspect umbilicus for hernia, fistulas, discharge, odor, and hygiene (Fig. 27-17).<br>b. Observe for inguinal hernia by sliding little finger into external inguinal ring at base of scrotum. Inguinal hernia will be felt as bulge when child coughs, laughs, or cries.<br>c. Observe for femoral hernia by palpating femoral canal, located below inguinal ligament medial to femoral artery. Note any bulging, swelling, or tenderness.<br>d. Palpate hernia for abdominal contents, if hernia noted. | Inguinal and femoral hernias require surgical repair. Incarceration, with irreducible swelling, tenderness, and pain, may result in intestinal obstruction and requires immediate referral.<br>***Special Considerations:*** *Umbilical hernias are common, particularly in black infants, and generally resolve spontaneously during first 1 to 2 years of life; if greater than 5 cm, child should be referred for medical evaluation.* |
| 6. Palpate femoral pulses by lightly placing tips of fingers midway between iliac crest and symphysis pubis. Note strength and equality bilaterally. | Absent or decreased femoral pulse is sign of coarctation of aorta. |
| ***Genitalia (Males)*** | |
| 1. Observe size of penis. Inspect for swelling, skin lesions, or inflammation of glans and shaft. Inspect prepuce. | Large penis may be sign of precocious puberty or testicular cancer. A small penis is common in many genetic syndromes (Drapo, 1989). Skin lesions and inflammation may indicate infection.<br>***Special Considerations:*** *In uncircumcised infants and young boys, prepuce may be tight; do not force retraction. By 3 to 4 years of age, foreskin should easily retract.* |
| 2. Inspect for placement of urethral meatus. Note any discharge or excoriation. If possible, observe strength and direction of urinary stream. | Location of meatus on ventral or dorsal surface of penis is termed hypospadias or epispadias and may be sign of ambiguous genitalia. Pinpoint urethral opening and poor urinary stream may indicate urethral stenosis. |
| 3. Inspect scrotum, noting size, color, location, symmetry, skin, hair distribution, masses, and lesions. Palpate testes using thumb and index finger. Cremasteric reflex, which causes retraction of scrotal contents, is prevented by warming hands before examination, having child sit in tailor fashion, and blocking path of ascent by placing thumb and index finger over upper part of scrotal sac along inguinal canal (Fig. 27-18). Procedure may be performed in warm tub of water, if necessary. | Scrotum that is small, close to perineum, and with midline separation may be sign of ambiguous genitalia. A medical referral is indicated for a child over 1 year of age with undescended testes.<br>***Special Considerations:*** *By 1 year of age, undescended testes will descend spontaneously in 75% of infants. Descended testes should always be documented, since they may not be palpated at next exam because of cremasteric reflex.* |
| 4. Assess development of secondary sexual characteristics using Tanner Stages (Fig. 27-19). | Precocious or delayed development should be referred for medical evaluation. |
| ***Genitalia (Females)*** | |
| 1. Inspect external genitalia by placing child in supine position with knees bent and soles of feet in apposition. Observe mons pubis, clitoris, labia majora, and labia minora for size, color, integrity, and lesions. Palpate labia for masses (Fig. 27-20). | Fusion of labia or enlargement of labia or clitoris may indicate ambiguous genitalia. Palpable masses may be testes. |
| 2. Inspect urethral meatus for location, color, and discharge. | This is common site for cysts and venereal warts. |
| 3. Inspect vaginal orifice for obvious opening and any discharge or odor. Inspect Bartholin glands surrounding vagina. | Excessive or foul-smelling discharge is sign of infection.<br>***Special Considerations:*** *Internal pelvic exam is usually not done in children.* |
| 4. Assess development of secondary sexual characteristics using Tanner stages (Fig. 27-21). Obtain history of menses. | Precocious or delayed development should be referred for medical evaluation. |
| ***Anus*** | |
| 1. Inspect anus for general firmness, intactness and condition of skin. Note presence of polyps, warts, or skin tags. Elicit anal reflex by pricking or scratching perianal area gently; this should produce quick contraction of external sphincter with no protrusion of rectum. | Irritation of skin may be caused by diaper rash or pinworms. Fissures, polyps, warts, or rectal prolapse may be identified on inspection. |
| ***Back and extremities*** | |
| 1. Inspect curvature and symmetry of spine, shoulders, and hips. Palpate spine, noting any dimpling. Screen for scoliosis by:<br>a. Having child stand erect while observing from behind for any asymmetry of shoulders or hips.<br>b. Having child bend forward at waist with arms dangling, observing from front, side, and back for any asymmetry or prominence of scapula, rib cage or iliac crest, or for any lateral curve (Fig. 27-22). | Scoliosis indicates musculoskeletal or neurologic disorders. Mild scoliosis with no rotation and that straightens in prone position may be related to poor postural habits. Dimpling in the spine can be associated with spina bifida occulta.<br>***Special Considerations:*** *Under 5 years of age, scoliosis is usually related to congenital anomalies or lung or chest pathology. In older children, it may be idiopathic or caused by skeletal or neuromuscular disorders. In infants under 3 months of age, spine is normally rounded; lumbar curve forms at 12 to 18 months. Lumbar lordosis is normal in young children.* |

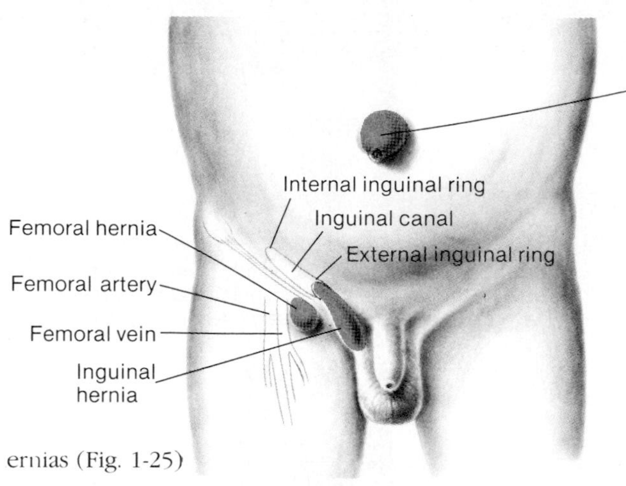


***FIG. 27-17*** Location of hernias.

From Wong DL and Whaley LF: Clinical manual of pediatric nursing, ed 3, St Louis, 1990, The CV Mosby Co.

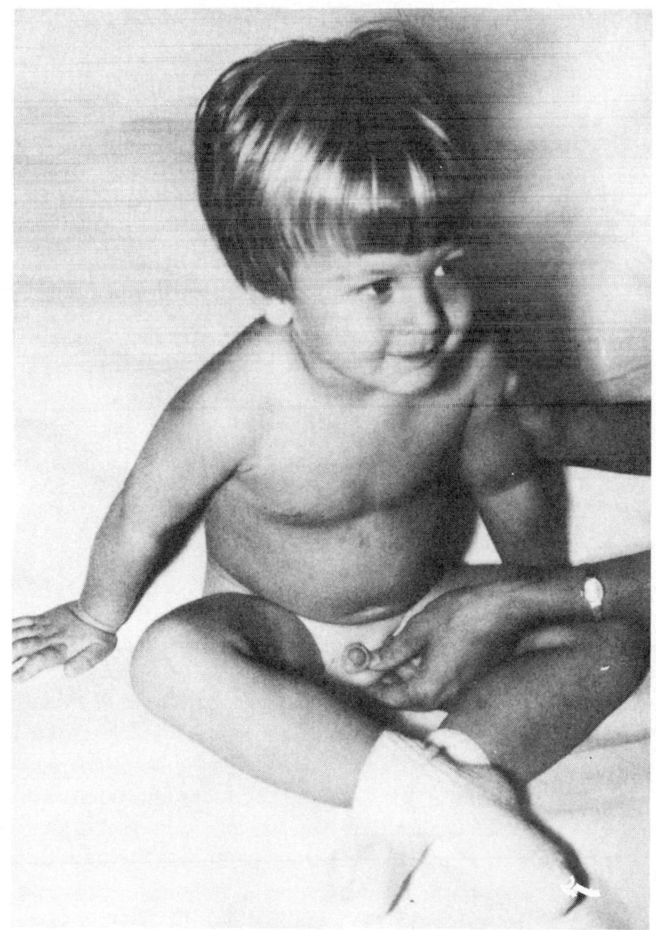


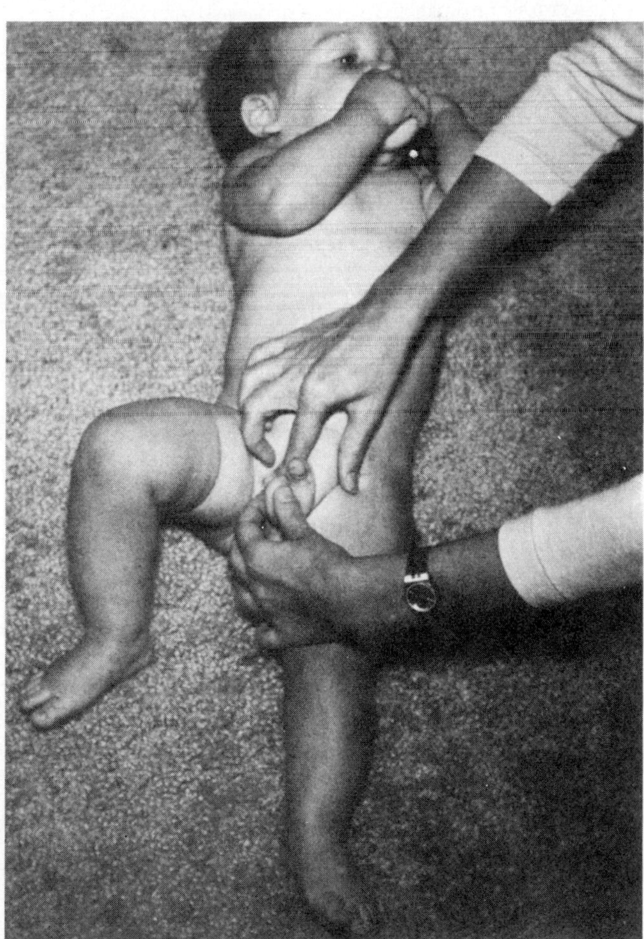


***FIG. 27-18*** **A,** Preventing cremasteric reflex by having child sit in "tailor" position. **B,** Blocking inguinal canal during palpation of scrotum for descended testes.

From Whaley LF and Wong DL: Nursing care of infants and children, ed 4, St Louis, 1991, The CV Mosby Co.

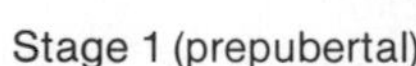


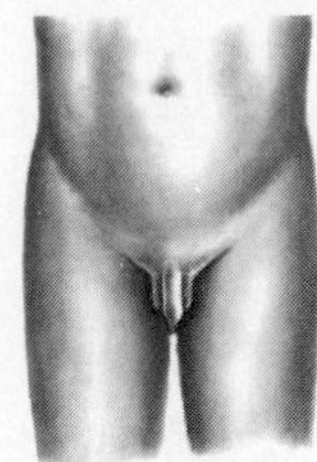


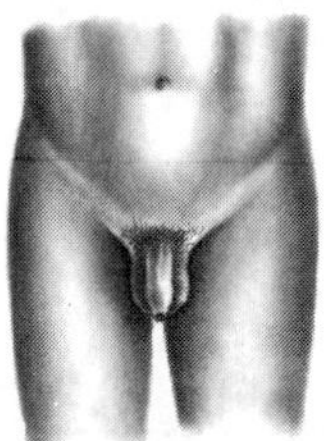


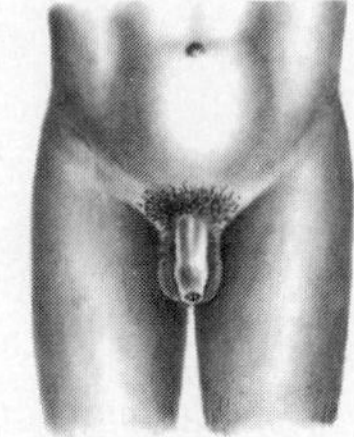


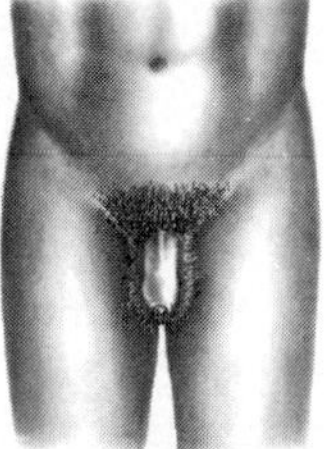


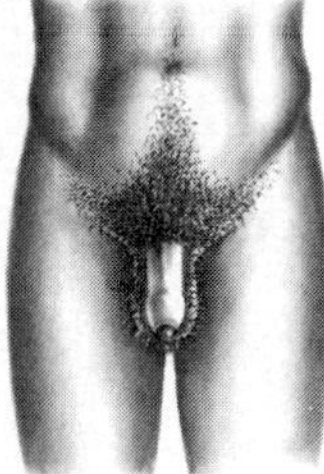


***FIG. 27-19*** Developmental stages of secondary sex characteristics and genital development in boys. Average age span is 12 to 16 years.

Modified from Marshall WA and Tanner JM: Arch Dis Child 45:13, 1970 and Daniel WA and Paulshock BZ: Patient Care, May 13, 1979, pp. 122-124.

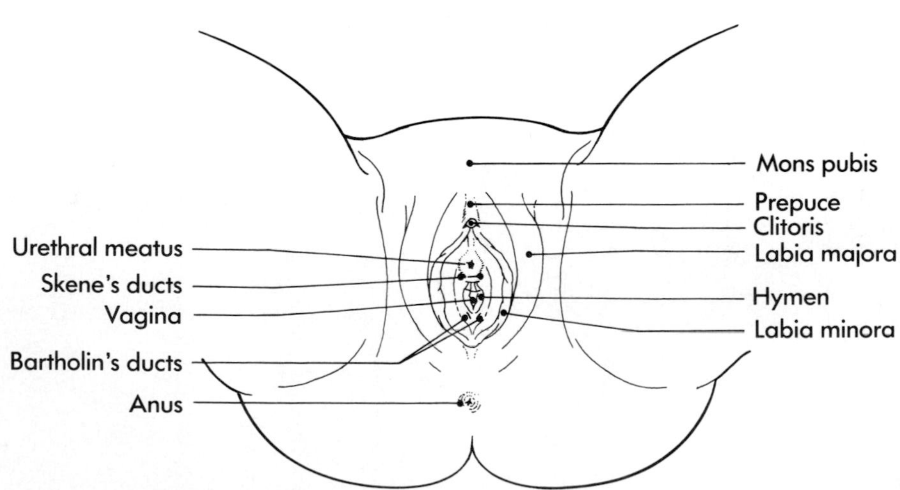


***FIG. 27-20*** External structures of female genitalia.

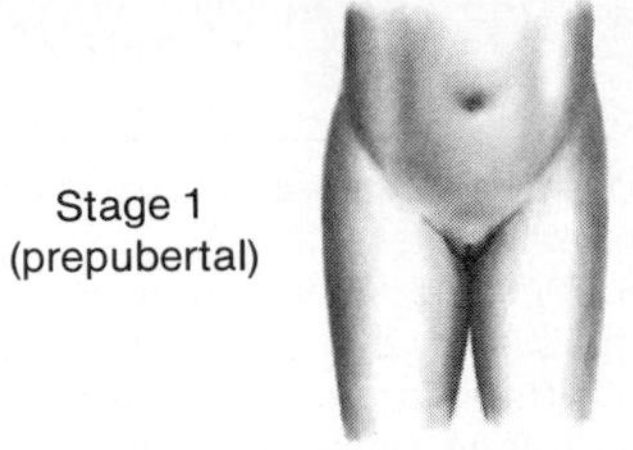


No pubic hair; essentially the same as during childhood; no distinction between hair on pubis and over the abdomen

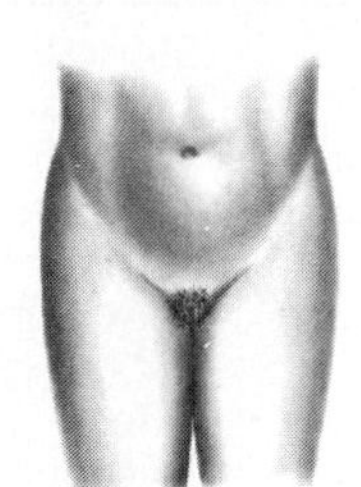


Sparse growth of long, straight, downy, and slightly pigmented hair extending along labia; between stages 2 and 3 begins to appear on pubis

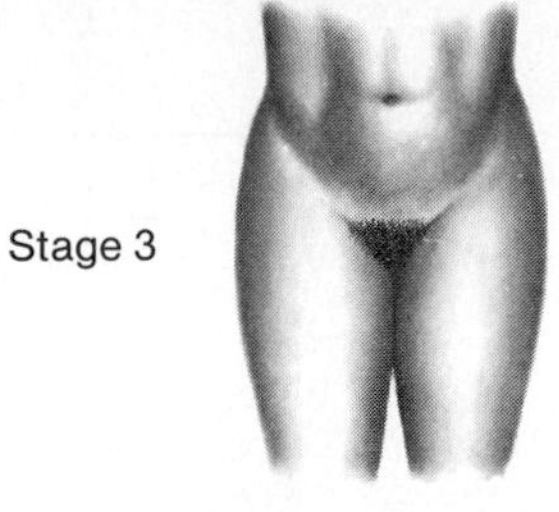


Hair darker, coarser, and curly and spread sparsely over entire pubis in the typical female triangle

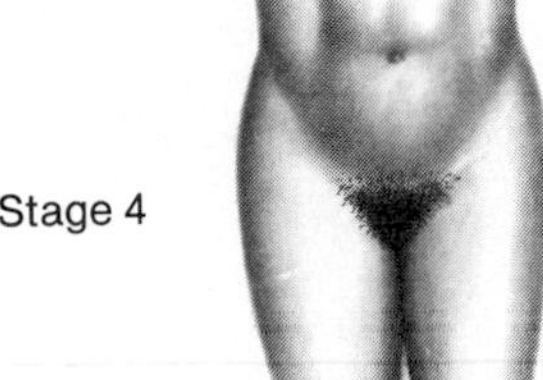


Pubic hair denser, curled, and adult in distribution but less abundant and restricted to the pubic area

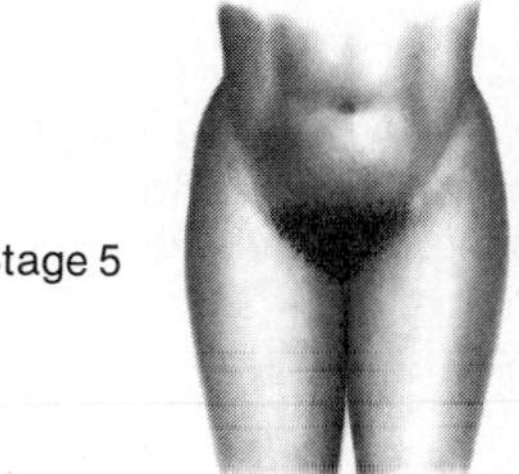


Hair adult in quantity, type, and pattern with spread to inner aspect of thighs

***FIG. 27-21*** Growth of pubic hair in girls. Average age span for stages 2 through 5 is 11 to 14 years.

Modified from Marshall WA and Paulshock BZ: Patient Care, May 13, 1979, pp 122-124.

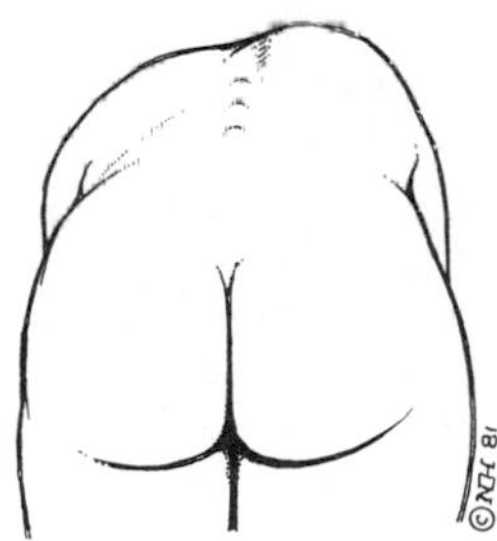

***FIG. 27-22*** Rib hump and flank asymmetry seen in flexion due to rotary component.

From Whaley LF and Wong DL: Nursing care of infants and children, ed 4, St Louis, 1991, The CV Mosby Co.

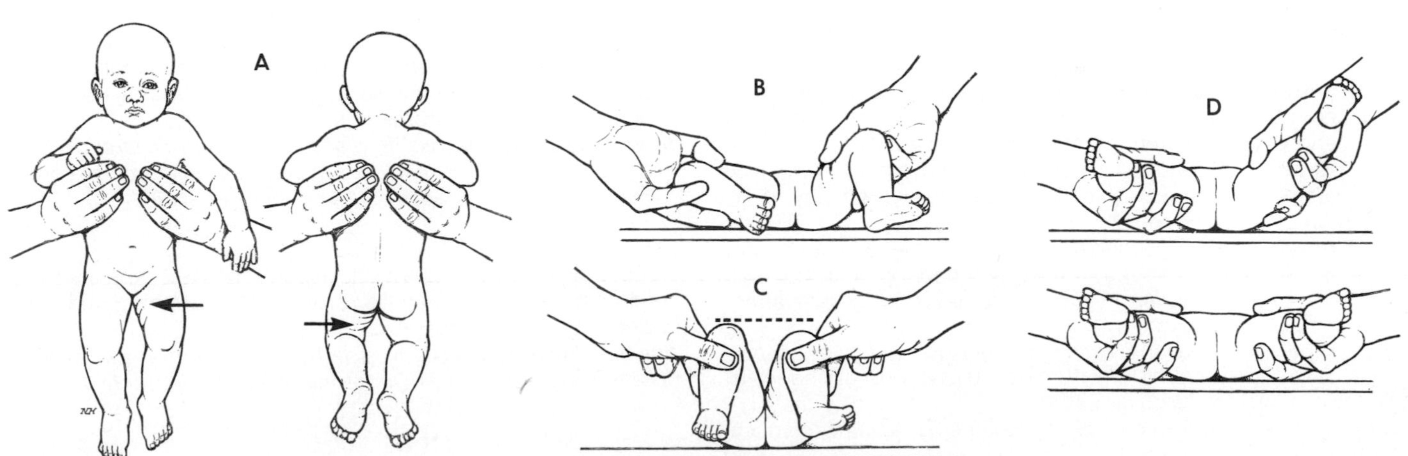


***FIG. 27-23*** Signs of congenital dislocation of the hip. **A,** Asymmetry of gluteal and thigh folds. **B,** Limited hip abduction, as seen in flexion. **C,** Apparent shortening of the femur, as indicated by the level of the knees in flexion. **D,** Ortolani click (if infant is under 4 weeks of age).

From Wong D and Whaley L: Clinical manual of pediatric nursing, ed 3, 1990, St Louis, The CV Mosby Co.

| Steps | Rationale |
|---|---|
| 2. Observe mobility of spine for flexibility and full range of motion. | Stiffness or pain on movement of back or neck indicates meningeal irritation and requires immediate evaluation. |
| 3. Inspect extremity joints for symmetry, size, temperature, color, mobility, and tenderness. Note correct number of digits. In infants, observe for dislocated hip.<br>a. Note any difference in length of legs or asymmetry of gluteal or leg folds (Fig. 27-23*A*). | Warmth, swelling, tenderness, and limited mobility of joints indicates inflammation. Limited mobility without pain may indicate congenital malformation. Differences in temperature of extremities is usually due to neurologic or vascular disorders. Children with genetic abnormalities often have extremity defects, especially in numbers of fingers, toes, and finger or toe length and appearance (Cohen, 1984). |
| b. Place infant supine with knees and hips flexed and feet flat on surface; knees should be equal in height (Fig. 27-23*C*). | ***Special Considerations:*** *Beyond 2 months of age, muscles surrounding the hip increase in strength and Ortolani sign disappears. Limited abduction becomes the most sensitive test for dislocated hip, as well as shortening of leg on affected side (Fig. 27-23B).* Congenital hip dislocation is more common in females and in breech presentations. It may be hereditary. |
| c. Perform Ortolani maneuver (Fig. 27-23*D*). While infant is in supine position with hips and knees flexed, place middle finger of each hand over greater trochanter and thumbs on inner thigh opposite lesser trochanter; abduct hips at least 70 degrees while applying forward pressure behind trochanter. If hip is dislocated, femoral head can be felt slipping into acetabulum; a "click" can sometimes be heard. | |
| 4. Observe shape of bones. Inspect for genu varum (lateral bowing of tibia) by having child stand with medial malleoli in apposition and measuring distance between knees; in child over 2 years of age, a distance greater than 2 inches indicates genu varum or bowlegs. Inspect for genu valgum by having child stand with knees together and measuring distance between malleoli; in child over 6 years of age, distance greater than 3 inches indicates genu valgum or knockknees. | Enlargement or swelling may indicate bone infection, nutritional disorders, bone cysts, or tumors.<br>***Special Considerations:*** *Genu varum is normally present for approximately 1 year after beginning to walk or until 2 to 3 years of age. Genu valgum is normal from 2 to 6 years of age as physiologic genu varum is correcting and overcompensation may occur.* |
| 5. Observe feet. Note position. In infants, scratch outside and then inside of lower border of foot; in self-correctable deformities, foot will assume right angle to leg. | Deformities that are inflexible or cannot be straightened need orthopedic evaluation.<br>***Special Considerations:*** *Because of fat pads under arch, feet may appear flat until child has been walking for 1 to 2 years.* |
| 6. Observe gait. Note any limp. | Waddling or scissor gait, toeing-in or broad-based gait in older children is indicative of musculoskeletal or neurologic disorder. Limp may be caused by muscle, nerve, bone, or joint disease or, more commonly, by trauma, fatigue, or hip pathology.<br>***Special Considerations:*** *A toddling, broad-based gait is normal until approximately 3 years of age.* |
| 7. Palpate pulses (see Skill 31). | |
| ***Neurologic function*** | |
| 1. Assess mental status. Observe behavior, mood, affect, general orientation to surroundings, and level of consciousness. Response to commands, speech, name, pinprick, and pain are useful in assessing degree of consciousness. In infants and young children, mental status is assessed through observation of position, spontaneous movements, and play activities. Note any irritability, hyperactivity, lethargy, delirium, stupor, or coma. | Alteration in a child's mental status may be related to acute febrile illness, poisonings, nutritional deficiencies, metabolic disorders, fluid electrolyte imbalances, central nervous system disorders, emotional disturbances, or brain injury.<br>***Special Considerations:*** *In infants and young children, onset of neurologic signs related to acute brain injury or bleeding may be delayed because of distensibility of skull.* |
| 2. Assess motor functioning.<br>a. Test muscle strength, tone, and development:<br>▪ Apply counterpressure while having child raise arms; repeat with legs.<br>▪ Have child squeeze your fingers as tightly as possible.<br>▪ Apply counterpressure to soles while having child plantar flex (Fig. 27-24).<br>These activities may be presented as a game to young children who are generally eager to show their strength. Responses should be equal bilaterally with increased tone during muscle contraction. | Atrophy, hypertrophy, spasticity, rigidity, or weakness indicate neuromuscular disorder. Spasticity and tetany may indicate electrolyte imbalance.<br>***Special Considerations:*** *Muscle hypertrophy in a young child can be an early sign of Duchenne muscular dystrophy.* |

**Steps** | **Rationale**

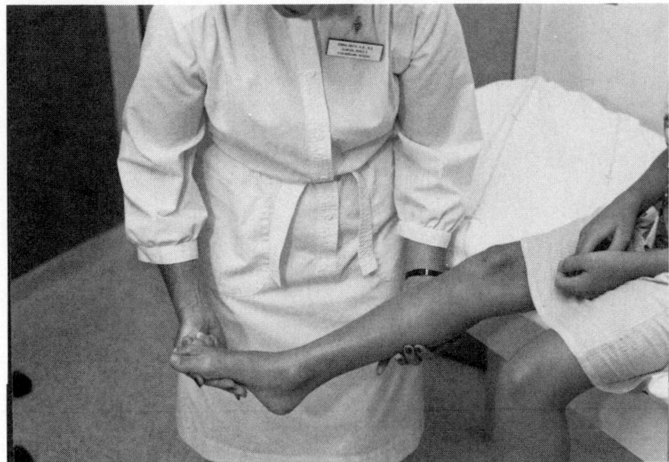

***FIG. 27-24*** Child performs plantar flex during assessment of motor function.

b. Test cerebellar functioning:
   - Have child touch tip of nose with index finger; repeat with other hand. Repeat with eyes closed.
   - Have child run heel of one foot down shin of other leg while standing. Repeat with eyes closed.
   - Perform Romberg test by having child stand with hands at sides, feet together, and eyes closed. Stand beside child in case he or she falls. Child normally should not lean or fall to side.
   - Have child touch tip of each finger with thumb of same hand in rapid succession.
   - Have child pat legs, first with palms and then back of hands in rapid sequence.

   These skills may be demonstrated to child by saying "Do as I do." Note any lack of coordination or awkwardness in performing these tests.

Difficulty in performing these tests indicates poor coordination, especially with eyes open, and poor sense of position, particularly with eyes closed. Cerebellar testing is particularly important in children with symptoms of hyperactivity or learning disability.

***Special Considerations:*** *Fine motor coordination is not fully developed until 4 to 6 years of age, and thus younger children will not be able to perform these tests. If preschooler can bring finger within 1 to 2 inches of tip of nose, it is generally considered normal.*

c. Test development (see Skill 25).

3. Assess sensory functioning.
   a. Test peripheral sensation.
      - Touch skin lightly with pin and have child point to stimulated area while keeping eyes closed.
      - Touch skin with pin or cotton and have child describe as sharp or dull while keeping eyes closed.
      - Touch skin with cold or warm object and have child differentiate temperatures; metal and rubber ends of reflex hammer work well.
      - Touch different parts of body simultaneously and have child localize both points.

Hyperesthesia (increased sensation) is found in central nervous system infection, diseases with increased intracranial pressure, and lesions of spinal cord. Decreased sensation may be due to spinal cord or peripheral nerve lesions, mental deficiency, or decreased consciousness.

***Special Considerations:*** *In children too young to cooperate, testing is limited to perception of pain.*

4. Assess reflexes.
   a. Deep tendon reflexes may be elicited using reflex hammer, finger, or side of hand; for younger children easily frightened by equipment, use of finger or hand is best. Because reflexes are inhibited by tensing of muscle, relaxation must be promoted through distraction with toys or talking to child; older children may be asked to grasp hands in front of them and pull to divert attention and promote involuntary relaxation of lower extremities; for testing of upper extremities, child may be asked to clench teeth or squeeze thigh with hand on side not being tested. Telling them to "act like Raggedy Ann" may be helpful. Reflexes normally elicited include:

Hyperactive or diminished reflexes indicate disturbance in neural pathways between muscle and spinal cord.

***Special Considerations:*** *Deep tendon reflexes may be difficult to elicit in neonates. Reflexes are commonly graded as:*

*4+ extremely brisk, hyperactive*
*3+ brisker than normal*
*2+ average, normal*
*1+ diminished*
*0 absent*

*Or they may simply be described as normal, hyperactive, hypoactive, or absent.*

| Steps | Rationale |
|---|---|
| ▪ Biceps—Hold child's arm by placing partially flexed elbow in hand with examiner's thumb over antecubital space. Striking thumbnail should cause partial flexion of forearm (Fig. 27-25). | |
| ▪ Triceps—Flex child's arm at elbow and rest his or her palm or forearm in hand. Striking triceps tendon just above elbow should cause partial extension of forearm (Fig. 27-26). | |
| ▪ Brachioradialis—Place child's forearm on his or her lap or abdomen with arm flexed at elbow and palm down. Striking radius approximately 1 inch above wrist should cause flexion of forearm and supination of palm (Fig. 27-27). | |
| ▪ Patellar—Have child sit with lower legs flexed at knee and dangling freely. Striking patellar tendon just below knee should cause partial extension of lower leg (Fig. 27-28). | |
| ▪ Achilles—Using same position as for patellar reflex, support child's foot lightly in hand. Striking Achilles tendon should cause plantar flexion of foot (Fig. 27-29). | |
| b. Test for signs of meningeal irritation.<br>▪ Kernig's sign is elicited by flexing child's leg at hip and knee while supine; normally there should be no pain or resistance (Fig. 27-30).<br>▪ Brudzinski's sign is elicited by flexing child's head while supine; normally there should be no pain or involuntary flexion of hip and knees (Fig. 27-31). | Positive signs indicate meningeal irritation. Immediate medical referral is essential. These signs are usually elicited only in children with upper respiratory infection or when there is suspicion of meningeal irritation. |
| 5. Assess functioning of cranial nerves. Testing may be done as part of neurologic assessment or integrated into each system or presented as game at beginning of assessment.<br>a. Olfactory (I)—Have child identify familiar odors, e.g., peanut butter, peppermint, or orange, with eyes closed. Test each nostril separately.<br>b. Optic (II)—Test visual acuity, peripheral vision, and light and color perception (see Skill 35).<br>c. Oculomotor (III)—Test extraocular movements by having child follow light or object moved to all 6 cardinal points of vision (Fig. 27-32). Check PERRLA (pupils equal, round, react to light, accommodation). Check placement of eyelid, noting any ptosis.<br>d. Trochlear (IV)—Have child look down and in without moving head, e.g., ask child to cross eyes and look at nose.<br>e. Trigeminal (V)—Test motor function by having child bite down hard; observe for symmetry and strength. Test sensory function by lightly touching forehead, cheeks, and jaws, with child's eyes closed. Test corneal and blink reflex by carefully touching cornea with wisp of cotton, approaching from side; both eyes should close.<br>f. Abducens (VI)—Have child look laterally or sideways without moving head.<br>g. Facial (VII)—Have child smile, make funny face, raise eyebrows, puff out cheeks, and show teeth; expression should be symmetrical. For infants, observe symmetry when crying and smiling. Test taste by placing salt and sugar on anterior portion of protruding tongue and having child identify each taste; rinse mouth or give drink of water between each taste.<br>h. Auditory, acoustic, or vestibular (VIII)—Test hearing (see Skill 34). Note any vertigo or loss of equilibrium.<br>i. Glossopharyngeal (IX)—Elicit gag reflex. Test taste by placing bitter and sour solution on posterior tongue. Rinse mouth or give drink between each test. | Inability to perform any item correctly indicates motor or sensory impairment of that nerve. Child should normally be able to perform all items.<br>***Special Considerations:*** *Cranial nerves are not usually tested below preschool age because child is not developmentally able to perform these tasks, although some can be tested by observation.* |

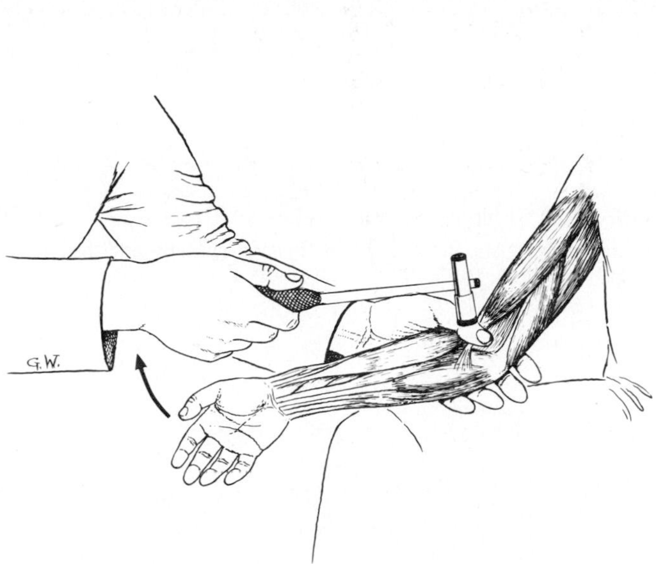


***FIG. 27-25*** Testing for biceps reflex.

From Whaley LF and Wong DL: Nursing care of infants and children, ed 4, St Louis, 1991, The CV Mosby Co.

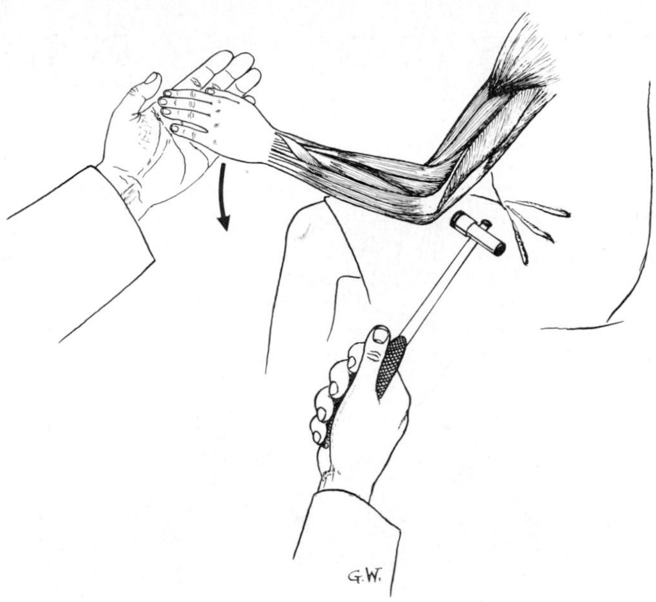


***FIG. 27-26*** Testing for triceps reflex.

From Whaley LF and Wong DL: Nursing care of infants and children, ed 4, St Louis, 1991, The CV Mosby Co.

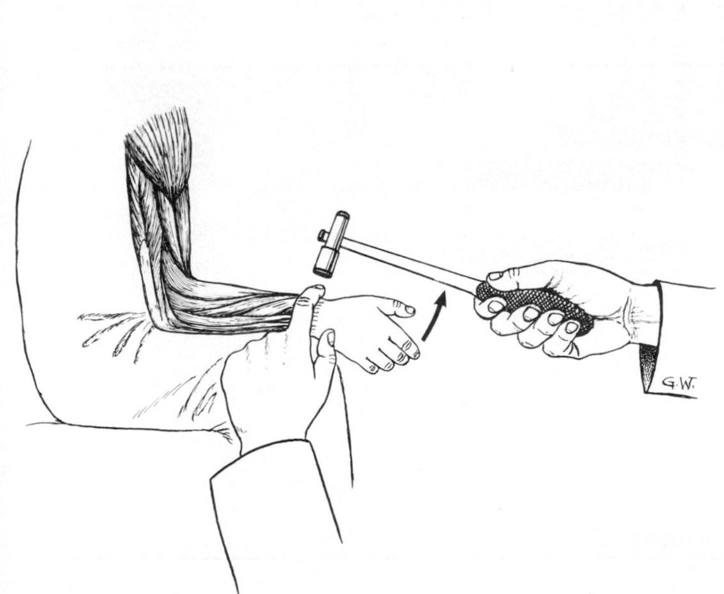


***FIG. 27-27*** Testing for brachioradialis reflex.

From Whaley LF and Wong DL: Nursing care of infants and children, ed 4, St Louis, 1991, The CV Mosby Co.

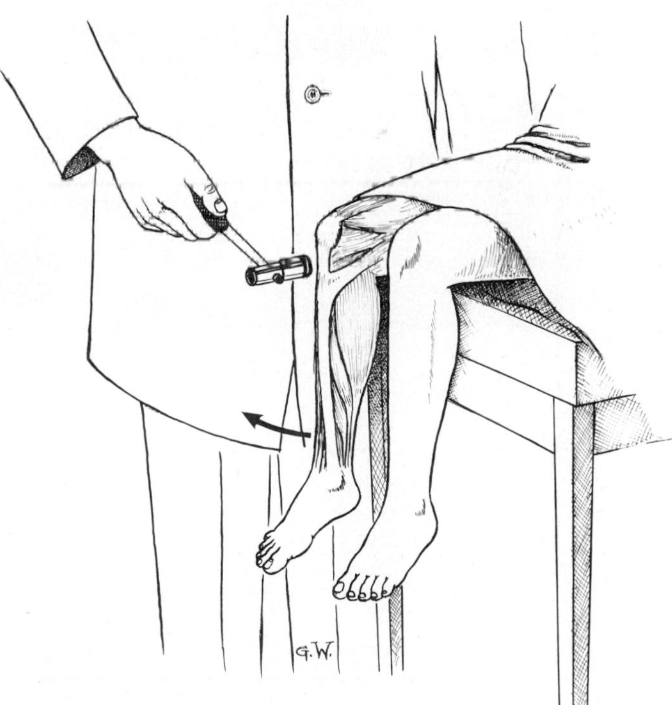


***FIG. 27-28*** Testing for patellar (knee jerk) reflex.

From Whaley LF and Wong DL: Nursing care of infants and children, ed 4, St Louis, 1991, The CV Mosby Co.

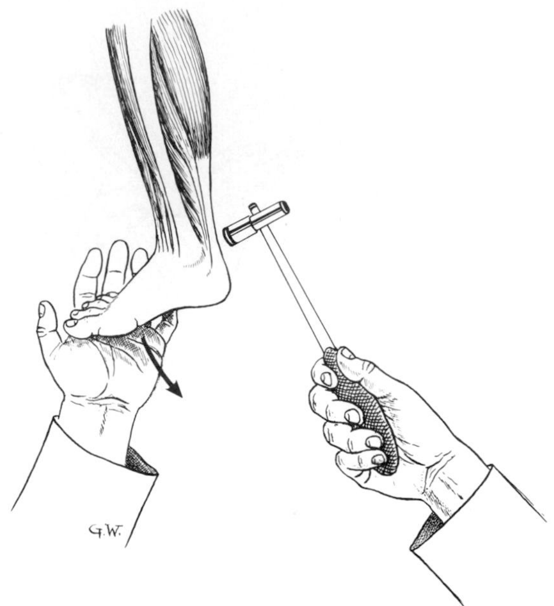


***FIG. 27-29*** Testing for Achilles reflex.

From Whaley LF and Wong DL: Nursing care of infants and children, ed 4, St Louis, 1991, The CV Mosby Co.

**A**

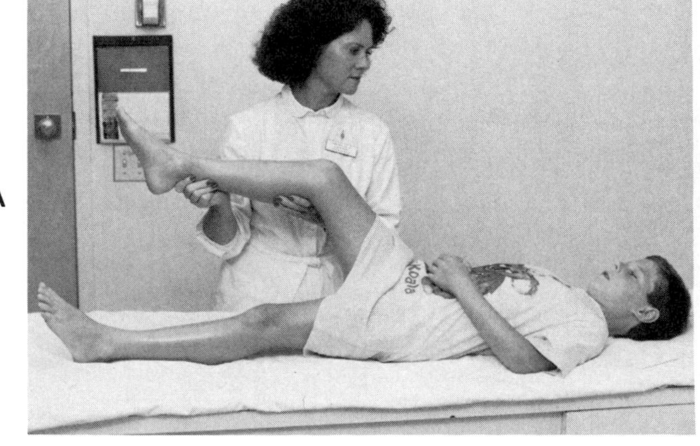

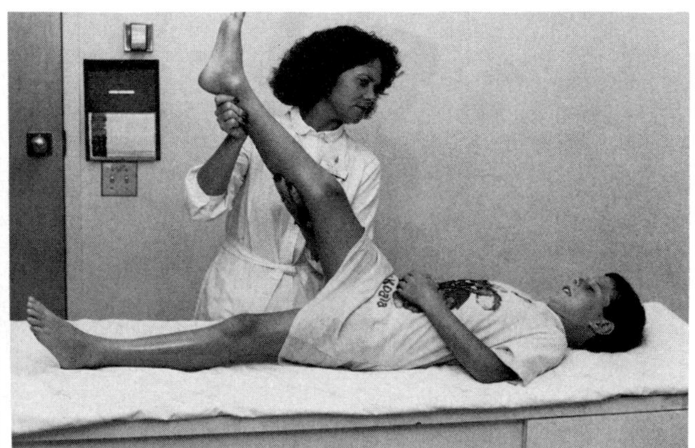

**B**

***FIG. 27-30*** Kernig's sign is elicited by flexing child's leg. **A,** At knee. **B,** At hip. Normally no pain or resistance is encountered upon flexion.

| Steps | Rationale |
|---|---|
| j. Vagus (X)—Elicit gag reflex. Have child swallow. Observe uvula for midline placement. Note any excessive drooling or hoarseness of voice. | |
| k. Accessory (XI)—Have child elevate shoulders while applying gentle counterpressure (Fig. 27-33). Have child turn head against opposing pressure on both sides. Note strength and symmetry of movements. | |
| l. Hypoglossal (XII)—Have child move tongue in all directions and protrude it as far as possible. Test strength by placing tongue blade on side of tongue and having child push it away. Note any tremors, twitching, or deviation from midline. | |

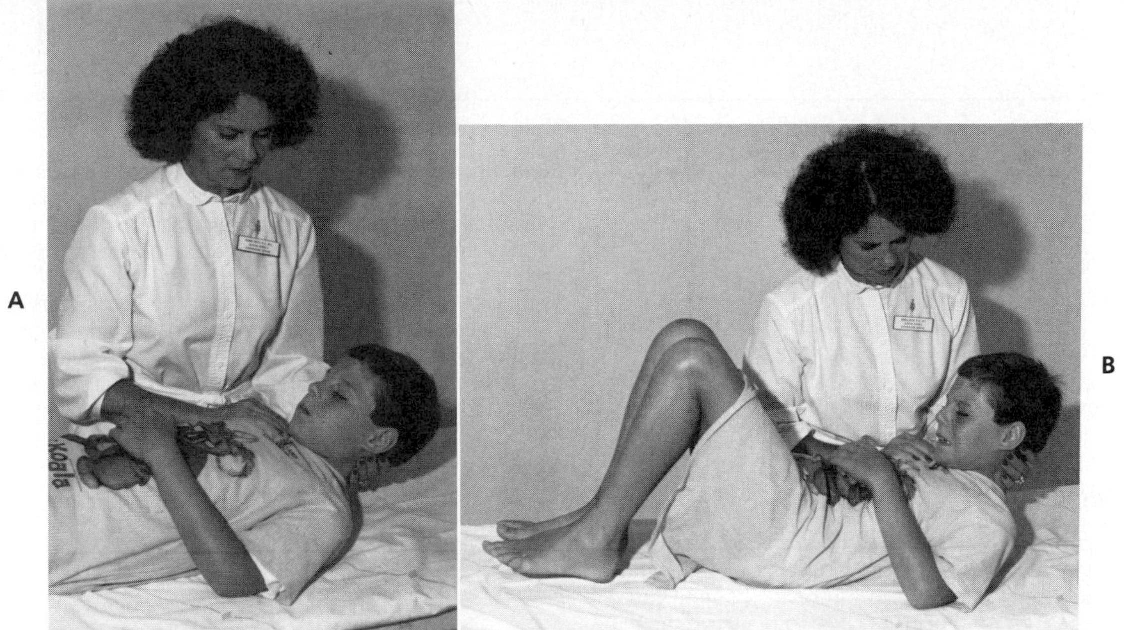


***FIG. 27-31*** **A,** Testing for Brudzinski's sign by having child flex head while supine. **B,** Pain or involuntary flexion of hip and knees is abnormal.

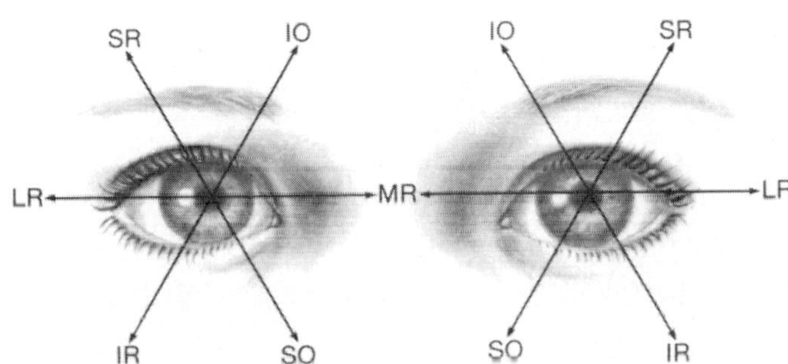


***FIG. 27-32*** Testing cardinal positions of gaze.

From Whaley LF and Wong DL: Nursing care of infants and children, ed 4, St Louis, 1991, The CV Mosby Co.

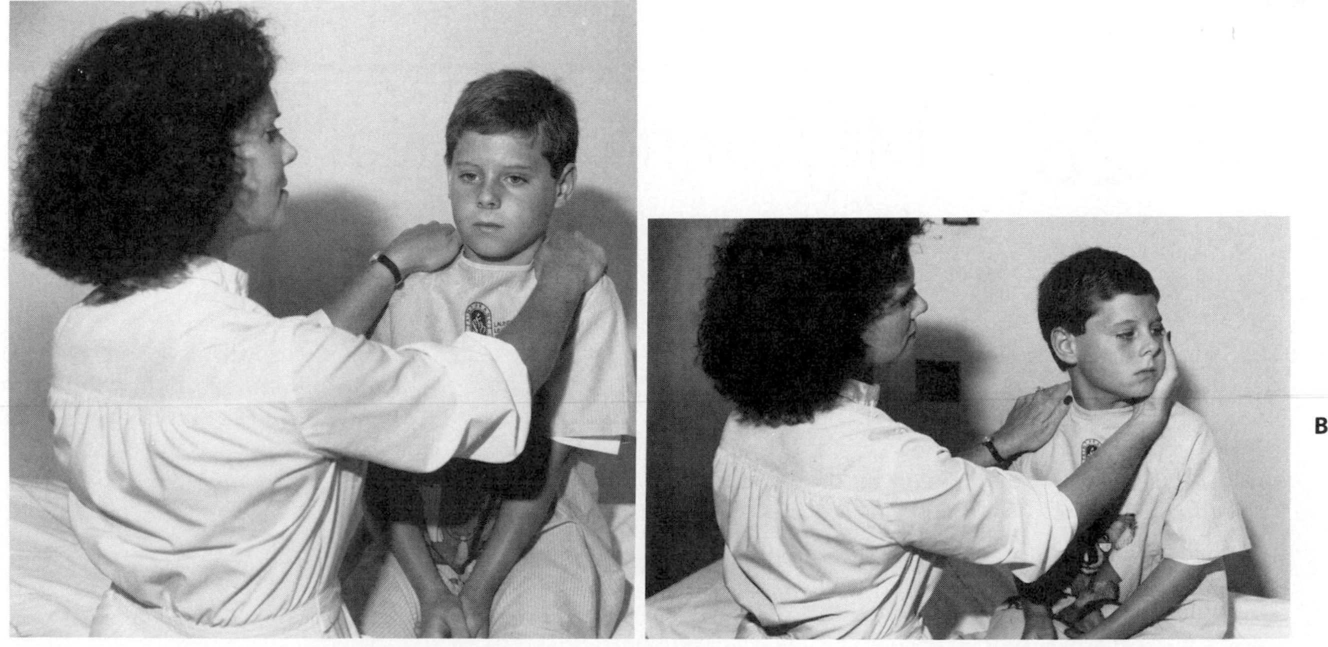


***FIG. 27-33*** Testing the accessory nerve. **A,** Child elevates shoulders while gentle counter-pressure is applied. **B,** Child turns head against opposing pressure.

| Steps | Rationale |
|---|---|
| **Evaluation Outcomes** | **Observational Guidelines** |
| 1. The approach is adapted to child's developmental level. | Age-appropriate procedures are completed. Child is able to adjust to procedures with minimal anxiety and remains cooperative, allowing examiner to touch him or her and accepting equipment. Family remains relaxed and willing to communicate. |
| 2. A systematic, organized approach to physical assessment is used. | Procedures are completed and findings documented in a logical sequence. Assessment is completed as planned or, if partial assessment is planned, all relevant procedures are completed. |
| 3. Variations from normal physical findings are identified, and referrals are made as appropriate. | Compare findings to normal assessment characteristics. Document abnormal findings and appropriate referral for further evaluation. |

### Documentation

Document findings of physical assessment for each system examined, recording all variations from normal and following head-to-toe sequence. Record actual observations and findings, not interpretations or conclusions, using objective rather than subjective statements. For example, say "Child is playing, talking, and smiling" instead of "Child appears comfortable." State specifically what is seen, heard, smelled, and felt during the physical assessment. Document referrals and follow-up.

### Child and Family Teaching

The physical assessment provides an excellent teaching medium from newborn through adolescent. The new mother can be taught normal infant characteristics and infant care, with the nurse demonstrating and modeling throughout the assessment. The physical assessment provides an opportunity to teach children and adolescents about their growing bodies and to address concerns that they may have. Likewise, the physical assessment provides an ideal opportunity for teaching signs of illness and discussing management of specific problems identified.

# *SKILL* 28 Measuring Physical Growth

*Sherry Baze*

Assessing physical growth is one of the most frequently used skills in pediatric nursing. Physical growth parameters include weight, height, head circumference, and chest circumference. By accurate completion and correct plotting on growth charts, a visual representation of growth emerges. Trends revealed through serial measurements are sensitive indicators of health and nutritional status in children.

### NURSING DIAGNOSES

Health-seeking behaviors (growth assessment) related to promotion of infant/child physical growth; Altered growth and development related to illness, stress, nutritional intake, and/or parental knowledge deficit.

| **Steps** | **Rationale** |
|---|---|
| **Assessment** | |
| 1. Determine presence of any physical anomalies. | Certain physical anomalies may interfere with accurate growth measurements. For example, deformities that prevent full extension preclude accurate measurement of height, or presence of a cast does not allow accurate weight measurement.<br>***Special Considerations:*** *If accurate measurement is not possible, that growth parameter can be deferred or omitted, or special techniques may be necessary, e.g., sitting height or crown-to-rump length.* |
| 2. Calculate child's age. Age is rounded to nearest month on birth to 36-month charts, or to nearest 3 months on 2- to 18-year charts. | Age determines which growth measurements are to be completed and assists in selection of proper measuring devices. Correct age is also essential for accurate plotting on growth charts.<br>***Special Considerations:*** *For premature infants, weeks of prematurity are subtracted from actual age before plotting on growth charts. Adjustments are made until 18 months of age for head circumference, 21 months of age for weight, and 36 months of age for length or stature.* |
| 3. Determine which growth measurements are to be obtained.<br>a. Weight is measured at all ages.<br>b. Recumbent length is measured for children under 24 months of age. Stature, or standing height, is measured for children over 36 months of age. Either measurement may be used from 24 to 36 months; recumbent length must be plotted on birth to 36-month charts, and stature must be plotted on 2- to 18-year charts. | The growth parameters to be measured will guide selection of equipment and growth charts needed for accurate determinations. |
| c. Head circumference is commonly measured up to 2 years of age. | ***Special Considerations:*** *The American Academy of Pediatrics recommends measurement of head circumference at each well child visit through 12 months. It is measured at any age if head size is questionable.* |
| d. Chest circumference may be measured for comparison with head circumference. | Marked disproportion between head and chest circumference is generally the result of abnormal head growth. |
| 4. Obtain family history relating to growth parameters, including heights, weights, and head circumferences of parents and siblings, if known. Information regarding general growth patterns of siblings may also be beneficial. | Growth is significantly influenced by genetic make-up. Thus tall parents tend to have tall children; small parents have small children. |
| **Planning and Goal Setting** | |
| 1. Assemble and prepare equipment. | Properly selected and maintained equipment is essential in achieving accurate growth measurements. |
| a. Balance beam scale, either pediatric or adult model, depending on child's age. Before use, balance scale by placing weights at zero position and adjusting screws as necessary until beam is in zero balance. Pediatric scales should be covered with clean paper that is changed after each use; if paper is to be used, scales should be balanced with paper in place. Scales should be cleaned with disinfectant daily or more often if contaminated. | ***Special Considerations:*** *Spring type scales do not produce an acceptable degree of accuracy for weights. It is preferable to have scales in same unit of measure, e.g., pounds or kilograms, used within agency to avoid calculation errors. Kilograms are generally used in calculating drug dosages. Digital readout scales are an acceptable alternative. As with balance beam scales, proper calibration is essential.* |
| b. Infant measuring board if recumbent length is to be measured or wall-mounted measuring board if stature is to be measured. Check to see that sliding headboards and footboards move easily, are not worn, loose, jagged, or broken, and are perpendicular to measurement surface. If measuring device is not available, a nonstretchable measuring tape or yardstick may be used. It should be attached to a rigid surface (door, wall without baseboard, table top) with "0" mark either at floor if child is to be measured standing, or at fixed headboard if recumbent length is to be measured; a right angle board is required to complete the measurement. | If measurements are to be compared with standardized norms, length or stature measurements must be accurate to ensure valid interpretation of findings.<br>***Special Considerations:*** *Measuring devices should be in same unit of measure, e.g., inches or centimeters, used within agency to avoid calculation errors. Movable measuring rods attached to platform scales are unstable and do not ensure accurate measurement of length or stature. Marking at child's head and feet as closely as possible, then measuring distance between marks, provides only an estimate of length or stature in absence of proper equipment. Caution must be used in interpreting such measurements by comparison with standardized norms.* |

| Steps | Rationale |
|---|---|
| c. Flexible, nonstretchable tape measure (paper or plastic) for measuring head and chest circumferences. | Cloth tape measures stretch, giving a falsely small measurement. Some metal tape measures may not be adequately flexible and may injure the child. |
| 2. Select appropriate National Center for Health Statistics (NCHS) growth chart. Choose the charts appropriate to the sex of the child.<br>a. From birth to 36 months:<br>▪ Chart showing norms for recumbent length by weight and age (for girls, Fig. 28-1; for boys, Fig. 28-2).<br>▪ Chart showing norms for head circumference by age and weight by recumbent length (for girls, Fig. 28-3; for boys, Fig. 28-4).<br>b. From 2 to 18 years:<br>▪ Chart showing norms for stature and weight by age (for girls, Fig. 28-5; for boys, Fig. 28-6).<br>▪ Prepubescent chart showing norms for stature by weight. Use only from age when begin measuring stature until child reaches Tanner I stage (for girls, Fig. 28-7; for boys, Fig. 28-8). | The correct standardized norms are essential for accurate interpretation. Growth norms may vary based on sex, age, measurement by recumbent length or stature, and pubertal status. The weight by age, recumbent length by age, stature by age, and head circumference by age charts compare the child's measurements to the same age children in the general population. The weight by recumbent length or weight by stature charts allow comparison of the proportions of the child's body measurements.<br>***Special Considerations:*** *NCHS growth charts are based on reference data from black and white children in the United States. Thus caution must be used in applying these norms to other ethnic groups; however, they may still be used effectively to monitor growth rate, since reference data is frequently not available for the particular group to which the child belongs. For example, children of Asian descent are commonly smaller, falling below the tenth percentile on weight and height for age; however, their growth rate should still follow the normal growth curve and weight for height should fall within normal range. It is unclear whether these differences result from nutritional factors, past illnesses or genetic factors.* |
| 3. Develop individualized goals of nursing care:<br>▪ Accurate, age-appropriate growth measurements will be obtained.<br>▪ Growth measurements will be correctly plotted on appropriate NCHS growth charts.<br>▪ Growth measurements falling outside normal parameters and child's own growth curve will be identified. | |

## Implementation

| Steps | Rationale |
|---|---|
| 1. Prepare child.<br>a. For infants and some toddlers, distraction may be necessary to keep them still during measurement. For cooperative toddlers and older children, age-appropriate explanations of procedures, equipment, and results are given. | By allaying anxiety and fear of unknown, child is better able to cooperate.<br>***Special Considerations:*** *If child is uncooperative and resistant, making accurate measurement impossible, postpone or omit measurement. Document reason.* |
| b. Remove child's clothing.<br>▪ Infants are completely undressed.<br>▪ For children, all but minimal indoor clothing is removed: coats, shoes, caps, etc. | Removal of clothing is required for accurate weight determination. Removal of shoes and headware is necessary to measure length or stature. Removal of headwear is also essential for accurate measurement of head circumference.<br>***Special Considerations:*** *Serial measurements will provide a more accurate picture if same approach is used each time child is measured, e.g., if infant is always nude.* |
| 2. Obtain height measurement.<br>a. To obtain recumbent length, place child supine on measuring board; have parent or attendant hold head firmly against headboard with child's line of vision straight up. Completely extend legs by gently pushing down on both knees while positioning footboard firmly against heels with toes straight up. Read measurement to nearest 1/8 inch (0.3 cm) (Fig. 28-9).<br>b. To obtain stature, have child stand with heels slightly apart, feet flat on floor, back straight, chin level, and eyes looking straight ahead; heels, buttocks, and shoulder blades should touch measuring surface. Lower headboard to rest firmly on child's head. Read measurement to nearest 1/4 inch (0.6 cm) (Fig. 28-10). | Along with weight, height is a good indicator of overall growth. Serial measurements provide good representation of growth rate. Shortness may be caused by chronic malnutrition, chronic disease affecting absorption or utilization of nutrients, or inadequate growth hormone; it may also be related to genetic factors and be a normal growth pattern. Tallness is generally related to genetic factors and a normal growth pattern, although excessively rapid growth may result from hormonal imbalance or accelerated maturation.<br>***Special Considerations:*** *A child normally grows approximately 10 inches (25 cm) in first year of life, 5 inches (13 cm) second year, 3 to 4 inches (8 to 10 cm) third year, and then 2 to 3 inches (5 to 8 cm) per year until pubertal growth spurt. Birth length is normally doubled by 4 years and tripled by 13 years. Greatest height gain usually occurs in spring, and least gain in fall (Kempe et al, 1987).* |

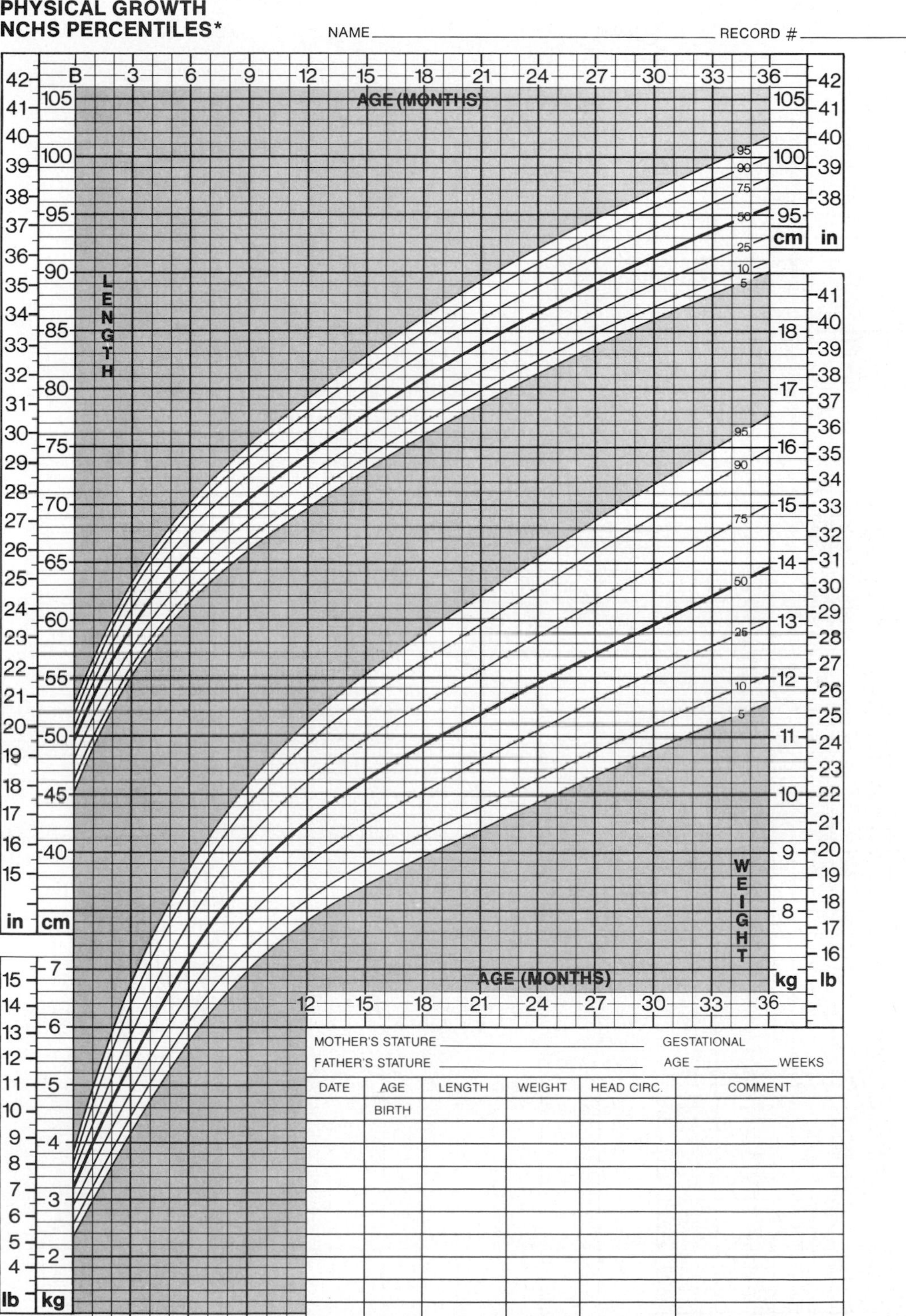


***FIG. 28-1*** Birth to 36 months physical growth NCHS percentiles (length, weight) for girls.

Adapted from Hamill PVV et al: Physical growth: National Center for Health Statistics percentiles, Am J Clin Nutr 32:607-629, 1979. Data from the Fels Research Institute, Wright State University School of Medicine, Yellow Springs, Ohio. Provided as a service of Ross Laboratories, 1982.

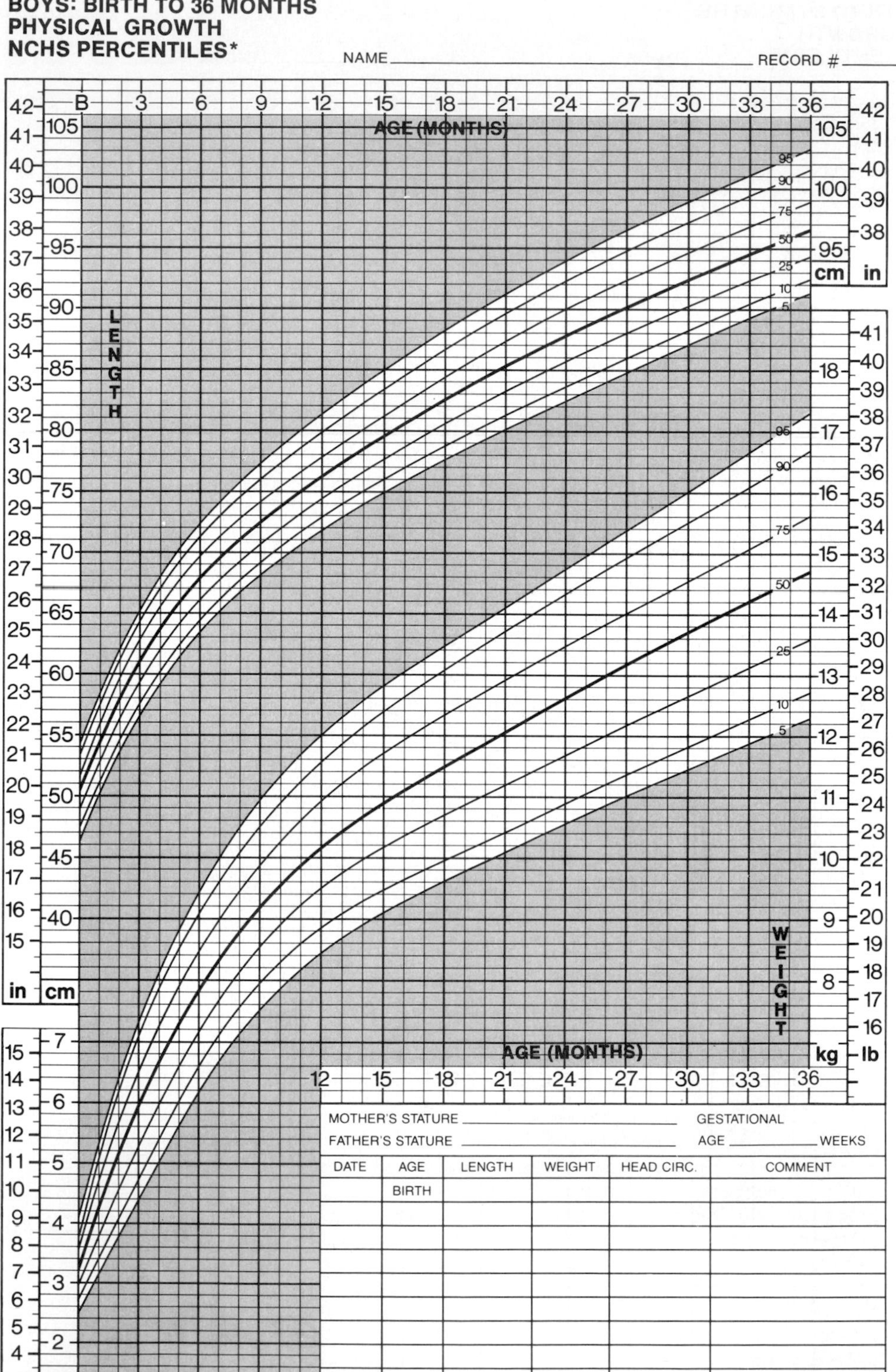


***FIG. 28-2*** Birth to 36 month physical growth NCHS percentile (length, weight) for boys.

Adapted from Hamill PVV et al: Physical growth: National Center for Health Statistics percentiles, Am J Clin Nutr 32:607-629, 1979. Data from the Fels Research Institute, Wright State University School of Medicine, Yellow Springs, Ohio. Provided as a service of Ross Laboratories, 1982.

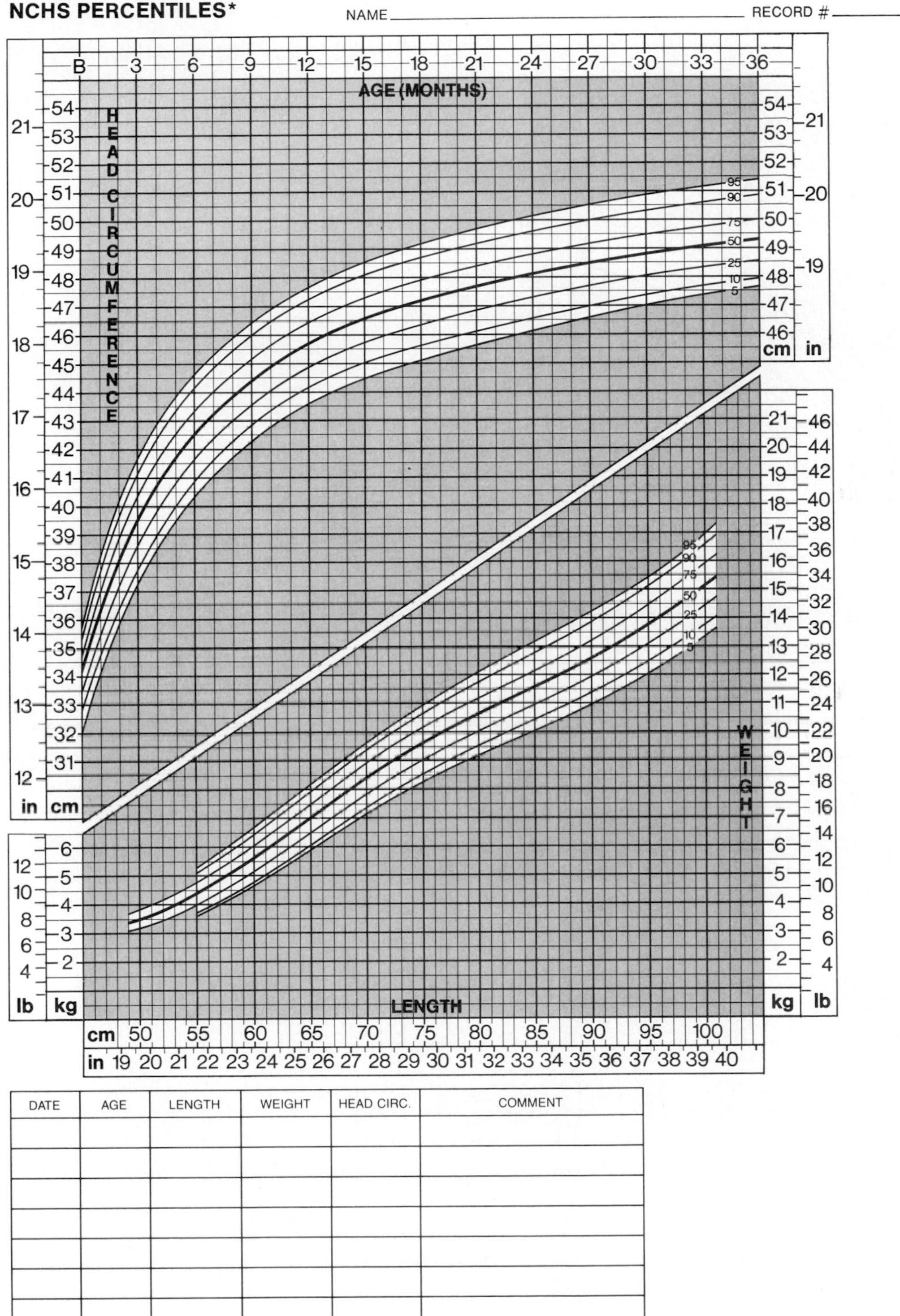


***FIG. 28-3*** Birth to 36 months physical growth percentiles (head circumference, length, weight) for girls.

Adapted from Hamill PVV et al: Physical growth: National Center for Health Statistics percentiles, Am J Clin Nutr, 32:607-629, 1979. Data from the Fels Research Institute, Wright State University School of Medicine, Yellow Springs, Ohio. Provided as a service of Ross Laboratories, 1982.

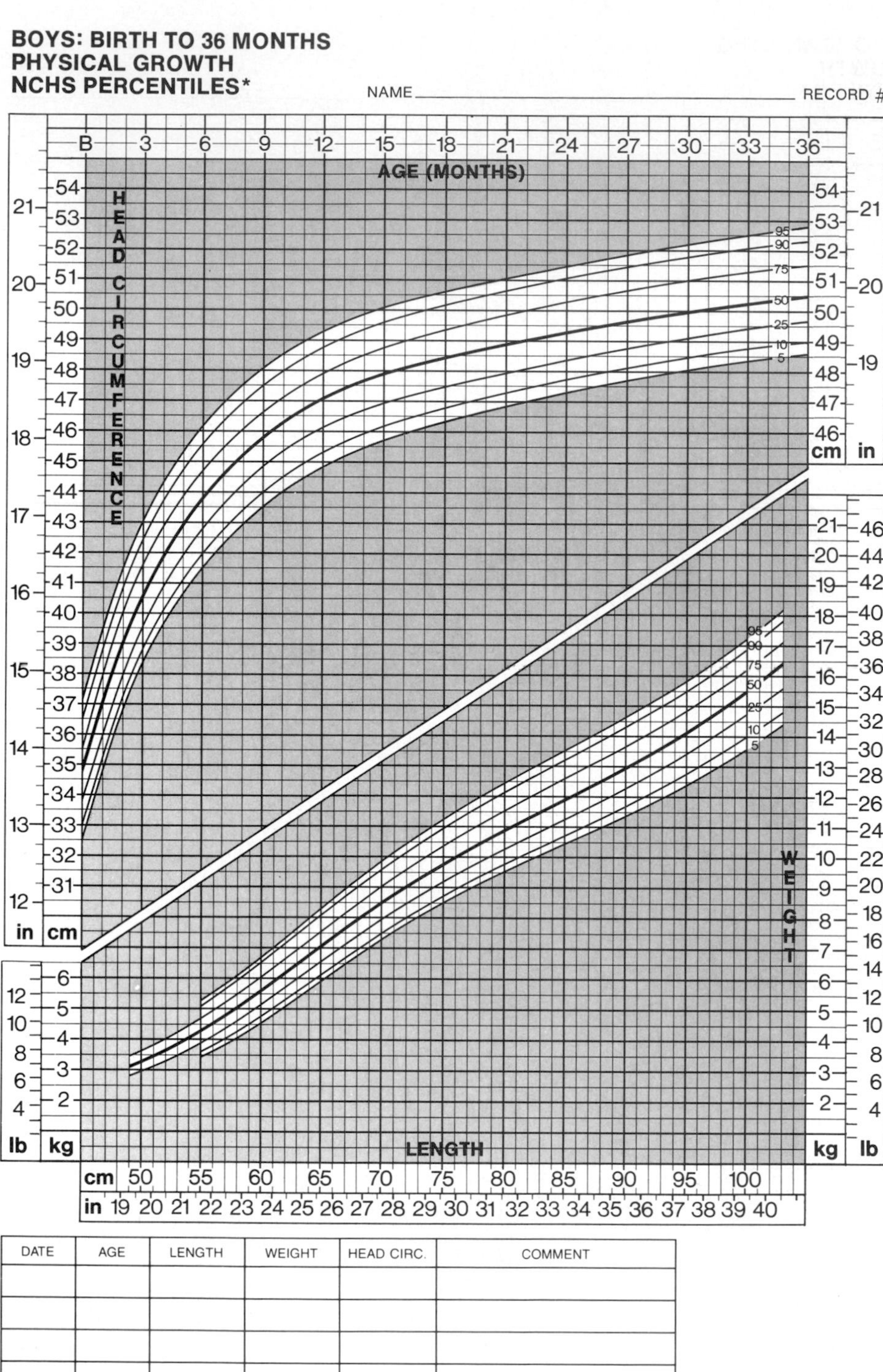


| DATE | AGE | LENGTH | WEIGHT | HEAD CIRC. | COMMENT |
|---|---|---|---|---|---|
| | | | | | |
| | | | | | |
| | | | | | |
| | | | | | |
| | | | | | |
| | | | | | |
| | | | | | |

***FIG. 28-4*** Birth to 36 months physical growth percentiles (head circumference, length, weight) for boys.

Adapted from Hamill PVV et al: Physical growth: National Center for Health Statistics percentiles, Am J Clin Nutr 32:607-629, 1979. Data from the Fels Research Institute, Wright State University School of Medicine, Yellow Springs, Ohio. Provided as a service of Ross Laboratories, 1982.

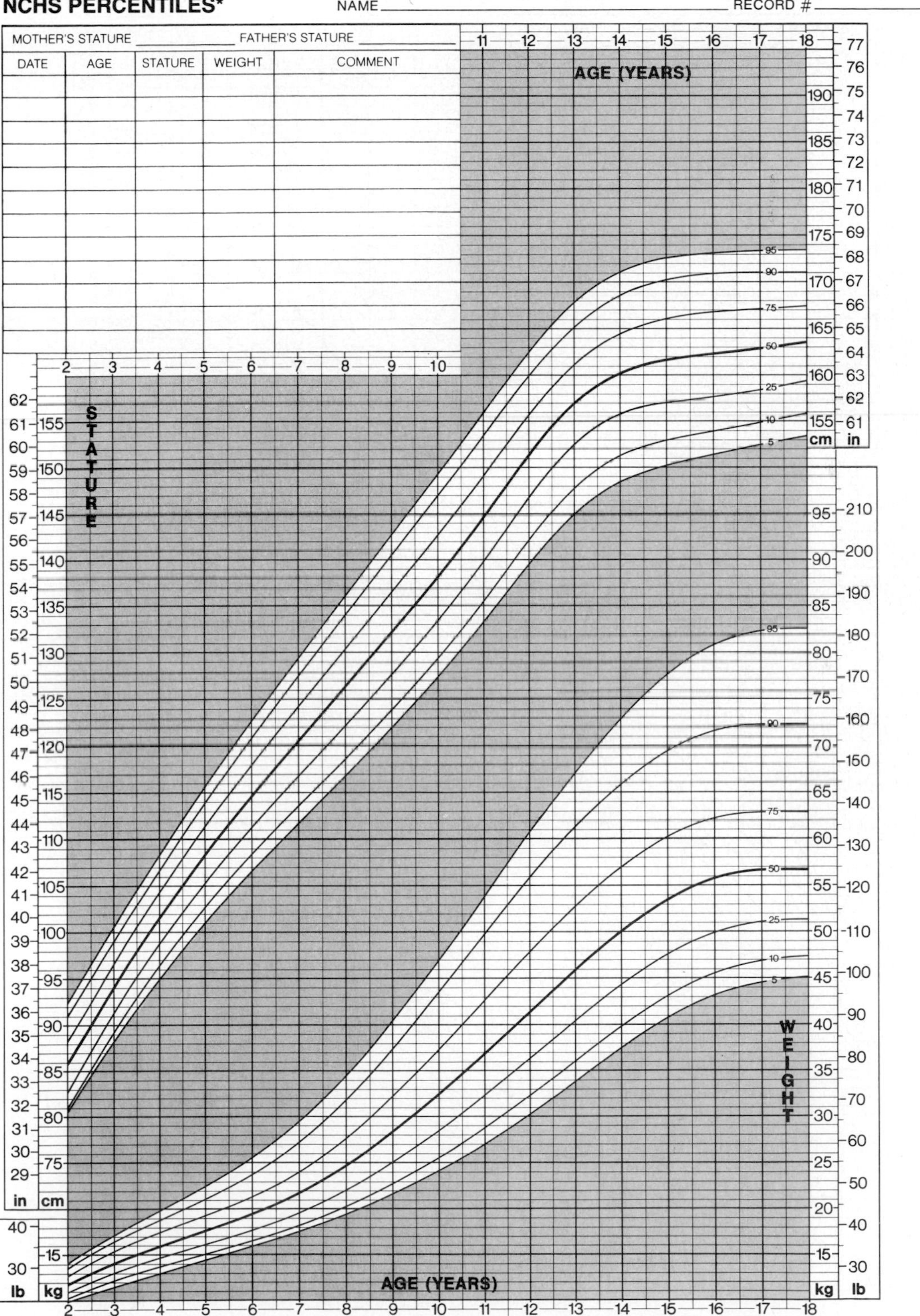


***FIG. 28-5*** 2 to 18 years physical growth NCHS percentiles (stature, weight) for girls.

Adapted from Hamill PVV et al: Physical growth: National Center for Health Statistics percentiles, Am J Clin Nutr 32:607-629, 1979. Data from the National Center for Health Statistics (NCHS), Hyattsville, MD. Provided as a service of Ross Laboratories, 1982.

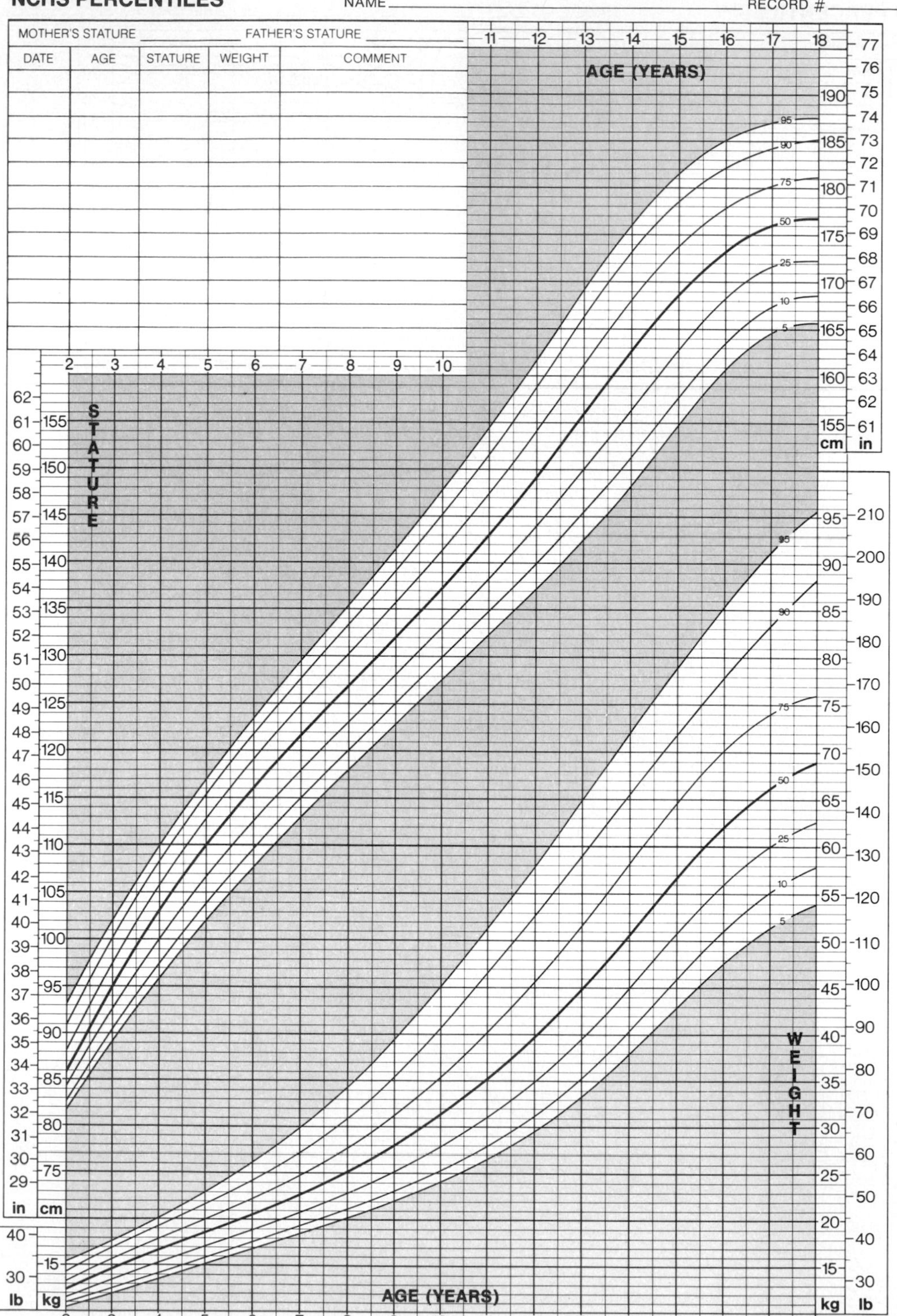


*FIG. 28-6* 2 to 18 years physical growth NCHS percentiles (stature, weight) for boys.

Adapted from Hamill PVV et al: Physical growth: National Center for Health Statistics percentiles, Am J Clin Nutr 32:607-629, 1979. Data from the National Center for Health Statistics (NCHS), Hyattsville, Md. Provided as service of Ross Laboratories.

**GIRLS: PREPUBESCENT PHYSICAL GROWTH NCHS PERCENTILES***

NAME________________ RECORD #________________

| DATE | AGE | STATURE | WEIGHT | COMMENT |
|---|---|---|---|---|
| | | | | |
| | | | | |
| | | | | |
| | | | | |
| | | | | |
| | | | | |
| | | | | |
| | | | | |
| | | | | |
| | | | | |
| | | | | |
| | | | | |
| | | | | |
| | | | | |
| | | | | |
| | | | | |
| | | | | |
| | | | | |
| | | | | |
| | | | | |

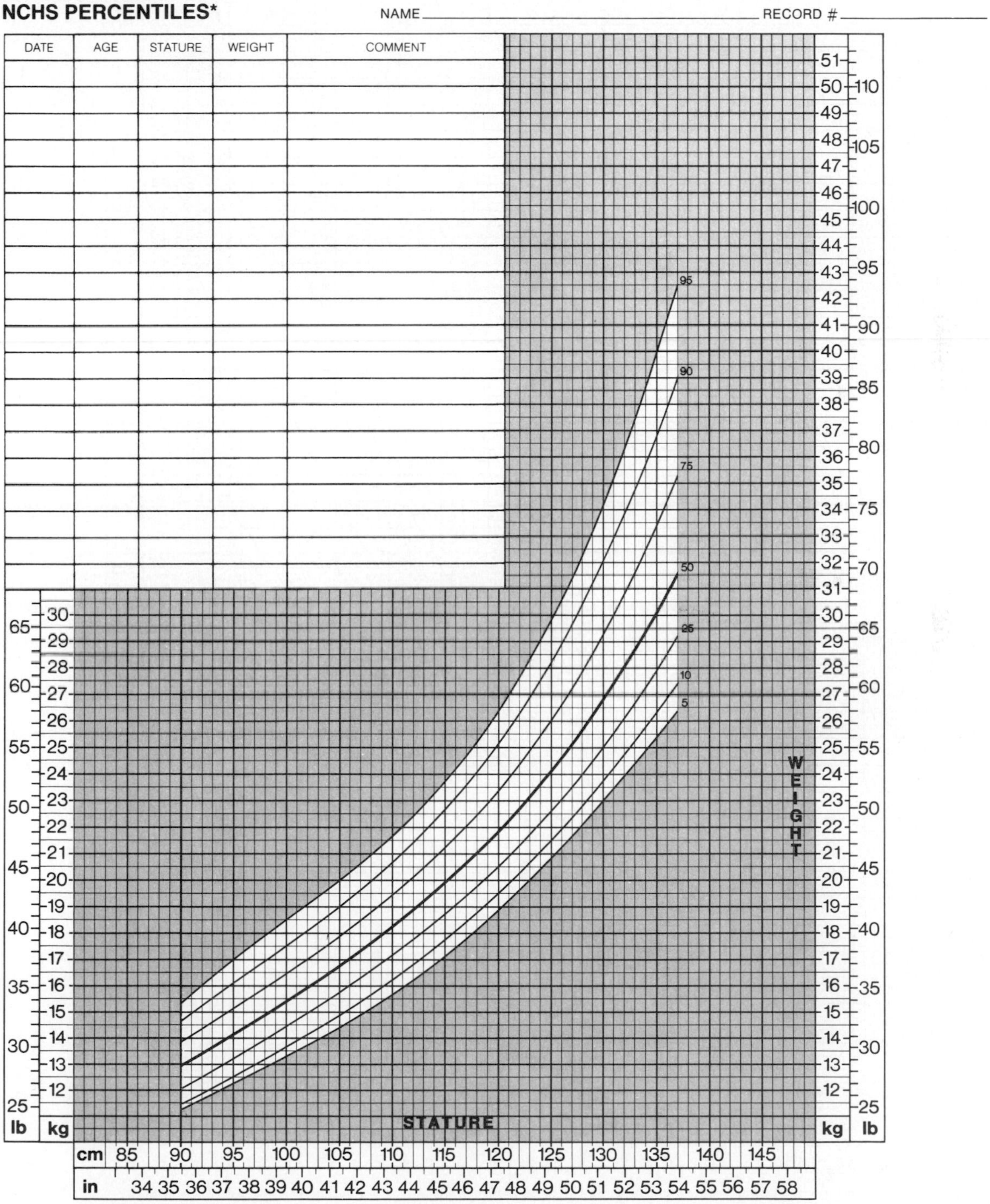

***FIG. 28-7*** Prepubescent physical growth NCHS percentiles (stature, weight) for girls.

Adapted from Hamill PVV et al: Physical growth: National Center for Health Statistics percentiles, Am J Clin Nutr 32:607-629, 1979. Data from the National Center for Health Statistics (NCHS), Hyattsville, MD. Provided as a service of Ross Laboratories, 1982.

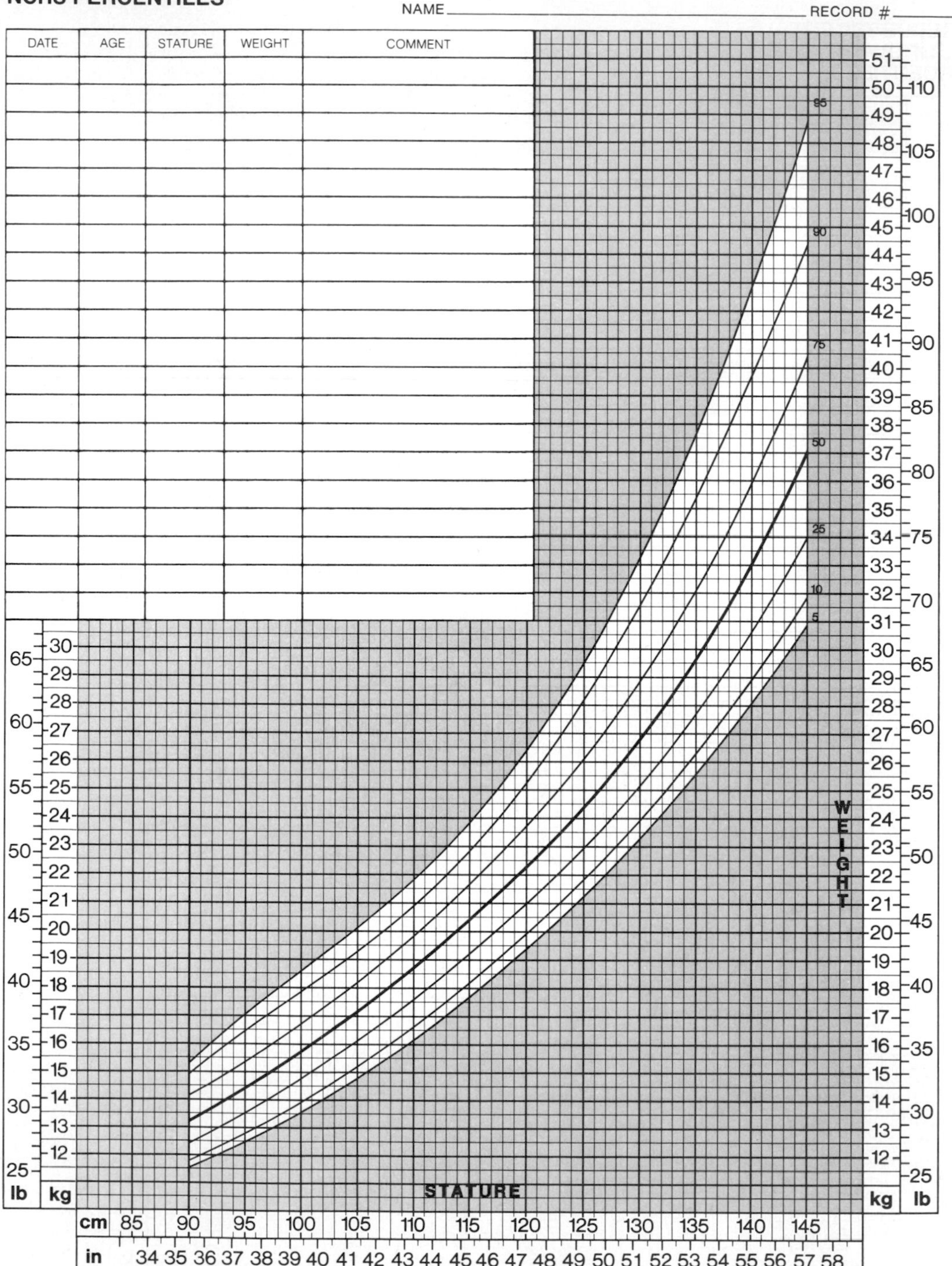


***FIG. 28-8*** Prepubescent physical growth NCHS percentiles (stature, weight) for boys.

Adapted from Hamill PVV et al: Physical growth: National Center for Health Statistics percentiles, Am J Clin Nutr 32: 607-629, 1979. Data from the National Center for Health Statistics (NCHS), Hyattsville, MD. Provided as a service of Ross Laboratories, 1982.

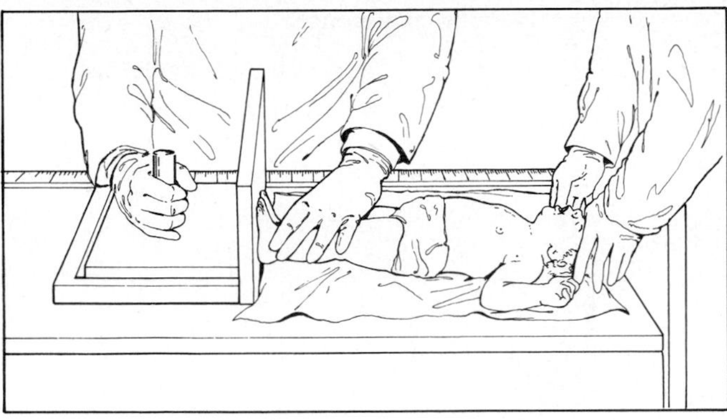

***FIG. 28-9*** Measuring recumbent length.

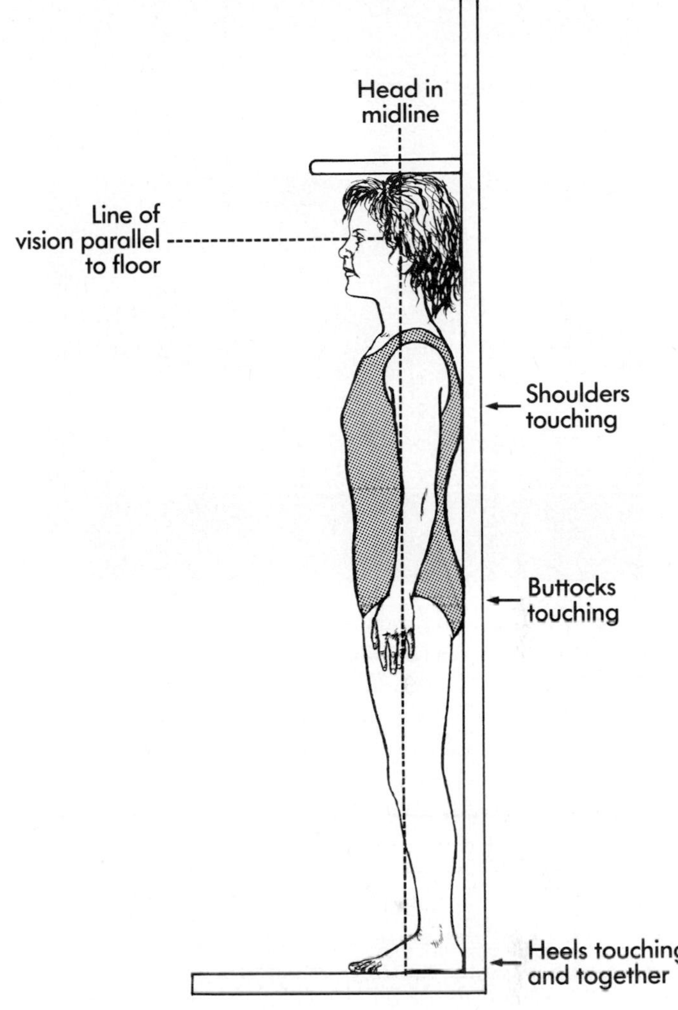


***FIG. 28-10*** Measuring height.

From Whaley LF and Wong DL: Nursing care of infants and children, ed 4, St Louis, 1991, The CV Mosby Co.

| **Steps** | **Rationale** |
| --- | --- |
| 3. Obtain weight measurement. Place undressed child in middle of weighing surface. Infants and young children are weighed while lying or sitting on pediatric scales; keep hand close to but not touching child to prevent accidental falls. Children over 2 to 3 years of age may be weighed standing on adult scales. Adjust beam weights on scale until horizontal beam is balanced at zero. Read weight to nearest 1/2 ounce (15 gm) on pediatric scales or 1/4 pound (0.1 kg) on adult scales (Fig. 28-11). | Serial weight measurements provide a good indicator of growth rate. Rapid or sudden weight loss suggests serious, acute disease or dehydration. Gradual weight loss suggests chronic disease or malnutrition. Underweight with normal growth rate may be caused by inadequate nutrition or may be related to genetic factors and normal for a specific child. Rapid weight gain usually indicates overfeeding, but may be a sign of fluid retention. Generalized overweight or obesity is generally due to overeating and/or underactivity but may be caused by endocrine disorders.<br>***Special Considerations:*** *Birth weight is normally doubled by 5 to 6 months, tripled by 12 months, and quadrupled by 2 to 2 1/2 years. During first 3 months, infants gain about 1 ounce (30 gm) per day or 2 pounds (1 kg) per month; between ages 3 to 12 months, weight gain is about 1 pound (0.5 kg) per month. During second year of life, weight gain is approximately 1/2 pound (0.25 kg) per month. After 2 years of age, weight gain averages 5 pounds (2.25 kg) per year until puberty, when growth spurt occurs. Greatest weight gain usually occurs in fall, least gain in spring (Kempe et al, 1987).* |

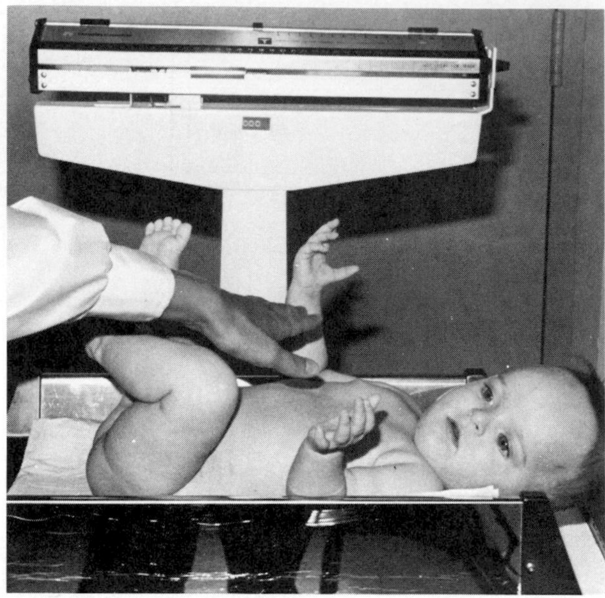

*FIG. 28-11* Infant being weighed on scale.

From Whaley LF and Wong DL: Nursing care of infants and children, ed 4, St Louis, 1991, The CV Mosby Co.

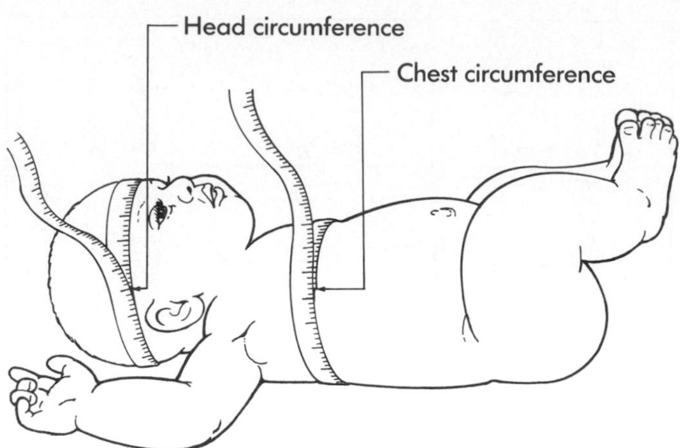


*FIG. 28-12* Measuring chest and head growth.

| Steps | Rationale |
|---|---|
| 4. Measure head and chest circumference.<br>a. Place tape measure around largest part of head, the frontal-occipital circumference (FOC), passing it over forehead just above eyebrows, above ears, and around occipital prominence. Place tape 3 times to ensure accuracy; record greatest circumference (Fig. 28-12).<br>b. Measure chest circumference at nipple line midway between inspiration and expiration. | Head circumference is an indicator of head and brain growth. Chest circumference is measured primarily for comparison with head circumference; marked disproportion between head and chest circumference is generally due to abnormal head growth rather than abnormal chest growth. A large head circumference suggests hydrocephalus. Small head suggests microcephaly, craniostenosis, or genetic disorders.<br>***Special Considerations:*** *FOC normally increases about 12 cm (5 inches) during first year of life, and another 10 cm (4 inches) from 1 to 16 years. Average chest circumference at birth is 1 cm (0.75 inches) less than FOC. Chest remains about same circumference as head until approximately 2 years of age. During childhood chest circumference exceeds FOC by 5 to 7 cm (2 to 3 inches), although it may be greater in children with chronic respiratory problems, e.g., asthma or cystic fibrosis.* |
| 5. Plot growth measurements on appropriate NCHS growth chart. Find child's age on horizontal scale and growth measurement on vertical scale; make dot or cross where two lines intersect. Repeat for each measurement obtained. On weight-by-length or weight-by-stature graphs, find length or stature on horizontal scale and weight on vertical scale; use this graph only on prepubertal children regardless of chronologic age. Age is plotted to nearest month on birth to 36-months chart and to nearest quarter year on 2- to 18-years chart. | Accurate plotting on appropriate charts is required for comparison with norms and interpretation.<br>***Special Considerations:*** *For premature infants, weeks of prematurity are recorded on growth chart and then subtracted from actual age before plotting on growth charts. Adjustments are made until 18 months of age for FOC, 21 months for weight, and 36 months for length or stature (Moore and Roche, 1983). A growth plotting aid, e.g., the Accuplot, promotes accuracy and makes plotting of growth measurements easier.* |
| 6. Interpret measurements by comparison with percentiles on charts. In general, normal measurements for height, weight, and head circumference should fall between the 5th and 95th percentiles after making any indicated adjustment for prematurity. Serial measurements should follow the normal growth curve. | If accurate measurements have been obtained, measurements falling about 95th percentile or below 5th percentile or serial measurements showing marked change in percentile levels are suggestive of health or nutrition problems. A change from one edge of percentile zone to other edge of that zone or shift across percentile zones away from 50th percentile is significant. The greater the change in growth percentile since previous measurements, the quicker the change has occurred, and the younger the age of child, the greater the reason for concern. |

| Steps | Rationale |
|---|---|
| | ***Special Considerations:*** *Exclusively breast-fed infants may exhibit a more rapid growth during the first 3 months of life, then a slower rate from 3 to 6 months as compared to NCHS 50th percentile (Wood et al, 1988). Additional techniques for assessment of growth are available, e.g., skinfold thickness measurements, water-resistance measure for percent of body fat, ultrasound methods, and incremental growth measurements. These tools may be used for more accurate assessment of children falling outside of normal range on general growth parameters.* |
| **Evaluation Outcomes** | **Observational Guidelines** |
| 1. Accurate, appropriate growth measurements are obtained. | Accuracy may be confirmed by repeating all measurements three times. Weight is obtained on all children. Recumbent length is measured if child is under 24 months and stature is measured if over 36 months; between 24 and 36 months, either measurement is acceptable. FOC is measured if child is under 12 to 24 months of age. Other measurements are completed on an individual basis. |
| 2. Growth measurements are correctly plotted on appropriate NCHS growth chart. | Confirm accuracy by rechecking plot points on chart. Recumbent length is graphed on birth to 36-months chart; stature is plotted on 2- to 18-years chart. Weight by stature is not used for postpubertal children. Adjustments are made for prematurity, if indicated. |
| 3. Growth measurements falling outside range of normal are identified. | Measurements above 95th percentile or below 5th percentile, or serial measurements showing significant change in percentile are documented and referrals are made as appropriate. |

## Documentation

Date and actual numerical values of all measurements completed are recorded and plotted on appropriate NCHS growth charts. Any factors that may affect accuracy or interpretation of measurements, e.g., clothing, prosthesis, casts, prematurity, physical anomalies, or an uncooperative child, are documented. Nursing diagnoses and plan of care, including referrals, are documented.

## Child and Family Teaching

Results of physical growth assessment should always be reviewed with family and child. Growth charts are shared and meaning of plotted points are explained. For example, if child falls at 25th percentile on weight for age, explain that if 100 children of the same age were compared, approximately 75 would weigh more and 25 less than this child. Normalcy is important to family and child and can be reassuring. This is particularly important to adolescents for whom body image is a primary concern. For those falling outside norms, sharing growth charts can provide an opening for developing intervention plans with family and child, e.g., discussing nutrition in more detail or referring family to nutritionist.

# SKILL 29 Assessing Nutritional Status

*Rosemary Liguori*

Nurses are in a key position to assess and educate the family on how nutrition influences cognition, learning, growth, and development. Nutritional status reflects the general health of the child. Nutritional intake can be influenced by culture, economics, genetic disorders, and environment. Good nutrition is difficult to maintain in modern society with the increasing influence of fast foods, hectic lifestyles, snack foods, and high pressure advertising.

## NURSING DIAGNOSES

Health-seeking behaviors (nutritional assessment) related to promotion/maintenance of child's health; Altered nutrition: less than body requirements related to inadequate caloric intake; Altered nutrition: more than body requirements related to excessive caloric intake; Altered growth and development related to inadequate nutritional intake.

| Steps | Rationale |
|---|---|
| **Assessment** | |
| 1. Assess characteristics of the child:<br>a. Age.<br>b. Activity level.<br>c. Food allergies. | Basic nutritional requirements vary according to age (see Skill 58). Usual activity level influences the amount of calories above basic requirements needed for growth and development. Allergies to an essential food may require dietary modification to ensure a balanced intake.<br>***Special Considerations:*** *Milk, egg, nuts, and chocolate are a few foods that frequently cause systemic reactions, e.g., hives, headaches, and difficulty breathing.* |
| d. History of prematurity or small for gestational age. | Infants that are small for gestational age have experienced poor fetal nutrition, which affects growth. Premature infants have increased nutritional needs because of immature body systems. |
| e. Past medical history, especially failure to thrive, cystic fibrosis, Crohn's disease, galactosemia, lactose intolerance, gastrointestinal anomalies (Hirschsprung's, tracheoesophageal fistula, gastroesophageal reflux, biliary atresia), neurologic defects, and physical disabilities. | These are some common conditions that affect nutrient intake, retention, absorption and growth.<br>***Special Considerations:*** *Often the initial step to identifying nutritional problems are indicators noted during a well-child visit. Potential problems noted in a brief history signal a need for a more thorough nutritional assessment.* |
| f. History of recent gastrointestinal disorders, e.g., pyloric stenosis, nausea and vomiting, indigestion, diarrhea, and constipation. | Recent gastrointestinal dysfunction can influence current nutritional status and may indicate an undiagnosed disorder. |
| g. History of frequent infections (more than 6 per year). | Frequent infections are often associated with chronic malnutrition, because the cell mediated immune response is depressed (Rosenthal and Padron, 1989). |
| h. History of emotional problems related to food intake or digestion: anorexia nervosa, bulimia, and gastrointestinal ulcers. | Emotion, self-esteem, and the struggle for independence can influence food intake. |
| i. Medications child receives. | Medications may affect absorption, metabolism, and excretion of nutrients. For example, anticonvulsants decrease vitamin D, folic acid, and riboflavin absorption. Antimicrobials may cause decreased vitamin K synthesis and reduced lactose, folate, and $B_{12}$ levels. Mineral oil may interfere with absorption of fat-soluble vitamins (Rosenthal and Padron, 1989). |
| 2. Assess characteristics of the family:<br>a. History of family growth patterns. Ask height/weight of family members. | Short stature family members usually indicate smaller size in children (Patterson et al, 1986). |
| b. Family history of heart disease before 60 years of age. | The American Academy of Pediatrics (1986) recommends blood cholesterol screening on children with a family history of early heart disease. |

| Steps | Rationale |
|---|---|
| | ***Special Considerations:*** *Davidson et al (1989) reported 10% of 420 9- and 10-year-olds in a mass screening had blood cholesterol levels greater than the desirable adult level (200 mg/dl). Only one third of these had a family history of heart disease.* |
| c. Cultural background (Fig. 29-1). | Culture and religion provide a significant influence on types of food eaten, patterns of eating, and preparation methods. ***Special Considerations:*** *The Hispanic, Native American, and black population have a high intake of vegetables and starches and a low intake of protein (Whaley and Wong, 1991). Mexican children are allowed considerable freedom in food choices and eating habits (Suitor and Crowley, 1984).* |

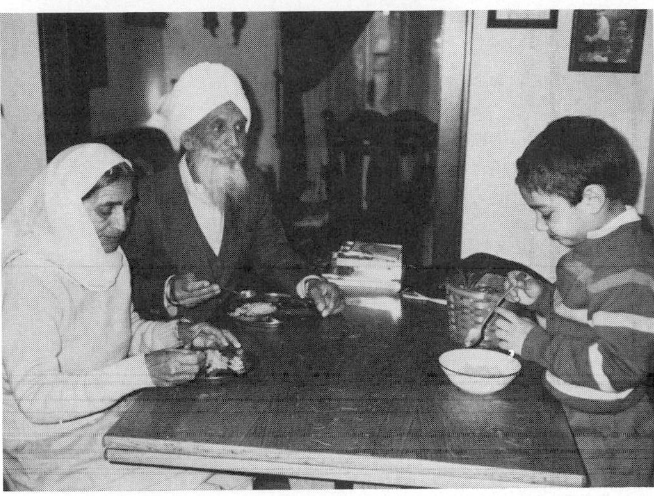

***FIG. 29-1*** Cultural background influences nutritional status.

| Steps | Rationale |
|---|---|
| d. Religion. | Some religious practices dictate food intake, although individual families may vary in their adherence to the rules. ***Special Considerations:*** *Hinduism prohibits eating beef and strict Judaism prohibits eating pork or shellfish. Seventh-Day Adventists are vegetarians who refrain from eating meat or shellfish (some may avoid dairy foods and eggs); consumption of highly spiced foods is also discouraged (Suitor and Crowley, 1984).* |
| e. Socioeconomic status. | Lower socioeconomic groups tend to have diets with higher concentrations of salt, calories, and nonnutritional foods (Brown et al, 1986). |
| f. Family stability (see Skill 38). | A cohesive family usually maintains better eating patterns. Members encourage children to try new, nutritional foods (Venters and Mullis, 1984). |
| g. Family's knowledge of the child's nutritional needs. | Determining present nutritional knowledge provides a baseline for teaching needs. |
| 3. Ask the parents if they have any concerns about the way their child is eating. | Determining parental concerns assists in identifying actual or potential problems of nutrition, as well as needed areas of teaching. It also assists in establishing a collaborative relationship with the parent. ***Special Considerations:*** *If the parent digresses with open-ended questioning, then direct questions may be needed.* |

## Planning and Goal Setting

| Steps | Rationale |
|---|---|
| 1. Allot sufficient amount of time to collect data. | A thorough nutritional assessment often requires considerable time to complete. |
| 2. Determine an appropriate method to collect data, depending on the time available, the nature of the potential problem, and cooperation of the family/child: | ***Special Considerations:*** *Assessing nutritional intake can: (1) provide information about the diet and feeding patterns of the child to identify potential or existing nutritional problems; (2) assist in planning individualized treatment; and (3) establish a baseline to evaluate future progress.* |
| a. Thorough diet history, including family patterns and developmental history. | A thorough diet history is necessary to gain complete nutritional intake information during the interview. It provides a large amount of detailed data, although one disadvantage is the amount of time needed to acquire the information. |
| b. A 24-hour recall, in which the parent or older child review what was eaten, the quantity, and when it was eaten. | A 24-hour recall is a quick and easy nutritional assessment method. Disadvantages are that recall is not always accurate, and it may not have been a typical day. |

**Steps** **Rationale**

## FOOD DIARY FOR CHILDREN

### Instructions

1. Record all foods and beverages immediately *after* they are consumed.
2. Measure the amounts of each food carefully with standard measuring cups and spoons. Record meat portions in ounces or as fractions of pounds, e.g., 8 oz of milk, 1 medium egg, ¼ lb of hamburger, 1 slice of bread, white; ½ small banana.
3. Indicate method of preparation, e.g., medium egg, fried, ½ cup baked beans with a 2-inch slice of salt pork, 4 oz of steak, broiled.
4. Be sure to record any condiments, gravies, salad dressings, butter, margarine, whipped cream, relishes, e.g., ¾ cup of mashed potatoes with 3 tbsp of brown gravy, ¼ cup of cottage cheese salad with 2 olives, ½ cup of cornflakes with 1 tsp of sugar and ⅓ cup of 2% milk.
5. Be sure to record all between-meal foods and drinks, for example coffee with 1 oz of cream, 12 oz of cola, 4 sugar cookies, 1 candy bar (indicate brand name).
6. If you eat away from home, please put an asterisk (*) in the food column beside the food listing.

**Day 1**

Date ______________ Day of week ______________ Weight ______________

| Time | Food | Amount | How prepared |
|---|---|---|---|
| | | | |
| | | | |
| | | | |
| | | | |
| | | | |
| | | | |
| | | | |
| | | | |
| | | | |
| | | | |
| | | | |
| | | | |

***FIG. 29-2*** The 3- or 7-day food diary for children.

c. A 3-day diary (Fig. 29-2). This is a written log of all meals/snacks (vitamin, liquid, and solid) in a 3-day period. The family records the quantity, type of food, how it was prepared, when eaten, and with whom. The child's feelings when eating are noted also, if appropriate.

A written record as the food is consumed is more accurate than attempting to recall intake. The process of keeping the diary may be an intervention itself, e.g., when a parent concerned that a child has a poor intake is surprised about how much the child actually eats. A food diary may hamper accurate assessment since people tend to select more nutritious food knowing the diary will be read by a health care professional.

***Special Considerations:*** *If possible, observing food preparation helps to identify inaccuracies, e.g., underestimating amount of salt added to food (Lierman et al, 1987).*

| Steps | Rationale |
|---|---|
| d. A 7-day diary (Fig. 29-2) notes the same information as on the 3-day diary, extending data collection to 1 week. | A longer diary is useful when an extensive history is required to review eating patterns. It creates greater awareness of patterns and more active involvement, especially with teenagers and older school-age children, who are at greater risk for fad diets, fast foods, anorexia nervosa, or obesity. |
| e. Food Frequency Questionnaire (Fig. 29-3) is a form that the child/parent may complete. It is a record of the amount and times in a day, week, or month that a child eats a food from the major food groups (Wong and Whaley, 1990). | An advantage of the questionnaire is that it may be used in combination with a 24-hour history for a more complete view of nutritional intake and can target particular nutrients, e.g., carbohydrates, protein, iron, vitamins C and A, and calcium (Moore, 1988). Food amounts and information about emotional aspects of food intake are not noted and are limitations of the questionnaire (Moore, 1988). |

ASSESSMENT OF FOOD FREQUENCY

| Food group | Number of servings per day or week | Approximate servings size (Indicate amount of liquids, fruits, and vegetables in cup portions; proteins in tablespoons or ounces) |
|---|---|---|
| MILK/CHEESE | | |
| Milk | | |
| Cheese | | |
| Yogurt | | |
| Pudding | | |
| Ice cream | | |
| Other | | |
| PROTEIN FOODS | | |
| Meat | | |
| Fish | | |
| Poultry | | |
| Egg | | |
| Peanut butter | | |
| Legumes (dried beans, peas) | | |
| Nuts | | |
| Other | | |
| BREADS/CEREALS | | |
| Bread, tortilla | | |
| Cooked pasta, rice, hot cereal | | |
| Dry cereal (not presweetened) | | |
| Crackers | | |
| Muffins | | |
| Other | | |
| VEGETABLES | | |
| Yellow or orange | | |
| Green/leafy | | |
| Other | | |
| FRUIT | | |
| Juice, citrus (orange, grapefruit, tangerine) | | |
| Juice, noncitrus | | |
| Other | | |
| FATS (butter, oil, margarine, salad dressing) | | |
| SWEETS | | |
| Soda, punch | | |
| Cake/cookie, etc. | | |
| Candy | | |
| Presweetened cereal | | |

***FIG. 29-3*** The food frequency questionnaire.

From Wong DL and Whaley LF: Clinical manual of pediatric nursing, ed 3, St Louis, 1990, The CV Mosby Co.

| Steps | Rationale |
|---|---|
| 3. Identify nutritional requirements according to child's age (see Skill 58). | As the child grows, nutritional needs change, e.g., the infant under 1 year and the emerging adolescent require increased calories for adequate growth and development. |
| 4. Develop nursing goals of care:<br>▪ Complete a nutritional assessment.<br>▪ Identify nutritional needs for the child. | |

## Implementation

| | |
|---|---|
| 1. Use the selected dietary assessment tool(s). | Assessment of dietary intake is part of a complete nutritional assessment. The selected tool should be suitable to the needs of the situation, available time, and cooperation of the child and parent.<br>***Special Considerations:*** *Caregivers of underweight infants tend to overestimate amounts of food eaten, and caregivers of overweight infants tend to underestimate the amounts of food eaten (Austin, 1989).* |
| *Dietary history:*<br>a. For infants, ask the questions in the box below left.<br>b. For children 1 year and older, ask the questions in the box below right. | Responses provide significant information for a complete nutritional assessment and may uncover gaps or misperceptions in nutritional knowledge. Direct questions may help conserve time. |

### *DIETARY HISTORY FOR INFANTS*

What was the infant's birth weight? When did it double, triple?
Was the infant premature?
Are you breast-feeding or have you breast-fed your infant? For how long?
If you use a formula, what is the brand? How long has the infant been taking it? How many ounces does the infant drink per day?
Are you giving the infant cow's milk (whole, low-fat, skimmed)? When did you start? How many ounces does the infant drink per day?
Do you give your infant extra fluids (water, juice)?
If the infant takes a bottle to bed at nap or nighttime, what is in the bottle?
At what age did you start cereal, vegetables, meat or other protein sources, fruit juice, finger food, table food?
Do you make your own baby food or use commercial foods, e.g., infant cereal?
Does the infant take a vitamin supplement? If so, what type?
Has the infant shown an allergic reaction to any food(s)? If so, list the foods and describe the reaction.
Are there any feeding problems (excessive fussiness, spitting up, colic, difficulty sucking or swallowing)?
Does the infant spit up frequently, have unusually loose stools, or have hard, dry stools? If so, how often?
How often do you feed your infant?
How would you describe your infant's appetite?

From Whaley LF and Wong DL: Nursing care of infants and children, ed 4, St Louis, 1991, The CV Mosby Co.

### *DIETARY HISTORY FOR CHILDREN (1 YEAR AND OLDER)*

What are the family's usual mealtimes?
Do family members eat together or at separate times?
Who does the family grocery shopping and meal preparation?
How much money is spent to buy food each week?
How are most foods prepared—baked, broiled, fried, other?
How often does the family or your child eat out? What kinds of restaurants do you go to? What kinds of food does your child typically eat at restaurants?
Does your child eat breakfast regularly?
Where does your child eat lunch?
What are your child's favorite foods, beverages, and snacks? Average amounts consumed or usual size portions? Special cultural practices, e.g., does the family only eat ethnic food?
What foods and beverages does your child dislike?
How would you describe your child's usual appetite (hearty eater, picky eater)?
What are your child's feeding habits (breast, bottle, cup, spoon, eats by self, needs assistance, any special devices)?
Does your child take vitamins or other supplements; do they contain iron or fluoride?
Are there any known or suspected food allergies; is your child on a special diet?
Has your child lost or gained weight recently?
Are there any dental problems or appliances, e.g., braces that affect eating?
What type of exercise does your child do regularly?
Is there a family history of cancer, diabetes, heart disease, high blood pressure, or obesity?

From Whaley LF and Wong DL: Nursing care of infants and children, ed 4, St Louis, 1991, The CV Mosby Co.

| Steps | Rationale |
|---|---|
| c. Determine the child's developmental history significant to feeding and nutrition. For example, ask:<br>▪ Does your child drink from a bottle/cup? Is he or she able to use a fork/knife/spoon?<br>▪ Is the child able to feed self or is assistance required?<br>▪ Does your child have coordination problems (developmental delays) that make eating difficult? | Asking questions about feeding and developmental milestones allows delays to be identified and anticipatory guidance to be offered. |
| ▪ Does the child take a bottle to bed or walk around with one during the day? | Bottles in bed may cause tooth decay and middle ear infections and increase upper respiratory infections. Constant drinking from a bottle may reflect excessive dependency and instant gratification in the older child. |
| ▪ Some children use food as a means of control, or for a power struggle. Does your child sometimes do that? | Children/parents may be caught in power struggles, especially with toddler or adolescents who are developing independence. |
| d. Determine the influence of geographic/societal food trends. For example, ask:<br>▪ Is your home located in a city, town, or in the country?<br>▪ What percent of the time does your family eat at a fast food restaurant?<br>▪ What percent of your family meals are convenience foods? | Fast foods and convenience foods often contain high levels of sodium and fat. Also factors such as geographic locale and urban or rural settings influence types and availability of foods. |
| e. Determine family food preferences, e.g., frequency of red meat consumption, snack food choices, or practice of vegetarianism. | Dietary practices may indicate specific nutrient deficiencies or excesses. For example, strict vegetarians may be at risk for rickets, vitamin $B_{12}$ deficiency, and riboflavin deficiency (Rosenthal and Padron, 1989).<br>***Special Considerations:*** *The father may influence family eating preferences (Venters and Mullis, 1984). Strict vegetarians (vegans) do not eat meat, dairy products, fowl, or fish; they only eat foods from plants. Vegetarians that eat eggs and dairy products are lactoovovegetarians. Some families eat fish or poultry, but avoid red meat (Suitor and Crowley, 1984).* |
| f. Determine patterns of food purchase and preparation. For example, ask:<br>▪ Does your child help select food when you are shopping?<br>▪ Who prepares the meals?<br>▪ Is the child involved in meal preparation?<br>▪ Is the child involved with cleanup tasks? | Allowing children to shop with parents fosters nutritional knowledge, socialization, and self-esteem. Knowledge of which family members prepare food gives clues to family dynamics and education. Allowing the child to participate in meal preparation encourages family growth and increases nutritional knowledge. |
| g. Determine family eating patterns. For example, ask:<br>▪ Where are the meals eaten?<br>▪ Are there regular mealtimes? | Having a regular mealtime and place where meals are eaten, e.g., kitchen or dining room, creates a safe and stable environment.<br>***Special Considerations:*** *Eating meals regularly in front of the television inhibits family interaction.* |
| ▪ With whom are the meals eaten? | Eating together as a family enhances socialization, a sense of belonging, and love (Venters and Mullis, 1984). |
| ▪ What kind of feelings are experienced around mealtime? Is it a time of confrontation, pleasure, smiles, or a sharing time? | Fostering a pleasant environment at meals enhances nutrition and family cohesiveness (Liguori and Wong, 1989). |
| h. Determine if food is used as a form of behavior modification. For example, ask:<br>▪ If your child is well behaved, do you treat him or her with cookies or other sweets?<br>▪ If your child misbehaves does he or she get sent to his or her room without supper? | Food may be misused as a reward, punishment, or comfort.<br>***Special Considerations:*** *Richardson (1988) found that 70% of parents give food as a reward for good behavior.* |
| i. Determine if child engages in pica behavior (eating nonfood substances). For example, ask:<br>▪ Does your child eat paint chips, dirt, or clay, or chew on window sills? | Pica may or may not be harmless, depending on the substance. For example, eating lead-based paint chips can have serious and irreversible effects (Whaley and Wong, 1991). |

| Steps | Rationale |
|---|---|
| *24-hour recall* | |
| a. Ask parent to describe the child's intake on a typical day. If the parent has difficulty responding, ask, for example: ▪ Was yesterday a typical day for Jimmy? If yes, proceed with: | An open-ended question allows parents to tell about nutritional intake at their own pace and in their words. Some parents need a more direct approach, thereby giving guidance in replying. |
| ▪ What does he do first in the morning? What and where does he eat/drink and how much (in terms of ounces)? ▪ Ask similar questions for lunch, dinner, and snacks. | It is more appropriate to ask when the child begins to eat for the day, instead of asking a leading question such as "Does he eat breakfast at 8 AM?" (Pipes, 1981). |
| *3- or 7-day food diary:* | |
| a. Provide a form for the parent/child. b. Discuss the purpose of the diary. c. Review information to be recorded and indicate placement on the form, e.g., the time food was eaten, type and amount of food, and how food was prepared (e.g., fried, baked, broiled). For the purpose of behavior modification, also record where the food was eaten and feelings at that time. d. Instruct to complete recordings immediately after eating or drinking. | Food diaries are time consuming and require commitment to recording the necessary information. Clarifying the process and reason for it and making the form easy to complete enhances compliance. Immediate recording of intake prevents accidental omissions. ***Special Considerations:*** *For a 3-day diary, recording two weekdays and 1 weekend day will obtain a typical pattern for most people (Whaley and Wong, 1991). If desired, ask family to mail the diary after completion for careful review and analysis to facilitate planning for the next session. Provide an addressed, stamped envelope.* |
| ▪ Encourage the older child to assume responsibility for recording intake. | When the child has input into the process of recording, compliance is fostered. |
| *Food frequency questionnaire:* | |
| a. Provide a form for the parent/child. b. Discuss the purpose of the frequency record. c. Review information to be recorded and indicate placement on the form, e.g., number of servings per day or week and amount of serving. | Understanding the reason for the questionnaire and having an easy-to-use form enhances compliance. ***Special Considerations:*** *A frequency questionnaire is most useful in combination with other assessment methods to validate or enhance data. It may be difficult for the user to categorize combination foods (Moore, 1988). If desired, have parent return form by mail as with the Food Diary.* |
| 2. Determine anthropometric measurements (see Skill 28). | Serial growth data and plotting a growth curve helps identify deviations early. Height and head circumference reflect past nutrition, while weight, skinfold thickness, and arm circumference reflect present nutritional status, especially of protein and fat reserves (Whaley and Wong, 1991). |
| a. Weight and height. | Growth delays may be caused by disorders in which food and nutrients are improperly absorbed (e.g., cystic fibrosis, celiac disease, diabetes) or by poor nutrient intake. |
| b. Body fat percentages. | Excess body fat percentage results from excess food intake and/or inadequate activity. ***Special Considerations:*** *Body fat percentage can be determined by various methods, e.g., skinfold thickness and water resistance measures. These methods generally require special training, therefore referral may be indicated to obtain an accurate measure.* |
| c. Arm muscle circumference. | This measure indirectly assesses total muscle mass. Muscle serves as the body's major protein reservoir, therefore, muscle mass indicates adequacy of these stores (Whaley and Wong, 1991). |
| 3. Assess for physical signs of nutritional deficiencies (Table 29-1). | Prolonged nutritional deficiencies will be reflected by physical characteristics. |
| 4. Review laboratory data. | Laboratory tests can confirm or detect nutritional deficiencies or problems and provide information about general nutritional status. ***Special Considerations:*** *Specialized biochemical analyses of body tissue and fluids, e.g., plasma, liver, bone, and hair, are also available and may be indicated in an extensive nutritional assessment.* |
| a. Hematocrit (hct)/hemogloblin (hgb). | Low levels of hct/hgb may indicate anemias: iron, vitamin B, or folate deficiency. |
| b. Albumin. | A low level may indicate liver or kidney disease, or inflammation of the gut, and is a late sign in protein malnutrition. |

| Steps | Rationale |
|---|---|
| c. Urine urea nitrogen. | A low level indicates decreased protein intake. |
| d. Urine creatinine. | An increased level may indicate a growth in muscle mass or high protein intake. |
| e. Blood urea nitrogen (BUN). | BUN is increased with high levels of protein metabolism, decreased when protein metabolism is inhibited, e.g., negative nitrogen balance (Dickey, 1988). |
| f. Lead. | Excessive amounts as measured in blood serum may be present with pica, batteries in the mouth, inhaling gasoline fumes, drinking water containing lead, or eating cigarette butts. |
| g. Glucose. | Elevated levels are present in shock, burns, dehydration, and acidosis (Simko, Cowell, and Hreha, 1989). |
| h. Blood cholesterol. | Elevated total blood cholesterol levels (greater than 200 mg/dl) in children are probably a mixture of genetic and environmental factors, e.g., diet (Davidson et al, 1989). For the child over 2 years of age with an elevated blood cholesterol, dietary counseling is recommended to limit fat and cholesterol intake (Davidson, Smith, and Qaqundah, 1990). |

***TABLE 29-1*** Clinical Signs Associated with Nutritional Deficiencies

| Body Area | Normal Appearance | Clinical Sign(s) | Nutritional Deficiency Indicated |
|---|---|---|---|
| Hair | Shiny, firm, not easily plucked | Hair dull and dry, lack of shine, thinness and sparseness, depigmentation (flag sign), straightness of previously curly hair, easy pluckability | Kwashiorkor; less commonly, marasmus protein-calorie |
| Face | Uniform skin color, smooth, healthy appearance, not swollen | Depigmentation: skin dark over cheeks and eyes, moon face | Protein-calorie, protein |
| | | Scaling of skin around nostrils, nasolabial seborrhea | Riboflavin or niacin pyridoxine |
| Eyes | Bright, clear, shiny, healthy pink moist membranes, no prominent blood vessels | Pale conjunctiva | Anemia: iron, folate, or $B_{12}$ |
| | | Bitot's spots, night blindness, conjunctiva and corneal xeroxis (drying), keratomalacia | Vitamin A |
| | | Redness and fissuring of eyelid corners (angular palpebritis) | Riboflavin, pyridoxine, niacin |
| Lips | Smooth, not chapped | Redness and swelling of mouth or lips, especially at corners of mouth (cheilosis) and angular stomatitis, angular scars | Riboflavin, niacin, iron, pyridoxine |
| Mouth | | Ageusia, dysgeusia | Zinc |
| Tongue | Deep red in appearance, not smooth or swollen | Glossitis | Niacin, folate, riboflavin, iron, vitamin $B_{12}$ |
| | | Scarlet and raw | Nicotinic acid |
| | | Magenta tongue | Riboflavin |
| Teeth | Bright, no cavities, no pain | Pitted, grooved teeth | Vitamin D |
| | | Missing or erupting abnormally, gray or black spots (fluorosis) mottled | Fluoride |
| | | Cavities | Poor hygiene and fluoride |
| | | Mottled enamel | Excess fluoride |
| Gums | Healthy red, do not bleed, not swollen | Spongy, bleeding gums, swollen | Ascorbic acid (vitamin C) |
| Glands | Face not swollen | Thyroid enlargement | Iodine |
| | | Parotid enlargement | Starvation (protein-calorie) |

*Continued.*

**TABLE 29-1** Clinical Signs Associated with Nutritional Deficiencies—cont'd

| Body Area | Normal Appearance | Clinical Sign(s) | Nutritional Deficiency Indicated |
|---|---|---|---|
| Skin | No signs of rashes, swelling, dark or light spots | Dryness of the skin (xerosis), sandpaper feel of skin (follicular hyperkeratosis) | Vitamin A or essential fatty acid |
| | | Petechiae ecchymoses | Ascorbic acid and vitamin D |
| | | Red, swollen pigmentation of exposed areas (pellagrous dermatosis) | Nicotinic acid and tryptophan |
| | | Flakiness of the skin, lack of fat under skin | Kwashiorkor, essential fatty acid |
| | | Increased fat | Obesity |
| | | Scrotal and vulvar dermatosis | Riboflavin |
| Nails | Firm, pink | Nails spoon shaped (koilonychia) | Iron |
| Muscles and skeletal system | Good muscle tone, some fat under skin, can walk or run without pain | Muscle wasting | Starvation, kwashiorkor, marasmus |
| | | Knock knees or bow legs | Vitamin D |
| | | Thoracic rosary | Vitamin D, ascorbic acid |
| | | Musculoskeletal hemorrhage | Ascorbic acid |
| **ORGAN SYSTEMS:** | | | |
| Gastrointestinal | No palpable organs or masses | Hepatomegaly (fatty infiltration) | Protein |
| Cardiovascular | Normal heart rhythm, no murmur, normal blood pressure for age | Cardiac enlargement, tachycardia | Thiamin |
| Nervous system | Psychological stability, normal reflexes | Psychomotor changes, mental confusion | Kwashiorkor, protein, thiamin, nicotinic acid |
| | | Sensory loss, motor weakness, loss of vibration, loss of ankle movement, knee jerks, calf tenderness | Thiamin, vitamin $B_{12}$ deficiency |

From Simko M, Cowell C, and Hreha M: Practical nutrition: a quick reference for the health care practitioner, Rockville, Md, 1989, Aspen Publishers; data contributed by George Christakis, Kathleen Mammel, Susan Rosenthal, and Celia Padron.

| Steps | Rationale |
|---|---|
| 5. Observe feeding of a child/infant by family if possible. Note:<br>a. Comfortable position of child, especially infant/child with disabilities.<br>b. Parent-child interaction.<br>c. Cues of the child to parent.<br>d. Atmosphere (pleasant, relaxed, tense). | Direct observation validates, clarifies, and/or enhances assessments. Actual or potential problems and causes may also be highlighted. |
| 6. Review all collected data.<br>a. Compare dietary intake records to age-appropriate calorie requirements and recommended servings of the basic food groups (see Skill 58).<br>b. Identify growth problems.<br>c. Identify behavior or family problems.<br>d. Identify intake problems, e.g., overeating.<br>e. Identify specific nutritional deficiencies and allergies.<br>f. Determine any additional nutrition-related problems, actual or potential. | Collaboration with the parents as to their child's diet, nutritional needs, and potential or actual problems fosters compliance. |
| 7. Discuss basic nutrition, normal developmental feeding patterns and selection of age-appropriate foods with the family and child, appropriate to assessed knowledge level (see Skill 58). | Family and child knowledge about nutrition needs, normal development, and appropriate food selection provides a basis for adequate nutrition, as well as intervening with potential or existing problems. |
| 8. Counsel the family regarding nutritional concerns and findings identified in assessment. For example:<br>a. Interpret results of laboratory data. | Diet history, clinical assessment, and anthropometry will help identify potential or actual problems. Each component is necessary to provide a complete picture of nutritional status, as well as clues to deficiencies/disorders (Whaley and Wong, 1991). |

| Steps | Rationale |
|---|---|
| b. Identify a lack of a specific food group or abundance of nonessential food, e.g., candy, soda, cookies, or excessive fried foods, as reported in history. | Lack of or excessive intake of specific foods may be noted and questions asked as to why and when these foods are offered. For example, "When do you tend to eat cookies?" or "I see that there are no vegetables in the diet, is there a reason for this?" |
| c. Discuss disharmony during mealtime. | Identifying and discussing the importance of a pleasant atmosphere at meals increases awareness of the need to improve interaction. |
| d. Formulate an appropriate dietary plan in collaboration with the child/parent (see Skill 58). | Collaboration will strengthen compliance with the diet.<br>***Special Considerations:*** *For low-fat, low-cholesterol dietary planning, see Davidson, Smith, and Qaqundah (1990).* |
| 9. Refer to other health professionals of a multidisciplinary team, if problem is not within scope of practice, e.g., dietician, social worker, physician, psychologist, or speech therapist. | Assessment, identification of nutritional concerns, counseling with families, and referrals to other members of the team when appropriate are nursing responsibilities. A dietician can work with the child and family to plan meals according to needs and provide a more in-depth nutritional consultation. A social worker can assist the family to obtain special formulas, e.g., for phenylketonuria (PKU), and financial aid. The physician treats the medical concerns, e.g., dehydration, food allergies, cystic fibrosis, or diabetes. A psychologist works with the family to solve problems that are caused or affected by behaviors, e.g., poor maternal-child interaction or failure to thrive. A speech therapist can assist the child with oral motor problems, e.g., poor swallow, cleft lip/palate (Lierman et al, 1987).<br>***Special Considerations:*** *Children with complex nutritional problems (e.g., developmental disabilities, cleft palate, anorexia, or failure to thrive) will greatly benefit from a multidisciplinary approach.* |

| Evaluation Outcomes | Observational Guidelines |
|---|---|
| 1. A nutritional assessment is completed. | Review documentation of interview: completion of 24-hour recall, 3- or 7-day food diary, or food frequency questionnaire; physical assessment findings; anthropometric measurements and laboratory results. |
| 2. Actual or potential nutritional problems are identified. | Review developed nursing diagnosis(es) and care plan. Compare with assessment documentation. |
| 3. A referral to other health care professionals or a multidisciplinary team is initiated, if necessary. | Review referral documentation, follow up on referral, and/or participate in multidisciplinary health team. |

## Documentation

Document all pertinent nutritional history; include any data collection tool used. Also, chart and plot on the serial growth grid the height, weight, and head circumference of the child. If plotting body fat percentages, compare previous measurements. Describe teaching content and child/family response.

# SKILL 30 Measuring Body Temperature

*Nancy Valentine Stevens*

Temperature is one of the oldest and most basic body measurements recorded in medical literature (Korones, 1981). Temperature regulation is a balance between heat production and heat loss or dissipation. Control of temperature is homeostatic, regulated by the hypothalamus to maintain the body's core temperature within 1 degree Fahrenheit except during illness. After an initial period of temperature instability in neonates, humans are considered homeothermic, capable of maintaining a fairly constant core temperature of 98 to 100°F (36.7 to 37.8°C) through thermal equilibrium. Skin surface temperature, however, varies more readily with environmental conditions (Guyton, 1986).

Temperature may fluctuate more readily in infants and children because of external and internal causes, e.g., activity, environment, infection, dehydration, and immaturity of temperature regulating mechanisms. Control of body temperature is enhanced as the child develops increased adipose tissue to provide insulation and muscles acquire the ability to shiver. The infant exhibits a higher than average body temperature that gradually decreases with age as the capability to prevent heat loss increases (Guyton, 1986).

Body temperature should be measured on all health care visits, any time a child appears lethargic or ill, or routinely on hospitalized children. A temperature elevation may be an early sign of illness in a young child who continues to play and perform daily activities even though ill. Since seizures may accompany fever in some infants and toddlers, early identification of an increasing temperature is important (see Skill 84). Identification of hypothermia, especially in the susceptible neonate, is also important because oxygen needs increase, stressing the infant (Merenstein, Gardner, and Blake, 1989).

Temperature measurement may be obtained by various methods, including glass or electronic thermometers; skin, rectal, esophageal, or tympanic membrane probes; and temperature sensitive skin strips. The glass or electronic thermometers and the tympanic membrane probes are most commonly used for acute care or home measurements, whereas the skin, rectal, and esophageal probes are often used for continuous temperature monitoring, e.g., in neonatal intensive care units and during surgery. This skill does not detail use of these continuous monitoring methods. Skin strips are less reliable for accurate temperature measurement and therefore are discussed only as an alternative method.

## NURSING DIAGNOSES

Health-seeking behaviors (temperature measurements) related to early identification of infection and prevention of seizures due to fever; Potential altered body temperature related to infection, dehydration, or environmental exposure; Ineffective thermoregulation related to prematurity.

| Steps | Rationale |
|---|---|
| **Assessment** | |
| 1. Determine the need for temperature measurement. | Temperature measurement is a basic assessment performed at office and home visits, as well as routinely on the hospitalized infant/child. |
| 2. Assess for behaviors that reflect temperature alterations, both hypo- and hyperthermia (e.g., whining, fretfulness, lethargy, restlessness, irritability, shivering, sweating, flushing, and poor feeding)(see Skills 83 and 84). | Physical and emotional behaviors may indicate temperature changes in the child.<br>***Special Considerations:*** *The child with an elevated temperature from an ear infection may rub his or her head on a pillow or pull at the ear.* |
| 3. Assess for factors that influence body temperature (e.g., illness, age, activity, environmental temperature, circadian rhythms, crying, amount of clothing worn, and nutritional intake). | Body temperature is affected by a variety of internal and external factors related to the body's ability to maintain homeostasis. Identification of factors possibly influencing the obtained measurement permits appropriate interpretation.<br>***Special Considerations:*** *A normal daily temperature fluctuation occurs, with the lowest value occurring in the early morning and the highest in the late afternoon (Erickson, 1980). Normal body temperature is higher in infants and gradually decreases with age (Table 30-1). Neonates are especially temperature labile and sensitive to environmental conditions (see Skills 83 and 84). It is important to differentiate between temperature alteration because of immaturity of temperature regulating mechanisms or as initial evidence of an infectious process.* |

**TABLE 30-1** Average Body Temperatures in Well Children under Basal Conditions

| Age | Temperature F | Temperature C |
|---|---|---|
| 3 months | 99.4 | 37.5 |
| 6 months | 99.5 | 37.5 |
| 1 year | 99.7 | 37.7 |
| 3 years | 99.0 | 37.2 |
| 5 years | 98.6 | 37.0 |
| 7 years | 98.3 | 36.8 |
| 9 years | 98.1 | 36.7 |
| 11 years | 98.0 | 36.7 |
| 13 years | 97.8 | 36.6 |

From: Whaley LF and Wong DL: Nursing care of infants and children, ed 4, St Louis, 1991, The CV Mosby Co; adapted from Lowrey GH: Growth and development of children, ed 8. Copyright © 1986 by Year Book Medical Publishers, Inc., Chicago. (Modified and reproduced with permission.)

| Steps | Rationale |
|---|---|
| 4. Assess for site of temperature measurement most appropriate for age, developmental and cognitive level, and other influencing factors. | Selecting the appropriate site will help minimize the risk of injury, enhance accuracy of the measurement, and may lessen distress for the child.<br>***Special Considerations:*** *Any alteration of the preferred site, e.g., an infection, surgical incision, tissue injury, or recent intake of hot or cold food or drink, may necessitate choosing another site. In addition to the traditional oral, axillary, and rectal sites, other sites exist related to specific measurement devices (see Planning, step 1).* |
| a. Oral—The child must be dependable and capable of following simple directions. Oral measurement may be contraindicated in a child following oral surgery/trauma/infection. | The child will need to be cooperative to obtain an accurate measurement and prevent injury from breakage when a glass thermometer is used. The oral site is usually more acceptable to children than the rectal since it is visible, easily accessible, nonpainful, and less invasive (Wong, 1988). Oral readings correlate well with internal or core temperature readings and reflect changes more rapidly than rectal readings, because the rich blood supply of the sublingual area is derived from the carotid arteries (Erickson, 1980).<br>***Special Considerations:*** *Factors that may temporarily affect the accuracy of the oral measurement include hot or cold food/fluid intake, smoking, rapid mouth breathing, and possibly oxygen administration (Tandberg and Sklar, 1983; Neff et al 1989; and Whaley and Wong, 1989). For these situations, select an alternative site or delay measurement.* |
| b. Axillary—This site is the recommended site for infants and young children. It is an alternative site to oral measurement in the older child. | Temperature measurement in the axilla is considered the safest, most accessible and least invasive method. Accuracy correlates well with the oral and rectal methods, with variations being less than 0.4° C in young children (Martyn et al, 1988).<br>***Special Considerations:*** *Metabolism of brown fat may make axillary readings misleadingly high in the cold stressed neonate (Merenstein, Gardner, and Blake, 1989).* |
| c. Rectal—This site is an alternative when the oral or axillary sites are unacceptable or unsafe. The rectal site is contraindicated in the neonate, a child who has rectal disease or surgery, is having diarrhea, or is in a spica cast. | Although the rectal site has traditionally been considered less affected by ambient factors, core or deep body temperature is not obtained unless the thermometer is inserted to a depth of at least 5 cm, which incurs a risk of rectal perforation. This risk is especially high in the neonate less than 3 months of age, since the colon curves significantly at a depth of 3 cm. (Merenstein, Gardner, and Blake, 1989).<br>***Special Considerations:*** *A 70% mortality rate is associated with rectal perforation in the neonate (Merenstein, Gardner, and Blake, 1989). A risk for perforation also exists in an older child who is uncooperative or difficult to hold securely, since penetration depth can not be controlled. Presence of stool in the rectum may affect accuracy of the temperature measurement (Whaley and Wong, 1991). Rectal measurement may stimulate defecation.* |

| Steps | Rationale |
|---|---|
| **Planning and Goal Setting** | |
| 1. Select temperature measuring device based on site selection and/or equipment availability. | ***Special Considerations:*** *Cost of the electronic devices is high compared to the traditional glass thermometer.* |
| a. Glass mercury thermometer, oral or rectal. | ***Special Considerations:*** *Oral and rectal thermometers differ only in the bulb shape; the oral thermometer has an elongated tip or bulb, the bulb on the rectal thermometer is rounded.* |
| b. Electronic thermometers (e.g., IVAC). | Electronic thermometers sense temperature with a small, solid-state electronic component called a thermistor mounted at the tip of a plastic and stainless steel probe, which is connected to an electronic recorder. The obtained measurement appears on a digital display (Erickson, 1980).<br>***Special Considerations:*** *The electronic thermometer is accurate for oral, axillary, and rectal sites, and the unbreakable plastic probe cover and short measurement time (generally under 60 seconds) make it especially useful with children (Whaley and Wong, 1989). Telethermometers are electronic instruments to which a long, soft, flexible probe is attached. The probe can be inserted in the rectum, esophagus, or be attached to the skin to provide a direct temperature reading in approximately 2 minutes (Eoff, Meier, and Miller, 1974). These devices are most often used for continuous temperature monitoring, e.g., in intensive care areas and with servocontrolled incubators (see Skill 83).* |
| c. Tympanic membrane sensor (e.g., FirstTemp, Ototemp). | Tympanic membrane sensors measure infrared energy emitted by the membrane. A temperature reading is obtained in 1 to 2 seconds by placing the sensor at the external auditory canal opening. Tympanic membrane sensors reflect cerebral blood temperature and are sensitive to subtle changes. Clinical accuracy has been demonstrated (Hancock, 1987; Shinozaki, Dean, and Perkins, 1988).<br>***Special Considerations:*** *The presence of cerumen does not affect readings (Hancock, 1987). Although it has been suggested that the presence of otitis media may cause a falsely high temperature reading, Weir and Weir (1989) reported only a 0.1°C difference between infected and noninfected ears.* |
| d. Other devices, e.g., forehead or skin strips, and pacifiers with a temperature sensitive dot. | ***Special Considerations:*** *Skin strips are primarily used by parents or in schools or day-care centers as a screening device. An elevated reading on a skin strip should be verified with a more accurate device, since the strips generally read high (Martyn et al, 1988). The pacifier has proven unreliable, failing to detect temperatures of 102°F and higher (Banco, Jayashekaramurth, and Giaffam, 1988).* |
| 2. Assemble additional supplies: | |
| a. Water-soluble lubricant, if using rectal method. | Lubricant allows safer and less traumatic probe or thermometer insertion. |
| b. Tissue, if using glass thermometer. | Tissue can be used to wipe the thermometer clean after use to aid in reading degree increments. |
| c. Writing instrument and paper. | Prompt recording facilitates accurate documentation. |
| d. Disposable gloves (optional). | Use of gloves will decrease the chance of transmitting infection, especially when taking rectal temperatures. |
| e. Watch with a second hand if using a glass thermometer. | Accurate timing provides a reliable measure. |
| f. Disposable probe cover for electronic devices. | Electronic devices are intended for multiple patient use and therefore require a clean cover for each child to prevent transmission of infection. |
| 3. Inspect temperature measuring device for proper functioning and/correct reading. For example, a glass thermometer should read at or below 95°F prior to insertion. | A nonfunctioning device or elevated reading before use may result in an inaccurate measurement.<br>***Special Considerations:*** *Refer to product operating manual for instructions on calibration and operation of electronic measuring devices.* |
| 4. Determine a position of comfort and safety appropriate for site and child. | Appropriate positioning ensures the child's safety and comfort during the procedure. |
| 5. Plan diversional activities to use during the procedure, e.g., singing songs or telling stories. | Diversional activities will facilitate the child's cooperation and allow completion of the procedure. |
| 6. Develop goals of nursing care:<br>▪ Obtain an accurate measurement of body temperature.<br>▪ Prevent complications of temperature measurement. | |

| Steps | Rationale |
|---|---|

## Implementation 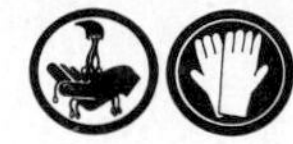

1. Prepare child for the procedure (see Skill 1).

Preparation decreases anxiety, enhances cooperation, and increases safety for a procedure.

2. Position child as planned and restrain if necessary.

Proper positioning facilitates cooperation and safety.

***Special Considerations:*** *For the rectal site, the child should be on his or her side, prone, or supine, with the knees flexed toward the abdomen. A small child may be placed prone across a parent's lap.*

3. Place thermometer or probe in proper position for the selected site.
   a. Oral: Place to one side in posterior sublingual pocket, under the tongue to the back, avoiding the frenulum (Fig. 30-1).

These pockets have a rich blood supply from the carotid arteries, which are located close to the thermal regulating center of the brain (Erickson, 1980).

   b. Axillary: Place under arm with the tip in the center of the axilla. Lower child's arm, and hold it firmly, being sure the tip is in contact with the skin and not clothing.

The center of the axilla is closest to the blood supply in this area and permits the least exposure to environmental effects. Holding the arm firmly maintains close contact of the tip with the skin.

   c. Rectal: Place well-lubricated tip not more than 2.5 cm (1 inch) into rectum. Securely hold the thermometer close to the rectum (Fig. 30-2).

Lubrication assists insertion of thermometer and decreases trauma to delicate tissues of the rectum. Secure positioning of the thermometer minimizes the risk of rectal perforation or breakage should movement occur.

***Special Considerations:*** *Rectal temperature measurement with a glass thermometer or rigid plastic probe is contraindicated in neonates (see Assessment section). In the past, a glass thermometer was used to detect imperforate anus in neonates. This condition can be assessed more safely using a well-lubricated, flexible, soft rubber catheter (Merenstein, Gardner, and Blake, 1989).*

   d. Other methods: Follow manufacturer's directions for placement.
4. Hold thermometer/probe in place for an adequate length of time.
   a. Glass thermometers: oral 2 to 3 minutes; axillary, 3 to 4 minutes; rectal, 3 to 5 minutes.
   b. Other devices: until reading is complete according to manufacturer's instructions.

Inadequate time exposure may provide an inaccurate reading. Time exposure varies with each method because of proximity to blood vessels and the thermal regulating center of the brain.

***Special Considerations:*** *The appropriate length of time a glass thermometer should remain in place for an accurate measure is controversial and research results vary. Follow facility policy.*

5. Maintain the child in a safe position, keeping one hand on the thermometer.

Maintenance of a safe position prevents dislodging the thermometer and avoids possible injury to the child.

6. Provide diversional activities, if needed.

Diversional activities facilitate the passage of time and enhance cooperation.

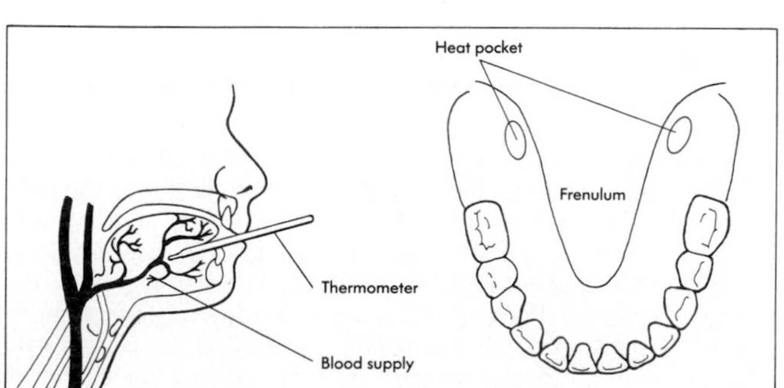


***FIG. 30-1*** Placement for measurement of oral temperature.

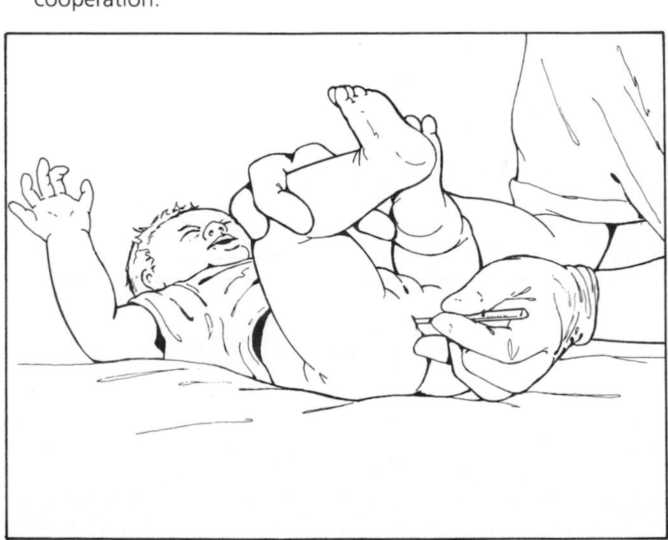

***FIG. 30-2*** Placement of thermometer for rectal temperature measurement.

| Steps | Rationale |
|---|---|
| 7. When reading is obtained, remove thermometer/probe. | Prompt removal of the thermometer minimizes discomfort to the child. |
| 8. For a glass thermometer, wipe with tissue beginning at the top and working to the tip (clean to dirty). | Wiping the glass thermometer decreases the spread of bacteria and facilitates visualization of the numbers for accurate reading. ***Special Considerations:*** *If the rectal site was used, wipe excess lubrication from the rectal area to promote comfort.* |
| 9. Determine measurement/read display and record (see inside cover for temperature conversion factors). | Immediate reading of a glass thermometer prevents exposure to the environment, which may alter measurement. |
| 10. Discard gloves, tissue, and probe covers, if used. | Proper disposal prevents transmission of infection. |
| 11. Redress or assist child to redress and resume previous position or activities. | Assistance facilitates the child's comfort and cooperation. |
| 12. Praise the child for cooperation and effort. | Praise enhances self-esteem and encourages continued positive behavior. |

| Evaluation Outcomes | Observational Guidelines |
|---|---|
| 1. An accurate measurement of temperature is obtained. | Note temperature and compare to baseline, norms, and clinical behaviors. |
| 2. Possible complications of temperature measurement are prevented. | Rectal perforation does not occur and, if a glass thermometer is used, it is not broken. |
| 3. Potential temperature changes are identified, as well as possible influencing factors. | Note child's behavior and trend of temperature changes; correlate with environmental and physical factors. |

## Documentation

Immediately record time, measurement obtained, method and site used, any possible influencing factors, child's behavior, and any pertinent verbalizations.

# *SKILL* 31 Measuring Pulses

*Nancy Valentine Stevens*

The pulse reflects the heart beat or ventricular contraction of the heart because of the wave of blood created by contraction of the left ventricle. Pulse rates are relatively simple to obtain. Pulsation is helpful in assessing the overall health of the child and is important to the specific assessment of the cardiovascular system. Pulse rates decrease with age, reaching adult levels at about 9 to 11 years of age. Determining rate, rhythm, and character is an essential part of assessing the pulse.

### NURSING DIAGNOSES

Impaired tissue integrity related to altered circulation; Altered tissue perfusion related to interruption of arterial/venous flow.

| Steps | Rationale |
|---|---|
| **Assessment** | |
| 1. Determine purpose for pulse measurement. | Pulse rate is one of the easiest to obtain and most accessible of basic measurements. Rate, rhythm, and character of the pulse is routinely assessed on home and office visits, with more in-depth assessment with suspected or known cardiovascular problems (e.g., congenital heart disease) and with certain drug therapies (e.g., digoxin, and some chemotherapeutic agents). |
| 2. Assess for influencing factors such as age, sex, cardiovascular fitness, activity, sleep, fever, anxiety, crying, stress, disease conditions, obesity, medications, blood volume, oxygenation status, electrolyte imbalance, and position change. | Pulse measurements are susceptible to physical, emotional, and environmental influences that may increase or decrease rate. Rhythm and character are not as easily influenced by outside factors. |

**Steps** | **Rationale**

**TABLE 31-1** Normal Heart Rates for Infants and Children

| Age | Heart rate (beats/min) | | |
|---|---|---|---|
| | **Resting (awake)** | **Resting (sleeping)** | **Exercise (fever)** |
| Newborn | 100-180 | 80-160 | Up to 220 |
| 1 week to 3 months | 100-220 | 80-200 | Up to 220 |
| 3 months to 2 years | 80-150 | 70-120 | Up to 200 |
| 2 years to 10 years | 70-110 | 60-90 | Up to 200 |
| 10 years to adult | 55-90 | 50-90 | Up to 200 |

From Gilette PC: Dysrhythmias. In Adams FH and Emmanouilides GC, editors: Moss' heart disease in infants, children, and adolescents, ed 3, Baltimore, 1983, Williams & Wilkins.

***Special Considerations:*** *An increase of 1° F of temperature increases pulse rate 8 to 10 beats/minute (Alexander and Murphy, 1979). As a child's age and heart size increase, the pulse correspondingly decreases to adult rate (Table 31-1).*

3. Assess for associated symptoms of cardiovascular alterations.

Symptoms such as dyspnea, fatigue, cyanosis, pallor, chest pain, peripheral pulse differences, and syncope suggest cardiovascular disease.

4. Assess for factors that may interfere with selection of a site for pulse measurement, e.g., a cast, wound, dressing, IV, or arterial line.

The site of choice may be inaccessible and a second site may need to be selected for easier access.

5. Determine previous pulse rate as a baseline, if available.

Comparison of previous assessments can reflect changes that may be significant.

***Special Considerations:*** *An athletic adolescent may have a normal pulse rate below 60 beats/minute. This slow rate may be misconstrued as abnormal if baseline rate is not available.*

## Planning and Goal Setting

1. Gather needed equipment:

Ready availability of supplies facilitates efficient interventions.

   a. Watch with second hand.
   b. Stethoscope with appropriate size bell and diaphragm.
   c. Pen and paper, or appropriate form from child's record.
   d. Electronic stethoscope or doppler, if needed.

The rapid, soft pulse of the young child and infant may be easier to count with the assistance of electronic amplification.

2. Plan time for pulse measurement when child is calm or involved in quiet activities, if possible. If child is taking medication that may affect pulse rate (e.g., digoxin), assessment before medication is necessary.

Activity, exercise, and anxiety can increase pulse rate.

3. Select position of comfort and accessibility, allowing the child to remain in the parent's arms or on their lap, if appropriate.

Comfortable positioning enhances cooperation during procedure and decreases anxiety.

4. Determine site for pulse measurement, considering age and physical state of child (Fig. 31-1).

Pulse sites include temporal, carotid, apical, brachial, radial, femoral, popliteal, posterior tibial, and dorsalis pedis or pedal. Radial pulses are used most often, with apical pulses usually obtained before 2 years of age.

***Special Considerations:*** *If abnormalities are noted or there is a history of cardiovascular disease or potential perfusion problems, apical pulses should be assessed regardless of age, as well as comparison of pulses in upper and lower extremities. Radial and femoral pulses should be measured and compared at least once during the first year of life to assess for cardiovascular problems, e.g., coarctation of the aorta. In an emergency, femoral or carotid pulses are usually assessed because they are easy to locate. When palpating carotid pulses, avoid excessive pressure that can cause vagal nerve stimulation, inducing a bradycardia reflex. Only palpate one side at a time when assessing the carotid pulse to minimize interference with cerebral circulation.*

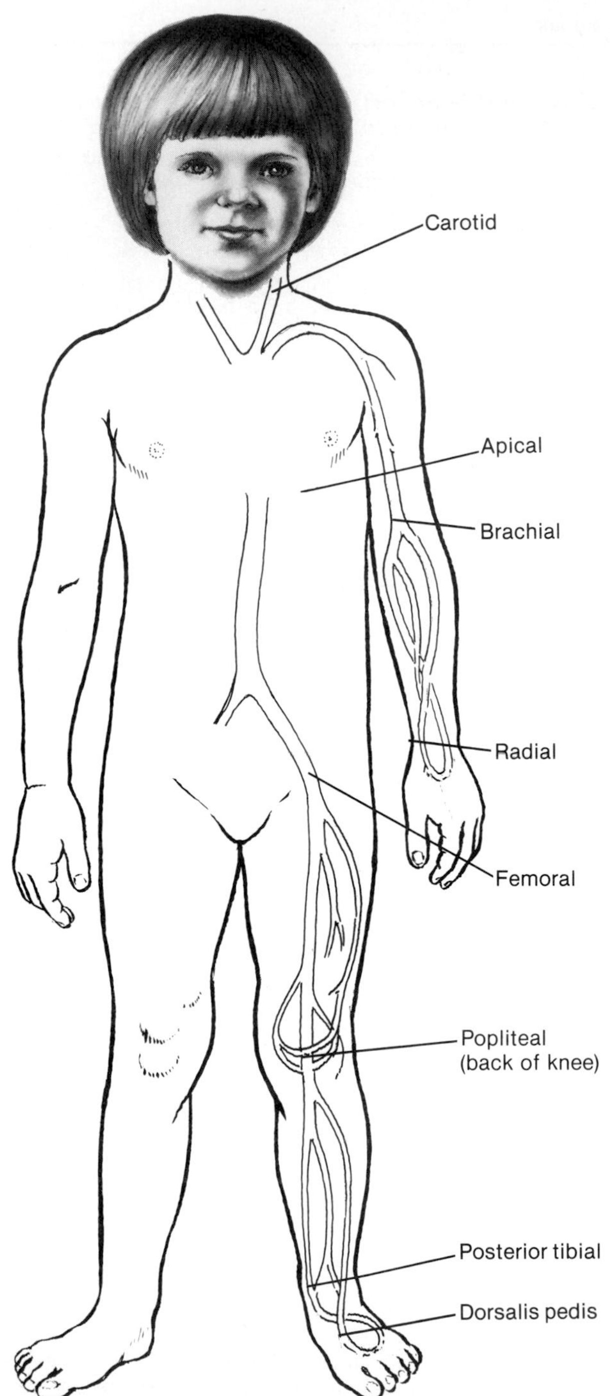


***FIG. 31-1*** Location of pulses.

From Whaley LF and Wong DL: Nursing care of infants and children, ed 4, St Louis 1991, The CV Mosby Co.

5. Plan diversional activities appropriate for the child, e.g., a bright mobile to watch or a parent present to tell a story.

Diversional activities facilitate cooperation and decrease anxiety during procedure.

6. Develop individualized nursing goals of care:
   - Obtain an accurate pulse measurement.
   - Identify abnormalities of rate, rhythm, or character of pulse.
   - Detect changes in rate, character, or rhythm from baseline.

## Implementation

1. Explain procedure to child and family. For a toddler or preschooler, for example, have child place hand on chest to feel heartbeat. Tell child, "I am going to count the number of times a minute I can feel (or hear) this beat."

Understanding the process enhances cooperation and decreases anxiety.

***Special Considerations:*** *It may be helpful to demonstrate the procedure on a doll or stuffed toy.*

| Steps | Rationale |
|---|---|
| 2. Allow child to touch and play with equipment, if desired. May practice on doll or toy. | Familiarity and involvement with equipment dispels fears and encourages participation during procedure. |
| 3. Position child to provide access to selected pulse site. | Proper positioning facilitates cooperation, safety, and accurate measurement. |
| 4. Locate the pulse point previously selected, using one of the following three methods (Fig. 31-1). | Appropriate site selection enhances accurate assessment. |
| a. Place one to three fingertips lightly over pulse point. | Proper placement of fingertips maximizes correct calculation of pulse. Fingertips are used instead of the thumb because the pulse in the thumb may be mistaken for the child's pulse. Also, the fingertips are the most sensitive parts of the hand for palpation of vibration. |
| b. If taking an apical pulse, place the diaphragm of the stethoscope over the point of maximum impulse (PMI) on the child's chest. The site of the PMI will vary, but stabilizes at the 4th to 5th intercostal space (ICS) midclavicular line at about 7 years of age (Fig. 31-2). | Placing the diaphragm at the PMI allows for maximal sound to be heard. The PMI is usually at the apex of the heart, and the change in location reflects the rotation of the heart as the child grows and matures. |
| c. If using a doppler, apply gel to the pulse point, then place the bell over the pulse point. Turn on the machine. | Proper placement maximizes sound transmission and accurate calculation. The gel enhances transmission of ultrasound waves that do not transmit well through air. |
| 5. When second hand of watch is on a number, begin to count pulse for 1 full minute. | The pulse should be counted for 1 full minute in children for accuracy since rate irregularities are common and may be missed if using a 10- or 15-second multiplication rate. |
| 6. Identify rhythm and character. Pulse character includes volume, which is described from 0 to 4: 0-absent, 1-thready or weak, 2-obliterated with pressure, 3-normal, and 4-bounding (Table 31-2). | Certain disease conditions affect cardiac output, reflected by changes in pulse rhythm and character.<br>***Special Considerations:*** *Physiologic sinus arrhythmia, an increase of pulse rate with inspiration and a decrease with expiration, is common in many children (Whaley and Wong, 1991).* |
| 7. When finished with measurement, assist child to return to comfortable position and previous activity. | This promotes a sense of well-being and comfort. |
| 8. Praise cooperation. | Praise for cooperative behavior enhances self-esteem. |

***TABLE 31-2*** **Various Patterns of Heart Rate or Pulse**

| Term | Description |
|---|---|
| Tachycardia | Increased rate |
| Bradycardia | Decreased rate |
| Pulsus alternans | Strong beat followed by weak beat |
| Pulsus bigeminus | Coupled rhythm in which beat is felt in pairs because of premature beat |
| Pulsus paradoxus | Intensity or force of pulse decreases with inspiration |
| Sinus arrhythmia | Rate increases with inspiration, decreases with expiration |
| Water-hammer or Corrigan pulse | Especially forceful beat caused by a very wide pulse pressure (systolic blood pressure minus diastolic blood pressure) |
| Dicrotic pulse | Double radial pulse for every apical beat |
| Thready pulse | Rapid, weak pulse that seems to appear and disappear |

From Whaley LF and Wong DL: Nursing care of infants and children, ed 4, St Louis, 1991, The CV Mosby Co.

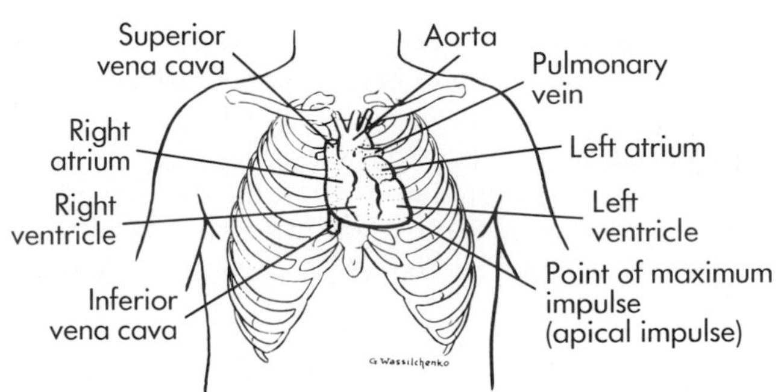


***FIG. 31-2*** Diaphragm of stethoscope is placed over point of maximum impulse (PMI).

From Wong D and Whaley L: Clinical manual of pediatric nursing, ed 3, St Louis, 1990, The CV Mosby Co.

| Steps | Rationale |
|---|---|
| **Evaluation Outcomes** | **Observational Guidelines** |
| 1. An accurate pulse measurement is obtained. | Note pulse rate obtained. Note existence of factors that may have influenced rate. Correlate with clinical appearance. |
| 2. Abnormalities of rate, rhythm, or character are identified. | Compare rate to normals for age, sex, and influencing factors with baseline rate, if available. Review observations of rhythm and character; compare to previous assessments, if available. |

### Documentation

Immediately record time, site, rate, rhythm, and character of pulse, as well as child's behavior, emotional state, and influencing factors immediately before and during procedure. Include any verbalizations or influencing stimuli assessed during pulse measurement.

### Child/Family Teaching

1. Demonstrate pulse measurement for parents or caregivers.
   a. For emergency situations, demonstrate use of femoral or carotid site.
   b. For digoxin administration, demonstrate apical pulse measurement.
2. Discuss features, prices, and source of stethoscopes, if needed.
3. Discuss use and care of stethoscope, include placement on chest, where to store when not in use, checking for cracks in earpieces, tubing, or diaphragm, and cleaning.

# *SKILL* 32 Measuring Respirations

*Nancy Valentine Stevens*

Respiration, one of the basic body functions, is the gaseous exchange of oxygen and carbon dioxide between the child's lungs and the environment. An adequate supply of oxygen is essential for life and maintenance of vital body organs.

Measuring respiratory effort involves assessing chest and abdominal movement and breath sounds, including rate, depth, symmetry, and pattern. (For in-depth assessment of respiratory system, see Skill 27.)

Assessment of respirations is a routine part of pediatric examination because the respiratory tract is a common site of infections in children. The respiratory system is involved in many chronic disorders, e.g., asthma, bronchopulmonary dysplasia, and cystic fibrosis. Nutritional deficits also frequently manifest as respiratory behaviors.

## NURSING DIAGNOSES

Health-seeking behaviors (respiration measurements) related to prevention of respiratory disorders; Ineffective breathing pattern related to pain, anxiety, decreased energy, or inflammatory process; Ineffective airway clearance related to tracheobronchial infection, obstruction, or secretions.

| Steps | Rationale |
|---|---|
| **Assessment** | |
| 1. Determine need for respiratory assessment. | Respiratory assessment is a basic technique performed in all child health settings. Respiratory alterations are often the earliest signs of underlying infections and illnesses in the child, especially upper respiratory infections. |
| 2. Assess for behaviors reflective of respiratory alteration, e.g., restlessness, apprehension, fear, pallor, cyanosis, nasal flaring, weak cry, and retractions. | Physical and emotional behaviors may indicate respiratory changes in the child prior to actual manifestation of the disease/infectious process. ***Special Considerations:*** *Correlate behaviors, e.g., color, cry, or restlessness with respiratory rate.* |
| 3. Assess for factors influencing respiratory functioning, e.g., age, exercise, body temperature, emotional and physical state, posture, medications, infection, prematurity, diet, and environmental conditions, including extremes in weather and barometric pressure. | Respiratory functioning is affected by various physical and environmental factors that cause changes in rate and characteristics. Respiratory rate decreases with age, sleep, and certain drugs, e.g., narcotics and anesthetics. Respiratory rates increase with fever, exercise, and anxiety or fear. |
| 4. Assess relevant laboratory data and monitor readings reflecting oxygenation: | |
| a. Complete blood count (CBC). | CBC measurements include concentration of hemoglobin and number and volume of red blood cells, all reflective of the body's capacity to carry oxygen. |
| b. Blood gases—capillary and arterial. | Blood gases reflect oxygenation status by measuring blood pH, oxygen saturation, and partial pressure of oxygen and carbon dioxide. |
| c. Pulse oximetry (see Skill 91). | Oximetry measures the arterial hemoglobin oxygen saturation percentage. This percentage correlates approximately with arterial $PO_2$ values on an oxyhemoglobin dissociation curve. |
| 5. Review previous measurement of respiratory status for baseline, if available. | Establishment of a baseline aids in identifying any changes of status. |
| **Planning and Goal Setting** | |
| 1. Gather all needed equipment.<br>a. Wristwatch with second hand.<br>b. Pen and paper. | Ready availability of supplies facilitates efficient interventions. |
| 2. Select time to assess respirations when child is calm. If child has been active or emotionally upset, wait 5 to 10 minutes, if possible. Assess respirations before invasive or painful procedures. | Activity or emotional disruptions may cause invalid respiratory assessment by yielding false highs, lows, or irregular patterns. |
| 3. Select a position of comfort and safety appropriate for child, e.g., in the parent's arms or on their lap. | Positioning ensures child's safety and comfort during procedure. Closeness to a parent may minimize anxiety, which may cause an increase in respiratory rate. |
| 4. Plan diversional activities to use during procedure, e.g., using a finger puppet to explain the procedure. | Diversional activities facilitate child's cooperation, lessen anxiety, and decrease self-consciousness that may alter normal pattern. |
| 5. Assess respirations as first vital sign in infant or child. | Respirations are best done when child is as quiet as possible and before procedures that may increase anxiety and cause changes in respirations. |
| 6. Develop individualized nursing goals of care:<br>▪ Obtain an accurate measurement of respiratory rate, rhythm, and depth.<br>▪ Identify abnormal respiratory patterns.<br>▪ Detect changes in respirations from the baseline and correlate with influencing physical and environmental factors. | |
| **Implementation** | |
| 1. Explain procedure to child and family. | Understanding the process enhances cooperation. ***Special Considerations:*** *This step may be delayed to observe and count respirations without the child being aware of procedure to minimize unnatural respiratory pattern.* |
| 2. Allow child to touch and play with stethoscope, if desired. The child may like to try to count or listen to own or parents' respirations or practice on a doll or stuffed toy. | Involving the child with equipment dispels fear and encourages involvement in the procedure. Including parents or favorite toys can also lessen fears. |

| Steps | Rationale |
|---|---|
| 3. Position child as planned with chest visible to facilitate observation of respiratory efforts. | Proper positioning facilitates cooperation and safety. |
| 4. Observe and listen to a complete respiratory cycle of one inspiration and one expiration. | Observing one cycle allows the assessment to begin with the inspiratory phase. ***Special Considerations:*** *Children under 7 years of age are primarily diaphragmatic breathers, so observe the rise and fall of the abdomen versus chest movements in older children. When assessing respirations in infants and young children, it may be helpful to place fingers below the xiphoid to feel inspiratory rises (Engel, 1989).* |
| 5. Focus on second hand on watch and begin to count respiratory rate when second hand is on an easily remembered number. | It is easier to keep track of time if counting begins on a number instead of a mark on the watch. |
| 6. Count respirations for 1 full minute (Table 32-1). | Since children's respirations are quite irregular, 1 full minute allows variations in respirations to be counted and not estimated. |
| 7. Observe pattern (regular, irregular, or periodic) (Table 32-2); depth (shallow, normal, or deep); quality (labored, effortless, difficult); and symmetry of chest wall movement (bilaterally symmetrical and coordinated with breathing) (for more detailed information on respiratory assessment, see Skill 27). | Observation of all facets of respiratory effort allows for more complete assessment than only counting the rate. |

***TABLE 32-1*** **Average Respiratory Rates at Rest (Breaths/Minute)**

| Age | Rate (breaths/minute) |
|---|---|
| Newborn | 35 |
| 1-11 months | 30 |
| 2 years | 25 |
| 4 years | 23 |
| 6 years | 21 |
| 8 years | 20 |
| 10 years | 19 |
| 12 years | 19 |
| 14 years | 18 |
| 16 years | 17 |
| 18 years | 16-18 |

From Whaley LF and Wong DL: Nursing care of infants and children, ed 4, St Louis, 1991, The CV Mosby Co.

***TABLE 32-2*** **Various Patterns of Respiration**

| Term | Description |
|---|---|
| Tachypnea | Increased rate |
| Bradypnea | Decreased rate |
| Dyspnea | Distress during breathing |
| Apnea | Cessation of breathing |
| Hyperpnea | Increased depth |
| Hypoventilation | Decreased depth (shallow) and irregular rhythm |
| Hyperventilation | Increased rate and depth |
| Kussmaul breathing | Hyperventilation, gasping and labored respiration, usually seen in diabetic coma or other states or respiratory acidosis |
| Cheyne-Stokes respirations | Gradually increasing rate and depth with periods of apnea |
| Biot breathing | Periods of hyperpnea alternating with apnea (similar to Cheyne-Stokes except that the depth remains constant) |
| Seesaw (paradoxic) respirations | Chest falls on inspiration and rises on expiration |

From Whaley LF and Wong DL: Nursing care of infants and children, ed 4, St Louis, 1991, The CV Mosby Co.

| Steps | Rationale |
|---|---|
| 8. Finish other vital signs, if needed. | Usually vital signs are measured at the same time to observe relationship between them and for efficiency. |
| 9. Assist child to redress, if necessary, and return to previous activity. | Facilitates comfort and enhances self-esteem. |
| 10. Praise child for cooperation. | Positive reinforcement enhances nurse/child interactions for the present and the future. |

| Evaluation Outcomes | Observational Guidelines |
|---|---|
| 1. An accurate rate of respirations is obtained. | Note rate of respirations and compare to baseline and norms for age. |
| 2. Abnormalities of respiratory quality, depth, pattern, symmetry, and effort are identified. | Note observations of respiratory characteristics. Compare to baseline, if available. |
| 3. Changes from the baseline are identified and correlated with influencing factors. | Compare present findings with baseline data, correlating with clinical observations and environmental factors. |

| Steps | Rationale |
|---|---|

### Documentation

Record time, rate, depth, rhythm, quality, symmetry, and effort on appropriate record.

Record respiratory alterations in appropriate record. Report abnormal findings to physician.

# SKILL 33 Measuring Blood Pressure by Indirect Methods

*Nancy Valentine Stevens*

Blood pressure (BP) is the measurement of the force exerted in the large arteries at the height of the pulse wave. As left ventricular resistance increases with age and growth in size, BP values rise correspondingly, reaching adult values around puberty. Indirect BP measurement is obtained in clinics and most hospital settings by noninvasive methods such as auscultation, palpation, and oscillometry. Less commonly used noninvasive methods are ultrasonography and flush technique. Direct BP measurement is obtained with invasive methods such as arterial catheters and is used primarily in emergency and intensive care settings. This skill will address only noninvasive measurement.

Assessing BP in children facilitates early detection of potentially serious disorders, e.g., hypertension with no identifiable cause and hypertension secondary to renal problems, congenital heart disorders (particularly coarctation of the aorta), and certain metabolic disorders. There is evidence that essential hypertension in adults may begin in childhood (Report of the Second Task Force, 1987). Parameters for classification of elevated BP are (Report of the Second Task Force, 1987):

- Normal BP—systolic and diastolic pressure below the 90th percentile for age and sex.
- Normal high BP—average systolic and/or average diastolic BP between 90th and 95th percentile for age and sex.
- High BP—average systolic and/or average diastolic BP at or greater than the 95th percentile for age and sex with measurements obtained on at least three occasions.
- Significant hypertension—persistent measurements between the 95th and 99th percentile for age and sex.
- Severe hypertension—persistent measurements at or above the 99th percentile for age and sex.

Conversely, the detection of hypotension commonly associated with circulatory shock is actually a late sign. As cardiac output decreases, the body compensates by increasing peripheral vascular resistance, thereby maintaining fairly normal blood pressure. Hypotension does not occur until this compensation mechanism fails, usually suddenly, with cardiopulmonary arrest likely to follow (Chameides, 1988).

## NURSING DIAGNOSES

Health-seeking behaviors (blood pressure measurements) related to prevention of cardiovascular, renal, or metabolic disorders; Altered tissue perfusion related to interruption of arterial/venous blood flow.

| Steps | Rationale |
|---|---|

### Assessment

1. Determine need for blood pressure measurement—measure routinely for well and sick child clinic visits on children over 3 years of age and according to facility policy or clinical status on hospitalized child.

BP determination is indicated in the management of acutely ill children, in detecting secondary hypertension that may be amenable to cure, and in early detection of essential hypertension (Park and Guntheroth, 1989).

***Special Considerations:*** *Many authorities believe BP readings should be obtained routinely from birth. Children with previously elevated readings or cardiovascular, genitourinary, and neurologic problems should have routine blood pressure checks regardless of age.*

| Steps | Rationale |
|---|---|
| 2. Assess for patient variables that may influence true BP (not the obtained reading), e.g., age, size of child, medications, recent exercise, and presence of pain (Table 33-1 and Fig. 33-1; see inside book cover for normal blood pressure readings). | Physical, emotional, and environmental factors can increase or decrease BP, especially the systolic reading. For example, larger children have higher blood pressures than smaller children of the same age. (Report of the Second Task Force, 1987). |
| 3. Assess potential sites for blood pressure measurement considering age, development, and possible contraindications to the use of a particular extremity (Fig. 33-1). | Consideration of site selection based on contraindications and other factors enhances accurate readings and prevents injury or pain. |
| a. Preferred site:<br>▪ Upper arm (brachial artery).<br>Other acceptable sites include:<br>▪ Lower arm (radial artery).<br>▪ Thigh (popliteal artery).<br>▪ Lower leg (dorsalis pedis or posterior tibial). | BP normative studies are based on brachial artery determinations, therefore use of that site allows accurate comparison. Measurements vary by site because of the physiologic concept of systolic pressure amplification. Systolic pressure is lowest in the ascending aorta (central aortic pressure) and tends to increase peripherally from the heart. The systolic pressure in the brachial artery is about 10 mm Hg higher than the central aorta; the radial may be slightly higher; the femoral is about the same as the radial; the pedal artery averages 20 mm Hg higher. The diastolic pressures remain equal. This systolic amplification usually does not appear until after 1 year of age. Before that time, thigh and arm systolic pressure are equal (Park and Guntheroth, 1989).<br>***Special Considerations:*** *BP measurements in the leg that are lower than those in the arm are diagnostic of coarctation of the aorta, since these findings are the opposite of the expected findings based on systolic pressure amplification. With electronic devices, the thigh site is reserved as a last choice since it is the most uncomfortable (Wong and Whaley, 1990).* |
| b. Contraindications include:<br>▪ Injury.<br>▪ Surgical incision.<br>▪ Intravenous cutdown site.<br>▪ Central venous or arterial line.<br>▪ Poor perfusion.<br>▪ Antecubital tenderness from venipunctures. | The pressure from the inflated cuff could cause pain or injury in these situations. Also, pain and poor perfusion will alter the obtained reading.<br>***Special Considerations:*** *A peripheral IV infusion is not a contraindication to BP measurement proximal to the site. BP measurement in the left arm is contraindicated following coarcectomy, because vessel repair may affect arterial circulation to that arm.* |
| 4. Assess for appropriate cuff size (cuff refers to the inner inflatable bladder, not the cloth or plastic covering). For cuff width and length, two recommended methods of measurement exist:<br>a. Report of the Second Task Force (1987)—cuff width approximately 75% of the length of the extremity, between the top of the shoulder and the olecranon. The cuff width should allow sufficient room to avoid impinging on the axilla, and to place the bell of the stethoscope at the antecubital space. The cuff length should be sufficient to completely encircle the arm, overlapping if necessary.<br>b. American Heart Association (Frolich et al, 1988)—cuff width 40% to 50% of limb circumference measuring midway between the top of the shoulder and the olecranon. The cuff length should be sufficient to completely or nearly completely encircle the limb without overlapping. | All methods of BP measurement use an occluding cuff. The child's size (rather than age) should determine cuff selection. The proper width and length of cuff ensures the proper pressure on the arterial wall for accurate measurement. Pressure within the cuff is transmitted toward the artery in a wedge shape (Fig. 33-2) and if the cuff is correctly sized, the pressure exerted on the arterial wall will be equal to the amount of pressure registered on the manometer (Park and Guntheroth, 1989). If a cuff is too small, it tends to produce false high readings because the artery is never completely occluded (Fig. 33-2*A*). A cuff that is too large may yield false low readings because it affects an excessive length of the artery (Fig. 33-2*B*).<br>***Special Considerations:*** *If a choice must be made between a too large or too small cuff, the larger cuff is suggested. Another option is to use a site that better accommodates the cuff size, e.g., a large cuff around the thigh or a small cuff placed above the wrist (Darnall, 1985). Using the Task Force method for selecting cuff width may produce satisfactory readings in children with average weight for height, but inaccurate readings in children with thick extremities; using limb circumference for selecting cuff width more accurately reflects arterial blood pressure readings than using length (Park and Guntheroth, 1989).* |
| 5. Determine previous measurement, if available. | Baseline measurement(s) facilitate interpretation of the obtained reading. |

**TABLE 33-1** Factors Influencing Blood Pressure in Children

| Higher BP Readings | Lower BP Readings |
|---|---|
| **PATIENT VARIATIONS** | |
| Age and size (older and larger) | Diurnal variations (evening/night) |
| Sex—male (rare) | Medications (narcotics, anesthetics, diuretics) |
| Diurnal variations (morning/afternoon) | Dehydration |
| Emotions—fear, anxiety, apprehension | Severe anemia |
| Activity (exercise) | Coarctation (legs < arms) |
| Distended urinary bladder | Hemorrhagic shock (late sign) |
| Stress | |
| Medications—vasoconstrictors (e.g., nose drops) and corticosteroids | |
| Smoking (temporary vasoconstriction) | |
| Immobility (especially orthopedic traction) | |
| Fever | |
| Acute pain | |
| Coarctation of aorta (arms > legs) | |
| Renal disease | |
| Increased intracranial pressure | |
| Weather extremes, especially with increases in barometric pressure | |
| **TECHNIQUE VARIATIONS** | |
| Cuff size—too small | Cuff size—too large |
| Rapid cuff deflation | Upper extremity site |
| Bladder not centered over artery | Palpation method |
| Cuff applied too loosely | Auscultation method |
| Unsupported arm | |
| Lower extremity site | |
| Oscillometry method | |
| Doppler method | |

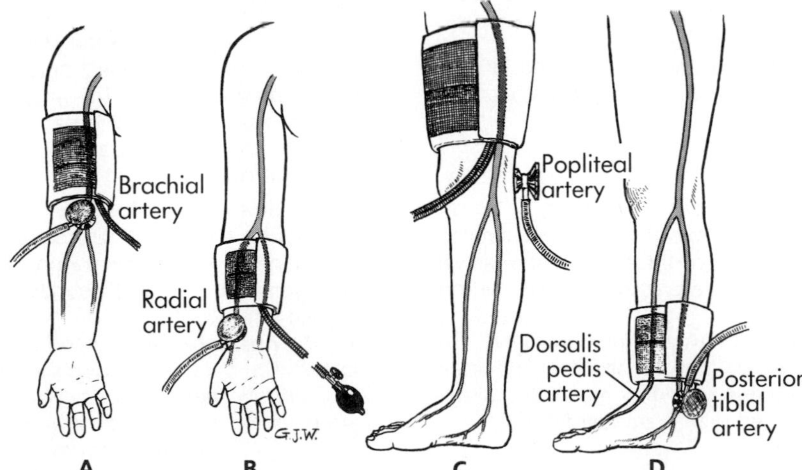


***FIG. 33-1*** Sites for measuring blood pressure. **A,** Upper arm. **B,** Lower arm or forearm. **C**, Thigh. **D,** Calf or ankle.

From Wong D and Whaley L: Clinical manual of pediatric nursing, ed 3, St Louis 1990, The CV Mosby Co.

**Steps** | **Rationale**

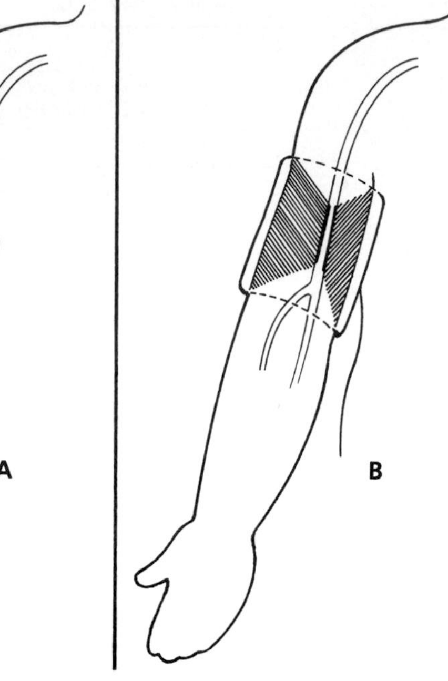


***FIG. 33-2*** Effects of cuff size on blood pressure measement. **A,** A cuff that is too small may yield false high readings. **B,** An excessively large cuff produces false low readings.

## Planning and Goal Setting

1. Determine the method for blood pressure reading, considering assessment data and availability of equipment.

Selecting the appropriate method will enhance accurate readings.

   a. Auscultatory.
   Inflating a cuff and listening with a stethoscope for characteristic systolic and diastolic pressure sounds (Korotkoff) correlated to the manometer readings as the cuff deflates.

The most traditional method of BP measurement uses auscultatory sound waves created by the arterial pulse as counterpressure from the cuff is decreased.

***Special Considerations:*** *Korotkoff sounds are faint in infants/small children and those in circulatory shock. Environmental noises may also make them difficult to hear (Park and Guntheroth, 1989).*

   b. Palpation method.
   Palpating for pulse return distal to a deflating BP cuff, correlated to manometer reading. Only a systolic pressure is determined.

This method is especially useful with infants when unable to hear Korotkoff sounds and electronic devices are not available.

***Special Considerations:*** *The systolic measurement obtained by palpation is consistently lower than other methods (Park and Guntheroth, 1989). Pulsations will be difficult to detect if the child is in circulatory shock.*

   c. Electronic devices.
   - Oscillometry (Dinamap)—Pressure changes create oscillations that are transmitted through the arterial wall and detected by a sensitive pressure indicator in the cuff (Table 33-2).
   - Doppler ultrasound—Changes in ultrasound frequency caused by blood movement within the artery are translated to audible sound by means of a transducer. It is usually used with a standard cuff.

Electronic devices are generally reliable and easy to use, especially with young children. These devices are particularly useful to determine BP during circulatory shock, when brachial artery pulsations and Korotkoff sounds may be diminished or absent (Frolich et al, 1988).

***Special Considerations:*** *Blood pressure readings using oscillometry or doppler are usually higher than those taken by auscultatory methods, but correlate better with direct radial artery blood pressure than auscultation readings (Park and Menard, 1987). Electronic devices are much more costly than sphygmomanometer methods. Other disadvantages of the ultrasound method include: diastolic pressure not discerned; unable to measure continuously; and transducers are easily broken. The other disadvantage of oscillometry is the need for the child to be still to avoid erroneous readings (Darnall, 1985). Electronic devices have largely replaced the "flush" method that involved wrapping the hand or foot to blanch it and observing for the return of color (flush) to obtain an approximate mean BP. The flush method is less reliable than other methods, because it depends on the quality of peripheral perfusion and the skill of the nurse, and is also uncomfortable for the child.*

**Steps** | **Rationale**

***TABLE 33-2*** Normative Dinamap (Oscillometry) BP Values (Systolic/Diastolic, Mean in Parentheses)

| Age Group | Mean | 90th Percentile | 95th Percentile |
|---|---|---|---|
| Newborn (1-3 days) | 65/41(50) | 75/49(59) | 78/52(62) |
| 1 month to 2 years | 95/58(72) | 106/68(83) | 110/71(86) |
| 2-5 years | 101/57(74) | 112/66(82) | 115/68(85) |

From Park M and Menard S: Normative oscillometric blood pressure values in the first five years in the office setting, Arch Dis Child 143(7): 860-864, 1989.

***TABLE 33-3*** Recommended Bladder Dimensions for Blood Pressure Cuffs

| Arm Circumference at Midpoint (cm) | Cuff Name* | Bladder Width (cm) | Bladder Length (cm) |
|---|---|---|---|
| 5-7.5 | Newborn | 3 | 5 |
| 7.5-13 | Infant | 5 | 8 |
| 13-20 | Child | 8 | 13 |
| 24-32 | Adult | 13 | 24 |
| 32-42 | Wide adult | 17 | 32 |
| 42-50 | Thigh | 20 | 42 |

From Frohlich ED et al: Recommendations for human blood pressure determination by sphygmomanometers: report of a special task force appointed by the Steering Committee, American Heart Association, Circulation 77:501A, 1988.

*Cuff name does not guarantee that the cuff will be appropriate size for a child within that age range.

2. Gather needed equipment:
   a. Appropriate size BP cuff (see Assessment, step 4; Table 33-3).
   b. Sphygmomanometer.
   c. Stethoscope.
   d. Pen and paper.
   e. Optional electronic devices.

Ready availability of supplies facilitates efficient interventions.

***Special Considerations:*** *Sphygmomanometers are either mercury-gravity (with a mercury reservoir) or aneroid (with an internal metal bellows). The metal parts of the aneroid type are subject to temperature expansion and contraction and require calibration if the needle does not point to zero, so the aneroid type may be less reliable (Perry and Potter, 1990).*

3. Plan to measure BP before other stressful procedures or wait 15 to 20 minutes for the child to calm.

Stress and anxiety can cause falsely elevated BP measurements.

4. Plan appropriate diversional activities, e.g., musical mobile or book.

Appropriate diversional activities enhance cooperation and decrease anxiety, thus increasing accuracy in BP measurement.

5. Develop individualized nursing goals of nursing care:
   - Obtain an accurate BP measurement.
   - Detect changes in present BP measurements from previous readings.
   - Prevent pain or injury from BP measurement.

## Implementation

1. Explain procedure to child and family. Use phrases such as "Fill up a balloon around your arm," "Watch the silver rise," or "See how strong your muscles are."

Understanding the process enhances cooperation.

2. Allow the child to touch and play with the equipment, if desired, or practice on a toy or doll.

Familiarity and involvement with the equipment dispels fears and may encourage participation during the procedure.

3. Remove clothing surrounding the selected site. Assist the child to the appropriate position of comfort or allow the parent to hold the child securely, maintaining access to the selected extremity. A sitting position is usually easiest for use of the arms in a child, whereas a supine position facilitates access in infants or for the use of the lower extremities.

Clothing will interfere with the accurate transmission of pressure and auscultation of sounds. Proper positioning facilitates accuracy, cooperation, and safety.

***Special Considerations:*** *If using a wall-mounted or table sphygmomanometer, position the child so that visibility of the gauge or mercury column is clear and at eye level.*

4. Extend the extremity and place it securely on a flat surface that maintains it level with the heart. For the infant, securely hold the arm.

Extension allows easier and better exposure to needed site. Providing support is more comfortable and less stressful for the child. Placement of the arm above the level of the heart may cause a false low reading, and positioning below heart level may add gravity pressure, resulting in a falsely high reading (Britton, 1981).

5. Center the cuff over the brachial (or other) artery. Wrap the appropriate cuff smoothly and securely around the extremity, allowing a single fingertip to slide under the edge.

If the cuff is not centered over the artery, the reading may be falsely elevated (Frolich et al, 1988). A smooth, securely wrapped cuff facilitates accuracy and comfort during the procedure. Too tight of a cuff can cause venous congestion and discomfort, whereas a cuff that is too loose can produce a falsely elevated BP measurement (Ramsey, 1980).

***Special Considerations:*** *The center of the cuff can be found by folding it in half lengthwise. The covering marking for artery placement may not be accurate (Frolich et al, 1988).*

| Steps | Rationale |
|---|---|
| ***Auscultatory method*** | |
| a. Palpate the selected pulse immediately distal to the cuff. | Locating the artery determines proper placement of the stethoscope bell, to enhance maximum sound retrieval. |
| b. Place the stethoscope bell using light pressure over the skin at the pulse site. | The stethoscope bell is recommended instead of the diaphragm to allow better detection of the low frequency sounds generated by the blood vessels (Frolich et al, 1988). Heavy pressure on the stethoscope bell over the brachial artery may generate misleading Korotkoff-like sounds (Frolich et al, 1988) |
| c. Close the control valve with dominant hand and repeatedly compress the bulb to inflate cuff quickly to approximately 20 mm Hg above point at which pulse disappears. | Complete closure of the valve allows inflation to the proper level. Excessive pressure may cause discomfort.<br>***Special Considerations:*** *If tapping sounds are heard, continue to inflate cuff until no sounds are heard.* |
| d. Open control valve slowly to release the pressure at the rate of 2 to 3 mm Hg/second. | The cuff is released slowly to allow proper detection of sounds. If pressure is released too fast, sounds may be missed or distorted and an inaccurate low reading obtained. If pressure is released too slowly, venous distension can occur, attenuating Korotkoff sounds, resulting in a falsely elevated diastolic reading (Ramsey, 1980). |
| e. Listen for Korotkoff sounds.<br>▪ Systolic: sharp, clear tapping sound—onset is first Korotkoff sound (K1).<br>▪ Diastolic for infant or child up to age 12 years: muffling of sound—fourth Korotkoff sound (K4).<br>▪ Diastolic for adolescent 13-18 years: tapping sound disappears—fifth Korotkoff sound (K5). | These are the sounds heard over the artery as the pressure from the cuff is lowered. Using the correct diastolic reading for the child's age (K4 or K5) ensures accuracy when comparing to normal BP standards (Report of the Second Task Force, 1987).<br>***Special Considerations:*** *Standard practice for adult diastolic is the measurement of the fifth Korotkoff sound (disappearance of sound), while pediatric practice has favored the 4th sound, or muffling. Record both to provide consistency, e.g., 120/70-40 (Park and Guntheroth, 1989).* |
| ***Palpation and doppler methods*** | |
| a. Using one or two fingertips, palpate pulse immediately distal to the cuff. For the doppler method, apply conducting gel at the pulse site, and place the transducer over the gel. Relocate the pulse by listening for the flow signal, a "whooshing" sound. | Return of the pulse provides the systolic measurement for the palpation/doppler methods.<br>***Special Considerations:*** *Doppler devices are available with the transducer incorporated in the cuff, e.g., Arteriosonde. Follow manufacturer instructions for use.* |
| b. Maintaining fingertip/transducer placement, use the other hand to inflate quickly (as described in auscultation method) to approximately 20 mm Hg above point where pulse disappears. | Inflation of cuff above the pressure that occludes blood flow allows detection of pulsation when pressure is released. |
| c. Open control valve and slowly release pressure at the rate of 2 to 3 mm Hg/second. | Slow release of control valve allows blood flow to resume at normal pressure. |
| d. Note reading at which pulse return is detected by fingertips (palpation method) or sound (doppler method). | Detection of pulse return indicates systolic pressure.<br>***Special Considerations:*** *The systolic pressure is recorded as the reading over P for palpation, or over D for doppler, e.g., 90/P or 90/D.* |
| ***Oscillometry method*** | |
| a. Inflate cuff according to manufacturer's instructions. | ***Special Considerations:*** *The cuff must be completely deflated before placement for accurate readings.* |
| b. Gently stabilize the limb during automatic cuff deflation. | Movement or forcible restraint (causing isometric muscular contraction) interferes with the device's ability to measure blood pressure accurately (Ramsey, 1980). |
| c. Observe/record obtained readings on the display. | ***Special Considerations:*** *Oscillometric devices provide systolic and diastolic pressures and mean arterial pressure (MAP) based on characteristic changes in the magnitude of oscillation; heart rate is also measured (Table 33-2).* |
| 6. Release all pressure and remove cuff. | Release of pressure prevents venous congestion and allows removal of cuff. |
| 7. Return equipment to usual storage area. | Proper storage decreases chances of breakage or misplacement of equipment. |
| 8. Assist child to return to comfortable position and to resume activities. | Assistance measures restore dignity and comfort. |
| 9. Compare obtained reading to norms (see inside book cover) and baseline measurements, considering technique and patient. | Consideration of all influencing factors facilitates determination of the accuracy of the measurement. |

| **Steps** | **Rationale** |
|---|---|

***TABLE 33-4*** Classification of Hypertension in the Young by Age Group

| Age | ≥95th Percentile (mm Hg) | ≥99th Percentile (mm Hg) |
|---|---|---|
| Newborns | | |
| 7 days | SBP ≥ 96 | SBP ≥ 106 |
| 8-30 days | SBP ≥ 104 | SBP ≥ 110 |
| Infants | SBP ≥ 112 | SBP ≥ 118 |
| (≤2 years) | DBP ≥ 74 | DBP ≥ 82 |
| Children | SBP ≥ 116 | SBP ≥ 124 |
| (3-5 years) | DBP ≥ 76 | DBP ≥ 84 |
| Children | SBP ≥ 122 | SBP ≥ 130 |
| (6-9 years) | DBP ≥ 78 | DBP ≥ 86 |
| Children | SBP ≥ 126 | SBP ≥ 134 |
| (10-12 years) | DBP ≥ 82 | DBP ≥ 90 |
| Children | SBP ≥ 136 | SBP ≥ 144 |
| (13-15 years) | DBP ≥ 86 | DBP ≥ 92 |
| Adolescents | SBP ≥ 142 | SBP ≥ 150 |
| (16-18 years) | DBP ≥ 92 | DBP ≥ 98 |

From Report of the Second Task Force on Blood Pressure Control in Children, Pediatrics, 75:1-25, 1987.

| **Steps** | **Rationale** |
|---|---|
| 10. If elevated readings are obtained during well child visit, repeat measurement later during visit when child may be less anxious. Also document need in child's record to repeat measurements at least three times during subsequent visits (Wong and Whaley, 1990). | Hypertension should not be diagnosed on the basis of a single measurement. Repeated measurements are needed to determine the stability or lability of BP elevation (Report of the Second Task Force, 1987).<br>***Special Considerations:*** *See Table 33-4 for classification of hypertension.* |
| 11. Report significant deviations or differences between upper and lower extremity readings to physician. | Documented hypertension should be evaluated medically. The higher the blood pressure and the younger the child, the greater the possibility of hypertension secondary to another disorder (Report of the Second Task Force, 1987). Hypotension, even mild, in a clinically unstable child can signal cardiovascular decompensation and must be treated promptly (Chamcides, 1988). Significant differences in readings between upper and lower extremities, e.g., a calf pressure in newborns less than 6 to 9 mm Hg of upper arm pressure, could indicate coarctation of the aorta (Park and Lee, 1989). |

| **Evaluation Outcomes** | **Observational Guidelines** |
|---|---|
| 1. Accurate blood pressure measurement is obtained. | Note blood pressure obtained using correctly sized cuff. Note factors that may have influenced measurement. Compare serial measurements. |
| 2. A significant deviation from baseline or norms is identified. | Compare BP with norms for age, sex, race, and other influencing factors with previous readings, if available. |
| 3. Injury or pain from BP measurement is prevented. | Note venous congestion, adequacy of pulse, color of extremity, patency of IV, comfort level of child, and avoidance of contraindicated sites. |

## Documentation

Record date, time, blood pressure reading, extremity(ies) used for measurement, child's position, method used, cuff size, child's behaviors, and any pertinent verbalizations or stimuli during the procedure.

# SKILL 34 Audiometric Screening

*Rosemary Liguori*

It is estimated that 12% to 20% of children in our society have a hearing impairment. Children with a hearing impairment are at risk for school problems, learning disabilities, and behavior problems. Screening is essential for early identification, referral, and treatment. The cost of screening is far less than the cost of long-term remediation, therapy, loss of self-worth and self-esteem. Most deafness in adulthood could have been avoided if hearing impairment had been detected and treated early in childhood. Hearing assessment and audiometric screenings are easy to implement. Audiometric tests measure the acuity of hearing for the various frequencies of sound waves (see box for definitions). There are several screening tests that nurses may administer using an audiometer. The Air Conduction Sweep Check Test is a pure tone test performed at a fixed level of 25 decibels (dB) with different frequencies. A more sensitive variation is the Threshold Acuity Test (see box), which measures hearing thresholds at each frequency with decibel adjustments. Another test, Play Audiometry, is used for the child younger than 30 months and for the hard to test child (see box on p. 219 for this and other measures for use with young or hard to test children).

## NURSING DIAGNOSES

Sensory perceptual alteration (auditory) related to disease, trauma, congenital defect, or medication; Impaired verbal communication related to auditory impairment; Impaired social interactions related to hearing deficit and language barrier; Ineffective individual coping related to auditory impairment.

| Steps | Rationale |
|---|---|
| **Assessment** | |
| 1. Determine the child's age and cognitive ability. | These factors will influence the child's ability to understand the instructions of the various tests and therefore may determine which test to use. |
| 2. Review child's history and interview parent for factors that may influence hearing. | The child's history will indicate risk factors for hearing loss. |
| a. Antepartal history: maternal infections during pregnancy, e.g., rubella, chicken pox, rubeola, or syphilis; maternal drug use, e.g., alcohol use, ototoxic drugs (streptomycin), salicylates, and quinine. | ***Special Considerations:*** *Sensorineural hearing loss is caused by disease, drugs, or an inner ear defect that affects the cochlear hair cells or the cochlear lymph system and the acoustic nerve and is nearly irreversible. These insults to the ear may occur during gestation, especially in the first trimester when the ear is developing (Bower, 1980).* |
| b. Neonatal history: prematurity; low birth weight; congenital rubella; hypoxia; neonatal infection, e.g., septicemia; ear, nose, and throat or physical abnormalities; ventilator care; hyperbilirubinemia and exposure to sounds associated with incubator and intensive care units. | These conditions typically place the child at risk for hearing deficits from insult to the ear (DiChiara, 1985). Premature infants are often exposed to excessive dB levels and are at risk for hearing loss (Whaley and Wong, 1991). |
| c. History of acute or serous otitis media; frequent upper respiratory infections or excessive cerumen. | Cerumen, foreign bodies in ear canal, and serous otitis media are common causes of hearing loss in 5- to 9-year-old children (DiChiara, 1984). The loss is a conductive one and often may be corrected by surgery or medical treatment (Bower, 1980). |
| d. Use by the child of an ototoxic medication, e.g., neomycin or streptomycin. | These drugs can cause sensorineural hearing loss (Bower, 1980). |
| e. Exposure to excessive repeated loud noises, underwater swimming, or participation on a diving team. | These activities reduce the number of sensory hairs lining the organ of Corti, which is the direct pathway to cranial nerve VIII (Grimes and Iannopollo, 1982; DiChiara, 1984). |
| f. Family history of hearing problems. | Several hearing disorders have a genetic component, e.g., Streacher-Collins Klippel-Feil syndrome, Waardenburg syndrome, and chromosomal abnormalities (D & F trisomies) (Robinson, 1986). |
| 3. Observe the child's behavior for the following:<br>a. Head tilting or turning when listening.<br>b. Poor attention span.<br>c. Inability to follow spoken directions. | Head tilting or turning toward sound is a compensatory mechanism to enable the sound to be "caught" by the ear. Children with a mild-to-moderate hearing loss often exhibit these subtle behaviors, which may go unrecognized because they respond to sound in general. They may be "labeled" slow, lazy, a daydreamer, or a discipline problem (Whaley and Wong, 1991). |

## TERMINOLOGY

*Auditory testing*—Hearing can be screened by various methodologies: behaviors indicating hearing loss (no response to loud noises); not turning to sound; the Colorado testing; Crib-O-Gram; Infant Hearing Kit; Play Audiometry; Rinne and Weber and audiometric testing with machine, e.g., the Maico or Belltone.

*Audiometers*—Various electronic machines that produce pure tones of intensity (loudness) in headsets. Frequencies and intensity of sounds may be regulated. Examples of audiometers include Maico and Belltone.

Features include:

1. On/off button.
2. Output selector that directs sound to the right or left ears.
3. Threshold lever regulates loudness (dB) 0 to 100.
4. Frequency lever regulates frequency 250 to 8000 Hz, ½ to 1 octave increments.
5. Earphones: blue—left ear; red—right ear (the center of the phones are color coded).

*Decibel* (dB)—A unit to express the ratio of one sound (loudness) intensity to another.

*Frequency* (high or low sounds)—Normal range of speech is 300 to 3000, but the human ear may hear the range of 20 to 20,000 Hz.

*Hertz* (Hz)— A unit of frequency equal to one cycle per second. It is the number of times the objects vibrate, e.g., the middle string on the piano moves back and forth 256 times every second, therefore it is said to have 256 Hz (Bower, 1980).

## ADDITIONAL AUDITORY SCREENING TESTS

Some authorities believe that screening should begin in the newborn nursery. Early identification is essential to promote appropriate intervention for normal speech development.

*Colorado Testing:* Appropriate for infants from 6 months to 2½ years of age. The child faces the examiner. A sound is introduced to either side of the child through speakers. The frequencies tested are 500 to 3000 Hz. When the child looks to the sound, a bear lights up as a reward (Fig. 34-1) (see Product References and Teaching Resources).

*Crib-O-Gram:* This method may be used in the newborn nursery to identify hearing loss without interfering with the nursery care or requiring cooperation of the infant. A motion sensitive transducer is placed in the bassinet. During a 24-hour period, sound is introduced at preset intervals, with the transducers picking up and recording the movement, heart rate, respiratory rate, and motor activity of the baby. Activity before, during, and after the test is compared.

*Infant Hearing Kit:* This kit consists of various calibrated toys. The first testing is done at 2 weeks to 2 months. Have the baby sit on the mother's lap, ensuring that baby has freedom to move head. Kneeling at a 45-degree angle, attract the baby's attention to the front with a bright colored toy. Then squeeze a horn held 3 feet away on the child's right side (Fig. 34-2). The baby's eyes should widen, or the infant should startle or stop present activity. Repeat the test for the other ear. At 6 months, the infant's response is tested with high-, middle-, and low-pitched frequencies.

*Play Audiometry:* Is used to detect a hearing loss in a child younger than 30 months, a child with a developmental delay, or one who does not understand English. Play audiometry evaluates pure tone hearing. An audiometer, blocks, and a box are needed for the test.

Procedure:

1. Demonstrate for the child putting a block in the box (or a ring on a ring stacker) when the sound (at 6000 Hz and 50 dB) is heard on the headset. Repeat the demonstration several times.
2. Place headset on the child's head and introduce the sound at a loudness of 40 dB and a frequency of 1000 Hz (Fig. 34-3). Guide the child's hand holding the block to the box. Allow the child to place the block alone. Repeat this procedure several times.
3. If the child hears the sound, indicated by placing the block in the box, lower the loudness to 20 to 25 dB, introducing other frequencies: 500, 2000, 4000.
4. Test both ears.
5. If the child does not understand the testing, the parent may practice the response with child at home. Reschedule the test when a response pattern is established.

*Threshold Acuity Test:* Is another audiometric test usually done when the child fails the air conduction sweep test. It is more definitive in screening to determine the frequency and decibel levels of the child's hearing. It provides information as to severity of a hearing loss, and possible location of the defect (Whaley and Wong, 1991). The test must be performed in a soundproof room. The decibel levels are lowered to zero and all frequencies are tested.

*Tympanometry:* Assesses the mobility or compliance of the tympanic membrane in response to air pressure variations (Bower, 1980). Perforation of the membrane or serous otitis media will decrease mobility of the membrane. The testing may also follow the progress of acute otitis media and assesses the patency of ventilation tubes present in the tympanic membrane.

Compliance information provides possible causes of a hearing deficit, but does not assess the extent of a hearing loss. Tympanometry is quite reliable when combined with an otoscopic examination and pure tone audiometry testing. To cooperate, the child need only to remain still for a few seconds. Sucking on a pacifier or bottle can change the compliance of the membrane, so a bright colored object should be used to provide momentary distraction. A soft rubber cuff is placed in the external ear canal, causing an airtight seal. Reading of the air pressure is done by a hand-held probe (Fig. 34-4). The compliance of the tympanic membrane is recorded on a graph called a tympanogram.

*Verbal Auditory Screening for Children (VASC):* Is a speech reception-based screening audiometer. A series of 12 two-syllable words are introduced on a prerecorded tape. The child points to the corresponding object on the picture board. The words are presented in descending decibel increments, beginning at 51 dB down to 15 dB. Failure is based on inability to respond correctly to two to three 15 dB words (Hamill, 1988).

It is easy to administer, taking about 3 minutes. The disadvantage is that it does not pick up high-frequency losses outside the speech range. In a study by Hamill (1988), the VASC was superior to pure tone audiometry in detecting hearing deficits in a preschool-kindergarten screening program.

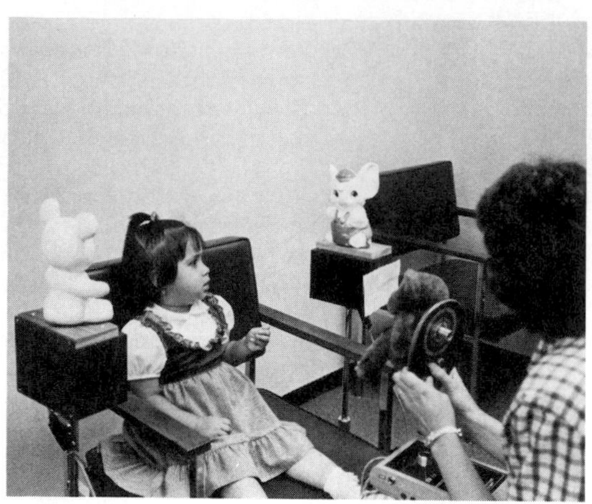

***FIG. 34-1*** Colorado Testing is used to conduct audiometric screening.

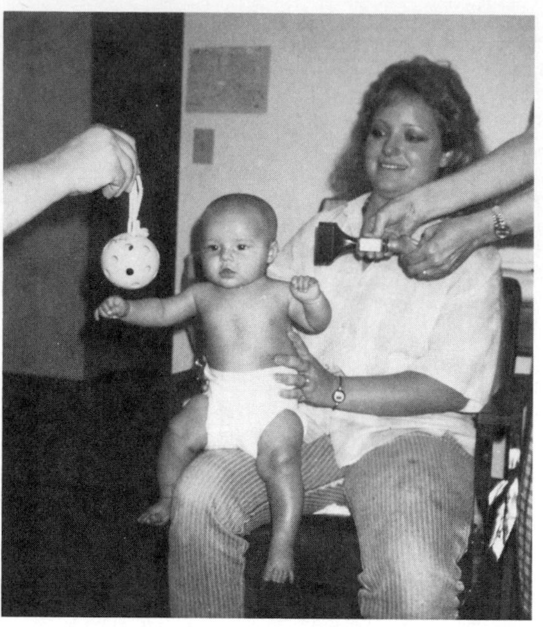

***FIG. 34-2*** The Infant Hearing Kit.

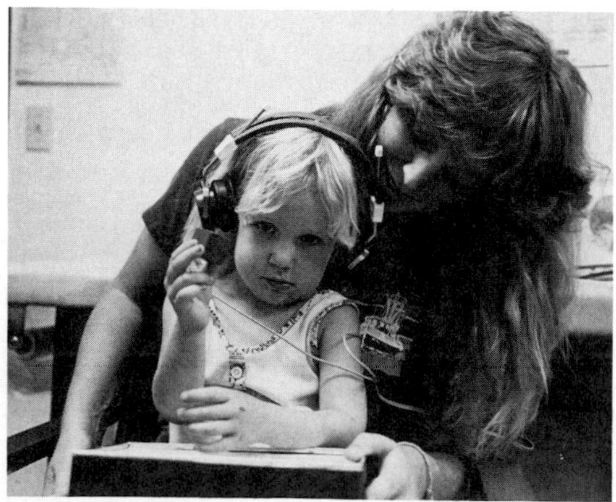

***FIG. 34-3*** Child listens to sound during play audiometry.

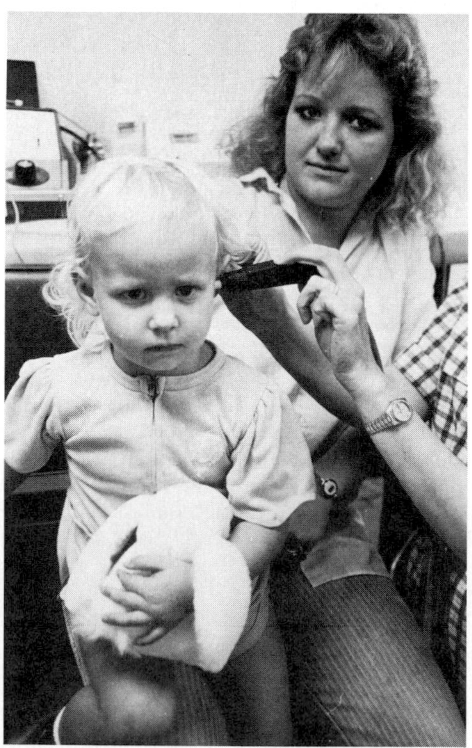

***FIG. 34-4*** Audiometric screening using tympanometry.

| Steps | Rationale |
|---|---|
| d. Limited speech or no speech. | A hearing impairment affects speech development. Speech may be flat or monotone. |
| e. Use of an inappropriately soft or a loud voice. | A child with a conductive hearing loss will often speak in a loud voice. A child with a sensorineural loss will often speak with a soft, inaudible voice because of an articulation problem (Whaley and Wong, 1991). |
| f. No response or limited response to environmental sounds. | This lack of response may be the first indication that an infant suffers a hearing loss. |
| 4. Assess the child's present health status that may affect hearing: viral or bacterial infection; allergy; excessive cerumen; foreign body in the canal or upper airway congestion. | Fluid, infection, rhinitis, rhinorrhea, an ear canal occluded with cerumen, or a foreign body will temporarily impede even normal hearing because these conditions interfere with sound waves being transmitted from the external ear to the inner ear through the middle-ear pathway (Bower, 1980). |
| 5. For group testing such as in a school setting:<br>a. Review school records.<br>b. Mail questionnaires home for parents to complete and return to school. | In schools, audiometric screening is done according to district policy (e.g., every other year). It is essential to have a current history on all the children to screen effectively. |

## Planning and Goal Setting

| Steps | Rationale |
|---|---|
| 1. Assemble and prepare equipment.<br>a. Audiometer with headset: red coded earpiece for right ear and blue coded earpiece for left ear.<br>b. Pen and audiogram form.<br>c. Two chairs and a table. | Having equipment available will facilitate testing and decrease anxiety.<br>***Special Considerations:*** *Inspect audiometer for proper functioning. Audiometers should be calibrated at least every 2 years to ensure accurate measurement.* |
| 2. Select a quiet area for testing. | Children may become distracted and ambient noise interferes with hearing ability at 0 to 15 dB. |
| 3. Develop individualized goals of nursing care:<br>▪ To accurately screen hearing ability.<br>▪ To identify any hearing loss.<br>▪ To refer to nurse practitioner or family doctor, if necessary. | |

## Implementation

| Steps | Rationale |
|---|---|
| 1. Explain the procedure to the child and family (if present). | Preparing the child will increase accuracy of the results (Sullivan, 1988). |
| 2. Explain that the purpose of the test is for general screening, not a diagnostic evaluation. | An awareness of the screening nature of the test will minimize anxiety and prevent misunderstanding of the results.<br>***Special Considerations:*** *If screening will be for a group, explain initially to all and then reinforce the purpose during individual screening.* |
| 3. Explain the testing procedure. If testing a group of children, demonstrate the procedure with a volunteer. | Audiometric screening is often done with groups of children in school settings. A group demonstration of how a test will be done can save time and minimize anxiety. Only a quick review is usually needed before individual testing. |
| 4. Perform an air conduction sweep check test at a fixed 25 dB level. Refer to audiometer manual. | For a sweep check, 25 dB is within normal range (0 to 25 dB). Screenings are not done in a soundproof room, so it would be hard to hear 0 to 5 dB. Pure tone is standardized and is accurately measured. As frequencies tested have anatomical counterparts in the organ of Corti, an audiometer can locate the loss and its degree (Bower, 1980). |
| 5. Test the following frequencies in each ear at 25 dBs: 1000 Hz, 2000 Hz, 4000 Hz, 6000 Hz, 8000 Hz, 500 Hz, and 250 Hz. Test all frequencies in one ear and then the other or alternate between the two ears. Vary the time interval between introducing the different sounds. | Normal speech is between 300 to 3000 Hz; these frequencies test for the most common hearing range. The time interval should vary so the child does not anticipate a pattern, thus giving inaccurate responses. |
| 6. Observe child's face for confusion. | Many false responses may be caused by lack of understanding and improper preparation (DiChiara, 1985). |
| 7. Determine results:<br>▪ Positive: pass.<br>▪ Negative: fail. | Pass is defined as correct responses to all or all but one frequency in one or both ears. Failure is defined as two or more failed responses to frequencies in one or both ears. |

| Steps | Rationale |
|---|---|
| 8. Record results for audiometric sweep as:<br>Pass: date, ANSI Rt 25S<br>Lt 25S<br>Fail: record the ear(s) and the frequencies not responded to.<br>For example: Left ear, failed 2000 Hz and 4000 Hz. | The American National Standards Institute (ANSI) sets the standards for hearing screening (DiChiara, 1985). 25S means that the audiometer remains at 25 dB and S indicates audiometric sweep screening. |
| 9. If child fails, inspect the ear to identify possible causes of failure. | Infection, excessive cerumen, acute or serous otitis, or a foreign body may impede hearing.<br>***Special Considerations:*** *If excessive or hardened cerumen is present, suggest the use of mineral oil or half strength hydrogen peroxide for removal. Do not do this if there are signs of infection or perforation of the tympanic membrane.* |
| 10. Refer to health care provider for evaluation if signs of serous or acute otitis media or a foreign body. | These conditions require medical intervention by a nurse practitioner or physician. |
| 11. If there is no obvious cause for hearing loss, reschedule for screening in to 2 to 3 weeks. | A recheck allows for resolution of the problem if apparent. The child may have been ill, shy, or may have misunderstood testing. |
| 12. Perform a Threshold Acuity Test at the rescheduled visit if possible (see box on p. 219). | A Threshold Acuity Test provides a more sensitive evaluation of hearing threshold than the Air Conduction Sweep Check Test, but a soundproof room is required, and one is frequently not available. |
| 13. Refer for further evaluation if the child still does not pass. | A referral to the family doctor or nurse practitioner is essential for diagnosis and treatment of the cause of the hearing failure on the screening. |
| 14. Notify the school nurse or the child's teacher of the hearing screening results. | Proper classroom placement is essential for learning. The child's education program may be altered based on the evaluation and possible hearing loss. |

| Evaluation Outcomes | Observational Guidelines |
|---|---|
| 1. An accurate hearing screening is completed. | Note completion of screening forms. Note rescreening scheduled and completed if child failed initial screening. |
| 2. Abnormal hearing screening results are identified. | Note failing results and compare to established criteria. |
| 3. Potential causes of failure are identified. | Using an otoscope, inspect external canal for cerumen and foreign bodies; inspect the middle ear for fluid or infection. Note documentation of findings and recommendations or referrals. |
| 4. Referral is made to family doctor or audiologist for further evaluation. | Written letter and/or audiogram form are provided for the referral. A written or verbal report is obtained following evaluation. |
| 5. The child's school and teacher are notified of a documented hearing loss. | Review documentation of official contact. Verify with child and family that steps were taken to meet educational standards. |

## Documentation

On the child's record, document the results of the screening, e.g., passed all frequencies at 25 dB or failed initial screening in right ear 40 dB in 1000 and 2000 frequencies; rescreen in 2 weeks at 9:30 AM. Note if the child passes or fails the rescreening and document referral to the family health care provider. Follow-up care should be noted, e.g., the family made and kept appointment with a doctor, and the results of the evaluation should be listed.

# *SKILL* 35 Screening for Visual Acuity

*Rosemary Liguori*

Problems with visual acuity, the ability to see near and far objects clearly, may cause significant learning impairment. Studies indicate that as much as 25% of the school-age population may have some visual problem. Vision screening is most often used to identify far visual acuity problems, e.g., the inability to read words on a chalkboard. However, screening is not diagnostic and should not be substituted for a thorough vision examination by an ophthalmologist or optometrist. Every child should have a professional evaluation before the age of 4 to 5 years (Sullivan, 1988) and again during school years, preferably at puberty. The cost of screening and time involved are minimal compared to the possible permanent visual and learning impairment. Early identification and intervention can often lessen or correct the visual problem.

The Snellen tests are commonly used to detect problems in visual acuity such as myopia, strabismus, ptosis, and amblyopia (Holland, 1982). Screening with the Snellen E or the Snellen chart for visual acuity identifies the majority of children who need eye treatment (National Society for the Prevention of Blindness, 1988).

## NURSING DIAGNOSES

Sensory perceptual alterations (visual) related to disease, trauma, or congenital defect; Altered growth and development related to visual impairment; Potential for injury related to visual impairment; Impaired social interaction related to visual defect; Ineffective individual coping related to visual impairment.

| Steps | Rationale |
|---|---|
| **Assessment** | |
| 1. Determine the child's age:<br>Normal vision by age:<br>a. Newborn—20/200 to 20/400 | Normal visual acuity varies by age. Newborns will focus on a face, track briefly, turn toward light, and widen their eyes when they see an object/face. Visual acuity in newborns is estimated at 20/200 to 20/400 by special tests developed for infants and difficult to test children (Whaley and Wong, 1991). |
| b. 2 months | A 2-month-old infant is able to track beyond midline, demonstrate a responsive smile and follow objects 6 feet away. |
| c. 3 months | A 3-month-old infant is able to track eyes and head 180 degrees. |
| d. 4-6 months—20/200 | A 4 to 5 month-old infant is able to reach for objects. By 3 to 6 months, the infant should develop binocular vision, the ability to fixate on visual images with both eyes.<br>***Special Considerations:*** *The infant should not exhibit strabismus (crossed eyes) after 6 months (see Skill 36).* |
| e. 1 year and up—20/40-60 to 20/20 | Special infant visual acuity tests have estimated achievement of 20/20 to occur from 6 to 30 months (Whaley and Wong, 1991). |
| 2. Observe for the following vision-related behaviors or ask if the family has noted the following:<br>*Young infant:* | |
| a. Nystagmus: fast or slow horizontal movement of the eyes. If present, note if the motion was induced (by shining a light or assessing extraocular movement) or spontaneous (without known external stimulation). | Spontaneous nystagmus may indicate hypothyroidism, blindness, brain tumors, or degenerative disease. Fast jerky eye movements indicate a vestibular disease or a severe refractory error (Barness, 1981). |
| b. Not following objects.<br>c. Not fixating on a face or objects. | These signs may indicate a visual acuity problem. |
| d. "Setting sun" sign (sclera is exposed above the iris). | This is normal in prematurity and to some extent in normal newborns; if marked, hydrocephalus, increased intracranial pressure, or kernicterus is suspected (Barness, 1981). |
| e. Ptosis (drooping of the upper eyelid). | Unilateral lid closure may increase the axial length of the eye, causing amblyopia (Nelson et al, 1984). |
| f. Marked hemangiomas of the eyelid and orbit. | There is an increased occurrence of refractive errors in children with hemangiomas (Nelson et al, 1984). |

| Steps | Rationale |
|---|---|
| *6 months or older:* | |
| a. Not able to track when looking at a toy or a face to the side, up, or down. | This may be an indication of a visual loss. |
| b. Tilting head to the side. | Turning or tilting the head is a compensatory mechanism that allows the child to block double vision with nose. |
| c. Excessive blinking.<br>d. Squinting.<br>e. Crossed eyes.<br>f. Excessive tearing.<br>g. Eye pain. | These behaviors are indicative of possible visual disturbances requiring a referral to an eye specialist (Whaley and Wong, 1991). |
| h. Recurrent styes. | Styes may be caused by excessive eyestrain (Barness, 1981). |
| i. Holding a book or toy close.<br>j. Stumbles or trips frequently. | When a child holds a book or toy close to the face, he or she is attempting to focus on the image. |
| 3. Review the child's history for factors that may have an influence on visual acuity: | |
| a. Prematurity. | Prematurity predisposes the child to visual disturbance because concentrated oxygen may be used to treat respiratory distress (Whaley and Wong, 1991). Myopic refractive errors are common in premature infants (Nelson et al, 1984). |
| b. Birth injuries. | Tiny hemorrhages during birth trauma may cause strabismus (Windsor and Hurtt, 1974). |
| c. Previously diagnosed vision problems: glasses for myopia or hyperopia; eye patches for amblyopia; surgery for strabismus. | Visual acuity may change as the child matures despite previous corrective therapy. An awareness of these measures provides a baseline for evaluation. |
| d. Family history of: blindness, albinism (lack of melanin), retinoblastoma, strabismus, and cataracts. | These conditions are genetic and may signify a higher risk for visual disorders in the child. |
| 4. Review indicators for screening for visual acuity:<br>a. Preschool children 3 to 5 years.<br>b. Kindergarten pupils.<br>c. 2nd grade pupils.<br>d. 5th grade pupils.<br>e. 8th grade pupils.<br>f. 10th or 11th grade pupils.<br>g. Any child with signs and symptoms of eye problems.<br>h. All new pupils in a school.<br>i. Teacher referrals. | Ideally every child should be annually screened. Because of the lack of school personnel, the National Society for the Prevention of Blindness recommends these guidelines for screening.<br>***Special Considerations:*** *Volunteers can be instructed to administer the screening test.* |
| j. Children who have a potential or identified learning disability. | Vision should be assessed for a complete evaluation of a learning disability. |
| k. Children who have a change in behavior. | Children who have difficulty in seeing may exhibit behavioral changes, e.g., acting out or withdrawal from the group or activities. |
| l. Children who are under medical care for a refractive error, e.g., myopia or hyperopia. | The eye continues to grow during childhood, especially at puberty; visual changes occur and need to be reevaluated periodically (e.g., every 6 to 12 months).<br>***Special Considerations:*** *Encourage the child to continue prescribed eye treatment.* |
| m. Children with eye pathology such as cataracts or amblyopia. | Amblyopia needs to be followed closely to ensure success of treatment. When a cataract is extracted a refractive error such as hyperopia and a potential for amblyopia may occur. Continued evaluation by an ophthalmologist is needed (Nelson et al, 1984). |

## Planning and Goal Setting

| Steps | Rationale |
|---|---|
| 1. Select a quiet, well-lit room with at least 20 feet of space for the testing. Twenty to thirty footcandles of light is required; room should be free from glare and shadows. | Adequate spacing, lighting and undisturbed environment allows for accuracy in testing.<br>***Special Considerations:*** *For testing in an area less than 20 feet, alternate, but less accurate, methods include use of the 10-foot Snellen chart or a 20-foot chart placed between the examiner and the child and a mirror placed 10 feet in front to simulate the distance of 20 feet (Bower, 1980).* |
| 2. Select the appropriate test for this child. | Testing will be more accurate when it is appropriate to the child's developmental level. |
| a. Informal visual acuity screening. | The child younger than 3 years can be tested informally by light perception and tracking, and observation for specific signs. Special tests are available if further evaluation is indicated (Nelson et al, 1984; Friendly, 1987). |

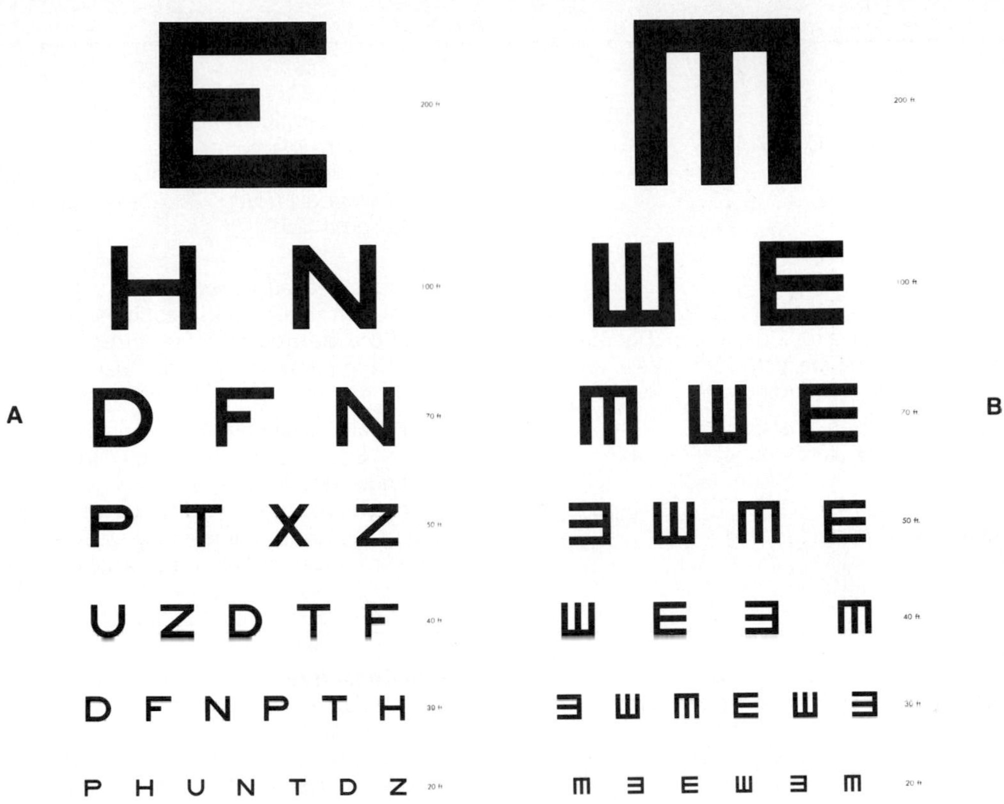


***FIG. 35-1*** Snellen Chart. **A,** Letter (alphabet) chart. **B,** Symbol E chart.

From National Society to Prevent Blindness, Inc., New York.

### *ADDITIONAL VISION SCREENING TESTS*

*Blackbird Vision Screening System:* Modification of the Snellen E using a blackbird symbol. The test uses flashcards instead of a chart. The kit includes disposable, child-sized glasses that say "I just had my eyes checked." This system fosters cooperation by the child. A chart version has also been developed (Holland, 1982). Available from:

Blackbird Vision Screening System
P.O. Box 7424
Sacramento, CA 95826

*HOTV:* A four-figure letter chart that may be used for a child as young as 3 years old. The child responds by naming the letter or matching a response on the "response panel." The letters are based on the Snellen standards and are manufactured by the:

Good-Lite Company
1540 Hannah Ave.
Forest Park, IL 60130

| Steps | Rationale |
|---|---|
| b. Snellen E (Fig. 35-1). | This test is accurate with children 3 to 8 years of age. Knowledge of the alphabet is not required. It is also appropriate for non-English speaking individuals. |
| c. Snellen Letter Chart (Fig. 35-1). | The letter chart is accurate and used with children above the second grade and adults who know the alphabet. **_Special Considerations:_** *For other visual acuity screening tests, see box on p. 225.* |
| 3. Gather materials to be used: | |
| a. Penlight. | A penlight is needed to assess infants for tracking, blink reflex, corneal light reflex, and nystagmus induction. |
| b. Occluder: a 3-by-5 inch card, a paper cup (Fig. 35-2) or a commercially made occluder (Fig. 35-3). Use a separate occluder for each child, discarding after use. | **_Special Considerations:_** *A fish, turtle shape, or a "pirate patch" made from construction paper may be used for younger children.* |
| c. Snellen E Chart or Snellen Chart. | The charts are standardized and reliable (Bower, 1980). |
| d. A large E card (teaching card). | The large "E" is used to allow the child to become familiar with the various positions. |
| e. A pointer. | The pointer will be used to indicate which letter is to be identified. |
| f. Recording paper and pencil. | Recording the results immediately assures accuracy. |
| g. Light meter. | The proper footcandle light is essential to ensure accuracy of the screening. **_Special Considerations:_** *A light meter can usually be borrowed from local power company.* |
| h. Two window cards (optional)—one with a centered slot to show a line of letters at a time and one with a centered square to show one symbol at a time. | **_Special Considerations:_** *The National Society to Prevent Blindness (1988) recommends the use of window cards as the younger child may have a difficult time focusing on one symbol when all the lines are exposed. However, Bower (1980) cautions that amblyopia may be missed if the symbols are isolated.* |
| 4. Hang/tape E chart on the wall. | **_Special Considerations:_** *The chart should be placed at the child's eye level to ensure accuracy of test.* |
| 5. Measure a 20-foot distance from chart to where the child will stand. | Snellen charts are drawn to an exact scale for use at 20 feet. Because rays of light at this distance are almost parallel when they reach the eye, a minimum amount of accommodation is needed to focus them on the retina. This distance causes the least strain on the eye (National Society for the Prevention of Blindness, 1972). |

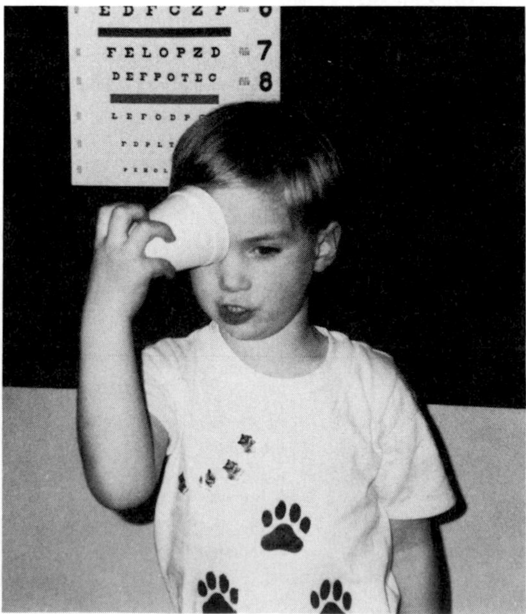


***FIG. 35-2*** Child using paper cup occluder.

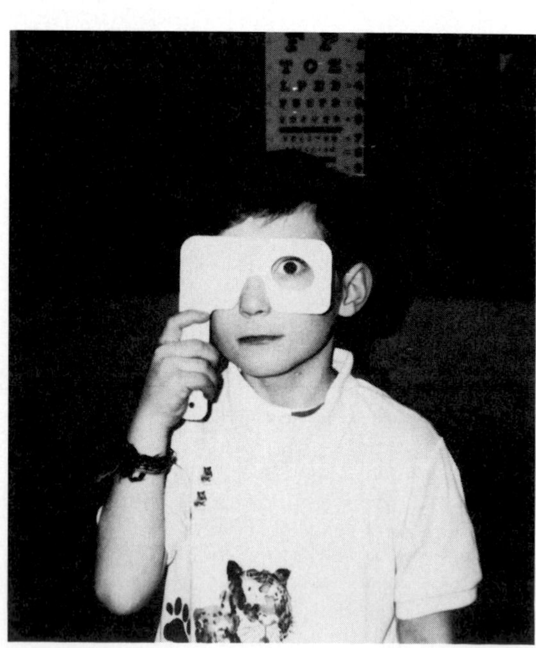

***FIG. 35-3*** Child using commercially made occluder.

| Steps | Rationale |
|---|---|
| 6. Tape child-sized paper feet to floor. Position the footprints so the heels will touch the 20-foot line (Whaley and Wong, 1991). | Footprints will help remind children of the proper position for testing. |
| 7. Develop individualized goals of nursing care:<br>▪ Screen the child for age-appropriate vision.<br>▪ Identify any abnormal findings.<br>▪ Educate the family as to the purpose of screening.<br>▪ Refer to eye doctor for further evaluation if indicated. | |

## Implementation

### *Assessment of infants*

| Steps | Rationale |
|---|---|
| 1. Newborn to 6 months.<br>a. Blink reflex: shine a light in infant's eyes, observe blink response.<br>b. Tracking: move the light slowly, observe eyes following the light for a short distance.<br>c. Nystagmus: If present, note if it is induced (by the presence of light or during the assessment of extraocular movement) or if it is spontaneous (present without any stimulation). | Informal testing for visual acuity, e.g., the presence of the blink reflex, the absence of nystagmus, and the ability to elicit a pattern of fixation is considered adequate to note presence of central vision. |
| d. Criteria for referral.<br>▪ Failure in the blink response.<br>▪ Child does not track.<br>▪ Nystagmus is spontaneous and continuous. | Abnormal findings in these tests may indicate visual problems, e.g., blindness, tumors, or severe refractive errors (Windsor and Hurtt, 1974; Barness, 1981). |
| 2. 6 months and older.<br>a. Strabismus assessment (see Skill 36). | Strabismus should not occur after the age of 6 months. Early identification is essential to prevent the development of amblyopia (Friendly, 1987). |
| b. Tracking: move a light or object in various positions; observe eye movement. | A cursory assessment of vision is to observe a child track an object. |

### *Snellen and Snellen E Screening*

| Steps | Rationale |
|---|---|
| 1. Explain screening procedure to child and family. | Understanding the procedure facilitates cooperation and accuracy of screening. |
| 2. Explain the visual acuity terminology, e.g., 20/20.<br>a. The numerator 20 is the distance from the testing chart.<br>b. The second number is the distance in feet at which the letter (or the direction of the E) is readable by a person who has normal eyesight. Each line has a distance value assigned to it. | Understanding the terminology and results of the screening fosters compliance.<br>***Special Considerations:*** *For example, a child with 20/100 vision is standing 20 feet from the chart, but is only able to read a line that a child with normal vision could read clearly at 100 feet.* |
| 3. For the younger child to be tested with the Snellen E chart, demonstrate how the E may be up, down, to either side by using the E teaching card.<br>a. Equate the E with fingers or say, "Pretend the E is a table and has three legs. Which way are the legs pointing?"<br>b. Ask the child to show with a hand or fingers how the E is pointing. | The "illiterate E" is presented in various positions to prepare the child for the test and verify if the child is able to accurately respond for testing. Comparison of the E to the legs of a table may help the younger child know how to respond. |
| c. Allow the child to manipulate E card. | Allowing the child to handle the card may lessen anxiety. |
| 4. If using the Snellen Alphabet Chart, point to the letters on the top and next line, asking the child to name each letter. | Using larger letters validates child's understanding of the testing procedure without prematurely screening their vision. |
| 5. General test guidelines for the Snellen E or Snellen Chart.<br>a. Have the child stand the premeasured distance from the chart. | Twenty feet is the standard distance for accuracy of the test. |
| b. Test both eyes; then use the occluder to test each eye individually. | Testing both eyes first allows the child to use his or her eyes in a normal fashion and standardizes the routine to avoid confusion and facilitate recording the results. |
| c. When using the occluder, the older child may hold it. Cup it slightly to avoid touching the eye or lashes. Instruct the child to keep both eyes open, even though one eye is covered. | The eye not being tested must be covered to detect problems such as amblyopia.<br>***Special Considerations:*** *If holding the occluder for a younger child, an assistant will be needed to point to the chart.* |
| d. If applicable, test first without glasses and then with glasses. | Testing without glasses provides the actual acuity level of the child. Testing with glasses may indicate if vision is adequately corrected or if there is a need to be reevaluated by the eye specialist. |

| Steps | Rationale |
|---|---|
| e. Expose the entire line being tested for 6 years and older. For 3 to 5 years old, an isolated letter is recommended. | Isolation of letters prevents confusion by the young child in response to the symbol for testing (National Society to Prevent Blindness, 1988). However, Bower (1980) cautions that isolating letters may allow problems such as amblyopia to be missed. |
| f. Observe behaviors indicative of eye problems during testing: rubs eyes; holds items close; crossing eyes or wandering eye; eye pain; squints; tilts or thrusts head; blinks excessively. | Children may pass the vision screening but should be referred if these symptoms are present. |
| 6. Procedure (for Snellen and Snellen E). | |
| a. Point to E or letter on the 20/200 line.<br>b. For Snellen E, ask the child which way the E is pointing (see Step 3 on previous page).<br>If using the alphabet chart, ask child to name the letter. | This is the largest E and allows the examiner to validate that the child understands the testing. Also, it allows the child to feel some success in responding correctly and knowing the expectations of the test. |
| c. For a 3-year-old child, begin with the 20/50 line. Point to the symbols one at a time, moving from left to right. If the child identifies more than half of the E directions correctly, proceed to the next line, but change the reading direction from right to left ("snake" pattern). Continue to the 20/20 line if the child passes the previous lines. | For 3-year-olds, the referral line is the 20/50 and the passing line is the 20/40. These are the most important lines to test at this age. The child is tested to the 20/20 line, if possible, to establish a baseline for future screening. The "snake" pattern makes it difficult to memorize responses (National Society to Prevent Blindness, 1988).<br>***Special Considerations:*** *Some authorities recommend that all the lines should be evaluated, but this may fatigue a 3-year-old with a short attention span.* |
| d. For a child 4 years of age or older, start with the 20/40 line, then follow the same procedure as above if the child identifies more than half of the letters or E directions correctly. | For children four years of age and up, the referral line is 20/40 and the passing line is 20/30. |
| e. If the child fails a line (correctly responds only half or less of the time), repeat the line in reverse order. | Retesting a failed line ensures accuracy of the screening. |
| f. If the child fails twice on the first line presented, move up the chart to the next larger symbols and continue until the ability to identify at least one more than half the symbols is reached. | Testing until the child passes a line is necessary to complete testing and to provide information for the referral. |
| g. Repeat the procedure in the order outlined above, testing the right eye and covering the left eye.<br>h. Repeat the test, testing the left eye and covering the right eye.<br>i. Repeat the entire test with glasses, if applicable. | Testing the eyes separately will help to detect problems such as amblyopia. |
| j. Criteria for failing the vision screening is:<br>▪ Not being able to read the majority of letters on the referral line:<br>(a) 3-year-old—20/50 or less.<br>(b) 4 years and older—20/40 or less. | Criteria is based on the child's failure to identify accurately more than half of the symbols on a given line of the test chart at the distance of 20 feet.<br>***Special Considerations:*** *The National Society to Prevent Blindness recommends this criteria. Local advisory committees may recommend more stringent criteria.* |
| ▪ A difference of 2 or more lines between the two eyes (e.g., 20/20 right eye [O.D.] and 20/40 in left eye [O.S.]). | A difference in vision between the eyes indicates pathology such as amblyopia, myopia, or hyperopia (Bower, 1980). |
| 7. Test for hyperopia: Repeat procedure for testing eyes with the child wearing plus or convex lens glasses. This should be done routinely from the age of 7 years and up (National Association for the Prevention of Blindness, 1971). | The plus lens make the images cloudy, and the child normally should not be able to read the 20/30 or 20/40. If the child reads the appropriate line, refer child for evaluation for hyperopia (farsightedness).<br>***Special Considerations:*** *Children under 8 years of age may have hyperopia normally.* |
| 8. Record findings, including visual fraction, time of day; unusual behavior, e.g., ill, fatigued, busy; results of the test; signs and symptoms of possible visual problems. | Findings should be documented for the referral. Fatigue, illness, and behaviors may influence the testing. |
| 9. If a young child does not pass the screening the first time, allow the child to take the teaching card home to become more familiar with it. | Familiarity of test materials facilitates cooperation and accuracy when retesting. The child could be unsure of self because of the new concepts or may be shy. |
| 10. Retest the child in a morning within a week. | Children are usually more cooperative and alert in the morning. Retests are necessary to prevent overreferral. |
| 11. If child fails screening again, using the same criteria in 6j, refer to ophthalmologist or optometrist for evaluation. | There is a high correlation with failing the screening test and eye problems.<br>***Special Considerations:*** *Even if the child passes the screening, refer for any behaviors indicative of visual problems.* |

| Steps | Rationale |
|---|---|
| 12. Contact the family to determine the time and day of the referral appointment. | Contact will encourage the family to seek an evaluation. It demonstrates an interest in the child by the health care provider and reinforces the importance of further evaluation. ***Special Considerations:*** *If there are financial problems, community agencies, e.g., the Lion's Club, are known to assist families with eye care.* |
| 13. Confirm with the eye specialist that the appointment was kept. Ask for a written report. | Unkept appointments may indicate disinterest or financial problems. A written report confirms the results of the screening and guides collaboration with the educational system. |

| Evaluation Outcomes | Observational Guidelines |
|---|---|
| 1. An accurate and appropriate vision screening is completed. | Note completion of screening using age-appropriate test. |
| 2. Abnormal findings are identified. | Using established criteria, failing responses are noted. |
| 3. Rescreening occurs as appropriate in 1 week. | Review documentation of scheduled rescreening for failures. |
| 4. A referral is initiated for further evaluation when indicated. | Note documentation of referral for failing results or behaviors indicating eye problems. Note that written results are sent to selected physician. |
| 5. Family teaching on the purpose and procedure of eye screening is completed. | The family verbalizes the purpose of vision screening as it differs from a medical evaluation. |
| 6. The child's vision is evaluated by an ophthalmologist or optometrist. | A written or oral report is received from the examiner. |
| 7. Resources are provided for families in financial need. | Ask family if assistance was obtained from any of the provided resources. |

## Documentation

On the child's record document the results of the screening, e.g., rt 20/30, lt 20/20, passed hyperopia, or rt 20/50, lt 20/70, passed hyperopia. Document referral to optometrist or ophthalmologist. Also record any behaviors noted. Note follow-up actions taken to ensure compliance with referral. Record referral report when received. Document referral to community agencies that assist families with eye care (e.g., Lion's Club).

## Home Care Modifications

The National Society for the Prevention of Blindness, Inc., provides and distributes an eye test for preschoolers in the How's Your Vision?—Family Home Eye Test (see Product References and Teaching Resources). This test may be administered by the parents or may be used to prepare the child for vision screening by health care providers. Educational information is provided for the parents.

# *SKILL* 36 Screening for Strabismus

*Rosemary Liguori*

Seventy-five percent of eye muscle disorders (malalignment) occur after the first year of life, especially between the ages of 2 and 3-1/2 years. It is believed that the child at this age is developing focusing power and visual interest at various distances. It is at this time that the retina is fully developed to receive images properly (Windsor and Hurtt, 1974).

Screening for strabismus (cross eye) is easily done during a physical examination at any age. Early identification of strabismus is essential to prevent amblyopia (lazy eye), which may lead to permanent vision loss and behavior and learning difficulties. In strabismus, one eye deviates and cannot focus along with the other eye on an object. This malalignment can be categorized by severity as a tropia or a phoria (see box). A tropia is more severe and more likely to result in amblyopia than a phoria. Two tests commonly used to detect malalignment are presented in this skill: the corneal light reflex test (Hirschberg) and the two-part, cover-uncover test. The corneal light reflex test and the cover portion of the cover-uncover test detect tropias; the uncover portion detects phorias.

Strabismic amblyopia results from malalignment; the two eyes are unable to fuse the object as one, so diplopia (double vision) and visual confusion (seeing the same object in two different locations) occur (Friendly, 1987). The weaker eye becomes "lazy" (less functional) and the brain eventually suppresses the image in the deviating eye. Failure to identify and correct this condition by 4 to 6 years of age may result in permanent blindness in the weak eye.

## NURSING DIAGNOSES

Sensory perceptual alteration (visual) related to disease, trauma, congenital defect, or medication; Impaired social interactions related to visual deficit; Ineffective individual coping related to visual impairment.

### *CLASSIFICATION OF STRABISMUS*

Tropia: Constant or intermittent malalignment, usually obvious, of the eye.

Phoria: Tendency toward malalignment of the eye that is not obvious until fusion is prevented. This is also called a latent tropia.

Tropias and phorias are described as:

- Esotropia (esophoria)—eye turns inward
- Exotropia (exophoria)—eye turns outward
- Hypertropia—the visual axis of one eye has a permanent upward deviation
- Hypotropia—the visual axis of one eye has a permanent downward deviation

Hypertropia and hypotropia are more difficult to correct.

Adapted from Windsor C and Hurtt J: Eye muscle problems in childhood, St Louis, 1974, The CV Mosby Co.

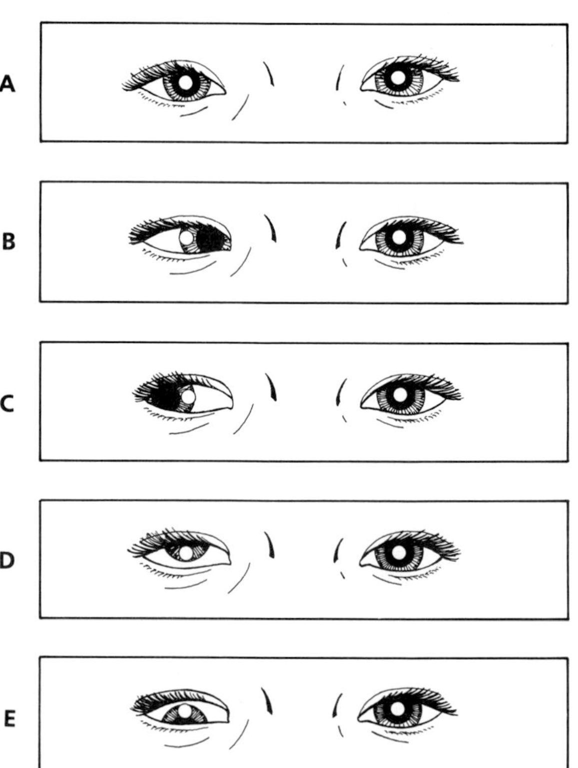


Types of strabismus. **A,** Normal alignment. **B,** Esotropia (right eye turned in toward nose). **C,** Exotropia (right eye turned toward temple). **D,** Hypertropia (right eye turned upward). **E,** Hypotropia (right eye turned downward).

## Assessment

| Steps | Rationale |
|---|---|
| 1. Determine the child's age: | |
| a. Less than 6 months. | Babies under 6 months of age frequently have an alternating strabismus because of immature eye muscle development. |
| b. 6 months and older. | If strabismus is identified from screening after 6 months of age, a referral is indicated to rule out pathologic cause, e.g., tumor or optic atrophy (paralytic strabismus). |
| 2. Question the family: | Family observations are essential because the family may have noted behavior that will not be evident during the examination. |
| a. "Have you noticed your child's eyes crossing, especially when fatigued or ill?" | During an acute illness or at the end of the day, the eye muscles tend to relax and the eyes will cross (nonparalytic strabismus). Childhood diseases, e.g., measles, interfere with the development of eye fusion (Windsor and Hurtt, 1974). |
| b. "Do your child's eyes seem to move together when following an object or person?" | Some children's eyes will cross when focusing on a moving object. |
| c. "Does your child squint or tilt head to the side?" | In an attempt to focus on an object, children will squint or turn their heads to see with the better eye. |
| d. "Does your child maintain eye contact?" | If a child is seeing two images, it is uncomfortable to maintain eye contact. |
| e. "Is your child able to judge when and where to return a ball when playing catch?" | The brain normally fuses the images seen from the two eye angles to provide depth perception. In strabismus or amblyopia only one eye is functioning, therefore depth perception is not obtained. |
| f. "Does your child complain of double or blurred vision?" | When two images are seen and not fused, double or blurred vision results. |
| g. "Does your child complain of dizziness or headache?" | Constant malalignment of the eyes will cause a headache or dizziness. |
| h. "Is there any history of eye muscle problems or crossed eyes in the family?" | The extraocular muscles may deviate in length, strength, or the way that they are attached to the eyeball. These deviations can be an inherited factor (Windsor and Hurtt, 1974). |
| i. "Was your labor or delivery long and difficult? Were forceps used?" | Tiny hemorrhages may occur in the baby's eyes because of a difficult labor or delivery and may cause permanent eye damage. ***Special Considerations:*** *If the baby is born with constant crossed eyes, refer to an eye doctor because the eyes may not improve by 6 months of age.* |
| j. "Does your child have any neurologic problems?" | Children with neurologic deficits have a higher risk of exotropia or esotropia. |

## Planning and Goal Setting

| Steps | Rationale |
|---|---|
| 1. Select a quiet area to perform assessment. | An environment with minimal distraction enables the child to concentrate on the task. |
| 2. Gather equipment.<br>a. Penlight or otoscope.<br>b. Finger puppet or small toy.<br>c. Pencil and paper. | Having equipment ready promotes efficiency in performing the assessment. |
| 3. Develop individualized goals of nursing care:<br>▪ To identify deviations from normal alignment of the eyes.<br>▪ To refer to an eye doctor for further evaluation of deviations, if noted. | |

## Implementation

| Steps | Rationale |
|---|---|
| 1. Explain to child and family the reason for the screening. | Explaining the procedures to the family and the child facilitates understanding, gains cooperation, and decreases anxiety. |
| 2. Perform the examination. | |
| a. Observe:<br>▪ The alignment of the eyes for symmetrical appearance. | ***Special Considerations:*** *Some cases of strabismus will be readily observable (see box on p. 230 for descriptive terms).* |
| ▪ Nasal bridge. | *Oriental children normally have epicanthal folds and a delay in nasal bridge development, giving the appearance of crossed eyes (pseudostrabismus)(Fig. 36-1).* |

| Steps | Rationale |
|---|---|
| 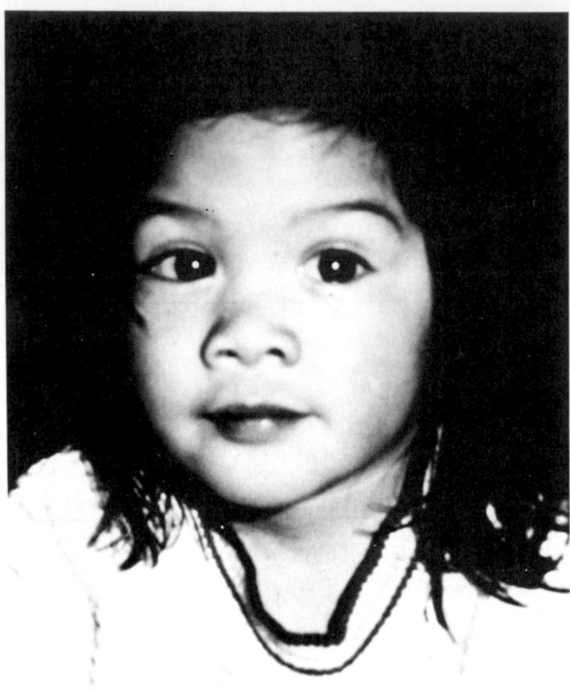 | ***FIG. 36-1*** Pseudostrabismus. Inner epicanthal folds cause eyes to appear malaligned; however, corneal light reflexes fall symmetrically.<br>From Whaley LF and Wong DL: Nursing care of infants and children, ed 4, St Louis, 1991, The CV Mosby Co. |
| b. Perform the corneal light reflex, also called Hirschberg test. | |
| ▪ Stand 14 inches to 16 inches in front of the child. | This distance allows clear observation of the child. |
| ▪ Hold the penlight and the puppet or toy directly in front of the child. | The puppet or toy will catch the child's interest, encouraging child to gaze straight ahead. |
| ▪ Allow the child to blow out the light if old enough to follow directions. | Allowing the child to blow out the light encourages participation, decreasing anxiety. |
| ▪ Hold the chin to steady the head, if needed. | Holding the chin steadies the head so the alignment of the eyes may be seen. |
| ▪ Shine the penlight (or otoscope light) into both pupils. The light should be in the center of the pupils as it is reflected back. | If the light reflex is not symmetrical, strabismus is suggested: esotropia if the light reflex is off to the medial position of the pupils, and exotropia if the light reflex is off to the lateral position of the pupils. |
| ▪ Record the results. | |
| c. Perform the cover test: | |
| ▪ Have the child focus on an object 14 inches away, e.g., a puppet, for the near point testing. | Near point alignment, the ability to focus at a close object, is tested from a distance of 14 inches. |
| ▪ Cover one eye completely with hand or small card, but do not touch the eyelid or lashes. | Complete occlusion of the eye is needed for an accurate test. Touching the eyelid or lashes may distract or cause inattention, causing the eye to move toward the area being touched. |
| ▪ Observe the uncovered eye for any movement when covering the other eye. | If the uncovered eye moves, it indicates a tropia (Bower, 1980). The stronger eye is temporarily covered and the weaker eye is trying to focus on object (Whaley and Wong, 1991). |
| ▪ Have the child focus on an object 20 feet away for far point testing. Repeat procedure as for near point testing. | The eye may turn outward when the child is asked to look at something at a distance, yet the eyes look straight when using near vision (Windsor and Hurtt, 1974). |
| ▪ Repeat the cover test procedure for both near and far point testing with the other eye. | |
| ▪ Record findings. Normal finding is no movement of the uncovered eyes. Abnormal finding is deviation in or out of the uncovered eye. | |
| ▪ Refer for further evaluation if abnormal findings. | If a tropia is not corrected, eventually vision will be diminished, perhaps permanently. |
| d. Perform the uncover test (also called the alternate test). | This test determines if there is a deviation of the eye (the muscles relax and turn in or out) when it is covered, known as a phoria. |
| ▪ Have the child focus on an object 14 inches away for near point testing. | |
| ▪ Cover one eye for 5 to 10 seconds with a hand or small card. | This time allows the eye muscles to relax, letting the eye deviate in or out. The vision has to be completely occluded to ensure accuracy. |

| Steps | Rationale |
|---|---|

A

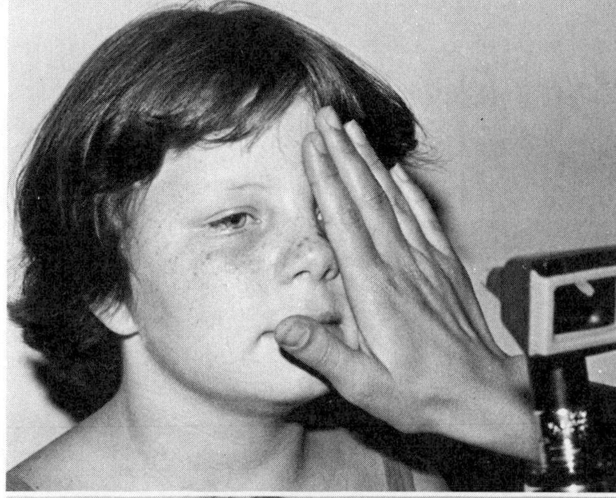

B

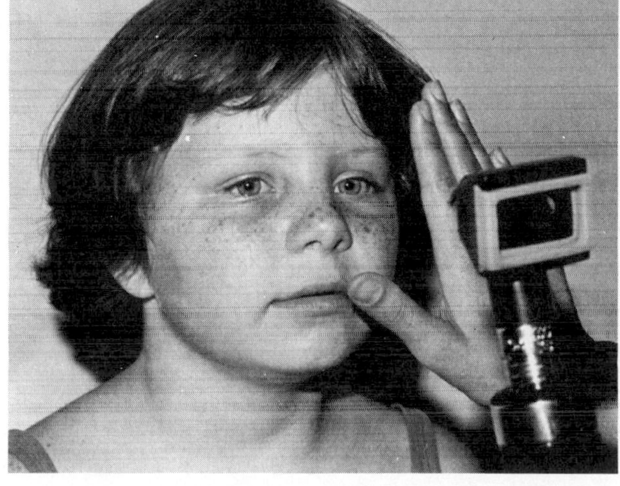

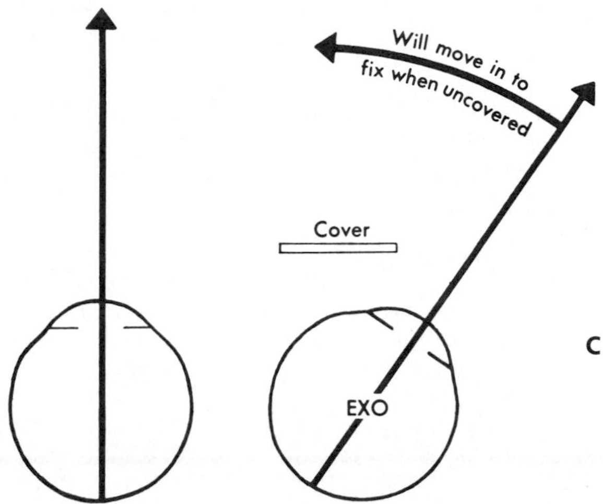


***FIG. 36-2*** Uncover test for strabismus. **A,** Eye is occluded, child is fixating on light source. **B,** If eye does not move when uncovered, eyes are aligned. **C,** Exophoria. As eye is uncovered, it shifts to fixate on object.

**A** and **B** from Whaley LF and Wong DL: Nursing care of infants and children, ed 4, St Louis, 1991, The CV Mosby Co. **C** from Prior JA: Physical diagnosis: the history and examination of the patient, ed 6, St Louis, 1981, The CV Mosby Co.

| Steps | Rationale |
|---|---|
| ▪ Uncover the eye and cover the other eye quickly. | ***Special Considerations:*** *This test takes practice to move quickly and to simultaneously watch the eye being uncovered.* |
| ▪ Observe the covered eye as it is being uncovered. If malalignment is present, the eye will move from its covered position to a straight position when uncovered (Fig. 36-2). | Eye movement as it is being uncovered indicates a phoria that is not obvious until fusion is disrupted by covering the eye. In a nonphoric eye, the eyes remain constant and do not deviate. |
| ▪ Repeat the procedure with the child focusing on an object 20 feet away for far point testing.<br>▪ Test the other eye, both near and far point. | |
| ▪ Repeat test several times. | Repeating the test confirms the results, because eye movement is more difficult to detect with the uncover test. |
| ▪ Record findings. Normal finding is no movement as the eye is uncovered. Abnormal finding is deviation of the eye as it is uncovered. | ***Special Considerations:*** *An eye that has deviated in (esophoria) or out (exophoria) while covered will move to fixate when uncovered.* |
| 3. Discuss the findings with the family. Refer the child for further evaluation if abnormal findings are obtained. | An explanation of the results provides a teaching opportunity with the family.<br>If a referral is made, the importance of follow-up can be stressed. |

| Evaluation Outcomes | Observational Guidelines |
|---|---|
| 1. Strabismus screening will be accurately completed. | Review recorded findings. Note completion of corneal light reflex test, and near and far point testing of both eyes with the cover and uncover tests. |

| Steps | Rationale |
|---|---|
| 2. Normal or abnormal findings are identified. | Review recorded findings. For normal findings, note that: (1) pupil reflections were equal in both eyes and (2) the eyes did not deviate, covered or uncovered. For abnormal findings, note that: (1) pupil reflections were unequal or (2) eyes deviated inward or outward during the cover or uncover tests. |
| 3. A referral is made for further evaluation if abnormal. | Observe documentation of written or phone contact with eye doctor. Contact family or doctor for report of evaluation. |

## Documentation

Note the time of day, date, results of the test, and if the child was cooperative or not, ill, understood procedures, or any other behaviors pertinent to the examination. Document if a referral was made and whether teaching with the family was conducted about the importance of follow-up.

# *SKILL* 37 Screening Language and Speech Development

*Rosemary Liguori*

Screening speech and language in children during a nursing assessment is a valuable activity since it takes only a few minutes and early identification may diminish or eliminate a lifetime communication disorder. Approximately 2.6% of all preschool and school-age children have a speech/language problem, in addition to 26% of handicapped children (American Speech-Language-Hearing Association, 1983). There are many causes of language delay, e.g., hearing loss, autism, environmental deprivation, or emotional disorders. Few pediatricians routinely screen language or speech, confirming the need to include speech and language assessment in the nursing assessment. Speech and language skills are essential for the child's social and educational development.

## NURSING DIAGNOSES

Impaired verbal communication related to auditory, cerebral, or neurological impairments, oral deformities, cultural barriers, or emotional disorders; Impaired social interaction related to verbal communication barrier; Self-esteem disturbance related to speech or language disorders.

| Steps | Rationale |
|---|---|
| **Assessment** | |
| 1. Review medical history or question the family as to: | |
| a. Significant prenatal events such as maternal infection and medication usage. | Prenatal conditions such as rubella or toxoplasmosis are associated with speech/hearing problems (Ruben, 1987). |
| b. Characteristics of infancy, e.g., cry or poor sucking, and achievement of developmental milestones, e.g., babbling, first words and sentences. | There is an association between high-pitched cry and poor sucking and speech problems later in life (Bower, 1980). |
| c. Presence of medical problems such as: | |
| ▪ Otitis media; acute or serous. | By the age of 3 years, two thirds of all children will have had at least one ear infection and one third will have three or more (NAHSA, 1985). Children with chronic middle ear effusion often perform below age norms on speech evaluation (Dyson, Holmes, and Duffitt 1987). |
| ▪ Allergies. | Allergies may produce fluid in the middle ear. If present at a crucial period of speech and language development, a temporary or minimal hearing loss may result. |
| ▪ Chronic upper respiratory infections (URI). | URI cause blockage of the eustachian tubes from edema or fluid. |

| Steps | Rationale |
|---|---|
| ▪ Cleft palate (see also Implementation, step 3c). | Cleft palate causes speech problems not only from the orofacial defect, but it may result in ineffective eustachian tube function, contributing to middle ear effusion and ear infections (Ruben, 1987). |
| ▪ Hearing loss. | A hearing loss will interfere with speech development because the child cannot imitate sounds he or she does not hear. |
| ▪ Mental retardation. | Expressive language delays are associated with mental retardation (Fischel, 1989).<br>***Special Considerations:*** *This is the most common cause of speech problems. The child's language should correspond with his or her mental age.* |
| 2. Determine the child's age. Note correlation between age and expected speech/language development (Table 37-1). | A comparison of the child's speech with expected age development can indicate delays. |
| 3. Assess for negative factors in the family relationships, e.g.,: | The presence of certain negative factors within the family have the potential to lead to speech development problems. |
| a. Overprotective or overanxious family. | By anticipating every vocalization or gesture, parents and siblings may not be encouraging expressive language. |
| b. Excessive tension/stress. | Excessive stress in the family may cause stuttering, withdrawal, or regression in speech patterns. |
| c. Recent significant changes, e.g., a birth of a sibling, divorce, death, or entering a new school. | These changes may precipitate a disturbance in speech, e.g., refusal to speak or stuttering. |
| 4. Determine family constellation: | Family constellation has a significant influence on speech and language development. |
| a. Presence of twins or triplets. | Multiple births tend to influence speech as the need for social communication with people other than the twin is decreased. |
| b. Birth order. | Children with older siblings tend to develop speech later because their needs are often met by communicating through prelinguistic behavior (by pointing or grunting without using words); the social impetus appears later. |
| c. Number of preschool children in the home. | It has been noted that when the number of preschoolers in the home increases, there is a delay in speech. The need for socialization with other people outside the home is lessened because the children communicate with each other (Bower, 1980). |
| 5. Assess if the child has bilingual exposure; ask, "What is the primary language spoken in the home?" | Two languages in the home may initially delay the child's speech development because he or she must learn linguistic systems simultaneously (Saville-Troike, 1979). |

***TABLE 37-1*** Normal Speech and Language Development

| Age range | Verbal ability |
|---|---|
| 12-14 months | one word |
| 18 months | 10-50 words |
| 24 months | 2-3 word phrases |
| 36 months | communicative speech (statements, questions, and commands); more than 1000 word vocabulary |
| 48 months | language is developed |

| Age range | Specific sounds | Sentence length | Intelligibility to a stranger |
|---|---|---|---|
| 2 years | | | 50% |
| 2½ years | p,b,m | 3 word | 75% |
| 3 years | p,b,m,n, 14 vowels in total | 5 word | 85% |
| 4 years | 10 vowel/blends<br>ng,w,h,t,d,k,g | | 100% |
| 4½ years | | 6 word | 100% |
| 5 years | f,v,y,th,l,wh | | 100% |
| 6 years | r,s,z,ch,j,sh,zh,<br>consonant blends | | 100% |
| 8 years | most 2 and 3 sound blends<br>such as spl and spr | | 100% |

| Steps | Rationale |
|---|---|
| 6. Assess the characteristics of the child's voice by engaging in a conversation. Listen to pitch, quality, and volume. | By 7½ years, the voice should be pleasant and well modulated. If the voice is too persistently harsh, soft, loud, high, low, or nasal, a referral should be made to a speech pathologist (Shanley and Gagliardi, 1988). Misusing of the voice such as excessive screaming may cause a temporary paralysis of a vocal fold. Nodules and polyps on the vocal cords may cause a voice change (Goldberg, 1984). |
| 7. Assess the fluency of speech:<br>a. Repetitions (st-stuttering).<br>b. Prolongations (sssstuttering).<br>c. Hesitations (no sound). | Normal dysfluency (pseudostuttering) is the repetition of words when children are developing speech between 24 months and 5 years (Biro and Thompson, 1984). It usually lasts about 3 months if the speech pattern is not focused on. Pseudostuttering occurs in 90% of children in this age range. True stuttering occurs in 1% of children. The cause of true stuttering may be from pressuring a child to improve speech or it may be genetic (Schmitt, 1987). |
| 8. Assess competence in use of language in speaking. | Language is how humans communicate with others. Speech is the spoken language (NAHSA, 1983). |
| a. Ability to express self. | In an expressive language disorder, the child has difficulty in explaining self, naming things properly, or asking questions (Biro and Thompson, 1984). |
| b. Ability to understand what is said. | In a receptive language disorder, the child has difficulty knowing what is expected and may ask for instructions to be repeated. |
| 9. Assess articulation ability.<br>a. Observe child's manipulation of the lips and tongue when talking.<br>b. Observe how the child forms words. | Articulation ability is needed for proper speech development. It is the formation of sounds by the tongue, lips, teeth, jaw, and palate as they alter the air stream coming from the vocal cords (NAHSA, 1983). |
| 10. For an infant, assess prelinguistic behavior (Table 37-2). | The actual importance of prelinguistic behavior is not known, but the child progresses through these stages (Caputo, Shapiro, and Palmer, 1987). Nonprogression is a strong indicator of later speech or language problems. |

## Planning and Goal Setting

| | |
|---|---|
| 1. Locate a quiet area to interview family and child. | A quiet location prevents distractions and permits hearing the child's speech. |
| 2. Gather materials:<br>a. Paper and pen.<br>b. Normal speech development chart (Table 37-1). | |
| c. Speech screening tests, e.g., the Denver Articulation Screening Exam (DASE); Early Language Milestone (ELM); Clinical Linguistic and Auditory Milestone Scale (CLAMS); or the Pre-School Language Scale (Biro and Thompson, 1984). | Screening tests help to identify speech and language delays, however, familiarity with the test is necessary (Castiglia, 1987).<br>***Special Considerations:*** *The ELM is a valid measure of language development in hearing children (Walker, 1989). The CLAMS may be used in screening with children from birth to 3 years old and has been standardized and validated (Ruben, 1987; Caputo, Shapiro, and Palmer, 1987). The language sector on the DDST is commonly used to identify a speech delay because it is easily available. It may be less sensitive than these other screening tests since it contains a limited number of items (Biro and Thompson, 1984).* |

***TABLE 37-2*** Prelinguistic Behaviors

| Age | Behaviors | Age | Behaviors |
|---|---|---|---|
| 1st 4-6 weeks | Reflexive sounds characterizing this period include: crying, gurgling, quiet vowels sounds. | 7-8 months | Da-da occurs before ma-ma, even in the absence of a father figure (Caputo, Shapiro, and Palmer, 1987). |
| 2-3 months | Cooing (long vowel sounds produced in a melodylike manner) begins (Caputo, Shapiro, and Palmer, 1987). | 6-10 months | Social babbling occurs when the infant interacts with individuals in the environment. |
| 4 months | Ah-goo sound occurs. | 10 months | Jargon stage where the child talks to people/toys in 4 or more syllables. |
| 5-6 months | Babbling begins. Even deaf infants will babble until 6 months when babbling ceases because of lack of self-reinforcement (Ruben, 1987). | | |

**Steps** | **Rationale**

3. Develop individualized goals of nursing care:
   - To assess the development of the child's speech and language.
   - To identify speech/language delays.
   - To refer for further evaluation.
   - To encourage families to promote speech development.

## Implementation

1. Question the family about speech development and hearing loss behaviors.

Hearing is necessary for normal speech development.
***Special Considerations:*** *If a hearing loss is suspected, implement audiometric screening, or refer to an audiologist.*

   a. Ask about speech milestones, e.g., "At what age did cooing begin? Babbling? Da-da? First word?"

   b. Ask, "How does your child let you know what he wants? Points? Speaks?" "Does your child look at you when you speak to him?" "Does your child startle with loud noises?" "Does he turn to you when he hears his name?" "Do siblings interpret for the child?"

Children may reach a milestone and then regress, e.g., a deaf child begins babbling, then ceases at about 6 months because of the lack of self-reinforcement (Ruben, 1987). Children will attempt to cover up deficiencies by nonverbal gestures. Children who do not look towards sound or attend when others speak may have a hearing loss. When older siblings and family members speak for the child or anticipate needs, there is no motivation to speak.
***Special Considerations:*** *Avoid asking, "How is the child's hearing?" Children with hearing loss may compensate by using visual cues or anticipating certain situations, which may make families believe that they can hear.*

   c. For the child between 12 and 24 months:
      - Ask, " How many words does the child say?"

***Special Considerations:*** *Differentiate between repetitions and spontaneous speech. Many children will "parrot" speech, but not use the words on his or her own.*

      - Ask if there is a history of echolalia (repeating like an echo).

Echolia is normally present in the child from 8 months to 30 months and is usually most prominent at 24 months. If it is still present after 30 months, it is indicative of a receptive language disorder or infantile autism (Caputo, Shapiro, and Palmer, 1987).

2. Listen to the child's articulation in speech:
   a. Observe how the child manipulates his or her lips and tongue when forming words.

When forming a word one or more speech sounds may be used.

   b. Identify errors of articulation.

Recognizing errors helps to determine the need for further evaluation.

      - An example of the error of substitution is "dirl" instead of saying the sound of "girl."

Substitution is the most common error and is easily identified.

      - An example of the error of omission is "at" instead of "cat".
      - An example of addition is "broux" instead of "box".
      - An example of distortion is "yesterday" sounding as "letssay."

Distortion occurs when blends of "r," "s," or "sh" are used causing a "fuzzy" sound (Frankenburg, 1973).

   c. Identify speech patterns as normal or abnormal by listening carefully to the child.

Normal speech can be characterized as the message being attended to rather than the way the person is speaking. Abnormal speech is defined as speech with many errors that makes the way the child speaks more noticeable than the message being expressed (Frankenburg, 1973).

   d. Observe for delays in speech (see box on p. 239).

***Special Considerations:*** *No words by 18 months or no phrases by 24 months, or distortion of speech should be evaluated (Resnick, Allen, and Rapin, 1984).*

3. Inspect for presence of orofacial structure defects.

Congenital orofacial defects may interfere with formation of words and subsequent speech development.

   a. Note excessive drooling.

Inappropriate swallowing, characterized by drooling, can interfere with speech.

   b. Assess for the presence of tongue thrust (reversed swallowing).
      - Place fingers on masseters (the muscles that close the jaw).
      - Break the lip seal with thumb.
      - Ask the child to swallow. If masseter movement is slight or absent, tongue thrust is present.

***Special Considerations:*** *Controversy exists as to how tongue thrust interferes with the development of certain sounds, how to treat it and the prognosis (Bower, 1980). A Nuk nipple or breast-feeding may help prevent tongue thrust, as the infant uses the tongue in a backward movement when swallowing (Bower, 1980).*

| Steps | Rationale |
|---|---|
| c. Assess for cleft palate. | |
| ■ Overt cleft: obvious upon inspection. | Overt cleft palate is one of the most common anatomical defects causing speech problems. |
| ■ Submucous cleft palate: palpate the upper hard palate. If submucous cleft is present, there will be a notch in the hard palate. Have the child say "ah," the notch can be seen in the hard palate. Note if a bifid uvula is present. | Submucous cleft may go undetected. Children with a bifid uvula frequently have a submucous cleft (Bower, 1980). |
| 4. Observe for "motherese," the mother-child language pattern of communication. | Castiglia (1987) states that "motherese" is universal, spontaneous, and crucial to language development. |
| a. Note the use of "motherese": restricted vocabulary, short simple sentences, paraphrasing, repeating words, slow rate of speech, long pauses, and present time orientation ("here and now"). | ***Special Considerations:*** *Mothers should encourage alternate caregivers to talk to the child in simple well-formed sentences and implement "motherese" techniques (Castiglia, 1987).* |
| b. Observe nonverbal interaction between mother-child: | |
| ■ Initiated by eye-to-eye contact. | Nonverbal interaction stimulates speech. |
| ■ Gaze is approximately 30 seconds.<br>■ Facial expressions are exchanged. | These behaviors signal the baby's readiness for an interaction with the mother (Lombardino, 1987). |
| 5. Ask the child the wh-type questions (why, what, who, when):<br>■ "Where is your nose?"<br>■ "What happened to the doll?"<br>■ "Why are you coloring?"<br>■ "When will you be in school?" | These types of wh questions are complex and are reached at a developmental sequence (Resnick, Allen, and Rapin, 1984).<br>***Special Considerations:*** *Avoid gestures when assessing language comprehension.* |
| 6. Engage the child in a conversation. Ask the child:<br>■ "What is your favorite TV show?"<br>■ "What do you do for fun with your friends?"<br>■ "How is school, your dog, cat, etc.?" | Asking open-ended questions allows the child to respond at his or her level and provides information about the child's ability to formulate answers, articulation, fluency, vocabulary, knowledge, and thought process (Goldberg, 1984). |
| 7. If the child will not speak, have the family tape his or her speech at home. | The child may refuse to speak because of shyness, illness, unfamiliarity, etc. Taping the child's voice allows completion of screening. |
| 8. Identify speech distortions by listening to the child speak (see box on p. 239 on Clues to Delayed Speech). | Engaging the child in a conversation allows for identification of speech distortions (Goldberg, 1987). |
| 9. Perform the 30-second test for intelligibility: | |
| a. Ask parents what percentage of the time are their children easily understood by strangers:<br>■ Less than half<br>■ About half<br>■ Three quarters<br>■ All or almost all | A quick test developed to screen speech problems, the pilot study reported that 95% of referred children had significant disorders (Coplan and Gleason, 1988). |
| b. Compare results to intelligibility norms for age group on Table 37-1. | |
| 10. Perform a Denver Articulation Screening Exam (DASE). | The DASE, a quick and valid screening test, identifies speech and language delays (Frankenburg and Drumwright, 1973). |
| 11. Perform audiometric screening (see Skill 34). | A hearing loss may be responsible for speech and language delay. |
| 12. Discuss significant history findings and actual/noted speech or language problem with family. | ***Special Considerations:*** *It is important to stress the screening nature of the assessment and the need for further evaluation, if problems noted.* |
| 13. Refer to a certified speech language pathologist if: | Identification of one or more of these conditions is indication for referral. |
| a. Speech is unintelligible. | Unintelligible speech is that in which more attention is focused on how it is being said than what is being said. |
| b. Speech is delayed by 1 year or more (see Table 37-1 and box on clues on p. 239). | Although children develop at different paces, a year delay is indication for a referral. |
| c. Inconsistent responses to environmental sounds during the first 2 years. | Hearing may be being affected by middle ear effusion. |
| d. Not speaking at all by 2 years. | |
| e. Not using sentences by 3 years. | |
| f. History of cleft lip/palate, significant prenatal events, recurrent otitis media, chronic respiratory infections, allergies. | Delays in speech-language can be the result of other disorders. (Resnick, Allen, and Shapiro, 1984: Sande and Billingsley, 1985; Ruben, 1987; and Shanley and Gagliardi, 1988). |
| g. History of hearing loss or failure of audiometric screening. | |
| h. Parent's intuition that child is not being understood. | Parents are with child constantly and are aware of development. |
| i. Stuttering lasting longer than 6 months. | Stuttering may normally be present for 3 months. |

### CLUES TO DELAYED SPEECH AND LANGUAGE DEVELOPMENT

- Not talking by 2 years of age.
- Omission of initial consonants after 3 years of age.
- Difficulty in being understood when speaking by 3 years of age.
- Substituting easy sounds for difficult ones after 5 years of age.
- Omission of word endings after 5 years of age.
- Abnormal rhythm, rate, and inflection after 5 years of age; monotone, nasal, loud, harsh or soft quality in speaking.
- Faulty sentence structure after 5 years of age.
- Distortions, omissions, or substituting sounds after 7 years of age.
- Embarrassment about speech by child, at any age.

## Evaluation Outcomes

1. The child's speech and language are assessed.
2. Speech and language actual and potential delays are identified.
3. The child is referred to a speech pathologist if indicated.

## Documentation

Indicate the method of screening used, specific problems or delays noted, and if speech was characteristic for this child. Note significant history for speech/language development, e.g., otitis media, congenital birth defects (e.g., cleft palate, cleft lip), recent birth of a sibling, or other significant events.

## Child and Family Teaching

Discuss techniques to help develop good language and speech patterns with family. Family should:

a. Talk naturally to the child, avoiding "baby talk."
b. Listen and talk frequently to the child from birth on, even if the child is too young to understand, e.g., "Mommy is going to give you a bath."
c. Provide listening experiences for the child, e.g., music, animal sounds, singing, reading stories, tape recorders, records, clapping hands, and musical instruments.
d. Revise and complete the child's speech, e.g., "Doggy gone." Parent may respond, "Yes, the doggy went home for his dinner."
e. Be a good role model for the child by speaking clearly and avoiding slang and jargon.
f. Avoid asking child to talk slowly, to repeat what has just been said, or to "start over," especially if stuttering.
g. Not laugh at what the child is saying; it is demeaning to self-esteem.

## Observational Guidelines

Review written notes, results of interview, observations, and testing.

Compare results to normal speech and language development guidelines. Note conditions that can potentially cause problems, e.g., serous otitis and existing delays.

Review written records for potential or existing problem and documentation of a referral. Follow up results of referral.

UNIT III

**PRODUCT REFERENCES AND TEACHING RESOURCES**

**Books**

Healthy Lifestyles
Suite 1200
4500 Park Ave South
New York, NY 10016

Strive for five: healthy lifestyles—Leaflet that contains menus and tips to help children learn to eat a healthy diet. For a free copy, send a self-addressed, stamped envelope.

Lansky V: Feed me, I'm yours, New York, 1981, Bantam Books.

Lansky V: The taming of the C.A.N.D.Y. monster, New York, 1982, Bantam Books.

Satter E: Child of mine: feeding with love and good sense, Palo Alto, Calif. 1986, Bull Publishing Co.

Toddler Nutrition
Suite 1900
40 West 57th Street
New York, NY 10019

Nutritional FUNdamentals leaflet—For a free copy, send a self-addressed, stamped envelope.

**Products**

Colorado Testing Materials
Colorado Hearing Systems, Inc
PO Box 20324
Denver, CO 80121

Crib-o-gram
Telesensory Systems, Inc
Palo Alto, CA 94304

DDM, Inc
PO Box 6919
Denver, CO 80206-0919
(303) 355-4729
Offers DDST Materials and Instruction Manual. Provides materials for the DASE.

FirstTemp
Intelligent Medical Systems
2233 Faraday Ave, Suite K
Carlsbad, CA
1-800-535-5188
1-800-628-1414 (in California)

Hearing Testing Guidelines
National Association of School Nurses
PO Box 1300
Scarborough, ME 04074

Infant Hearing Kit
BAM World Markets Inc
PO Box 10701
University Park Station
Denver, CO 80121

NCAST
University of Washington, WJ-10
Seattle, WA 98195
(206) 543-8528
Provides the following instruments for those interested in more sophisticated developmental assessment techniques: The Nursing Child Assessment Satellite Training and the Washington guide.

OTOTEMP
Omega Medical
1221 Turner Street #206
Clearwater, FL 34616
1-800-447-6010

Perspective Enterprises
7622 Sprinkle Road
Kalamazoo, MI 49001
Offers recumbent infant length board, stature measurement board, and balance beam scales.

Ross Laboratories
625 Cleveland Avenue
Columbus, OH 43216
Offers NCHS growth charts and Accuplots, also available through local Ross Laboratories representatives.

Total Engineering and Marketing (TEAM)
938 Michigan National Tower
Lansing, MI 48933
Offers infant recumbent length board.

### Organizations

American Council of the Blind
1010 Vermont Ave, NW
Suite 1100
Washington, DC 20005
1-800-424-8666
(202) 393-3666 in Washington, DC
The Council provides information on blindness and referrals to clinics, rehabilitation organizations, research centers, and local chapters.

American Speech-Language-Hearing Association (ASHA)
10801 Rockville Pike
Rockville, MD 20852
or call
National Association for Hearing and Speech Action (NAHSA)
1-800-638-TALK

March of Dimes Birth Defects Foundation
1275 Mamaroneck Ave
White Plains, NY 10605
(914) 997-4523
The March of Dimes provides research grants and education for public and professional persons. Their computer information system readily provides genetic/birth defect information to professionals. Pamphlets and other audiovisual materials are available to enhance public awareness about birth defects.

National Society for the Prevention of Blindness, Inc
500 Remington Rd
Schaumburg, IL 60173
1-800-331-2020

Quick Communications
PO Box 27891
St. Louis, MO 63141
Offers an information sheet on "How to Check Your Child's Speech," "How to Improve Your Child's Speech," and "If You Think Your Child Stutters."

## REFERENCES


Alexander MM and Brown MS: Pediatric history taking and physical diagnosis for nurses, ed 2, New York, 1979, McGraw-Hill Book Co.

Alexander MM and Brown MS: Pediatric physical diagnosis, ed 2, New York, 1979, McGraw-Hill Book Co.

Als H et al: Individualized behavior and environmental care for the very low birth weight preterm infant at high risk for bronchopulmonary dysplasia: neonatal intensive care unit and developmental outcome, Pediatrics 78:1123-1132, 1985.

American Academy of Pediatrics Committee on Nutrition: Prudent lifestyle for children: dietary fat and cholesterol, Pediatrics 78:521-525, 1986.

American Academy of Pediatrics: Impedance bridge tympanometer as a screening device in school, Pediatrics 79(3):472, 1987.

Banco L, Lavashekaramurth S, and Giaffam J: Usefulness of a temperature-taking pacifier, Am J Dis Child, 142:171-172, 1988.

Barness L: Manual of pediatric physical diagnosis, ed 5, Chicago, 1981, Year Book Medical Publishers, Inc.

Bates B: A guide to physical examination, ed 3, Philadelphia, 1983, JB Lippincott Co.

Biro P and Thompson M: Screening young children for communication disorders, MCN 9:410-413, 1984.

Bower F: Health screening, New York, 1980, John Wiley & Sons, Inc.

Brazelton TB and Lester BM, editors: New approaches to developmental screening of infants, New York, 1983, Elsevier Science Publishing Co, Inc.

Britton CV: Blood pressure measurement and hypertension in children, Pediatr Nurs 7(4):13-17, 1981.

Brown J et al: Ethnic group differences in nutritional status of young children from low-income areas of an urban county, Am J Clin Nutr 44:938-944, 1986.

Cadman D et al: Evaluation of public health preschool child developmental screening: the process and outcomes of a community program, Am J Public Health 77:45-51, 1986.

Caputo AJ, Shapiro BK, and Palmer FB: Marking the milestones of language development, Contemp Pediatr 4:24-41, 1987.

Casey PH et al: Developmental intervention: a pediatric clinical review, Pediatr Clin North Am 33(4):899-923, 1986.

Castiglia P: Speech-language development, J Pediatr Health Care, 1(3):165-167, 1987.

Castiglia PT and Petrini MA: Selecting a developmental screening tool, Pediatr Nurs 11(1):8-17, 1985.

Chamcides L: Textbook of pediatric advanced life support, Dallas, 1988, American Heart Association and American Academy of Pediatrics.

Chow MP et al: Handbook of pediatric primary care, ed 2, New York, 1984, John Wiley & Sons, Inc.

Cohen FL: Clinical genetics in nursing practice, Philadelphia, 1984, JB Lippincott Co.

Coplan J and Gleason JR: Unclear speech: recognition and significance of unintelligible speech in preschool children, Pediatrics 8(3 pt 2):447-452, 1988.

Darnall RA: Noninvasive blood pressure measurement in the neonate, Clin Perinatol 12(1):31-47, 1985.

Davidson DM et al: School based blood cholesterol screening, J Pediatr Health Care 3(1):3-8, 1989.

Davidson DM, Smith RM, and Qaqundah PY: Cholesterol screening in children during office visits, J Pediatr Health Care 4(1):11-17, 1990.

DiChiara E: A sound method for testing children's hearing, Am J Nurs 84(9):1104-1106, 1984.

Dickey S: A guide to the nursing of children, Baltimore, 1988, Williams & Wilkins.

Drapo P: Protocol for genetic assessment: physical examination of the child. In Foster R, Hunsberger M, and Anderson J, editors: Family-centered nursing care of children, Philadelphia, 1989, WB Saunders.

Dyson A, Holmes A, and Duffitt D: Speech characteristics of children after otitis media, J Pediatr Health Care 1(5):262-265, 1987.

Emans SJ and Goldstein DP: Pediatric and adolescent gynecology, ed 3, Boston, 1989, Little, Brown & Co, Inc.

Engel J: Pocket guide to pediatric assessment, St Louis, 1989, The CV Mosby Co.

Eott MJ, Meier RS, and Miller C: Temperature measurement in infants, Nurs Res 23(6):457-458, 1974.

Erickson E: Childhood and society, ed 2, New York, 1963, WW Norton & Co, Inc.

Erickson R: A sourcebook for temperature taking, San Diego, 1980 IVAC Corporation.

Fisheel J et al: Language growth in children with expressive language delay, Pediatrics 82(2):218-227.

Fleming J: An evaluation of the use of the DDST, Nurse Res 30(5):290-293, 1981.

Fomon SJ: Nutritional disorders of children: prevention, screening and followup. Bureau of Community Health Services. DHEW, Publication No (HSA) 77-5104, Washington, DC, 1977, US Government Printing Office.

Francis PL, Self PA, and Horowitz FD: The behavioral assessment of the neonate: an overview. In Osofsky JD, editor: Handbook of infant development, New York, 1987, John Wiley & Sons, Inc.

Frankenburg W and Dodds J: The Denver Developmental Screening Test, J Pediatr 71:181-191, 1967.

Frankenburg W and Dodds J: Denver Developmental Screening Test Manual, Denver, 1975, Ladoca.

Frankenburg W and Drumwright A: Denver articulation screening exam, Denver, 1973, University of Colorado Medical Center.

Frankenburg W et al: The Denver Prescreening Developmental Questionnaire (PDQ), Pediatrics 57:744-753, 1976.

Frankenburg W et al: Validation of Key Denver Developmental Screening Test items: a preliminary study, J Pediatr 112(4):560-566, 1988.

Frankenburg W, Fandal A, and Thornton S: Revision of the Denver Prescreening developmental questionnaire, J Pediatr 110(4):653-657, 1987.

Frankenburg W, Goldstein A, and Cole B: The revised Denver Developmental Screening Test: its accuracy as a screening instrument, J Pediatr 79(6):988-995, 1971.

Frankenburg W and Thornton S: Denver developmental activities, Dev Behav Pediatr 10(1):22-26, 1989.

Fraser F: Genetic counseling, Am J Hum Genet 26:636-659, 1974.

Friendly D: Amblyopia: definition, classification, diagnosis, and management considerations for pediatricians, family physicians, and general practitioners, Pediatr Clin North Am 34(6):1390-1401, 1987.

Frolich ED et al: Recommendations for human blood pressure determination by sphygmomanometers: Report of the special task force appointed by the Steering Committee, American Heart Association, Circulation, 77:501A-514A, 1988.

Gallagher T: Medical care of the adolescent, ed 3, New York, 1976, Appleton, Century, Crofts.

Gilette PC: Dysrhythmias. In Adams FH and Emmanouilides GC, editors: Moss heart disease in infants, children and adolescents, ed 3, Baltimore, 1983, Williams & Wilkins.

Goldberg R: Identifying speech and language disorders in children, Pediatr Nurs 10(4):252-259, 1984.

Gordon H: The family history and the pedigree chart, Postgrad Med 52(2):123-125, 1972.

Grimes J and Iannopollo E: Health assessment in nursing practice, Monterey, Calif, 1982, Wadsworth, Inc.

Guide to testing distance visual acuity, Schaumberg, Ill, 1988, National Society to Prevent Blindness, Inc.

Guyton C: Body temperature: temperature regulation and fever, Textbook of medical physiology, Philadelphia, 1986, WB Saunders.

Hall P and Wick B: Simple procedures for comprehensive vision screening, J School Health 58(2):58-61, 1988.

Hamdan JA, Taleb YA, and Ahmed MS: Traction induced hypertension in children, Clin Orthop 185:87-89, 1984.

Hamill B: Comparing two methods of preschool and kindergarten hearing screening, J School Health 58(3):95-97, 1988.

Hancock LS: FirstTemp, J Pediatr Health Care 1(3):163-164, 1987.

Hartman A: Diagrammatic assessment of family relationships, Soc Casework, 59:465, 1978.

Hayes C, editor: Risking the future: adolescent sexuality, pregnancy and childbearing, Washington, DC, 1986, National Academy Press.

Hohn AR and Loadholt C: Which blood pressure? J Pediatr 104(1):89-91, 1984.

Holland SH: 20/20 vision screening, Pediatr Nurs 8(2):81-87, 1982.

Irwin R: Attentional deficit disorder presentation, Tulsa, Okla, 1986.

Johnson SH: Nursing assessment and strategies for the family at risk: high risk parenting, Philadelphia, 1986, JB Lippincott Co.

Jolly W, Froom J, and Rosen M: The genogram, J Fam Pract 10(2):251-255, 1980.

Jones DA, Lepley MK, and Baker BA: Health assessment across the life span, New York, 1984, McGraw-Hill Book Co.

Joyner M: Hair care in the black patient, J Pediatr Health Care 2(6):281-287, 1988.

Kempe C et al: Current pediatric diagnosis and treatment, ed 9, Norwalk, Conn, 1983, Appleton and Lange.

Korones S: High-risk newborn infants, St Louis, 1981, The CV Mosby Co.

Lawhon G: Management of stress in premature infants. In Angelini DJ, Knapp C, and Gibes R, editors: Perinatal/neonatal nursing: a clinical handbook. Boston, 1984, Blackwell Scientific Publications, Inc.

Lierman C et al: Multidisciplinary treatment of feeding disorders in the home, Pediatr Nurs 13(4):266-271, 1987.

Lombardino L, Stapell JB, and Gephardt K: Evaluating communicative behaviors in infancy, J Pediatr Health Care 1(5):240-246, 1987.

Maheady D: Health concepts of preschool children, Pediatr Nurs 12(3):195-197, 1986.

Marino BL: Assessment of infant play: applications to research and practice, Issues Comp Pediatr Nurs 11:227-240, 1988.

Martyn KK et al: Comparison of axillary, rectal and skin-based temperature assessment in preschoolers, Nurse Prac 13(4):31-33, 1988.

Meer P: Using play therapy in outpatient settings, MCN 10(6):378-380, 1985.

Merenstein GB and Gardner SL: Handbook of neonatal intensive care, ed 2, St Louis, 1989, The CV Mosby Co.

Merenstein GB, Gardner SL, and Blake WW: Heat balance. In Merenstein GB and Gardner SL, editors: Handbook of neonatal intensive care, ed 2, St Louis, 1989, The CV Mosby Co.

Moore M: Pocket guide to nutrition and diet therapy, St Louis, 1988, The CV Mosby Co.

Moore M and Roche F: Pediatric anthropometry, ed 2, Columbus, Ohio, 1983, Ross Laboratories.

Morton PG: Health assessment in nursing, Springhouse, Penn, 1989, Springhouse Corp.

Muscari ME: Obtaining the adolescent sexual history, Pediatr Nurs 13(5):307-310, 1987.

National Association for Hearing and Speech Action: Hearing impairment and the audiologist, Rockville, Md, 1985, NAHSA.

Nelson LB et al: Developmental aspects in the assessment of visual function in young children, Pediatrics 73(3):375-381, 1984.

Neff J et al: Effect or respiratory rate, respiratory depth and open versus closed mouth breathing on sublingual temperature, Res Nurs Health 12(3):196-202, 1989.

O'Brien EI: Clinical thermometry in need of nursing research, J Pediatr Nurs 3(3):207-208, 1988.

O'Pray M: Developmental screening tools: using them effectively, MCN 5(2):126-130, 1980.

Orchik DJ et al: Intensity and frequency of sound levels from cordless telephones: a pediatric alert, Clin Pediatr 24:688-690, 1985.

Owen GM: Measurement, recording and assessment of skinfold thickness in childhood and adolescence: report of a small meeting, Am J Clin Nutr 35(3):629-638, 1982.

Park MK and Guntheroth WG: Accurate blood pressure measurement in children, Am J Noninvas Cardio 3:297-308, 1989.

Park MK and Lee DH: Normative blood presure values in the arm and calf in the newborn, Pediatrics 83:240-243, 1989.

Park MK and Menard SM: Accuracy of blood presure measurement by the Dinamap monitor in infants and children, Pediatrics 79:907-914, 1987.

Patterson R et al: Factors related to obesity in preschool children, J Am Diet Assoc 86(10):1376-1380, 1986.

Perry AG and Potter PA: Clinical nursing skills and techniques, ed 2, St Louis, 1989, The CV Mosby Co.

Petrillo M: Preventing hospital trauma in pediatric patients, Am J Nurs, 68(7):1468-1473, 1968.

Petrillo M and Sangar S, editors: Emotional care of the hospitalized child, ed 2, Philadelphia, 1980, JB Lippincott Co.

Piaget J: Play, dreams, and imitation in childhood, New York, 1962, WW Norton & Co, Inc.

Pillitteri A: Child health nursing, Boston, 1987, Little, Brown & Co, Inc.

Pipes PL: Assessing food and nutrient intake. In Erickson M: Assessment and management of developmental changes in children, ed 2, St Louis, 1981, The CV Mosby Co.

Pipes PL: Nutrition in infancy and childhood, ed 4, St Louis, 1989, The CV Mosby Co.

Poland R, Wells D, and Ferlauto J: Methods of detecting hearing impairment in infancy, Pediatrics Ann 9(1):31-44, 1980.

Powell ML: Assessment and management of developmental changes in children, ed 2, St Louis, 1981, The CV Mosby Co.

Ramsey M: Noninvasive blood pressure monitoring methods and validation. In Gravenstein J et al, editors: Essential noninvasive monitoring in anesthesia, New York, 1980, Grune and Stratton.

Resnick T, Allen D, and Rapin I: Disorders of language development: diagnosis and intervention, Pediatr Rev 6(3):85-92, 1984.

Richardson S: Child health promotion practices, J Pediatr Nursing 2(2):73-78, 1988.

Robertson J: Young children in hospitals, New York, 1958, Basic Books.

Robinson T: Early identification of vision and hearing problems, Pediatrics, nursing update, 1(12):1-8, 1986.

Roeser RJ and Downs MP: Auditory disorders in school children, New York, 1981, Thieme-Stratton.

Ruben RJ: Diagnosis of deafness in infancy, Pediatric Rev 9(5):163-166, 1987.

Sande D and Billingsley C: Language development in infants and toddlers, Nurse Pract 10(9):39-47, 1985.

Saville-Troike M: First-second language acquisitions. In Trubea HT and Barnett-Mizrahic A, editors: Bilingual multicultural education and the professional from theory to practice, Rowley, Mass. 1979, Newbury House Publishers, Inc.

Schmitt BD: Your child's health, Toronto, 1987, Bantam Books.

Schneider E: Parent questionnaires: a useful tool to pediatric practice, Pediatr Nurs 13(3):193-197, 1987.

Seidel HM et al: Mosby's guide to physical examination, St Louis, 1987, The CV Mosby Co.

Shanley DA and Gagliardi D: The nurse's role in identifying children with communicative disorders, J Sch Health, 58(2):75-77, 1988.

Shinozaki T, Dean RS, and Perkins F: Infrared tympanic thermometer: evaluation of a new clinical thermometer, Crit Care Med, 16(2):148-150, 1988.

Simko MD, Cowell C, and Hreha MS, editors: Practical nutrition: a quick reference for the health care practitioner, Rockville, Md, 1989, Aspen Publishers, Inc.

Smith S and Duell D: Clinical nursing skills, ed 2, Norwalk, Conn, 1989, Appleton & Lange.

Steele S: Assessing developmental delays in preschool children, J Pediatr Health Care 2(3):141-145, 1988.

Suitor C and Crowley M: Nutrition: Principles and application in health promotion, Philadelphia, 1984, JB Lippincott Co.

Sullivan L: How effective is preschool vision, hearing and developmental screening? Pediatr Nurs 14(3):181-183, 1988.

Tandberg D and Sklar D: Effect of tachypnea on the estimation of body temperature by an oral thermometer, N Engl J Med 308(16):945-946, 1983.

Venters M and Mullis R: Family-oriented nutrition education and preschool obesity, J Nutr Educ 16(4):159-161, 1984.

Vision screening of children, New York, 1971, The National Society for the Prevention of Blindness.

Walker D et al: Early language milestones scale and language screening of young children, Pediatrics 83(2):284-292, 1989.

Weighing and measuring children: a training manual for supervisory personnel, Atlanta, 1980, US Department of Health and Human Services, Public Health Service Centers for Disease Control, Nutrition Division.

Wen MR and Weir TE: Are hot ears really hot? Am J Dis Child, 143(7):763-764, 1989.

Whaley LF and Wong DL: Essentials of pediatric nursing, ed 3, St Louis, 1989, The CV Mosby Co.

Whaley LF and Wong DL: Nursing care of infants and children, ed 4, St Louis, 1991, The CV Mosby Co.

Windsor C and Hurtt J: Eye muscle problems in childhood, St Louis, 1974, The CV Mosby Co.

Wong DL: Measuring temperatures accurately in children, Child Nurse 5(2):15-17, 1988.

Wong DL: Taking accurate blood pressure in children, Child Nurse 6(3):1-4, 1988.

Wong DL and Whaley LF: Clinical manual of pediatric nursing, ed 3, St Louis, 1990, The CV Mosby Co.

Wood CS et al: Exclusively breast-fed infants: growth and caloric intake Pediatr Nurs 14(2):117-124, 1988.

Yoos L: A developmental approach to physical assessment, MCN, 6(3):168-180, 1981.

Zitelli BJ and Davis HW: Atlas of pediatric physical diagnosis, New York, 1987, Gower Medical Publishing Ltd.

# UNIT IV The Family, Environment, and Culture

# SKILL 38 Conducting a Psychosocial Assessment of the Family

*Deborah Kay Brantly*

Assessing the psychosocial component of family relationships is important to providing comprehensive and individualized family-centered care. The family is the primary system affecting the child. In some instances the family is viewed as the client. Psychosocial assessment of the family is a complex process and demands discriminating analytical skills. The genogram and sociogram are two formats through which the practitioner can obtain much of this information. In this skill the family assessment process is refined to its essential components: structure, roles, basic rules, discipline methods, boundaries, decision-making and problem-solving, communication, developmental needs of members, reactions to stress, support, nurturing, and the home environment.

## NURSING DIAGNOSES

Health-seeking behaviors related to family health promotion/maintenance; Altered family processes related to situational/developmental transition or crisis; Ineffective family coping (compromised or disabling) related to unrealistic role expectations or unmet psychological needs.

| Steps | Rationale |
|---|---|
| **Assessment** | |
| 1. Identify the indications for a psychosocial assessment of the family, e.g., to determine family strengths, need for social support, level of current and potential future stress, or the need for improved family communication. | Reasons for the family assessment guide the methods of assessment and focus of information gathered.<br>***Special Considerations:*** *Psychosocial needs of the family may be identified that were not part of the original indications. When this occurs, implementation can be tailored to the needs identified in the interview.* |
| 2. Determine the most appropriate person to interview the family. | The indications for and depth of assessment needed will determine the most appropriate provider. Persons with more training offer a more comprehensive psychosocial assessment of the family.<br>***Special Considerations:*** *On initial assessment, the admitting nurse or primary nurse may wish to interview the family. When specific problems are present or more thorough assessment is needed, a nurse specialist who is skilled in family therapy would be an appropriate interviewer.* |

**TABLE 38-1** Duvall's Development Stages of the Family

| Stages | Tasks |
|---|---|
| **STAGE I:** Marriage and an independent home: the joining of families | Reestablish couple identity.<br>Realign relationships with extended family.<br>Make decisions regarding parenthood. |
| **STAGE II:** Families with infants | Integrate infants into the family unit.<br>Accommodate to new parenting and grandparenting roles.<br>Maintain the marital bond. |
| **STAGE III:** Families with preschoolers | Socialize children.<br>Parents and children adjust to separation. |
| **STAGE IV:** Families with school children | Children develop peer relations.<br>Parents adjust to their children's peer and school influence. |
| **STAGE V:** Families with teenagers | Adolescents develop increasing autonomy.<br>Parents refocus on midlife marital and career issues.<br>Parents begin a shift toward concern for the older generation. |
| **STAGE VI:** Families as launching centers | Parents and young adult establish independent identities.<br>Renegotiate marital relationship. |
| **STAGE VII:** Middle-aged families | Reinvest in couple identity with concurrent development of independent interests.<br>Realign relationships to include in-laws and grandchildren.<br>Deal with disabilities and death of older generation. |
| **STAGE VIII:** Aging families | Shift from work role to leisure and semiretirement or full retirement.<br>Maintain couple and individual functioning while adapting to the aging process.<br>Prepare for own death and dealing with the loss of spouse, siblings, and/or other peers. |

From Whaley LF and Wong DL: Nursing care of infants and children, ed 4, St. Louis, 1991, The CV Mosby Co.; Modified from Wright LM and Leahey M: Nurses and families: a guide to family assessment and intervention, Philadelphia, 1984, FA Davis Co.

| Steps | Rationale |
|---|---|
| 3. Determine developmental level of the family using a model such as Tapia (1975) or Duvall (Wright and Leahey, 1984). Tapia compares the family's functioning with developmental life stages. Duvall defines the family's developmental stage depending on the family composition and age of family members (Table 38-1). | Tapia (1975) states that a "family's level of functioning is an indication of its state of health" and that nursing activities will be more effective based on the level of functioning the family has achieved.<br>***Special Considerations:*** *Several other developmental models exist, and can be quite divergent in focus.* |
| 4. Assess cultural and spiritual variables that may affect the family's functioning (see Skills 41 and 42). | Culture and religion are transmitted largely through the family unit. Cultural and/or spiritual values influence family belief and norms that may be different from those of the health care provider. When values differ, misunderstandings can occur unless information is taken within the context of the child/family values. |
| 5. Determine need to assess the home environment. Commonly assessed features of the home include its physical/structural characteristics as well as the material, financial, and human resources within the environment. | The home environment plays a central role in children's health and development. Behaviors of individuals and family systems are inseparable from the physical and psychological features of the environment. |

## Planning and Goal Setting

| | |
|---|---|
| 1. Plan the time and place of the interview with the family and determine who will attend. | Interviewing the family when all family members are present yields more data and opportunity to observe total family functioning. |

| Steps | Rationale |
|---|---|
| | ***Special Considerations:*** *Not all family members may be willing or able to participate in the family assessment interview, e.g., infants and toddlers, the index case, a sick child, or a working parent. Recognize that when family members are absent, views and behaviors expressed in the assessment may not be reflective of missing family members and that the presence of those members may elicit different behaviors from those present.* |
| 2. Prepare the environment (see Skill 10). | Prearranging a comfortable environment enhances the interview process. |
| 3. Develop individual goals of nursing care:<br>▪ To conduct a psychosocial assessment of the family.<br>▪ To identify psychosocial strengths and areas of need. | |

## Implementation

| Steps | Rationale |
|---|---|
| 1. Introduce self to all family members if not already acquainted. Identify name and explain role. | Introducing self provides all members with clear understanding of who the nurse is and clarifies the nurse's role. This helps break the ice and can establish the warm environment needed for trust development. |
| 2. Discuss the purpose of the interview and assure confidentiality. The following example may be used as a guide: "I am here to talk to you about your family. Your presence here shows your willingness to participate in your child's care. I value that and hope we can work together to plan your child's care. Feel free to let me know your concerns or needs. Some of the things I will be asking may seem somewhat personal. I am not here to invade your privacy and I want you to know that what you decide to share is confidential and will only be used to help plan care for your child and family." | Defining the purpose in the beginning of the interview provides direction for all family members. Assuring confidentiality provides safe parameters for the family to share information. Since psychological information is often private, feelings of invasion can be allayed by an initial discussion of purpose. |
| 3. Become familiar with each family member by inquiring about:<br>a. Name.<br>b. Interests.<br>c. Individual schedules (e.g., work, school, and hobbies).<br>d. Comment about the person as appropriate, e.g., "I see you have on a St. Louis Cardinals T-shirt. Are you a Cardinals fan?" | Addressing all family members assures that each is included in the interview. Commenting on interests and observations about the person assures the individual's importance to the interviewer, increases knowledge of each person, and establishes rapport in a nonthreatening manner.<br>***Special Considerations:*** *If some members seem hesitant to share, say, "It helps me to know a little about each of you since I will be directly involved with (the child's name)."* |
| 4. Diagram a family genogram (see box). | The genogram is an effective assessment tool for the purpose of delineating interpersonal family relationships, and identifying familial coping patterns and family history of mental illness.<br>***Special Considerations:*** *If time is limited, a 5-minute family APGAR instead of the genogram can reveal some of the needed information.* |
| 5. Determine family roles, tasks, and rules.<br>a. How are daily tasks delineated (e.g., house cleaning, grocery shopping, and child care)?<br>b. What are the most important family rules? List three or four. If the family seems unsure of how to respond, say "For example, some families have a rule of not watching TV during the evening meal." | Families who have consistent, developmentally appropriate rules with consequences, tasks, and roles provide more stability for their members. A parental decision-making style that is authoritative (has firm parental expectations coupled with responsiveness to the changing needs of the family), rather than authoritarian (rigid expectations) or democratic (expectations decided by majority rule of family members) provides security and direction for the child. Family rituals are rich ground for positive family bonding. |
| c. How did the family decide these rules?<br>d. What happens when one of these rules is broken and who provides consequences for rules being broken?<br>e. What kind of consequences/methods of discipline are used in the family?<br>f. How are family disagreements solved?<br>g. Are there any special family rituals? | ***Special Considerations:*** *Begin with more concrete information, then couple it with less concrete. For example, move from "What are your rules," to "How did the family decide on these rules?"* |

### THE GENOGRAM

The genogram is similar in structure and procedure to the pedigree (see Skill 24). The symbols developed for the genogram are somewhat different, however, and delineate selected psychosocial data symbolically (see accompanying figure). Familial patterns that affect psychosocial status of the family can be revealed through the genogram, e.g., divorce or alcoholism, as well as mental illness.

When diagramming the genogram, follow the same procedure as the pedigree, using the genogram symbols. To obtain information about relationships, ask, e.g., "What kind of relationship do you and ________ have?" or "How do ________ and ________ get along" or "How does ________ interact with the rest of the family?"

For an example of a completed genogram, see the genogram of Jenny below.

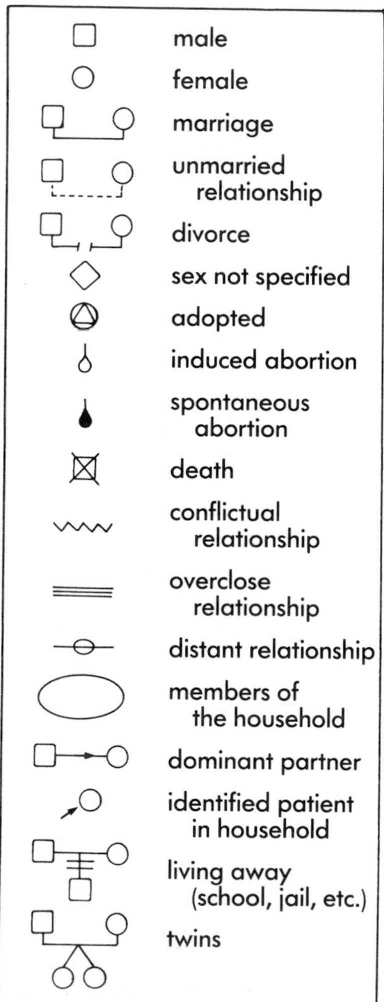


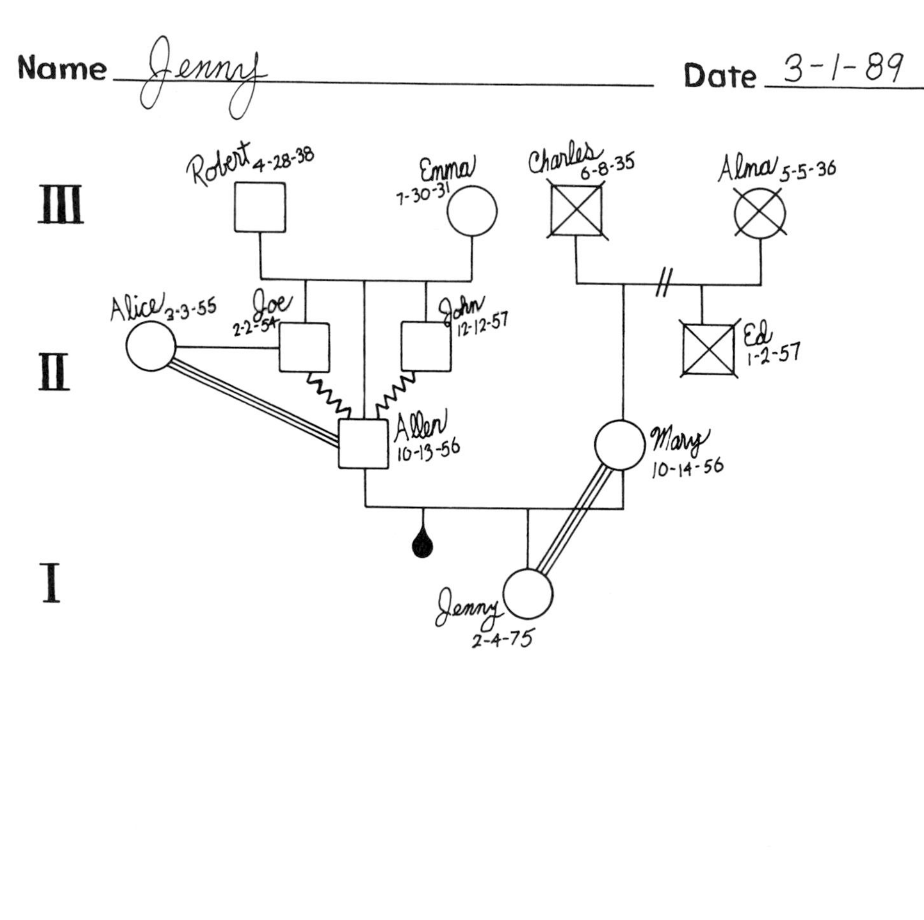

| Steps | Rationale |
|---|---|
| 6. Determine allocation of power and decision-making in the family. One way to do this is to give the family a situation to handle, e.g., a child in the family has failing grades; observe how the family solves the problem (Whaley and Wong, 1991).<br>Other questions to include: Directed to child—"If one parent makes a decision, can you appeal to the other parent to change it?" Directed to the parents—"What input do the children have in making decisions or discussing rules?" (Whaley and Wong, 1991). | The allocation of power will give an indication of each individual's sense of personal power. Decision-making in the family unit prepares the children in the family for problem-solving.<br>***Special Considerations:*** *A family who perceives the health care professional as having power or control over the ill family members may adapt to the health care professional's standards and not reveal psychosocial information/needs (Satariano and Briggs, 1989).* |
| 7. Assess family communication patterns. Consider:<br>a. Who answers interview questions?<br>b. Who talks to whom?<br>c. Who gives positive or negative reinforcement and to whom?<br>d. Which siblings talk with one another?<br>e. Are expressions of feelings, opinions, and beliefs allowed? For example, ask, "Is it O.K. to get angry/sad in your house? Who gets angry/sad most of the time? What do they do?" (Whaley and Wong, 1991).<br>f. Are problem-solving behaviors present? | Families that are functional have flexible and interactive communication patterns that respect opinions of all members, encourage expression of feelings, and promote mutual problem-solving. Satir (1964) calls the communication patterns of functional families "congruent" and proposes that congruent communication patterns enhance self-esteem. |
| 8. Assess the manner in which each family member is allowed to grow and change, e.g.:<br>a. Solutions to individual needs are provided in the family.<br>b. Individual members are warmly accepted and not labeled as "bad." Behavior changes are encouraged in a caring manner, and all family members accept some responsibility for family problems.<br>c. As children enter each developmental stage they are encouraged to master the tasks of that stage. | Functional families negotiate relationships so that individual needs are met. They view each member as an important and dynamic individual.<br>***Special Considerations:*** *Dysfunctional families often label one member as "the problem" (family scapegoat) with little hope for that individual to change; they give unrealistic labels and roles to its members, and take sides against another member (family triangles) (Bullock and Thompson, 1979).* |
| 9. Determine how stress affects the family.<br>a. For example, ask, "What is it like when the family is under a lot of stress?"<br>b. Determine individual members' coping strategies. | Individual family members may cope with stress differently, and the family may employ strategies as a unit to cope with a stressor impinging on all members. Lack of or limitations in coping can affect family interaction patterns, nurturance, and self-esteem of its members. |
| 10. Determine family support.<br>a. Ask each member who is the most help (support) to them in the family.<br>b. Note who sits next to whom, e.g., Do parents sit next to one another? Where do individual children sit with respect to the parents? (Bullock and Thompson, 1975).<br>c. Note presence and components of nurturing behaviors expressed: Who expressed them and to whom?<br>d. Ask how often the family uses persons outside of the family (friends, neighbors, relatives, church members, or support organizations) for verbal support and ventilation of feelings; and how often they use these persons for physical assistance, e.g., bringing in food or running errands.<br>e. Ask if each person, or the family as a whole, believes more support (or help) is needed. | Support within and without the family system can affect coping ability and family dynamics. |
| 11. Analyze family strengths and delineate identified psychosocial needs of the family. | Determining strengths and needs provides a foundational list that can be used when planning care. |
| 12. Incorporate needs and strengths into the plan of care. For example, if the child's mother is a primary source of nurturing for the child, encourage interactions that are nurturing (rocking chair available, private times for the child to be held and sung to, etc.), or if family supports are scarce, introduce the family members to other families that are experiencing similar problems. | The family's psychosocial needs are an important part of the plan of care. Strengths can be fostered to enhance coping and build self-esteem in the family. |
| 13. Refer the family to family therapy, if indicated. | When psychosocial needs are significant, referral to a family therapist can assist the family in developing coping skills and strength and improving the level of functioning. |

| Steps | Rationale |
|---|---|
| 14. Determine family boundaries by using the assessment information already gained. Examples of appropriate boundaries are:<br>a. Inside the family unit the parents mainly confide in one another or in a peer, not one of the children.<br>b. Individual family members' task performances are consistent with developmentally appropriate expectations. | Clear generational boundaries provide stability in families. In times of stress (e.g., hospitalization of a child) it is imperative that boundaries be clear and appropriate because the instability created by inappropriate boundaries may cause undue pressure on certain family members. |
| 15. Assess features of the home environment using one or a combination of the following methods: | The home environment plays a central role in children's health and development. Assessment of the environment provides a way to identify contextual and functional influences of environment on behavior. It yields information different from that obtained in other family assessments and complements findings on such family characteristics as needs, resources, and relationships. |
| a. Graphic representation (a drawing, photograph, or other method of presentation). | A graphic representation by means of pictures, drawings, or schematics is a simple, uncomplicated method of assessing the family's physical environment. For example, if the purpose is to determine wheelchair accessibility, doorways can be measured and the distance recorded.<br>***Special Considerations:*** *Not only can a graphic representation portray the environment unique to a family, it can also reflect change, providing evaluation of an intervention.* |
| b. Systematic observation (an alert and focused eye on behaviors and interactions between family members). | This approach could be used to demonstrate that environmental factors contributed to current health status or change in behavior. For example, systematic observation could reveal a child's interest in peeling lead-based paint or mother's and father's lack of parenting skills. |
| c. Formal measurement using home environment assessment tools (see boxes on pp. 249 and 250). Some tools are completed by the observer, others by the family. Some tools assess the home environment indirectly, without an actual visit to the home. | A growing number of valid and reliable tools provide a comprehensive means to assess certain features of the home environment accurately and with ease. The relationship of environment to behavior is usually assessed in the actual environment. While many tools overlap in content, some focus on children and others focus on families (Simeonsson, 1988).<br>***Special Considerations:*** *Tools typically have clear and complete directions for use.* |

| Evaluation Outcomes | Observational Guidelines |
|---|---|
| 1. Accurate psychosocial family assessment data is obtained. | A completed genogram or family APGAR is obtained. Charting reflects the family structure, nurturing behaviors observed, family decision-making and parenting style, rules, methods of discipline, roles of family members, family communication patterns, family boundaries, and ability to cope with stress. |
| 2. The plan of care reflects psychosocial family strengths and needs. | Psychosocial family information is reflected on the plan of care, e.g., psychosocial problems are identified and strengths are incorporated to facilitate coping of the child. |
| 3. Referrals are implemented as appropriate. | Review documentation for referral. Confer with therapist and/or family following initial visit. |

## Documentation

Document family genogram, family structure and developmental level, and psychosocial factors identified in the assessment. Nursing plan of care reflects psychosocial needs, as well as uses psychosocial data to enhance interventions with the child and family. Document any referrals initiated.

### *MEASURES FOR ASSESSMENT OF CHILD ENVIRONMENTS*

| | |
|---|---|
| Home Observation for the Measurement of the Environment (HOME)<br>Bureau of Educational Research<br>University of Arkansas<br>33rd Street & University Ave.<br>Little Rock, AK 72204 | The HOME is perhaps the best known instrument for assessing environments of infants (birth to 3 years) and young children (3 to 6 years). There is now a third level for assessing environments in the early elementary grades, (6 to 10 years) (Bradley and Caldwell, 1988). The HOME consists of a number of true/false items. There are two levels involving such subscales as emotional and verbal responsivity of the mother; avoidance of restriction and punishment; organization of physical and temporal environment; provision of appropriate play materials; maternal involvement with child; and opportunities for variety in daily stimulation. Items tap both the physical features (child has a push or pull toy) and the psychological features (mother spontaneously praises child's qualities or behavior twice during visit) of the environment. These measures can provide appropriate means for examining the relationship of the environment to the development progress of infants with disabilities (Caldwell, 1972). |
| Home Screening Questionnaire (HSQ)<br>Denver Developmental Materials, Inc.<br>P.O. Box 20037<br>Denver, CO 80220 | The HSQ was developed using HOME as a guide. For children 0 to 3 years old, there are 30 items plus a checklist of toys available to the child in the home. There are 34 items and a similar toy list for assessing the environment for children 3 to 6 years. Questions are at a third to sixth grade reading level. For each age group there is a minimum score for determining suspect or nonsuspect results. The HSQ can be completed by parents in any setting, taking about 15 to 20 minutes, contrasting with an hour home visit to administer HOME (Whaley and Wong, 1991). |
| Early Childhood Environment Rating Scale<br>Teachers College Press<br>1234 Amsterdam Ave.<br>New York, NY 10027 | Items are rated on a 7-point scale in the areas of personal care routines of children; furnishings and display for children; language-reasoning experiences; fine and gross motor activities; creative activities; social development; and adult needs. This measure is useful for assessing the day care or preschool setting (Harms and Clifford, 1980). |
| Purdue Home Stimulation Inventory<br>Feffer & Simons<br>1114 Avenue of the Americas<br>New York, NY 10036-7794 | Scores are based on questions and observations in three areas: aspects of child's rearing environment; stimulus characteristics of home; and state of the home. Measure includes items that document specific physical features (mobile over crib) as well as a range of psychological characteristics (rate of maternal speech) (Wach, Francis, and McQuiston, 1978). |
| Characteristics of the Inanimate Environment<br>Hemisphere Publishing<br>79 Madison Ave., Suite 1110<br>New York, NY 10016 | This observational measure documents the environment of the child in terms of responsiveness, complexity, and variety. Ratings are based on observations (time sampling) (Yarrow, Rubenstein, and Pedersen, 1975). |

Adapted from Simeonsson RJ: Assessing family environments. In Bailey DB and Simeonsson RJ, editors: Family assessment in early intervention, Columbus, Ohio, 1988, Merrill Publishing Co.; Bradley R and Caldwell B: Using the HOME inventory to assess the family environment, Pediatr Nurs 14(2):97-102, 1988; Busch-Rossnagel N: Review of the children's version of the family environment scale, Supplement to the ninth mental measurements yearbook, Lincoln, Neb, 1988, The Buros Institute of Mental Measurements; Whaley LF and Wong DL: Nursing care of infants and children, ed 4, St Louis, 1991, The CV Mosby Co.

### *MEASURES FOR ASSESSMENT OF FAMILY ENVIRONMENTS*

| | |
|---|---|
| Henderson Environments Learning Process Scale (HELPS)<br>Arizona Center for Early Childhood Education<br>The University of Arizona<br>1515 East First Street<br>Tucson, AZ 85719 | The HELPS measures the perceived characteristics of the home relative to child aspiration level, parental reinforcement practices, and educational opportunities. The measure uses a structured interview format employing a Likert-type scale (Henderson, Bergan, and Hurt, 1972). |
| Home Quality Rating Scale<br>UCLA/Neuropsychiatric Institute<br>760 Westwood Plaza<br>Los Angeles, CA 90024 | This scale was developed to portray the psychological climate of families of disabled children as it pertained to child-rearing attitudes and practices. A factor analysis of the scale items yields five main factors: harmony of the home and quality of parenting, concordance in parenting and marriage, openness and awareness of respondent, quality of the residential environment, and quality of the residential area. Interviewer ratings employ a variable format including 5-point rating scales and fixed choice responses (Myers, Mink, and Nihira, 1977). |
| Family Environment Scale (FES)<br>Consulting Psychologists Press, Inc.<br>577 College Ave.<br>Palo Alto, CA 94306 | FES was developed by drawing on the concept of environmental press as a determiner of behavior. In this instance environmental press means that the environment exerts its influence in several ways. Moos, Insel, and Humphrey (1974) emphasize that environments, like people, can be distinguished by their personalities. These environments could be described in terms of these following family dimensions: independence, structure, achievement, expression, moral/religious emphasis, or conflict. Items are answered in a true/false manner using pencil-and-paper method. |
| Children's Version of the Family Environment Scale (CVFES)<br>Slosson Educational Publications, Inc.<br>P.O. Box 280<br>East Aurora, NY 14052 | A downward extension of the Family Environment Scale (FES), Pino, Simons, and Slawinowski developed the CVFES to provide a measure of young children's subjective appraisal of their family environment. The 30-item test enables children ages 5 to 12 years to provide self-reports of family relationships. Their perceptions of 10 dimensions in three general areas of family functioning are assessed: Relationship Dimensions (Cohesion, Expressiveness, and Conflict); Personal Growth Dimensions (Independence, Achievement Orientation, Intellectual-Cultural Orientation, Active-Recreational Orientation, and Moral-Religious Emphasis); and System Maintenance Dimensions (Organization and Control). Each item has 3 pictures; each picture is a cartoonlike drawing of a mother, father, son, and/or daughter. The child is asked to select the picture from each grouping that "looks like your family" (Busch-Rossnagel, 1988). |

Adapted from Simeonsson RJ: Assessing family environments. In Bailey DB and Simeonsson RJ, editor: Family assessment in early intervention, Columbus, Ohio 1988, Merrill Publishing Co.; Bradley R and Caldwell B: Usingthe HOME inventory to assess the family environment, Pediatr Nurs 14(2):97-102, 1988; busch-Rossnagel N: Review of the children's version of the family environment scale, Supplement to the ninth mental measurements yearbook, Lincoln, Neb, Neb, 1988, The buros Institute of Mental Measurements; Whaley LF and Wong DL: Nursing care of infants and children, ed 4, St Louis, 1991, The CV Mosby Co.

# SKILL 39 Administering a Kinetic Family Drawing

*Judy Holt Rollins*

The Kinetic Family Drawing Test (KFD) is a projective test to be used with interviews and other therapy techniques. An age-independent measure for persons approximately 4 years old and above, the tool is useful for gathering information about a family system for the purpose of planning treatment and evaluation. It is helpful when additional information is needed to supplement other family assessment tools and techniques. It can be used with any family member, not just children.

## NURSING DIAGNOSES

Altered family processes related to situational/developmental transition or crisis; Ineffective family coping (compromised or disabling) related to unrealistic role expectations or unmet psychologic needs; Ineffective individual coping related to situational/maturational crises, inadequate family support, or unmet expectations; Impaired social interactions related to separation or loss of family member.

| Steps | Rationale |
|---|---|
| **Assessment** | |
| 1. Review information about subject.<br>a. Age.<br>b. Willingness to participate.<br>c. Suitability of this test for providing needed information. | The use of a method of nonverbal expression will often result in information unobtainable from verbal tools (Fig. 39-1).<br>***Special Considerations:*** *Offering a nonverbal means of expression is particularly helpful for young children and other family members who have difficulty communicating verbally. The KFD reflects the subject's perceptions at that moment in time.* |
| **Planning and Goal Setting** | |
| 1. Choose a convenient time that is free of interruptions to be alone with the subject. | People often become distracted or self-conscious when other people are in the room.<br>***Special Considerations:*** *Most children and adults will complete a KFD in 5 to 10 minutes. Commonly, all members produce KFD's together during the same session. The emphasis of such a session usually concerns the interaction between family members rather than the individual drawings themselves.* |
| 2. Develop an individualized client or family member goal:<br>▪ To complete a drawing of everyone in the family doing something. | |
| **Implementation** | |
| 1. Seat subject on a chair at a table of appropriate height. Place a sheet of plain white 8½ × 11 inch paper and a number 2 pencil with an eraser on the table directly in front of the subject. Instruct subject, "Draw everyone in your family doing something. Try to draw whole people, not cartoons or stick people. Remember, make everyone DOING something." | Young children usually express themselves more naturally and spontaneously through actions rather than through words. Drawing tests are simple to administer, normally nonthreatening, and can be used where other techniques are limited by language barriers, cultural deprivation, and inability to communicate verbally.<br>***Special Considerations:*** *If subject asks, "Should I draw myself?" repeat, "Draw everyone in your family." Should the subject continue to ask, say, "That is up to you." Stress that there is no right or wrong way to construct the drawing. It is simply a "quick way to get to know you better." Discontinue the test if the subject becomes unduly anxious or refuses to draw.* |

| Steps | Rationale |
|---|---|

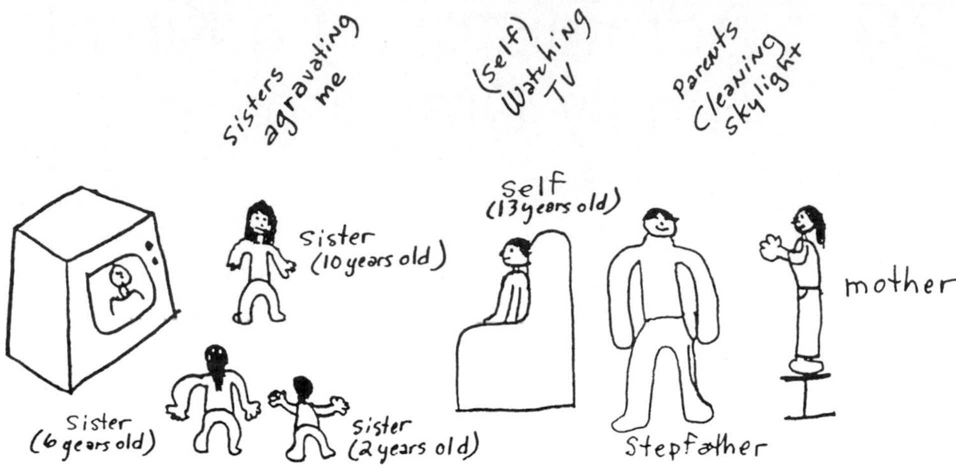


***FIG. 39-1*** The Kinetic Family Drawing (KFD) of a 13-year-old male with acute lymphoid leukemia. Note that everyone in the drawing is active, while the subject portrays himself in a passive activity—watching television. The mood of the drawing is rather sad, which, because later KFD's were cheerful, is probably because the subject was about to undergo a lumbar puncture.

2. Tell subject, "I will be making some simple notes while you are drawing. We will talk about your drawing and my notes when you are finished."

Information may be obtained from the subject's running narrative, the chatter that often accompanies the drawing process with children.

***Special Considerations:*** *Adults, teenagers, and older children may be more comfortable alone. They may be instructed to write thoughts and comments directly on the drawing.*

3. Note: Who was drawn first? Last? Was there any hesitation? Heavy pressure applied? Was heavy pressure used with all family members, or just certain ones? Also note any comments the subject makes while drawing.

Observations of the drawing process often reveal feelings such as anger toward a particular family member or jealousy.

***Special Considerations:*** *Be sure to note any erasures. Try to save questions until after the drawing is completed, but if a subject begins to "open up" while drawing, do not lose the opportunity for discussion.*

4. Wait for an indication that the subject has finished drawing.

Allow subject to proceed at natural pace for a reasonable period of time.

***Special Considerations:*** *Subjects usually announce when the drawing is complete. If no announcement is made, ask, "Are you finished?"*

5. When subject has completed drawing, first look for omission of family members.

Subject will often omit someone they wish were not in the family, or even omit self if not feeling a part of or wanting not to be in the family.

***Special Considerations:*** *If subject has omitted a family member or self, ask, "Is this everyone in your family?" Ask about missing family members. Subject may include them or explain omission, e.g., "Well, I am in the hospital."*

6. Ask subject to explain what each family member is doing. Add this data to notes.

Because individuals attach different meanings to symbols and activities, it is important to learn what the subject intended.

***Special Considerations:*** *Younger children will often present information in a story format. Much additional information can be gathered at this time through pertinent questions.*

7. Thank subject and offer praise for a job well done.

Showing appreciation for the subject's sharing information may encourage future expression of feelings and raise level of self-esteem.

***Special Considerations:*** *At this time children often ask for the drawing. A copy may be made or children may want to produce another drawing of choice.*

**Steps** | **Rationale**

### *ANALYZING A KINETIC FAMILY DRAWING*

What is your first impression?
Who and what do you see?
What is happening?
How do you feel about what is happening?
What do you notice about physical intimacy or distance?
Is the KFD warm or cold, soft or hard, pleasant or unpleasant?
Are people touching or are they shut off from each other?
Who is facing whom?
How do people in the KFD feel about their bodies?
- Are they using their bodies to show off?
- To hide?
- To be seductive?
- Are they proud of their bodies?
- Ashamed?

Who's ascendant? (Near the top of the page)
Who's descendant? (Near the bottom of the page)

Are the KFD "people":
- Happy?
- Sad?
- Sadistic?
- Suffering?
- Blank?
- Bored?
- Rigid?
- Strong?
- Involved?
- Detached?
- Angry?
- Subservient?
- Trusting?
- Satisfied?

How does the group relate?
Are they tense or relaxed?
What are their messages toward each other?
Do you feel love present?
Is it a family you would like to be a member of?

Adapted from Burns RC: Self-growth in families: kinetic family drawings (KFD) research and application, New York, 1982, Brunner/Mazel Publishers.

8. Analyze the drawing. For a simple analysis, see box.

Drawings may be analyzed on many levels, depending upon knowledge of projective drawing techniques.

***Special Considerations:*** *Avoid overinterpretation. Seek the opinion of an art therapist or clinical psychologist when meaning of drawing is unclear.*

## Evaluation Outcomes

1. The subject successfully produces a family drawing providing information for assessment in the diagnostic areas listed above.

## Observational Guidelines

Observe subject's ability to follow instructions and complete the drawing.

## Documentation

Record observations about drawing from notes and subject's behavior before, during, and after the test. Include in notes any verbal information subject added. Document interpretations based on personal level of knowledge of projective drawing techniques.

# SKILL 40 Promoting Bonding Between Parents and Children

*Lynn B. Clutter*

A close relationship between parent and child is healthy and occurs when bonding is adequate. Bonding is defined as the growth and maintenance of responsiveness between members of a parent-child dyad. Other qualities are inherent within bonding, including specificity in person, persistence over time or separation, and the existence of affectional aspects. The terms attachment and bonding are often used synonomously. Since this skill is applicable to a wide age range, developmental changes in the dyad are highlighted.

Identifiable characteristics can be assessed to determine the extent of or to foster bonding within a specific relationship. Critical times for fostering close family relationships occur with the addition of a family member, illnesses, or hospitalization. Development and maintenance of bonding during these times can significantly improve health, enhance well-being, and enrich a family. For infants, absence of this type of close, consistent relationship has been shown to result in abnormal development, increased susceptibility to disease, personality changes and even death. Similar but perhaps less severe results have been noted in people of other ages. The purpose of this skill is to provide descriptions of the characteristics and process of bonding, to facilitate accurate assessment, then strengthen the parent-child bonding through appropriate goals and interventions.

## NURSING DIAGNOSES

Altered family process related to addition of a new family member, maturational crisis, or separation from family members; Altered parenting related to change in family unit, interruption in bonding process, lack of knowledge about parenting, or unrealistic expectations of self, infant or family; Health seeking behaviors (bonding) related to infant—child health promotion.

| Steps | Rationale |
|---|---|
| **Assessment** | |
| 1. Assess situational characteristics.<br>a. Age of family members.<br>b. Developmental stage of children, parents, and family.<br>c. Other (e.g., health status, adoption, family constellation, social support systems, culture, etc.). | Situational variables affect the type of bonding characteristics displayed. For example, a parent will demonstrate bonding in different ways with an infant as compared to a school-age child. |
| 2. Assess for general characteristics of bonding.<br>*Dyad assessment:* | Some qualities of bonding and attachment are evident in all parent-child relationships. |
| a. Observe for sensory expressions of bonding and attachment. | Although bonding has important internal aspects, the physical aspects are most easily identified; specifically the visual, tactile, vocal, and auditory senses. |
| ▪ Visual: Eye-to-eye contact (looking at the other). | Unless culturally inappropriate, frequent eye contact is prevalent in close dyad relationships. |
| ▪ Tactile: Physical contact. | Physical contact is a hallmark of bonding in any relationship. The type and amount of contact will vary with age and is culturally influenced. |
| ▪ Vocal/auditory communication: Mutuality; talking directly to the other person; affectional tones and content; presence of specialized communications, e.g., pet names; attentive to the other's communications. | Vocal and verbal expressions are another primary means of demonstrating and developing bonding. These features are characteristic of bonded dyads. |
| b. Observe body language while interacting. | Nonverbal messages that occur during interactions reflect the depth of bonding. |
| ▪ Entrainment, or a reciprocity in communication. | Sensitivity to one another will be evident in communications through a "back and forth" nature of talk and body posture. |
| ▪ Positive affect with interactions (e.g., warmth, smiling, facial brightening). | Positive affect is common during interactions of those with close dyad bonding. |
| ▪ Specific displays of affection: type, frequency, and mutuality. | Some form of affectional actions are present between those with adequate bonding, demonstrating that the other is a uniquely valued person. Expressions are especially common with greetings and separations. Culture, family, individual, and relationship differences exist. |

| Steps | Rationale |
|---|---|
| c. Assess behavior during stress, threat of or actual separation (i.e., proximity seeking, separation avoidance). | Dyad members may seek proximity and resist separation, sometimes with great protest, especially during times of stress. The presence of this behavior is stable, although the frequency of expression reduces with age. Dyads with adequate bonding experience a measure of comfort after closer proximity is gained. |
| *Parent toward child assessment*: | Some behaviors are typically parental.<br>***Special Considerations:*** *Differences in maternal and paternal bonding have been identified, but it is unclear if differences are a result of gender, role with the child, or other variables.* |
| a. Responsiveness to child's cues that reflect needs or desires. | In dyads with adequate bonding, responsiveness and sensitivity to these cues are evident in the parent's actions.<br>***Special Considerations:*** *Some children may send cues that are vague and difficult to read. Assess for both clarity of cues and speed or adequacy of parental response.* |
| b. Availability: In time, emotional energy, attention, etc. | Type and amount of availability will vary, but the quality is important for adequate bonding.<br>***Special Considerations:*** *Parent may lack emotional availability during times of stress, fatigue, depression, or emotional conflict.* |
| c. General acceptance of child and behavior. | ***Special Considerations:*** *While specific behaviors may be unacceptable for a child, an overall acceptance of the child is characteristic.* |
| d. Nurturance, protection caregiving. | The types of activities demonstrated by the parent vary with the age of the child, but consistency, adequacy, and an underlying caring approach should be evident. |
| *Child toward parent assessment*:<br>a. Specific behaviors that are expressed for the purpose of obtaining and maintaining parental proximity or caretaking. | The actual behaviors may vary in type and effectiveness, but the purposes are generally stable. |
| b. Increase in proximity-seeking behaviors, especially when tired, hungry, upset, or alarmed (Bowlby, 1969). | The child with adequate bonding seeks proximity especially during stress, even with common situations such as naptime.<br>***Special Considerations:*** *Types of stress will change with age.* |
| c. Increased quieting or settling is evident with the parent present. | The presence of an attachment figure has a comforting effect. |
| d. Use of parent as a "secure base" from which to gain security and reassurance then to separate and explore. | Children tend to look to parent as a secure "touchpoint" or base. Young children demonstrate more frequent proximity seeking. |
| 3. Assess age-specific bonding characteristics (Table 40-1). | Progressive age and developmental status affect the expression of bonding. |
| 4. Assess verbalizations that reflect the person's internal thoughts, commitments, feelings, or values toward the relationship or the other person.<br>a. Listen for comments, e.g., a father of a hospitalized child states, "He's got to get better, he's my fishing partner." | Mind, will, emotions, and values are involved in bonding. Internal perceptions underlie outward expressions of bonding. These aspects may be assessed by verbalized comments. They are important because one can "perform" some of the actions without having the internal qualities necessary for adequate bonding. On the other hand, the internal qualities may be present but inadequately or inappropriately expressed. |
| b. Ask related questions or make statements, e.g., a nurse replies, "You seem to feel pretty close to him." | If adequate bonding is demonstrated, questions may not be necessary. If bonding adequacy is of concern, inquiries may reveal areas of needed growth. |
| 5. Assess factors that may hinder the bonding process (see box on p. 257). | Careful consideration of possible hindrances can provide valuable insights and directions for care. Hindrances may be subtle or readily evident. |
| 6. Observe for signs of negative interactions between parent and child. Note any behavior that is opposite to bonding characteristics (e.g., an infant may excessively display gaze aversion, a parent may lack sensitivity to a child's cues, or either may display excessive dependence or avoidance). | Consideration of observed negative interactions can help determine need for bonding or other types of interventions. Bonding inadequacies can be one of numerous causes for negative interactions.<br>***Special Considerations:*** *See the box on Attachment Disorders on p. 257 for signs of severe disorders indicating a need for referral.* |
| 7. Identify types and numbers of relationships with significant others. | Inappropriate types or numbers of relationships can reveal bonding inadequacies or hindrances. |
| 8. Note if any other family dyads appear to be stressful or poorly bonded. | Problems in one family relationship can affect bonding in other relationships.<br>***Special Considerations:*** *Divorce or separation has a strong impact on bonding between parents and children (see Skill 22).* |

**TABLE 40-1** Age-specific Bonding Characteristics

| Age | Dyad Interaction | Parent to Child | Child to Parent |
|---|---|---|---|
| Infant | Characterized by:<br>Monotrophy (attaching to one figure, usually the mother, and later to others); a cycle of infant cue, parental response, and infant contentment.<br>Assess:<br>Dyad interaction and communication; context in which attachment behaviors are manifested; entrainment (rhythmicity of body motions and vocalizations between parent and infant while interacting); affect (attention, facial brightness, amount of smiling, etc.). | Characterized by:<br>An underlying warmth and positive valuing of the infant. Sensitivity and consistent availability in seeing and meeting infant's needs.<br>Assess:<br>Visualization of infant (e.g., inspecting, attempts to gain eye to eye contact); presence, amount, and type of touching the parent displays (stroking, cuddling, enfolding, patting, hugging, kissing); observe gentleness of handling and provision of comfort measures; appropriateness of alerting actions (e.g., rocking or gently bouncing the infant); vocal interactions for content, extent of involvement, pitch, rhythm; degree of parental listening; adequacy and consistency of parenting skills. | Characterized by:<br>Attentiveness, facial brightening, visual alertness, eye contact and vocalizations during alert interactions; smiling, nestling, cuddling when held.<br>Assess:<br>Response to being held by parent; turning and searching to hear parent's voice; reaction to comforting; quality of alertness in response to parent; with older infants determine use of locomotion, grasping, and reaching to gain and maintain proximity to parent. |
| Toddler | Characterized by:<br>Frequent contact and affectional touches; greater reciprocity in the dyad relationship; frequent short cycles of separation and return.<br>Assess:<br>Presence of playful or affectional types of touch; verbal negotiation of goals to accommodate both parent and toddler needs; proximity seeking by toddler (especially during stressful and fearful events); separation resistance; level of contact seeking after separation. | Characterized by:<br>"Retrieval" behavior with aim of security and proximity maintenance; warmth and affectional content in verbal exchanges; visual and/or auditory tuning to child. Communication is animated and adapted to toddler's level; emotional availability but increased limit setting.<br>Assess:<br>Parent's continued availability for touchpointing (being accessible as a "secure base"); willingness to allow exploration; awareness of child's whereabouts; conversation for affect, animation of vocal tones, frequency of initiation, and content; affectional eye contact. | Characterized by:<br>A mix of exploration, then touchpointing upon return; regular proximity seeking; visual orientation toward and frequent observation of parent and parental responses.<br>Assess:<br>Proximity-seeking behavior (e.g., climbing on parent's lap or clinging); touchpointing with parent; frequent verbal and especially nonverbal expressions of affection and desire for proximity; increase in attachment behaviors when child is hungry, alarmed, or rebuffed, has strayed too far, or is separated from parent. |
| School-age | Characterized by:<br>Greater "give and take" in dyad relationship; reduction in frequency or length of affectional touches; greater reliance on verbal expression.<br>Assess:<br>Mutuality in affection, assistance, and communication; presence and amount of verbal and physical affectional expressions. | Characterized by:<br>Parents' continued primacy in influence, guidance, and emotional support; parental availability at special or critical times. Attachment is less tied to physical meeting of needs and more to emotional availability.<br>Assess:<br>Presence and adequacy of nurturance, responsiveness, and emotional availability; perceived adequacy of time spent with child; parent's presence during critical times for child; amount and style of parental training and discipline. | Characterized by:<br>Attachment behaviors, especially when away from peers and/or during stress; decreased direct affectional expression.<br>Assess:<br>Presence of direct attachment behaviors (e.g., contact seeking) and indirect behaviors (e.g., joking with parent). |

***TABLE 40-1*** **Age-specific Bonding Characteristics—cont'd**

| Age | Dyad Interaction | Parent to Child | Child to Parent |
|---|---|---|---|
| Adolescent | Characterized by:<br>Increase in reciprocity; sensitivity to respective needs; reduction in time spent together. | Characterized by:<br>Lessening of authoritative role, but continued availability for emotional support and guidance; acceptance of adolescent as preadult. | Characterized by:<br>Strengthened tie and internal perception of closeness to parent, despite possible differences in beliefs, values, and practices. Child may be outwardly less expressive. |
| | Assess:<br>Quality of relationship through individual inquiry; general tone and comfort level of dyad; communication for elements indicative of bonding (e.g., friendly kidding) or problems (e.g., yelling or ignoring). | Assess:<br>Compatibility and acceptance of adolescent even though differences may exist; willingness to work through changes that accompany adolescence; easing of parental limits; communication styles, especially in areas of problem solving and affectional qualities; continued eye contact and physical touch, though brief and less frequent; greater mutuality in decision making. | Assess:<br>Desire to maintain proximity and closeness; frequency of indirect attachment behaviors; adjustment to expectations of increased responsibility; desire to maintain relationship over time. |

### *GROUPS AT HIGHER RISK FOR DELAY OF OR INADEQUACIES IN BONDING**

**PARENTS**

Mothers with physical complications of birth
Single parent
Physical, mental or sensory disability
Critically ill
Chronic illness
Absence of social support systems
Family discord
Low self-image or negative emotional overtones
Overbearing or excessive in correction/punishment
Conflictual parental relationship with own parent

**INFANTS AND CHILDREN**

Unexpected or unwanted
Multiple births
Prematurity
Critically ill
Chronic illness
Physical, mental, or sensory disability
Developmental delay
In foster care or blended families
Born shortly after another sibling
Strong willed and/or rebellious to parent

**SPECIFIC DYADS**

Lack of temperament fit between parent and infant
Early and/or prolonged separation
Acute or chronic stress in the relationship
Those in dysfunctional families
Lower socioeconomic status without adequate emotional resources and social support

*Not all parents or children within these groups are genuinely at risk, however, it is important to consider the factors listed to determine presence of risk.

### *ATTACHMENT DISORDERS*

Children demonstrating some of the following symptoms may warrant referral to a mental health professional. Regular presence of most or all of the following symptoms warrants referral to a mental health professional or facility (see Product References) qualified to treat attachment disorders. (Treatment for severe attachment disorders is often controversial and may vary considerably with professionals.)

1. Lack of ability to give and receive affection (is not cuddly).
2. Abnormalities of eye contact, e.g., eye-to-eye contact avoidance.
3. Superficially engaging and "charming."
4. Phoniness.
5. Indiscriminately affectionate with strangers.
6. Destructive to self, others, and material things (accident-prone).
7. Cruelty to others or pets.
8. Obvious or absurd lying.
9. No impulse control (frequently acts hyperactive).
10. Learning lags or disorders.
11. Lack of cause and effect thinking.
12. Lack of conscience.
13. Abnormal eating patterns (food stealing, hoarding, or gorging).
14. Poor peer relationships (lack of long-term friendships).
15. Preoccupation with fire, blood, and gore.
16. Persistent nonsense questions and incessant chatter.
17. Inappropriately demanding and clingy.
18. Abnormal speech patterns.

Additional factors include:

1. Abnormalities in early history.
2. Parents may appear unreasonably angry or hostile.
3. Parent's relationship with other children seems generally healthy.
4. Parental reports about child's abnormal behaviors are consistent with those of teachers, care providers, and neighbors.

Adapted from Cline FW: Understanding and treating the severely disturbed child, Evergreen, Colo, 1979, Evergreen Consultants.

**Steps** | **Rationale**

### *SELECTED TOOLS FOR BONDING AND ATTACHMENT*

**MOTHER-INFANT**

Cropley C et al: Assessment tool for measuring maternal attachment behaviors. In McNall L and Galeener J, editors: Current practice in obstetric and gynecologic nursing, St Louis, 1976, The CV Mosby Co.

Reiser S: A tool to facilitate mother-infant attachment, JOGNN 10(4):294-297, 1981.

Funke J and Irby M: An instrument to assess the quality of maternal behavior, JOGNN 7(5):19-22, 1978.

**SIBLING-INFANT**

Marecki M et al: Early sibling attachment, JOGNN 14(5):418-423, 1985.
*Not a complete tool but has a listing of characteristics.*

**FATHER-INFANT**

Greenberg M and Morris N: Engrossment: the newborn's impact upon the father, Am J Orthopsych 44(4):520-531, 1974.
*Not a complete tool but has a listing of characteristics.*

Peterson G et al: The role of some birth-related variables in father attachment, Am J Orthopsych 49(2):330-338, 1979.

Wieser MA and Castiglia PT: Assessing early father-infant attachment, MCN 9:104-106, 1984.

**MOTHER/FATHER-CHILD**

Ainsworth M and Wittig B: Attachment and exploratory behavior of one-year-olds in a strange situation. In Foss BM, editor: Determinants of infant behavior, vol 4, London 1969, Methuen.
*Primarily for mothers and 1-year-olds but has been used with other dyads and older ages.*

9. For further assessment of attachment and bonding within specific relationships, see list of suggested formal tools in the box above.

Tools used for research and practice are often quick, comprehensive, and have established validity and reliability.

## Planning and Goal Setting

1. Determine if bonding behaviors are progressing developmentally. If bonding is deemed adequate, affirm adequacy as appropriate.

If bonding is developmentally appropriate, interventions may be unnecessary. Affirmation can be beneficial acknowledgment, especially in times of stress.

2. Identify areas of teaching to promote bonding if inadequate.

If bonding is inadequate, teaching to promote it is essential, especially during a stressful event.

3. Set appropriate time and environment for specific interventions with parent and child.

Appropriate timing and situation can limit disruptions and allow for greater effectiveness.

***Special Considerations:*** *Spontaneous interactions can also be beneficial, especially when affirming bonding.*

4. Review bonding characteristics that are related to the specific culture and dyad. (For example: A Japanese father-infant dyad will demonstrate bonding in a different manner than will a Native American mother-child dyad.)

A knowledge of general tendencies or characteristics of bonding can provide a backdrop of information from which to determine specific bonding goals and care.

5. Develop individualized child/family goals:
   - Parent and child will demonstrate appropriate bonding behaviors.

## Implementation

### *General interventions*

1. Identify and encourage aspects of bonding strength. For example, say, "I noticed that you are really available for her when she comes to touch base with you. She seems to gain security, then is able to explore."

Encouragement strengthens the behavior. If changes are needed in some areas, identifying strengths can foster receptivity to further interventions for bonding deficits.

2. Describe and support any observed reciprocity of cues between the child and parent.

By identifying the cycles of reciprocity, growth of awareness and valuing of mutual responsiveness can occur.

3. Discuss own perceptions of the relationship and benefits of a close bond. For example, say, "I notice that when you praise her she seems to try harder to breathe deep for her respiratory treatments."

This type of discussion emphasizes and perhaps increases the internal valuing of bonding.

| Steps | Rationale |
|---|---|
| 4. Promote the value of parent-child bonding in general. For example, say, "Having a close relationship with a parent can often help a child cope with a chronic illness." | Two important presuppositions to this intervention are that the valuing of dyad bonding can be imparted and that greater valuing of bonding will lead to greater bonding in the dyad. |
| 5. Discuss with parent developmentally appropriate and age-appropriate bonding characteristics, needs, behaviors, and abilities. | Awareness of appropriate characteristics for a child and for the parent-child relationship assists a parent in developing reasonable expectations. Inappropriate expectations can hinder bonding. |
| 6. Identify specific behaviors that would improve bonding, e.g., gaining eye contact before talking with a toddler. Then do one or more of the following as appropriate:<br>a. Discuss importance of the behavior.<br>b. Model the behavior.<br>c. Teach, then demonstrate, the behavior.<br>d. Teach, then observe, the behavior in dyad interaction. | Multiple reasons could explain the lack of appropriate bonding behaviors by dyad members. One is simply a lack of information. Teaching bonding behaviors is informative. It does not necessarily increase internal aspects of bonding (feelings, commitment, etc.) but can promote dyad communication of bonding. |
| 7. Mention observed behaviors that could be interfering with bonding, e.g., chronic infant crying with limited consolability or excessive parental anger; then intervene accordingly. | Numerous behaviors delay development and hinder the maintenance of bonding.<br>***Special Considerations:*** *Additional teaching may be indicated on observed behaviors, and/or referral to support groups or other health professionals.* |
| 8. Address specific bonding needs within families who are at higher risk (see box on p. 257). For example, a blended family dyad may benefit from receiving a list of strategies to improve step relationships. | Offering specialized interventions that address risk factors can reduce hindrances to bonding. |
| ***Interventions for dyads with a hospitalized child*** | |
| 1. Have parent describe how they and their child show their love to each other. | Identifying usual behaviors provides information for further interventions and indirectly emphasizes the importance of maintaining closeness. |
| 2. Encourage close proximity and usual displays of affection. Offer suggestions for new methods of expression toward one another when usual ones are not possible. For example, if a hug is not possible, holding a hand might be encouraged; if ongoing presence is not possible, recording a message or reading a story on tape may be helpful. | The parent or older child may be embarrassed or feel inhibited expressing affection in front of others. Encouraging such behavior and providing suggestions for restrictive situations communicates both that the behavior is acceptable and important.<br>***Special Considerations:*** *The potential for growth of dyad bonding exists during hospitalization. The threats of harm or loss can serve to put the relationship in a different perspective, strengthening it.* |
| 3. Promote parental caregiving and presence. | Presence fulfills a child's desire for proximity during a stressful situation. Caregiving invites further expressions of bonding and acts to reduce the threatening nature of the situation. |
| 4. Encourage parental expressions of bonding before, during, or following stressful procedures. Give the parent and child (if old enough) the choice of parental presence during and immediately following procedures (see Skill 1). | Since attachment behavior is more frequently demonstrated and needed by a child during times of stress, opportunity should be available for its expression. |
| 5. Teach the older child new ways of giving cues for parental presence or care. Demonstrate nonverbal cues or state possible wording for verbal cues, e.g., "Sometimes it helps to have your mom be near. When you want her to come close, you can pat the bed and smile or can say, Mom, sit with me please." | The child has the capacity to learn positive behaviors that foster bonding. Sending clear cues leads to a greater chance of having needs met.<br>***Special Considerations:*** *Usual cues may need to be modified while in the hospital.* |
| 6. Provide strategies to reduce separations and separation stress. For example:<br>a. Limit frequency and length of separations.<br>b. Encourage use of the telephone, pictures, tape recordings, or exchange of special items that represent the person. | Separation stress may go unnoticed but can diminish a child's coping resources.<br>***Special Considerations:*** *If a child gives a parent a gift such as a personal drawing, a snapshot of the parent holding the drawing while at home or at work can be meaningful.* |
| ***Interventions for clinic or home visits*** | |
| 1. Verbally identify parent-child bonding behaviors. | Supporting strengths fosters healthy behaviors. |
| 2. When a problem is observed, use an indirect approach to address the issue but avoid verbalizing the problem. For example:<br>a. "Occasionally a child of this age can resist a parent's affection. Have you noticed anything like that?"<br>b. "Let's talk about family relationships."<br>c. "A good time to seek outside help is when a (parent, child, or family) is experiencing ________. A (nurse, pediatrician, psychologist, etc.) may help." | An indirect approach is less threatening and can promote further dialog. |

| Steps | Rationale |
|---|---|
| 3. Use a direct approach to verbalize and confront a specific problem, e.g., "You and Timmy seem to avoid looking at each other." | A direct approach is helpful for deeper problems that are hidden or are blind spots. |
| ***Interventions with the parent-newborn dyad*** | |
| 1. Encourage and model bonding behaviors with the infant during routine care. | Modeling allows opportunity for learning the techniques of infant caretaking. |
| 2. Highlight attributes that parent views as positive (e.g., If a father proudly states, "He has my eyes," positive comments about the infant's eyes can promote bonding). | When a parent already sees a "special" quality in the infant, having another appreciate the quality can further the development of bonding. |
| 3. Address variables that may be hindering early bonding (e.g., if a difficult labor and delivery was experienced, encourage discussion of experiences and feelings). | ***Special Considerations:*** *The time surrounding birth can be filled with hindrances to bonding. Resolution of hindrances allows bonding to occur and is often more effective with early intervention.* |
| 4. Teach parent behavioral characteristics and responses of the infant including:<br>a. Infant states, especially quiet alert.<br>b. Cues of readiness for attention and of overstimulation.<br>c. Care eliciting behaviors and distress signals.<br>d. Reflexes and positive individual characteristics of infant.<br>e. Positive responses that infant demonstrates toward parent. | Once understood, infant behavioral characteristics can be powerful forces in promoting caretaking and bonding (Brazelton, 1984; Nugent, 1985). With a greater understanding of their child, parents can provide more sensitive and appropriate care. It is essential that the parent realize the importance of responding to an infant's distress. Early relief of distress fosters trust, vital for bonding. Positive results from care can increase both parent to infant and infant to parent bonding.<br>***Special Considerations:*** *Adoptive parents especially benefit from instruction on specific and general infant characteristics.* |
| 5. Teach parent appropriate timing and methods of engaging infant's attention, e.g.:<br>a. Darken the room.<br>b. Maintain infant's body temperature by having a warm room temperature or skin to skin contact.<br>c. Provide vestibular stimulation such as swaying, rocking or gently bouncing if infant is drowsy.<br>d. Provide swaddling or hold limbs if baby is active or crying.<br>e. Hold infant so eye contact can be gained.<br>f. Talk rhythmically with infant.<br>g. If inattentive, postpone interaction or reduce stimulation.<br>h. Interact after physical needs are met and while alert. | When interactions take place during quiet alert periods, greater chance of mutual responsiveness is possible. Learning methods of alerting and interacting can lead to more frequent interactions and thus greater bonding potential. |
| 6. Stress importance of responding to infant's signals of distress such as fretfulness, crying. | Early responsiveness fosters bonding and the establishment of trust. |

| Evaluation Outcomes | Observational Guidelines |
|---|---|
| 1. Physical expressions of bonding (visual, tactile, vocal, auditory, etc.) are displayed by each dyad member toward the other. | Observe during times of greeting, interaction, or departure. Expressions such as eye contact, hugs, words of affection, etc. indicate bonding. |
| 2. Expressions of bonding are appropriate for age, developmental status, and type of relationship. | Compare observed behaviors to established age-appropriate attachment behaviors. |
| 3. Parents and child maintain internal aspects of bonding (feelings, commitment, thoughts toward and about the other). | Listen for statements or actions that reflect internal bonding. An example is a child who cries for Daddy in the night, or a parent who misses work to be with a child during a stressful procedure. |
| 4. Infant and parent develop and demonstrate adequate early bonding characteristics. | Infant displays proximity seeking and maintaining activities such as crying and cooing, comfort to parent's presence and caretaking. Parent displays physical characteristics such as eye and skin contact, warm and expressive communication. |
| 5. Usual bonding behaviors are maintained (if possible) while hospitalized. | Parent and child have comfortable, close contact and proximity. Displays of affection are present. |
| 6. While hospitalized, alternate bonding behaviors are developed when usual ones are not possible. | Behaviors such as hand holding, patting and verbal expressions are demonstrated. |

## Documentation

Documentation should include an assessment of the relationship (e.g., mother-infant) and the physical characteristics of bonding observed while parent and child were interacting (e.g., touch, eye contact, alerting of infant etc.). Record statements that especially demonstrate presence of internal commitment, depth of loving feelings or thoughts toward the other person.

Note any lack in bonding characteristics and indicate variables that appear to be interfering with bonding. Document other relationships that appear to be significant. Record the content of parent/child teaching, the type of instruction, and the outcome. Document all supportive and affirmative interventions used.

# SKILL 41 Providing Culturally Sensitive Care

*Janice S. Hayes and Melanie C. Dreher*

Culture is defined as "an acquired knowledge people use to interpret experience and generate behavior." When attempting to understand behavior, one should consider the family's heritage. There is variation in health care practices and beliefs among and even within different cultures. Effective health care and nursing care require knowledge of and sensitivity to cultural variation in beliefs and customs, health care practices, language, child rearing methods, dietary practices, and physical differences. While general information about a culture can be helpful, variations are numerous even within specific cultural groups. For this reason, individual and family assessments are vital.

A culture is composed of individuals with a common set of values, beliefs, practices, and information that is learned, integrative, social, and satisfying. Cultural variables can exert great influence on the family's acceptance or rejection of care. Culturally informed planning, implementation, and evaluation can increase effectiveness and acceptability of care.

## NURSING DIAGNOSES

Spiritual distress related to conflict between cultural beliefs and prescribed health regimen; Altered health maintenance related to cultural beliefs; Anxiety related to unconscious conflict about essential values; Decisional conflict related to perceived threat to value system; Impaired verbal communication related to language or cultural barriers.

| Steps | Rationale |
|---|---|
| **Assessment** | |
| 1. Assess the family structure by discussion and direct observation.<br>a. Determine who is considered to be family members.<br>b. Identify the decision maker regarding the child's care.<br>c. Identify the child's caregivers.<br>d. Determine who is the primary caregiver.<br>e. Determine what roles each family member plays. | The concept of family varies among cultures. Family ties within some cultures or subcultures may be especially strong. Family groups rather than the parents may be decision makers or decisions may be concentrated in one or two specific family members such as a grandfather or maternal uncle. |
| 2. Review the beliefs and customs of the child's culture.<br>a. Talk with individuals of the cultural group to learn about general beliefs and customs.<br>b. Review literature and maintain a file of written information related to specific ethnic or cultural groups. | There is wide variation among different cultures in health care beliefs and practices, e.g., the concept of illness as a result of opposing forces within the body is held by some cultural groups while other cultures may attribute illness to witchcraft and the manipulation of evil spirits. Conflicts may arise with the dominant culture because the family may feel that the child is not receiving the correct treatment. |
| c. Ask the child and family about their beliefs and customs: "What do you think causes illness?" "How do you usually treat illness?" "What do you think will help you get well?" "What things would you like us to do?" | Gaining an awareness of culturally related views can increase sensitivity of care.<br>***Special Considerations:*** *Beliefs about causes of illness may be inconsistent with scientific information. Religious beliefs and health care practices are frequently intertwined.* |
| 3. Assess the health care practices of the family:<br>a. Determine what the family usually does about particular illnesses or problems.<br>b. Ask family members how they usually maintain health. | There is variation in health care practices in different cultural groups.<br>***Special Considerations:*** *Use of folk healers and folk medicines is common among some groups. It is not uncommon for Western medicine to be used in conjunction with folk remedies.* |
| 4. Determine the primary language or form of communication used by the family. | Language barriers may exist when the child/family is not fluent in the language of the health care giver. Subtle variations in the meaning and interpretation of words may occur even within a language.<br>***Special Considerations:*** *Interpreters must be well-versed in both languages and understand clearly the message being conveyed. They must also be carefully selected because different dialects within a language may contribute to misunderstanding.* |

| Steps | Rationale |
|---|---|
| 5. Determine the family's dietary patterns and preferences:<br>a. Ask about a typical day's diet.<br>b. Ask about food preferences and dislikes.<br>c. Ask if certain foods are regarded as having special benefits. | Food selection and preparation often vary from culture to culture.<br>***Special Considerations:*** *Beliefs about curative and restorative effects of food may exist; some groups use specific food to restore body imbalances, especially for "hot" and "cold" diseases.* |
| 6. Assess the child in accordance with known information about physical differences (see Skills 27 and 28). | A knowledge base of physical differences is necessary for accurate assessments.<br>***Special Considerations:*** *Growth patterns for different racial groups may reflect norms that are different from standard norms of height and weight charts established in North American populations. Risk factors for different groups also should be recognized and considered, e.g., sickle cell and thalassemia.* |
| 7. Review cultural taboos and sanctions of this culture.<br>a. Use information from review of cultural beliefs.<br>b. Ask if there are any special limitations or proscriptions for pregnant women or children. | These may affect acceptance or rejection of a treatment or intervention as well as of the health care provider.<br>***Special Considerations:*** *For example, in some Caribbean societies it is considered dangerous for someone to stare at a baby or young child. Certain dietary restrictions may apply to pregnant women, infants, and children. Violations of these taboos are believed to adversely affect their health and well-being.* |
| 8. Determine the family's degree of adherence to cultural heritage. | General patterns may not apply to any individual in a group as cultural groups are not homogeneous. Stereotyping should be avoided. For example, it would be incorrect to assume that if a family is from Latin America, the members necessarily endorse the hot-cold theory of disease. |

## Planning and Goal Setting

| | |
|---|---|
| 1. Develop a plan of care in collaboration with the child and family including the designated decision maker. | Goals and plans must be acceptable to the family and the designated decision maker who will carry them out. If such plans are not culturally informed, they are unlikely to be fulfilled. |
| 2. Make special arrangements as required to meet cultural needs, e.g., obtain a qualified interpreter or consult with a dietician. | Implementing culturally sensitive care may require resources not readily available. |
| 3. Develop an individualized goal of nursing care:<br>▪ To incorporate the family's cultural beliefs and practices in providing care. | |

## Implementation

| | |
|---|---|
| 1. Incorporate use of cultural practices related to health care that are not detrimental to the child, e.g., allow child to wear amulet or religious relics during procedures. | Adapting existing practices rather than attempting to change long-standing beliefs will be more acceptable to the child and family and will foster compliance. |
| 2. Accept the family's use of folk healers and folk remedies when not contraindicated by health state, safety, or treatment intervention. | The integration of these practices may increase acceptance of the health care. |
| 3. Plan diet and dietary changes around food preferences. Allow family to bring food from home. | Planning diet around preferred and acceptable foods will increase adherence to the regimen. Some groups prefer highly seasoned foods or types of food that may not be available in the hospital. |
| 4. Arrange for caregiver who speaks the same language or a translator if possible. | Communication is necessary to validate understanding.<br>***Special Considerations:*** *See Skill 13.* |
| 5. Interpret behavior nonjudgmentally in relation to culture but avoid labels. | Behavior that may seem unusual may be understandable within the framework of a specific culture, but not all families adhere to all practices prescribed by the culture. For instance, there are variations in the way or degree to which emotions are expressed. |
| 6. When conflict occurs between cultural practices and the health, safety, and treatment intervention, explain why the practice is considered harmful and encourage the family to seek less harmful ways of treating the problem. | Some cultural practices may conflict with the dominant culture's beliefs and values regarding health and safety or there may be potentially harmful interactions with the medical intervention. Some folk remedies may be contraindicated because of pharmacologic prescriptions. It is important to explain why a familiar and tried remedy may now be harmful. Sensitivity to the importance of cultural practices must be balanced with concern for the child's welfare, health, and safety. |

| Steps | Rationale |
|---|---|
| | ***Special Considerations:*** *Some child care and childrearing practices that are accepted by a cultural group may be viewed as abusive by the dominant culture. For example, some Southeast Asian groups treat enuresis and temper tantrums by burning small areas of skin. Some Caribbean groups use child discipline measures such as forced kneeling for long periods of time. It is important that the family understand how such practices can place them in jeopardy with child protective services and explore alternative measures that are more acceptable to the dominant culture.* |

### Evaluation Outcomes

1. Health care is accepted by the child and the family.
2. The family is satisfied that care provided respects their cultural beliefs.

### Observational Guidelines

The family carries out the health care regimen.

The family seeks health care for follow-up or for new health care needs. The family states that they are pleased with the care and the caregivers.

### Documentation

Communicate the plan of care to co-workers by recording it on Kardex or patient's record. Document special considerations such as dietary preferences. Make notation regarding decision makers in family and communicate variation in family structure that should be considered in care, e.g., visitation and rooming-in policy adjustments that may be needed. Note areas of continued noncompliance with care that should be reexamined in light of continuing assessment of cultural factors.

# *SKILL* 42 Fostering Spiritual Care for the Child and Family

*Lynn B. Clutter*

Spirituality extends beyond religion (an organized set of beliefs and practices), affecting the whole person: mind, body, and spirit. Spiritual care, important for everyone, is any act that touches the spirit of another person (Carson, 1989). Sense of meaning and purpose in life, a means of forgiveness, and a source of love and relatedness are aspects of spiritual care. Nurses attend to the spiritual dimension in order to promote health and encourage healing (Shelly and Fish, 1988). Assessment of spirituality enhances understanding of the child and family. Spiritual beliefs affect attitudes and behaviors. On a less observable level, these beliefs are often foundational for the code of morality, values, and standards for behavior. During times of crisis or change, spirituality can be a strength to mobilize in care since reliance on one's source of strength can enhance coping, hope, and self-esteem. Spirituality can also be an area of distress where belief systems are challenged and disrupted. This distress can negatively impact health and therefore become an important aspect for assessment and intervention. Finally, during illness or hospitalization, the nurse present at the time may be called upon to provide immediate spiritual support. Willingness to discuss spiritual matters and an ability to accept and respect beliefs or values different from one's own are necessary for effective spiritual care. Maintenance of a warm, caring, nonjudgmental approach is vital.

### NURSING DIAGNOSES

Spiritual distress related to separation from own religious/cultural ties or challenged belief/value system; Impaired adjustment related to inadequate spiritual support; Family coping, potential for growth (spiritual well-being) related to congruency of values and beliefs with behavior.

| Steps | Rationale |
|---|---|
| **Assessment** | |
| 1. Determine child's age and developmental level. | Spiritual care differs for the various ages and developmental levels. |
| 2. Read chart/Kardex for listing of religious affiliation and cultural heritage. | Spiritual and cultural sensitivity begins with knowledge of religious affilitation and heritage. **Special Considerations:** *Absence of formal religious affiliation also provides insight into spiritual status.* |
| 3. Observe for spiritually related resources among personal effects: books, pictures, religious cards, cassette tapes, objects, etc. | Presence of resources can indicate importance of spiritual aspects. |
| 4. Observe for spiritually related activities such as prayer. | Knowledge of meaningful spiritual practices can be helpful for developing appropriate interventions |
| 5. Listen for mention of spiritually related comments by child or significant others. | Comments that are made can provide a natural beginning point to spiritual assessment. **Special Considerations:** *Children will rarely announce a spiritual need (Still, 1984). Indirect comments such as "God doesn't care about what happens to people" can reveal concerns.* |
| 6. Note visitation from spiritual leaders and significant others (pastor, minister, prayer partner, priest, rabbi, etc.). Observe responses during or after visit. | The number and type of visitors can provide information related to spiritual environment. Responses can be positive or negative and can be helpful in determining the course of spiritual care. |
| 7. Observe for expressions of spiritual strengths or difficulties through: | Spiritual strengths or difficulties are often detected indirectly through observation. Once expressions are observed, they can be interpreted and validated. Early validation with verifiable information is necessary to prevent personal orientation or viewpoint from interfering with spiritual care (Still, 1984). |
| a. Behavior such as "acting out", self-destructive actions, apathy, or anger toward participation in spiritual activities versus those such as calm assurance in the midst of difficulty. | |
| b. Verbal expressions such as voicing spiritual concerns, questions, struggles, difficult feelings, or those of confidence and strength. | **Special Considerations:** *The dying child, or any child at critical moments, may have deeper spiritual questions such as "What is heaven like?"* |
| c. Emotional overtones such as fear, hopelessness, guilt, (Shelly, 1982) or those of peace, hope, courage, and will. | |
| d. Spiritually related themes demonstrated within artwork or play. | Drawings, artwork, or play of the preschool or school-age child may reveal spiritual content. |
| 8. Consider the relationship of the observed spiritual expressions (those from step 7) to each of the following areas: | The spiritual component of a person has been described as including these three aspects (Shelly and Fish, 1988). |
| a. A sense of meaning and purpose of life.<br>b. A means of forgiveness.<br>c. A source of love and relatedness. | Spiritual expressions often have links to deeper areas that once identified can be strengthened or supported. Strengths in these areas can positively impact health status, e.g., by providing a sense of hope and a positive outlook. In like manner, difficulties in any one area can have a negative impact on the healing process. |
| 9. Determine religious involvements. | Questions related to religious involvements are less threatening topics of direct spiritual assessment (Betz, 1981). A discussion of activities rather than internal beliefs tends to be beneficial for developing trust. **Special Considerations:** *Religious assessment is only a part of spiritual assessment. A person may have a spiritual need such as one for meaning and purpose that is not directly related to religious involvements or activities (Peterson, 1987). Questions listed in the box may be useful.* |
| a. Religious preference: the group, extent of participation of family and children, child's choice in type and extent of participation. | Knowledge of religious groups and activities can be helpful for planning daily routines of the hospitalized child. **Special Considerations:** *The child and family may differ in the amount and type of religious participation desired.* |
| b. Home religious practices of the family, parents, and child. | Religious practices may directly impact receptivity to certain types of care, e.g., food types. Furthermore, knowledge of usual home activities is necessary for adapting care during hospitalization. **Special Considerations:** *Omission of prayers or reading from a favorite Bible story book before bed can be especially distressing to some children, though they seldom will say anything unless asked directly.* |

## AGE-APPROPRIATE QUESTIONS RELATED TO SPIRITUALITY

**PRESCHOOL***

Who is God?
Tell me about God. What is God like?
Do you think about God?
How does God help you?
What helps you when you are scared?
Tell me about someone who loves you (or, . . . who you love).
Tell me about when you have felt closest to God.
What happens when you do something "bad"?
Where is God? (Young children often name a building.) Do you go there?
Do you pray? How does God answer your prayers?
How does God help you stay well?
What does God think about ________ (your illness)?
Tell me what you think caused your illness (made you sick)?
Do you think God can help you get better?

**SCHOOL-AGE**

What things come to your mind when I mention the word "God"?
Some people feel that God helps people get well. What do you think about that?
How does God help people get well?
What does God do for you?
How can a person get help from God if they want it?
Who do you turn to when you are ________ (scared, worried, etc.)? (If the answer is, "My parents," ask, "Is there anyone else?")
What does it mean to be forgiven?
Do you go to church (or other appropriate term)?
Are there any religious things you do (or, things about God or church things) that are important to you? Would you tell me about them? OR ask specific questions such as, "Do you pray? When? How?"
Are there things you do besides going to church that have something to do with God (or are related to God)? (e.g., read spiritual book, listen to spiritual music, watch religious programs on television, pray). How does doing this help you?
Are there special books that help you learn about God? Which ones help the most?
Are there any songs about God/Jesus that you like?
What does God mean to you?
Do you think prayers help people?
What about your faith is most important to you right now?
Are there things that can keep someone from getting well? What are they?
What caused your illness (or injury or "you to get sick")?†
What do you think dying is like?
How does God answer your prayers?

**ADOLESCENT‡**

Who, if anyone, would you say is in control?
Is religion or God important to you? If yes, describe how.
What were your thoughts about God when you were younger?
When stressed (or When something like this happens), do you rely on any kind of a "higher power"?
What have you found that gives you an inner peace?
What is your biggest source of strength and hope?
What is your source of strength right now?
Do you have a source of inspiration when you feel down?
What helps you feel good about yourself?
What hopes and dreams do you have for your life?
Has there ever been a time in your life when you felt you really needed God?
In what ways do you express your faith (or spiritual beliefs)?
Do you (e.g., meditate, read religious books, or pray)?
Do you belong to any group that meets regularly? (Encourage elaboration if answer is "yes.")
How much satisfaction do you get from your spiritual life?
Do you feel your faith (or religion) is helpful to you? If yes, would you tell me how?
Is prayer helpful to you? What happens when you pray?
Do you ever wonder how God is involved in this situation?
Being sick can sometimes change what a person believes about God. Has that happened to you? Has being sick made any difference in your religious practices?
Often a person who is ill thinks more about his relationship with God. Is that true with you?
Do your beliefs differ from those of your parents? If so, how?
What helps you when you feel ________ (a difficult emotion such as fear, guilt, shame, bitter, etc.)?

**ADULT/PARENT**

How would you describe God?
How is God involved in your life?
What sorts of things provide meaning in your life?
In times of crisis, where do you find comfort and solace?
What gives you the strength to go on?
What or who are you living your life for?
What is of most importance in your life?
What do you spend most of your time doing?
How happy are you with your life?
Are there changes in your life-style you would like to see take place?
What dreams and hopes do you have for yourself? (Your family? Your child?)
In what way do you attempt to gain freedom from ______ (a difficult emotion) when you are aware of its presence?
What kinds of spiritual support have helped you in the past?
Is there a particular spiritual practice that has meaning for you?
Are you aware of any spiritual needs that have emerged since your child's (hospitalization, illness, injury)?
Has your child's condition affected your relationship with God?
Sometimes people struggle with spiritually related difficulties like fear, bitterness, anxiety, or hopelessness. Is anything like that affecting you?
Sometimes in the midst of a crisis, spiritual strengths (love, peace, trust, contentment, acceptance, ability to cope, sense of belonging, hope, etc.) can be uncovered. (Pause for a response.)
What religious practices are significant to your child when he or she is not ill?
What meaning do these practices have for your child?

Note: The items listed in the younger categories can be used for older ages as well.
* Christian preschoolers may relate better to the use of "Jesus" than the term "God."
† Children, especially of school age, may causally link their own "bad behavior" to their illness or other difficult situation, e.g., child disobeyed parent and thinks it caused the disease. Careful assessment is necessary.
‡ Crisis or illness often cause even late adolescents to revert to concrete thinking. Abstract questions are inappropriate. Chronic illness, however, may lead to abstract, philosophical considerations.

| Steps | Rationale |
|---|---|
| c. Religious support groups used by the family or individuals within the family. | Groups that can lend true support during times of illness, injury, or hospitalization can be valuable resources that help the child and family maintain strength. ***Special Considerations:*** *Family members themselves are often the most available spiritual support group.* |
| 10. Discuss personal aspects of spirituality | |
| a. If indicators of spirituality are noted, comment or ask a question. For example, "I noticed you were reading your Bible earlier." (Pause for response or ask a related question.) | Comments about observable signs of spirituality provide a comfortable opening. |
| b. If no indicators are noted, use a general question to initiate conversation (see box on p. 265). | Sensitivity is required in deciding appropriate questions. Nonverbal aspects of communication are equally as important. |

## Planning and Goal Setting

| Steps | Rationale |
|---|---|
| 1. Review general practices of the child's organized religion (Note: For a comprehensive overview of religious groups, see Carson, 1989; Pumphrey, 1977; or Whaley and Wong, 1991). | Knowledge about the religion may increase awareness of assessment factors and provide sensitivity helpful for trust development. |
| 2. Review cultural variables that could affect beliefs (see Skill 41). | Religious beliefs shape cultures, but with children the culture can shape spiritual practices and beliefs. |
| 3. Review age-related developmental information (see box below) to determine nursing approach. | Awareness of development may affect communication approaches and intervention measures that are selected. |
| 4. Decide who should be present during spiritual interactions. | Presence or absence of parents and other family members can affect interactions. When this decision can be made before an interaction, a more directed approach can take place. |
| 5. Select a time when an uninterrupted discussion can occur. | Interruptions can be disruptive to spiritual care. |
| 6. Obtain any materials (pamphlets, books, tapes, videos, etc.) that may be helpful. | If possible, resources should be obtained before the discussion to avoid disruption. ***Special Considerations:*** *Careful consideration of the child and family beliefs is necessary for appropriate selection of materials.* |
| 7. Gain a comfortable but close proximity: a. Eye level with child. b. Touch, if appropriate. c. Sensitive to child's cues about comfort with close proximity. | Close proximity is possible after trust has been established. It is desirable for demonstrating concern and allows for eye contact, handholding, a hug, or touch as appropriate. ***Special Considerations:*** *Cultural and individual variables exist that will influence proximity.* |

### *FOWLER'S SEVEN STAGES OF FAITH*

Primal faith (infancy): A prelanguage disposition of trust forms the mutuality of one's relationships with parents and others to offset the anxiety that results from separations that occur during infancy.

Intuitive-projective faith (early childhood): Imagination, stimulated by stories, gestures, and symbols and not yet controlled by logical thinking combines with perception and feelings to create long-lasting images that represent both the protective and threatening powers surrounding one's life.

Mythic-literal faith (childhood and beyond): The developing ability to think logically helps one order the world with categories of causality, space, and time; to enter into the perspectives of others; and to capture life meaning in stories.

Synthetic-conventional faith (adolescence and beyond): New cognitive abilities make mutual perspective-taking possible and require one to integrate diverse self-images into a coherent identity. A personal and largely unreflective synthesis of beliefs and values evolves to support identity and to unite one in emotional solidarity with others.

Individuative-reflective faith (young adulthood and beyond): Critical reflection on one's beliefs and values, understanding of the self and others as part of a social system, and the assumption of responsibility for making choices of ideology and life-style open the way for commitments in relationships and vocation.

Conjunctive faith (midlife and beyond): The embrace of polarities in one's life, alertness to paradox, and the need for multiple interpretations of reality mark this stage. Symbol and story, metaphor and myth (from one's own traditions and others'), are newly appreciated as vehicles for grasping truth.

Universalizing faith (midlife or beyond): Beyond paradox and polarities, persons in this stage are grounded in a oneness with the power of being. Their visions and commitments free them for a passionate yet detached spending of the self in love, devoted to overcoming division, oppression, and brutality.

From Carson VB: Spiritual dimensions of nursing practice, Philadelphia, 1989, WB Saunders Co.

| Steps | Rationale |
|---|---|
| 8. Develop individualized child/family goals:<br>▪ Spiritual concerns and needs will be addressed and supported.<br>▪ Spiritual distress will have adequate resolution.<br>▪ Spiritual well-being and positive coping will be supported.<br>▪ Spiritual beliefs will be reinforced so they may serve as a source of strength during times of need. | |

## Implementation

### *General Measures*

| Steps | Rationale |
|---|---|
| 1. Provide supportive behavior such as a cheerful, kind, and caring approach; empathy; concern; genuineness; and active listening. | Adult patients viewed these supportive behaviors as being especially appropriate spiritual care from nurses (Shelly and Fish, 1988). They also apply for children and make up the majority of spiritual interventions. They are foundational for further discussions of spiritual needs. |
| 2. Maintain normal spiritual activities such as bed or mealtime prayer and reading. For example, in the absence of a parent, learn the child's special prayer or have the parent bring the favorite Bible storybook. | Maintaining usual spiritual activities, especially during parental absence, reduces stress and promotes normalcy. |
| 3. When usual routines such as church attendance are not possible, offer alternatives such as hospital chapel services or clergy visitation in room. | Alternative routines may help maintain a sense of normalcy and spiritual strength. |
| 4. Maintain availability to discuss spiritual matters when readiness is apparent. | Being available at critical times is important. Since timing of spiritual communications is often determined by the child, assessing, planning, goal setting, and implementing can occur at one time. When readiness is demonstrated, care can be productive and beneficial.<br>***Special Considerations:*** *Bedtime and nighttime can be difficult for hospitalized children, and thus can be critical times for communicating spiritual matters (Still, 1984).* |
| 5. Ask, "How can I help you carry out your spiritual practices or maintain your relationship with God?" (Shelly, 1978). | When identification of appropriate interventions takes place with the child or parent, acceptance of resultant care is increased. |
| 6. If a specific spiritual need has been identified, ask, "What would help you meet this need?" Offer additional suggestions if desired. | Often personally identified solutions are most effective.<br>***Special Considerations:*** *When solutions are not named, additional options or spiritual resources may be suggested. If unable to provide appropriate spiritual care (e.g., strong belief differences or magnitude of need is greater than personal expertise), referral to another nurse or care provider is necessary.* |
| 7. Offer to: (1) summon a spiritual resource person such as a clergy member or hospital chaplain, or (2) make provision for rituals and sacraments if so desired. | Many believe this should be routine in nursing care (Shelly and Fish, 1988). In times of confusion or distress, presence of clergy can have a positive impact. If in-depth spiritual counseling is needed, clergy members may be the appropriate providers.<br>***Special Considerations:*** *A paradoxical effect can occur if imminent death is feared because of the arrival of clergy. A comment such as, "Sometimes having a spiritual leader can be helpful during times of stress. Would that help you now?" can clarify intent and prevent concerns. Awareness of functions and services of a facility's spiritual care department should be known before delivery of patient care.* |
| 8. Provide direct spiritual care. Some resources available include: | Because of presence at critical times of need, the nurse is a likely provider of spiritual care after having already developed a trusted relationship and met other personal needs. Furthermore, clergy members may not always be desired or available. |
| a. Use of self (Shelly and Fish, 1988).<br>▪ Listen nonjudgmentally, empathize, and offer opportunities to communicate. | Supportive listening alone can often diminish or alleviate spiritual needs and allow working through of own spiritual distress. |
| ▪ Maintain caring "presence" during times of stress or crisis. | Being present and available conveys support and fosters strength (Lane, 1987). |
| ▪ Offer compassionate touches at appropriate times. | A warm and caring touch, holding of a hand, or sitting close can promote trust, provide comfort, and open a route for needed verbalization. |

| Steps | Rationale |
|---|---|
| ▪ Give names to feelings observed, for example, "I see you're holding your bear tightly. Are you afraid?" | Personal awareness of or vocabulary of feelings may not be fully developed even though feelings exist. |
| ▪ If death is imminent, listen to a review of child's life from the parent or child (see Skill 21). | A review of life can assist with preparedness for death. ***Special Considerations:*** *A review is often initiated spontaneously, but if not, ask, "I would like to hear more about you (or child's name). Will you share some of your memories?" Much internal strength and support is necessary for this type of spiritual and emotional care.* |
| b. Use of prayer or meditation. ▪ Ask, "Would praying help you now?" | Personal prayers or those received by others at times of need can provide comfort, counteract loneliness, increase hope, and deepen trust. |
| ▪ Ask, "What should we pray about?" | Sometimes the requested prayer is quite different from what would be expected and reflects actual patient needs versus those perceived by the nurse. |
| ▪ Offer simple, direct prayer with a clear theme. Prayer can include requested content but can also include areas such as hope, fears, or needs, as well as God's ability to comfort, guide, meet needs, and care (Shelly and Fish, 1988). | Since concentration abilities may be limited, simplicity and clarity are important. |
| c. Use of scripture. Use wording that is easily understood by the child. Scriptures may be written or verbalized. | Scriptures are especially meaningful when they are familiar or have content specific to the situation. ***Special Considerations:*** *Verbal and environmental clues are helpful in determining appropriate use of scriptures (Wessman, 1978).* |
| d. Use of spiritual resources such as written (prayer books, poetry, etc.), audio, visual, or audiovisual materials. | Often a child may not be able to articulate spiritual needs but will welcome resources of this nature. |
| 9. Ask other questions as appropriate for further intervention (see box on p. 265). | Questions used should be developmentally appropriate, comfortable, and appropriate to the level of trust that has developed. ***Special Considerations:*** *If the child is uncomfortable with a question, a common reaction is to guard further communication. Inappropriately deep questions may also be offensive and limit communication.* |
| 10. Be alert to overt and covert concerns and fears e.g., fear of the dark, animals, bad people, the supernatural (Miller, 1979). | Children of various ages have spiritually related fears that can be diminished through verbalization, changes in the environment, explanations, or comforting. Fears that are not directly spiritual may also be relieved through spiritual interventions. |
| 11. If spiritual strength has been identified, acknowledge strength or say, "Your faith seems to help you in this situation." Encourage continued use of spiritual strength. | Verbally linking spirituality with the current stress can strengthen existing coping skills. |
| ***Developmentally specific measures*** | |
| *Infant:* | |
| 1. Assist parent in becoming a source of trust and strength for infant by promoting: a. Bonding and attachment (see Skill 40). b. Sensitivity to the infant's individuality. c. Loving, consistent caretaking. | Assisting the parent benefits the infant since the most significant relationship for the infant involves the parent, especially the mother. |
| 2. Build infant trust, especially when parent is not able to be present, through the following: warm and gentle care, holding, cuddling, eye contact, talking directly to the infant, responding to physical and behavioral cues, and prompt meeting of needs. | Trust is necessary for the development of relationships and of spiritual beliefs. Consistent, competent, and gentle care builds trust and minimizes separation anxiety. |
| *Preschool:* | |
| 1. Use the child's usual religious rituals or customs such as mealtime and bedtime prayers. | Beliefs and basic trust in God can originate in preschool years and are often expressed through rituals. Rituals are of primary importance, providing meaning and comfort. |
| 2. Assist expression of spiritual concerns through play or symbolic language. | |
| a. Story telling. Tell or have parent tell a story with one clear theme and warm feeling tones or have child develop a story related to a given topic. Use stuffed animals or puppets. | Stories can provide comfort and direction appropriate for dealing with the current, difficult situation (Hahn, 1987). Puppets and stuffed animals visually enhance learning (Gustafson, 1980). |

| Steps | Rationale |
|---|---|
| b. Directed play. Use dolls or puppets along with directed comments to elicit spiritual perceptions. For example, "The doggie is sick and in the hospital. The kitty is the doggie's Mommy and the horse is God. What does the doggie say to his Mommy? How about to God? What does God think about the doggie being sick? If the doggie felt afraid (or mad, or any other emotion) what would he do?" | Directed play can be specific to the situation but less threatening than a direct verbal approach. |
| 3. Guide play sessions to offer indirect spiritual support. For example, using the situation in 2b, a question may be asked, "Does God love the doggie? I think God loves the doggie when he's sick and loves him when he's well. Do you?" | Offering such comments during play may provide the child with positive spiritual feelings and encourages verbalizations by the child. |
| 4. When praying, use simple, concrete sentence prayers. | The preschooler grasps information easier when messages are simple, concrete, and short. |
| 5. Role model and assist parent in demonstrating unconditional love, positive reinforcement, and realistic discipline. | These qualities form a healthy environment for spiritual development (Shelly, 1982). |
| *School-age:* | |
| 1. Provide opportunities for directed drawing, e.g., "Draw a picture of God." Have the child tell about the picture. | Spiritually related drawings can reveal feelings that can later be explained verbally.<br>***Special Considerations:*** *Since a common belief is that God punishes for bad behavior, punishment themes may be expressed in drawings. A safeguard against misinterpretation of a drawing is to verbally summarize and verify the child's comments (Still, 1984).* |
| 2. If unhealthy perceptions are present (e.g., the child may perceive himself as bad or feel he is being punished for some transgression), provide opportunities for projective drawing or play sessions (see Preschool intervention step 3). | The school-age child is often receptive to different perceptions when presented in play. Further, play can help the child work through feelings. |
| 3. Use third-person technique (e.g., "Some children like to pray when . . . ") or story telling for communicating interventions. | Spiritually related assistance is difficult for some to receive when stated directly but is accepted more easily when presented indirectly. |
| 4. Promote use of prayer or other rituals if child is accustomed to these practices. | The school-age child usually views the relationship with God as a personal and helpful one; much benefit can be derived from spiritual activities that strengthen the bond with God. |
| 5. Be sensitive to feelings of guilt, fear, or anger. If negative feelings are perceived, ask, "What do you think is making you sick (or in the hospital, or hurt, etc.). | Awareness regarding sin, punishment for wrongdoing, forgiveness, conscience, and moral decision making is developing. Negative, spiritually related feelings may occur during stressful experiences. |
| *Adolescent:* | |
| 1. Explore the adolescent's interpretation of reasons for current stress. Determine if feelings relate to God. Clarify confused information and focus on reality in interpretation. | Adolescents commonly formulate unconventional or imaginative explanations of causality in stressful situations. |
| 2. If trust is gained and feelings are shared, use therapeutic listening skills. | Listening is one of the most effective spiritual interventions since much weighing of beliefs, values, and behaviors takes place. Opportunities for self-expression are appreciated. |
| 3. Maintain an open, nonjudgmental, and accepting attitude. Be sensitive to age-appropriate independence/dependence and security/insecurity issues. | Various defense mechanisms are commonly used in dealing with stress and are often evident in spiritually related discussions. An understanding approach with careful attention to attitude, verbal, and nonverbal communications can diminish defensive reactions. |
| 4. Use age-appropriate written, audio, or visual spiritual materials. | Resources of this nature allow for the private introspection and self-determination of beliefs that is especially important to adolescents.<br>***Special Considerations:*** *Use of the Spiritual and Religious Concerns Questionnaire (Silber and Reilly, 1985) can be especially beneficial for hospitalized adolescents.* |
| 5. Promote use of peer spiritual support. | Parents and other authority figures may be rejected at this time. Peer relationships hold much influence. |
| 6. Promote open discussions between adolescent and parent(s) regarding beliefs and values. | Communication increases understanding of viewpoints. |
| 7. Explore with adolescent and family how beliefs might differ and mediate to foster workable solutions that tolerate differences. | Clarifying and raising tolerance level of spiritual belief differences can reduce intergenerational stress. |

| Steps | Rationale |
|---|---|
| *Young adult and parent:* | |
| 1. Actively listen, allow for expression of feelings, and be attentive for spiritual comments or overtones. | When stressed, young adults may be searching for truth and meaning. When a child is stressed, a parent carries an additional sense of responsibility and often a sense of guilt or helplessness. Verbalization can reduce negative feelings. |
| 2. Offer empathy, support, or reassurance about verbalized feelings. Restate comments when more feelings may be underlying, for example, "You feel like Billy's injury may be a punishment?" | Since spiritually related issues are commonly difficult to discuss, trust may be slow to form. A supportive response may lead to greater inner strength, trust, and further sharing of concerns. |
| 3. Acknowledge parent's valuable parenting skills and provision of spiritual support (if present) for the child. | Providing acknowledgment can be meaningful and can diminish the feelings of helplessness that are common when a child is stressed. ***Special Considerations:*** *Parents may need to sense acceptance to maintain spiritual support while the child is hospitalized.* |
| 4. Teach or coach parent in facilitating child's spiritual strength. For example, say, "Mrs. Moreno, explaining the Bible verse on this card in words that your daughter understands might mean a lot to her." | Teaching the parent spiritual support not only helps the child, but also encourages an active role in the midst of a difficult situation. The spiritual perspective may strengthen coping abilities. |
| 5. Promote parent's spiritual growth or strength. | A parent's spiritual growth and strength can positively affect other aspects of life and foster the child's strength. |

| Evaluation Outcomes | Observational Guidelines |
|---|---|
| 1. Usual spiritual practices are maintained (as possible) while hospitalized. | Observe for prayer, spiritual reading, or other usual spiritual practices. |
| 2. Alternate spiritual practices are exhibited when usual ones are not possible. | Note substitutions such as chapel attendance instead of church attendance. |
| 3. Child/family receives additional spiritual assistance as desired (prayer, sacraments, etc.) during time of stress. | Observe for visit from spiritual leader, addition of prayer or sacraments, etc. |
| 4. Child's spiritual distress is reduced or relieved. | Manifested behaviors of spiritual distress, e.g., statements of despair, are diminished or eliminated. |
| 5. Child gains strength from spiritual relationship. | Evidence of hope, peace, comfort, etc., is verbalized or demonstrated behaviorally. |

## Documentation

Quote verbatim any overt or covert statements that relate to spirituality (e.g., patient stated, "Why is God letting this happen?"). Nurse's responses can be included. A summary of spiritual assessment data should be recorded, along with any verbalized concerns. Nonverbal communication that could relate to spiritual condition (e.g., patient sighs frequently, speaks slowly, and looks at the floor when discussing present injury) is documented, as is pertinent physical or emotional assessment information. Record nursing diagnoses and interventions. Note referrals, presence of spiritually related people or resources, and resultant patient outcomes.

## UNIT IV

### PRODUCT REFERENCES AND TEACHING RESOURCES

**Organizations**

Attachment Center at Evergreen
28000 Meadow Drive
PO Box 2764
Evergreen, CO 80439
(303) 674-1910

### REFERENCES


Ainsworth MDS: Attachments across the life span, Bull NY Acad Med 61(9)792-812, 1985.

Ainsworth MDS: Object relations, dependency, and attachment: a theoretical review of the infant-mother relationship, Child Dev 40:969-1025, 1969.

Ainsworth MDS and Wittig B: Attachment and exploratory behavior of one-year-olds in a strange situation. In Foss BM, editor: Determinants of infant behavior, vol 4, London, 1969, Methuen.

Betz CL: Faith development in children, Pediatr Nurs 7(2):22-25, 1981.

Bowen SM and Miller BC: Paternal attachment behavior as related to presence at delivery and preparenthood classes: a pilot study, Nurs Res 29(5):307-311, 1980.

Bowlby J: Attachment and loss, vol 1, New York, 1969, Basic Books, Inc.

Bowlby J: The making and breaking of affectional bonds, Br J Psychiatry 130:201-210, 1977.

Boyle JS and Andrews MM: Transcultural concepts in nursing care. Boston, 1989, Scott, Foresman & Co.

Bradley R and Caldwell B: Using the HOME inventory to assess the family environment, Pediatr Nurs 14(2):97-102, 1988.

Brazelton TB: Behavioral competence of the newborn infant, Semin Perinatol 3(1):35-44, 1979.

Brazelton TB: Neonatal behavioral assessment scale, ed 2, Philadelphia, 1984, Spastics International Medical Publications.

Bullock D and Thompson B: Guidelines for family interviewing and brief therapy by the family physician, J Fam Pract 9(5):837-841, 1979.

Burns RC: Self-growth in families: kinetic family drawings (KFD) research and application, New York, 1982, Brunner/Mazel Inc.

Burns RC and Kaufman SH: Kinetic family drawings (KFD): an introduction to understanding children through kinetic drawings, New York, 1970, Brunner/Mazel Inc.

Busch-Rossnagel N: Review of the children's version of the family environmental scale. Supplement to the ninth mental measurements yearbook, Lincoln, Neb, 1988, The Buros Institute of Mental Measurements.

Caldwell B: HOME inventory, Little Rock, Ark, 1972, University of Arkansas.

Carson VB: Spiritual dimensions of nursing practice, Philadelphia, 1989, WB Saunders Co.

Chrisman N and Kleinman A: Health beliefs and practices. In Thunstrom S, editor: Harvard encyclopedia of American ethnic groups, Cambridge, Mass, 1980, Harvard University Press.

Cline FW: Understanding and treating the severely disturbed child. Evergreen, Colo, 1979, Evergreen Consultants.

Cranley MS: Development of a tool for the measurement of maternal attachment during pregnancy. Nurs Res 30(5):281-284, 1981.

Cropley C et al: Assessment tool for measuring maternal attachment behaviors. In McNall LK and Galeener JT, editors: Current practice in obstetric and gynecologic nursing, St Louis, 1976, The CV Mosby Co.

DeSantis L: Childrearing beliefs and practices of Cuban and Haitian parents: implications for nurses. In Carter MA, editor: Proceedings of the tenth annual transcultural nursing conference, Salt Lake City, 1985. Transcultural Nursing Society.

DeSantis L: Cultural factors affecting newborn and infant diarrhea, Pediatric Nurs 3(6):391-398, 1988.

DiLeo JH: Interpreting children's drawings, New York, 1983, Brunner/Mazel Inc.

Egeland B and Farber E: Infant-mother attachment: factors related to its development and changes over time, Child Dev 55:753-771, 1984.

Feldman KW: Pseudoabusive burns in Asian refugees, Am J Dis Child 138:768-769, 1984.

Fong CM: Ethnicity and nursing practice, Top Clin Nurs 7(3):1-10, 1985.

Fowler JW: Stages of faith, San Francisco, 1981, Harper & Row.

Funke J and Irby M: An instrument to assess the quality of maternal behavior, JOGNN 7(5):19-22, 1978.

Gay J: A conceptual framework of bonding, JOGNN 10:440-444, 1981.

Grace JT: Does a mother's knowledge of fetal gender affect attachment? MCN 9(1):42-45, 1984.

Greenberg M and Morris N: Engrossment: the newborn's impact upon the father, Am J Orthopsych 44(4):520-531, 1974.

Gustafson M: Puppets in the nursing process, Supervisor Nurse 11(11):33-35, 1980.

Hahn K: Therapeutic storytelling: helping children learn and cope. Pediatr Nurs 13(3):174-178, 1987.

Harms T and Clifford RM: Early childhood environment rating scale, New York, 1980, Teachers College Press.

Hartman A: Diagrammatic assessment of family relationships, Social Casework 59:465, 1978.

Henderson RW, Bergan JR, and Hurt J Jr: Development and validation of the Henderson environmental learning process scale, J Soc Psychol 88:185-196, 1972.

Jolly W, Froom J, and Rosen M: The genogram, J Fam Pract 10(2):251-255, 1980.

Klaus MH and Kennell JH: Maternal-infant bonding, St Louis, 1976, The CV Mosby Co.

Lane J: The care of the human spirit, J Prof Nurs 3(6):332-337, 1987.

Leahey M and Wright L: Families and psychosocial problems, Springhouse, Penn, 1987, Springhouse Corp.

Lipson JG and Meleis AI: Culturally appropriate care: the care of immigrants, Top Clin Nurs 7(3):48-56, 1985.

Low SM: The cultural basis of health, illness, and disease, Soc Work Health Care 9(3):13-23, 1984.

McCown D: Moral development in children, Pediatr Nurs Jan/Feb 1984, pp. 42-44.

Marecki M et al: Early sibling attachment, JOGNN 14(5):418-423, 1985.

Miller SR: Children's fears: a review of the literature with implications for nursing research and practice, Nurs Res 28(4):217-223, 1979.

Moos RH, Insel PM, and Humphrey B: Family, work and group environment scales manual, Palo Alto, Calif, 1974, Consulting Psychologists Press.

Myers CE, Mink I, and Nihira K: Home quality rating scale, Pomona, Calif, 1977, UCLA/Neuropsychiatric Institute-Pacific State Hospital Research Group.

Niederhauser BP: Health care of immigrant children: incorporating culture into practice, Pediatr Nurs 15(6):569-574, 1989.

Nugent JK: Using the NBAS with infants and their families, White Plains, NY, 1985, March of Dimes Birth Defects Foundation.

Oster G and Gould P: Using drawings in assessment and therapy, New York, 1987, Brunner/Mazel Inc.

Overfield T: Biological variation in health and illness: race, age, sex differences, Menlo Park, Calif, 1985, Addison-Wesley.

Peterson EA and Nelson K: How to meet your clients' spiritual needs, J Psychosoc Nurs 25(5):34-39, 1987.

Peterson GH and Mehl LE: Some determinants of maternal attachment, Am J Psychiatry 135(10):1168-1173, 1978.

Pumphrey JB: Recognizing your patients' spiritual needs, Nursing 7(12):64-70, 1977.

Reiser SL: A tool to facilitate maternal-infant attachment, JOGNN 10(4):294-297, 1981.

Roberts C and Feetham S: Assessing family functioning across three areas of relationships, Nurs Res 31(4):231-235, 1982.

Rubin J: Child art therapy, ed 2, New York, 1984, Van Nostrand Reinhold Co, Inc.

Satariano H and Briggs N: The good family syndrome, Pediatr Nurs 15(3):285-286, 1989.

Satir V: Conjoint family therapy: a guide to theory and technique, Palo Alto, Calif, 1964, Science and Behavior Books.

Shelly JA: Spiritual care workbook, Downers Grove, Ill, 1978, Inter Varsity Press.

Shelly JA: The spiritual needs of children, Downers Grove, Ill, 1982, Inter Varsity Press.

Shelly JA and Fish S: Spiritual care: the nurse's role, ed 3, Downers Grove, Ill, 1988, Inter Varsity Press.

Silber T and Reilly M: Spiritual and religious concerns of the hospitalized adolescent, Adolescence 20:217-220, 1985.

Sodestrom K and Martinson M: Patients' spiritual coping strategies: a study of nurse and patient perspectives, Oncol Nurs Forum 14(2):41-46, 1987.

Spector RE: Sociocultural influences on children's health. In Scipien G et al: Comp Pediatr Nurs, ed 3, New York, 1986, McGraw-Hill Book Co.

Spinetta JJ and Spinetta PD: Living with childhood cancer, St Louis, 1981, The CV Mosby Co.

Spiritual assessment questions, NUR 302 course handout, Oral Roberts University, Anna Vaughn School of Nursing, Tulsa, Okla, Oct 9, 1985.

Still JV: How to assess spiritual needs of children and their families, J Christ Nurs 1(1):4-6, 1984.

Stoll R: Guidelines for spiritual assessment, Am J Nurs 79(9):1574-1577, 1979.

Tapia J: The nursing process in family health. In Spradley B: Contemporary Community Nursing, Boston, 1975, Little, Brown & Co.

Tripp-Reimer T, Brink PS, and Saunders JM: Cultural assessment: content and process, Nurs Outlook 32:78-82, 1984.

Wach TD, Francis J, and McQuiston S: Psychological dimensions of the infant's physical environment. Paper presented to the Midwestern Psychological Association, Chicago, 1978.

Wessman J: Scripture in intervention, The nurses lamp XXIX(3):2-3, 1978.

Whaley LF and Wong DL: Nursing care of infants and children, St Louis, 1991, The CV Mosby Co.

Whall A: Nursing theory and the assessment of families, J Psych Nurs Ment Health Serv 19:30-36, 1981.

Whall A: The family as a unit of care in nursing: a historical overview, Public Health Nurs 3(4):240-249, 1986.

Wieser MA and Castiglia PT: Assessing early father-infant attachment. MCN 9(2):104-106, 1984.

Wright LM and Leahey M: Nurses and families: a guide to family assessment and intervention, Philadelphia, 1984, FA Davis.

Yarrow LJ, Rubenstein JL, and Pedersen FA: Infant and environment: early cognitive and motivational development, Washington, DC, 1975, Hemisphere Publishing.

# UNIT V Health and Wellness with Children and Families

# SKILL 43 Teaching Children and Their Families

*Rosemary Liguori*

Children learn differently than do adults. An adult has the ability to understand abstract ideas, whereas a child's thinking involves more of the use of concrete concepts. Effective teaching of children must therefore be grounded in a knowledge of cognitive maturation and developmental readiness to learn.

Teaching children requires creativity and an awareness of their ability, needs, and developmental level. It is a collaborative process between the child, the family, and the health care professional. Information to be taught may range from simple handwashing methods to a complex procedure such as self catheterization. Approaches to the teaching process may involve: the cognitive domain, which relates to facts and knowledge that need to be comprehended; the affective domain, which involves feelings, values, and emotions; and/or the psychomotor domain, which combines knowledge and physical activities.

Because of changes in the health care delivery system in the past few years and the increased scope of nursing practice, patient teaching and health education have become essential components of nursing. This professional responsibility also involves a legal duty to provide written, along with verbal, instructions and careful documentation of the teaching process (Cushing, 1984).

## NURSING DIAGNOSES

Altered health maintenance related to lack of knowledge about child's health or illness; Anxiety related to unmet informational needs about health care facility, policies, and procedures; Altered parenting related to lack of knowledge about creating an environment to promote child's growth and development: Ineffective family coping related to inadequate information about child's illness and treatment regimen.

| Steps | Rationale |
|---|---|

## Assessment

1. Assess the characteristics of the child:
   a. Age.

The child's age indicates general guidelines of cognitive capability. The ability to reason and development of fine motor skills have an impact on how the child will be able to participate in the teaching process.

   b. Developmental level.
      - Sensorimotor (0-2 years): learns through senses and interaction with the environment.
      - Preoperational (2-7 years): learns through symbols in a concrete mode.
      - Concrete operational (7-12 years): logical concrete problem solving.
      - Formal operational (12 years and older): logical abstract reasoning.

Children learn by experience. New ideas can be added to the child's knowledge base if it can be compared to something that is familiar.

***Special Considerations:*** *When the child is developmentally delayed, teaching is addressed to his or her developmental level rather than chronological age (see Skill 25).*

   c. Previous knowledge regarding content area being taught. For example, ask, "What usually causes you to start wheezing? Is there anything you can do to prevent it?"

Building on what the child already knows gives a sense of security and confidence that strengthens the foundation of learning and allows for individualization of the teaching process. For example, if a child has asthma and knows that exercise may precipitate an attack but doesn't know how to prevent it, teaching can be geared to the use of medication before exercise.

   d. Readiness. Note if the child seems interested by asking questions, expressing curiosity, and talking freely.

If a child is not ready for or receptive to teaching, the situation will not be conducive to learning.

   e. Attention span.

The time allotted for teaching must be geared to the child's attention span to be effective, e.g., 5 to 10 minutes for a preschooler and 20 to 30 minutes for the school-age child.

***Special Considerations:*** *The younger the child, the more limited the attention span, so plan the length of teaching sessions accordingly.*

   f. State of health: presence of illness or condition requiring adaptation by the child. Determine level of adaptation.

Perceptual or motor difficulties, e.g., visual impairment or cerebral palsy will influence teaching methods. Adaptation will influence readiness and motivation.

2. Assess characteristics of the family:
   a. Ability to provide emotional support and communicate well with the child (see Skill 38).

It is essential to assess the emotional strength of the family to determine if the child will have the support needed to do or learn the necessary task or information.

   b. Readiness to be involved in care of the child.

As parents will often be required to give care at home, their readiness to participate in learning needs to be determined.

***Special Considerations:*** *Many children are discharged from the hospital requiring highly technical care. Parental motivation is essential to assume major responsibility for a child with special needs and coordinate multidisciplinary involvement, consistent with the concept of family-centered care.*

   c. Knowledge level regarding information or skill to be taught.

Knowledge level guides preparation for teaching.

***Special Considerations:*** *The family of a child with a chronic illness may have considerable knowledge about it. Accurately determining their present level is essential.*

   d. Ability to comprehend:
      - Diagnosis.
      - Treatment.
      - Home care.
      - Nutrition.
      - Medications.
      - Exercise.

Various factors (e.g., the grieving process, cognitive abilities, language barriers, fears and vulnerability in an unfamiliar environment) may interfere with the family's ability to comprehend. Recognition of these factors can guide planning for effective teaching methods.

## Planning and Goal Setting

1. Determine teaching needs and content based on assessment, a review of the medical records, and collaboration with the health care team.

Defining the specific content to be taught is essential to an effective and organized teaching plan.

***Special Considerations:*** *Teaching often occurs in spontaneous interactions with the child and family. For tips on taking advantage of those teachable moments, see box.*

2. Develop objectives and goals for teaching collaboratively with child/family.

Objectives and goals provide direction and a means of evaluating achievement.

| **Steps** | **Rationale** |
|---|---|

### *INFORMAL TEACHING OPPORTUNITIES*

Avenues of teaching available to the nurse include structured teaching sessions (as addressed in this skill) and informal, spontaneous teaching. A planned teaching session offers structure through the use of a prepared format. Unscheduled opportunities provide chances to identify and use teachable moments to meet child and family learning needs.

**Identify teachable moments**

- Administration of routine care (e.g., taking vital signs, giving medications) offers opportunities to teach.
- A health behavior is observed in the child or family that requires modification or reinforcement.
- The family's experience of crisis increases receptivity to teaching.
- A family member initiates conversation about the child's care or illness.
- The parent/child actually asks for information.
- Verbal statements and/or nonverbal body language indicates concerns, questions, uncertainty, or confusion.
- The child demonstrates a readiness to talk/play with the nurse.

**Make the best use of the moment**

- Recognize the opportunity to teach.
- Teach while performing tasks by describing what is being done and why.
- Take time to play or talk with the child who has expressed interest.
- Listen to the family and ask questions to set the stage for effective teaching.
- Initiate activities conducive to learning (e.g., explanations that incorporate doll play for the preschooler, drawing pictures for the school-age child, or conversing with the adolescent).
- Allow family to model behavior by being aware that the child/family is always observing and learning, and by taking advantage of opportunities to explain and demonstrate proper technique, methods, and/or care priorities.

**Recognize blocks to learning**

- Parent/child may perceive a busy nurse as not wishing to be bothered. Pause, direct attention to them, and show availability for discussion or questions.
- Excess people in the room, such as visitors or staff, can be distracting and/or inhibiting.
- Avoid teaching during a time of stress or pain.
- Be aware when the teachable moment has passed—child will change the subject, act disinterested, or get very quiet.

Courtesy Kathryn A. Perry, Tulsa, Okla.

| Steps | Rationale |
|---|---|
| 3. Organize information in a logical manner.<br>a. Simple to complex.<br>b. Essential to less essential. | Subgrouping the information in a progressive fashion facilitates the learning process.<br>***Special Considerations:*** *Depending on the age of the child and amount of the content, several sessions may be indicated.* |
| 4. Plan cognitive, affective, and/or psychomotor methods as developmentally appropriate, e.g., audiovisuals, games, and role playing (see box on Developmental Approaches on following page). | Teaching needs are more likely to be met using developmentally appropriate strategies. |
| 5. Write out plan step by step. (see box containing sample teaching plan on following page). | A written plan prevents accidental omission of information, facilitates presentation and provides documentation. |
| 6. Obtain teaching tools: pamphlets, audiovisuals, dolls, and information sheets. | Learning is enhanced using a variety of methods and tools to reinforce teaching (Fig. 43-1).<br>***Special Considerations:*** *Many health related organizations and support groups provide literature and audiovisuals that may be beneficial to the family teaching process.* |
| 7. Select a private and comfortable area with adequate lighting. | Privacy and comfort facilitate an open exchange necessary for effective teaching. |
| 8. Determine a time conducive to learning. Avoid sessions before mealtimes, naptime, or when child is uncomfortable or preoccupied. Collaborate with child/family to coordinate with other activities. | Selecting a time to meet that is convenient and not distracting for the participants facilitates the teaching/learning process. |
| 9. Rehearse the plan in front of the mirror, or with peers or family. | Rehearsal refines the presentation and builds confidence. |
| 10. Develop an individualized goal of nursing care:<br>■ To provide developmentally appropriate teaching of defined knowledge and skills to the child and family. | |

## *DEVELOPMENTAL APPROACHES TO TEACHING*

**SENSORIMOTOR—(0-2 YEARS)**

- Direct teaching to the parent who can use the information to stimulate the child's learning.
- Provide age-appropriate toys to stimulate normal development.

**PREOPERATIONAL (2-7 YEARS)**

- Be aware that logic may not be understood. The child is unable to understand multiple concepts.
- Use role playing, puppet play, and doll play to validate understanding. Directing the attention toward a puppet or doll also takes the focus away from the child, which may be less stressful.
- Use visual aids such as videos, films, books, models, and puppets. Visual methods of teaching are especially productive at this age.

**CONCRETE OPERATIONS (7-12 YEARS)**

- Gear teaching for the present. The child is concerned only with what is happening "now." The future has little meaning or importance.
- Use a variety of activities for learning.

1. Puppets, models, and audiovisual materials promote learning by using more than one sense.
2. Coloring books, booklets, and information sheets are useful to take home and reinforce what was taught.
3. Small groups encourage interaction with peer input to aid in problem solving.

**FORMAL OPERATIONS (12 YEARS-ADULTHOOD)**

- Teaching can be more detailed because the capacity for logic and reasoning is developed.
- Include the adolescent in goal planning for learning. The more involvement the adolescent has in the decision-making process, the greater the possibilities for active participation and compliance.
- Be prepared to answer underlying reasons and causes of problems. Understanding why something occurs gives the teaching credibility and maintains the adolescent's interest.
- Address questions honestly and in a nonjudgmental manner. This helps to develop a sense of trust in the teacher that may provide opportunities for the adolescent to address other questions of concern.

## *SAMPLE TEACHING PLAN*
### *Safety: What To Do for Choking*

Purpose: To teach children and parents about preventing choking in small children, and what to do if choking occurs.

**SHORT SESSION CONTENT**

a. General safety: e.g., picking up toys.
b. Specific safety: e.g., What to do for an airway obstruction.

**Steps**

1. Gather demonstration doll, small items (e.g., a Lego block), a pamphlet from the American Heart Association on choking, a poster on choking placed on the wall.
2. Introduce topic. "Good morning, Mrs. Linn and Tommy. Today we will talk about the importance of keeping small items such as Lego blocks or money away from 11-month-old Judy. Tommy, you can help by keeping your toys up. Do you know why it is important to keep your small toys away from your sister?" (Allow response.) "Mrs. Linn, I will show you what to do if one of your children chokes."
3. Discuss prevention measures, e.g., say, "Until Judy can chew her food completely avoid giving her:"
   - carrot sticks, celery, grapes, apples with peels
   - peanut butter (unless thin spread on a cracker/bread)
   - hot dog with casing on it (you may cut hot dogs in small pieces)
   - popcorn and peanuts (until 4 to 5 years old)
   - hard candies, gum

   Discuss prevention measures with Tommy (age 6 years), e.g., say, "Until Judy is able to understand that Lego blocks are not for eating, please keep out of her reach:"
   - small objects like Lego blocks
   - metal cars, tanks, and trucks
   - toys with moveable and small parts
   - marbles, jacks
   - pennies, dimes, nickels
4. Use visual aids such as the No-Choke Testing Tube to determine if a small part of a toy could pose a choking hazard. (Available from Toys to Grow On, 2695 E. Dominquez St., Long Beach, Ca, 90801.)
5. Discuss the indications for clearing an airway obstruction.
   a. If the child is able to speak, cry, or make noise, allow the child to attempt to clear own airway.
   b. Perform airway obstruction maneuver if the child is doing any of the following:
      - choking
      - not able to cough
      - producing high-pitched noises
      - turning cyanotic
6. Demonstrate procedure on a doll.
7. Allow mother to return a demonstration on the doll.
8. Praise her for her efforts.
9. Validation: Do you have any questions?
10. Give a pamphlet on choking to post at home.

Plans for future sessions: Child proofing the home; Plants, drugs; Garage and tool safety.

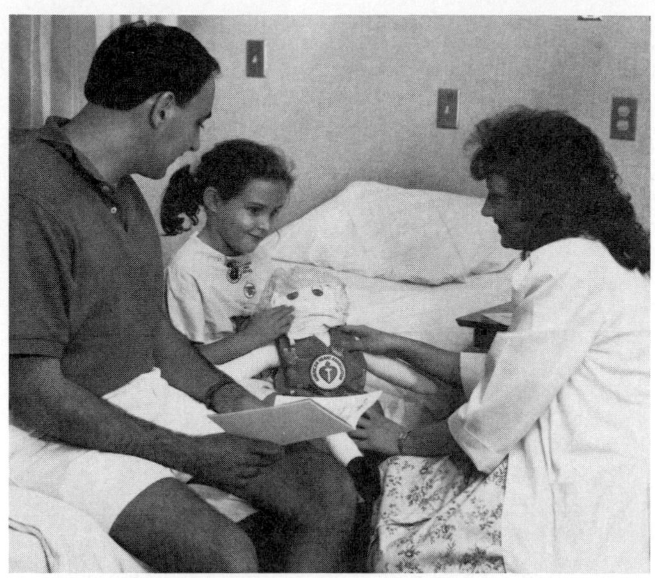

***FIG. 43-1*** Teaching tools reinforce learning.

| **Steps** | **Rationale** |
|---|---|
| **Implementation** | |
| 1. Introduce the topic and share a brief outline of the content of the session. "Good morning, Mrs. Linn, today I will demonstrate what to do if your child chokes. Here is a guide, What to do for choking, that may be posted on a bulletin board at home for reference" or "Tommy, we will talk about how you can keep your small toys away from your little sister." | Initially defining the topic and content provides a focus for the session. |
| 2. Follow the teaching plan (content may be given in several short sessions). | Following the developed plan facilitates organization and ensures complete coverage of the needed information. ***Special Considerations:*** *While following the teaching plan, be flexible and sensitive to other concerns or needs that may arise and require attention.* |
| 3. Ask for validation of understanding at short intervals if possible. Be alert for signs of confusion or noncomprehension. For example, say, "You seem a little confused by what I just said." | Validating understanding frequently during teaching permits for clarification of content and provides reinforcement before the child and family become overwhelmed. |
| 4. Repeat information as needed and provide written information. | Repeating information enables the child/family to process the concept. ***Special Considerations:*** *Learners often become overwhelmed with new information and retain best what is repeated and/or reinforced in written materials for later review. Legally it is more difficult to substantiate in court that teaching occurred if written instructions were not provided for reinforcement (Cushing, 1984).* |
| 5. Demonstrate patience and reassure child/family that their learning pace is appropriate. Maintain a relaxed approach and commend their efforts by saying e.g., "That was a good demonstration of what to do for choking." | Learning will be hampered if the child/family senses impatience, or feels rushed and not able to proceed at own pace. |
| 6. Observe for decreased attention span and boredom (fidgets, wanders, or changes the subject). Stop the session and complete at a later time. | Learning will not take place if the child is not paying attention. ***Special Considerations:*** *If more sessions are needed, break information into smaller segments, and/or plan ways to make the learning more fun to keep the child's interest.* |

| Steps | Rationale |
|---|---|
| 7. Monitor child for fatigue. | A child's endurance level will vary, especially when ill. |
| 8. Encourage child/family's participation in the session. For example, say, "It is really frightening when a child chokes on a small item such as a Lego. How do you feel about handling a future emergency?" | Using the skills, asking questions, and sharing their thoughts and feelings, will expand and increase their competencies (Braga and Braga, 1976). |
| 9. Provide reinforcement and praise during and at the conclusion of the session. | |
| a. Give positive feedback such as a smile, a touch, or a gesture. Verbal reinforcers or special privileges (e.g., a sticker, marking on a chart, or going to the playroom) are especially helpful for children. | When the child/family is rewarded positively for their participation, motivation for additional learning is fostered. |
| b. Describe the behavior observed, e.g., say: "That is a good job" or "You are really working hard at following directions." | Reflecting positive attention to behavior that should be reinforced fosters learning. Mentioning the desired behavior rather than labeling the child as "good" avoids a source of stress. |
| 10. Revise plans if needed based on evaluation of goals and objectives. | If goals are not achieved, they must be reevaluated and new ones developed. |

| Evaluation Outcomes | Observational Guidelines |
|---|---|
| 1. The content of the teaching plan is defined. | Review nursing care plan or prioritized list of teaching needs. |
| 2. The goals and objectives are developed in collaboration with the child/family. | Review written goals and objectives; note presence of evaluation criteria. Validate agreement with child/family. |
| 3. A teaching plan is developed, incorporating a variety of developmentally appropriate methods. | Review written teaching plan, note use of variety of methods, compare child's developmental level to planned methods. |
| 4. The teaching plan is implemented. | Review documentation of teaching session and written materials provided. |
| 5. Achievement of goals and objectives is evaluated and revised if necessary. | Note written evaluation using established criteria. If not achieved, note revision of goals and additional teaching employed. |

## Documentation

Document date, time of teaching, content methods, and written instructions given on the chart. Document whether or not the child and family understood the information and their response to teaching session. Include progress or revision of teaching plan.

# SKILL 44 Instructing Families in Child Safety

*Rosemary Liguori*

Injury is the leading cause of death among young children. Most injuries can be prevented, therefore it is essential that child safety is stressed at every opportunity. Health care providers have a responsibility to educate parents in injury prevention, including the selection of safe and developmentally appropriate toys.

## NURSING DIAGNOSES

Health-seeking behaviors (child safety) related to child health promotion and maintenance; Altered health maintenance related to lack of knowledge about child safety needs; Potential for injury related to household/environmental hazards; Decisional conflict related to infant/child toy selection.

| Steps | Rationale |
|---|---|
| **Assessment** | |
| 1. Assess characteristics of the child: | Knowledge of characteristics of the child is essential in determining the appropriate safety concepts to discuss with family. |
| a. Age. | Children from the ages of 1 to 4 years, and adolescents have the highest injury death rate (Whaley and Wong, 1991). |
| b. Developmental level. | Potential hazards to a child's safety differ according to developmental abilities. For example, a toddler who is naturally curious and investigates by tasting, climbing and exploring is at risk for ingestion of hazardous substances or burns. |
| c. Temperament. | A child's temperament influences activity level, injury incidence, toy selection, and amount of exploration. Some children are prone to greater risk taking. Others may be influenced by siblings or peers to push beyond their own cautions. |
| 2. Determine the number of adults and children in the family. | A high ratio of children to adults, especially when the children are close in age, poses safety concerns because of difficulties in supervision. |
| 3. Assess parental knowledge regarding injury prevention:<br>a. Existing safety practices. For example, ask, "What measures have you taken to childproof your home?" | Assessing parental knowledge provides a baseline and indicates priority concepts for teaching needs. Also, asking questions about safety reinforces its importance to the family. |
| b. Selecting and maintaining safe and age-appropriate toys. For example, ask: | Selecting age-appropriate safe toys fosters development and helps protect the child from harm. Toys also need to be properly maintained to decrease the potential for injury. |
| ▪ "How do you select your child's toys?"<br>▪ "How helpful are the age recommendations listed on the toy label for you in obtaining safe and appropriate toys for your child?" | ***Special Considerations:*** *When selecting toys, safety, durability, sensory appeal, age range, independent play, and variety should be considered (Rothenberg et al, 1981).* |
| 4. Identify parental concerns related to safety. For example, ask, "Do you have any concerns about your child's swimming lessons?" | Addressing parental concerns fosters communication and encourages additional questions. It may reveal a past incident in relation to safety (e.g., a neighbor child drowning in a family pool), which makes the parent especially receptive to teaching. |
| 5. Assess the older child's knowledge about safety rules. For example, ask a school-age child, "What safety rules do you use when riding your bike?" or "Do you wear a helmet?" | Obtaining the child's knowledge base of safety rules, encourages greater safety and fosters a dialogue between the child and the professional.<br>***Special Considerations:*** *In the United States, 650 children die annually from bike injuries. The majority of the deaths are from head injuries (Weiss and Duncan, 1986). Use of bicycle helmets reduced the risk of head injury by 85% in one study (Thompson, Rivara, and Thompson, 1989). The American Academy of Pediatrics (1989) strongly urges wearing a safety helmet when riding a bicycle.* |

| Steps | Rationale |
|---|---|
| 6. Determine if the child lives in an urban or rural area. | Living in a rural area increases the risk for injury morbidity and mortality because of the inaccessibility of immediate medical care and the severity of injuries. The rate of unintentional deaths in rural areas is about twice that of larger cities: 75 per 1000 deaths (rural) and 37 per 1000 deaths (city) (Pediatrics, 1988). |
| 7. Assess the child's home environment for actual/potential hazards by visiting the home and/or using a questionnaire, e.g., the Framingham Safety Survey (Fig. 44-1). | Observation or identification of actual/potential hazards allows development of an individualized teaching plan. A developed tool provides an organized framework for thorough assessment and future teaching. |

## Planning and Goal Setting

| Steps | Rationale |
|---|---|
| 1. Allot time at each well-child visit, during hospitalization, or in the home for discussing safety issues. | Teachable moments afford an opportunity to discuss safety concepts. Regularly scheduling a discussion of safety concepts helps ensure the information is timely and in manageable amounts.<br>***Special Considerations:*** *The American Academy of Pediatrics "TIPP" Injury Prevention Program is a set of parent information sheets designed to be given during well-child visits. Information is age related. Topical information sheets such as "Safe Bicycling" are also available through the American Academy of Pediatrics (see Product References and Teaching Resources).* |
| 2. Gather written teaching handouts/publications (see Product References and Teaching Resources). | Written materials reinforce concepts and provide information for reference.<br>***Special Considerations:*** *Many agencies and manufacturers supply pamphlets and information free or at a nominal cost.* |
| 3. Include the children, if age-appropriate, in injury prevention education. | Children become more accountable for their own safety when given information to prevent injuries. |
| 4. Develop individualized child and family goals:<br>▪ The home environment will be appropriately childproofed.<br>▪ Available toys will be age-appropriate, safe, and maintained.<br>▪ The child/family will consistently practice injury prevention.<br>▪ Parents will have plans of action for emergencies. | |

## Implementation

| Steps | Rationale |
|---|---|
| 1. Instruct child and family on age-appropriate injury prevention measures. | Anticipatory guidance is essential to alert parents to potential hazards that develop in relation to the child's growth in abilities. |
| *Infancy/toddlers:*<br>Potential topics: cribs, water safety, changing tables, pacifiers, strollers, choking, poisoning, burns, and car safety (see Skill 45). | Many hazards exist even for the young, immobile infant such as falls or inadequate restraint during a motor vehicle collision. An infant is entirely dependent upon the caregiver for protection. As mobility is gained the infant, unaware of the danger, may create a hazardous situation, e.g., climbing out of a high chair. |
| *Early childhood:*<br>Potential topics: climbing, poisoning, stranger awareness, handling or mouthing hazardous objects, water safety, use of seatbelts, pedestrian safety rules, and fire safety. | Variables contributing to the potential for injury at this age include the inability to read, development of new motor skills, natural curiosity, and ignorance of danger (Whaley and Wong, 1991).<br>***Special Considerations:*** *Drowning is the number one cause of death between the age of 1 to 2 years and remains high through preschool years (Baker, 1984). Since the advent of childproof caps in 1973, the incidence of poison ingestion has decreased from 2.2 per 1000 children in 1960 to 0.5 per 1000 children in 1980 (Baker, 1984).* |
| *School-age years:*<br>Potential topics: being home alone, playground safety, burn prevention, bicycle and skateboard safety, helmet use, use of seatbelts, water safety, drug abuse prevention and sport safety. | Although the school-age child is cognitively able to recognize hazards in the environment, adult supervision usually decreases, therefore education of the child and family is an effective means of injury prevention (Whaley and Wong, 1991). |

## FRAMINGHAM SAFETY SURVEY
### From Toddlers through School (Part 1)

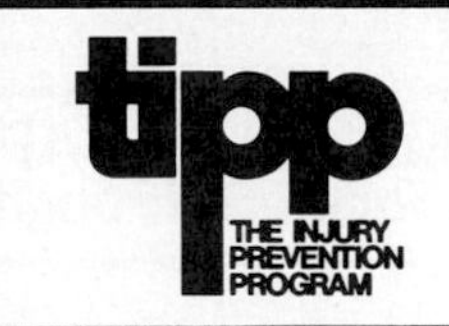


SAFETY IS YOUR BEST PRESCRIPTION

Name ______________________ Date ______________

| | Please X through one answer | | | |
|---|---|---|---|---|
| 1. Do you leave your child alone in the house? | Frequently | Occasionally | Never | |
| 2. Are any of your babysitters less than 13 years old? | Yes | No | Don't know | |
| 3. Do you keep plastic wrappers, bags and balloons, peanuts and other small objects out of the reach of your children? | Always | Sometimes | Never | |
| 4. Do you know how to prevent your child from choking? | Yes | No | | |
| 5. Do you have mechanical garage doors or hideaway beds? | Yes | No | | |
| 6. Do you keep guns or air rifles in your house? | Yes | Don't know | No | |
| 7. Are your window screens or guards in good condition? | All windows | Some windows | None | |
| 8. Is your child in the yard while the lawn mower is in use? | Never | Sometimes | Have no mower | |
| 9. Do you keep your child in an enclosed area when alone and not being watched by an adult? | Always | Sometimes | Never | |
| 10. Do you place gates at the entrance to stairways? (for children less than 3 years of age) | Always | Sometimes | Never | All children 3 or older |
| 11. Have any of your children ever had an accident requiring a visit to the doctor or hospital? | Yes ______ How many visits | Don't remember | No | |
| 12. Do you check for safety hazards in homes of friends or relatives where your child may play? | Always | Sometimes | Never | |
| 13. Do you keep household products, medicines (including aspirin and iron) and sharp objects out of reach and in locked cabinets? | Always | Sometimes | Never | |
| 14. Do you dispose of old medicines? | Always | Sometimes | Never | |
| 15. Do you store household products in empty soda bottles, glasses or jars? | Always | Sometimes | Never | |
| 16. Do you have safety caps on all bottles of medicine? | Always | Sometimes | Never | |
| 17. Does your child chew on paint chips or windowsills? | Frequently | Occasionally | Never | |
| 18. Do you have Ipecac in the house? | Yes | Don't know | No | |
| 19. Do you know how to use Ipecac? | Yes | No | | |
| 20. Have you checked your yard and house for poisonous plants and wild mushrooms? | Yes | No | | |
| 21. How frequently do you check the heating system in your home? | Never | At least once/year | Every few years | |

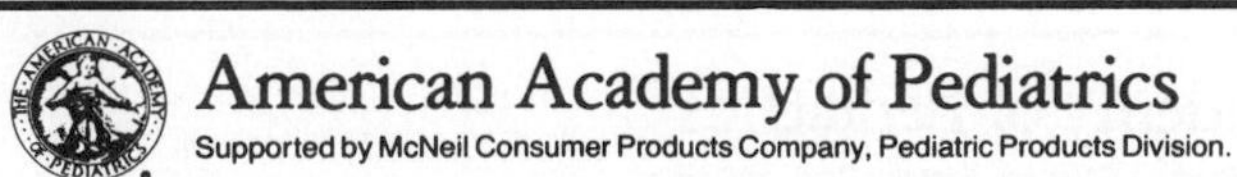


*Continued.*

***FIG. 44-1*** A sample safety questionnaire.

Adapted with permission from TIPP Framingham Safety Survey: From Toddlers through School, copyright © 1988, American Academy of Pediatrics.

## FRAMINGHAM SAFETY SURVEY
### From Toddlers through School (Part 2)

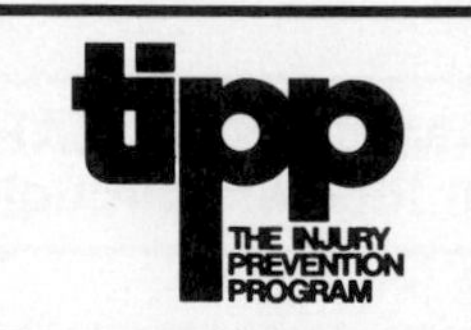


SAFETY IS YOUR BEST PRESCRIPTION

**Name** ______________________ **Date** ______________

| | **Please X through one answer** | | |
|---|---|---|---|
| 1. Do you have safety plugs on unused electrical outlets? | All outlets | Some outlets | None |
| 2. Do you use electrical appliances in the bathroom? | Yes | Don't know | No |
| 3. Do you keep electrical appliances and cords out of reach? | Always | Sometimes | Never |
| 4. Do you keep matches out of reach of your children? | Always | Sometimes | Never |
| 5. Do you smoke in bed? | Frequently | Occasionally | Never |
| 6. Do you have a plan for escape from the house in the event of fire? | Yes | No | |
| 7. Do you have working fire extinguishers in the house? | Yes | Don't know | No |
| 8. Do you have a screen for the fireplace? | Yes | No Fireplace | No |
| 9. Do you have smoke or fire detectors in the house? | Yes | No | |
| 10. Have you checked the temperature of the hot water in your house? | ______ Indicate temperature | | Don't know |
| 11. Do you keep handles of pots and pans out of reach when on the stove? | Always | Sometimes | Never |
| 12. Do you leave your child alone in the bath? | Frequently | Occasionally | Never |
| 13. Do you take your child on a boat? | Frequently | Occasionally | Never |
| 14. Do you allow your child to swim unsupervised? | Frequently | Occasionally | Never |
| 15. Does your child ride on your bicycle with you? | Always | Sometimes | Never |
| 16. Have you taught your child about watching for cars in the street or driveway? | Yes | No | |
| 17. What type of car seat do you use when your children ride in a car? | ______ Indicate Brand | | None used |
| 18. Do you leave your child alone in the car? | Always | Sometimes | Never |
| 19. Where do you seat your children in the car? | Front | Rear | Front or Rear |
| 20. Do you lock the car doors before driving? | Always | Sometimes | Never |
| 21. Do you check your child's toys for safety hazards? | Always | Sometimes | Never |
| 22. Does your child ever play with darts or bows and arrows? | Frequently | Occasionally | Never |

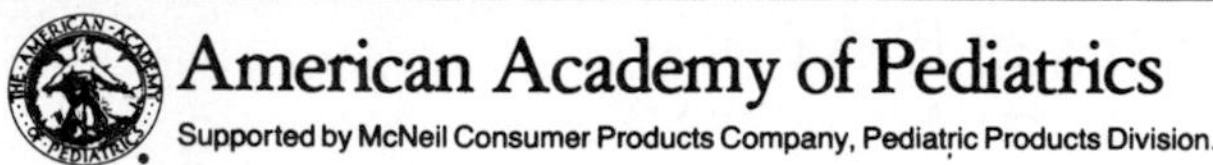

| Steps | Rationale |
|---|---|
| | ***Special Considerations:*** *A significant risk for this age is head injuries involving the use of bicycles, roller skates, skateboards and all-terrain vehicles (ATVs) (Whaley and Wong, 1991). Playground injuries are also likely to occur; in a study of 57 playgrounds in two suburban communities, 99% of the equipment was unsafe and the personnel supervising were unqualified to provide first aid (Ridenour, 1987).* |
| *Adolescence:* Potential topics: Motor vehicles/driving safety; advanced water safety; drug abuse prevention and suicide prevention. | Adolescents are prone to risk-taking behaviors and feelings of invulnerability. These characteristics contribute to physical injury being the single greatest cause of death in this age group (Whaley and Wong, 1989). |
| 2. Provide parents with appropriate information specific to identified concerns. | Parents are likely to be especially receptive to information regarding a specific concern. Addressing their concerns communicates respect for their parenting abilities. |
| 3. Demonstrate appropriate safety measures, e.g., holding a hand on an infant who is on an examining table or buckling a child being discharged from the hospital in a car seat for transport home. | Role modeling demonstrates and reinforces safe practices. |
| 4. Assist parents in developing a plan of action for an emergency, e.g., calling 911, having a Poison Control Number near the phone, performing the Heimlich maneuver for a choking child, and having a fire escape plan. | Having a plan for an emergency empowers the family. During a crisis people may panic and feel immobilized. However, a written number and developed plan fosters control of the situation. ***Special Considerations:*** *The Heimlich maneuver can be easily taught in a few minutes. Provide infant CPR training (see Skill 126 or recommend a convenient class).* |
| 5. Provide an inventory checklist to assist in childproofing the home (see box on following page). | The checklist provides an organized way for the parents to make the home a safe environment. |
| 6. Discuss safe toy selection. | Evaluating the safety of a toy is a parental responsibility (Whaley and Wong, 1991). |
| 7. Involve the child in safety awareness/education, e.g., teaching the child in front of the parent how to keep small objects away from younger children and discussing stranger awareness. | The child should become knowledgeable in safety and injury prevention measures, as independence from the parents increases. ***Special Considerations:*** *A 1984 survey revealed that 2.1 million children between the ages of 5 to 13 were left unattended after school (Padilla and Landreth, 1989). A program such as "Kid Safe" teaches self-care and survival skills for these children (Moore et al, 1988).* |

| Evaluation Outcomes | Observational Guidelines |
|---|---|
| 1. The home is age-appropriately childproofed. | Visit the home and/or interview the family regarding potential hazards identified and corrective measures taken. |
| 2. Toys are age-appropriate and safe. | Inspect toys or ask family to describe toy selection criteria and maintenance procedures. |
| 3. Family consistently practices injury prevention measures. | Observe and/or question family regarding age-appropriate measures such as using car restraints system, removing hazards in a new environment, not propping bottles, raising crib side rails, etc. |
| 4. Child demonstrates safe practices. | Observe or question child regarding helmet use, water safety, stranger awareness, etc. |
| 5. The family has developed plans for action in emergencies. | Interview family, asking them to describe plans for fire escape, calling emergency personnel, or poison control. Ask for a demonstration or verification of class attendance for CPR training, first aid, and choking relief measures. |

## Documentation

Document safety concepts taught, by whom, the family's response, and actions taken. Note referrals and/or special training provided, e.g., CPR. Document any safety concerns that require further assessment or interventions.

## *SAFETY AND INJURY PREVENTION*
## *Child Safety Home Checklist*

### SAFETY: FIRE, ELECTRICAL, BURNS

- Guards in front of or around any heating appliance, fireplace, or furnace (including floor furnace)*
- Electrical wires hidden or out of reach*
- No frayed or broken wires
- No overloaded sockets
- Plastic guards or caps over electrical outlets, furniture in front of outlets*
- Hanging tablecloths out of reach and away from fires*
- Smoke detectors tested and operating properly
- Kitchen matches stored out of child's reach
- Large, deep ashtrays throughout house (if used)
- Small stoves, heaters, and other hot objects (cigarettes, candles, coffee pots, slow cookers) placed where they cannot be tipped over or reached by children
- Hot water heater set 49° C (120° F) or lower
- Pot handles turned toward back of stove
- No loose clothing worn near stove
- No cooking or eating hot foods or liquids with child standing nearby or sitting in lap
- All small appliances, such as iron, turned off, disconnected, and placed out of reach when not in use
- Cool, not hot, mist vaporizer used
- Fire extinguisher on each floor and checked periodically
- Electrical fuse box and gas outlet accessible
- Family escape plan in case of a fire and practiced periodically; fire escape ladder available on upper level floors
- Telephone number of fire or rescue squad and address of home with nearest cross street posted near phone

### SAFETY: POISONING

- Toxic substances placed on a high shelf and preferably in locked cabinet
- Toxic plants hung or placed on high surface rather than on floor*
- Excess quantities of cleaning fluid, paints, pesticides, drugs, and other toxic substances not stored in home
- Used containers of poisonous substances discarded where child cannot obtain access
- Telephone number of local poison control center and address of home with nearest cross street posted near phone
- Syrup of ipecac in home with 2 doses per child
- Medicines clearly labeled in childproof containers and stored out of reach
- Household cleaners, disinfectants, and insecticides kept in their original containers, separate from food and out of reach

### SAFETY: FALLS

- Non-skid mats, abrasive strips, or textured surfaces in tubs and showers
- Exits, halls, and passageways in rooms kept clear of toys, furniture, boxes, or other items that could be obstructive
- Stairs and halls well lighted, with switches at both top and bottom
- Sturdy handrails for all steps and stairways
- Nothing stored on stairways
- Treads, risers, and carpeting in good repair
- Glass doors and walls marked with decals
- Safety glass used in doors, windows, and walls
- Gates on top and bottom of staircases and elevated areas, such as porch, fire escape*
- Guardrails on upstairs windows with locks that limit height of window opening and access to areas, such as fire escape*
- Crib side rails raised to full height; mattress lowered as child grows*
- Restraints used in high chairs, walkers, or other baby furniture; walker not used near stairs*
- Scatter rugs secured in place or used with nonskid backing
- Walks, patios, and driveways in good repair

### SAFETY: SUFFOCATION AND ASPIRATION

- Small objects stored out of reach*
- Toys inspected for small removable parts or long strings*
- Hanging crib toys and mobiles placed out of child's reach*
- Plastic bags stored away from young child's reach; large plastic garment bags discarded after tying in knots*
- Mattress or pillow not covered with plastic or in manner accessible to child*
- Crib design according to federal regulations with snug-fitting mattress*†
- Crib positioned away from other furniture or window*
- Portable playpen gates up at all times while in use*
- Accordion-style gates not used*
- Button-size batteries stored safely and discarded properly, where child will not have access*
- Bathroom doors kept closed and toilet seats down*
- Faucets turned off firmly*
- Pool fenced with locked gate
- Proper safety equipment at poolside
- Electric garage door openers stored safely and adjusted to raise when door strikes objects
- Doors of ovens, trunks, dishwashers, refrigerators, and frontloading clothes washers and dryers closed at all times*
- Unused appliance, such as a refrigerator, securely closed with lock or doors removed*
- Food served in small noncylindric pieces to young children*
- Toy chests without lids or with lids that securely lock in open position*
- Pails, buckets, and wading pools kept empty when not in use*
- Clothesline above head level
- At least one member of household trained in basic life support (CPR), including first-aid for choking

### SAFETY: BODILY INJURY

- Knives, power tools, and unloaded firearms stored safely or placed in locked cabinet
- Garden tools returned to storage racks after use
- Pets properly restrained and immunized for rabies
- Swings, slides, and other outdoor play equipment kept in safe condition
- Yard clear of broken glass, nail-studded boards, and litter
- Cement birdbaths placed where young child cannot tip them over*
- Telephone number of ambulance and address of home with nearest cross street posted near phone

*Safety measures are specific for homes with young children. All safety measures should be implemented in homes where children reside and visit frequently, such as those of grandparents or babysitters.

†Federal regulations available from U.S. Consumer Product Safety Commission 1-800-638-CPSC; teletypewriter service for the hearing impaired is available at 1-800-638-8270 ( in Maryland, 1-800-492-8104).

From Wong D and Whaley L: Clinical manual of pediatric nursing, ed 3, St Louis, 1990, The CV Mosby Co.

# SKILL 45 Instructing Parents in the Use of Car Restraint Systems

*Kristie S. Nix*

Motor vehicle accidents are the most preventable killer of infants and young children. While motivated parents may seek information independently, nurses can promote safety seats through classes for parents of newborns, community awareness classes, discharge teaching, health fairs, and radio and television programs, including closed circuit hospital systems.

## NURSING DIAGNOSES

Health-seeking behaviors (automobile safety seats) related to infant/child safety needs; Altered health maintenance related to demonstrated lack of knowledge regarding automobile safety seats; Potential for injury related to motor vehicle accident; Decisional conflict related to safety seat choices.

| Steps | Rationale |
|---|---|
| **Assessment** | |
| 1. Determine child's age, height, weight, and developmental status; history of safety seat use including model(s); and parent's use of seat belts. | Assessment provides information for determination of appropriate safety seat and past parental experience and attitudes. ***Special Considerations:*** *Health history forms or hospital admission records should include questions regarding the use of safety seats.* |
| 2. Ascertain parental knowledge level of the following by written or verbal report or return demonstration:<br>a. Correct model for age, height, and weight.<br>b. Correct placement within safety seat.<br>c. Correct installation of safety seat in vehicle. | Knowledge level guides plan for teaching. |
| **Planning and Goal Setting** | |
| 1. Determine appropriate safety seats to discuss based on assessment. | Correct model is determined by age, height, and weight of child. The child's developmental status, particularly related to head control, should also be considered. |
| 2. Gather necessary equipment for teaching session: safety seat(s), dolls for demonstration, locking clip, audiovisual aids (literature, films). | Hands-on experience with actual equipment reinforces teaching. ***Special Considerations:*** *A variety of audiovisual materials are available including literature and videotapes from safety seat manufacturers and groups that promote child passenger safety.* |
| 3. Select an optimal time and place for teaching and encourage both parents or other culturally significant family members to attend. | Compliance with use is improved if significant family decision-makers attend sessions and understand the importance of using safety seats on every trip (Faber, 1986). |
| 4. Develop individualized child and family goals:<br>▪ Correctly uses safety seats for all trips in vehicles.<br>▪ Parents use seat belts. | |
| **Implementation** | |
| 1. Identify benefits of safety seats:<br>a. Prevent injury or death in accidents or when attempting to avoid an accident. | It is estimated that safety seats reduce the death rate by 80% to 90% and injury rate by 60%. Children who are in safety seats are also less likely to be victims of noncrash accidents such as quick stops, swerves, or opening and falling out of vehicle doors. |
| b. Child is a better behaved passenger, thus less distracting for driver (see box on following page). | An often unrecognized benefit of safety seats is that children who are buckled up are better behaved than unrestrained children (Christopherson and Gynlay, 1984). |

Steps | Rationale

### TIPS FOR PARENTS FOR GOOD BEHAVIOR

1. Praise children frequently for good behavior while riding in the car.
2. Insist that others who transport your child (babysitters, daycare workers, grandparents) also follow safety seat rules.
3. Never allow children to ride unrestrained or to climb out of seats. Older infants and young children (usually between 9 and 30 months) test parents regarding the habitual use of restraints by fussing or even climbing out of the seat. If such happens, stop the car and say, "You must put on your seat belt." Do not resume travel until the child has done so. Be firm.
4. Buckles may be wrapped with a cloth cover secured by velcro as a means of discouraging a child from unbuckling (Gunnip et al, 1987).
5. Make certain the seat is comfortable: carry a damp cloth to cool vinyl and metal parts that can become extremely hot in an enclosed vehicle. Commercial or homemade covers increase the seat's comfort.
6. A young child who has not been required to ride in a safety seat can be taught to do so. Giving the child the seat as a special present is a good introductory technique. Let the child help put the seat in the car, then try it out for a ride around the block. Let the child personalize the seat with stickers. Some children enjoy pretending they are astronauts, pilots, or firemen while in their seats. Be firm and patient when teaching a child this new seat habit.
7. A good example helps children learn: adults should also buckle their seat belts.

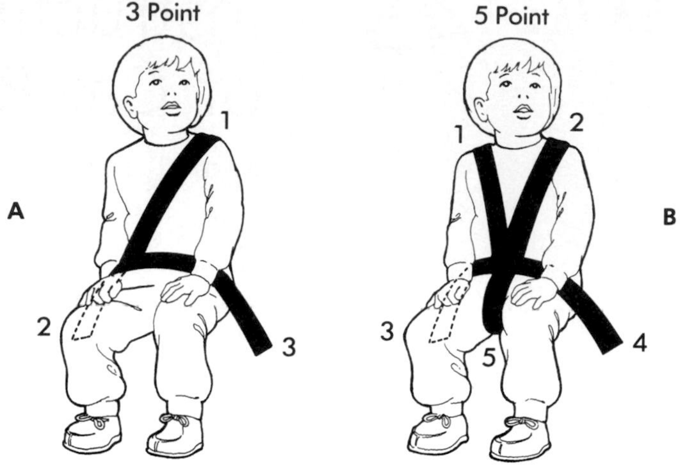


***FIG. 45-1*** Automobile safety seats with **A,** a three-point harness and **B,** a five-point harness.

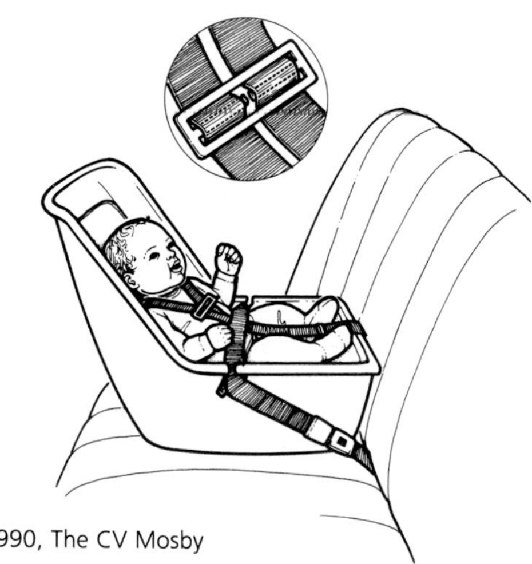

***FIG. 45-2*** Rear-facing infant car seat.

From Wong DL and Whaley LF: Clinical manual of pediatric nursing, ed 3, St Louis, 1990, The CV Mosby Co.

c. Child develops good safety habits at an early age.

2. Instruct family regarding appropriate models of safety seats.
   a. Seats may have:
      - A "5-point" safety harness with 1 crotch, 2 shoulder, and 2 hip straps.
      - A shield that covers the abdomen.
      - A combination of the two, with a 3-point harness for shoulders and crotch (Fig. 45-1).

There are many different models of safety seats that meet federal standards.

***Special Considerations:*** *A shopping guide for safety seats is available from the American Academy of Pediatrics (see Product References and Teaching Resources).*

   b. Seats vary according to child's age.
      - *Infant seats* (Fig. 45-2) are suitable for infants from birth to 17 to 20 pounds, 26 inches, or 9 months. *All infants ride in the rearward facing position.* Adaptations for premature infant's seat include:
      - crotch strap attached to the shell 4½ to 5½ inches from the back of the seat to prevent slouching;
      - lowest shoulder strap slots should be 10 inches or less above the seat bottom;
      - a harness retainer clip keeps harness in place at mid-chest position;
      - seats with shields or lap pads are unsuitable (Stroup, Weber, and Bull, 1987).

The rear-facing position permits crash forces to be absorbed by the back, the strongest part of the infant's body.

***Special Considerations:*** *Although some safety seats are designed to double as infant carriers, lightweight household carriers and beds do not provide the protection afforded by a safety seat that meets federal standards; they should never be used for travel. Infants who must lay prone to maintain respiratory functions may be transported safely in an Evenflo Swinger, a car bed that meets federal safety standards (Stroup, Weber, and Bull, 1987; Bull, Weber, and Stroup, 1988).*

**Steps** | **Rationale**

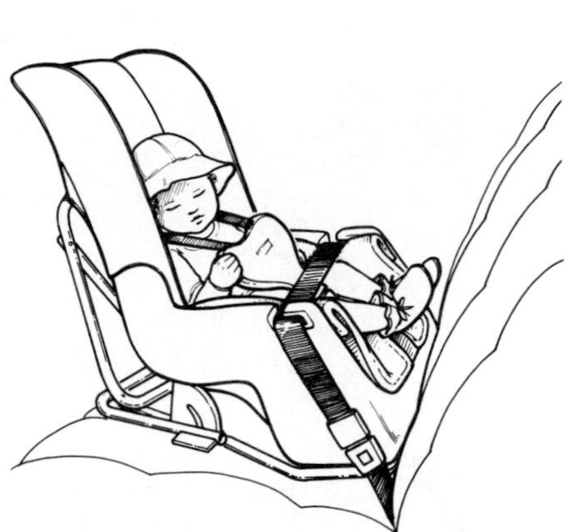

***FIG. 45-3*** Convertible seat in rear-facing position for use with infants.

From Wong DL and Whaley LF: Clinical manual of pediatric nursing, ed 3, St Louis, 1990, The CV Mosby Co.

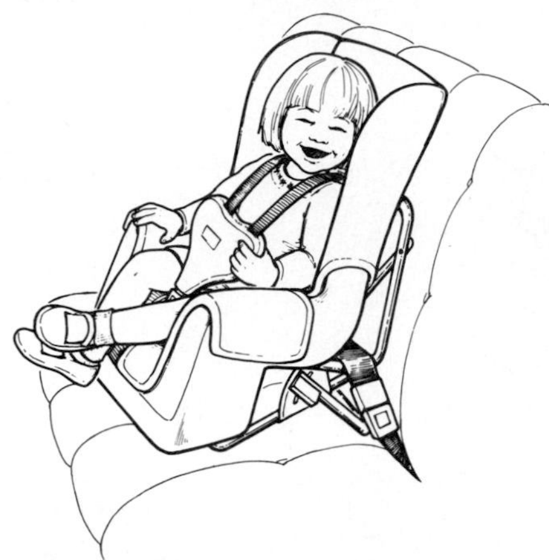

***FIG. 45-4*** Convertible seat in forward-facing position for older infants and children.

From Wong DL and Whaley LF: Clinical manual of pediatric nursing, ed 3, St Louis, 1990, The CV Mosby Co.

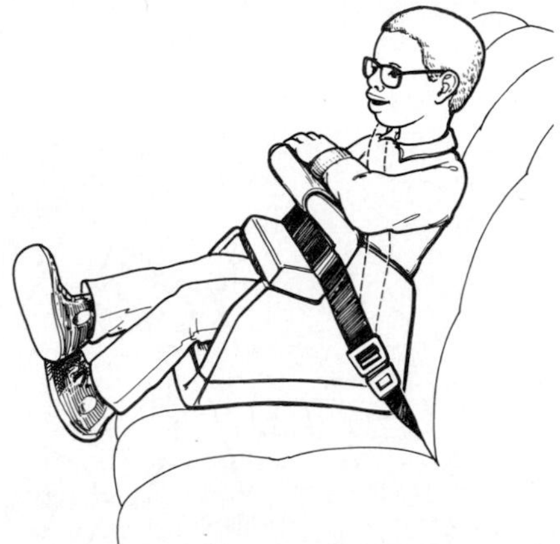

***FIG. 45-5*** Automobile booster seat. Dashed lines indicate placement of shoulder strap.

From Wong D and Whaley L: Clinical manual of pediatric nursing, ed 3, St Louis, 1990, The CV Mosby Co.

- *Convertible safety seats* (Figs. 45-3 and 45-4) may be used in a rearward position for infants, then faced forward as the child reaches 9 months or 20 pounds.
- *Toddler safety seats* face forward only, and are for children over 9 months or 20 pounds.

While more expensive than infant seats, convertible seats can be used until the child is approximately 4 years of age, 40 pounds, or 40 inches tall.

***Special Considerations:*** *When changing or rethreading the harness system to adjust for a child's growth, always refer to the manufacturer's instructions. In general, harness straps should be threaded through higher slots of the safety seat only when the child's shoulders are above the lower slots. Children with special needs, e.g., spica casts or handicapping conditions, may benefit from modified or specially designed safety seats, vests, or beds (see Product References and Teaching Resources) (Bull, Weber, and Stroup, 1986; Feller et al, 1986).*

- *Automobile booster seats* (Fig. 45-5) are intended for preschoolers and older children who weigh at least 30 pounds. The midpoint of the child's head must not exceed the height of the seat back; the child has outgrown the booster seat when this occurs.

***Special Considerations:*** *While some models are marketed for use by children who weigh 20 pounds, the National Passenger Safety Association (NPSA) (1986) strongly recommends that a child remain in a convertible or toddler seat as long as possible because of the lateral and upper torso protection provided by the design of those seats.*

3. Demonstrate proper placement of child within safety seat.
   a. Dress the child comfortably.

***Special Considerations:*** *Some types of clothing, e.g., buntings, prohibit fastening the buckle properly between the infant's legs, and should not be used. If blankets are needed, place them over the infant after the harness is fastened.*

   b. Place the child in the safety seat with buttocks and back flat against the seat.

***Special Considerations:*** *Infants may require special support until head and trunk control develop. Place rolled blankets around the head and sides to assist in keeping the infant upright. Commercially available products may be purchased for this purpose.*

   c. Follow seat manufacturer's instructions for placement of straps, harness and/or shields. Shoulder harness straps should go through slots on the safety seat level with or just above shoulders. Many seats have a harness retainer (clip) that is used to keep shoulder straps from slipping off the shoulders (see insert Fig. 45-2). After buckling, check that straps are comfortably snug so that two fingers fit between strap and child. Harness webbing must lie flat, not twisted. The crotch strap should be kept short.

For the seat to perform properly in the event of a crash, the child must be secured according to manufacturer's instructions.

**Steps** | **Rationale**

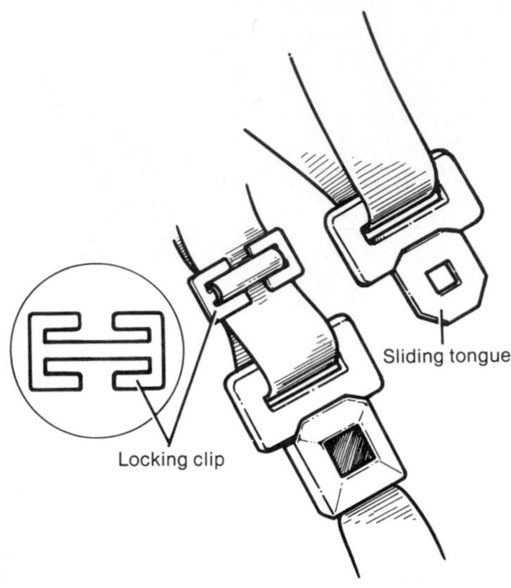


***FIG. 45-6*** Use of a locking clip.

From Wong D and Whaley L: Clinical manual of pediatric nursing, ed 3, St Louis, 1990, The CV Mosby Co.

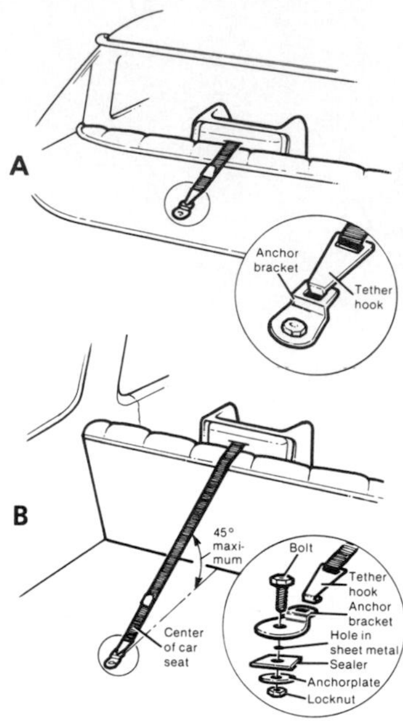


***FIG. 45-7*** Tether straps. **A,** Rear window shelf installation for sedans. **B,** Floor mount installation for hatchback or station wagon.

From Wong D and Whaley L: Clinical manual of pediatric nursing, ed 3, St Louis, 1990, The CV Mosby Co.

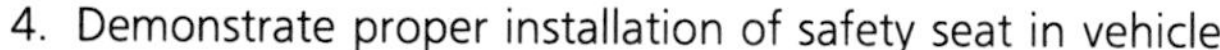

4. Demonstrate proper installation of safety seat in vehicle.

The safest place in the car for the safety seat is the back seat, center position.
***Special Considerations:*** *While the back seat is preferred, this position may not be practical when the driver is alone and unable to see the child without taking his or her eyes from the road. In this case a frontseat position is acceptable.*

   a. Follow seat manufacturer's instructions regarding correct threading of the vehicle's seat belt to secure the safety seat. Newer models have instructions and red arrows that adhere to the seat to illustrate proper use and seat belt threading through the metal base or shell of the seat.

Improperly secured safety seats reduce intended protection. Surveys show that only 55% of all children riding in safety seats are fully protected (National Highway Traffic Safety Administration, 1988).

   b. Buckle the belt and pull snugly. The vehicle's seat belt should remain snug and keep the safety seat in place.
   c. Locking clips are recommended for use with lap/shoulder belts with a "sliding tongue" (Fig. 45-6).

A locking clip holds the lap and shoulder belts together.
***Special Considerations:*** *Locking clips are available from safety seat manufacturers, automobile dealers' parts departments, and retailers of safety seats.*

   d. Some safety seat models, particularly older models and models for disabled children, require use of a tether (anchor) strap that must be bolted to a sturdy metal panel (Fig. 45-7).

Tethering provides an extra measure of protection by anchoring the top portion of the seat. Unfortunately, tether systems have an extremely high misuse rate and have been substantially discontinued.
***Special Considerations:*** *Emphasize the correct use of tether systems and reinforce that tether strap and bolt system must be in place in each vehicle in order to use the seat properly.*

5. Discuss common areas of parental concern regarding safety seats.
   a. Discuss costs of safety seats and suggest alternatives to purchasing.

***Special Considerations:*** *To be familiar with prices, check with local merchants. If family cannot afford to purchase a seat, refer to local safety seat rental programs that offer inexpensive long-term rentals of infant/and or toddler seats. Rental programs may be located through the local or state health department, hospital, or state highway safety office.*

| Steps | Rationale |
|---|---|
| b. Parents often ask what to do when no safety seat is available. There is no safe alternative for infants. In an emergency, toddlers and young children may use the vehicle's seat belt. The lap belt should be positioned low on the child's pelvic area and not over the abdomen. The shoulder belt should cross the child's chest; if it cannot be adjusted to fit properly, place the shoulder belt behind the child's back (University of North Carolina Highway Safety Research Center, 1988). | While a safety seat should be used on each trip, there may be an occasion when no safety seat is available. In this situation, use of the vehicle's seat belt is better than no restraint. ***Special Considerations:*** *Encourage parents to anticipate safety seat needs and plan accordingly (such as when traveling by air and safety seat will be needed at destination). Children should never ride buckled up with someone, as that person's weight could crush the child in the event of an accident.* |
| c. Parents should be encouraged to choose a seat that is simple to operate and to practice with the harness straps, shield, or other seat features. | Parents are more likely to misuse safety seats that are inconvenient to use and are not comfortable for the child. A seat that is difficult to use may cause misuse that may cancel or negate the safety seat's effectiveness in a crash. ***Special Considerations:*** *Recommend against buying or borrowing a used safety seat unless the seat's safety status is known.* |
| 6. Emphasize that parents and all other persons riding in the vehicle should buckle up. | Children learn by the examples set by their role models. Parents provide an excellent beginning to a good safety habit each time they buckle themselves and their children with safety belts. |

| Evaluation Outcomes | Observational Guidelines |
|---|---|
| 1. Parent demonstrates correct use of safety seats. | Have the parent provide return demonstration or ask questions to validate knowledge of safety seats, e.g.: ▪ What model of seat are you using? ▪ Does the seat face forward or rearward? ▪ How do you adjust the harness straps in the seat to fit your child? ▪ Where are you threading the seat belt? |
| 2. Parent uses car safety seats for all trips in vehicles. | Ask the parent: ▪ Are you having any problems with your safety seat? ▪ Does your child always stay in the seat? |
| 3. Parent uses seat belt for self. | Ask the parent about consistent use of seat belts. |

## Documentation

Document the following: date, time, assessment information, family members present, place and time where teaching occurred, teaching and type of educational aids provided, return demonstration by parents, parent reaction or statements, and suggestions for future teaching.

# *SKILL* 46 Fostering Healthy Sleep Patterns in Children

*Lynn B. Clutter*

Sleep habits change as children grow and develop. Sleep patterns emerge early in life, and by 6 months a healthy child should sleep through the night. Often, however, families struggle with sleep problems for much longer, or problems emerge at later ages. Sleep problems with infants can be so intense that the family is severely disrupted. Other sleep problems are common in older ages. Lack of adequate daytime and nighttime sleep interferes with normal growth, development, and health.

Sleep patterns are largely learned behaviors. A child is affected by internal factors that change slowly, e.g., the circadian rhythm. Numerous external factors, however, have significant influence as well and can be changed over a short period of time. Daytime and nighttime routines that foster healthy sleep patterns can be taught to parents who can help their children develop enjoyable and healthy habits. Knowledge about these patterns and about methods for teaching them to families is necessary to promote, maintain, or restore children's sleep. This skill provides assessment and intervention for those with existing sleep disruptions. Anticipatory guidance to prevent sleep problems is outlined in the Child and Family Teaching section.

## NURSING DIAGNOSES

Sleep pattern disturbances related to anxiety, depression, disruptions in life-style or environmental changes due to illness or hospitalization; Altered parenting related to lack of knowledge about methods to promote, maintain, or restore child's sleep.

| Steps | Rationale |
|---|---|
| **Assessment** | |
| 1. Determine age and developmental status of child. | Age and developmental status affect daytime and nighttime sleep requirements. Length and frequency of periods of sleep vary with age. |
| 2. Identify any neurologic deficits. | A child with neurologic deficits is more prone to sleep disorders that are organically based.<br>***Special Considerations:*** *More extensive evaluation or referral may be necessary for these types of sleep disorders.* |
| 3. Identify the presence of any physical causes of sleep disruption such as ear infections, teething, colic, or sleep apnea. Make referrals as necessary. | Physical causes can go unnoticed and should always be considered first. When treatment is possible, the sleep problem usually resolves itself. Some causes such as teething or colic are time limited, so sleep disruptions may be easier for a parent to accept.<br>***Special Considerations:*** *If loud snoring or periods of apnea are present, referral for a medical evaluation is a priority. Infant apnea is defined as: (1) cessation of breathing for 20 seconds or more; or (2) apnea less than 20 seconds but with bradycardia, cyanosis, or pallor (Whaley and Wong, 1991).* |
| 4. Identify family, social, or emotional factors that may be affecting sleep patterns. Pay special attention to family and individual stress levels. | Numerous social factors affect sleep. For example, sleeplessness in adolescence is common with depression or anxiety. Families and individuals with increased stress also have sleep difficulties related more to the causes of stress than the sleep problems.<br>***Special Considerations:*** *When other factors such as adolescent depression become evident, referral may be necessary.* |
| 5. Conduct a thorough sleep history (see box on p. 294). Include the following:<br>a. General history of chief complaint.<br>b. 24-hour sleep history.<br>c. Past sleep history. | A thorough history provides the detailed information necessary for an accurate plan of care. Many sleep problems and causes become clear once the problem is fully described.<br>***Special Considerations:*** *A parent who is sleep deprived may have difficulty concentrating on extensive questioning. Initially, focus on the chief complaint, providing ample opportunity to discuss feelings and concerns.* |

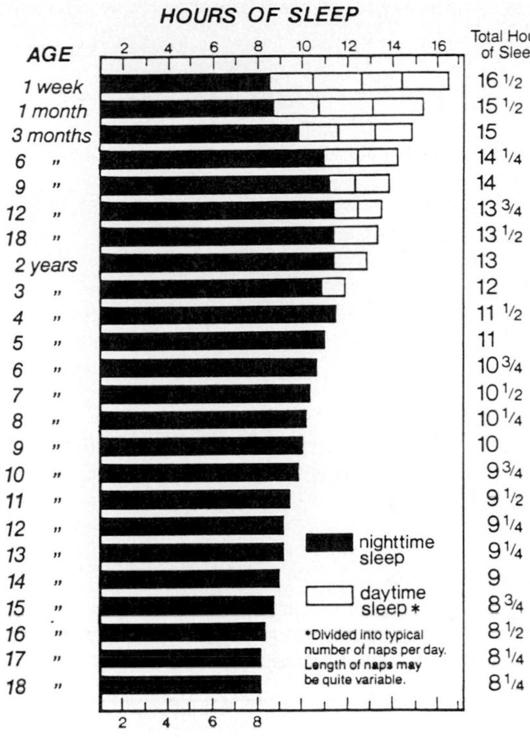


***FIG. 46-1*** Typical sleep requirements in childhood.

From Ferber R: Solve your child's sleep problems, New York, 1985, Simon and Schuster.

| Steps | Rationale |
|---|---|
| 6. Determine typical patterns of sleep for the child's age group (Fig. 46-1). | A knowledge of usual lengths and frequencies of daytime and nighttime sleep can assist in identifying problems and determining appropriate interventions.<br>***Special Considerations:*** *Variations in sleep patterns exist between individual children.* |
| 7. If additional home assessment data is needed from the family, ask the family to record actual sleep patterns for 2 weeks including bedtimes, night wakings, morning awakening, and naptime and additional observations. | Parents may not have organized routines or be aware of the child's actual sleep/wake patterns. Completing a sleep diary can increase awareness and may spontaneously lead to improvement. |

## Planning and Goal Setting

| Steps | Rationale |
|---|---|
| 1. Review common sleep disturbances (Table 46-1), identify disorder, review literature for specific information and management recommendations. | Common sleep disturbances are numerous and management regimes differ. If problems are not common and are outside the scope of nursing, referral may be necessary. |
| 2. Obtain or devise written materials (see Product References and Teaching Resources). | Parents who are distracted or sleep deprived may not fully remember suggested strategies, so they may benefit from additional materials for home use. |
| 3. Choose a time to be with appropriate family members when disruptions are limited. | Disruptions can hinder communication and comprehension.<br>***Special Considerations:*** *Recognize that their decision-making capacity, attention span, etc., may be altered because of sleep deprivation.* |
| 4. Develop individualized child and family goals:<br>▪ The child will learn to fall asleep alone.<br>▪ Parental intervention will not be required during child's routine night waking (after 6 months of age).<br>▪ The older child will stay in bed all night.<br>▪ Appropriate day, sleep and pre-sleep routines will be developed. | |

**TABLE 46-1** Selected Sleep Disturbances During Infancy and Childhood

| Disorder/Description | Management |
|---|---|
| **NIGHTTIME FEEDING** | |
| Child has a prolonged need for middle-of-night bottle- or breast-feeding.<br>Child goes to sleep at the breast or with a bottle.<br>Awakenings are frequent (may be hourly).<br>Child returns to sleep after feeding; other comfort measures (e.g., rocking or holding) are usually ineffective. | Increase daytime feeding intervals to 4 hours or more (may need to be done gradually).<br>Offer last feeding as late as possible at night; may need to gradually reduce amount of formula or length of breast-feeding.<br>Offer no bottles in bed.<br>Put to bed *awake*.<br>When crying, check at progressively longer intervals each night; reassure child but do not hold, rock, take to own bed, or give bottle or pacifier. |
| **DEVELOPMENTAL NIGHT CRYING** | |
| Child aged 6-12 months with undisturbed nighttime sleep now awakes abruptly; may be accompanied by nightmares. | Reassure parents that this is temporary phase.<br>Enter room immediately to check on child but keep reassurances brief.<br>Avoid feeding, rocking, taking to own bed, or any other routine that may initiate trained night crying. |
| **TRAINED NIGHT CRYING** | |
| Child typically falls asleep in place other than own bed, e.g., rocking chair or parent's bed, and is brought to own bed while asleep; upon awakening, cries until usual routine is instituted, e.g., rocking. | Put child in bed when *awake*.<br>If possible, arrange separate sleeping area from other family members.<br>When crying, check at progressively longer intervals each night; reassure child but do not resume usual routine. |
| **REFUSAL TO GO TO SLEEP** | |
| Child resists bedtime and comes out of room repeatedly.<br>Nightime sleep may be continuous, but frequent awakenings and refusal to return to sleep may occur and become a problem if parent allows child to deviate from usual sleep pattern. | Evaluate if hour of sleep is too early (child may resist sleep if not tired).<br>Assist parents in establishing consistent before-bedtime routine and enforcing consistent limits regarding child's bedtime behavior.<br>If child persists in leaving bedroom, close door for progressively longer periods.<br>Use reward system with child to provide motivation. |
| **NIGHTTIME FEARS** | |
| Child resists going to bed or wakes during the night because of fears.<br>Child seeks parent's physical presence and with parent nearby, falls asleep easily, unless fear is overwhelming. | Evaluate if hour of sleep is too early (child may fantasize when nothing to do but think in dark room).<br>Calmly reassure the frightened child; keeping a nightlight on may be helpful.<br>Use reward system with child to provide motivation.<br>Avoid patterns that can lead to additional problems, e.g., sleeping with child or taking child to parent's room.<br>If child's fear is overwhelming, consider desensitization, e.g., progressively spending longer periods of time alone; consult professional help for protracted fears.<br>Distinguish between nightmares and sleep terrors (confused partial arousals); best approach with sleep terrors is to remain uninvolved and allow child to stay asleep. |

From Wong DL and Whaley LF: Clinical manual of pediatric nursing, ed 3, St Louis, 1990, The CV Mosby Co.; Adapted from Ferber R: Behavioral "insomnia" in the child, Psychiatr Clin North Am 10(4):641-653, 1987.

| Steps | Rationale |
|---|---|
| **Implementation** | |
| 1. Isolate and describe the problematic behavior. | Clarity is improved when the problem is specifically isolated and reviewed. |
| 2. Determine potential causes of sleep problem from the sleep history. | The sleep history should reveal clusters of behaviors that are causes or results of a problem. For example, in early infancy, night feeding is necessary. If night feedings become a habit but are not required (generally after 6 months) they can cause sleep disruption because of digestive activity. |
| 3. Validate sleep problem and potential causes with family members. | Once sleep problems and potential causes are perceived, they should "ring true" to the family. If either is not validated, often information previously overlooked will be provided at this time. |

| **Steps** | **Rationale** |
|---|---|
| 4. Determine family members' willingness to work together in implementing planned changes. | Sleep pattern changes require a coordinated effort to be effective. Differences from one parent to the other are quickly perceived. Changes can best occur when all family members understand and work together toward the desired goals. Consistency is vital. |
| 5. Discuss potential origins of sleep problems such as those arising from the parent, child, or environment. For example:<br>a. Parent:<br>▪ Insufficient knowledge, e.g., number of average hours of sleep for age.<br>▪ Practices that hinder child's sleep.<br>▪ Lacks in schedule structuring.<br>▪ Lacks in behavioral limitations on child.<br>b. Child:<br>▪ Schedule inconsistencies.<br>▪ Strong desires such as staying up late to watch television.<br>▪ Problematic day, presleep, or nighttime habits.<br>c. Environment:<br>▪ Changes in noise, lighting, temperature, etc.<br>▪ Presence of people who are awake. | This information can distinguish problem clusters and shed light on intervention strategies (Table 46-1). |
| 6. Discuss any misconceptions parents may have about normal sleep or sleep problems. | Misconceptions and misunderstandings are common when dealing with children's sleep problems. Early clarification can prevent complications. For example, a common misconception is that sleep terrors are caused by bad dreams (Ferber, 1985).<br>***Special Considerations:*** *Sleep terrors can be frightening to witness, but unlike nightmares, the child will usually not remember the episode. Parental support should be offered.* |
| 7. Identify and discuss any emotional reactions. Allow adequate ventilation of feelings. | Concerns related to children are often laden with emotion. Furthermore, if sleep disruption to the parents has been great, it can lead to emotional distress. If parents disagree on management of the problem, or if the responsibility for management has fallen on one parent, marital stress can magnify emotions (Ferber, 1987b).<br>***Special Considerations:*** *Since sleep problems can be a symptom of other difficulties, close attention to emotions can encourage a willingness to discuss these issues.* |
| 8. Discuss suggested pattern changes for the child, parent, or both, e.g.:<br>a. The child changes associations of falling asleep from those of being rocked and with a parent, to going to sleep alone and in a crib/bed.<br>b. Once a child is in bed but begins to cry, the parent progressively lengthens the amount of time before intervening.<br>c. The parent learns to delay contact and the child learns to return or initiate sleep alone (Ferber, 1985). | Family members must take part in and be fully aware of changes that are to occur. Active involvement increases compliance with the plan.<br>***Special Considerations:*** *Some families that have lived with a child's sleep problem for a long time are very motivated to change. Others may feel that changes will require greater effort and lengths of time than they feel capable of giving. In these cases, discussions of actual time and effort necessary may be beneficial.* |
| 9. Discuss other recommended strategies that relate to the specific sleep problem (see Table 46-1 and References). | Some sleep problems are brief and easily corrected. Others require in-depth or ongoing interventions. Literature on sleep can be a valuable information source on strategies for specific disorders. |
| 10. Establish a plan for a follow-up contact by phone or visit. | Some changes are often difficult and results can be variable; a follow-up contact is needed. Further, a plan will less likely be abandoned if a follow-up contact is expected. |

| **Evaluation Outcomes** | **Observational Guidelines** |
|---|---|
| 1. The child goes to sleep alone. | The child is put to bed while awake and is asleep when checked on. The child uses comfort measures to put self to sleep. |
| 2. The child's usual pattern is to stay in bed all night except for bathroom trips when night toilet trained. | No evidence of the child having been up is seen. Parent is not awakened. |
| 3. The child does not require intervention once asleep. | Protests or pleas for parental presence stop. After normal, brief night wakings, the child returns to sleep without crying. |
| 4. Adequate day, presleep, and sleep patterns are present. | The child is alert in the daytime. Naps are appropriate in length. Presleep regime is not resisted and seems to be enjoyed. Night sleep is not disrupted. |

### ASSESSMENT OF SLEEP PROBLEMS IN CHILDREN*

**GENERAL HISTORY OF CHIEF COMPLAINT**

Ask parents/child to describe sleep problems; record in their words.

Inquire about onset, duration, character, frequency, and consistency of sleep problems:

- Circumstances surrounding onset (birth of sibling, start of toilet training, death of significant other, move from crib to bed).
- Circumstances that aggravate problem, e.g., overtiredness, family conflict, or disrupted routine (visitors).
- Remedies used to correct problem and results of interventions.

**24-HOUR SLEEP HISTORY**

Time and regularity of meals:†

- Family members present.
- Activities afterward, especially evening meal.

Time of nighttime and daytime sleep periods:

- Hours of sleep and waking.
- Hours of being put to bed and taken out of bed.
- How bedtime is decided (when child looks tired or at a time decided by parent; do both parents agree on bedtime).

Pre-bedtime or nap rituals (bath, bottle or breastfeeding, snack, television, active or quiet playing, story):

- Mood before nap or bedtime (wide awake, sleepy, happy, cranky).
- Which parent(s) participates in nap or bedtime rituals?

Nap and bedtime rituals:

- Where is child allowed to fall asleep (own bed or crib, couch, parent's bed, someone's lap, other)?
- Is child helped to fall asleep (rocked, walked, patted, given pacifier or bottle, placed in room with light, television, radio, or tape recorder on, other)?
- Are patterns consistent each time or do they vary?
- Does child awake if sleep aids are changed or taken away (placed in own bed, television turned off, other)?
- Does child verbally insist that parents stay in room?
- Child's behaviors if refuses to go to sleep or stay in room.
- If child complains of fear, how convincing are the fears?

Sleep environment:

- Number of bedrooms.
- Location of bedrooms, especially in relation to parent(s)' room.
- Sensory features (light on, door open or closed, noise level, temperature).

Nightwakings:

- Time, frequency, and duration.
- Child's behavior (call out, cry, come out of room, appear frightened, confused or upset).
- Parent(s)' responses (let child cry, go in immediately, take to own bed, feed, pick up, rock, give pacifier, talk, scold, threaten, other).
- Conditions that reestablish sleep.
  Do they always work?
  How long do the interventions take to work?
  Which parent intervenes?
  Do both parents use same or different approach?

Daytime sleepiness:

- Occurrence of falling asleep at inappropriate times (circumstances, suddenness, and irresistibility of onset, length of sleep, mood on awakening).
- Signs of fatigue (yawning, lying down, as well as overactivity, impulsivity, distractibility, irritability, temper tantrum).

**PAST SLEEP HISTORY**

Sleep patterns since infancy, especially age when slept during the night, stopped daytime naps, later bedtime.

Response to changes in sleep arrangements (crib to bed, different room or house, other).

Sleep behaviors (restlessness, snoring, sleepwalking, nightmares, partial wakings, [young child may wake confused, crying, and thrashing, but does not respond to parent; falls asleep with intervention if not excessively disturbed]).

Parent(s)' perception of child's sleep habits (good or poor sleeper, light or deep sleeper, needs little sleep).

Family history of sleep problem (sibling behavior imitated by child; some sleep disorders, e.g., narcolepsy and enuresis, tends to recur in families).

*Not all of these areas need to be assessed with every family. For example, if night wakings are not a problem, this section of the interview can be eliminated.

†A convenient point to start the 24-hour history is the evening meal.

From Wong DL and Whaley LF: Clinical manual of pediatric nursing, ed 3, St Louis, 1990, The CV Mosby Co.; Adapted from Ferber R: Assessment procedures for diagnosis of sleep disorders in children. In Noshpitz J, editor: Sleep disorders for the clinician, London, 1987, Butterworth Publishers.

## Documentation

Record detailed sleep history as needed (see box above); times of sleep and feedings; patterns of presleep behavior; and any usual presleep rituals. Describe problematic night waking and behaviors. Document interventions that are changes in habits, along with child and family members' responses. Record any intended future changes.

**Child and Family Teaching:**
***General strategies for prevention of sleep problems****

1. Maintain a consistent schedule. The child uses environmental cues such as daylight, dark, meals, school, activities, bedtime, presleep rituals, and times of waking to keep a 24-hour cycle.
2. In general, eliminate long daytime naps. Keeping nap length to 3 or less consecutive hours helps ensure prolonged sleep at night.
3. Limit excessive daytime and environmental stresses where possible.
4. Develop a consistent presleep bedtime routine that is peaceful, quiet, shared with a parent, and enjoyable. Reading, talking together, singing, playing quietly in bed, or saying prayers is appropriate.
5. Provide transitional presleep objects not associated with the parent but ones that can remain with the child to ease separation anxiety. Items such as a special blanket or stuffed animal are appropriate.
6. Put the child in bed while awake. The child must learn to go to bed alone, self-quiet, and put own self to sleep. This will help the child return to sleep without crying after normal, brief night wakings. When the child is old enough to understand, say "You're learning to go to sleep alone."
7. Establish the limit that once put to bed, the child will stay in bed. Parents should ignore ongoing questions, requests, demands, or protests and leave the room. If the child comes out of the room, they should be returned quickly and without conversation or affection. Consistency will prevail.
8. When a night visit is necessary, do not pick up the child. Offer brief (1 to 2 minutes) comfort, keep the room dark, act sleepy, whisper, and avoid eye contact. Give gentle reassurances but absolutely avoid secondary gains such as rocking, playing, prolonged presence, etc.

*Adapted from Schmitt BD: Your child's health, New York, 1987, Bantam Books and Ferber R: Solve your child's sleep problems, New York, 1985, Simon & Schuster.

9. Nightmares and bedtime fears differ from manipulative behavior. When experienced, brief parental presence and reassurance is provided.
10. Amount of sleep required varies, however, daytime naps usually reduce to one nap that is less than 2 hours. A common progression from ages 1-5 is from 2 naps, to 1 afternoon nap, to an afternoon "rest period."
11. Switch from crib to bed at 2 to 2½ years, or sooner with the first climbing out of the crib (when the crib springs are at the lowest setting).
12. In general, avoid the following:
    - Giving a bottle in the crib or bed.
    - Nursing, feeding, or rocking to sleep (these may be done while the child is drowsy but not asleep).
    - Disturbing the child as he or she moves around, makes noises, talks, sucks, or even cries out briefly as these often accompany light sleep or brief waking. The child is learning to put himself or herself back to sleep.
    - Providing entertainment at night.
    - Changing diapers (unless the diaper is soiled or a rash is present).
    - Taking the child to the parent's bed.
    - Returning to the crib to make the child lie down if he or she stands up as parent leaves.

***Selected guidelines for infants***

1. Make nightime feedings brief and boring.
2. Place infant in the crib when sleepy but awake. Allow time for self-quieting.
3. Try to keep the infant awake for the 2 hours before bedtime. Choose a late and consistent bedtime hour (10 or 11 p.m.) for the final feeding.
4. Interact, hold, and play with the infant during the daytime, wakeful periods. Providing daytime stimulation improves nighttime sleep.

# *SKILL 47* Instructing Parents in Day-care Selection

*Donna Phillips Smith*

With at least half of the mothers of young children employed outside the home, the impact of the day-care environment is considerable. Parents often have little knowledge to guide them in selecting alternative care that will be safe for their child emotionally, developmentally, and physically. Pediatric nurses can serve as a valuable resource to guide parents in this important decision.

## NURSING DIAGNOSES

Impaired home maintenance management related to lack of knowledge about evaluating child-care environments; Altered family process related to adjustment to child care; Potential for infection related to contact with contagious illnesses from other children.

| Steps | Rationale |
|---|---|
| **Assessment** | |
| 1. Assess the characteristics of the child.<br>a. Age.<br>b. State of health.<br>c. Physical or developmental impairments.<br>d. Temperament. | Child-care options vary considerably in the type of children served, and individual children vary in which option is most suitable for them.<br>***Special Considerations:*** *Many child-care options do not accept infants or nontoilet-trained toddlers. Parents of children with chronic health problems or physical/developmental impairments should seek centers specializing in this type of care (Briggs, 1987). The child's temperament must be considered (e.g., activity level, interaction with other children, need for consistency, maturity).* |
| 2. Assess family characteristics and needs.<br>a. Two working parents or a single parent.<br>b. Ability to pay for care.<br>c. Religious/cultural beliefs.<br>d. Hours during which care is needed and importance of flexibility.<br>e. Flexibility of job.<br>f. Availability of family member to provide care.<br>g. Prefer care to be located close to home or work. | The family characteristics, needs, and type of job must be considered to find an option that will be satisfactory.<br>***Special Considerations:*** *A single parent may need a more flexible arrangement in case of overtime, illness, or overnight travel. Quality child care is costly. Low-cost care may be unsafe and detrimental to the child. Investigate community resources if the family needs assistance to pay for quality care. Family may prefer a center with similar religious/cultural ties or philosophies. Hours and days of operation can vary considerably in day-care centers and group homes. Family and home sitters are usually more flexible. Type of care and job flexibility are considerations in case of illness of the child or the caregiver. Breastfeeding mothers may prefer care close to work.* |
| 3. Determine parental knowledge regarding evaluating child-care options and feelings and fears regarding child care. | An awareness of parental knowledge, fears, and feelings helps determine which issues to focus on in teaching.<br>***Special Considerations:*** *Parental fears, feelings, and prior experiences will strongly influence their decision as to the type of care they choose.* |
| **Planning and Goal Setting** | |
| 1. Select a quiet time to talk with the parent(s) without distractions. | Day-care issues can be sensitive and emotional. Providing privacy and freedom from distraction is helpful.<br>***Special Considerations:*** *Arrange for the child to not be present, if possible. The child may sense the parent's anxiety.* |
| 2. Investigate community resources based on assessment of the child and family's needs. | Focusing on facilities and types of care that will best meet needs saves time.<br>***Special Considerations:*** *State licensing agencies, which are usually affiliated with the state welfare or health department, often provide names of licensed centers and homes. Other resources are local child-care councils, family service agencies, churches, United Way, Community Chest, Junior League, a community helpline, the library, and other parents (Wong, 1986).* |
| 3. Obtain pamphlet or checklists for reference following discussion. | Written materials will reinforce the information presented.<br>***Special Considerations:*** *See Product References and Teaching Resources. Local welfare or health departments, or child-care councils may have materials.* |
| 4. Develop individualized child and family goals:<br>▪ To select a suitable child care arrangement.<br>▪ To prepare the child for the selected situation. | |
| **Implementation** | |
| 1. List the options generally available. Discuss the advantages and disadvantages of the types. See Table 47-1. | Parents may not be aware of options, and how various choices meet different needs. |
| 2. Suggest that parents personally visit several types of child care during normal hours of operation, with or without an appointment. | Observing several types of child care during operation will provide a basis for evaluating them.<br>***Special Considerations:*** *Parents should avoid any child-care option that refuses to tour parents without an appointment. An appointment may be needed, however, to meet the director.* |

***TABLE 47-1*** **Comparison of Child-care Arrangements**

| Type of Care | Advantages | Disadvantages |
|---|---|---|
| In-home sitter—Relative or person employed to provide child care in the child's home. | Consistent caregiver; undivided attention; maintenance of usual daily routines; no extra daily travel time; low infectious disease risk; illness of child does not necessitate other arrangements; caregiver may help with household duties; hours of care based on need. | Expensive; no contact with other children; quality of care and developmental stimulation will vary with caregiver; caregiver illness will require alternative care arrangement; abuse/neglect potential. |
| Family day care—In one caregiver's home with five or less children, including the caregiver's. | Small family setting; consistent caregiver; slight infectious disease risk; playmates for child, may be close to child's home; usually lower cost; child may already know caregiver. | Quality of care and developmental stimulation will vary with caregiver; may not be licensed; facilities may be less than adequate (e.g., sharing cribs); caregiver illness may require alternative care arrangement; no backup in case of emergency situation with one child; may have safety hazards such as unlocked cleaning materials; abuse/neglect potential. |
| Group day care—More than one caregiver (often family) and six or more children in the primary caregiver's home. | Home setting; fewer children than day-care centers; playmates available; usually lower cost. | Quality of activities may vary considerably; facility may be crowded and inadequate for variety of age groups; infectious disease risk; quality of care and developmental stimulation will vary with caregivers; may not be licensed; abuse/neglect potential. |
| Day-care centers—Larger numbers of children cared for in a facility designed for child care with staff, and a director | Planned daily activities and curriculum; staff more likely to be educated in child development and health and safety practices; age groups segregated; facilities usually more suitable; usually licensed, hot meals generally served; parent committees may be encouraged; social skill development fostered; abuse/neglect potential minimized because of supervision. | Quality of planned activities varies; caregivers may change; stimulation may be overwhelming to some chldren; more infectious disease risk depending on center practices; less individual attention; cost can vary considerably depending on quality of program and external funding. |

| Steps | Rationale |
|---|---|
| 3. Discuss factors parents can consider when visiting or interviewing a center, home, or caregiver. | |
| a. Licensing and accreditation status.<br>b. Availability of references. | Most states have licensing requirements for day-care homes and centers. Day-care centers may meet voluntary standards for accreditation through various organizations (Wong, 1986).<br>***Special Considerations:*** *Enforcement of state requirements varies considerably. Licensed facilities will have reports and records on file in regard to health, safety, qualifications of employees, and complaints. In-home sitters and family day care should provide references.* |
| c. Policies and philosophies, e.g., hours, fees, ages served, toilet-trained requirements, types of discipline practiced, religion and moral practices, personnel policies, and staff turnover rates. Also, for-profit or nonprofit status and sources of funding. | Characteristics and needs of the child and parents must be compatible with the facility's policies and philosophies. |
| d. Staff performance. Consider factors such as qualifications of staff and administrator, continuing education requirements, use of substitutes and volunteers, ratio of staff to children (the usual is 1:4 infants; 1:6 toddlers; 1:8-12 preschoolers; requirements vary state to state), and class size. Also, signs of caring staff include holding babies to bottle-feed, greeting children by name in the morning, and providing written or verbal comments on the child's day when the parent arrives. | Warm, nurturing and qualified staff are essential to a good child-care environment. |

| Steps | Rationale |
|---|---|
| e. Daily activities. Babies should be out of their cribs when awake; activities should vary between active/quiet, structure/free, group/individual and indoor/outdoor; television viewing should be selective; and independence in daily living skills should be encouraged. | A flexible daily schedule of a variety of activities will promote growth and development. **Special Considerations:** *The focus should be developmental rather than custodial, especially by age 3.* |
| f. Parental involvement, such as parents are allowed to visit at any time without notice; there are periodic meetings, newsletters, and evaluation; parents are encouraged to bring the child to and pick them up from the classroom rather than dropping them off at the door. | Alert, involved parents ensure quality child care (Wong, 1986). |
| g. Physical arrangement, e.g., separation of age groups; rooms should have adequate space with different areas or "centers" to play; each child should have an individual storage area for hats, coats, etc.; each child should have a crib or sleeping mat for naps. | Adequate space and pleasant surroundings will be enjoyable and healthier for children. |
| h. Health and safety. The playground should be safe and well-supervised; menus should be available and feature a variety of balanced foods with hot entrees, two snacks a day, and limited sweets; age-appropriate safety restraints should be used during vehicle transportation; poisonous plants should not be accessible on the playground; staff should wash hands frequently (especially after each diaper change) and encourage hand washing among the children; the diaper-changing table should have a washable covering that can be wiped with disinfectant after each change; older children should not help change diapers; infant and toddler toys should be cleaned frequently with disinfectant; and policies should exist regarding administering medications and excluding sick children and "drop-ins," who may be sick children not accepted at their regular center (Smith, 1986). | The health and safety practices of caregivers can have a significant effect on the child's physical safety and exposure to infectious diseases in day care settings. Chang, Hill-Scott, and Kassim-Lakka (1989) identified that day-care providers have definite health training and information needs. |
| 4. Serve as a resource for questions after parents have made visits or conducted interviews, and for decision-making. | Parents may feel confused and overwhelmed about the best situation for the child and their own needs. **Special Considerations:** *Ambivalence and guilt over working, even if there is no alternative, may intensify confusion.* |
| 5. Encourage the parents to prepare the child for the new care situation. Suggest parents visit the center or home with the child to meet the caregiver(s) and become familiar with the surroundings; talk enthusiastically about the new friends, toys, and activities the child will encounter; allow the child to bring a favorite toy or blanket; talk and behave confidently (Wong, 1986). Arrange for a new sitter to spend some time with the child while the parent is at home before the first day of care. | Children will adjust easier to the change if they are adequately prepared. **Special Considerations:** *Despite adequate preparation, the adjustment may be difficult for the parents and child.* |
| 6. Encourage the parents to make alternate plans between themselves or with family before illness of the child or a home caregiver. | When a child is ill, the parents must obtain or provide alternate care. **Special Considerations:** *For mild or prolonged illnesses (e.g., chicken pox), other options include private-duty nurse aides or sitters and "mildly ill child" care centers located on hospital pediatric units or close to day-care centers. A few day-care centers provide mild illness care for their regular enrollees (Harrison et al, 1987).* |
| 7. Provide guidelines to parents for continuing evaluation of the child-care situation. The best indicator of the quality of the services is a happy child who separates fairly easily from the parent when attending. | Continuing evaluation of the child-care situation will provide feedback as to their decision, alert the parents to potentially harmful situations, and indicate when the needs of the child change. **Special Considerations:** *Parents should investigate any unusual or suspicious incidents, accidents, bruises, behavioral changes, or remarks by the child (Wong, 1986). Advise the parent to provide sexual abuse awareness education to the child (Whaley and Wong, 1991).* |
| 8. Encourage parents to seek another arrangement if the situation is not satisfactory. | Even with careful investigation and decision-making a situation may not work. |

### Evaluation Outcomes

1. Parents identify their child-care needs.
2. Parents evaluate specific child-care situations.
3. Parents select a suitable child-care situation.
4. Parents prepare the child for the new situation.
5. Parents evaluate the success of the new arrangement.

### Observational Guidelines

Interview parents to determine the types of options they believe are most suitable for their needs.

Ask parents to share the questions and observations they are planning for their visits and interviews.

Ask parents to share their decision when made.

Ask parents to share what activities they have planned to ease the transition.

Have parents identify behaviors by the child or situations they might observe that would indicate an undesirable or unsafe situation.

### Documentation

Document in facility record teaching done, parental concerns expressed, and decision made by parents. Attendance at child care should also be documented on facility records to alert heath care professionals to potential infectious disease contact or neglect/abuse situation.

# *SKILL* 48 Instructing Parents in Child Sexuality and Sex Education

*Sylvia Kerr*

Instructing parents in childhood sexuality and sex education requires some specific skills related to the nurse's knowledge base, communication techniques, teaching/learning process and teaching methodologies.

Many parents are not prepared to discuss sexual matters with their child. Parents may lack information, be embarrassed, or not know how to begin. Therefore it may be easier for them to say, "I'll answer the questions as they arise." However, some children receive the message early on that it is "not O.K." to discuss sexual matters, so they do not ask questions. The nurse has an opportunity to assist the parents and the child with sex education.

### NURSING DIAGNOSES

Altered sexuality patterns related to absence of sexual education; Parental anxiety related to unmet informational needs regarding child's sexual development and strategies for teaching sexuality; Altered parenting related to inability to communicate with child about sexuality.

| Steps | Rationale |
|---|---|
| **Assessment** | |
| 1. Assess parents' knowledge of sexual anatomy, physiology, and vocabulary. For example, ask, "When you were a child where did you get information about sexual matters? As an adult? What did you learn to call the various parts of the genitalia? As a child, were you able to figure out how everything worked? What did you learn as an adult?" | Information obtained from parents will be helpful in developing the teaching plan. Sensitivity to parent's religious, ethnic, and cultural background is essential in dealing with sexuality. Parental experiences with sex education need to be taken into consideration. |
| 2. Determine parents' knowledge about sexual development. For example, ask, "Have you had the opportunity to learn about sexual development in children? Can you share with me what sexual activity you might expect from your child?" | |

| Steps | Rationale |
|---|---|
| 3. Gather information concerning the communication process between parents and child. For example, ask, "Who is responsible for talking with your child? Do you have a special time to talk with your child? Mom and child? Dad and child? Mom and Dad and child? What topics do you talk about? Who usually starts the discussion? How do you handle a situation in which your child disagrees with you? What kinds of questions has your child asked you about sexual matters?" | |
| 4. Ask parents to relate previous experiences with teaching this or another child. | This information will be helpful in choosing teaching methods that parents are comfortable using. |

## Planning and Goal Setting

| Steps | Rationale |
|---|---|
| 1. Prepare necessary materials, e.g., books, pamphlets, diagrams, models, films. | Being organized facilitates the teaching/learning process. **_Special Considerations:_** *See Product References and Teaching Resources for books for parents and children. Parent should read or review any material before using with a child.* |
| 2. Select an optimal time and place for educational interventions. | Learning is more likely to occur in a calm environment with minimal interruptions. |
| 3. Develop individualized child and family goals:<br>▪ Demonstrate knowledge of sexual vocabulary and expected sexual development through adolescence.<br>▪ Develop effective age-appropriate communication and teaching techniques for sex education. | |

## Implementation

| Steps | Rationale |
|---|---|
| 1. Review sexual anatomy and physiology using correct terminology. | It is necessary for parents to have an understanding of anatomy and physiology and know correct terminology to teach their child. Using the correct terminology will increase the parents' comfort with the vocabulary. |
| 2. Describe expected sexual development from infancy to adolescence.<br>a. Emphasize development for specific age of child.<br>b. Concentrate on development from specific age of the child through adolescence. | Parents will have an understanding of what "normal" sexual development entails as it relates to both their immediate and future parental needs. |
| 3. Describe the teaching process (see Skill 43). | Parents need to understand the basics of teaching for their efforts to be effective. |
| a. Choose the right time and place or use "teachable moments." The moments include when:<br>▪ Child notices Mom has breasts and pubic hair.<br>▪ Child notices Mom is pregnant.<br>▪ Child notices Dad has a penis.<br>▪ Child notices males and females urinate differently.<br>▪ Child walks in on adults having intercourse.<br>▪ Child sees sexually oriented programs and advertisement on television, in movies, and in magazines.<br>Additional opportunities that can be created by the parents:<br>▪ Newspaper, TV, and magazine stories.<br>▪ Bring up situations that you have heard about.<br>▪ Use books and pamphlets. | Parents must have the child's attention. |
| b. Determine what the child knows and thinks. For example, ask, "Can you explain that to me? What do you think about that? Would you describe that for me?" | Asking these questions identifies misconceptions the child might have. This allows the parent to begin teaching at the appropriate level. |
| c. Supply age-appropriate information with honesty. | Child will only understand if information is provided using a vocabulary with which he or she is familiar. Child will detect dishonesty and communication links will be destroyed. |
| d. Evaluate child's understanding of information presented:<br>▪ Ask child to repeat explanations.<br>▪ If using a book or pamphlet, go over it again and let child describe the content to you.<br>▪ Ask questions about the content.<br>▪ Say to the child, "If you were going to tell ________ about this, how would you explain it? What would you tell ________ if he/she asked (questions related to content)?" | Child can misinterpret or only pick up on certain parts of what is presented. The parent needs to know what the child's understanding is so that clarifications and corrections can be made. **_Special Considerations:_** *Evaluation does not need to be in the same session as the teaching. It can be done later and/or a little at a time.* |

| Steps | Rationale |
|---|---|
| 4. Discuss effective teaching techniques that parents may use. | Parents must be comfortable with teaching methods selected or they will not use them. |
| a. Use age-appropriate printed and audiovisual materials (books, pamphlets, models, diagrams, films, TV programs) with *discussion*. | Many teaching aids can be used, but the most effective teaching will include a discussion of the materials. |
| b. When no materials are available, simply discuss the topic with the child. | |
| 5. Facilitate communication between parents and child. | |
| a. Assist parents in planning their first experience in teaching their child. | This activity gives parents confidence in their ability to plan a teaching session. |
| b. Role play teaching session with parents, if necessary. | Role playing provides an opportunity for practice and helps to ease parental discomfort. |

| Evaluation Outcomes | Observational Guidelines |
|---|---|
| 1. The parents use sexual vocabulary accurately. | Ask questions and note vocabulary used in discussions and role play situations to validate use of accurate vocabulary. |
| 2. The parents correctly describe expected sexual development through adolescence. | Ask questions and note developmental information included in parental teaching plan to validate correct expected sexual development. |
| 3. The parents select age-appropriate teaching techniques. | Ask questions and note choices for teaching plan. |
| 4. The parents demonstrate age-appropriate communication techniques. | Ask questions and note techniques used in role playing activities. |

## Documentation

Record all pertinent assessment information obtained and any special concerns identified. Note parental response to sexuality topics (e.g., talks freely, evasive answers, or refuses to discuss). Document information presented, both verbal and written materials regarding child's sexual development and teaching techniques. Record parental plans to discuss topics with child and any special methods used, e.g., role playing. On follow-up visits, document reported interactions and outcomes and any additional teaching or referral provided.

UNIT V

### PRODUCT REFERENCES AND TEACHING RESOURCES

### Books

Berenstain S and Berenstain J: How to teach your children about sex . . . without making a complete fool of yourself, New York, 1979, Ballantine Books.
A funny, illustrated cartoon book depicting the humorous aspects of discussing sexuality with children.

Brazelton TB: Working and caring, Reading, Mass, 1985, Addison-Wesley Publishing Co, Inc.

Calderone M and Johnson E: The family book about sexuality, New York, 1989, Harper & Row, Publishers Inc.
A book for parents with a comprehensive discussion of the nature and development of human sexuality from birth to death. Emphasizes the importance of sexuality in a family setting.

Comfort A and Comfort J: The facts of love: loving, living and growing up, New York, 1979, Crown Publishers.
Sensitive, honest book about sexuality for teens and their parents. Provides information, dispels fears, discusses sexual behavior within a loving and responsible framework. Sets limits without being "preachy." Realistic line drawings.

Ferber R: Solve your child's sleep problems, New York, 1985, Simon & Schuster.
This book includes in-depth, easy-to-understand guidelines for solving numerous sleep problems.

Gordon S: Girls are girls and boys are boys: so what's the difference? Fayetteville, NY, 1979, Ed-U Press.
Briefly explains human reproduction, the physical differences between boys and girls, and that these differences have no effect on a person's choice of career or other interests.

Gordon S: You would if you loved me, New York, 1978, Bantam Books.
Collection of "sex lines" heard and used by youth and responses to them.

Gordon S and Gordon J: Did the sun shine before you were born? Fayetteville, NY, 1979, Ed-U Press.
A book that parents can read with their preschool or primary school-age children. In addition to answering the questions "Where do babies come from?" clearly and directly, it deals with other aspects of how different kinds of families live and grow.

Madaras L: What's happening to my body? A growing up guide for mothers and daughters, New York, 1983, Newmarket Press; What's happening to my body? Book for boys: a growing up guide for parents and sons, New York, 1984, Newmarket Press.
Separate books for boys and girls designed to be read with a parent. Includes information on puberty in girls and boys.

McCoy K: The teenage body book guide to sexuality, New York, 1983, Simon & Schuster.
Provides answers to teens' questions about sexuality. Designed to enable teens to better understand themselves, their sexual feelings, actions, and alternatives, and to help them make the right choices. Quotes from teens highlight points being made. Illustrations supplement text.

Miller JA and Weissman S: The parent's guide to day care, New York, 1986, Bantam Books.

Ross Laboratories: Your child and sleep, Columbus, Ohio, 1987, Ross Laboratories.
A pamphlet and poster are available with a chart of typical hours of required sleep, and a guide for learning to fall asleep with proper associations.

Schmidt BD: When your child refuses to go to bed, Contemp Pediatr 6(7):70-71, 1989.
A parent information aid on bedtime refusal that may be photocopied and distributed to parents and patients without permission of the publisher.

### Products

Toys to Grow On
2695 E. Dominquez St
Long Beach, CA 90801
No Choke Testing Tube (to determine if small parts of toys pose a choking hazard to children under 3).

### Organizations

American Academy of Pediatrics
141 Northwest Point Blvd
PO Box 927
Elk Grove Village, IL 60009-0927
1-800-433-9016 or 1-800-421-0589 (IL)
Items available from AAP:
Pamphlets addressing safety concepts related to trampolines, school buses, car safety, skateboard injuries, rural injuries, and general injury prevention. Send a self-addressed, stamped envelope with request to obtain one free copy. These include:
Child safety slips—Safety guidelines cover infant furniture, playground equipment, safe swimming
TIPP (The Injury Prevention Program)—Framingham Safety Survey questionnaires and age-related safety sheets
Traffic Safety Education Program Catalogue—Publications and services for pediatric health care professionals
Offers the following:
A family shopping guide for infant child safety seats; Children and car safety: making friends with a safety seat
Child safety seat check up
Premature infants and car seats
Safety seat use for children with hip dislocation
Also offers:
Tips on selecting the "right" day care facility
Day care: finding the best child care for your family

Automotive Safety for Children Program
James Whitcomb Riley Hospital for Children
Indiana University School of Medicine
702 Barnhill Drive, P-121
Indianapolis, IN 46223
(317) 274-2977
The Program is a resource and network for information on transporting infants and children who cannot use regular safety seats.

National Center for Missing and Exploited Children
1-800-843-5678
The Missing Child Network 1-800-235-3535

National Safe KIDS Campaign
Sk-2. 111 Michigan Avenue NW
Washington, DC 20011
Free magazine for children on traffic safety.

National Safety Council
444 North Michigan Ave
Chicago, IL 60611
1-800-621-7619
(312) 527-4800 (IL)
Resources such as videos, films, booklets and pamphlets.

Planned Parenthood Federation of America, Inc
810 Seventh Ave
New York, NY 10019

Sex Information and Education Council of the United States
80 Fifth Ave
Suite 801
New York, NY 10011

U.S. Consumer Product Safety Commission
Washington, DC 20207
Hotline 1-800-638-2772—For safety questions and to report an unsafe consumer product or product-related injury.
Safety News—Free monthly publication of safety alerts and news releases.

U.S. Department of Health and Human Services
Washington, DC 20201
Offers the Parents checklist for day care, DHHS Publication No. (OHDS) 84-30270.

## REFERENCES


American Academy of Pediatrics, Committee on Accident and Poison Prevention: Bicycle helmets, Elk Grove Village, Ill, 1989, American Academy of Pediatrics.

American Academy of Pediatrics: Health in day care: a manual for health professionals, Elk Grove Village, Ill, 1987.

Baker S, O'Neill B, and Karp R: The injury fact book, Lexington, Mass, 1984, DC Health and Co.

Braga J and Braga L: Children and adults: activities for growing together, Englewood Cliffs, NJ, 1976, Prentice-Hall.

Briggs N: Day care for medically fragile children, Pediatr Nurs 13(2):120-121, 1987.

Bull MJ and Stroup KB: Premature infants in car seats, Pediatrics, 75(2):336-339, 1985.

Bull MJ, Weber K and Stroup KB: Safety seat use for children with hip dislocation, Pediatrics 77(6):873-875, 1986.

Bull MJ, Weber K, and Stroup KB: Automotive restraint systems for premature infants, J Pediatr 112:385-388, 1988.

Chang A, Hill-Scott K, and Kassim-Lakka S: Health training and information needs of child day care providers, Children's Health Care 18(2):96-101, 1989.

Christopherson ER and Gynlay ME: Parental compliance with car seat usage—a positive approach with long-term follow-up, J Pediatr Psych, 6:301-311, 1981.

Cushing M: Legal lessons on patient teaching, Am J Nurs 84(6):721-722, 1984.

Cynecki MJ and Goryl ME: The incidence and factors associated with child safety seat misuse, US Department of Transportation Report, No DOT HS 806-676, Washington, DC, 1984, National Highway Traffic Safety Administration.

DiMario F and Emery ES III: The natural history of night terrors, Clin Pediatr 26(10):505-511, 1987.

Dorman L and Rebelsky F: Growing children, Monterey, Calif, 1976, Brooks Cole Publishing Co.

Edgil A et al: Sleep problems of older infants and preschool children, Pediatr Nurs 11(2):87-89, 1985.

Eiden H, Thomas M, and Fosarelli P: A teaching tool for children in self care, J Pediatr Health Care 1(6):292-296, 1987.

Faber MM: A review of efforts to protect children from injury in crashes, Fam Comm Health 9(3):25-41, 1986.

Ferber R: Solve your child's sleep problems, New York, 1985, Simon & Schuster.

Ferber R: Assessment procedures for diagnosis of sleep disorders in children in Noshpitz J, editor: Sleep disorders for the clinician, London, 1987a, Butterworth Publishers.

Ferber R: Behavioral insomnia in the child, Psych Clin North Am 10(4):641-653, 1987b.

Ferber R: Sleeplessness, night awakening, and night crying in the infant and toddler, Pediatr Rev 9(3):1-14, 1987c.

Ferber R: Sleep disorders in children, Pediatr Consult 7(2):1-12, 1988.

Fisher B et al: Children's sleep behavior scale; normative data on 870 children in grades 1 to 6, Percept Mot Skills 68(1):227-236, 1989.

Green M: Helping parents make the right child-care choice, Contemp Pediatr 3(6):40-49, 1986.

Greensher J: How anticipatory guidance can improve control of childhood "accidents," Pediatric Consult 3(2):1-8, 1984.

Guilleminault C, editor: Sleep and its disorders in children, New York, 1987, Raven Press.

Gunnip A et al: Car seats: helping parents do it right! J Pediatr Health Care 1(4):190-195, 1987.

Hancock L: Safe biking: A bike helmet, J Pediatr Health Care 1:334, 1987.

Hancock L: Product alert, J Pediatr Health Care 2:155, 1988.

Harrison L et al: Establishing and evaluating a children's sick room program, MCN 12(3):204-206, 1987.

Knafle K, Cavallari K, and Dixon D: Pediatric hospitalization: family and nurse perspectives, Glenview, Ill, 1988, Scott, Foresman & Co.

Masters WH, Johnson VE, and Kolodny R: Human sexuality, ed 3, Glenview, Ill, 1988 Scott, Foresman & Co.

Mims FH and Swenson M: Sexuality: a nursing perspective, New York, 1980, McGraw-Hill, Inc.

Moore E et al: Protecting our children through kid safe, Pediatr Nurs 14:32-36, 1988.

National Highway Traffic Safety Administration, Notices, Federal Register, 53(124):24395, 1988.

National Passenger Safety Association, Child Safety Seat Shopping Guide, Washington, DC, 1986, National Passenger Safety Association.

Nix KS: Guidelines for car safety. In Wong DL and Whaley LF: Clinical manual of pediatric nursing, ed 3, St Louis, 1990, The CV Mosby Co.

Padilla ML and Landreth GL: Latchkey children: a review of the literature, Child Welfare 68:445-454, 1989.

Pagel J: Nightmares, Am Fam Phys 39(3):145-148, 1989.

Pontius S: Practical Piaget: helping children understand, Am J Nurs 82(1):114-117, 1982.

Poorman S: Human sexuality and the nursing process, Norwalk, Conn, 1988, Appleton and Lange.

Potter PA and Perry AG: Fundamentals of nursing concepts, process and practice, ed 2, St Louis, 1989, The CV Mosby Co.

Rickert V and Johnson CM: Reducing nocturnal awakening and crying episodes in infants and young children: a comparison between scheduled awakenings and systematic ignoring, Pediatrics 81(2):203-212, 1989.

Ridenour MV: Elementary school playground: safe play areas or inherent dangers, Percept Mot Skills 64:446-451, 1987.

Rothenberg B et al: A practical handbook for teaching parent classes about babies and toddlers. Menlo Park, Calif, 1981, The Banister Press.

Rural Injuries, Pediatrics, 81:902, 1988.

Schmit B: When your child refuses to go to bed, Contemp Pediatr 6(7):70-71, 1989.

Shesser LK: Car seat modification for children under treatment for congenitally dislocated hips, Orthop Nurs 4(6):11-13, 1985.

Smith D: Myths about day care: fact or fantasy? Pediatr Nurs 10(4):278-280, 1984.

Smith DP: Common day care diseases: patterns and prevention. Pediatr Nurs 12(3):175-179, 1986.

Statistical abstract of the US national data book and guide to sources, Washington, DC, 1987, US Department of Commerce.

Stroup KB, Weber K, and Bull MJ: Safe transportation solutions for children with special needs, American Association of Automotive Medicine, Thirty-first annual conference proceedings, New Orleans, Sept 28-30, 1987.

Taylor R: Making the most of your time for patient teaching, RN 12:20-21, 1987.

Thompson RS, Rivara FP, and Thompson DC: A case-control study of the effectiveness of bicycle safety helmets, N Engl J Med, 320(21):1362-1367, 1989.

University of North Carolina Highway Safety Research Center: Restraint options for the older child, Highway Safety Directions 1(2):12-19, 1988.

Weber K and Allen NP: Factors affecting consumer acceptance and use of child restraint systems, University of Michigan Highway Safety Research Institute Report No. UM-NSRI-82-1, 1982.

Weiss B and Duncan B: Bicycle helmet use by children, Am J Public Health 76:1022-1023, 1986.

Whaley L and Wong D: Nursing care of infants and children, ed 4, St Louis, 1991, The CV Mosby Co.

White BL: Educating the infant and toddler, Lexington, Mass, 1988, DC Heath & Co.

Wintemute GJ et al: Drowning in childhood and adolescence: a population based study, Am J Public Health 77:830-832, 1987.

Wishon P and Oreskovich M: Bicycles, roller skates and skateboards: safety promotion and prevention, Children Today, May/June, 1986, pp. 11-15.

Wong DL: Helping parents select daycare centers, Pediatr Nurs 12(3):181-187, 1986.

Wong DL and Whaley LF: Clinical manual of pediatric nursing, ed 3, St Louis, 1990, The CV Mosby Co.

Young K and Zigler E: Infant and toddler day care: regulations and policy implications, Am J Orthopsychiatry 56(1):43-55, 1986.

Younger J: The managements of night waking in older infants, Pediatr Nurs 8(3):155-158, 1982.

# UNIT VI Safety and Comfort

# SKILL 49 Providing a Safer Hospital Environment

*Kathryn A. Perry*

Accidents are the major cause of morbidity and mortality in childhood. Health professionals teach parents about safety hazards in the home, in cars, near water and at play. Health care facilities, however, are another source of potential environmental hazards that must be evaluated. Assessment of developmental age and level of mobility is crucial in defining potential risks for injury. Implementing an individualized plan for a safer hospital environment is more than good patient care or risk management; it also provides the opportunity to demonstrate injury prevention skills to parents.

## NURSING DIAGNOSES

Potential for injury related to hospital environmental hazards, unfamiliar surroundings, and/or developmental age; Altered health maintenance related to lack of parental knowledge about child safety needs.

| Steps | Rationale |
|---|---|
| **Assessment** | |
| 1. Assess child's age, developmental level, and physical development (see Skills 25 and 27). | The risk factors for injury potential are determined by developmental stage. Many of these factors are different at each developmental stage and also vary from child to child. ***Special Considerations:*** *Child may attain a new developmental task for the first time while in the hospital. Anticipate development to reduce risk (e.g., infant who rolls over for the first time or child who learns to climb).* |
| 2. Assess normal daily activities and patterns. | Knowledge of usual patterns is helpful when developing an individualized plan of care. As the plan of care reflects progress toward normal activities, the safety factors for these activities must also be included. For example, an active child may be at greater risk for injury than a lethargic child expending little energy. |
| 3. Assess level of mobility. | Mobility is assessed so that hazards may be anticipated. ***Special Considerations:*** *During the hospitalization, the level of mobility may change as the child feels better. There should be an ongoing assessment of these risk factors.* |
| 4. Assess medical history and therapies for potential safety risks such as physical limitations, past injury history, and conditions predisposing to injury risk (e.g., seizures, altered mentation, drug therapy). | These factors may increase injury risk, although Banco and Powers (1988) reported few falls during ambulation related to preexisting medical problems. Unsafe play was a more common reason for falls. Presence of sedation, confusion, or disorientation indicate a need for precautions such as raised side rails for an older child. |
| 5. Review physician activity orders/restrictions. | Although a child may be capable of activity and mobility, it may not be permitted for therapeutic reasons. |

| Steps | Rationale |
|---|---|
| 6. Assess physical environment such as the flow of the room, equipment within the child's reach, unnecessary clutter, and potential hazards on the unit outside the room. | Unfamiliar surroundings create the potential for injury. A careful evaluation of the environment from the viewpoint of the child can reveal many hazards. |
| 7. Observe parent/child interaction: parents' awareness of safety hazards and parents' limit-setting abilities. | Family may need additional information regarding potential hazards in the hospital environment. Parents who do not safely restrict their child's activity need additional teaching and role modeling of safe limits. |

## Planning and Goal Setting

| Steps | Rationale |
|---|---|
| 1. Gather age-appropriate equipment. Inspect equipment and furniture. | Developmental considerations for equipment used for a child are vital to providing a safe environment. |
| 2. Inspect electrical equipment and sources for potential hazards. | Electrocution and burns are major concerns for the curious child. |
| 3. Inspect toys that are available on the unit and toys that are brought from home or given by visitors. | Toys should be in good repair and age appropriate. |
| 4. Develop individualized goals of nursing care:<br>▪ Injury during hospitalization will be prevented or minimized.<br>▪ Hospital environment will be assessed for potential hazards throughout hospitalization. | |

## Implementation

### *General measures*

| Steps | Rationale |
|---|---|
| 1. Explain safety measures to family and child. | Family and child awareness of safety measures and reasons for them may foster cooperation.<br>***Special Considerations:*** *Role modeling is an effective means to communicate the importance of safety measures.* |
| 2. Remove excess equipment and furniture from rooms and hallways, e.g., wheelchairs, chairs, extra cribs/beds, wagons, and carts. | Excess clutter increases the risk for falls and is a hazard in case of emergency evacuation. Unused wheelchairs stored in hallways are also a hazard because children, including visitors, are tempted to play with them.<br>***Special Considerations:*** *Removal of excess furniture is also important to prevent injury during a seizure (see Skill 85).* |
| 3. Avoid highly waxed floors. Wipe liquid spills on the floor immediately. | Floors that are slick from liquid or polish increase the risk for falls.<br>***Special Considerations:*** *The child with unsure footing or the toddler with newly acquired walking skills is at risk for falls.* |
| 4. Prevent access by the child to tubs, laundry chutes, and medication rooms/carts. | A potential for drowning, falls, and poisonings exists with unimpeded access to these areas (Banco and Powers, 1988). |
| 5. Secure windows if ventilating type; check for screens and guards. If window coverings have an operating cord, shorten it or secure cord out of reach. | Windows that will open pose a fall risk. Operating cords for window coverings pose a strangulation hazard for young children. |
| 6. Place bed or crib out of reach of heating units, equipment, and dangling cords or IV lines. | Burns, strangulation, or injury from falling equipment may occur. |
| 7. Coil and secure excess electrical cord on equipment. | Cords on the floor may cause a fall or other injuries should equipment be caught and turned over. |
| 8. Place locked sharps (needles, lancets, and blades) disposal boxes in a location inaccessible to the child but easy for staff to use (see also Skill 50). | Locked sharps disposal boxes that are properly placed and secured prevent needle stick and laceration injuries. |
| 9. Properly dispose of other waste items such as glass and tubing. Do not use plastic bags in trash containers without adequate supervision. | Young children often explore trash containers for "play" items. Plastic bags pose a suffocation hazard, and other risks exist specific to the discarded item. |

### *Infants and toddlers*

| Steps | Rationale |
|---|---|
| 1. Keep crib side rails up at all times unless direct care is being given. Maintain hand contact if turning away to obtain an item. Use a bubble top or crib netting if child may be capable of climbing over raised rails (see Skill 51). | Raised side rails are an important fall prevention measure. Banco and Powers (1988) found in a survey of incident reports that in all cases of crib-related falls, the side rail of the crib had been left down, generally by parents or visitors.<br>***Special Considerations:*** *The contact surface and height of the fall are variables determining the severity of injury (Nimityongskul and Anderson, 1987).* |
| 2. Inspect crib mattress/frame fit for gaps at the top or bottom when the mattress is level, and when the head or knee gatch is engaged. | Gaps between the mattress and crib frame could result in entrapment or strangulation. |

| Steps | Rationale |
|---|---|
| 3. Avoid using pillows and excess linen in an infant's crib. | These items could result in accidental suffocation. |
| 4. Use infant seats, highchairs, strollers and swings with adequate restraints and in good repair. High chairs should balance. | Inadequate restraint or unsafe use of these items is a commonly identified hazard (Banco and Powers, 1988). **Special Considerations:** *Baby walkers pose a hazard for burns, falls down stairs, and other injuries by providing access the child would not otherwise have to hazards (Child Health Alert, 1988).* |
| 5. Inspect playpens for broken sides that may suddenly collapse. | If lowered, the playpen side becomes a hazard for entrapment and strangulation. |
| 6. Cover all electrical outlets that are not in use. | Exposed electrical outlets present a hazard for electrocution/electrical burns. |
| 7. Provide only commercially made, one-piece pacifiers. Do not tie a pacifier around a child's neck. | Fatal aspirations have been reported with use of "makeshift" pacifiers (bottle nipples stuffed with cotton and taped) (Millunchick and McArtor, 1986). |
| 8. Use metal or unbreakable spoons when feeding. | Plastic spoons may splinter if a child bites down forcefully. |
| 9. Allow only safe and age-appropriate toys. Avoid toys with small parts, balloons, bean bag toys, and toy boxes without safe hinges. | Toys with small parts, balloons, and beans pose an aspiration risk. Aspirated beans may also swell as moisture is absorbed, increasing airway obstruction. Toy boxes without safe hinges may cause head entrapment. **Special Considerations:** *Use only nonfriction toys in an oxygen tent.* |
| 10. Keep cleaning agents stored out of reach of children, including those on housekeeping carts. Mop buckets containing liquid should also be inaccessible. | Cleaning agents are usually hazardous if ingested. A filled bucket can be a drowning hazard for toddlers who are prone to lose balance and fall head first. |
| 11. Provide adequate playroom supervision by child life staff, volunteers, or family members. | Supervision of young children helps prevent injuries from unsafe play and age-inappropriate toys. |
| ***Preschool and older children*** | |
| 1. Maintain beds in low position with wheels locked in place. Electric beds should not have "walk away down controls" (once activated, bed automatically descends to low position) or the feature should be disabled. | Low position and locked wheels help to prevent or minimize injury from falls. Fatalities have occurred when children became trapped under a descending bed with a "walk away down control" feature (Merz, 1983). **Special Considerations:** *A high bed position permits easier access for care with a critically ill or comatose child not at risk for climbing out of bed.* |
| 2. Raise side rails for younger child, or if indicated by assessment of risk or physician order. | **Special Considerations:** *In most cases of falls from beds, the rails were in the raised position (Banco and Powers, 1988).* |
| 3. Use only wheelchairs appropriately equipped with restraints, footrests, and wheel locks. | Restraints and wheel locks reduce the risk for falls. Footrests help prevent entrapment or other foot injuries. |
| 4. Provide nonskid surfaces in showers/tubs. | Wet, smooth surfaces increase the risk for falls. |
| 5. Place shoes with nonskid soles on the child for ambulation (see Skill 71). | Nonskid soles help prevent falls. |

| Evaluation Outcomes | Observational Guidelines |
|---|---|
| 1. Hallways and rooms remain free of the clutter of extra furniture or equipment. | Continually observe for potential hazards, e.g., equipment or excess furniture that may be carelessly left in hallways or rooms. |
| 2. No injury occurs because of faulty equipment or furniture. | Inspect beds, cribs, wheelchairs, highchairs for broken parts, malfunctions, or missing restraints. |
| 3. Environmental hazards are not present. | Observe for potential hazards in storage of supplies, open doors and on floors. |
| 4. Toys are age-appropriate and safe. | Inspect toys for broken parts or multiple pieces that could become aspirated. |
| 5. Family demonstrates proper safety precautions and use of equipment. | Note family's observation of safety precautions, e.g., keeping crib/bed rails up, proper use of bed, keeping hazardous objects out of reach. |

## Documentation

Document behaviors or conditions that may place the child at risk for injury. Document any changes that are made to accommodate the potential risks. Document teaching done with the family on crib/bed safety, ambulation restrictions, or additional precautions taken for safety.

# SKILL 50 Preventing Transmission of Infection in an Acute Care Setting

*Donna Phillips Smith*

Preventing the transmission of infectious microorganisms in an acute care setting requires consistent and effective infection control practices. The chain of infection within this setting requires three elements: a source of infecting organisms, a susceptible host, and a means of transmission (Centers for Disease Control, 1983). The source of organisms and the susceptible host elements are difficult to control, so efforts to interrupt the chain are usually aimed at transmission: from patient to patient, from staff to patient, and from patient to staff.

Traditionally, two types of infection control measures have been implemented to achieve this purpose (Lynch et al, 1987). One type is routine patient care practices such as handwashing, sterile needles for injections, and sterile catheter insertion. Used with all patients, these measures are *procedure driven*. The second type, *diagnosis-driven* measures, dictate the use of special isolation precautions for those patients diagnosed or suspected of having a particular infectious disease. These precautions consist of various barriers such as nonsterile gloves, gowns, masks, and/or private rooms.

The Centers for Disease Control (CDC) 1983 Guideline for Isolation Precautions in Hospitals reflected commonly used diagnosis-driven measures with two recommended systems. First, the *category specific* system of isolation precautions was a revision of the CDC's 1970 recommendations, and included seven categories: Strict, Respiratory, Enteric, Contact, Tuberculosis, Drainage-Secretions, and Blood-Body Fluids. The alternative *disease specific* isolation precautions system was tailored to the transmission peculiarities of different infectious organisms. The CDC encouraged adoption of one of the two systems, or the hospital could design their own system (CDC, 1983).

Growing concern that diagnosis-driven precautions left a gap in coverage when infection was not suspected or diagnosed led one medical center to develop their own system over a period of 3 years (McPherson and Jackson, 1987). This system recognized that a large majority of infectious and communicable diseases are undiagnosed, and of the diagnosed ones, most are communicable before the onset of symptoms (Lynch and Jackson, 1986). Additionally, hospitalized patients may have colonized body substances such as tracheostomy secretions that can serve as a reservoir for multiple drug-resistant organisms yet not be considered as "infectious." The new system, called *body substance isolation* (BSI), targets isolation of potentially infectious body substances through the use of appropriate barrier precautions with all patients. This system is *interaction driven,* since all interactions that could result in contact with blood or body fluids require barrier precautions such as gloves, plastic apron/gown, goggles, and/or masks. The only exception is a diagnosis-driven precaution for diseases transmitted by the airborne route; a mask is required based on a determination of susceptibility to the particular agent.

In response to the increasing risk and fear of transmission of HIV, hepatitis B, and other blood-borne pathogens, especially in undiagnosed patients, the CDC revised its guidelines in 1987 (CDC, 1987). The recommendations included application of the precautions outlined in the "Blood and body fluid" category to all patients, subsequently known as *universal precautions* (UP). The remaining six categories would still apply to patients diagnosed as requiring such precautions.

The previously developed body substance isolation (BSI) system, a similar system of universal precautions, has been endorsed by the American Hospital Association. Whether the CDC's universal precautions or a variation such as BSI is adopted by the hospital, these newer guidelines encourage individual judgment in applying the appropriate barriers. Nurses who work with children experience substantial contact with communicable diseases, body secretions, and exposure to blood during procedures. This skill provides guidelines to implement appropriate infection control measures to protect both the child and the nurse in an acute care setting.

## NURSING DIAGNOSES

Potential for infection related to inadequate host defenses (broken skin, immunosuppression, malnutrition); Diarrhea related to gastrointestinal irritation due to infection.

| Steps | Rationale |
|---|---|
| **Assessment** | |
| 1. Determine infection control policies of facility: | Facility policies vary based on many factors such as local disease prevalence. Familiarity with the appropriate policies allows informed decision-making in patient care. |
| a. Isolation system: universal precautions, with category or disease specific system; BSI; or other developed system. | A consistent, effective system of appropriate barrier precautions prevents the transmission of potentially infectious agents. ***Special Considerations:*** *Combining elements of the category and disease specific systems, or BSI with either category or disease specific systems is not recommended as it is confusing and sends unclear directives to the staff (CDC, 1983 and Jackson et al, 1987).* |
| b. Room assignment. | Facility policies vary on room assignment, with decisions based on patient diagnosis, type of isolation system used, type of rooms available, ventilation system, and priority protocol for assigning rooms. |
| c. Playroom privileges. | In some facilities a practitioner's order may be necessary for a child to be allowed to visit the playroom, although infection control may not be the only factor. In others, nursing judgment is sufficient. |
| d. Toy cleaning procedure—playroom toys and toys from patient rooms. | Policies on toy cleaning and the type of toys allowed vary based on the type of isolation precautions employed by the facility, and the age of the child. |
| 2. Review patient information as known: | |
| a. Diagnosis. | A known or suspected diagnosis of infectious disease has implications for appropriate barrier precautions. Other diagnoses may indicate that the child is at increased risk for infection, e.g., surgical incision, nonintact skin, immunosuppression. |
| b. Health history—Significant information to elicit includes congenitally acquired infectious disease (HIV, rubella, cytomegalovirus [CMV]), immunization status, exposure to infectious disease at home or in the community, transfusion recipient, travel out of the country, presence of blood in normally blood-free body fluids (stool, urine, vomitus), and persistent cough (see also Skill 23). | A health history may elicit significant information that will influence nursing care, diagnosis, and treatment. For example, a newborn with congenital rubella syndrome will shed the virus for months (Berenson, 1985). However, a medical history will not reliably identify all patients capable of transmitting infectious agents. |
| c. Physical assessment—Significant signs and symptoms to observe include fever and alterations in vital signs, enlarged lymph nodes, skin rashes and lesions, inflammation (redness, warmth, swelling, pain), unusual discharge, lethargy, respiratory symptoms, and anorexia. Also note the presence of invasive devices, surgical incision, or trauma wound or burn. Review laboratory data (see Skill 27). | Identification of an infectious process aids in diagnosis and therapeutic treatment and determination of appropriate barrier precautions. Identification of invasive devices or altered protective mechanisms that increase host susceptibility also allows appropriate observation and intervention. |
| d. Physician orders such as need for private room or special diagnostic tests. | A review of physician orders assists in planning additional precautions and routine nursing care. ***Special Considerations:*** *If physician orders are not consistent with facility policy, follow appropriate procedure to resolve.* |
| 3. Determine own health status. | Nursing staff can serve as a reservoir for infectious agents, as well as being susceptible hosts. An evaluation of these factors to determine appropriate barrier precautions should be based on anticipated contact. |
| a. Intact skin. | Nonintact skin serves as a portal of entry for potentially pathogenic microorganisms. Minor cuts and areas of breakdown may go unnoticed. |
| b. Immune status for rubella, measles, poliomyelitis, influenza, and hepatitis B (Williamson et al, 1988). | Nursing personnel are at risk for exposure to and possible transmission of vaccine-preventable diseases, so maintenance of appropriate immunity is an essential part of occupational health and infection control programs (Williamson et al, 1988). ***Special Considerations:*** *Previous varicella and cytomegalovirus (CMV) exposure should also be considered. Self-report of immune status and communicable disease history may frequently be inaccurate (Williamson et al, 1988).* |

| Steps | Rationale |
|---|---|
| c. Localized infectious process such as herpes simplex or whitlow, varicella zoster infection (shingles), exudative lesions, or weeping dermatitis. | In some cases, direct patient care should not be given during an acute infective episode. For example, a person with an active case of zoster can transmit the virus by direct contact to a susceptible child (one who has never had chicken pox or is immunocompromised), causing a primary varicella infection. Also, gloving is not known to be adequate during an active case of herpetic whitlow. Those with oral herpetic lesions should avoid neonates, and severely burned or immunocompromised children (CDC, 1983). |
| d. Pregnancy. | The infectious diseases that pose the greatest reproductive threat are rubella and cytomegalovirus (CMV). Congenital acquisition of either of these diseases can lead to fetal death or serious birth defects/developmental disorders. Acquiring an HIV infection during pregnancy compounds the devastation by placing the fetus at risk for congenital transmission (CDC, 1987). |

## Planning and Goal Setting

| Steps | Rationale |
|---|---|
| 1. Review the barrier precaution policies of the facility. | A review of the facility policies permits effective planning and implementation to prevent transmission of infection. |
| 2. Gather equipment needed: gloves, gowns, masks, aprons, isolation cards/BSI decals, sterile supplies for appropriate procedures, disinfectant cleaner, etc. | Easily accessible supplies encourage adherence to the appropriate precautions.<br>***Special Considerations:*** *Regardless of the system adopted by the facility, point-of-use sharps/needles disposal containers should be prominently labeled and inaccessible to children.* |
| 3. Develop an individualized goal of nursing care:<br>▪ To prevent cross transmission of infectious agents. | |

## Implementation

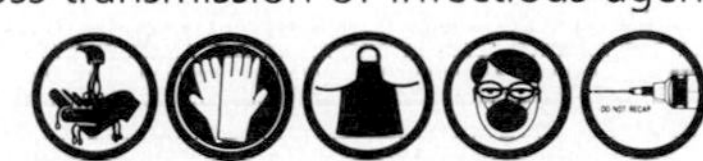

| Steps | Rationale |
|---|---|
| 1. Explain barrier precaution measures to child and family. Also explain if any precautions such as masks are necessary for family members and visitors, based on susceptibility. | Explaining that precautions may be used with all children regardless of diagnosis and are intended to protect both the child and staff will enhance cooperation and decrease feelings of alienation and uncleanliness. |
| 2. Follow barrier system as appropriate. | ***Special Considerations:*** *Facility policy, which may vary from these recommendations, should be followed.* |
| ***Universal precautions (UP)***<br>▪ Use when contacting the following body substances: blood, semen, vaginal secretions, and internal fluids (cerebrospinal, synovial, pleural, peritoneal, pericardial, and amniotic).<br>▪ Not necessary when contacting the following body substances unless they contain visible blood, or are included in additional precautions for this child, (e.g., enteric precautions): feces, nasal secretions, sputum, sweat, tears, urine, and vomitus. | Universal precautions derive from the view that all patients are potentially infectious only for blood-borne pathogens, because blood is the most significant source of HIV, HBV, and other blood-borne pathogens in the occupational setting (MMWR, 1988). The risk of transmission of HIV and HBV from the body substances not included in the precautions is extremely low or nonexistent (MMWR, 1988). Nonblood-borne pathogens may be transmitted in these substances however, e.g., pseudomonas and salmonella. Additional precautions, category- or disease-specific may be necessary based upon diagnosis (or suspicion).<br>***Special Considerations:*** *Breast milk does not require precautions unless frequent exposure occurs, e.g., staff in breast milk bank. Saliva also does not require precautions unless likely contamination with blood, e.g., oral surgery or dental procedures.* |
| ***Body substance isolation (BSI)***<br>▪ Use when contacting all body substances including blood, feces, urine, vomitus, wound and other drainage (nonintact skin), and oral secretions. | Under BSI precautions all patients are assumed potentially infectious for all pathogens. Use of BSI depends upon the interaction between the caregiver and the child. Organisms, both normal flora and potentially pathogenic, are always present in feces, oral secretions, sputum, pus, wound drainage, and genital secretions. Organisms may be present in cerebrospinal fluid, blood, and urine, and are usually present in the urine of catheterized patients (Jackson and Lynch, 1984). |

| Steps | Rationale |
|---|---|
| Follow the appropriate steps according to BSI or UP. | |
| a. Handwashing:<br>▪ UP—Between patient contact and after gloves removed, immediately and thoroughly wash hands and other skin surfaces that are contaminated with blood and applicable body fluids.<br>▪ BSI—Anytime the hands are visibly soiled and between most patient contacts even if gloves are worn; wash for 10 seconds with soap, running water and friction.<br>▪ Both systems—Handwashing is not necessary between sequential low-risk patient contact involving intact skin, e.g., taking vital signs or administering medications. | Handwashing is the single most important strategy to break the chain of transmission, i.e., transient colonization by potentially pathogenic microorganisms.<br>***Special Considerations:*** *An antimicrobial soap may be more effective than plain soap in reducing skin surface bacterial count, and with repeated use leaves an antimicrobial residue to further inhibit transmission. Frequent use of emollients following handwashing helps to prevent irritation and skin breakdown.* |
| b. Gloves:<br>▪ UP and BSI—Use when contact with blood or applicable body fluids is likely to occur or own skin is not intact; change between patient contacts. | Gloves reduce the possibility of transmission of infective organisms from patient to staff, transmission of own endogenous or infective flora to child with reduced protective mechanisms (e.g., surgical wound), and transient colonization that permits transmission of organisms to others (CDC, 1983). Changing gloves is recommended; washing or disinfecting them reduces effectiveness and may increase penetrability (MMWR, 1988).<br>***Special Considerations:*** *During routine bathing, gloves are only needed if washing genital areas (UP and BSI) or rectal areas and stool soiling (BSI). Gloves are indicated for the initial bath of a newborn because of presence of bloody amniotic fluid. General guidelines to guide glove use in anticipation of blood exposure during phlebotomy procedures: high community prevalence, lower skill level, uncooperative child, finger and/or heel stick (MMWR, 1988).* |
| c. Gown/plastic apron:<br>▪ UP and BSI—Gown or plastic apron should be worn when it is likely that blood or body substances to which UP/BSI apply would soil clothing; change between patient contacts. | Gowns/plastic aprons prevent soiling of clothing with potentially infectious blood or body substances. Cloth gowns are not impervious, and do not keep clothing dry (McPherson and Jackson, 1987).<br>***Special Considerations:*** *Clothing is rarely shown to be a significant factor in the transmission of infectious agents (Lynch and Jackson, 1986). Plastic aprons do not provide adequate protection when burping infants in the shoulder position. In the UP system, emesis is not an applicable body substance unless visible blood is present. In BSI system, wear a plastic gown or apron or burp the child in the lap position (see Skill 59). Routine use of cover gowns in newborn care for visitors was demonstrated to have no significant effect on neonatal infection rates (Campbell, 1987).* |
| d. Masks and/or eye protection (eyeglasses, goggles, or face shields):<br>▪ UP—Worn when it is likely that the eyes and/or nose and mouth will be splashed with blood or applicable body substances or when working directly over large, open skin lesions; wear masks for respiratory/AFB (Acid Fast Bacillus) isolation category.<br>▪ BSI—Same as UP except masks are worn if susceptible to diagnosed airborne infection. | Masks and/or eye protection provide safety from direct splashes or splatter of blood or body substances to the mucous membranes of the eyes, nose, and mouth.<br>***Special Considerations:*** *It is unclear whether masks adequately filter inspired air to prevent airborne droplet nuclei transmission. However, few diseases are actually transmitted this way, primarily chicken pox and tuberculosis. When a cough or sneeze occurs within 3 feet, droplet contact is the more common means of transmission; even with a mask, the conjunctiva are unprotected. Use a mask only once or until wet, then discard. Also, never lower the mask around the neck, then reuse.* |
| e. Needles/syringe units and other sharps:<br>▪ UP and BSI—Used needles/sharps are directly discarded in a rigid, puncture-resistant container; do not remove from disposable syringe, recap or break/cut needle. Containers should be located near common use areas (point-of-use) such as patient rooms, treatment rooms, and medication preparation areas. | Needle stick injuries, especially when attempting to recap the needle, are a leading cause of nosocomial transmission of blood-borne pathogens. As gloves cannot prevent these injuries, proper handling of sharps is essential.<br>***Special Considerations:*** *If recapping is unavoidable, use no touch method: lay the syringe/needle unit on a table and using one hand, slide the needle into the cap.* |
| f. Trash and linen:<br>▪ UP and BSI—Single bag securely in leakproof containers and disposed of or clean according to institutional policy. Handle linens minimally; avoid shaking. | Unless the bag or container is visibly soiled on the outside or leaking, a single bag is sufficient to prevent transmission of infectious agents on trash or linens. Although linens are not a common means of transmission, minimal handling and agitation prevents gross microbial contamination of the air, environment, and self (MMWR, 1987). |

| **Steps** | **Rationale** |
|---|---|
| g. Private room:<br>▪ UP—Not necessary unless required by category or disease specific isolation precautions pertinent to child's diagnosis.<br>▪ BSI—Preferable for child who soils the environment with body substances; required for child diagnosed with a disease transmitted by airborne route.<br>▪ Both systems—Can share with a roommate known to be immune to diagnosed disease, or cohort (one infected with the same agent). | A private room is especially necessary to prevent respiratory transmission of an infectious agent. In the BSI system, adherence to appropriate precautions is a sufficient barrier for disease transmitted by direct contact. Indirect transmission through the environment or objects is not a major source of transmission (Jackson, 1986).<br>***Special Considerations:*** *A forced air incubator is not a substitute for a private room for a neonate, because it does not filter the air returned to the environment (AAP Committee on Infectious Disease, 1988). Diseases affecting children transmitted by airborne route requiring special precautions in either system are: measles, mumps, rubella, varicella (chicken pox), epiglottitis, meningitis or pneumonia (caused by* Haemophilus influenzae, *meningococcal organisms), meningococcemia, or tuberculosis.* |
| h. Specimens.<br>▪ UP and BSI—Place specimens containing blood or body fluids in a well-constructed container with a secure lid. All specimens should be treated as potentially infectious, therefore no additional labeling is required (CDC, 1987; Jackson et al, 1987). | Labeling some specimens as potentially infectious promotes a false sense of security for personnel when handling specimens not so labeled.<br>***Special Considerations:*** *Facility policy may vary regarding labelling requirements.* |
| 3. General infection control measures: | These measures are appropriate in all patient care situations. |
| a. Emergency resuscitative equipment such as a pocket mask or resuscitation bag should be readily available. | Resuscitative equipment provides an appropriate barrier precaution, by eliminating the need for mouth-to-mouth resuscitation. |
| b. Allow playroom attendance based on facility policy or practitioner's orders. If none available, some general guidelines include afebrile or on antibiotics for at least 24 hours, no excretion of body substances that soil the environment (feces, wound drainage), and no suspected or diagnosed infectious disease that is transmissible. | Children interacting in playrooms are not protected by barrier precautions, therefore exclusion practices must consider contact sources of transmission. |
| c. Clean toys in the playroom or following use in a patient room according to facility policy if available, or day-care guidelines: clean and sanitize infant/toddler toys when visibly soiled and before use by another child by washing in a soap and water solution, rinsing in a sanitizing solution, and allowing to air dry (AAP Committee on Early Childhood, 1987). | Infectious agents can be transmitted on toys by children with inadequate hygiene practices, and especially infant/toddlers who frequently place objects in their mouth.<br>***Special Considerations:*** *For cleaning, use a commercial disinfectant spray or a sanitizing solution of a 1 : 10 dilution of household bleach with water. This solution must be made fresh daily (AAP Committee on Early Childhood, 1987). Stuffed toys that cannot be washed are not suitable as common playroom toys; a child's personal stuffed toy poses no risk to other children.* |
| d. Assist or wash a child's hands after toileting and before eating. | Assisting a child to maintain good hygiene practices can interrupt the transmission chain, and stress the importance of these practices to the child.<br>***Special Considerations:*** *Disposable food trays are no longer recommended for isolation precautions as the risk of transmission of infection on eating utensils is negligible and washing the child's hands before eating is a more effective means of interrupting transmission (CDC, 1983, and Jackson, 1986).* |
| e. Guidelines to transporting children: transport personnel should follow UP or BSI for all patients according to facility policy. Additional precautions include masks for the child with an infection transmissible by the airborne route and for susceptible transport personnel. | Adherence to appropriate barrier precautions during transport maintains effectiveness of the system. |
| f. Follow recommended practices for sterile technique related to procedures, e.g., catheterization, suctioning. (Refer to specific skills in this text for sterile technique recommendations.) | Procedures that disrupt normal protective mechanisms such as entering a normally sterile body orifice or disrupting skin integrity provide a means of entry for potentially pathogenic organisms. Sterile technique minimizes this risk.<br>***Special Considerations:*** *Some procedures that are performed in the hospital using sterile technique, can be performed in the home using clean technique because the transmission risk is significantly reduced for sources of infectious agents (other patients) and modes of transmission (staff hands).* |
| 4. Specific infection control measures: | These measures are indicated in certain situations.<br>***Special Considerations:*** *Many other specific measures are addressed in specific skills in this text.* |

| Steps | Rationale |
|---|---|
| a. Avoid assigning children at increased risk for infection (e.g., having a surgical incision or immunosuppression) to a room with a child who has a known or suspected infectious process or colonization of body secretions. | Although the consistent practice of appropriate barrier precautions is adequate to interrupt transmission, infected patients should not share a room with a patient who is likely to become infected or in whom consequences of infection are likely to be severe (CDC, 1983). Also, in general, hygiene practices of children cannot be considered adequate. Separate/private room assignments are no more effective than the same room if barrier precautions are inconsistent.<br>***Special Considerations:*** *The category of protective (reverse) isolation was discontinued in the CDC's 1983 guidelines because Nauseef and Maki (1981) found it to be of no value in preventing nosocomial infections in immunocompromised patients.Often the source for an infection in these patients is normal flora or existing colonization.* |
| b. Use an individual urine measuring container to empty the collecting bag of an indwelling catheter. | Shared urine measuring containers have frequently been implicated as the source of retrograde urinary tract infections with indwelling catheters (Jackson and McPherson, 1986). |
| 5. Personnel infection control measures: | In addition to appropriate barrier precautions, these measures can minimize transmission risks for the child and staff. |
| a. Do not provide direct patient care or expose susceptible co-workers if infectious. | Professional responsibility includes avoiding exposing others to potentially infectious agents.<br>***Special Considerations:*** *Infections of the most common concern include enteric pathogens, HBV, active varicella zoster, oral HSV, herpetic whitlow, and respiratory viruses.* |
| b. Wash hands after toileting and before eating, in addition to situations recommended in relation to patient contact. | Handwashing is the single most effective means of interrupting transmission of infectious agents. |
| c. Avoid touching the conjunctiva of the eye and mucous membranes of the nose and mouth. | These are common portals of entry for infectious agents. The conjunctiva is especially significant in the transmission of respiratory viruses, yet is unprotected by face masks. |
| d. If possible, avoid direct patient care of child with an infectious disease if personal susceptibility increases risk. | Susceptibility related to immune status or pregnancy increases the risk and/or serious consequences of acquiring the infection.<br>***Special Considerations:*** *Although avoidance of patients with known CMV infection during pregnancy is suggested, the prevalence of asymptomatic children excreting the virus, especially among those who attend day care, may be over 50%. Viral excretion is prolonged and has been isolated in saliva, tears, breast milk, semen, urine, and feces. Universal precautions and careful handwashing are indicated to minimize the risk of contracting CMV (Williamson et al, 1988).* |

| Evaluation Outcomes | Observational Guidelines |
|---|---|
| 1. Nosocomial infection is prevented or minimized. | Monitor temperature; assess for other signs and symptoms of infection, e.g., wound drainage or urinary tract infection. Correlate with length of hospitalization. Review infection control chart audits. |
| 2. Occupational acquisition of infectious disease is prevented or minimized. | Review records related to needle-stick injuries or other blood exposures, employee follow-up testing on seroconversion, TB skin test, or other testing to determine occupational exposure to infectious agents. Observe employee compliance with protective system. Review employee illness records. |

## Documentation

Document all assessment information pertinent to diagnosis or suspected diagnosis of infectious disease or colonization. Note possible community exposure and stage of potential incubation period. Document use of appropriate barrier precautions, and use of isolation system if appropriate. Document all applicable child/family explanations and teaching.

# *SKILL* 51 Applying and Maintaining Restraints and Restraining for Procedures

*Deborah Kay Brantly*

The use of restraints with the pediatric client requires knowledge of multiple applications, techniques, and ethical responsibilities. Restraints are used when the child's movement might be harmful during a procedure or with a therapy, when constant immobility of a body part is necessary, when the child is unaware of surroundings and needs protection, or—as a last resort—when the child is aggressive or out of control. Although applications for restraints vary, principles are essentially the same. Various attitudes exist about using restraints with children. For this reason, use of a restraint must have a clear rationale. Restraints are to be used as a protection for the child and never to be used because of insufficient staffing, convenience, as a substitute for observation or as a punishment. In all situations restraining a child should be done only when safety needs deem it necessary. Constant monitoring is of paramount importance to: (1) determine the need for continued restraints; (2) assure proper positioning of restraints; (3) maintain skin integrity and circulation because of the restraints; and (4) decrease complications of immobility.

## NURSING DIAGNOSES

Potential for injury related to altered cerebral function, altered mobility, impaired sensory function, or pain; Potential for violence related to mental retardation, suicidal behavior, perceived threat to self-esteem, or feelings of helplessness; Impaired physical mobility related to musculoskeletal restraint; Potential for impaired skin integrity related to physical immobilization by restraints.

| Steps | Rationale |
|---|---|
| **Assessment** | |
| 1. Determine the child's size and developmental level. | Different restraint techniques and materials are used depending on the child's size, developmental level, and part of body to be restrained (see box on following page).<br>***Special Considerations:*** *Infants generally need more protection. For example, because of more involuntary movement, stabilization of an IV is of paramount importance. Softer restraining materials are needed to protect fragile neonate skin.* |
| 2. Review pertinent information such as medical history, medications given (or illicit drug use), and psychosocial behaviors, e.g., the presence of fear, anxiety or anger. | Reviewing information about the child directs individualized care and provides a basis for the decision to use restraints or alternative interventions, planning type of restraint needed, length of time restraint will be engaged, and psychosocial needs while restraints are being applied and/or maintained.<br>***Special Considerations:*** *Be alert to medical conditions, especially circulation problems, skin disorders or orthopedic or neurological states. Restraints may compromise or worsen these conditions and require extra monitoring if restraints are essential.* |
| 3. Determine the situation and/or behaviors that necessitate the need for restraints, e.g., protection during procedures, protection of an indwelling device (e.g., catheter, IV, or nasogastric tube), immobility of body part, and/or protection of the disoriented or aggressive child. | Documenting specific behaviors which indicate the need for restraints validates the intervention.<br>***Special Considerations:*** *Documentation of exhibited behaviors is extremely important. For example, a chart entry for a child who is unaware of the surroundings and needs self-protection might read: The child "was unresponsive to vocal stimuli, however, was forcefully moving arms and legs from one side of the bed to another in an agitated manner."* |

## *PROTECTIVE RESTRAINTS*

### CHEST OR JACKET RESTRAINT

The chest or jacket restraint is a cloth, wraparound restraint with armholes. Although not frequently used in most settings, it can be used for children of all ages. The restraint prevents gross movement but permits some mobility.

Step 1
Place closed side of the chest restraint over the front of the child. Put arms through arm holes.

Step 2
Cross the ends of the restraint in the back.

Step 3
Place one end of the restraint through the back slit of the other side.

Step 4
Secure the chest restraint to the underneath side of the bed or back of chair or wheelchair by tying the ends together with a bow or slipknot. If the child gets out of the chest restraint easily, place two on—one backwards and one forwards. Long ties on each side are to be secured to the bed frame, if child is in bed.

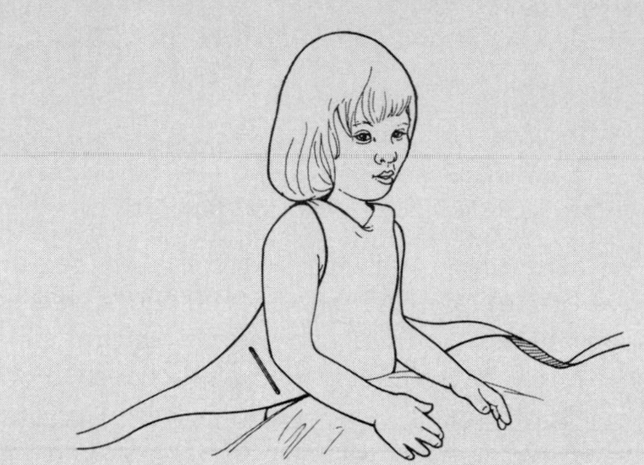

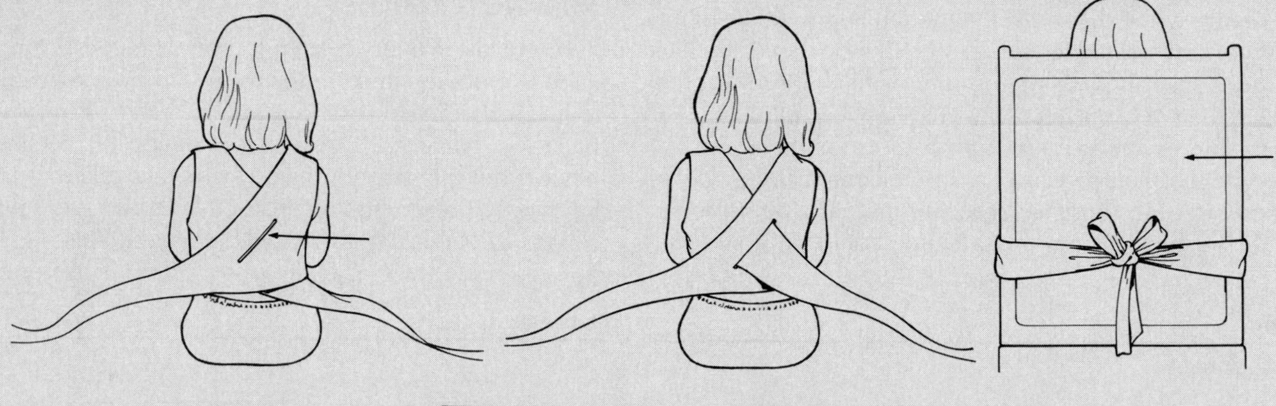

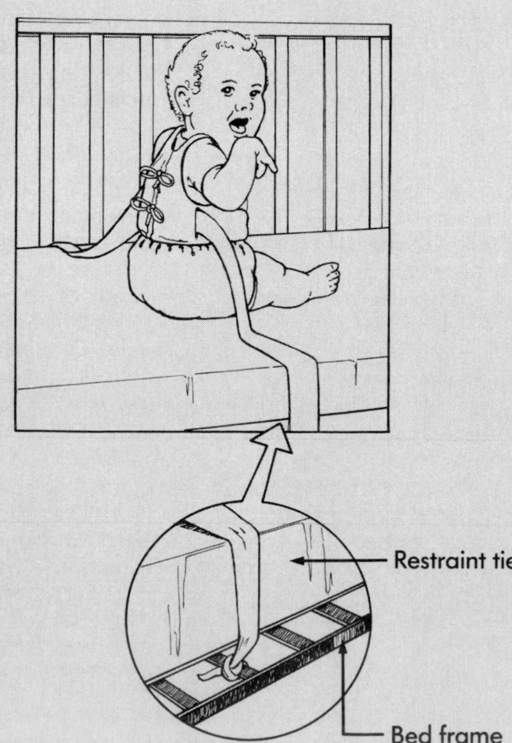

## *PROTECTIVE RESTRAINTS—cont'd*

### EXTREMITY RESTRAINTS

#### Clove hitch restraint

The clove hitch restraint, normally used on the wrists, is a simple-to-make soft restraint.

Step 1

Wrap an ACE bandage around the area to be restrained (use soft gauze for infant). Make a clove hitch with soft gauze. (Illustration from Whaley L and Wong D: Nursing care of infants and children, ed 4, St Louis, 1991, The CV Mosby Co.)

Step 2

Place the clove hitch over the wrapped area of the child's extremity and tighten to secure. (Illustration from Whaley L and Wong D: Nursing care of infants and children, ed 4, St Louis, 1991, The CV Mosby Co.)

Step 3

Tie the ends of the clove hitch to the bed frame, as with jacket restraint.

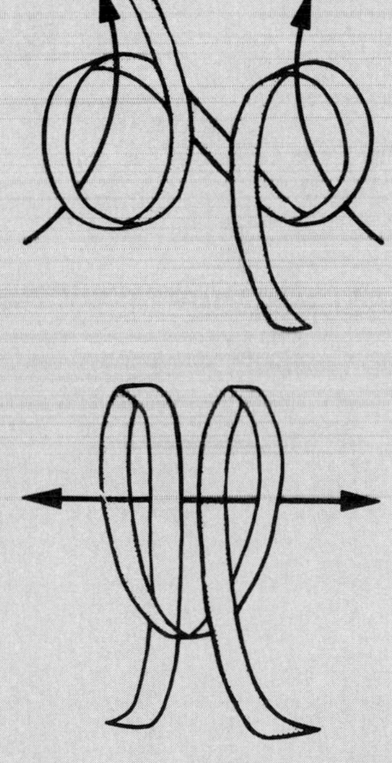

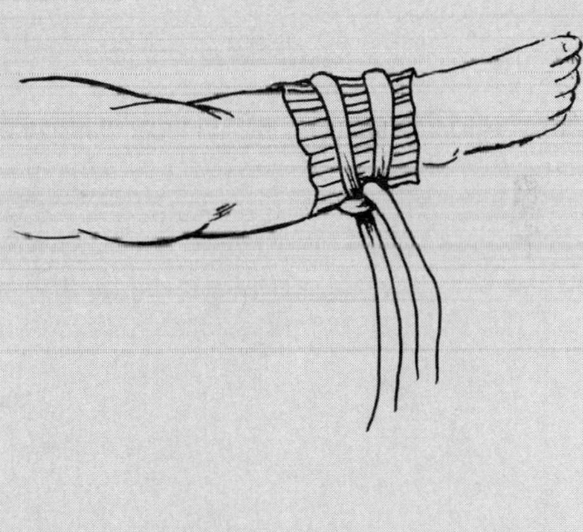

*Continued.*

### *PROTECTIVE RESTRAINTS—cont'd*

**Cloth restraint**

The cloth restraint is a commercially prepared soft restraint that can be used for the wrists or ankles.

Step 1
Wrap padded area of the restraint around the wrist (or ankle).

Step 2
Slip the strap through the slit in the restraint securely.

Step 3
Tie the ends of the restraint to the bed frame.

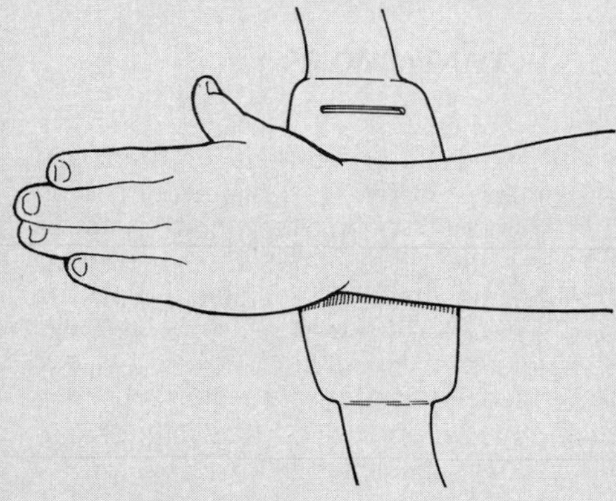

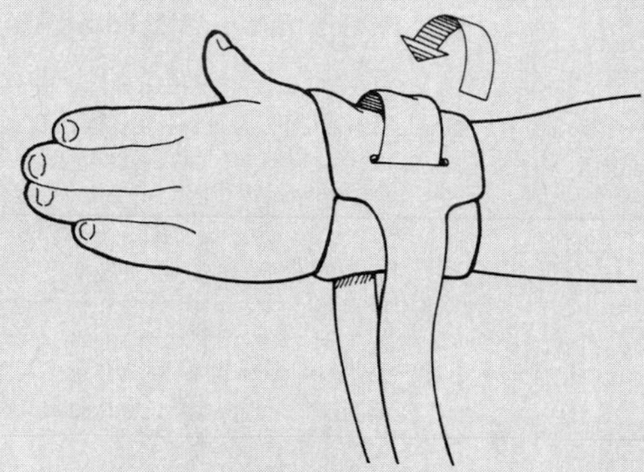

**Mitt restraint**

The mitt restraint is used with the younger child to prevent irritating an area with the hand.

Step 1
Wrap gauze around the child's fingers, if necessary, to absorb moisture or protect the restrained area.

Step 2
Place the mitt over the gauze and tighten. Tie the straps at the wrist or to the bed frame.

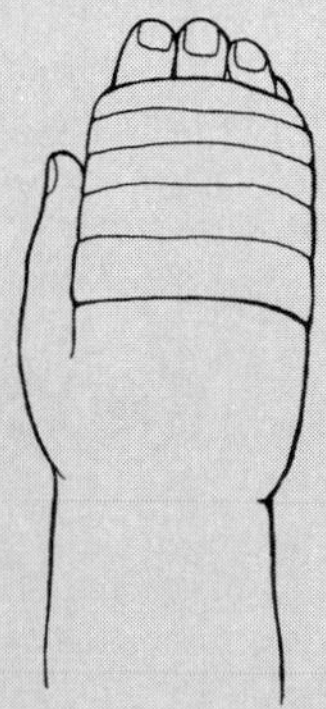

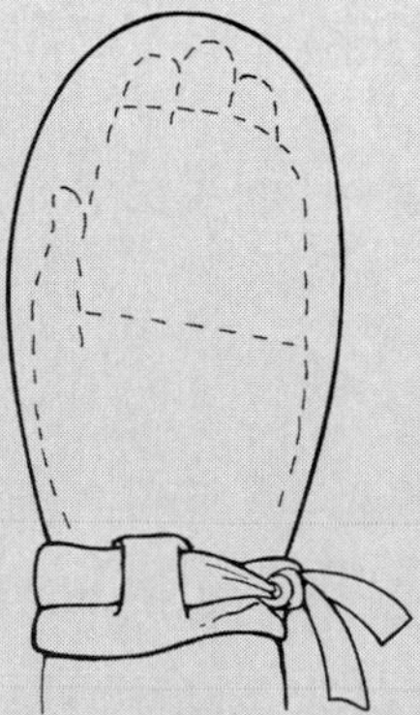

## PROTECTIVE RESTRAINTS—cont'd

### Elbow restraint

The elbow restraint is used to prevent the young child from dislodging indwelling devices or touching the face with the hand(s) by preventing flexion of the elbow.

Step 1

Place tongue blades in the pockets of the restraint. (Illustration from Whaley LF and Wong DL: Nursing care of infants and children, ed 4, St Louis, 1991, The CV Mosby Co.)

Step 2

Place elbow restraints over elbow of one or both arms and wrap around. If long-sleeved clothing is to be worn, pull the sleeve, wrinkle free down to the child's wrist and wrap restraint around the sleeve. Tie restraint ends. (Illustration from Whaley LF and Wong DL: Nursing care of infants and children, ed 4, St Louis, 1991, The CV Mosby Co.)

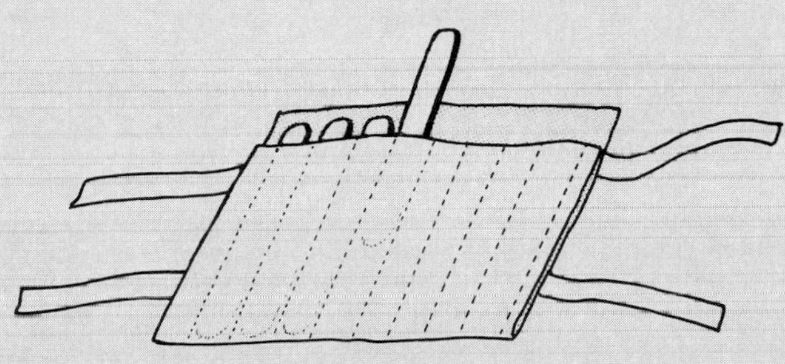

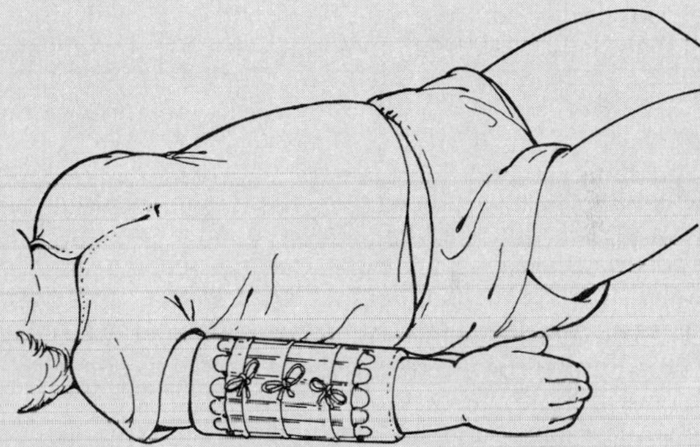

### Leather or plastic restraints

Leather or plastic restraints are extremely durable, commercially prepared, locking restraints that can be used for the wrists or ankles.

Step 1

Wrap the restraint around the child's wrist (or ankle).

Step 2

Slip the end of the restraint into the locking device until the end is secure. Close the lock. (Some need to be locked with a key.) Keep the key accessible, e.g., tape it to the head of the child's bed.

Step 3

Pull the leather or cloth tiedown straps through the opening on the side of the restraint. Tie the straps to the bedframe.

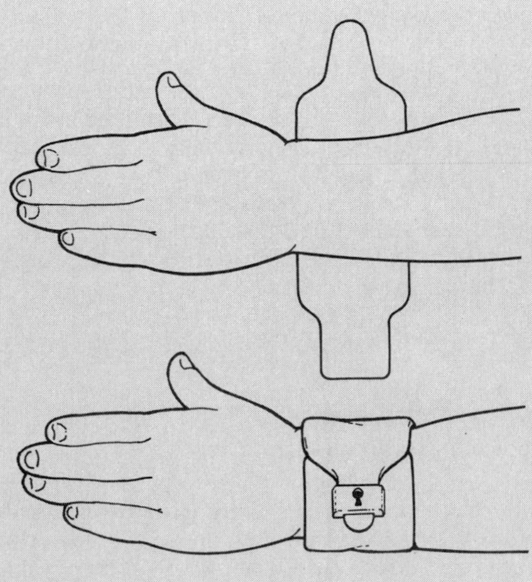

*Continued.*

## PROTECTIVE RESTRAINTS—cont'd

**Bubble top crib/net top crib**

The hard, plastic bubble top and net top are used to prevent older infants and the young child from falling or climbing out of the crib.

1. Place the child in the crib and the rails all the way up.
2. Place the bubble top (shown here) on the crib and secure it to the ends of the crib frame with clamps. (When using net instead of bubble top, place straight on top, drawn tight and secured to the legs and frame.)

4. Determine previous interventions to avoid restraints. Initiate least restrictive interventions before using a restraint. Least restrictive interventions include: talking, reading, play, diversion, 1:1 supervision, holding by a parent or staff member, room near the nurses' station, time out, or medications.

Restraining the child restricts mobility, which is necessary for developmental needs. Restraints should be initiated only when less restrictive interventions are not effective.

5. Assess the family's understanding of the need for the restraint.

In addition to the parents' legal right to know what is occurring, being told a restraint is needed or seeing their child in a restraint can be a frightening experience for the parents.

6. Determine the type of restraint needed, the extremities to be restrained, and the approximate amount of time restraint is likely to be used. Restraint of one extremity is called a one-point restraint, both hands or both feet a two-point restraint, and all four extremities a four-point restraint (see box on p. 320).

Determining the type of restraint needed and the specific parts to be restrained assists in preparation.

***Special Considerations:*** *The least restrictive form of restraint is always to be attempted first; when the need for restraint is no longer necessary, it is to be discontinued. For example, the use of elbow restraints to prevent flexion may be all that is needed to keep an infant from dislodging a scalp infusion. Thus, the infant's hands are still free. Restraints may only be necessary during certain times, e.g., at night.*

## RESTRAINING FOR SPECIFIC PROCEDURES

### EXTREMITY VENIPUNCTURE

Position the child supine on the bed or examination table, with the extremity to be used in the procedure outstretched to the side. The clinician performing the procedure is positioned on the side of the extremity to be used in the procedure. The adult holding the child positions self on the opposite side of the bed or table across the child's upper body to contain the chest and then stabilizes the extremity above the procedure site by placing the child's free arm behind his or her back, while placing arm underneath the child and firmly grasping the child's upper arm (Fig. 51-1). The free arm is used to grasp the child below the puncture site.

### FEMORAL VENIPUNCTURE

Place the child on back with legs in the frog-leg position to expose the groin area. The adult stands over the child's head, grasping the child's knees while allowing elbows to hold the child's arms (Fig. 51-2). Place a cloth diaper over the infant's perineal area and tuck in under buttocks with procedure site exposed in case the child urinates during the procedure.

### JUGULAR PUNCTURE

Place the child in a mummy restraint (see p. 323), lying in the supine position and allowing enough room on the top edge of the restraint to permit easy access to the jugular vein. (If the mummy restraint is not used, request an adult hold the arms and legs of the child during the procedure.) The child's head is held hyperextended to the side opposite the procedure site over the edge of a table or a small pillow (Fig. 51-3). Care should be taken with the infant to avoid excessive hyperextension that might cause airway collapse.

### LUMBAR PUNCTURE

See Skill 124.

### SUBDURAL OR VENTRICULAR TAP

See Skill 86.

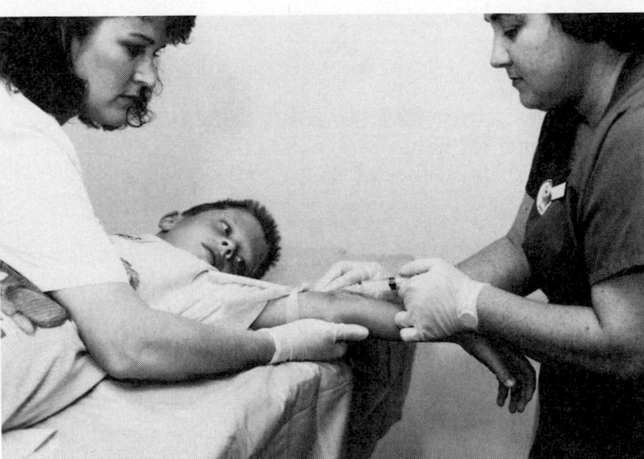

***FIG. 51-1*** Extremity is stabilized for venipuncture.

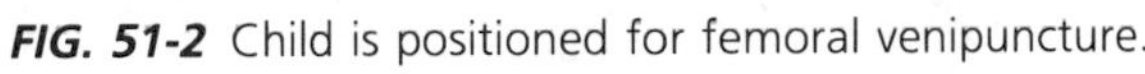


***FIG. 51-2*** Child is positioned for femoral venipuncture.

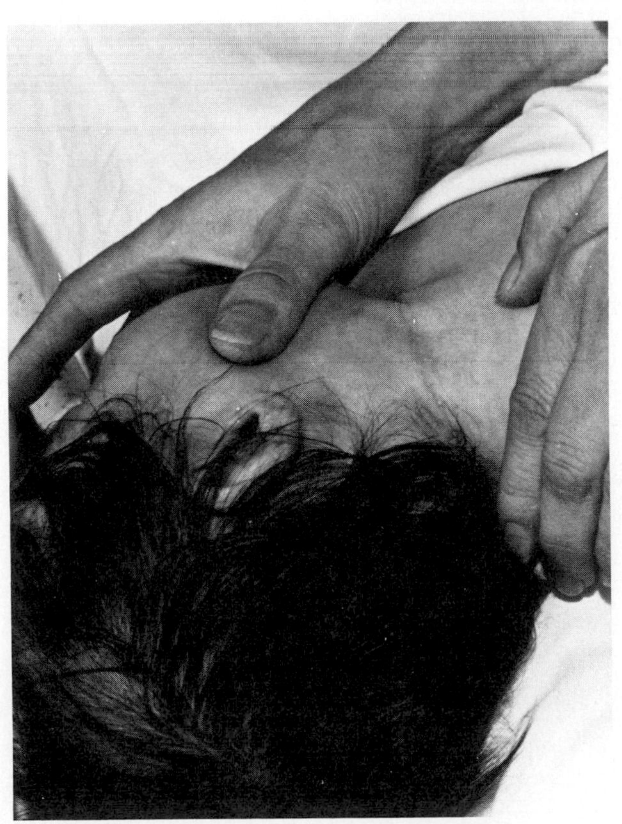

***FIG. 51-3*** Restraining child for jugular vein puncture.

From Whaley LF and Wong DL: Nursing care of infants and children, ed 4, St Louis, 1991, The CV Mosby Co.

## EXTREMITY IMMOBILIZATION

### UPPER EXTREMITY WITH BOARD RESTRAINT

**Palm up method**

1. Place arm palm up on an armboard. (For full extremity restraint, use armboard that extends from beyond the fingertips to under the scapula. For distal extremity restraint, use armboard that extends from the fingertips to the elbow.)
2. Place two adhesive strips across the hand in an X fashion, allowing the thumb full range of motion and fingers to move freely. (Use 5-cm adhesive tape for the child, 2-cm for the infant.)
3. Make a double adhesive strip by using one long and one short piece of tape. Attach them to one another, adhesive sides together. With the short strip touching the child's arm, tape the arm to the armboard at the edge of the antecubital fossa. Tape does not need to be secured directly to the arm.
4. A final double adhesive strip may be placed midway between the hand and the antecubital fossa or above the antecubital fossa, depending on the greatest need for stabilization.

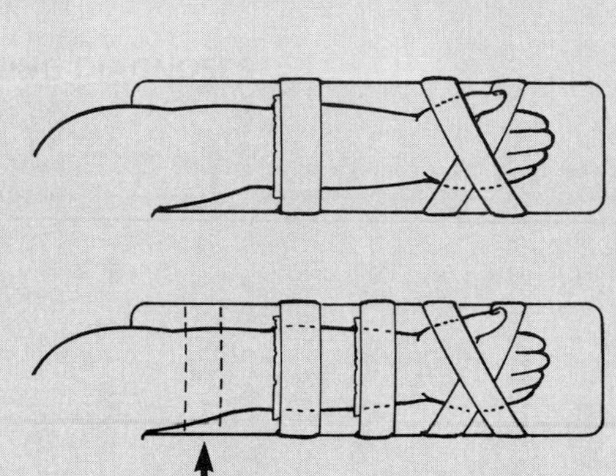

**Palm down method**

1. Place the arm palm down on the armboard. Place the first adhesive strip over the wrist. (Use 5-cm width adhesive for the child, 2-cm width for the infant.)
2. Secure the second adhesive strip across the proximal end of the phalanges, leaving the thumb mobile.
3. Using a double adhesive strip (see Step 3 under palm up method), secure the arm just under the elbow.
4. The final piece of tape is placed obliquely over the thumb and, for security, over the second strip.
5. Adhesive placement for the infant: it may be necessary to start with at least one strip on the fingers to prevent movement during the rest of the procedure.

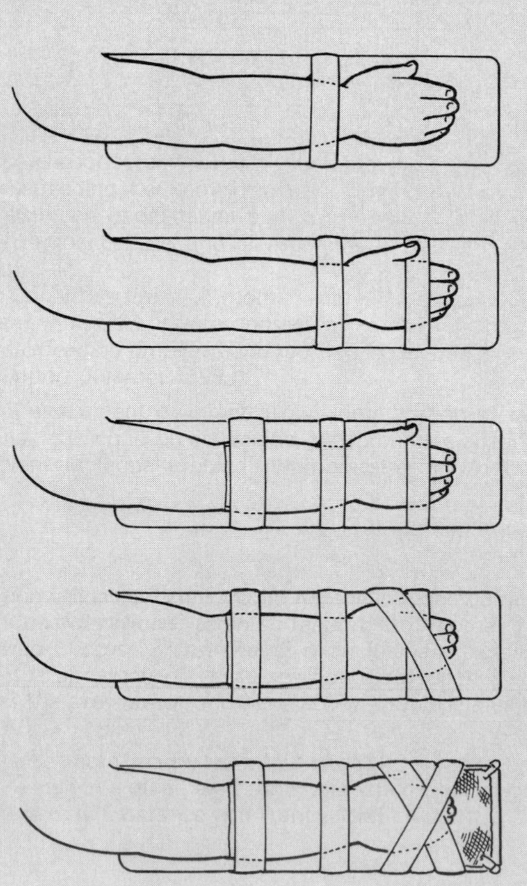

### *EXTREMITY IMMOBILIZATION—cont'd*

**LOWER EXTREMITY WITH BOARD RESTRAINT**

1. With the child in a supine position, leg in full external or internal rotation on the restraint board, place a 5-cm piece of adhesive (2-cm for infants) diagonally across the foot. For a full leg restraint, choose restraint board that extends from beyond the end of the foot to the mid-portion of the buttock.
2. The second piece of adhesive is placed securely over the heel and across the foot in an X formation. (The medial malleolus remains exposed on external rotation.)
3. Using a double strip of adhesive (see Step 3 of Upper Extremity with Armboard Restraint, palm up method), tape the third strip above the knee. (On the infant, place one additional strip midway between the knee and ankle.)

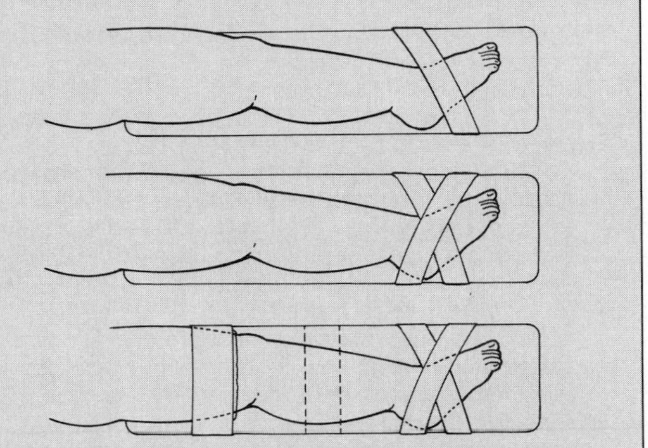

| Steps | Rationale |
|---|---|
| 7. Assess the area dorsal, ventral, proximal, and distal to the restraint site for adequate circulation and absence of lesions or compromised skin integrity. | Restraints increase the risk of compromised skin integrity, skin breakdown, and musculoskeletal weakness. Restraints should be avoided in an area where skin integrity or circulation is already compromised.<br>***Special Considerations:*** *If the danger to the child makes the restraints imperative, softer materials may be selected and greater observation of the compromised/restrained area is required.* |

## Planning and Goal Setting

| Steps | Rationale |
|---|---|
| 1. Obtain physician's order to follow facility protocol for restraint. | Some restraints, e.g., leather, must be legally ordered by the physician, although others do not need a physician order and are a nursing judgment.<br>***Special Considerations:*** *Refer to facility policy and procedure manual for approved protocol.* |
| 2. Gather needed materials according to the type of restraining needed, e.g., adhesive tape, board, gauze, cloth restraints, mummy board, etc. | Gathering materials before the restraint is efficient and facilitates a smoother procedure.<br>***Special Considerations:*** *Using clear adhesive tape may aid in assessment of skin integrity and neurological status when taping an extremity to a board. Many types of commercial restraints are available or can be made easily, especially for small children.* |
| 3. Recruit an assistant to apply restraints, if needed. | Having assistance available when needed facilitates procedure. |
| 4. Develop nursing goals of care:<br>▪ Apply and maintain restraints properly.<br>▪ Protect the child from harm. | |

## Implementation

### *General guidelines*

| Steps | Rationale |
|---|---|
| 1. Approach the child/family in a calm, confident manner to discuss planned use of restraint. Review the reasons restraint is needed. Explain the procedure. | Remaining calm and confident while discussing planned use of restraint prepares the child/family. Parents have a legal right to know why the child is being restrained and are generally more cooperative when the reasons for restraint are explained to them.<br>***Special Considerations:*** *If restraints are to be used for an extended period of time, frequently reinforce the reason for the restraint (Whaley and Wong, 1991).* |

### TIPS ON RESTRAINING FOR A PROCEDURE

1. Restraining the infant and young child can be accomplished by an adult holding the child astride his or her lap in a face-to-face position. The child can then be held firmly against the adult's body to provide comfort, as well as restraint (Whaley and Wong, 1991).
2. When holding the infant or young child on his or her back on a flat surface, the adult can be positioned to use arms or body to hold the child's arms and legs still.
3. When restraining for procedures, be sure the child's extremities cannot invade the procedure site. More than one person may be needed to restrain the child. The use of mummy or papoose restraints are effective when all extremities need to be still while performing procedures on the upper body or head (Fig. 51-4).
4. Stabilize the child both above and below the procedure site when possible. Stabilize joints when possible because they can give the child leverage to escape from a hold, e.g., child who is on back may need to be held or stabilized at the knee joints, as well as ankles, and the child who is on his or her stomach can be held above the knee joints to prevent pelvic movement.
5. Ensure that adequate visualization of the procedure site is maintained.
6. Maintain psychosocial integrity of the child and family, e.g., by giving choices about positioning when appropriate, talking to the child, maintaining parental presence (if the parents wish). Avoid asking parents to restrain a child for a painful procedure because the parent may feel guilt and the child may feel betrayed.
7. Monitor the child during the procedure for respiratory distress or excessive pressure on restraint or holding site; provide the most comfortable position possible for the child.

| Steps | Rationale |
|---|---|
| 2. Provide psychosocial support before and during application of the restraint as appropriate, e.g., reassuring the child he or she will not be harmed, talking to the child, etc. | Attending to the psychosocial needs during a procedure provides integration of care and elicits cooperation from the child/family during an unpleasant procedure. |
| 3. Invite the child's participation by showing how he or she may help. | Participation gives the child an opportunity to control some aspect of care. |
| 4. Use other professionals to assist in holding the child during the application of restraints (see box above). | Additional help during the application of restraints maintains an added element of safety. |
| 5. Lower the siderails of bed or crib; if the child is in a hospital bed, raise the bed. | Raising the bed and lowering the siderails places the child in a more accessible position. |
| 6. If appropriate to the type of restraint, wrap soft gauze around the restraint site and tape securely. | Soft materials provide cushioning while making a firm foundation for the restraint. |
| 7. Apply the restraint in a safe and efficient manner. Position the restraint to allow for the greatest safety while maintaining developmental needs, e.g., allow the infant sufficient mobility to comfort self by sucking thumb when restraint is prolonged (Evans and Hansen, 1985). (See box on protective restraints on p. 314.) | Restraints applied carefully, yet quickly, can serve to hasten the child's adjustment to the restraint or completion of the procedure to be done. ***Special Considerations:*** *Ensure that there is easy access to the child in case of an emergency (Wong and Whaley, 1990).* |
| 8. If the restraint needs to be tied to a secure object, tie it to the bed frame if lying; if sitting, tie to the back of the chair/wheelchair, using a slipknot. | Tying the restraint to the bed frame provides stability. Slipknots are easy to remove. ***Special Considerations:*** *Never tie restraints to bed rails because of the mobility of the bed rail and resulting potential for injury, e.g., dislocated shoulder.* |
| 9. Place one finger under the restrained area to ensure one finger's breadth space between the restraint and the skin. | Adequate space between the child's skin and restraint allows for proper circulation. |
| 10. After application of restraint, check the child's capillary refill, skin color, or peripheral pulses to assess peripheral circulation. Recheck in 15 minutes after initial application. | Normal capillary refill, pulse, and skin color indicate restraint is not restricting the child's circulation and skin integrity will not be compromised. |
| 11. Continue to evaluate the need for restraints. | Nursing care standards promote least restrictive interventions. Periodic evaluation validates the continued need for restraints or updates the care plan for alternative interventions. As soon as the need for restraints is no longer supported through assessment, they should be discontinued. ***Special Considerations:*** *The type of restraint needed may change as the child's response to care changes, e.g., a small child who was restrained with cloth restraints directly after surgery to protect an IV site may later only need an armboard to protect the site.* |

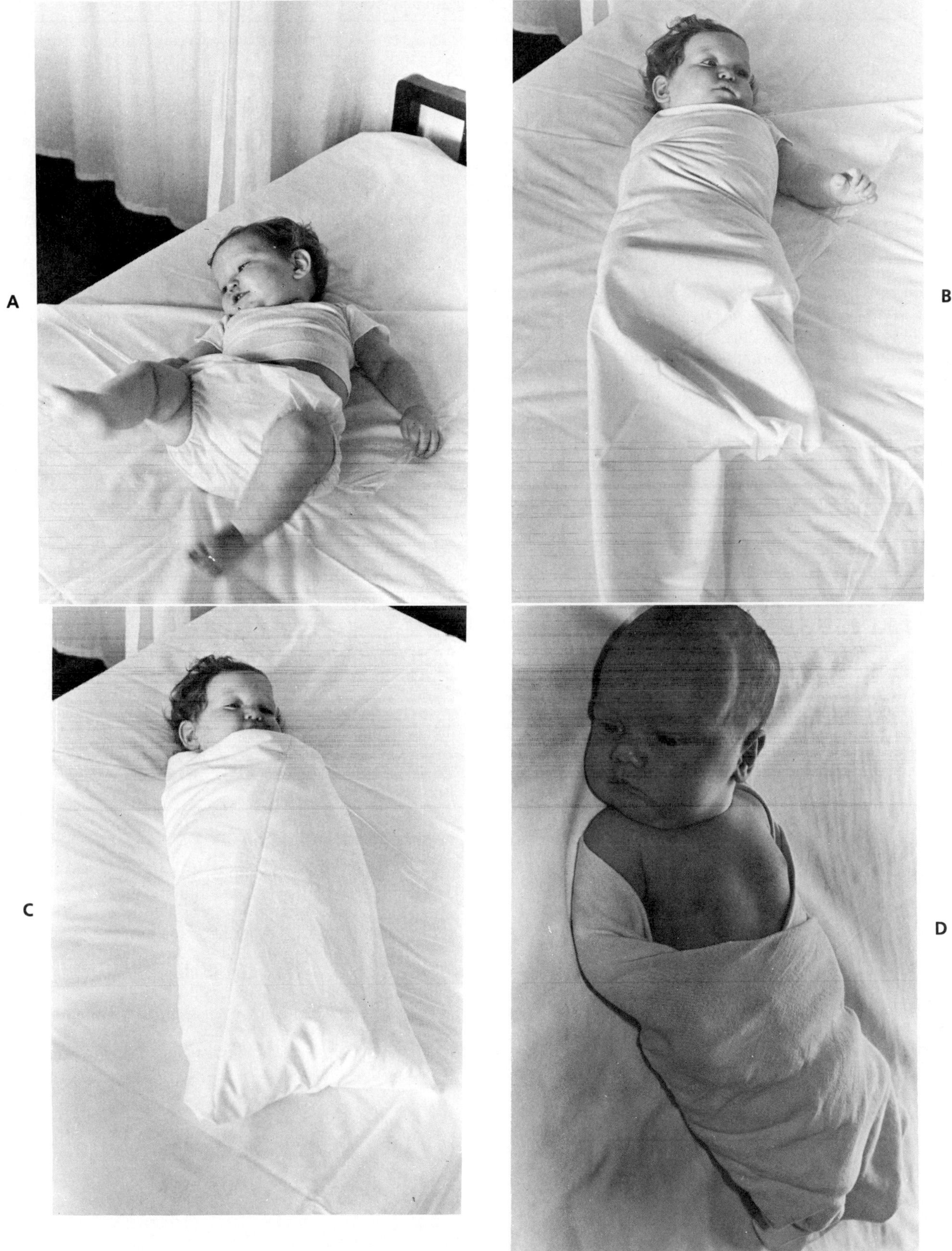


***FIG. 51-4*** Application of mummy restraint. **A,** Infant placed on folded corner of blanket. **B,** One corner of blanket brought across body and secured beneath body; **C,** Second corner brought across body and secured, and the lower corner folded and tucked or pinned in place; **D,** Modified mummy restraint with chest uncovered.

From Whaley LF and Wong DL: Essentials of pediatric nursing, ed 3, St Louis, 1989, The CV Mosby Co.

| Steps | Rationale |
|---|---|
| 12. Encourage parental participation, especially if using restraint for an extended period of time. | Both parents and the child can feel comforted by parental participation. |
| a. Encourage interaction with the child. | Parents may hesitate to get close to or interact with the child because of fear of dislodging indwelling devices or restraints (Evans and Hansen, 1985). |
| b. Teach parents how to remove and apply restraints that can be periodically untied. | Parents feel more involved in their child's care when they can remove restraints when needed. |
| c. Teach the parents how to monitor for signs of circulatory or musculoskeletal impairment, and appropriate actions to take. | Parents who remain with their child may notice excessive stress on restraints or other complications between nursing evaluation points. The parent will know to change the child's position or notify the nurse. Early detection of complications can diminish/eliminate their effects. |
| ***Maintaining restraints*** | |
| 1. Check restraints at least every hour: ensure proper positioning of child and restraints, assess circulation and sensation, and determine condition of the skin. | Frequent checking of restraints prevents or minimizes complications. ***Special Considerations:*** *When restraining the aggressive child, 1:1 supervision is imperative. If the child is pulling the restraints forcefully, check the restraints/restrained extremity thoroughly every 15 minutes.* |
| 2. Release the restraints one at a time, every 2 hours to allow for range of motion exercises, massage of the area under the restraint and repositioning. When parents are involved with direct care, teach them when and how to release the restraints and how to provide care and comfort to the child while restraints are released. | Exercise, massage, and repositioning decrease the incidence of joint stiffness or contractures and skin breakdown. Releasing one restraint at a time diminishes the incidence of injury or dislodging of indwelling devices. |
| 3. If appropriate, offer the child a bathroom break and food every 2 to 4 hours. | The child in restraints must maintain basic needs. |
| 4. Place the call light in an accessible location to the child, if appropriate for child's age. | The child must be provided with a means to summon assistance. ***Special Considerations:*** *If the child is developmentally or physiologically unable to use the call light, check the child more frequently.* |
| 5. Provide the child who is restrained for a long period of time with diversionary play and stimulation (see Skill 15). | Restraining can increase a child's frustration. Play activities will provide diversion from restraints and allow the child an emotional outlet. ***Special Considerations:*** *If active play activities are not possible, provide stimulation with music, story tapes, mobiles, colorful surroundings, etc.* |

| Evaluation Outcomes | Observational Guidelines |
|---|---|
| 1. Restraints are properly and securely applied. | Observe for proper positioning of the restraint and one finger breadth space between the restraint and the child's skin. Pulses should be strong distal to restraint with good capillary refill. |
| 2. Restraints are properly maintained. | Check restraints at least every hour for proper positioning. Restraints are released every 2 hours for massage, exercise, and repositioning of the child. The need for restraints is reevaluated with each check. |
| 3. The child remains safe. | The child does not injure self or dislocate indwelling instrumentation. |
| 4. The child's skin integrity is maintained. | The child's skin remains warm, moist, and pink, without abrasions or signs of skin irritation. |

## Documentation

Document specific behavioral observations regarding need for the restraint. Document physician notification and approval, if applicable. Document the time of the application and removal of restraints. Note the condition of the skin and capillary refill before and just after application and removal of restraints, materials used for the restraint, type of restraint used, and position of the restraint. Document maintenance care received and specific times given, along with current description of skin condition, capillary refill, pulse, and restraint position. Note the child's emotional response to the restraint and play or stimulation activities provided.

# *SKILL* 52 Managing Pain

*Donna L. Wong*

Pain management involves assessment and control of pain through pharmacologic and nonpharmacologic methods. Pain has been defined as "an unpleasant sensory and emotional experience associated with actual or potential tissue damage, or described in terms of such damage. Pain is always a subjective experience" (International Association for the Study of Pain, 1986). An operational definition that is useful with verbal children is "pain is whatever the experiencing person says it is, existing whenever he says it does" (McCaffery and Beebe, 1989). Both definitions imply that the assessment of pain and the effectiveness of pain reducers must be inferred from the child and cannot be directly measured. Until recently, management of pain in children has received little attention. Research conducted on the use of analgesics to control pain in pediatrics have found gross undermedication of children (see box). Several reasons may account for undertreatment of pain in children by professionals: misconceptions about pain (Table 52-1), complexities of pain assessment, lack of information regarding effective analgesic use, and unrealistic fears about respiratory depression and addiction from narcotic analgesics.

## NURSING DIAGNOSES

Pain related to biological, chemical, physical, or psychological injuring agents; Chronic pain related to chronic physical and/or psychological disability; Constipation related to narcotic medications; Anxiety related to lack of pain relief.

### *UNDERMEDICATION OF CHILDREN FOR PAIN*

Several studies have examined the pattern of pain medication for children as compared with adults. One study found that of 25 hospitalized children, 12 children received a total of 24 doses of analgesics postoperatively; the remaining children received no pain medication. In contrast, 18 adults with identical diagnoses received 671 doses of analgesics (Eland and Anderson, 1977).

The situation is even more serious with infants and young children. One analysis of anesthetic practices with newborns undergoing surgical ligation of patent ductus arteriosus found that 76% of the infants received only a muscle relaxant and nitrous oxide (Anand and Aynsley-Green, 1985). In a survey of nurses working in neonatal intensive care units, 79% of the respondents believed that infants are undermedicated for pain. The same study found that more than one-half of the medications used for pain relief had no analgesic properties (Franck, 1987).

Practices such as these have prompted the American Academy of Pediatrics and the American Society of Anesthesiologists (1987) to publish a joint statement on neonatal anesthesia that encourages the use of local or systemic pharmacologic agents "according to the usual guidelines for the administration of anesthesia to high-risk, potentially unstable patients." If medication is withheld, the decision should be based on the same medical criteria used for older patients not on the infant's age or perceived degree of cortical maturity.

***TABLE 52-1*** Fallacies and Facts about Children and Pain

| Fallacies | Facts |
|---|---|
| Infants do not feel pain. | Infants demonstrate behavioral, physiologic, and hormonal indicators of pain (Anand, Phil, and Hickey, 1987). |
| Children tolerate pain better than adults. | Children's tolerance to pain actually *increases* with age (Haslam, 1969). |
| Children cannot tell where they hurt. | Children beyond infancy can accurately point to the body area or mark the site on a drawing; by 3 years of age, children can use simple pain scales, e.g., faces (Beyer, 1988; Wong and Baker, 1988; Savedra et al, 1989). |
| Children always tell the truth about pain. | Children may not admit to having pain to avoid an injection; because of constant pain they may not realize how much they are hurting (Eland, 1985). |
| Children become accustomed to pain or painful procedures. | Children do not demonstrate decreased behavioral signs of discomfort with repeated painful procedures (Katz, Kellerman, and Siegel, 1980). |
| Behavioral manifestations of pain reflect pain intensity. | Behavioral manifestations do not necessarily correlate with pain intensity. Developmental level, coping skills, and temperament influence children's behavioral responses to pain (Wallace, 1989; Broome et al, 1990). |
| Narcotics are dangerous drugs for children. They cause addiction and respiratory depression. | Narcotics are no more dangerous for children than adults. Addiction from narcotics used to treat pain is extremely rare in adults, and no reports substantiate narcotic addiction in children (see p. 336); reports of respiratory depression in children are rare (see p. 336). |

| Steps | Rationale |
|---|---|

## Assessment

1. Determine child's age, developmental level, weight, and height.

Information on age and development is needed to determine types of pain assessment tools to use. Weight and sometimes height are needed to calculate drug dosage, although age alone may also be used.

2. Assess pain using a variety of pain assessment strategies.

Because pain is a sensory and emotional experience, using several assessment strategies provides qualitative and quantitative information about pain.

a. Question the child and parents regarding previous pain experiences, child's coping strategies, and understanding of pain (see box on p. 330).

Children's verbal statements and descriptions of pain are the most important factor in assessing presence of pain. Parents are valuable sources of information about their child's usual behavior when in pain and what measures help relieve child's discomfort.

***Special Considerations:*** *Some parents have never seen their child in pain and may need assistance in recognizing signs of pain such as behavioral changes.*

- If possible, take pain history before pain is expected such as on admission to hospital or preoperatively.

Children are more likely to communicate about experiences with pain when they are not distressed.

- Use a variety of words to describe pain such as "owie," "boo boo," "feel funny," or "hurt."

Young children may not know what the word pain means and may need help to describe pain.

- Inquire about duration, type, and location of current pain.

These characteristics of pain help determine the general severity of pain.

(1) Have child locate pain by marking body part on a human figure drawing (Fig. 52-1). Point to area, with one finger on self, doll, stuffed animal, or "where Mommy or Daddy would put a Band-Aid."

Children as young as toddler age or any child who has difficulty understanding pain scales can usually locate pain on a drawing or on their body.

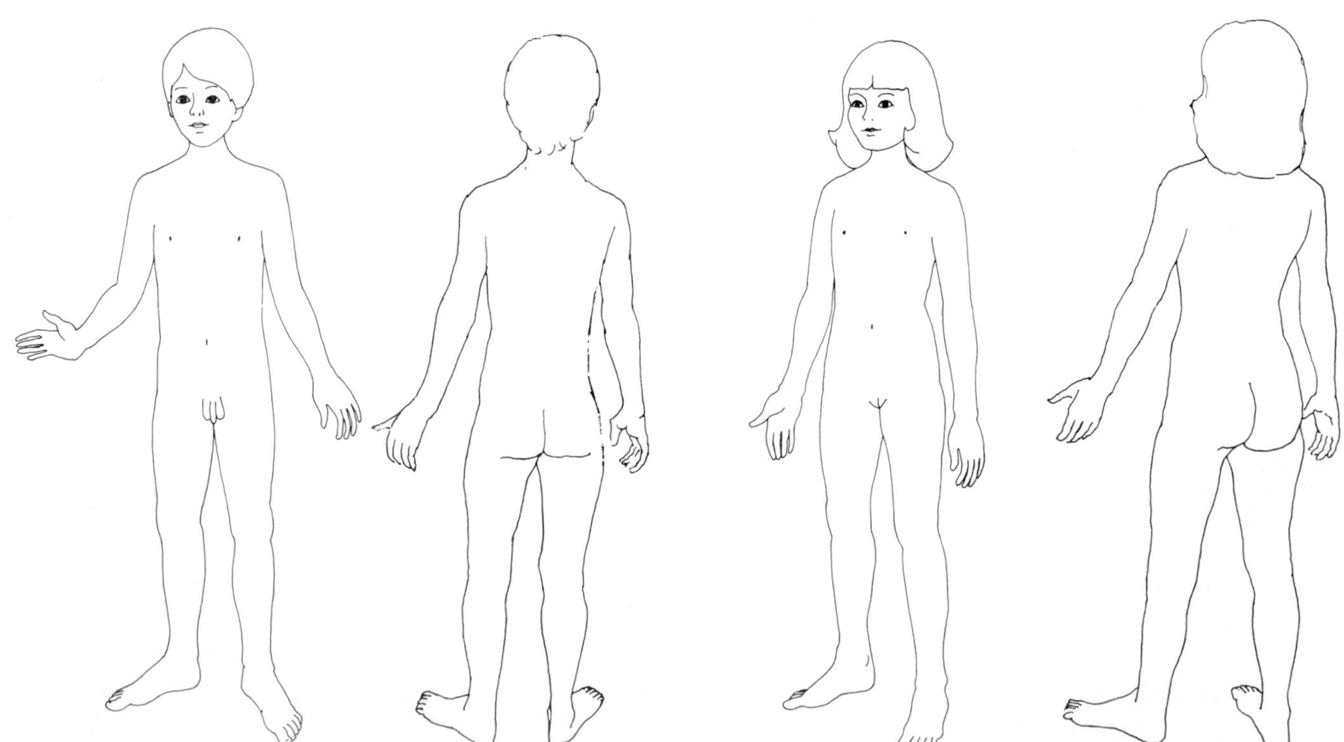

***FIG. 52-1*** Human figure drawings for preparing children for procedures and for assessing pain.

From Wong DL and Whaley LF: Clinical manual of pediatric nursing, ed 3, 1990, St Louis, The CV Mosby Co.

| Steps | Rationale |
|---|---|
| (2) Have parent or child describe pain in terms of interruption of daily activities. | Describing pain in terms of how it affects the child's daily activities is much more informative than global statements such as "He feels really miserable." **_Special Considerations:_** *Children may deny pain for fear of receiving an injection if they admit to discomfort or because they believe they deserve to suffer (e.g., punishment for some misdeed). They may also deny pain to a stranger but will readily admit to parent that they are hurting. This should not be interpreted as seeking attention from the parent but as a valid indication of pain.* |
| b. Use pain rating scale (see box below). | Pain rating scales provide a subjective quantitative measure of pain. |
| ▪ Select a scale that is suitable for the child's age, abilities, and preferences. | The selected scale must be suited to the individual child to be a valid and reliable tool. **_Special Considerations:_** *Faces and Oucher scales can be used with children as young as 3 years old. Chips and color scales can be used with children as young as 4 to 4½ years old. Numeric, simple descriptive, and visual analog scales may be appropriate for children 5 years old and older. Children who cannot count may not be able to use scales that employ numbers. Children who do not know colors or who are color blind may not be able to use the color scale. Some scales such as the color scale require construction, which takes more time and may be difficult if child is already in pain. Reliability and validity for faces, horizontal numeric, simple descriptive, and modified versions of the color and chips scales have been shown to be fairly consistent, but children prefer faces scale (Wong and Baker, 1988).* |

## *PAIN RATING SCALES*

### FACES SCALE

Explain to child that each face is for a person who feels happy because he has no pain (hurt) or sad because he has some or a lot of pain. Face 0 is very happy because he doesn't hurt at all. Face 1 hurts just a little bit. Face 2 hurts a little more. Face 3 hurts even more. Face 4 hurts a whole lot, but Face 5 hurts as much as you can imagine, although you don't have to be crying to feel this bad. Ask child to choose face that best describes how he is feeling (Wong and Baker, 1988).

From Whaley LF and Wong DL: Nursing care of infants and children, ed 4, St Louis, 1991, The CV Mosby Co.

### OUCHER SCALE

Comprises six photographs of child's face representing "no hurt" to "biggest hurt you could ever have." Child chooses face that most nearly describes his pain. Also includes a vertical numeric scale with numbers from 0 to 100 for children who can count to 100 by ones. Child chooses number that best describes his pain (Beyer, 1988).

### POKER CHIP TOOL

Use four red plastic (poker) chips. Explain to child that these are "pieces of hurt." One piece is a "little bit of hurt" and four pieces is the "most hurt you can have." Ask child to choose number of pieces he feels describes his pain. If child replies "no pain," record a 0 (Hester, 1979; Hester, Personal communication, 1989).

### COLOR TOOL

Ask child to identify things that have hurt in the past and what has hurt the worst. Give child 8 crayons or markers (yellow, orange, red, green, blue, purple, brown, and black) in random order. Ask child which color is like the worst pain experienced. Place that crayon or marker aside and ask child to identify crayon that is like a hurt not quite as bad as the worst hurt. Place that crayon aside and ask which other crayon is like something that hurts just a little. Place that crayon with the others and ask child which crayon is like no hurt at all. Show four crayon choices to child in order from worst hurt color to no hurt color. Ask child to show on body outline where he hurts using crayon of color that most nearly is like the pain he feels. When colors are ranked, assign them a numeric value of 0 to 3 (Eland, 1985).

*Continued.*

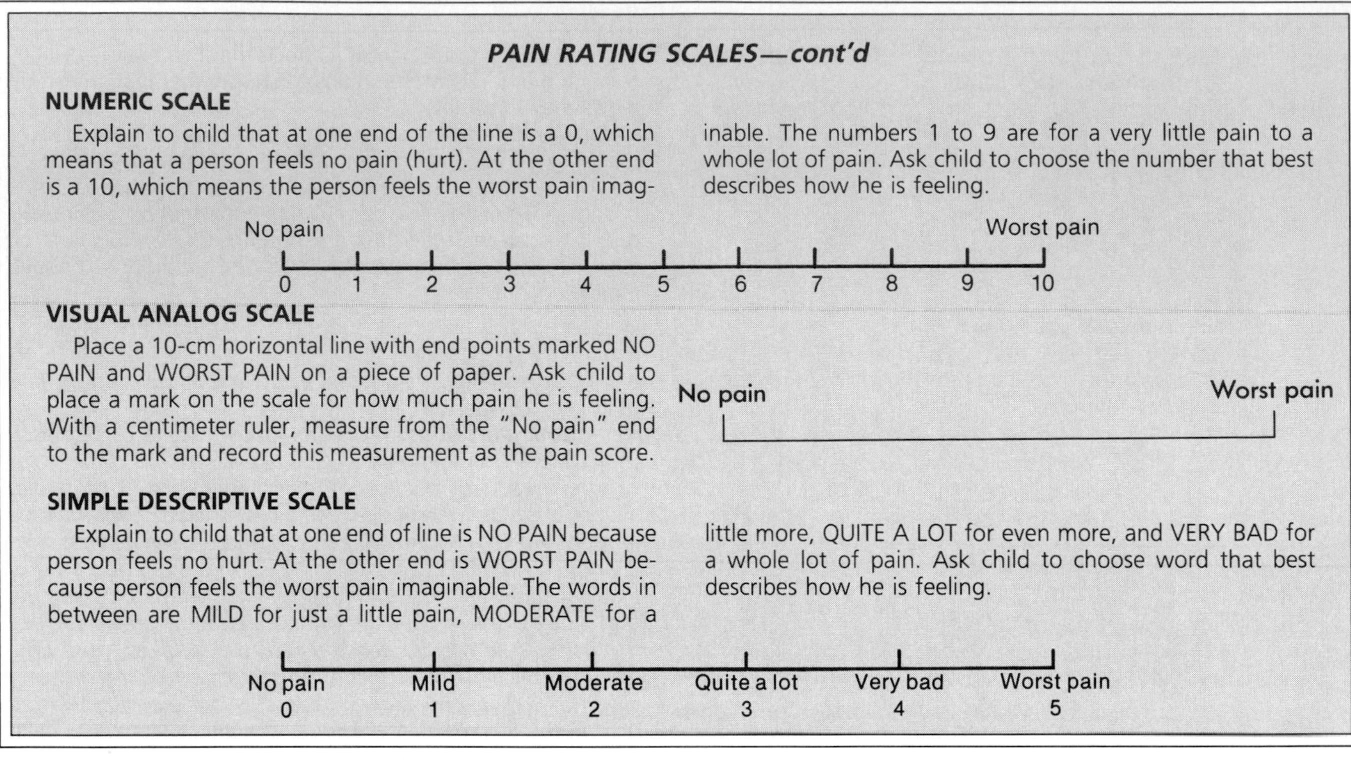

## *PAIN RATING SCALES—cont'd*

### NUMERIC SCALE

Explain to child that at one end of the line is a 0, which means that a person feels no pain (hurt). At the other end is a 10, which means the person feels the worst pain imaginable. The numbers 1 to 9 are for a very little pain to a whole lot of pain. Ask child to choose the number that best describes how he is feeling.



### VISUAL ANALOG SCALE

Place a 10-cm horizontal line with end points marked NO PAIN and WORST PAIN on a piece of paper. Ask child to place a mark on the scale for how much pain he is feeling. With a centimeter ruler, measure from the "No pain" end to the mark and record this measurement as the pain score.



### SIMPLE DESCRIPTIVE SCALE

Explain to child that at one end of line is NO PAIN because person feels no hurt. At the other end is WORST PAIN because person feels the worst pain imaginable. The words in between are MILD for just a little pain, MODERATE for a little more, QUITE A LOT for even more, and VERY BAD for a whole lot of pain. Ask child to choose word that best describes how he is feeling.



From Wong DL and Whaley LF: Clinical manual of pediatric nursing, ed 3, St Louis, 1990, The CV Mosby Co.

| Steps | Rationale |
|---|---|
| ▪ Use same scale with child each time pain is assessed. | Using same scale avoids confusing child with different instructions. **Special Considerations:** *Use pain assessment scale for pain only. Multiple uses of scale, e.g., a general measure of the child's feelings, can cause child to lose interest in the scale.* |
| ▪ Teach child to use scale before pain is expected, such as preoperatively. | Teaching child to use the scale before expected pain occurs facilitates its use during actual pain. |
| c. Evaluate behavioral characteristics and physiologic changes such as change in heart rate, blood pressure, and respirations (usually increase then return to normal); decreased oxygen saturation; dilation of pupils; flushing or pallor; nausea; muscle tension; sweating. | Behavioral changes are common indicators of pain in children and are especially valuable in assessing pain in nonverbal children. However, physiologic changes are primarily seen in acute pain and subside with continuing or chronic pain, making them unreliable indicators. **Special Considerations:** *Both behavioral and physiologic changes may indicate emotions other than pain such as fear or anxiety. No single behavioral or physiologic change is an absolute indicator of pain. Any change in behavior, e.g., an active child becoming quiet and withdrawn, is a cardinal sign of pain.* |
| ▪ Observe for specific behaviors that indicate local body pain, e.g., pulling ears, rolling head from side to side, lying on side with legs flexed on abdomen, limping, or refusing to move a body part. | Specific behaviors often indicate location of body pain. |
| ▪ Observe for improvement in behavior following administration of analgesic. Use pain assessment record to monitor effectiveness of interventions (Fig. 52-2). | Improvement in behavior such as less irritability or cessation of crying is an excellent clue that the child was experiencing pain. A pain assessment record provides documentation of behavior changes. |

## PAIN ASSESSMENT RECORD

Directions:

1. Record time of administering drug and assess analgesic effect 30 minutes later and then hourly.
2. State "Reason for drug administration" in behavioral terms, e.g., "child says he hurts" or "child crying and irritable."
3. Use column "Reason for drug administration" to record behavior during reassessment, e.g., "child says he feels better" or "child playing."
4. Use pain rating scale if child understands its use and only when child is awake. Name of scale: ____________________ ; Rating: No pain = ________ and Worst pain = ________ .
5. Suggested guidelines for safe minimal respiratory rates for children receiving narcotics are 10 to 16 breaths/minute. Consider child's age (with age respiratory rate decreases) and physiologic status (shallow respiration, decreased oxygen saturation, decreased consciousness) when evaluating respirations.

| Date | Time | Drug administered | Reason for drug administration | Pain rating | Respirations | Signature |
|---|---|---|---|---|---|---|
| | | | | | | |
| | | | | | | |
| | | | | | | |
| | | | | | | |
| | | | | | | |
| | | | | | | |
| | | | | | | |
| | | | | | | |
| | | | | | | |
| | | | | | | |
| | | | | | | |
| | | | | | | |
| | | | | | | |
| | | | | | | |
| | | | | | | |
| | | | | | | |
| | | | | | | |

***FIG. 52-2*** Record helps monitor effectiveness of interventions.

From Wong DL and Whaley LF: Clinical manual of pediatric nursing, ed 3, 1990, St Louis, The CV Mosby Co.

***PAIN EXPERIENCE INVENTORY***

**QUESTIONS FOR PARENTS**

Describe any pain your child has had before.
How does your child usually react to pain?
Does your child tell you or others when he is hurting?
How do you know when your child is in pain?
What do you do for your child when he is hurting?
What does your child do for himself when he is hurting?
Which of these actions work best to decrease or take away your child's pain?
Is there anything special that you would like me to know about your child and pain? (If yes, have parent[s] describe.)

**QUESTIONS FOR CHILD**

Tell me what pain is.
Tell me about any hurt you have had before.
What do you do when you hurt?
Do you tell others when you hurt?
What do you want others to do for you when you hurt?
What don't you want others to do for you when you hurt?
What helps the most to take away your hurt?
Is there anything special that you want me to know about you when you hurt? (If yes, have child describe.)

From Hester N and Barcus C: Assessment and management of pain in children, Pediatrics: Nursing Update 1(14):3, 1986.

| Steps | Rationale |
|---|---|
| ▪ Observe coping strategies child uses during painful procedure, such as talking, moaning, lying rigidly still, or squeezing hand. | Children who experience repeated painful procedures often develop effective coping strategies, which can be used with future experiences of pain. |
| ▪ Consider pathology associated with underlying condition or expected pain associated with a procedure. | Pathology may give clues to expected intensity and type of pain. For example, pain associated with vasoocclusive crises in sickle cell disease is severe (Schechter, Berrien, and Katz, 1988). Pain associated with procedures such as bone marrow tests, lumbar punctures, arterial punctures, and chest tube insertions is typically greater than discomfort from venipunctures, finger/heel punctures, or injections (Wong and Baker, 1988). |

## Planning and Goal Setting

| Steps | Rationale |
|---|---|
| 1. Select pain control strategies based on information from: | Information on pain guides planning regarding the use of effective pain-reducing strategies and developing an individualized plan of care. |
| a. Pain experience inventory (see box above). | Information from family and child promotes collaborative planning based on identification of previously successful strategies. |
| b. Pain assessment record (see Fig. 52-2) or initial pain rating. | Record allows for continuation or modification of actual or potential interventions. |
| c. Pathology or procedure. | Knowledge of the expected type and severity of pain allows for an appropriate starting strategy. Narcotic analgesics should be used if pain is typically severe. Brief pain may be lessened with nonpharmacologic methods with or without analgesics. However, nonpharmacologic methods should be used as adjuncts rather than as pharmacologic substitutes. |
| 2. For pharmacologic pain control strategies: | |
| a. Select an appropriate nonnarcotic, narcotic, or a combination of the two types of analgesics. | Nonnarcotic analgesics are suitable for mild to moderate pain. Narcotic analgesics are indicated for moderate to severe pain. Combination of the two analgesics attacks pain on two levels: nonnarcotics at the peripheral level and narcotics at the central nervous system. This allows for increased analgesia with decreased side effects.<br>***Special Considerations:*** *Commercially available combinations such as Tylenol with codeine have increasing doses of the narcotic but a constant dose of nonnarcotic. Therefore it may be better to increase the nonnarcotic component to the recommended dose, e.g., 650 mg of acetaminophen for children 12 years of age and older, before doubling the combination drug. For example, add one plain Tylenol 300 mg to Tylenol with codeine no. 3 before advancing to Tylenol with codeine no. 4. Safety of various narcotics differs. Morphine is considered the drug of choice. Meperidine is not recommended for chronic use because of the accumulation of metabolite normeperidine, a central nervous system (CNS) stimulant that can produce anxiety, tremors, myoclonus, and generalized seizures (American Pain Society, 1989). CNS excitation is not reversed with naloxone (see p. 332).* |

| Steps | Rationale |
|---|---|
| b. Select most effective and least traumatic route of administration: | Several routes of administration exist. Child should not have to endure pain such as from intramuscular injection to achieve pain relief. |
| ▪ Oral. | Oral administration is preferred because of convenience, cost, and relatively steady blood levels, but higher dosages of the oral form of narcotic analgesics are required to achieve equivalent analgesia provided by parenteral form. |
| ▪ Sublingual. | Sublingual route is highly desirable because its effects are more rapid than oral; many drugs can be compounded into a troche or lozenge (Wong, 1987). |
| ▪ IV bolus. | IV bolus provides the most rapid onset of effect, usually in about 5 minutes. May be administered via a programmable infusion pump that allows the child to self-administer predetermined boluses of medication; may be combined with a continuous infusion of narcotic, as well as intermittent boluses (referred to as *patient-controlled analgesia* or *PCA*). PCA is suitable for children as young as 4 years who can follow directions (Gaukroger, Tomkins, and van der Walt, 1989; Pauly-O'Neill, 1990). |
| ▪ IV (continuous). | Continuous IV infusion provides steady blood levels and ability to easily titrate dosage. |
| ▪ Intramuscular. | Intramuscular (IM) injection is readily available but has several disadvantages: painful, wide fluctuation in absorption of drug from muscle, shorter duration than oral administration, expensive, and time consuming for staff. |
| ▪ Subcutaneous (continuous). | Subcutaneous infusion may be used when oral and intravenous routes are not available and child requires continuous pain medication such as in terminal phase of cancer. Suitable analgesics include morphine and dilaudid, but not meperidine. |
| ▪ Intradermal. | A local anesthetic is injected over area to be accessed, e.g., for lumbar puncture, bone marrow aspiration, or arterial puncture.<br>***Special Considerations:*** *To avoid stinging sensation associated with lidocaine, buffer the solution by adding 1 part of sodium bicarbonate (1 mEq/ml) to 10 parts of 1% lidocaine (McKay, Morris, and Mushlin, 1987).* |
| ▪ Rectal. | Rectal route is an alternative to oral or parenteral routes but is disliked by children and has variable absorption rates. Many drugs can be compounded into rectal suppositories. |
| ▪ Topical. | Topical administration can be used for limited number of applications such as lidocaine/prilocaine cream (EMLA [eutectic mixture of local anesthetic] is pending approval by the Food and Drug Administration) for venipunctures (Juhlin and Evers, 1990) or tetracaine/adrenalin/cocaine (TAC) liquid dripped into wounds for suturing (Engebo, 1990). |
| ▪ Inhalation. | Use of anesthetics such as nitrous oxide, ketamine, or halothane can be used to produce partial or complete analgesia for painful procedures (Griffin, Campbell, and Jones, 1981; Perin and Frase, 1985). |
| ▪ Epidural or intrathecal. | Epidural or intrathecal administration is sometimes used postoperatively or in selected terminal care; a catheter is placed into the epidural or intrathecal space, and a narcotic is instilled via continuous drip or intermittent administration. Analgesia primarily results from drug's direct effect on opiate receptors in the spinal cord rather than in the brain, which is responsible for undesirable effects, e.g., sedation and respiratory depression (McCaffery and Beebe, 1989). However, there remains uncertainty about optimal drug choice and indications for choosing this route over other routes (American Pain Society, 1989). |
| ▪ Nerve blocks. | A local long-acting anesthetic (bupivavaine) is injected into site, most often at end of surgery, to provide prolonged analgesia postoperatively, e.g., following inguinal herniorrhaphy (Hinkle, 1987). Nerve blocks usually using lidocaine also provide local anesthesia for surgery such as dorsal penile nerve block for circumcision (Williamson and Williamson, 1983). |

**TABLE 52-2** Dosage and Therapeutic Activity of Selected Opioids for Children

| Drug (route) | Initial Dose (a) | Conversion Factor IM to PO (b) | Equivalent IM Dose (mg) (c) | Therapeutic Activity for IM Route Except as Noted (d) |
|---|---|---|---|---|
| Morphine (IV, IM, SC, PO) | 0.1-0.2 mg/kg IM | 3-6 | 10 | O = 15-60 min.<br>P = 0.5-1 hr.<br>D = 3-7 hr. |
| Fentanyl (Sublimaze) (IV) | 2-3 μg/kg IV | — | 0.1 | IV route:<br>O = 7-8 min.<br>P = No data<br>D = 1-2 hr. |
| Codeine (IM, PO) | 0.5-1 mg/kg PO | 1.5 | 130 | O = 15-30 min.<br>P = 0.5-1 hr.<br>D = 4-6 hr. |
| Methadone (Dolophine) (IM, PO) | 0.1-0.2 mg/kg PO | 2 | 10 | O = 30-60 min.<br>P = 0.5-1 hr.<br>D = 4-6 hr. (d) |
| Hydromorphone (Dilaudid) (IV, SC, PO) | 0.015-0.03 mg/kg IM | 5 | 1.5 | O = 15-30 min.<br>P = 0.5-1 hr.<br>D = 4-5 hr. |
| Levorphanol (Levo-Dromoran) (SC, IV, PO) | 0.02-0.04 mg/kg IM | 2 | 2 | O = 30-90 min.<br>P = 0.5-1 hr.<br>D = 4-8 hr. |
| Meperidine (e) (Demerol) (IV, IM, PO) | 1 to 2 mg/kg IM | 4 | 75 | O = 10-45 min.<br>P = 0.5-1 hr.<br>D = 2-4 hr. |

From Wong D and Whaley L: Clinical manual of pediatric nursing, ed 3, St. Louis, 1990, The CV Mosby Co; Principal reference: American Pain Society: Principles of analgesic use in the treatment of acute pain and chronic cancer pain, ed 2, Skokie, IL, 1989. American Pain Society.

(a) These dosages are considered initial starting doses for moderate to severe pain in children who have not developed tolerance to the drug. The optimal dose is determined by titration: increasing or decreasing the dose according to the child's response. Dosages for hydromorphone and levorphanol are based on the equianalgesic dose of parenteral morphine.

(b) To convert an IM dose to a PO dose, multiply the IM dose by the conversion factor. Based on clinical experience, IM and IV doses are considered equianalgesic. However, some clinicians suggest that ½ the IM dose equals the IV dose, especially for an initial IV bolus dose. For morphine a conversion factor of 3 is recommended for repetitive dosing.

(c) When converting from one drug to another drug, be certain that the dosages of the drugs are equivalent. For example, 5 mg of IV morphine is equal to 0.75 mg of IV or 4 mg of PO hydromorphone.

(d) O = onset; P = peak; D = duration. With IV administration, times may be shorter, and with PO administration, times may be longer. Times for all drugs are approximate and may be shorter in children due to their more rapid metabolism of the drug. With repeated dosing, duration of methadone and levorphanol increases. Sustained-release preparations of oral morphine are available (MS Contin, 8-12 hours: Roxanol-SR, 8 hours).

(e) Should not be used chronically, particularly in patients with compromised renal function or for treatment of sickle cell crisis pain, because of accumulation of the metabolite, normeperidine, which causes central nervous system irritability (anxiety, tremors, myoclonus, and generalized seizures).

| Steps | Rationale |
|---|---|
| c. Plan preventive schedule of medication around the clock (ATC), not as needed (PRN), when pain is continuous and predictable such as postoperatively. | A preventive schedule provides more effective pain control than with a PRN schedule because the ATC schedule avoids the low plasma concentrations that permit "breakthrough" pain. |
| d. Plan to administer analgesic before a scheduled procedure for its peak effect to coincide with inducement of pain (Table 52-2). | Maximum analgesia occurs at time of drug's peak effect.<br>***Special Considerations:*** *When pain can be predicted, the peak effect should be timed accordingly, e.g., with narcotics, the peak effect is approximately 30 minutes to 1 hour for the intramuscular or subcutaneous route (considerably less for the intravenous route) and for nonnarcotics about 2 hours after oral administration.* |
| e. Have emergency drugs and equipment available in case of respiratory depression from narcotics. | Respiratory depression is the most serious side effect of narcotics. Naloxone is drug of choice; it is a narcotic antagonist that rapidly reverses respiratory depression. Epinephrine may be required in the rare event of anaphylactic shock.<br>***Special Considerations:*** *Fear of respiratory depression is not a valid reason to withhold pain relief.* |
| 3. For nonpharmacologic pain management strategies: | |
| a. Select appropriate strategy. | General strategies (see box at right) are effective with most children, especially those who can benefit from explanations. However, specific nonpharmacologic strategies are more effective with certain children than others. Experimentation with several strategies that are suitable to child's age, pain intensity, and abilities is often necessary to determine most effective strategy. |

## *GUIDELINES FOR NONPHARMACOLOGIC PAIN MANAGEMENT*

### GENERAL STRATEGIES

Form a trusting relationship with child and family:
- Express concern regarding their reports of pain.
- Take an active role in seeking effective pain management strategies.

Use general strategies to prepare child for painful procedure.

Prepare the child before potentially painful procedures but avoid "planting" the idea of pain. For example, instead of saying
- "This is going to (or may) hurt," say "Sometimes this feels like pushing, sticking, or pinching and sometimes it doesn't bother people. You tell me what it feels like to you."
- Use "non-pain" descriptors when possible, e.g., "It feels like intense heat," rather than, "It's a burning pain."
- This allows for variation in sensory perception, avoids suggesting pain, and gives the child control in describing reactions.

Avoid evaluative statements or descriptions, such as "This is a terrible procedure" or "It really will hurt a lot."

Stay with the child during a painful procedure:
- Encourage parents to stay with child if child and parent desire; encourage parent to talk softly to child and to remain near child's head.
- Involve parents in learning specific nonpharmacologic strategies and assisting child in their use.

Educate the child about the pain, especially when explanation may lessen anxiety (e.g., that the pain the child is experiencing is expected after surgery and does not indicate that something is wrong; reassure the child that he is not responsible for the pain).

For long-term pain control give the child a doll that becomes "the patient" and allow child to do everything to the doll that is done to the child; pain control can be emphasized through the doll by stating, "Dolly feels better after the medicine."

### SPECIFIC STRATEGIES

#### Distraction

Involve parent and child in identifying strong distractors.

Involve child in play; use radio, tape recorder, record player; have child sing or use rhythmic breathing.

Have the child concentrate on yelling or saying "ouch" by focusing on "yelling loud or soft as you feel it hurt; that way I know what's happening."

Use humor, such as watching cartoons, telling jokes or funny stories, or acting silly with the child.

#### Positive self-talk

Teach child positive statements to say when in pain, e.g., "I will be feeling better soon," "When I go home, I will feel better," "Relaxing will make me hurt less."

#### Thought-stopping

Identify positive facts about the painful event, such as "It does not last long."

Identify reassuring information, such as, "If I think about something else, it does not hurt as much."

Condense positive and reassuring facts into a set of brief statements and have the child memorize them, e.g.: "Short procedure, good veins, little hurt, nice nurse, go home."

Have the child repeat the memorized statements whenever thinking about or experiencing the painful event.

#### Relaxation (See p. 78)

With an infant or young child:
- Hold in a comfortable, well-supported position, such as vertically against the chest and shoulder.
- Rock in a wide, rhythmic arc in a rocking chair or sway back and forth, rather than bouncing the child.
- Repeat one or two words softly, such as "Mommy's here."

With a slightly older child:
- Ask the child to take a deep breath and "go limp as a rag doll" while exhaling slowly, then ask the child to yawn (demonstrate if needed).
- Help the child assume a comfortable position (e.g., pillow under neck and knees).
- Begin progressive relaxation: starting with the toes, systematically instruct the child to let each body part "go limp" or "feel heavy"; if the child has difficulty with relaxing, instruct him to tense or tighten each body part and then relax it.
- Allow child to keep eyes open since children may respond better if eyes are open rather than closed during relaxation.

#### Guided imagery

Have the child identify some highly pleasurable real or pretend experience.

Have the child describe the details of the event, including as many senses as possible, e.g., "feel the cool breezes," "see the beautiful colors," "hear the pleasant music."

Have child write down or record script.

Encourage the child to concentrate only on the pleasurable event during the painful time; enhance the image by recalling specific details, such as reading the script or playing the record.

Combine with relaxation (see p. 78).

#### Behavioral contracting

Informal—May be used with children as young as 4 or 5:
- Use stars or tokens as rewards.
- Uncooperative or procrastinating children (during a procedure) can be given a limited amount of time (measured by a visible timer) to complete the procedure.
- Proceed as needed if child is unable to comply.
- Reinforce cooperation with a reward if the procedure is accomplished within specified time.

Formal—Use written contract, which includes the following:
- Realistic (seems possible) goal or desired behavior;
- Measurable behavior, e.g., agrees not to hit anyone during procedures;
- Contract written, dated, and signed by all persons involved in any of the agreements;
- Identified rewards or consequences are reinforcing;
- Goal can be evaluated.

#### Cutaneous stimulation

Includes simple rhythmic rubbing; use of pressure, electric vibrator; massage with hand lotion, powder, or menthol cream; application of heat or cold, such as an ice cube on the site before giving injection or application of ice to the site opposite the painful area (e.g., if right knee hurts, place ice on left knee).

A more sophisticated method is transcutaneous electrical nerve stimulation (TENS) (use of controlled low voltage electricity to the body via electrodes placed on the skin).

From Wong D and Whaley L: Clinical manual of pediatric nursing, ed 3, St. Louis, 1990, The CV Mosby Co.

| Steps | Rationale |
|---|---|
| | ***Special Considerations:*** *Most specific nonpharmacologic strategies require children's understanding and cooperation. Therefore try to match the strategy with the pain severity. Children in severe pain may not be able to devote the attention and effort necessary to learn the technique, and those with mild symptoms may not be motivated to learn; therefore these strategies may be most useful with midrange pain (Cleeland, 1986).* |
| ▪ Use strategy familiar to child, or describe several strategies and let child select one that appeals to him. | Child is more likely to comply when given choices about what strategies he or she believes may relieve pain. |
| ▪ Involve parent in selection of strategy. | Parent may be familiar with child's usual coping skills and can help identify potentially successful strategies. Involving parent in selection encourages participation in learning skill with child and acting as coach. |
| b. Select appropriate individual, preferably the parent, to assist child with strategy. | For maximum effectiveness in applying the method, only individuals familiar with the strategy should participate. ***Special Considerations:*** *If the parent cannot assist the child, other appropriate persons may include relatives such as grandparents or older siblings or staff such as a nurse or child-life specialist.* |
| 4. Assemble needed equipment for type of pain intervention employed. | The use of analgesics may require special devices or sophisticated equipment, such as computerized pumps, for certain routes of administration. Most nonpharmacologic interventions do not need special devices, although exceptions include audio devices for music, taped instructions for relaxation/guided imagery, ice, and transcutaneous electrical nerve stimulation (TENS). |
| 5. Collaborate with physician, supplying pain assessment data collected from child and family. | A physician's order or medical protocol is necessary to administer pharmacologic agents. ***Special Considerations:*** *Professional nursing expertise is often required in selecting from among ordered agents, determining dosages and timing from ordered ranges, and serving as an advocate if pain relief is not adequate.* |
| 6. Develop individualized child and family goals: ▪ Decreased pain. ▪ Increased use of coping strategies. | |

## Implementation

### *Pharmacologic*

| Steps | Rationale |
|---|---|
| 1. Administer analgesic. | ***Special Considerations:*** *Effective analgesia requires the appropriate strength analgesic for the severity of pain, sufficient dosage, and correct schedule of administration.* |
| 2. Titrate the dosage for maximum pain relief. | Titration refers to the gradual adjustment of drug dosage (usually by increasing the dose) until optimal pain relief is achieved without excessive sedation. |
| a. Begin with recommended dosage for age and weight (Tables 52-2 and 52-3). | Textbook recommendations are only safe starting dosages but are not optimal dosages. References, e.g., *Physician's Desk Reference* and package insert, do not necessarily represent the latest research on drugs. Also, children metabolize drugs more rapidly than adults. Studies have found that younger children (except infants under 3 months of age) require higher doses of narcotics than older children and adults to achieve same analgesic effect (Hertzka et al, 1989; Olkkola et al, 1988). Therefore therapeutic effect and duration of analgesia will vary. Children's dosages are usually calculated according to body weight or body surface area or, less precisely, as percentage of adult dose. ***Special Considerations:*** *General rules for children's starting dosages are: children 2-6 years: 20%-25% of adult starting dose; children 7-12 years: 50% of adult starting dose; children 12 years of age and older: full adult starting dose (American Pain Society, 1989).* |

***TABLE 52-3*** Nonsteroidal Anti-inflammatory Drugs (NSAIDs) Approved for Children*

| Drug (Trade Name) | Dose | Comments |
|---|---|---|
| Acetaminophen (Tylenol and other brands) | 10 to 15 mg/kg/dose every 4 to 6 hours not to exceed 5 doses in 24 hr. | Available in drops (80 mg/0.8 ml), elixir (160 mg/5 ml), tablets (80 mg), and swallowable caplets (160 mg)<br>Nonprescription |
| Choline magnesium trisalicylate (Trilisate) | Children 37 kg or less:<br>50 mg/kg/day divided into 2 doses<br>Children >37 kg:<br>2250 mg/day divided into 2 doses | Available in elixir 500 mg/5 ml<br>Prescription |
| Ibuprofen (PediaProfen) | Children 6 months to 12 years:<br>5 to 10 mg/kg/dose every 6 to 8 hours not to exceed 40 mg/kg/day for fever<br>Children over 12 years:<br>200 to 400 mg/dose every 6 to 8 hours | Available in suspension 100 mg/5 ml<br>Prescription<br>Recommended for fever reduction in children 6 months to 12 years but is also indicated for use in juvenile rheumatoid arthritis and mild to moderate pain in children over 12 years. |
| (Children's Advil) | Children 12 months and older:<br>30 to 40 mg/kg/day divided in 3 or 4 doses | Available in suspension 100 mg/5 ml<br>Prescription<br>Dosage is recommendation for juvenile rheumatoid arthritis; dosage for fever is same as for PediaProfen but for children 12 months and over. |
| Naproxen (Naprosyn) | Children >2 years:<br>10 mg/kg/day divided in 2 doses | Available in elixir 125 mg/5 ml<br>Prescription |
| Tolmetin (Tolectin) | Children >2 years:<br>20 mg/kg/day divided in 3 or 4 doses | Available in scored 200 mg tablets<br>Prescription |

* All NSAIDs in the table except acetaminophen have significant anti-inflammatory, antipyretic, and analgesic actions. Acetaminophen has a weak anti-inflammatory action and its classification as an NSAID is controversial. As analgesics, NSAIDs are effective for mild to moderate pain. Patients respond differently to various NSAIDs; therefore changing from one drug to another may be necessary for maximum benefit.
Acetylsalicylic acid (aspirin) is also an NSAID but is not recommended for children because of its possible association with Reye syndrome. The NSAIDs in the table have no known association with Reye syndrome. However, caution should be exercised in prescribing any salicylate-containing drug (e.g., Trilisate) for children with known or suspected viral infection.
Side effects of ibuprofen, naproxen, and tolmetin include nausea, vomiting, diarrhea, constipation, gastric ulceration, bleeding, nephritis, and fluid retention. Acetaminophen and choline magnesium trisalicylate are well tolerated in the gastrointestinal tract and do not interfere with platelet function. NSAIDs, with the exception of acetaminophen, should not be given to patients with allergic reactions to salicylates. All the NSAIDs should be used cautiously in patients with renal impairment.
From FDA-approved product information, 1989; Wong D and Whaley L: Clinical manual of pediatric nursing, ed 3, St Louis, 1990, The CV Mosby Co.

| Steps | Rationale |
|---|---|
| b. Increase dosage and/or decrease interval between doses if pain relief is inadequate. | Increasing the dosage provides greater analgesic effectiveness. Decreasing the interval provides more continuous pain relief.<br>***Special Considerations:*** *Nonnarcotics have ceiling effect, which means that doses higher than the recommended dosage will not produce greater pain relief. Most narcotics do not have a ceiling effect other than that imposed by side effects; therefore larger dosages can be given for increasing severity of pain.* |
| c. Decrease dosage if excessive sedation or decreased respiratory rate occurs. | Excessive sedation and/or decreased respirations can occur if dose is too high. Gradually lowering dose usually provides adequate analgesia without excessive sedation because analgesia occurs at lower doses than those required to produce sedation. However, lowering the dose sufficiently to prevent sedation and decrease respirations may interfere with optimal pain control. As an alternative, a stimulant, e.g., dextroamphetamine, can be given. |

| Steps | Rationale |
|---|---|
| | ***Special Considerations:*** *If a stimulant is given, the last dose should be administered at least 6 hours before bedtime to prevent insomnia (McManus and Panzarella, 1986). No research exists regarding safe minimal respiratory rates for patients on narcotics. However, guidelines include ranges of 13 to 16 (Dilworth and MacKellar, 1987) and 8 to 10 (Eland, 1988). Since respiratory rates decrease with age, the upper limits should be used with younger children and the lower limits for older children.* |
| 3. Monitor for side effects of analgesics, especially narcotics, which may include respiratory depression, sedation, constipation, nausea and vomiting, agitation or euphoria, mental clouding, orthostatic hypotension, pruritis, sweating, and miosis (sign of toxicity). | Respiratory depression is the most serious complication of narcotics, it is most likely to occur 7 minutes after intravenous infusion, 30 minutes after intramuscular administration, and 90 minutes after oral administration of morphine (Gilman et al, 1985).<br>***Special Considerations:*** *Respiratory depression is a side effect of narcotics, but is a rare occurrence; one study of adults found an incidence of 0.09% respiratory depression from parenteral meperidine and none from oral meperidine (Miller and Jick, 1978). Reports of respiratory depression are nonexistent or rare in children (Beasley and Tibballs, 1987; Dilworth and MacKellar, 1987). Children are no more likely to develop respiratory depression than adults (Olkkola et al, 1988). As tolerance to the drug develops, tolerance to side effects (except constipation) also occurs.* |
| a. Administer naloxone (Narcan) (IV or intratracheal) if severe respiratory depression occurs. Recommended dosage: 0.1 mg/kg from birth (including premature infants) until 5 years of age or weight of 20 kg, at which time use minimum dosage of 2 mg (American Academy of Pediatrics, 1989). | Naloxone is a narcotic antagonist that rapidly reverses respiratory depression. It also reverses analgesia, can precipitate withdrawal, and in the case of meperidine, can precipitate seizures (see p. 330). Therefore it must be used cautiously with frequent monitoring of child's condition.<br>***Special Considerations:*** *Since the duration of naloxone's action (about 1 to 4 hours) may be shorter than the duration of the narcotic, repeated doses may be required to prevent recurrence of respiratory depression.* |
| b. Administer stool softener or laxative to prevent constipation. | Constipation is a common side effect of narcotics, which decrease peristaltic activity and increase anal sphincter tone (Gilman et al, 1985). Prevention is more effective than treatment once constipation occurs.<br>***Special Considerations:*** *Dietary treatment such as increased fiber is usually not sufficient to promote regular bowel evacuation. However, dietary measures (e.g., increased fluid, juice, fruit, and bran), should be encouraged.* |
| c. Observe for signs of tolerance and physical dependence with use of narcotics. | Signs of tolerance and physical dependence may occur with continued use of narcotics but must not be confused with addiction. |
| ▪ Signs of tolerance include: decreasing pain relief and decreasing duration of pain relief.<br>▪ Signs of physical dependence include withdrawal symptoms once the drug is discontinued. Initial signs of withdrawal are lacrimation, rhinorrhea, yawning, and sweating; later signs are restlessness, irritability, tremors, anorexia, dilated pupils, and gooseflesh (Gilman et al, 1985; Miser et al, 1986). | *Tolerance* is the physiologic need for increased dosage; *dependence* is physiologic withdrawal when drug is discontinued abruptly; *addiction* is psychologic dependence on drugs (Gilman et al, 1985).<br>***Special Considerations:*** *Fears of addiction are unsupported, with an incidence of 0.03% among adults (Porter and Jick, 1980). Similar research is not available for children, although reports indicate no evidence of addiction in children receiving narcotics (Cole et al, 1986; Schechter, Berrien, and Katz, 1988).* |
| d. Treat tolerance and physical dependence appropriately. | Since tolerance and physical dependence are physiologic consequences (and never the child's fault), treatment of tolerance involves increasing the dosage or decreasing the duration between doses; treatment of physical dependence involves gradually reducing the dosage over 7 to 10 days to prevent occurrence of withdrawal symptoms (similar to tapering of steroid dosages after chronic steroid therapy); treatment of withdrawal includes the use of methadone in tapering doses over 5 days (Miser et al, 1986). |

| **Steps** | **Rationale** |
|---|---|
| 4. Monitor for allergic reactions to analgesics. | Allergic reactions to analgesics are uncommon. Mild reactions are usually manifested as skin rashes, especially urticaria. Anaphylactoid reactions to IV codeine and morphine are rare. Certain individuals may have allergic reactions to aspirin and most aspirin-like drugs. Symptoms range from vasomotor rhinitis to complete vasomotor collapse. While rare in children, such reactions occur in 20% to 25% of adults with asthma (Gilman et al, 1985). |
| 5. If using parenteral route, change to oral route as soon as possible, using equianalgesic dosages (see Table 52-2). | Oral form of narcotic analgesics requires higher dosages than parenteral form to provide equivalent analgesia because of "first-pass effect," in which drug is rapidly absorbed from gastrointestinal tract and enters portal circulation where it is partially metabolized before reaching the central circulation. |
| a. Convert directly by giving next dose of analgesic orally in equivalent dosage without any parenteral form of the same drug.<br>*OR* | Direct conversion is usually successful in children who do not associate the parenteral form of narcotic with superior pain relief. |
| b. Convert gradually to oral form using the following steps:<br>▪ Convert half of the parenteral dose to a PO dose.<br>▪ Administer half the parenteral dose and the PO dose.<br>▪ Assess pain relief.<br>▪ If pain relief is inadequate, increase the PO dose as needed.<br>▪ If sedation occurs, decrease the PO dose as needed.<br>▪ When the parenteral and PO doses are effective, discontinue the parenteral dose and give twice the PO dose. | Gradual conversion may be needed when the child associates the parenteral form with superior pain relief and doubts that an oral form will be as effective. It should also be used when large doses are given for severe pain because direct conversion to a large oral dose may be excessive. |
| 6. Avoid combining narcotics with so-called potentiators. | There is little evidence that any drug potentiates the analgesics effect of narcotics; rather, drugs such as promethazine (Phenergan) produce sedation that is erroneously equated with analgesia (American Pain Society, 1989; Howland and Goldfrank, 1986). Drugs such as hydroxyzine (Atarax or Vistaril) have analgesic properties of their own; 100 mg of hydroxyzine is equal in analgesic potency to 8 mg of morphine, offering a cumulative analgesic effect. However, it is only available in parenteral form (not IV) and is a painful IM injection. |
| 7. Avoid using placebos to verify if pain is real. | A positive response to a placebo such as a saline injection is common in patients who have a documented organic basis for pain. Therefore the deceptive use of placebos does not provide useful information about the presence or severity of pain (Goodwin, Goodwin, and Vogel, 1979). In addition, the use of placebos can destroy the child's trust in health care staff and raises serious ethical and legal questions. |
| 8. Use supportive statements when administering analgesics.<br>a. Reinforce effect of analgesic by telling child "the medicine will make the pain less" and that he or she will begin to feel better in x amount of time (according to drug used); can use a clock or timer to measure onset of relief with child. | By reinforcing the cause and effect of the medication and analgesic, child can become conditioned to expect pain relief.<br>***Special Considerations:*** *While this approach is helpful, it should only be used when there is reasonable assurance that the analgesic will be effective.* |
| b. Avoid saying "I am going to give you a shot for pain," since this is one pain in addition to existing pain; if child refuses an injection, explain that the little hurt from the needle will take away the big hurt for a long time. | Ideally, injections should not be given, but when they are, child needs to understand that the injection will result in pain relief. |
| c. Avoid statements, e.g., "this is enough medicine to take away anyone's pain" or "by now you should not need so much pain medicine." | Such statements belittle the child's feelings about his or her pain and discourage the child from communicating pain relief needs. |
| d. Never refer to child who is tolerant or physically dependent as addicted. | Because addiction is often a concern to the family, any statement that implies addiction must be avoided.<br>***Special Considerations:*** *If increasing the dosage of narcotics concerns the child or family, reassure them of extremely low incidence of addiction and ask them the question: "if you did not have this pain, would you want to take this medicine?" This can reassure them that the only reason for the narcotic is pain relief.* |

| Steps | Rationale |
|---|---|
| ***Nonpharmacologic*** | |
| 1. Use general nonpharmacologic strategies to reduce perception of pain and increase tolerance of pain (see box on p. 333). | General and specific nonpharmacologic strategies reduce fear and anxiety and may interfere with pain transmission. |
| 2. Use specific nonpharmacologic strategies to reduce perception of pain (see box on p. 333). | |
| a. Teach child to use specific nonpharmacologic strategies before pain occurs or before it becomes severe. | A child is more likely to learn strategies when not distressed. ***Special Considerations:*** *To reduce the child's effort in memorizing instructions for a strategy, e.g., distraction, present the steps on audio tape.* |
| b. Assist or have parent assist child with using strategy during actual pain. | A coach, especially a parent, can facilitate implementation of the strategy and help conserve the child's energy. |

| Evaluation Outcomes | Observational Guidelines |
|---|---|
| 1. Pain is eliminated or reduced to tolerable level. | Observe child's behavior for signs of pain and pain relief. Review pain assessment record for evidence of pain relief from analgesics. Question child and family regarding their satisfaction with pain management. |
| 2. Child learns effective coping strategies. | Observe child's behavior when in pain for evidence of use of specific nonpharmacologic strategies. Observe nurses' and other staff's interaction with child for evidence of use of general nonpharmacologic strategies. Question child regarding his satisfaction with nonpharmacologic strategies to relieve pain. |
| 3. Parent or other appropriate person learns effective coping skill with child and acts as coach. | Observe parent's behavior when with child for evidence of use of specific nonpharmacologic strategies during painful events. Question parent regarding satisfaction with learning strategy, acting as coach, and its effectiveness in reducing child's pain. |

## Documentation

Record factors substantiating initial assessment of pain, such as child's behavior, vital signs, or pain intensity rating in nurses' notes or progress notes. Record date, time, drug, dose, route of administration, and reason for giving analgesic. At 30 minutes after analgesic administration and then every hour for the drug's expected duration, record child's degree of pain relief and occurrence of any side effects on the medication sheet and/or pain assessment record. If nonpharmacologic interventions are employed, record date, time, type of strategy, reason for its use, person employing the strategy or serving as coach, and child's response to the intervention in nurses' notes, progress record, and/or pain assessment record.

UNIT VI

## PRODUCT REFERENCES AND TEACHING RESOURCES

### Books

Butler NB: How to raise professional awareness of the need for adequate pain relief for infants, Birth 15:38-41, 1988.
Questions parents and concerned professionals might ask of their local health care institutions. A one-page sheet that addresses questions that effectively raise awareness about infant pain control.

Wisconsin Cancer Pain Initiative
3625 Medical Sciences Center
University of Wisconsin Medical School
1300 University Avenue
Madison, WI 53706
(608) 262-0978
Booklets provide parents with facts about pain and its management in children with cancer. Titles include: Children's cancer pain can be relieved: a guide for parents and families; and Jeff asks about cancer pain.

### Products

Oucher
University of Colorado Health Sciences Center
School of Nursing
Campus Box C288
4200 East Ninth Avenue
Denver, CO 80262
(303) 270-1317
Includes Oucher pain scale, user's manual, and technical report.

The Purdue Frederick Company
100 Connecticut Avenue
Norwalk, CT 06850-3590
1-800-243-5667, ext. 4008 or 4010
Distributes Wong-Baker Faces Scale.

American Pain Society
5700 Old Orchard Rd.
Skokie, IL 60077
708-966-0050

Offers principles of analgesic use in the treatment of acute pain and chronic cancer pain, offers a booklet that describes most effective guidelines for treating pain.

## REFERENCES


American Academy of Pediatrics, Committee on Drugs: Emergency drug doses for infants and children and naloxone use in newborns: clarification, Pediatr 83(5):803, 1989.

American Academy of Pediatrics: Neonatal anesthesia, Pediatrics 80(3):446, 1987.

American Academy of Pediatrics, Report of the Committee on Infectious Diseases, ed 21, Elk Grove Village, Ill, 1988, American Academy of Pediatrics.

American Academy of Pediatrics: Task force on pediatric AIDS: Pediatric guidelines for infection control of Human Immunodeficiency Virus (Acquired Immunodeficiency Virus) in hospitals, medical offices, schools and other settings, Pediatrics 82(5):801-807, 1988.

American Pain Society: Principles of analgesic use in the treatment of acute pain and chronic cancer pain, ed 2, Skokie, Ill, 1989, American Pain Society.

Anand K and Aynsley-Green A: Metabolic and endocrine effects of surgical ligation of patent ductus arteriosus in the human preterm neonate: are there implications for further improvement of postoperative outcome? Mod Probl Paediatr 23:143-157, 1985.

Anand K, Phil D, and Hickey P: Pain and its effects in the human neonate and fetus, N Engl J Med 317(21):1321-1329, 1987.

Banco L and Powers A: Hospitals: unsafe environments for children, Pediatrics 82(5):794-797, 1988.

Beasley SW and Tibballs J: Efficacy and safety of continuous morphine infusion for postoperative analgesia in the pediatric surgical ward, Aust N Z J Surg 57:233-237, 1987.

Benenson AS, editor: Control of communicable disease in man, ed 14, Washington, DC, 1985, American Public Health Association.

Beyer JE: The oucher: a user's manual and technical report, Denver, 1988, University of Colorado.

Broome M et al: Children's medical fears, coping behaviors, and pain perceptions during a lumbar puncture, Oncology Nurs Forum 17(3):361-367, 1990.

Burns associated with baby walkers; Child Health Alert, Oct, 1988, p 4.

Butler NB: The ethical issues involved in the practice of surgery on unanesthetized infants, AORN J 46(6):1136-1144, 1987.

Campbell VG: In brief: covergowns for newborn infection control? MCN 12:54, 1987.

Centers for Disease Control: Guidelines for the prevention and control of nosocomial infections, Atlanta, 1983, Centers for Disease Control.

Centers for Disease Control: Recommendations for prevention of HIV transmission in health care settings, MMWR 36(25):3-18, 1987.

Centers for Disease Control: Update: Universal precautions for prevention of transmission of human immunodeficiency virus, hepatitis B virus, and other bloodborne pathogens in health-care settings, MMWR 37(24):377-382; 388-389, 1988.

Cleeland C: Behavioral control of symptoms, J Pain Sympt Manag 1(1):36-38, 1986.

Code for Nurses with Interpretive Statements, Kansas City, 1985, American Nurses' Association.

Cole T et al, Intravenous narcotic therapy for children with severe sickle cell crisis pain, Am J Dis Child, 140:1255-1259, 1986.

Committee on Early Childhood, Adoption and Dependent Care: Health in day care: a manual for health care professionals, Elk Grove Village, Ill, 1987, American Academy of Pediatrics.

Dilworth NM and MacKellar A: Pain relief for the pediatric surgical patient, J Pediatr Surg 22:264-266, 1987.

Eland JM: The child who is hurting, Semin Oncol Nurs 1(2):116-122, 1985.

Eland JM: Pharmacologic management of acute and chronic pediatric pain, Issues Comp Pediatr Nurs 11(2-3):93-112, 1988.

Eland J and Anderson J: The experience of pain in children, In Jacox A, editor: Pain: a source book for nurses and other health professionals, Boston, 1977, Little, Brown & Co, Inc.

Engebo D: Safe and effective use of tetracaine, adrenaline, and cocaine (TAC) solution anesthetic for anesthetizing of lacerations, J Emerg Nurs 16(2):100-101, 1990.

Evans M and Hansen B: A clinical guide to pediatric nursing, ed 2, Norwalk, Conn, 1985, Appleton-Century-Crofts.

Franck L: A national survey of the assessment and treatment of pain and agitation in the neonatal intensive care unit, JOGNN 16:387-393, 1987.

Gaukroger P, Tomkins DP, and van der Walt J: Patient-controlled analgesia in children, Anaesth Intens Care 17(3):264-268, 1989.

Gilman A et al: Goodman and Gilman's the pharmacological basis of therapeutics, ed 7, New York, 1985, Macmillan Publishing Co.

Haslam D: Age and perception of pain, Psychonomic Sci 15:86, 1969.

Hayman L and Sporing E, editors: Handbook of pediatric nursing, New York, 1985, John Wiley & Sons Inc.

Hertzka R et al: Fentanyl-induced ventilatory depression: effects of age, Anesthesiology 70:213-218, 1989.

Hester N: The preoperational child's reaction to immunization, Nurs Res 28(4):250-255, 1979.

Hester N: Personal communication, 1989.

Hinkle AJ: Percutaneous inguinal block for outpatient management of postherniorrhaphy pain in children, Anesthesiology 67:411-413, 1987.

Howland M and Goldfrank L: Meperidine usage in patients with sickle cell crisis, Ann Emerg Med 15(12):1506-1507, 1986.

Hughes W and Buescher ES: Pediatric procedures, Philadelphia, 1980, WB Saunders Co.

International Association for the Study of Pain: Pain terms: a current list of definitions and notes on usage, Pain 3:S216-S221, 1986.

Jackson MM: Rituals without reason. In Patterns in specialization: challenge to the curriculum, New York, 1986, National League for Nursing.

Jackson MM and Lynch P: Infection control: too much or too little? Am J Nurs 84(2):208-211, 1984.

Jackson MM and McPherson DC: Infection control: keeping current, Nurse Ed 11(4):38-40, 1986.

Jackson MM et al: Why not treat all body substances as infectious? Am J Nurs 87(9):1137-1139, 1987.

James S and Mott S: Child health nursing: essential care of children and families, Reading, Mass, 1988, Addison-Wesley Publishing Co.

Juhlin L, and Evers H: EMLA: a new topical anesthetic, Adv Dermatol 5:75-92, 1990.

Katz E, Kellerman L and Siegel S: Behavioral distress in children with cancer undergoing medical procedures: developmental considerations, J Consult Clin Psychol 18(3):356-365, 1980.

Lynch P and Jackson MM: Isolation practices: how much is too much or not enough? ASEPSIS: The Infection Control Forum 8(4):2-5, 1986.

Lynch P et al: Rethinking the role of isolation practices in the prevention of nosocomial infections, Ann Intern Med 107:243-246, 1987.

McCaffery M and Beebe A: Pain: clinical manual for nursing practice, St Louis, 1989, The CV Mosby Co.

McKay W, Morris R, and Mushlin P: Sodium bicarbonate attenuates pain on skin infiltration with lidocaine, with or without epinephrine, Anesth Analg 66:572-574, 1987.

McManus M and Panzarella C: The use of dextroamphetamine to counteract sedation for patients on a morphine drip, J Assoc Pediatr Oncol Nurs 3(1):28-29, 1986.

McPherson D and Jackson MM: Isolation precautions for a changing environment: a new approach, Journal of Healthcare Materiel Management 5(6):28-32, 1987.

Merz B: Hospital-bed deaths, injuries force down switch modifications, JAMA 250(7):871-872, 1983.

Miller R and Jick H: Clinical effects of meperidine in hospitalized medical patients, J Clin Pharmacol 18:180-189, 1978.

Millunchick EW and McArtor RD: Fatal aspiration of makeshift pacifier, Pediatrics 77(3):369-370, 1986.

Miser AW et al: Narcotic withdrawal syndrome in young adults after the therapeutic use of opiates, Am J Dis Child 140:603-604, 1986.

Nauseef WM and Maki DG: A study of the value of simple protective isolation in patients with granulocytopenia, N Engl J Med 304:448-453, 1981.

Nimityongskul P and Anderson LD: The likelihood of injuries when children fall out of bed, J Pediatr Orthop 7(2):184-186, 1987.

Olkkola K et al: Kinetics and dynamics of postoperative intravenous morphine in children, Clin Pharmacol Ther 44:128-136, 1988.

Olness K: Hypnosis in pediatric practice, Curr Probl Pediatr 12(2):1-47, 1981.

Pauly-O'Neill S: Children demand (PCA) pain relief, too, AJN 90(5):26, 1990.

Perin G and Frase D: Development of a program using general anesthesia for invasive procedures in a pediatric outpatient setting, J Assoc Pediatr Oncol Nurs 3(4):8-10, 1985.

Perry A and Potter P: Clinical nursing skills and techniques, ed 2, St Louis, 1990, The CV Mosby Co.

Pikl BH, editor: Massachusetts General Hospital manual of pediatric nursing practices, Boston, 1981, Little, Brown & Co.

Porter L and Jick H: Addiction rare in patient treated with narcotics, N Engl J Med 302:123, 1980.

Ross DM: Thought stopping: a coping strategy for impending feared events, Issues Comp Pediatr Nurs 7:83-89, 1984.

Savedra M et al: Pain location: validity and reliability of body outline markings by hospitalized children and adolescents, Res Nurs Health 12:307-314, 1989.

Schecter NL, Berrien FB, and Katz SM: The use of patient-controlled analgesia in adolescents with sickle cell pain crisis: A preliminary report, J Pain Sympt Manage 9(2):109-113, 1988.

Scipien G et al: Comprehensive pediatric nursing, ed 3, New York, 1986, McGraw-Hill, Inc.

Smith DP: Using humor to help children with pain, Child Health Care 14(3):187-188, 1986.

Smith S and Duell D: Clinical nursing skills, Los Altos, Calif, 1988, National Nursing Review.

Wallace M: Temperament: a variable in children's pain management, Pediatr Nurs 15(2):118-121, 1989.

Whaley LF and Wong DL: Essentials of pediatric nursing, ed 3, St Louis, 1989, The CV Mosby Co.

Whaley LF and Wong DL: Nursing care of infants and children, ed 4, St Louis, 1991, The CV Mosby Co.

Whitson B and McFarlane J: The pediatric nursing skills manual, New York, 1980, John Wiley & Sons.

Williamson KM et al: Occupational health hazards for nurses: infection, IMAGE: Journal of Nursing Scholarship 20(1):48-53, 1988.

Williamson PS and Williamson ML: Physiologic stress reduction by a local anesthetic during newborn circumcision, Pediatrics 71(1):36-40, 1983.

Wong DL: Lozenges can be "lifesavers," Am J Nurs 87(9):1129-1130, 1987.

Wong DL and Baker C: Pain in children: comparison of assessment scales, Pediatr Nurs 14(1):9-17, 1988.

Wong DL and Whaley LF: Clinical manual of pediatric nursing, ed 3, St Louis, 1990, The CV Mosby Co.

# UNIT VII Activities of Daily Living

# SKILL 53 Bathing the Newborn

*Krena Hunter White*

The primary objective of bathing the newborn is cleansing the skin of blood and amniotic fluid. The purpose of later baths is to maintain daily hygiene. In addition, bath time is an opportunity to observe the newborn, to teach the family about their newborn and bathing skills, and to simply enjoy interaction. Circumcision care is also discussed in this skill. Tips for giving care to an infant in a closed incubator and information for families considering circumcision for a male infant are included.

## NURSING DIAGNOSES

Altered health maintenance related to lack of parental knowledge about bathing a newborn; Hypothermia related to exposure and evaporation from skin in cool environment; Potential for infection related to tissue destruction at umbilical cord and circumcision sites.

| Steps | Rationale |
|---|---|
| **Assessment** | |
| 1. Assess body temperature. Bathe newborn after the temperature has stabilized at 37° C. | Delaying the first bath until after newborn's temperature has stabilized will help prevent hypothermia with inherent metabolic changes (Whaley and Wong, 1991).<br>***Special Considerations:*** *For tips on caring for the neonate in a closed incubator, see the box on p. 342.* |
| 2. Assess for signs and symptoms of respiratory distress, such as nasal flaring, retractions, increased respiratory rate, circumoral cyanosis, and mottling. | Respiratory distress is a contraindication for any of the following procedures. |
| **Planning and Goal Setting** | |
| 1. Gather all necessary supplies for bath, umbilical and circumcision care (if applicable) such as: clean washcloth and towel, mild soap, cotton balls, rubbing alcohol, petroleum jelly, and gauze. Also obtain a clean diaper and appropriate clothing to dress infant after bath. | There is risk of injury to the newborn if attention is diverted to obtain supplies. When supplies are immediately available, care can be more efficient with less risk of chilling the newborn. |
| 2. Plan baths according to the newborn's eating and sleeping patterns. | Bathing the newborn approximately midway between feedings has several benefits: the newborn will probably be more alert and content during the bath, and the feeding will be optimally retained. |
| 3. Provide room temperature of 24° to 25.5° C (75° to 78° F), with 40% to 50% humidity (Wong and Whaley, 1990). Also avoid drafts. | Appropriate warmth, humidity, and avoidance of drafts will prevent cold stress and chilling and promote the newborn's comfort during the bath. |
| 4. Develop individualized child and family goals:<br>▪ Newborn will not develop signs of hypothermia or restlessness.<br>▪ Newborn will remain injury free.<br>▪ Newborn will remain infection free.<br>▪ Newborn's skin will be free of excretions and other substances. | |

## TIPS FOR CARING FOR A NEONATE IN A CLOSED INCUBATOR

1. Maintaining a neutral thermal environment (NTE) is one of the most important reasons for using an incubator, and therefore it is a top care priority. An NTE is an environmental temperature that maintains the neonate's core temperature at a level where oxygen consumption and caloric expenditure are minimal (Merenstein and Gardner, 1989). For specific intervention guidelines to achieve this temperature (e.g., prewarming the incubator), see Skill 83.
2. Organize interventions to avoid excessive handling and provide maximum periods of rest. Caregiving activities such as diapering have been noted to markedly decrease $Pa_{O_2}$ (Hansen, 1982). When the neonate must expend energy to cope with such stimulation, less energy is available for growth and development (Whaley and Wong, 1991).
3. Place the neonate in the prone position to improve oxygenation (Martin et al, 1979; Wagaman et al, 1979).
4. Use the portholes to provide care as much as possible and to minimize heat and oxygen (if receiving) loss.
5. Cloth diapers produce more dust fibers inside an incubator than disposable diapers (Hashimoto, 1987).
6. When monitoring urinary output, consider that superabsorbent diapers have been noted to gain weight in the absence of urine output in warm, high humidity incubators (see Skill 64).
7. Maintain a quiet environment to decrease noise levels inside the incubator. The immature central nervous system of preterm infants can react with apnea or bradycardia to noises such as a tap on the incubator. Loud or prolonged noises can damage the cochlea (Thomas, 1989). Depress latches on portholes when closing them to avoid the loud click; use plastic trash containers rather than metal ones; do not write on top of incubators; and only speak in a soft voice around the incubator (Weibley, 1989).
8. Provide visual stimulation: mobiles, pictures, and other articles may be safely hung within the neonate's field of vision. Visual stimulation can facilitate development (see Skill 15).
9. Promote parent-infant bonding by demonstrating how to touch, caress, hold, and speak softly to the infant. Identifying ways to promote parent-infant bonding can help overcome some of the imposed barriers of the incubator.
10. Emphasize activities the family can do to provide a personal touch such as making or purchasing a special knit cap for the neonate's head.

| Steps | Rationale |
|---|---|

## Implementation 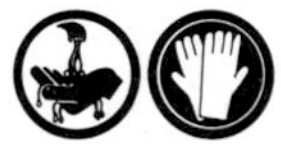

| Steps | Rationale |
|---|---|
| 1. Handle the newborn with clean gloves until after the first bath. | Wearing gloves prevents exposure to possible pathogens received by the newborn in utero or in the birth canal (Task Force, 1988). |
| 2. Maintain measures to prevent injury to newborn. For example, always maintain a secure hold, and avoid rough fingernails or jewelry that might scratch the newborn. Never leave a newborn unattended without the side guards up. | Constant vigilance will protect the newborn from possible falls or injury to the fragile integument. |

### *Bathing*

| Steps | Rationale |
|---|---|
| 1. Position the newborn comfortably in one arm or lying in a radiant warmer or incubator. | Appropriate positioning helps maintain comfort and safety. ***Special Considerations:*** *If a warmer is not available, wrap the newborn in a blanket while washing the hair and face to help maintain body temperature.* |
| 2. Adjust the water temperature by checking with a water thermometer or on outer aspect of own forearm. Water temperature should not be over 100° F. | The newborn's fragile skin can be severely burned by water that is too hot. ***Special Considerations:*** *If the bath is given near a water faucet, avoid bumping the newborn with the faucet handles because scalding injuries can result.* |
| 3. Run water into a clean basin, infant bathtub, or sink to a shallow depth of 3 to 4 inches. Do not place a newborn in the water until cord detachment, which usually occurs in a few weeks. Use the water for sponge bathing and shampooing the hair. | Bath container should be chosen according to convenience, safety, and ability to be cleaned thoroughly before and after each use. ***Special Considerations:*** *Bath time provides an opportunity to observe the newborn's behavior and to provide family teaching about newborn care.* |
| 4. At the beginning of the bath, wipe eyes from the inner to the outer canthus, using clean water and a different area of clean cloth for each wipe. | Wiping the eyes avoids introducing any organisms into the tear duct. The eye is normally sterile. ***Special Considerations:*** *Caution parents that rapidly lowering the newborn's head, sudden movements, or loud noises can cause the Moro reflex.* |

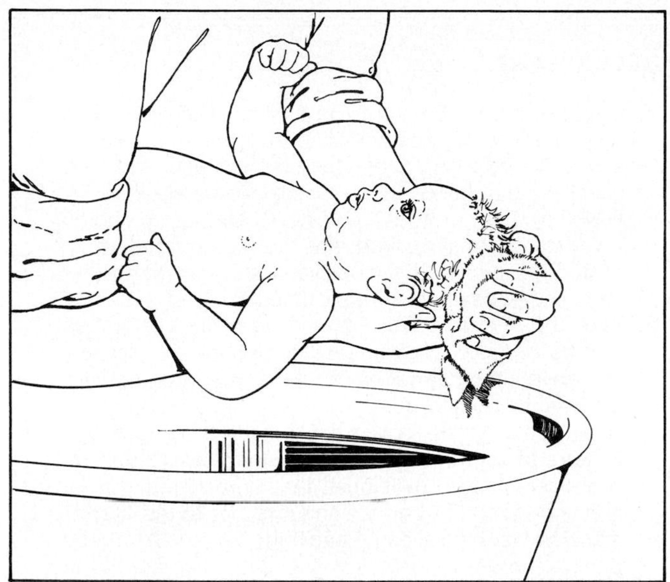

***FIG. 53-1*** Newborn is supported with football hold during shampoo.

| **Steps** | **Rationale** |
|---|---|
| 5. Gently wash face, using plain water (Whaley and Wong, 1991). | Washing the eye area first and then the face, follows the principle of cleansing in the direction from cleanest area to less clean area. Using plain water helps preserve skin's normal pH balance.<br>***Special Considerations:*** *Preserve the newborn's protective acid mantle (pH approximately 4.95 after delivery) by avoiding alkaline soaps, oils, lotions, and powders (Whaley and Wong, 1991). The acid mantle helps retard bacterial growth.* |
| 6. Shampoo hair:<br>a. With newborn in the "football hold," gently wet the hair with water (Fig. 53-1). | The "football hold" safely supports the newborn's body and allows one to carry out the procedure.<br>***Special Considerations:*** *It is not necessary to shampoo the hair with every bath—wiping the newborn's head with a wet cloth is often sufficient to keep the head and hair clean.* |
| b. Shampoo the newborn's hair with a cloth and nonalkaline soap (Whaley and Wong, 1991). | Shampooing removes dried material such as blood and amniotic fluid.<br>***Special Considerations:*** *To avoid "cradle cap" see Child and Family Teaching section.* |
| c. Rinse the hair completely and dry the scalp quickly and thoroughly. | Rapid drying prevents chilling because of heat loss through the head.<br>***Special Considerations:*** *If the newborn is crying, suggest to family that newborns typically do not enjoy baths as much as older infants and toddlers. For tips to calm infant during bath and at other times see the box on p. 344.* |
| 7. Wash external ears: use a clean part of the cloth rolled to a point to clean the external ear. Repeat with a different part of the cloth for the other ear. | Using different areas of a soft cloth prevents cross-contamination and possible injury to outer ear or tympanic membrane.<br>***Special Considerations:*** *Teach family to avoid using cotton-tipped applicators or hair pins to clean middle ear, since the tympanic membrane can be easily punctured. Explain that the ear canal is usually self-cleaning and removing ear wax from the external end of canal with a cloth is the only method needed.* |
| 8. Wash body and extremities:<br>a. After removing the newborn's blanket, wash the neck, chest, arms, legs and back in the same manner. | Bathing follows a cephalocaudal direction.<br>***Special Considerations:*** *Although complete baths are not necessary every day, it is important to keep the face and body skin folds, as well as the diaper area, clean to prevent irritation and preserve skin integrity. Do not attempt to remove the vernix caseosa. It will gradually be absorbed by the skin or will wear off. Excessive rubbing will irritate and traumatize the newborn's skin.* |

## *TIPS TO CALM A FUSSY INFANT*

Infants may fuss or cry for a number of reasons such as hunger, pain, colic, or for tension release. While an effort should always be made to discover a specific cause, the following suggestions may be helpful when a cause cannot be determined and/or remedied. Some suggestions are specific ideas for parents at home, others can also be used by a nurse trying to comfort an infant in the parent's absence.

1. First check to be certain that all the infant's basic needs are met: infant is not hungry (appetite may fluctuate considerably during the day); the diaper is clean and dry; he or she is not too hot or too cold; a pacifier, thumb, or finger is available to suck; and infant has been held and cuddled.
2. Infants respond to rhythm, motion, and soft, soothing sounds: rhythmically pat or rub the infant's back or buttocks; rock slowly and steadily in a rocking chair; with a wide stance, hold the infant, swaying slowly and rhythmically from side to side; bend the knees and rock up and down; carrying the infant, walk at a slow steady pace; talk, hum or sing softly, repeating notes or phrases such as "there, there it's alright." Use these techniques separately or in various combinations. Be patient if the infant does not respond immediately, it may take some time for the pattern to become soothing.
3. A reverse of the traditional horizontal infant hold may be comforting. Place the child face down with the abdomen along the length of the caregiver's forearm, with the head at the bend of the elbow and face turned to the outside. The infant's inside arm is securely tucked to the caregiver's abdomen. Securely hold the outside leg and bottom with the hand of the arm on which the infant is lying. This position frees the caregiver's other arm to perform other tasks or pat the infant's back or bottom (Creative Care Unit, 1982).
4. Newborns may respond to swaddling with a soft blanket (see Skill 51). Minimizing motor activity in this way is helpful for quieting. Another technique is to hold the newborn's hands close to his or her mouth or chest.
5. Place the infant in a wind-up swing. Prop the small infant using rolled blankets or towel. Always remain in attendance to prevent injury should the infant's position change.
6. Place the infant in a front-carrier sling. The close proximity is soothing, and the sling also minimizes motor activity as swaddling does. These devices allow the caregiver two free hands for shopping or household tasks.
7. Play soft music or a recorded heartbeat, or try singing a variety of songs to find one the infant responds to best. Tape record the caregiver's voice or any other sounds that have previously calmed the infant.
8. Take the infant outside for a stroller ride, or just sit outside because fresh air and the change of scenery and environmental noises can be soothing and relieve the infant's boredom.
9. A car ride is widely recognized to calm a crying infant. Be sure to use an appropriate infant restraint system. A device has been developed that simulates the vibration and sound of a car ride and attaches to the infant's crib. The device, called "SleepTight," has shown considerable promise in reducing crying associated with colic (Loadman et al, 1987).
10. A variety of unusual ideas to try include turning a ceiling fan on low in the infant's line of vision, running a vacuum cleaner, and placing restrained infant in an infant seat on top of a running clothes dryer, with the caregiver present and maintaining hand contact the entire time.
11. Some interventions specific to crying associated with colic include placing the infant on the lap over a warm water bottle or heating pad wrapped with a towel (Gillies, 1987). Always check the temperature to prevent burns. Also, using the shoulder carry, securely position the infant up higher so that the pressure of the shoulder on the infant's abdomen helps to expel gas.
12. If these measures are not effective, place the infant in a crib to ensure safety and allow infant to cry. Periodically hold and comfort the child, then return child to the crib if crying continues (Whaley and Wong, 1991). To provide relief and regain composure, take a shower, call a friend, walk around the house, or listen to music with earphones. However, frequently check the infant.

| Steps | Rationale |
|---|---|
| b. Wash each body part with mild soap and water, gently rinse and dry the part before moving to the next body part. | Drying each body part immediately after washing and rinsing prevents chilling the newborn. |
| 9. Clean the genitalia: | |
| a. Female: gently separate labia and carefully wash in posterior direction (front to back). | This helps prevent urinary tract infections (UTI) caused by fecal contamination.<br>***Special Considerations:*** *Stress this principle to the family. Teach/reinforce the rationale for this principle while relating to mother's self-care also.* |
| b. Male: In the uncircumcised newborn, gently retract the foreskin only as far as it will easily go (Whaley and Wong, 1991). Cleanse the tip of the glans in a circular motion with a moistened cotton ball or wash cloth. Replace the foreskin immediately after cleaning. See p. 346 for cleaning the circumcised newborn's glans. | The newborn's foreskin is usually tight and will gradually loosen with time. Forcefully retracting the foreskin can disrupt its normal adhesions. Failure to replace the foreskin can cause damage and painful swelling from a tourniquet effect.<br>***Special Considerations:*** *See the box at right for potential benefits and risks of circumcision for the family seeking this information.* |

## *POTENTIAL BENEFITS AND RISKS OF CIRCUMCISION*

The family considering circumcision for a newborn male needs a clear understanding of potential benefits and risks to make an informed decision. Since 1971 the American Academy of Pediatrics' (AAP) position has been that there are no valid medical indicators for circumcision in the neonatal period. This position was jointly reinforced in 1975 and in 1983 with the American College of Obstetrics and Gynecology. These statements also suggest that a program of good personal hygiene offers all the advantages of circumcision without the attendant surgical risk (Whaley and Wong, 1989).

In 1989 the AAP Task Force on Circumcision issued an update (AAP, 1989) presenting new information, both research and incidence statistics relevant to the issue. The summary of the update states that there are potential medical benefits and advantages, as well as disadvantages and risks, which must be explained to the parents. Many lay persons and professionals have misrepresented or misinterpreted this update as a reversal or endorsement of circumcision (Neifert, 1989; Tedder, 1989). Nurses have a responsibility to be knowledgeable about circumcision to provide accurate, rational information that the family can use in their decision-making process.

### POTENTIAL BENEFITS

Newborn circumcision prevents development of conditions related to foreskin retraction and inflammation of the glans and prepuce that may occur in the young males such as phimosis, paraphimosis, or balanoposthitis. A small percentage of uncircumcised males will require the procedure later for treatment of these conditions. Circumcision may be a more complicated procedure after the neonatal period.

Circumcision may also decrease the risk of UTI (Wiswell and Geschke, 1989), although there has been some question of the methodologic design of retrospective studies that have indicated a high association between uncircumcised males and UTI (AAP, 1989). Cancer of the penis, with an overall annual incidence of 0.7 to 0.9 per 100,000 men, occurs almost exclusively in uncircumcised men. However, adequate hygiene practices can play a significant role in prevention of penile cancer. Uncircumcised males must commit to a lifelong practice of good genital hygiene (AAP, 1989).

Some evidence exists regarding the relationship of circumcision to sexually transmitted diseases and cervical cancer; however, it is inconclusive and development of these diseases is known to be related to other factors as well.

### POTENTIAL RISKS

The most common complications of the procedure are hemorrhage and infection, with an approximate 0.2% to 0.6% incidence; attributable deaths are extremely rare (AAP, 1989). Other cited complications include dehiscence (separation of approximated skin edges), meatitis from the loss of protective foreskin, adhesions, urethral fistula, and meatal stenosis (Whaley and Wong, 1989). Poor surgical technique can result in dissatisfaction with the appearance of the penis after healing (Neifert, 1989).

A serious concern, often uppermost in the family's mind, is the pain associated with unanesthetized circumcision. Observed behavioral, cardiovascular, and hormonal responses associated with the procedure, lasting several hours, include a distress cry during the circumcision, activity changes such as irritability, altered sleep patterns, and an affected maternal-infant interaction pattern. Local anesthetic, especially dorsal penile nerve block, is being used with success. As with any local anesthetic, some risks exist, including hematoma, local skin necrosis, and systemic absorption of lidocaine. At present, the AAP does not endorse the penile nerve block pending greater numbers of reported experiences (AAP, 1989). Other anesthetic or analgesic options can be considered.

### ADDITIONAL CONSIDERATIONS

The social and cultural factors regarding circumcision are often at least as important as the medical ones to the family making a decision. For some cultures it simply is or is not accepted practice. In others, where either option is acceptable, the decision is more complex. Thought must be given to the inevitable comparison with other male family members such as fathers and brothers, as well as body image concerns with peer groups. The current circumcision rate for newborn American males is 60% (Neifert, 1989). This rate ensures a healthy mix of both circumcised and uncircumcised males in the coming years, whatever the family's ultimate decision.

| Steps | Rationale |
| --- | --- |
| 10. Wash and thoroughly dry perianal area after rinsing. | Leaving moist areas, especially enclosed areas, can foster microorganism growth and disrupt skin integrity. |
| 11. Avoid using powders, oils, or lotions on newborn's skin. | These alter the skin's normal protective pH balance and thereby encourage growth of microorganisms.<br>***Special Considerations:*** *Avoid using talcum powder since inhalation of talc can dry mucous membranes of the middle airways and interfere with cilia action. Its use has been reported in connection with several infant deaths (Wagner and Hindi-Alexander, 1984).* |
| 12. Liberally apply alcohol to the base of the umbilical cord stump using a cotton-tipped applicator. Lift the cord if necessary to clean adequately. | ***Special Considerations:*** *See Child and Family Teaching, Step 2.* |

| Steps | Rationale |
|---|---|
| 13. Apply diaper, folding the front below the cord so that the cord is exposed. | Leaving the cord exposed to air avoids irritation from urine and moisture against the cord stump.<br>***Special Considerations:*** *Family may be instructed that disposable diapers can have the upper front folded toward the caregiver (below the cord) to keep the area dry. Folding the disposable diaper in this way keeps the plastic away from the infant's skin, which may prevent sensitivity reactions and increased heat retention.* |
| 14. Dress the newborn in clothes appropriate to environmental conditions (see also box on Hints on Dressing Infants on p. 357). | Infants normally require approximately the same weight of clothes as adults in the same environment. |
| ***Circumcision Care*** | |
| 1. Provide care based on the type of circumcision method used. | Two basic methods of performing circumcision use Plastibell or Gomco clamp. The method used determines the type of care given afterward. |
| a. Hollister Plastibell: No dressing is applied to penis. Urine may be wiped with water and cloth, if needed; stool may be gently cleansed away from the penis. | This device helps prevent the diaper from adhering to the circumcision line. The yellowish-white exudate that forms is part of the healing process. The plastic ring will detach itself in a few days or weeks. It should not be removed by the family. |
| b. Gomco clamp: Apply petrolatum gauze loosely around circumcision site. Reapply gauze when soiled or as prescribed. | Gauze liberally spread with petrolatum helps prevent the diaper from adhering to circumcision line. |
| 2. Frequently assess the glans penis for bleeding, swelling, or foul odor. | Two potential complications of circumcision are excessive bleeding and infection. |

| Evaluation Outcomes | Observational Guidelines |
|---|---|
| 1. Newborn does not demonstrate signs of hypothermia. | Note signs of hypothermia such as mottling, increased respiratory rate and restlessness. Monitor body temperature. |
| 2. Newborn does not sustain injury during bath. | Note absence of falls or skin injury. |
| 3. Infection of the umbilical stump and circumcision line (if applicable) is prevented or minimized. | Note absence of purulent drainage, foul odor, redness, or swelling from the stump or circumcision line. |
| 4. Newborn's skin remains intact. | Inspect the skin for breaks in integrity. |
| 5. Newborn's skin is free of excretions and other substances. | The skin is clean, dry, free of odor, or stool. |

## Documentation

For the initial performance of the above procedures, record the time of the procedure, medications administered, dressings applied (Gomco clamp procedure), and newborn's reactions. Also note whether there were signs or symptoms of hypothermia or respiratory distress. If assessment shows any of these, thoroughly document the appearance of the newborn and other pertinent data.

## Child and Family Teaching

1. When washing eyes, wipe from the inner to the outer canthus.
2. The family may be instructed to apply rubbing alcohol to the cord after the newborn is discharged. Instruct in frequency of application, method of application (clean base of the cord thoroughly), signs and symptoms to watch for, such as those of infection or delayed cord detachment, and safety factors, such as keeping the cord dry, folding the diaper below the cord, and keeping the alcohol out of reach of other children.
3. Teach the family to wipe female newborn's genitalia from front to back. Remind them to teach this principle to the child as she is being toilet trained.

| Steps | Rationale |
|---|---|
| 4. The family of male newborns should be instructed to remove smegma from the infant's glans. In uncircumcised males, after the foreskin has naturally released and retraction is possible, the foreskin should be retracted for cleaning. The foreskin should then be replaced to avoid tissue damage from swelling. Teach this procedure to the child to incorporate into daily hygiene routine when he is cognitively able to learn it (see Skill 55). | |
| 5. Teach the family to avoid cradle cap by gently scrubbing the infant's scalp after shampooing with a fine-toothed comb or soft-bristled brush. | |
| 6. Reinforce checking the water temperature before bathing the infant. | |
| 7. Teach the family to avoid using soap on the infant's face. | |
| 8. Teach and demonstrate to the family that bath time is an ideal time to play and interact with the infant. | |
| 9. Instruct the caregiver that a towel may be placed in baby bath tubs to prevent the infant from slipping. | |
| 10. Clarify with the family that sponge baths (such as described in this skill) are given until the umbilical cord falls off. After that time, the infant can be placed in the water. Caution parents to fill the bathing container or sink only a few inches. | |
| 11. Reinforce avoidance of baby powder, which poses an aspiration hazard. | |

### Home Care Modifications

1. Encourage the family to problem solve to find a convenient location for bathing and related care that is free from drafts. Also avoid rugs that might cause slipping. The family should develop a habit of not answering the phone or door or make other arrangements during the infant's bath. Infants and young children should never be left alone around water.

# *SKILL* 54 Diapering and Skin Care

*Krena Hunter White*

One of the most frequently occurring skin problems in the infant is diaper dermatitis. Since diaper dermatitis is a common cause of infant discomfort and concern to families and nurses, skills such as diapering and skin care are important for the health of infants.

### NURSING DIAGNOSES

Potential for impaired skin integrity related to exposure to urine and fecal excretions, chemical irritation from soap, or occlusive diapers.

| Steps | Rationale |
|---|---|

## Assessment

1. Assess entire skin including diaper area, especially noting presence of reddened areas, rash, excoriation, pustules. Note characteristics such as color, size, shape, description of borders, and location of any abnormal skin areas.

   Assessment of the skin determines the most appropriate skin care. Healthy, intact skin is the body's first line of defense against infection. Description is a key factor in diagnosis of the skin problem. Diaper dermatitis may be seen mostly on convex surfaces or also in diaper area body folds. Chemical irritants usually result in dermatitis on convex areas (Whaley and Wong, 1991). Candidal infection produces perianal inflammation with sharply defined erythematous satellite lesions (Rasmussen, 1987; Whaley and Wong, 1991). Numerous other skin problems can occur in the diaper area.

   ***Special Considerations:*** *The peak age of diaper dermatitis is 9 to 12 months and occurs more frequently in formula-fed rather than breast-fed infants (Benjamin, 1987).*

2. Assess pattern and type of stools and frequency of urination.

   Some primary factors involved in the development of diaper dermatitis are wetness, increased pH on the skin, and the presence of fecal enzymes. Diarrheal stools are a strong irritant to the skin (Whaley and Wong, 1991). A positive relationship between incidence of diarrhea and diaper dermatitis has been documented (Benjamin, 1987).

3. Determine whether the infant is receiving antibiotic therapy.

   Studies also link oral antibiotic use and incidence of diaper dermatitis (Campbell, 1988).

## Planning and Goal Setting

1. Gather supplies needed for diapering and skin care. If possible, keep the supplies together in a convenient location. The supplies may include clean washcloths, mild soap, towels, diapers (cloth, disposable, or a combination), diaper pins for cloth diapers, and topical medication (if needed).

   Easy access to supplies will allow care to proceed more efficiently.

   ***Special Considerations:*** *It may be helpful to obtain a few appropriate toys for diversion or play purposes.*

2. Plan to change diaper and provide perineal skin care as soon as infant urinates or defecates.

   Immediate diaper changing controls the variables that are associated with diaper dermatitis such as wetness, pH, and presence of fecal enzymes (Whaley and Wong, 1991).

3. Develop individual child and family goals:
   - Skin in infant's diaper area will remain clean, dry, and intact without signs of inflammation or infection.

## Implementation

1. Clean urine from the perineal area by wiping with clean, warm water and washcloth.

   Plain water is usually sufficient to clean urine from the skin. Soap can be drying to the skin, possibly contributing to the skin's susceptibility to cracking.

   ***Special Considerations:*** *Ingredients in disposable wet towel products may lead to sensitivity in some infants (Whaley and Wong, 1991). Especially avoid use on already compromised skin.*

   a. Wipe female infant's genitalia gently in anterior to posterior direction (front to back), using a different part of washcloth for each stroke.

   Wiping in the front-to-back direction assists in preventing urinary tract infections by avoiding the introduction of fecal microorganisms into the urethra.

   b. Gently retract penile foreskin of uncircumcised male infant and cleanse in circular strokes starting at the urinary meatus and wiping toward body. Replace foreskin in original position.

   Wiping in this manner helps decrease the introduction of microorganisms into the urethra and also removes smegma.

   ***Special Considerations:*** *In the newborn, gently retract the foreskin only as far as it is easily retractable. Remember to replace foreskin, since swelling may occur, which could cause discomfort and interfere with circulation.*

2. Clean skin after defecation:

   a. Using a mild, less alkaline soap (e.g., Lowila, Aveeno, Basis, Neutrogena, Purpose or Oilatum brands) is preferable to using other, more alkaline soaps (Kuller, Lund, and Tobin, 1983).

   Factors associated with diaper dermatitis are increased skin hydration, occlusion, and fecal enzymes, especially when combined with urine, which results in increased pH as ammonia is produced (Campbell, 1987).

   ***Special Considerations:*** *Alkaline base soaps have been reported to increase the skin pH, inhibiting the natural bacteriocidal properties of skin (Kuller, Lund, and Tobin, 1983).*

| Steps | Rationale |
|---|---|
| b. Rinse area thoroughly with clean water. May use plastic squeeze bottle or bathe infant to cleanse gently and thoroughly. | Complete rinsing protects skin from chemical irritation associated with soap usage. |
| c. Always towel dry skin gently and thoroughly after cleaning diaper area, paying close attention to skin folds. Also, expose the skin to the air for short periods of time or during naps to achieve complete dryness before rediapering. A blow dryer used on a *cool* setting may help ensure dryness. | Complete drying prevents moisture in the diaper environment, which contributes to skin breakdown. **_Special Considerations:_** *Some disposable diapers contain nontoxic absorbent gelling materials (AGM) within their absorbent core that are composed of cross-linked sodium polyacrylate (Austin et al, 1988). AGMs (found in Ultra-Pampers disposable diapers, Proctor & Gamble, Cincinnati, Ohio) are helpful in preventing diaper dermatitis by absorbing water, buffering the skin pH, and helping prevent contact between urine and fecal material (Campbell, 1987). Studies have shown significantly less diaper dermatitis in infants wearing diapers with AGM under diarrheal conditions (Campbell, 1988) and when compared with other disposable diapers and cloth diapers (Campbell, 1987). Small quantities of AGM may transfer through the diaper material to the skin, where it may appear as a film or tiny beads, possibly giving the incorrect appearance of crystalluria (Davis, McKemis, and McEnery, 1988).* |
| 3. Do not apply baby powder to the infant's skin. | Accidental deaths from inhalation of talcum powder clouds puffed into the air have been documented (Wagner and Hindi-Alexander, 1984; Cotton and Davidson, 1985). |
| 4. If the infant has been diagnosed as having a candidal infection, apply anticandidal medication such as nystatin, topically (or orally) as prescribed. | |
| 5. Avoid use of hydrocortisone preparations unless specifically prescribed. | Hydrocortisone can suppress inflammation, while fungal infections continue to grow. Hydrocortisone can alter the appearance of fungal infections (causing increased redness) and other skin problems. Its use can make diagnosis of the problem more difficult (Tomovitch, 1981). **_Special Considerations:_** *In addition to considering potential side effects of oral medications, do not apply topical soaps, creams, lotions, or other products without evaluating the potential for systemic absorption of the product through inflamed skin. Also, it is important to be aware of the potency of topical steroids used in occluded, sensitive diaper area. Avoid use of products such as Lotrisone (combination clotrimazole and betamethasone diproprionate, a moderately high potency topical steroid) in children (see box on p. 509 in Skill 80).* |
| 6. A thin layer of zinc oxide may be applied to completely dry skin. | Based on the physiologic components involved in the diaper dermatitis cycle, occlusive ointments such as zinc oxide may create a barrier to protect the skin. If applied to slightly moist skin, however, the moisture is sealed in, contributing to skin breakdown. |
| 7. Place diaper on infant: | |
| a. In newborns, fold diapers below the umbilical stump until cord site has healed. | Contact with a wet diaper keeps the umbilical stump moist, which delays the healing process and encourages development of infection. |
| b. Fasten diapers loosely enough to allow full respiratory movement. | Infants are abdominal breathers. Tightly fastened diapers may prevent adequate inspiratory effort and add to occlusive effect. |
| c. Disposable diapers: | |
| ▪ After placing diaper under infant's buttocks with tabs on the back edge of diaper, expose sticky surface of tabs and fasten to diaper front, angling tabs slightly downward. | This method provides a secure fit. |
| ▪ When removing disposable diapers, fold tabs so they adhere to the diaper. | Loose tabs may adhere to the infant's skin during diaper removal, possibly causing discomfort or skin irritation. |
| d. Cloth diapers: | |
| ▪ Fold diaper as needed (Fig. 54-1). | This step helps ensure a neat, effective diaper fit. |
| ▪ Lap the back corner over the front corner on each side, keeping fingers between infant's body and diaper when pinning. | Lapping in this direction allows increased range of motion as infant flexes the hip. Protecting infant's skin with own fingers prevents accidental skin pricks. **_Special Considerations:_** *Keep pins closed and out of infant's or sibling's reach. Open pins can prick the skin or may be swallowed by infants and children.* |

| Steps | Rationale |
|---|---|

A

B

C

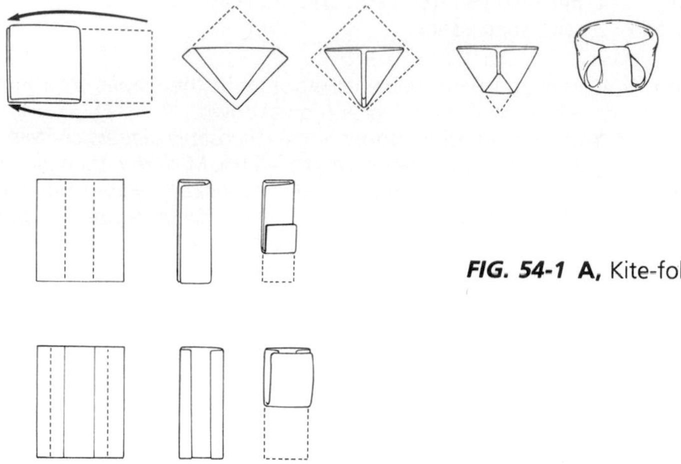

*FIG. 54-1* **A,** Kite-folded diaper. **B,** Rectangular folded diaper. **C,** Prefolded diaper.

| Steps | Rationale |
|---|---|
| ▪ Insert pins facing the infant's back. Fasten pins securely, making sure they are latched. | Facing the pin toward the back avoids possible abdominal puncture injury if the pin opens. Secure fastening helps prevent accidental opening. |
| ▪ Avoid plastic pants. May use double diapers, if desired, to increase absorbency. | Plastic coverings prevent evaporation of moisture. Increased moisture is one factor associated with diaper dermatitis. |

## Evaluation Outcomes

1. Infant's skin is clean and dry with no area of redness or other skin problem.

## Observational Guidelines

Observe infant's perineal area during diaper changes to determine the condition of the skin. Note frequency of diaper changes.

## Documentation

Record appearance of healthy skin. If redness, pustules, or other unusual skin manifestations are present, record location and description. For example, note whether the redness has a pinprick appearance or whether it has a solid red configuration, approximate shade of redness (pink to scarlet), and other precise descriptive assessment to aid in diagnosis and to provide baseline data.

## Child and Family Teaching

1. Explain the hazards associated with use of baby powder related to its action as a pulmonary irritant. If the family still wants to use a powder, cornstarch is recommended as an absorbent. Cornstarch is not associated with pulmonary complications, is somewhat more effective in reducing friction, tends to cake less on wet skin than talc, and does not support fungal growth under normal diaper conditions (Leyden, 1984). Its use, however, is still not recommended by some clinicians. Demonstrate how to use it safely by placing it in the caregiver's hand and rubbing it on the infant's skin, rather than shaking it in the air. Include other appropriate information such as avoiding caking of cornstarch in the skin folds.
2. Numerous skin problems may develop in the diaper area. If the skin care measures recommended in this skill do not result in improvement, consult a health care professional for advice.

## Home Care Modifications

1. The family may want to investigate various possibilities related to diaper type. Disposable diaper cost should be balanced with other factors such as expense of water, laundry products, and access to washer/dryer. Factors such as availability of laundering time should also be considered, as well as diaper service expenses.
2. Home laundering of cloth diapers should include soaking in a quaternary ammonium compound (e.g., Diaperene) or diluted bleach in hot water (Whaley and Wong, 1991). They should be washed in hot water with simple laundry soap and then rinsed twice to decrease the possibility of sensitivity to laundry product residue.

# *SKILL* 55 Assisting With or Bathing a Child

*Kelly Lannon Henderson*

Bathing an infant, child, or adolescent promotes cleanliness, stimulates circulation to the skin, provides exercise through joint range of motion, and may also help the child to relax and become more comfortable. There are two major types of baths that a nurse may provide: cleansing or therapeutic. Although traditionally the cleansing bath is given early in the morning before procedures and tests are started, the nurse should adapt the bathing procedure to the child's normal routine at home as much as possible. The therapeutic bath is ordered by the physician as an adjunct to various skin therapies. The type of cleansing bath selected will depend on the child's physical capabilities and the degree of hygiene that is required. It is the responsibility of the nurse to assess and determine the type of bath most appropriate for the child's needs to ensure safety.

## NURSING DIAGNOSES

Self-care deficit, bathing and hygiene related to age or to physical constraints; Potential for impaired skin integrity related to body secretions or physical immobilization; Altered health maintenance related to lack of knowledge about infant/child hygiene needs; Activity intolerance related to client's generalized weakness or immobility.

| Steps | Rationale |
| --- | --- |
| **Assessment** | |
| 1. Determine the child's age and developmental level. | Age and developmental level help determine the child's ability to perform self-care and the amount of assistance that will be needed. |
| 2. Assess child's activity tolerance, musculoskeletal function, and level of pain/discomfort. | Self-care can be therapeutic to the child, therefore the child should be encouraged to do as much as possible. However, the child should not be allowed to become fatigued, uncomfortable, frustrated, or aggravated in an attempt to bathe. |
| 3. Assess other conditions influencing type of bath given, e.g., recent surgical incision, casts, immobilizing traction, IV, NG tube, foley catheter, central IV line. | Assessment of these factors will also help to determine the type of bath and amount of assistance needed. |
| 4. Check the physician's orders for any instructions concerning the child's activity, movement, or positioning. Some examples of positioning restrictions might be spinal surgery, hip disorder, injuries or surgery to lower extremities, or externalized ventriculoperitoneal shunts. | Knowledge of activity, positioning, or movement restrictions will help to prevent an accidental injury or any unnecessary discomfort during the bath and help determine the level of assistance required for the bath. |
| 5. Assess risk for skin impairment such as: | Certain conditions will increase the chances for injury to the skin or for skin breakdown, therefore requiring more thorough hygiene. Although less common in children, they can occur. Dependent body parts exposed to underlying surfaces have an increased chance for pressure sores or skin breakdown. |
| a. Immobility, e.g., paralysis, large casts, traction, restriction to specific positions because of injury or disease, or inability to change positions. | |
| b. Decreased sensation, e.g., paralysis, circulatory insufficiency, or local nerve damage. | A decreased ability to sense ischemia or injury to the skin's surface can lead to skin breakdown. |
| c. Alterations in nutrition, e.g., protein loss or vitamin deficiency from poor intake, fever, burns, surgery, or draining wounds. | Limited protein intake or excessive protein loss can lead to impaired tissue synthesis. |
| d. Excessive secretions or excretion on the skin, especially on intertriginous areas such as under breasts, in the perineal area, and in skin folds. | Increased moisture on the skin's surface creates a medium for bacterial growth and also promotes softening of the epithelial cells. ***Special Considerations:*** *A child with a tracheostomy, excessive drooling, wound drainage, obesity skin folds, and who is non-toilet trained or incontinent is especially prone to moisture problems in intertriginous areas.* |

| Steps | Rationale |
|---|---|
| e. Insufficient vascular status such as with diabetes mellitus and peripheral vascular disease. | Poor peripheral perfusion may lead to ischemia and breakdown of the skin. |
| f. External devices applied to or around the skin, e.g., casts, bandages, dressings, tape, cloth restraints, identification bracelets, and urinary or drainage collection device tubing. | Many of the external devices used may cause friction, allow moisture to collect, or exert pressure on the skin's surface. |
| 6. Question the child/family regarding any existing skin conditions or problems such as lesions, dryness, or itching. If present, ask what treatment they have used and the effectiveness. | The family's responses provide direction to further assessment of skin during bath and can pinpoint misconceptions. **Special Considerations:** *Although a brief skin assessment is necessary to help determine the type of bath needed and products to select, a more thorough skin assessment can be done during the bath if preferred to save time and episodes of exposure.* |
| 7. Assess the child (or family's) bathing preferences such as time of day or assistance from family or staff person. | Determining the child/family preferences and planning collaboratively enhances cooperation and provides decision-making control. **Special Considerations:** *Children and adolescents often prefer to have a family member assist them with their bath instead of a staff member.* |
| 8. Determine whether child is allergic to any soaps, lotion, or other cleansing agents. | This information guides bath product selection. |
| 9. In infants and young children assess the parents' knowledge about bathing and skin characteristics. In older children/adolescents assess the child's knowledge. | An assessment of child/family knowledge indicates areas for teaching during the bath. **Special Considerations:** *Observing the family member performing the bath or involving them or the older child in the procedure is an ideal time to assess this information, as well as to engage in patient/family teaching.* |

## Planning and Goal Setting

| Steps | Rationale |
|---|---|
| 1. Determine the type of bath if not specifically ordered and level of assistance needed for this child. | Making a decision based on assessment information allows the safest and most beneficial bath possible for the current situation. |
| 2. Collect and prepare the equipment needed for the bathing procedure. | |
| a. Bed bath. | |
| ▪ Washbasin | **Special Considerations:** *A wash basin or a portable infant bath may be used to bathe infants at the bedside, if emersion is possible (Fig. 55-1).* |

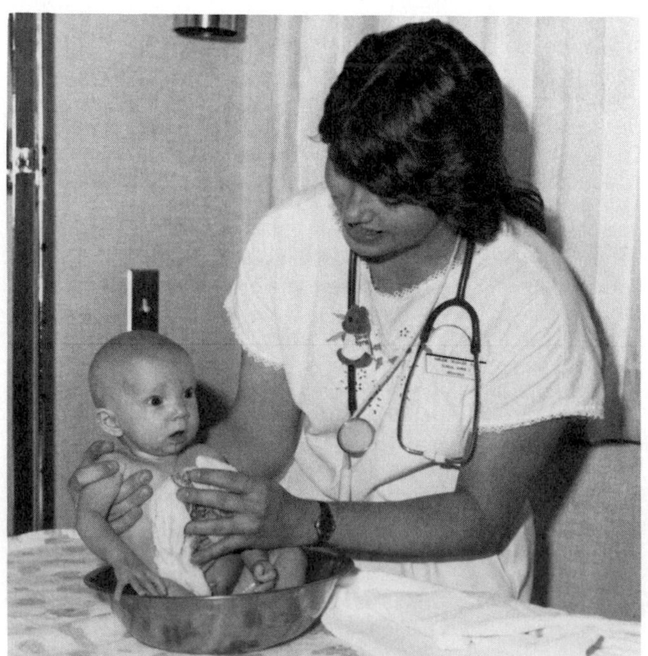

***FIG. 55-1*** Infant is slowly immersed, with proper support, into wash basin.

| **Steps** | **Rationale** |
|---|---|
| ▪ Mild soap, e.g., Dove, Ivory, Baby Magic. | Harsh soaps may irritate the skin. ***Special Considerations:*** *An antibacterial soap, e.g., Dial or Safeguard, provides some protection against gram-positive bacteria if used over several days. However, they are more drying to the skin because they remove the protective layer of sebum. If dry skin is a problem, use a superfatted soap such as Dove, Tone, or Basis, which removes less lipid from the stratum corneum.* |
| ▪ Two bath towels and two washcloths. | To enhance a feeling of cleanliness a separate washcloth and towel are used to clean the child's body and face. |
| ▪ Bath blanket. | This will help to maintain the child's body temperature during the bathing procedure. In infants or small children a bath towel may also be used. |
| ▪ Clean gown/pajamas, underwear, diaper, or other clean garments as appropriate. | |
| ▪ Optional supplies: cotton balls, lotion, deodorant for older children/adolescents, and gloves. | Cotton balls may be used to clean infants' eyes or in older girls may be used to remove make-up. Lotion may be used to help soothe dry skin and to provide a comforting tactile stimulation. Some lotions applied to the skin after bathing while the skin is still moist help increase the water-holding ability of the stratum corneum by retarding evaporation of water. ***Special Considerations:*** *Gloves do not need to be worn when bathing patients with intact skin; however, if there is an open lesion or when cleaning the genital or rectal areas, gloves may be preferred. Also, if the person assisting with the bath has any cuts or skin dermatitis, gloves should be worn (Jackson et al, 1987).* |
| b. Tub bath or shower. | |
| ▪ Disinfected tub or shower with the following safety features: rubber mat or nonslip strips, safety rail or bar, and nurse call signal. | The safety features will help to prevent accidental falls. Having the nurse call signal within reach allows the child to call for assistance if needed. ***Special Considerations:*** *Chairs/seats are also available to be used in the shower or bathtub for a child who is unable to stand or sit safely without assistance. When children share a bathtub, it should be cleansed with an antiseptic solution after each bath. An abrasive cleaning agent should also be used to help eliminate the microorganisms that survive the use of a disinfectant agent.* |
| ▪ Towels and wash cloths.<br>▪ Mild soap (see above). | |
| ▪ Bath mat or towel. | To prevent slipping on wet tile surfaces after a bath or shower, a mat or towel should be placed on the floor. |
| ▪ Clean garments—appropriate for the child's age.<br>▪ Optional supplies: lotion and deodorant (see above). | |
| 3. Adjust room temperature to a comfortable setting; control the ventilation in the room if possible by closing any doors and windows. | During the bathing procedure, the body can rapidly lose heat, especially in young children. |
| 4. Provide privacy for a bed bath by drawing the divider curtain and/or closing the door. | Providing privacy will make the older child more comfortable. Children and adolescents often feel shy and modest about a staff member bathing them. |
| 5. Develop individualized goals of nursing care:<br>▪ To maintain skin integrity.<br>▪ To maintain safety and comfort during bathing.<br>▪ To encourage activity, range of motion, and self-care as appropriate.<br>▪ To provide teaching of adequate hygiene measures to child and family. | |

## Implementation 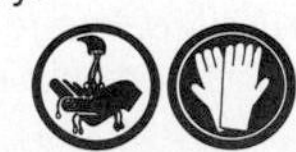

| | |
|---|---|
| 1. Prepare the child for the procedure appropriate to age. Explain the bathing procedure to the child/family. If a partial bed bath will be done, ask the child what part of the bath he or she would like to do. | This will encourage the child/family's participation, cooperation, and give them some control. It also lets the child/family know their role in the bathing procedure. Anxiety is decreased when individuals know what to expect. ***Special Considerations:*** *Although a younger child may need some direction, encourage child to assist with the bath and praise his or her efforts.* |

| Steps | Rationale |
| --- | --- |
| 2. Bathing in bed. | |
| a. Prepare wash basin with warm water. The water temperature should be 38° to 40.5° C (100° to 105° F) for infants and between 43° to 46° C (110° to 115° F) for older children. Test the water temperature by placing a couple of drops of the water on the inside surface of own forearm; it should feel comfortably warm. Ask the older child to test to see if it is comfortable for them. | Testing the temperature of the water prevents accidental burns to the child's skin. Infants cannot tolerate as warm a water temperature as an older child/adolescent. Warm water helps promote comfort for the child and also helps prevent chilling. Asking the older child to test the water promotes control and independence and allows for individual preferences. |
| b. Avoid adding liquid soap or leaving the bar of soap in the washbasin. | It is important to rinse all soap off the skin. If soap is added to the water or if the bar of soap is left in the water, then the water cannot be used for rinsing. ***Special Considerations:*** *All soaps, including liquid baby bath soaps, must be rinsed off the skin with fresh water.* |
| c. Lower side rail of bed and help child assume a comfortable position, close to the side of the bed from which the bath will be given. | This allows easier access to the child for bathing. Positioning the child to the side of the bed will alleviate having to reach across the bed. ***Special Considerations:*** *If demonstrating and teaching parents how to bathe an infant/small child, instruct them to arrange all equipment within close reach. Stress that the infant/small child should never be left unattended during a bath.* |
| d. Loosen the top covers at the foot of the bed. Place a bath blanket over the top sheet and then pull the top sheet from underneath the blanket. For the older child, ask them to hold the bath blanket while removing the top sheet. | Removing the top linens from the bed prevents them from becoming soiled or wet during the procedure if they are to be reused. The bath blanket will help provide warmth, prevent chilling, and also provide some privacy. |
| e. Raise the bed to a higher, more comfortable working position. | This will help minimize strain to the back muscles during this procedure. ***Special Considerations:*** *Traction, monitoring equipment, etc., may contraindicate a high bed position.* |
| f. Remove gown or other clothing except for diaper/underwear, keeping covered with a towel or bath blanket. | Use of a towel or bath blanket provides full exposure of the body parts for the bath while still preventing chilling. A diaper is handy should the child void before washing the perineum, and underwear preserves the child's modesty. |
| g. If an extremity is injured, has decreased mobility, or an IV, begin removing the clothing from the unaffected side. For IV tubing, unhook the fluid bag and slide the gown over the tubing and bag. Replace the IV bag back on the hook and check flow rate. | Undressing the unaffected side first will allow for easier removal of the clothing over the body part with decreased range of motion. ***Special Considerations:*** *Some agencies will have gowns with snaps on the sleeves for easier removal. Disconnecting the IV tubing when removing or putting on the gown increases the risk of introducing air or microorganisms.* |
| h. Wash each eye gently with plain water using a separate cotton ball or clean portion of the washcloth. Clean from the inner to the outer canthus. If there are any crustations on the eyelids, apply moistened cotton ball, gauze, or warm washcloth 1 to 2 minutes before cleaning. Ask the older child to close their eyes for cleaning. | This method of cleaning prevents microorganisms from entering the tear duct. Softening crustations allows for easy removal and prevents trauma to the eye. |
| i. Using no soap or a minimal amount, wash the forehead, cheeks, nose, neck, and ears. Rinse and dry well. Ask the older child if they wish to use soap. | Since the face is exposed to air more than the other body parts, soap has a tendency to dry the face more quickly. ***Special Considerations:*** *Adolescents generally have more active sebaceous glands, predisposing them to acne, and they may have a special soap or topical medication to apply to the face after it has been cleansed.* |
| j. With infants/small children, twist the end of a washcloth or roll a dampened cotton ball to clean the nares and ears. | Using this method will avoid causing any trauma to the mucous membranes and/or the internal ear structures. ***Special Considerations:*** *A cotton-tipped swab should never be used when cleaning an infant/small child's nose or ears. Sudden movements could potentially damage the eardrum or nasal mucosa. Also cotton swabs may embed ear wax.* |
| k. Pay special attention to the areas behind the ears and around the neck in infants. | The head and neck may become soiled with food or formula during feedings. Secretions may collect and irritate the skin. |
| l. With infants/small children, cleanse the hair and scalp with a washcloth. | |

| Steps | Rationale |
|---|---|
| m. Uncover child's far arm. Wash the arm with soap and water using strokes from the fingers to the axilla (distal to proximal). Raise and support arm over the child's head (if possible), then wash the axilla. Rinse and dry arm and axilla completely. | Bathing child's far side first prevents reaching over the clean area. Circulation is stimulated by washing with long, firm strokes. Moving arm over the child's head exposes the axilla and also exercises the joint using normal range of motion exercises. The skin needs to be thoroughly dried because moisture can cause breakdown and softening of the skin.<br>***Special Considerations:*** *If preferred to minimize back strain, move to the other side to wash the child's arm.* |
| n. If fingernails/cuticles are dirty, soak hand in basin for 3 to 5 minutes before washing hand and fingernails, or use a nail brush/nail stick. Dry hand well, especially between fingers. | Soaking hand helps soften cuticles and calluses of the hand and loosens any debris underneath nails.<br>***Special Considerations:*** *Trim or file the nails if indicated, e.g., ragged edges, or the child has a pruritic condition. Infants have soft thin nails that are best trimmed with thin-bladed nail or embroidery scissors. There is a risk of cutting the infant's fingertips with nail clippers.* |
| o. Repeat the last two steps to other arm. Apply deodorant or talcum powder to axilla, if child uses it. | ***Special Considerations:*** *The sebaceous glands become more active during puberty, prompting the use of antiperspirants and deodorants. More frequent bathing may also be needed to control body odors.* |
| p. For infants/small children, quickly and gently wash arms, axilla, the chest, abdomen, and back. Rinse, then dry thoroughly. Dress child in a clean shirt. | Infants/small children's skin is very sensitive therefore minimal friction should be used during the bath. It is difficult to keep infants covered during this time because they are usually active. Applying a clean shirt will help prevent chilling and make them more comfortable. |
| q. Check the temperature of the bath water and change if needed. | Fresh water may be needed to maintain proper temperature. |
| r. For older child/adolescents fold bath blanket down to umbilicus and cover chest with bath towel. With moistened wash cloth, clean chest using long firm strokes. Wash skinfolds under female adolescent's breasts, if indicated. Continue to keep child's chest covered as much as possible between washing and rinsing. Dry well.<br>Next, with one hand lift the bath towel and with the other bathe abdomen with moistened washcloth. Pay special attention to washing the umbilicus and any abdominal folds. Wash from side to side using firm strokes. Keep the abdominal/chest area covered between washing and rinsing. Dry well. | Keeping the area covered prevents chilling and promotes privacy and comfort. Moisture and sediment/dirt may collect in the skinfolds and may lead to skin irritations and/or breakdown of the skin.<br>***Special Considerations:*** *This is a time to observe the condition of the skin on the chest and abdomen for any rashes or breakdown. Inspect the skin between skinfolds, especially in the obese child.* |
| s. For infants use plain water or small amount of soap to wash their legs and feet. Dry thoroughly, especially between toes and skin folds. | The lower extremities in infants not yet crawling are less soiled than in mobile older children. |
| With older children/adolescents fold the bath blanket towards the midline to expose the far leg keeping the perineal area covered. Place a towel under the leg. With the child's leg bent at the knee, position foot flat on bed, or have the child do this. | A towel placed underneath the leg prevents soiling the bed linens or getting them wet.<br>***Special Considerations:*** *While bathing the lower extremities assess the skin carefully for dryness, cracks, and lesions. When positioning the child's leg, help support the knee joint and extremity while lifting to prevent strain.* |
| Using long, firm strokes, wash from the ankle to the knee to the thigh. Rinse and dry well. Clean the foot, washing carefully between the toes and rinse, then dry well. Repeat same procedure for other leg and foot. Apply lotion if indicated. | Cleaning the leg with long strokes promotes venous return.<br>Secretions and moisture may collect between the toes.<br>***Special Considerations:*** *Assess the condition of the feet for any skin irritation, breakdown, or sores, especially in a diabetic child. If no open sores or skin breakdown is noted, lotion may be applied to dry skin to retain moisture and soften skin.* |
| t. Check temperature of water and change if cooling off, or if soapy or soiled. | Clean water will help decrease transmission of microorganisms and allow adequate rinsing of soap.<br>***Special Considerations:*** *More water changes are generally needed when bathing an older child/adolescent than with the infants and smaller children.* |
| u. For older children/adolescents, help them move into a prone or side-lying position (if possible). Keep them covered as necessary to prevent chilling and avoid exposure of body parts. Wash, rinse, and dry the back from the neck to the buttocks using long, firm strokes. | ***Special Considerations:*** *Children with respiratory distress may not be able to tolerate the prone position. During this time assess the skin for the presence of any reddened areas or breakdown of the shoulder or sacral regions.* |

| Steps | Rationale |
|---|---|
| v. For older children/adolescents help the client into a supine or side-lying position (if possible), expose only the genitalia and then wash, rinse, and dry the genitalia. Give special attention to any skin folds in the perineal or buttocks/anus region. Children who are able to assist with their bed bath will usually prefer to wash their own genitalia, although it may be necessary to inspect the genitalia to ensure that all secretions have been removed. | Keeping the child covered as much as possible provides privacy and comfort. Allowing the child who is able to wash his own genitalia to do so minimizes embarrassment for the child. **Special Considerations:** *When cleansing females, clean from front to back to prevent spreading microorganisms to the urinary meatus. Gently retract the labia for thorough cleaning. In uncircumcised males, retract the foreskin and clean around the glans penis in circular motion, then return the foreskin to its normal position.* |
| w. When cleaning the genitalia of the infant/small child, first remove the diaper then: | |
| ▪ For females: | |
| (1) Wash the folds of the groin. | This is an area where secretions collect easily. |
| (2) Wash with washcloth or cotton ball from front to back as for older child. Use a different portion of the washcloth or a new moistened cotton ball for each wipe. | The direction of cleansing decreases the chance of spreading fecal organisms to the urethral meatus. |
| ▪ For males: | |
| (1) Cleanse with plain water around the penis and scrotum. | Soap may be irritating. |
| (2) In older uncircumcised infants and children, gently retract the foreskin only to the point where resistance is met. With a washcloth or moist cotton ball, cleanse around the glans in a circular motion, moving from the tip of the urethra outward. | As the foreskin loosens, it should be retracted to remove secretions that can be a source of irritation and possibly infection. The foreskin is usually not fully retractable until about four years of age (Krueger and Osborn, 1986). **Special Considerations:** *Good hygiene practices are integral to the American Academy of Pediatrics recommendations on circumcision (see box on p. 345 in Skill 53). Teaching is indicated for the parents and preschool or older boy on penile cleansing, especially if the condition of the glans indicates cleaning has not been adequate, such as accumulated smegma, inflammation, phimosis, or foreskin adhesions. Krueger and Osborn (1986) reported that 60% of uncircumcised males in a study (ages 2 weeks to 52 years) remembered (or the parent remembered) being instructed by a health care provider to attempt foreskin retraction for adequate cleansing. Regular cleansing with foreskin retraction significantly decreased the incidence of phimosis, adhesions, smegma accumulation, and inflammation. The authors also noted that in some cultures (such as Vietnamese and Cambodian) the foreskin is traditionally not retracted until adulthood.* |
| (3) Dry the area well and return foreskin to its normal position. | The foreskin may restrict blood flow to the penis if it remains retracted. |
| x. Apply clean diaper; dress infant in sleeper or gown (see box; also see Skill 54). Help the child/adolescent to get dressed in a gown or their own clothes. If an extremity is injured or immobilized, dress the affected extremity first. | Dressing the infant will help promote warmth and comfort. Dressing the affected side first promotes easier manipulation of the gown over the body part which has limited range of motion. |
| y. Assist the child/adolescent with other grooming such as combing hair and applying make-up. Encourage them to do what they are able to do. | Grooming habits help promote comfort and maintain body image. **Special Considerations:** *For tips on shampooing and hair care, see box at right.* |
| z. Change bed sheets. | Bed linens usually get damp, soiled, and wrinkled during the bath. |
| 3. Assisting with a tub bath or shower: | |
| a. Help child to the bathroom/tub room if assistance is needed. Slippers with non-skid soles and a robe should be worn to the bathroom/tub room. | Helping the child prevents accidental falls and provides reevaluation of the child's stability and need for assistance. Slippers and robe will help promote safety, warmth, and privacy. |
| b. Explain to the child and/or family member how to use the call signal if assistance is needed. Tell the child to expect frequent checks to assure they are all right. Provide as much privacy as possible while maintaining adequate supervision. | Adolescents prefer privacy for bathing, and children usually prefer a parent or family member to assist them. Knowing how to call for help and expecting frequent checks can allay fears. **Special Considerations:** *Placing an "occupied" or "in use" sign on the door will also help provide privacy.* |

## *HINTS ON DRESSING INFANTS AND TODDLERS*

### GENERAL MEASURES

1. Interact or provide diversion while dressing so that infant will be less active.
2. Use the fewest motions possible and have clothing items within reach.
3. A supine position is easiest for young infants. Older infants and toddlers can be seated in a chair, lap or floor, or can be standing.
4. Stretchy fabrics and loose fitting clothes facilitate ease in dressing.

### UNDERSHIRTS, SHIRTS, AND ONE-PIECE GARMENTS

1. For shirts with crew necks: have infant lying down or sitting. Grasp and gather the fabric into a circle at the neck, place over crown of infant's head so shirt tags are at the neck. Using both hands, gently ease over the head, then face.
2. For one-piece sleepers: gather material of leg on side without snaps. Position infant's foot then leg into sleeper leg. Repeat for the side with snaps. Stand child up or lift younger infant to complete dressing.
3. Sleeves for young infants: thread own hand through sleeve from hand to shoulder of shirt/sleeper. Grasp infant's hand and thread sleeve on infant's arms.
4. Sleeves for older infants/toddlers: same as for younger infants, or hold shirt by the shoulder exposing arm hole. Guide child's hand in the sleeve and gently push the elbow through while lifting the shirt.

### PANTS

1. Snaps, zippers, or Velcro that expose the leg and diaper area are preferable, since diapering is frequent.
2. Lay infant down. Put own hand through one pant leg from hem to waist, grasp child's foot, and thread the pant leg on child's leg. Repeat with the other leg. For the young infant, lift hips and pull pants to waist. For older infant or toddler, stand upright and pull pants to waist.

### SOCKS AND TIGHTS

1. Gather completely from top to toe; stretch gathered opening wide and position over child's toes, then foot and heel, then ankle and leg. Repeat for other foot. For tights, ease top over back of diaper, then front.

### SHOES

1. Velcro closures are preferred for ease.
2. Open shoe widely and pull tongue out firmly before placing on foot.
3. Shoes are needed when infant starts standing and walking for protection. Soles should be flexible; rigid soles are unnecessary.

### OUTER GARMENTS

1. Mittens that can be gathered for easy fingertip placement are preferable.
2. Have toddler hold cuff of shirt in hand, guide jacket or sweater into arm slowly.

Courtesy Lynn B. Clutter, Tulsa, Oklahoma.

## *TIPS ON SHAMPOOING AND HAIR CARE*

1. Children usually need hair shampooing once or twice weekly unless otherwise indicated (e.g., profuse sweating). Adolescents require more frequent shampooing because of increased sebaceous secretions.
2. Shampooing is generally contraindicated when pain, elevated temperature, unstable respiratory status, increased intracranial pressure, cerebral spinal fluid leak, or unstable cervical spine injuries exist.
3. Use hydrogen peroxide before shampooing to remove dried blood in the hair. Electrode gel is most easily removed by shampooing before the gel dries. Once the gel has dried, acetone may aid in removal.
4. Alternative shampooing methods for the immobilized child include transferring the child to a stretcher, which can be positioned under a utility sink faucet, and use of a shampoo basin, a specially constructed rigid plastic trough with an indentation for neck placement and a drainage spout on one side. To facilitate drainage from the basin when rinsing the hair, gently press down on the spout. A large container can be placed under the spout to collect rinse water. Another improvised method of shampooing hair that requires less neck movement is to remove the headboard from the bed and slide a large, open plastic trash bag under the child's neck up to the base of the neck (Wells and Trostle, 1984). Cut a hole in the sealed end of the bag, and place it into a large trash container to collect rinse water.
5. If the child is able to cooperate, provide a small towel or washcloth during shampooing to hold over his or her face to keep shampoo and water out of the eyes.
6. A blow dryer is recommended to prevent chilling after shampooing. Towel drying should be avoided to prevent discomfort or further injury to children with cervical injuries.
7. Black Americans use hair greases, oils, creams, or pomades to lubricate their hair to facilitate combing. This cultural practice should not be misinterpreted as evidence of poor grooming. Do not attempt to comb the child's hair before shampooing unless it has been straightened because it is much easier to comb when wet. Plaiting or braiding of the child's hair should be done with the hair damp, not wet. Hair draws and becomes shorter as it dries, putting tension on the scalp, which may lead to hair loss. Braiding the hair loosely will also help prevent excess tightening as the hair dries (Joyner, 1988).

Courtesy Patti J. Tombridge, Tulsa, Oklahoma.

| Steps | Rationale |
|---|---|
| c. Assist with filling the bathtub with warm water, generally about one-third full, depending on the age and size of the child. Test the water temperature as described on p. 354. Show the child or family which faucet is hot/cold. Start the shower with the correct temperature or explain and demonstrate for the older child. | Helping the client adjust the water temperature or explaining how the faucets and the shower work helps prevent any accidental burns. **Special Considerations:** *If bathing an infant or toddler who is very active and difficult to hold, it may help to cleanse eyes, ears, nose, face, and neck before placing them into the bath water. Caution parents of a child unable to sit up to fill the bathtub only a few inches.* |
| d. Undress the infant and slowly immerse into the bath water. To hold the infant/child using one hand, place it behind the child's neck and upper back, grasping the opposite arm (see Fig. 55-1). The older child/adolescent may or may not require assistance. Instruct the child to use any safety bars available when getting in and out of the tub or shower. | Slow immersion into the water will help decrease the chances of startling the infant. This position of holding will help prevent slipping and leaves a free hand to bathe the child. **Special Considerations:** *Commercial products are available that support the child in an upright position in a bathtub such as a platform ring with suction cups on the legs. Do not use bath or baby oil in the tub/shower. The oil causes tub/shower surfaces to become slippery and can increase the risk of accidental falls. Oil also makes the skin slippery, and it is difficult to maintain a secure hold on the infant/young child. Oil, if used, should be applied to the skin after the bath.* |
| ▪ Infants/young children: give the bath moving from the arms and shoulders then down to the lower extremities. Use soap as needed. Thoroughly rinse areas where soap is used. | Soiled areas and body creases are generally easier to clean because of the soaking effects of the bath tub. **Special Considerations:** *Do not soap up the entire body at one time because the skin becomes slippery and it is difficult to securely hold the infant. Avoid letting soap remain in the bath water because soapy water cannot be used for rinsing. Instruct the child/family in these precautions.* |
| ▪ If possible, allow toddlers/older children to have play time in the water with bath toys. Never leave the child unattended. | Play can make bathing a pleasurable experience. Bath toys may also entertain the child while the bath is completed. **Special Considerations:** *Stress to parents the significant drowning risk in a bathtub, even in just a few inches of water. The top-heavy infant/toddler can easily fall face down and drown within minutes.* |
| ▪ Do not leave the child in the tub for longer than 20 minutes. For the older child/adolescent left unattended, check at 5 minute intervals. | If the child remains in the tub for a prolonged period of time, the warm water may cause vasodilation and pooling of blood, which may lead to dizziness and/or lightheadedness. Frequently checking on the child will help assure their safety and make sure they have needed items. |
| ▪ If the child is bathing himself or herself, return to the bathroom/tub when signaled, knocking on the door before entering. | Knocking on the door prevents the child from being alarmed or surprised and provides a warning so they can cover themselves or dress. |
| ▪ Remove the infant/small child from the tub and wrap them with a large bath towel. Gently pat them dry, being sure to dry well in the body creases. With older children/adolescents, assist them with getting out of the tub/shower and with drying as needed. | Wrapping child with a towel prevents chilling and helps maintain warmth. Moisture left on the skin in intertriginous areas can lead to softening of the skin and skin breakdown. |
| ▪ If child has dry skin, or any skin areas that are dry or cracked, apply lotion while skin is still hydrated. | Applying lotion while the skin is still slightly damp slows evaporation, maintaining hydration. It also provides pleasant and beneficial tactile stimulation. |
| ▪ Help the child to dress in clothing appropriate for age and clinical status. Some children may prefer to put on a robe and slippers and return to the room to dress. | This maintains warmth and prevents chilling. Some children are more comfortable wearing their own clothing from home. If the child is having frequent examinations, or there is probability of blood/body fluid drainage, a hospital gown would be more practical. |
| ▪ Assist child back to the room as needed; help them into a comfortable position in bed (with rails up as appropriate) or in chair. For an infant/small child, place in crib with rails up unless family members are present, desiring to attend child. | Ensuring safety and comfort during transport and positioning promotes relaxation. |
| ▪ Clean tub or shower according to agency policy. | This will prevent transmission of microorganisms and infection from the moisture. |

| Steps | Rationale |
|---|---|
| **Evaluation Outcomes** | **Observational Guidelines** |
| 1. Bath/shower is completed without injury to the child. | Note that falls or scalding burns did not occur. Ask/observe if child felt dizzy or lightheaded. |
| 2. Skin integrity is promoted or maintained. | The skin is clean, dry, and free of crusted or malodorous secretions. The skin appears hydrated and less dry. |
| 3. Bathing is completed with a minimum of discomfort to the child. | The child is not observed chilling and does not complain of being cold, does not cry, smiles and plays during bath, or appears relaxed. The child does not exhibit fatigue. |
| 4. Range of motion to the joints is performed actively or passively. | Observe range of motion of joints performed. Note flexibility of joints and/or presence of pain or discomfort. |
| 5. Child's participation in the bath is fostered. | Note child's response to encouragement of self-care. Note child's efforts to wash self. |
| 6. The child/family is taught proper hygiene, skin care, and safety measures. | Observe family bathing child; note clean to dirty order, front to back cleaning of genitalia on female, and retraction and proper cleansing of foreskin on uncircumcised males. Note safety precautions such as a secure hold on the infant in the tub and avoiding oil or soapy water. |

## Documentation

Record the type of bath the child received, participation in the procedure, the level of assistance needed, and tolerance to the bath procedure. Document any changes in the child's skin condition or musculoskeletal system such as reddened areas, areas of breakdown, or muscle or joint pain or stiffness.

## Child and Family Teaching

For parents of young girls, discuss the frequent occurrence of vaginal irritation from bubble bath products. In addition, washing the child's hair while seated in the tub also has the potential for the detergents and perfumes in the shampoo to cause vaginal irritation (Brown, 1989). If irritation is a problem, wash the child's hair separately or at the conclusion of the bath with unscented soap.

## Home Care Modifications

Discuss safety modifications for the home such as nonskid tub and floor mats for the tub/shower areas. If the child's condition indicates, safety grab bars should be installed, e.g., for a child with juvenile rheumatoid arthritis.

# SKILL 56 Providing Oral Care for an Infant

*Caryn Stoermer Hess*

Good oral hygiene begins during infancy even though teeth have not erupted. Practices begun during this time can affect both the primary and permanent teeth.

## NURSING DIAGNOSES

Altered health maintenance related to demonstrated lack of knowledge about infant oral hygiene needs; Altered oral mucous membrane related to ineffective oral hygiene.

| Steps | Rationale |
|---|---|
| **Assessment** | |
| 1. Assess infant's mouth especially noting presence of teeth or teething and signs of infection such as oral candidiasis (thrush). (See Skill 27.) | Assessment of the mouth determines the appropriate oral care for the individual infant and identifies any potential health problems.<br>***Special Considerations:*** *The age of tooth eruption varies considerably in children. The general rule for estimating the number of primary teeth is the child's age in months minus 6 months equals the number of teeth. White, curdy patches or plaques that bleed when scraped are signs of oral candidiasis. In newborns "Epstein pearls" may be present, which are small, white epithelial cysts along both sides of the midline of the hard palate. They are insignificant and disappear in several weeks (Whaley and Wong, 1991).* |
| 2. Assess infant's nutrition (see Skill 29), especially type of feeding (bottle, breast, solid foods) and fluoride intake. | Nutritional assessment identifies infants at greater risk for dental caries, e.g., those who drink large amounts of juice from a bottle or eat many sugary foods. The type of feeding is especially important to determine fluoride intake. Sources of fluoride during infancy include drinking water and fluoride supplements. |

### Planning and Goal Setting

1. Gather supplies:
   a. Clean wash cloth.
   b. Small, soft toothbrush.
   c. Water.
   d. Fluoride supplements.
2. Develop individualized child and family goals:
   - Gums and teeth will be cleansed after feedings and at bedtime.
   - Infant will not sleep with a bottle of milk or juice or breastfeed while sleeping for a prolonged period of time.
   - Infant will receive recommended amount of fluoride.

### Implementation 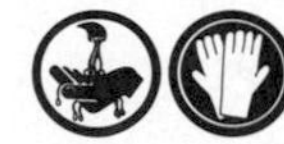

| Steps | Rationale |
|---|---|
| 1. Provide oral care after each feeding and at bedtime. | Bedtime cleansing is especially important so that plaque does not adhere to the teeth during the night, increasing the chance for dental caries. |
| a. If the teeth have not yet erupted, wrap a clean piece of cloth (e.g., washcloth) around the index finger, moisten it with water, and gently rub inside the mouth and gums. | Wiping removes any remaining milk or food.<br>***Special Considerations:*** *While there is no clear evidence that cleansing is necessary before eruption of teeth, it may have some value in decreasing moniliasis (Whaley and Wong, 1991) and in familiarizing the infant with toothbrushing in the future.* |

| Steps | Rationale |
|---|---|
| 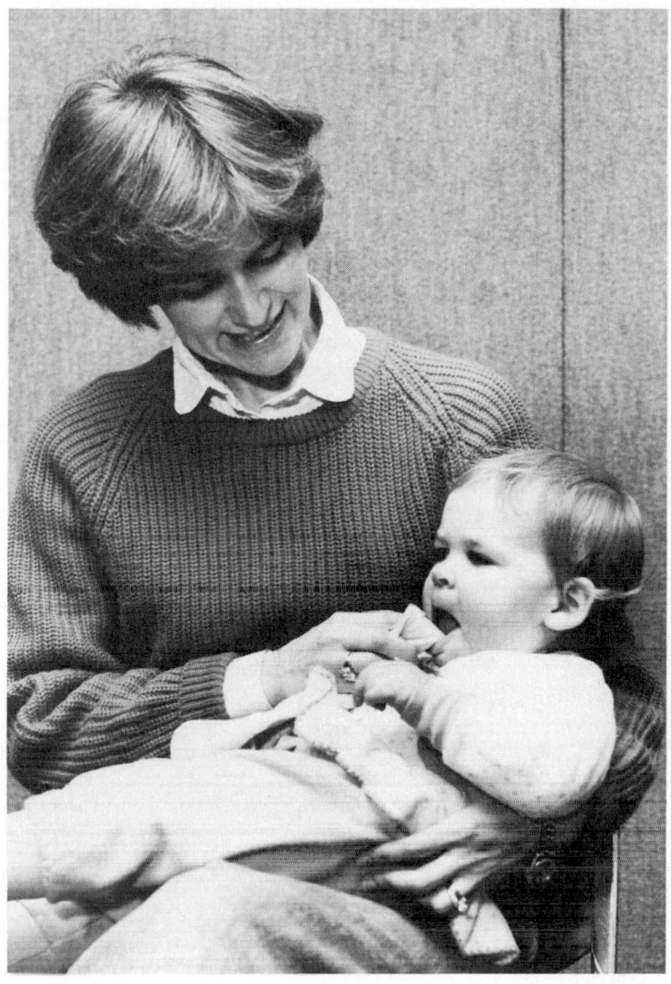 | ***FIG. 56-1*** A moist cloth is used to provide oral care. |
| b. If the teeth have begun to erupt, wipe them with a cloth moistened with water (Fig. 56-1). | Toothbrushing is too harsh for tender gingiva during infancy. |
| c. Toward the end of the first year, brush teeth gently with a small, soft toothbrush and water. The brush can be made softer by placing it in water for one minute before brushing. | There are no clear guidelines as to when toothbrushing should begin. Around 10 to 12 months of age many infants have 6 to 8 teeth. Sometimes it is several months until the next spurt of dentition occurs. Brushing can begin if the gums are not too tender so as to cause bleeding or discomfort. Water is used because many infants dislike the taste of toothpaste, and infants do not yet understand how to spit out toothpaste. Excessive ingestion of fluoridated toothpaste can cause fluorosis.<br>***Special Considerations:*** *Toothbrushing at an early age can be made fun or at least pleasant by singing, playing games, and talking to the infant. This may lead to greater compliance with oral hygiene as the child grows.* |
| d. If infant has oral candidiasis (thrush), rinse the mouth with plain water after each feeding and before applying the medication. | Rinsing the mouth removes any remaining milk without further irritating the affected mucous membranes that easily bleed and may be painful (Whaley and Wong, 1991). |
| 2. If the infant falls asleep during a feeding, remove the bottle or breast. Avoid letting infant go to bed with a bottle of milk or other liquid such as juice. | Bottle-mouth caries can develop when the teeth are constantly bathed with warm milk or other liquids containing sugar.<br>***Special Considerations:*** *Educate families to prevent or stop the habit of going to sleep with a bottle. A bottle of water can be substituted for milk or juice. Offer juice in a cup to avoid prolonging the bottle-feeding habit.* |

| Steps | Rationale |
|---|---|
| 3. Administer adequate amounts of fluoride to the infant. | When adequate amounts of fluoride are ingested before eruption of the teeth and to a lesser extent after tooth eruption, the enamel is more resistant to caries (Hess et al, 1984). |
| a. When local water is fluoridated, mix infant's formula, juice, and dry cereal with the fluoridated tap water. | ***Special Considerations:*** *The U.S. Public Health Service Drinking Water Standards has established the optimal level of fluoride in drinking water as 0.7 to 1.2 ppm (Driscoll et al, 1983). The city water department or health department can be contacted to determine if the local water is fluoridated.* |
| b. When local water contains excessive amounts of fluoride, use unfluoridated, bottled water instead of tap water. | Excessive natural fluoride is not very common. However, excessive fluoride ingestion results in fluorosis, which is characterized by an increase in the degree and extent of the enamel's porosity. Moderate and severe fluorosis occurs when the fluoride content of the water exceeds 4 ppm (Driscoll et al, 1983).<br>***Special Considerations:*** *In areas of the country where there is a natural level of fluoride in the water, the local water department or health department can be contacted to determine the level of fluoride in the water. Well water can also be analyzed for fluoride content.* |
| c. Give fluoride supplements (0.25 mg/day) as prescribed. Place the drops directly on the tongue. | This dosage schedule is recommended by the American Dental Association and the Nutrition Committee of the American Academy of Pediatrics (American Academy of Pediatrics, 1986). Placing the drops on the tongue allows it to mix with saliva and come in direct contact with any erupted teeth (Hess et al, 1984).<br>***Special Considerations:*** *Fluoride supplements are appropriate for:*<br>▪ *All infants 2 weeks of age or older who live in an area with suboptimum levels of fluoride in the local water supply.*<br>▪ *Exclusively breast-fed infants regardless of the fluoride content of the local water.*<br>▪ *Infants who consume relatively little or no fluoridated tap water such as those receiving ready-to-serve formula (Whaley and Wong, 1991).* |

| Evaluation Outcomes | Observational Guidelines |
|---|---|
| 1. Infant's gums and teeth are cleansed after feedings and at bedtime. | Inspect mouth for residue of milk or food and teeth for evidence of plaque. |
| 2. Family demonstrates proper cleansing of infant's gums and teeth. | Ask family to demonstrate cleansing of gums and teeth. |
| 3. Infant does not go to bed sucking on a bottle of milk or juice. | Observe infant while sleeping or interview family regarding bedtime bottle practices. |
| 4. Mother does not continue breastfeeding for a prolonged period of time after infant is asleep. | Observe mother and infant breastfeeding before bedtime or interview mother about breastfeeding practices. |
| 5. Infant receives adequate amounts of fluoride through either the ingestion of fluoridated water or fluoride supplements. | Determine fluoride intake and compare with recommended fluoride levels. |
| 6. Family demonstrates correct administration of fluoride supplements. | Observe family administering fluoride supplements. |
| 7. Family verbalizes importance of good oral hygiene, not sleeping with milk or juice in the mouth, and fluoride. | Interview and observe family for evidence of understanding the proper oral care of infants. |

## Documentation

Record assessment of mouth and current feeding practices, cleansing of teeth and gums, administration of fluoride supplements, and family teaching about oral care.

## Child and Family Teaching

1. Recommend that pacifiers not be coated with honey. Honey is not recommended in children under 12 months of age as a precaution against infant botulism (Turick-Gibson, 1988).
2. Counsel family about the detrimental effects of prolonged and frequent bottle feeding or breastfeeding during sleep when the milk or other liquid such as juice bathes the teeth. Discourage allowing the older infant to suck on a bottle as a pacifier. If a pacifier bottle is considered necessary by family, advise that only plain water should be given to the child in the bottle.
3. Encourage preventive dental health check-ups. Ideally, the child should see a dentist (or pedodontist) soon after the first teeth erupt and no later than by 2½ years when primary dentition is complete (Whaley and Wong, 1991).
4. Discuss with the family the role of fluoride in preventing dental caries.

# *SKILL* 57 Providing Oral Care for a Child

*Caryn Stoermer Hess*

Good oral hygiene is essential to preserving the teeth and maintaining healthy gums. Although tooth decay and gum disease is not life-threatening, the discomfort, tooth loss, appearance of the mouth, and cost of treatment create significant problems for children, as well as adults. Oral care needs to be consistent, continuous, and initiated at a very early age.

## NURSING DIAGNOSES

Altered health maintenance related to inadequate oral hygiene; Altered mucous membrane related to ineffective oral hygiene; Body image disturbance related to perceived oral imperfections or use of orthodontic appliances; Self-care deficit, oral hygiene related to cognitive, developmental, neuromuscular, or physical impairment.

| Steps | Rationale |
|---|---|
| **Assessment** | |
| 1. Assess mouth (see Skill 27), noting especially: | Assessment of the mouth determines the appropriate oral care for the individual child and identifies potential health problems. |
| a. Presence of primary and permanent teeth. | The age of tooth eruption varies considerably in children. The general rule for estimating the number of primary teeth is the child's age in months minus 6 equals the number of teeth. The shedding of primary teeth and eruption of permanent teeth generally occur between the ages of 6 and 12. |
| b. Appearance of teeth and gums. | The teeth are inspected for number, hygiene, and occlusion. Discoloration of tooth enamel with obvious plaque (whitish/yellowish coating on teeth) is a sign of inadequate oral care. Brown spots in the crevices of the crown of the tooth or between the teeth may be cavities. Healthy gums are coral pink with the surface texture stippled, similar in appearance to an orange peel. In dark-skinned children, the gums are more deeply colored and a brownish line is often observed along the gum line. With gingivitis, the gums are red, edematous, tender, and subject to bleeding at the slightest irritation. |
| c. Presence of orthodontic appliances (braces, retainers, or dentures). | Orthodontic appliances, common in school-age children and adolescents, require special oral hygiene since they encourage retention of food particles and plaque. Some children wear removable partial dentures either until permanent teeth erupt or a permanent bridge can be used. |
| d. Signs of infection such as oral candidiasis (thrush) and herpetic gingivostomatitis. | White, curdy patches of plaque on oral mucosa that bleed when scraped are signs of oral candidiasis (Whaley and Wong, 1991). Herpetic gingivostomatitis is the most common viral disease affecting children's oral mucosa. Symptoms include fever, an erythematous and edematous pharynx, possible lymphadenitis, and vesicles up to 10 mm that cause severe pain and a foul odor (Feldman and Aretakis, 1986). |
| 2. Assess nutritional intake including fluoride. | A well-balanced diet that promotes general health will also promote oral health and is necessary for the development of strong, healthy teeth during the formative years. Nutritional assessment identifies those children who are at greater risk for dental caries. Sugar intake and snack habits are of special concern. Fluoride is important in preventing tooth decay. Sources of ingested fluoride include drinking water and fluoride supplements. |
| 3. Assess for special oral care needs: | Some children have special oral needs related to their health. |
| a. Hemophilia. | With hemophilia, there is a potential for oral bleeding because there is a deficiency of one of the factors necessary for coagulation of the blood. |

| Steps | Rationale |
|---|---|
| b. Cancer and cancer treatments. | The decreased platelet production occurring with leukemia can cause oral bleeding. The child receiving radiation therapy or chemotherapy may also have special oral care needs. When the oral mucosa is exposed to radiation, there are changes in the character of the saliva and mucositis (inflammation of the oral tissues) results. A side effect of some chemotherapeutic agents is gastrointestinal mucosal cell damage. Red, eroded, painful oral ulcers can develop. Chemotherapy also impairs childrens' immune mechanisms. As a result, otherwise benign dental disease can become serious. |
| c. NPO (nothing by mouth). | When a child is NPO (e.g., unconscious or tube fed), the mouth tends to become dry or coated with mucus. |
| d. Vomiting. | Since vomiting exposes teeth to gastric acids that are highly corrosive to tooth enamel, dental caries are common in conditions with a high incidence of vomiting (e.g., bulimia, chemotherapy, or pregnancy). |
| e. Cognitive impairment/developmental disabilities. | Dental problems in mentally retarded children occur often as a result of neglected oral hygiene, excessive quantities of carbohydrates, and a side effect of some medications. |
| f. Neuromuscular/physical disabilities. | Children with neuromuscular/physical disabilities (e.g., cerebral palsy) may require special assistance with oral hygiene. |
| 4. Assess child's development. | A child's physical and cognitive development determines the amount and type of assistance needed for oral hygiene. Psychosocial development affects both the child's cooperation with and motivation for oral hygiene. |

## Planning and Goal Setting

| | |
|---|---|
| 1. Gather supplies:<br>a. Toothbrush.<br>b. Water.<br>c. Toothpaste.<br>d. Dental floss.<br>e. Fluoride rinse, supplements. | ***Special Considerations:*** *Select a toothbrush with soft, rounded nylon bristles that are not bent or frayed. This type of brush is less likely to injure gum tissue. Choice of brush design is primarily one of individual preference. Nylon bristles dry more rapidly after use and retain their shape better than natural bristles. Frayed or bent bristles are less effective in removing plaque. The younger the child, the smaller the toothbrush should be. Electric toothbrushes can be great motivational tools for children but require proper use to be effective in plaque removal. Consequently, electric toothbrushes should not replace parental involvement in child's oral hygiene (Kronmiller and Nirschl, 1985). Water is used to brush the very young child's teeth since the taste of toothpaste and its foaming action is often disliked at this age. When toothpaste is used, select a flavor the child likes to encourage a good brushing habit. Fluoridated toothpaste and mouth rinses that carry the seal (easily identified on package) of the American Dental Association Council on Dental Therapeutics are recommended. These products have been tested and proved effective in reducing cavities.* |
| 2. Develop individualized child and family goals:<br>▪ Teeth and gums will be cleansed after eating and at bedtime.<br>▪ Recommended amounts of systemic and topical fluoride will be received. | |

## Implementation

| | |
|---|---|
| 1. Brush and floss teeth after eating and before bedtime. | The primary method for preventing dental caries and gingivitis is regular plaque removal by brushing and flossing the teeth. Although thorough plaque removal once a day is generally recognized as being sufficient, cleansing 2 to 3 times per day increases the probability of cleaning teeth effectively (McDonald and Avery, 1987). Cleaning the teeth after eating reduces the amount of time sugars are in contact with the teeth. The most important time for oral care is following the last meal/snack of the day or at bedtime. This cleansing is critical to prevent the overnight interaction of carbohydrates and bacteria on the teeth. |

| Steps | Rationale |
|---|---|
| | ***Special Considerations:*** *At those times when brushing is impractical, the "swish and swallow" method of cleaning the mouth can be used. With a mouthful of water, the child swishes water to rinse the mouth and swallows repeating the procedure three to four times (Whaley and Wong, 1991). Some dentists recommend brushing the teeth before eating to remove the bacteria that can immediately convert sugars into acid. The time of brushing therefore may not be as important as the thoroughness of the cleaning.* |
| a. Brush primary teeth (in child under about age 10) using a horizontal scrub method. The tips of the bristles are placed firmly at a 45-degree angle against the teeth and gums and moved back and forth in a vibratory motion. The ends of the bristles should be wiggling but not moving forcefully back and forth. All the surfaces of the teeth are cleaned in this manner except the inner surfaces of the anterior teeth. To clean these surfaces, the toothbrush is placed vertical to the teeth and moved up and down. Brush a few teeth at a time, using six to eight strokes for each section (Whaley and Wong, 1991). | Several brushing methods are acceptable. This horizontal scrubbing technique is considered highly effective in removing plaque from primary teeth. Brushing too forcefully can damage the gums and tooth enamel, especially if there is gingival recession. A systematic approach is important so that all tooth surfaces are thoroughly cleaned.<br>***Special Considerations:*** *For toddlers and preschoolers the most effective cleaning is done by adults. Several positions can be used that facilitate access to the mouth and help stabilize the head for comfort: (1) Stand with child's back toward adult. (When done in front of a mirror, both child and adult can see what is being done in the mirror [Fig. 57-1].) (2) Sit on a couch or bed with the child's head resting in adult's lap. (3) Sit on a floor or stool with the child's head resting between adult's thighs. With all positions, use one hand to cup the chin and one to brush the teeth (Wong and Whaley, 1990). These positions are recommended because brushing the child's teeth from behind is similar to brushing one's own teeth and therefore easier. Toothbrushing at an early age can be made fun or at least pleasant by singing, playing games, and talking to the child. This may lead to greater compliance with oral hygiene as the child grows. When the child wants to begin brushing his or her own teeth, let the child do so before or after the parent. It is recommended that when children brush their own teeth, they brush for 3 full minutes (using an egg or special timer). This length of time increases the likelihood of cleaning all tooth surfaces. This fosters independence but ensures a complete cleansing, since the young child lacks the neuromuscular skills to clean his or her teeth thoroughly. Although the 6- to 10-year-old child can brush his or her own teeth, an adult needs to monitor the frequency and effectiveness of brushing.* |
| b. Brush permanent teeth as they begin to erupt, adding the roll method if desired. Hold toothbrush parallel to the long axis of the tooth with tips covering the gums. Using a gentle sweeping motion, pass bristles vertically along the gums and teeth (Kronmiller and Nirschl, 1985). | There is a more sophisticated technique recommended by some for the permanent teeth. There is, however, no conclusive evidence that one method is superior over another. The thoroughness of the cleaning is more important than the specific technique used (Whaley and Wong, 1991). The dentist can recommend the most appropriate brushing technique for the individual child. |

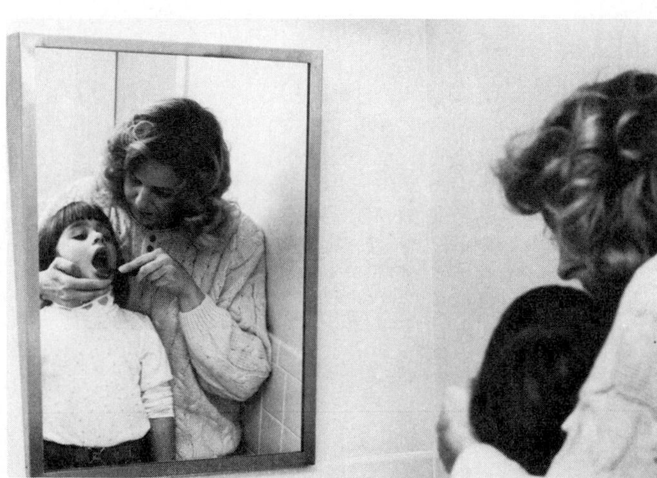

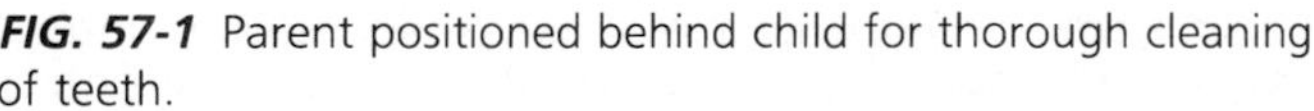

***FIG. 57-1*** Parent positioned behind child for thorough cleaning of teeth.

| Steps | Rationale |
|---|---|
| c. Use dental floss between contacting teeth. A length of dental floss about 12 to 18 inches can be either tied in a circle or wrapped around the fingers. With about 1 inch held tautly against the thumbs, the floss is gently inserted between two teeth, wrapped around the base of the tooth in a "C" shape, and directed below the gingival margin to remove plaque. The floss is then moved toward the biting surface of the tooth to also remove plaque between the teeth. Repeat this process between all teeth using a clean section of the floss (Whaley and Wong, 1991). | Flossing removes plaque and debris from between the teeth and below the gum margin where brushing is ineffective. ***Special Considerations:*** *The "circle or loop method" of holding the floss may be easier for some children to learn. Since young children lack the manual dexterity needed to floss teeth, an adult should do the flossing until the child is about 8 to 10 years old and can demonstrate ability to floss adequately. A plaque-disclosing agent, available through dental offices or commercially, can be used to identify those areas where plaque accumulates. This plaque-disclosing agent stains plaque red, allowing child to see the areas that are being inadequately cleansed. The child then brushes and flosses his or her teeth until the stained plaque is removed. This can be a useful tool in motivating children since they can actually see the effectiveness of their oral hygiene.* |
| d. Use water irrigating devices to remove large food particles from between the teeth and around fixed orthodontic appliances (braces). Cleanse removable appliances (dentures, retainers) by brushing with toothpaste or soaking in a denture cleaner for 15 minutes daily. Soak appliances in cleanser when not in use. | Irrigating devices are recommended by many dentists and orthodontists when children have orthodontic appliances that prevent the use of dental floss. Retainers and dentures require cleansing to remove food and bacteria adhering to the appliance. ***Special Considerations:*** *Since irrigation does not remove plaque, it is not a substitute for brushing. Brushing after every meal and snack is essential to remove plaque from the exposed teeth and under loose-fitting braces.* |
| 2. Provide oral care appropriate to the child with special needs. | Basic oral hygiene (i.e., brushing and flossing) needs to be adapted when a child has special health problems. Fluoride is important for children with special needs, especially because there is often a greater risk for dental caries in these children. |
| a. When a child is at risk for oral bleeding, cleanse teeth and gums using a small, soft-bristled toothbrush. Place the toothbrush in warm water for 1 minute before use. | Oral bleeding can be a problem for children with hemophilia and leukemia, as well as those receiving chemotherapeutic agents that lower platelet counts. A soft brush with small and flexible bristles will follow the contours of the teeth and reach into the gingival crevices without damaging sensitive tissues (Bersani and Carl, 1983). Soaking the brush in warm water will further soften the bristles. |
| b. If gentle brushing causes bleeding, cleanse the teeth using a water irrigating device adjusted to low pressure, a sponge-tipped toothbrush, a cotton-tipped applicator, or a gauze-wrapped finger. | Cleansing of the teeth must be done gently to prevent bleeding. Since these methods will only partially cleanse the teeth and gums, they should only be used temporarily when the threat of bleeding is severe (Bersani and Carl, 1983). |
| c. When the child has oral ulcers (mucositis, stomatitis), cleanse teeth with sponge-tipped toothbrush, cotton-tipped applicator, or gauze pads (2 X 2 or 4 X 4) and use frequent mouthwashes with normal saline. Mouth-care should be done routinely before and after eating and as often as every 2 to 4 hours (Whaley and Wong, 1991). | When a child has mucositis as a side effect of chemotherapy or radiation therapy, meticulous mouth care is important for comfort and to prevent bacterial and fungal infections. Cleansing the teeth needs to be done gently to prevent trauma to the irritated membranes. Frequent mouth irrigations clean the tissues, reduce local pain caused by dryness, and lubricate the membranes (Bersani and Carl, 1983). ***Special Considerations:*** *Agents recommended in the past such as lemon glycerin swabs, hydrogen peroxide, and milk of magnesia are avoided because of the drying effects on the mucosa (Whaley and Wong, 1991). Commerical mouthwashes are not recommended because they contain alcohol that can be irritating and drying to the mucous membranes. A variety of topical anesthetic agents can be applied to mouth lesions as prescribed. Dangers of topical anesthetics include depression of gag reflex, insensitivity to hot food, toxicity if ingested, and allergic responses.* |
| d. When a child is NPO, cleanse the teeth at least twice a day with a soft toothbrush moistened in water, a sponge-tipped toothbrush, or gauze saturated with saline. Apply a thin layer of petrolatum, glycerine, or similar product to the lips (Whaley and Wong, 1991). | Oral hygiene is especially important when fluids are withheld (e.g., in an unconscious or tube-fed child). Brushing the teeth and keeping the lips and mouth moistened will help to maintain the teeth and oral membranes until fluids by mouth and regular oral care can be resumed. |

| Steps | Rationale |
|---|---|
| | ***Special Considerations:*** *A very minimal amount of water or saline should be used to prevent ingestion or aspiration of the liquid. Suction equipment should always be available. When using a sponge-tipped toothbrush, be sure it is removed intact from child's mouth. When continuous suction (tonsil-tip) is available, as in long-term care situations, the teeth can be brushed in the usual manner with toothpaste and water, since all liquid can be safely removed from the mouth.* |
| e. Brush teeth after vomiting. | Brushing is important to remove gastric acids that can erode tooth enamel.<br>***Special Considerations:*** *If toothbrushing stimulates the gag reflex or if the child is too weak, rinse the mouth with water.* |
| f. When a child is cognitively, developmentally, or physically impaired, allow child to do whatever part of oral care he or she is capable of, e.g., put toothpaste on toothbrush, brush own teeth using "any direction" method (Whaley and Wong, 1991). | There is a wide variability in the amount of oral care the cognitively, developmentally, or physically impaired child is capable of doing. Encouraging the child to do as much as possible will foster independence, self-esteem, and compliance with oral hygiene.<br>***Special Considerations:*** *An adult may need to take the primary responsibility for oral hygiene, similar to the care of a young child. When a child has physical impairments that limit the ability to brush, special devices may be necessary such as a larger handle or a curved toothbrush. Electric toothbrushes may be helpful. It is also important to avoid the use of candy to reward behavior (Whaley and Wong, 1991). Because the needs of the special child often place great demands on the family's time, the oral hygiene program must be realistic or it will not be maintained (McDonald and Avery, 1987).* |
| 3. Administer appropriate amounts of systemic fluoride. | Fluoride is received systemically when any liquid or food containing fluoride is swallowed. When fluoride is absorbed by the teeth, they are stronger and more resistant to caries. Among the many groups recommending fluoride are the American Dental Association, the American Medical Association, the American Public Health Association, and The World Health Organization. |
| a. When local water is fluoridated, consume water and drinks prepared with tap water (e.g., juice, soups, or noncarbonated drinks). | The U.S. Public Health Service Drinking Water Standards has established the optimal level of fluoride in drinking water as 0.7 to 1.2 ppm (Driscoll et al, 1983). For a child to receive 1 mg of fluoride (1 ppm of fluoride is equivalent to 1 mg per liter), a liter of water a day must be consumed. In addition to drinking water, the child receives water from drinks and foods prepared with it. Carbonated beverages may contain fluoridated water, depending on the local water where the drink is manufactured (Hess et al, 1984).<br>***Special Considerations:*** *The local water department or health department can be contacted to determine the amount of flouride in the water. Well water can also be analyzed for fluoride content.* |

***TABLE 57-1*** Supplemental Fluoride Dosage Schedule*

| | Concentration (ppm) of Fluoride in Drinking Water | | |
|---|---|---|---|
| | | mg/day | |
| **Age** | **<0.3** | **0.3-0.7** | **>0.7** |
| 2 weeks-2 years | 0.25 | 0 | 0 |
| 2-3 years | 0.50 | 0.25 | 0 |
| 3-16 years | 1.00 | 0.50 | 0 |

*2.2 mg sodium fluoride contains 1 mg fluoride.
From American Academy of Pediatrics, Committee on Nutrition: Fluoride supplementation, Pediatrics 77(5):758-761, 1986.

| Steps | Rationale |
|---|---|
| b. When local water contains excessive amounts of fluoride, use unfluoridated, bottled water instead of tap water. | Although excessive natural fluoride is uncommon, it results in fluorosis, which is characterized by an increase in the degree and extent of the enamel's porosity. Moderate and severe fluorosis occurs when the fluoride content of the water exceeds 4 ppm (Driscoll et al, 1983). |
| c. When local water is unfluoridated (or contains less than 0.7 ppm), give fluoride supplements as prescribed. | See Table 57-1 for dosage recommended by both the American Dental Association and the Nutrition Committee of the American Academy of Pediatrics (American Academy of Pediatrics, 1986). |
| ▪ Fluoride drops (for infants and young children) are placed directly on the tongue. Fluoride tablets or lozenges (for older children) are chewed or sucked, then swished in the mouth for 30 seconds before swallowing. | Placing the drops on the tongue allows it to mix with saliva and come in direct contact with the teeth. Tablets or lozenges can be used when the child is old enough to safely chew or suck them to obtain the topical benefits in addition to the systemic benefits of fluoride (Hess et al, 1984). |
| ▪ Administer fluoride supplements on an empty stomach and do not give food or drinks (especially milk products) for 30 minutes. | Absorption is impaired when fluoride is not ingested on an empty stomach. Calcium especially inhibits absorption of fluoride. Fluoride supplements are absorbed in about 30 minutes (Hess et al, 1984). |
| ▪ Store fluoride supplements (in a labeled container) in a safe place away from small children and keep no more than a 4 month supply. | Acute toxicity and even death can occur from ingesting large quantities of fluoride. Safety precautions with fluoride supplements are necessary as with all medications.<br>***Special Considerations:*** *Fluoride toothpastes and rinses (see below) are also stored out of the reach of children.* |
| 4. Apply topical fluoride to the teeth. | Fluoride is absorbed by the teeth when it is applied topically with fluoridated toothpastes or mouthrinses.<br>***Special Considerations:*** *The chewing surfaces of children's teeth are most susceptible to decay and receive the least benefits from fluoride. Dentists can apply pit and fissure sealants to permanent teeth that anatomically are especially prone to caries (Starr and Gravits, 1985).* |
| a. Use a "pea-sized" amount of fluoridated toothpaste when brushing teeth. Avoid swallowing toothpaste. | A small amount of toothpaste is recommended to minimize the amount of fluoride ingested. Studies of toothpaste use and ingestion report that children may swallow up to 35% of their toothpaste. Swallowing this amount of excess fluoride could contribute to fluorosis (Hess et al, 1984).<br>***Special Considerations:*** *Studies have shown that swallowing toothpaste decreased with increased age; the highest ingestion was in children ages 2 to 4, but significant ingestion also occurred in children ages 5 to 7. Young children therefore require close supervision when brushing with fluoridated toothpastes and should be taught not to eat toothpaste. If this is not possible, use a nonfluoridated toothpaste until the child is older (Hess et al, 1984).* |
| b. Use a fluoridated mouth rinse daily for children over 6 years of age; use only the amount recommended, keep the solution in the mouth for 1 minute (timed by the clock) and then expectorate. Avoid food or fluid for 30 minutes. | The swallowing reflexes of young children are inadequate to prevent ingestion of the mouth rinse. As with toothpaste, excessive fluoride ingestion can occur if the mouthrinse is swallowed. Bathing the teeth in the solution for 1 minute allows all tooth surfaces to receive the topical fluoride.<br>***Special Considerations:*** *A good time to use the rinse is after the last meal or at bedtime. Topical fluoride solutions, pastes, and gels are also applied in dental offices after the child's teeth are cleaned. Some dentists recommend fluoride gels that contain more fluoride than rinses. These are available by prescription for home use.* |

| Evaluation Outcomes | Observational Guidelines |
|---|---|
| 1. Child's teeth are brushed and flossed after eating and at bedtime. | Inspect teeth and gums, looking especially for plaque. Use disclosing tablets. |
| 2. Child/family demonstrates proper cleansing of the teeth. | Ask child/family to demonstrate cleansing of teeth and to outline their brushing and flossing schedule. |

| Steps | Rationale |
|---|---|
| 3. Child receives adequate amounts of systemic fluoride either through the ingestion of fluoridated water or fluoride supplements. | Determine fluoride intake and compare with recommended levels. |
| 4. Child/family demonstrates correct administration of fluoride supplements. | Observe child taking fluoride supplements; interview family about administration of the supplements. |
| 5. Child's teeth receive adequate amounts of topical fluoride through fluoridated toothpastes and mouth rinses. | Inspect teeth for signs of dental caries. Interview family about use of fluoridated toothpaste and mouth rinses. |
| 6. Family verbalizes importance of storing fluoride supplements, toothpastes, and mouth rinses safely away from young children. | Interview family for evidence of understanding the safety precautions necessary with fluoride products. |

## Documentation

Record assessment of mouth and nutritional intake/practices, cleaning of teeth and gums, administration of systemic and topical fluoride, and child/family teaching about oral care.

## Child and Family Teaching

1. Teach family how to provide good oral care appropriate to individual child.
2. Discuss good nutrition and influence on dental health. This is especially important because habits begun during childhood tend to continue in later years. Specific nutritional recommendations include:
   a. Limit the amount of sugars eaten, especially sucrose. Read labels carefully to identify type and amounts of sugar. Common dietary sugars include sucrose, dextrose, maltose, fructose, lactose, glucose, corn syrup, maple syrup, molasses, corn sweeteners, and honey. (Dry cereals are a "hidden" source of sugar in many diets. For example, a cereal that is advertised as "low in sugar" because it has no sugar coating may still contain many types of sugar.)
   b. Limit frequency of sugar intake. When eating sweets, have them at mealtime rather than as a snack between meals. (How often children eat sweets is more important than the total amount eaten at one time. Every time a child eats sugar, the teeth are exposed for 20 minutes to the acids that demineralize tooth enamel. This explains why children who snack frequently have an inceased amount of cavities.)
   c. Avoid or limit retentive ("sticky" or "hard") sweets such as raisins, lollipops, and chewing gum. (Since these sugars remain in the mouth longer, they cause more cavities.)
   d. Select snack foods that do not encourage the development of cavities, e.g., popcorn, fresh fruits, nuts, cheese, cold meats, and peanut butter (without added sugars).
   e. If child routinely takes any medicine in sweetened liquid or chewable tablet form, clean the teeth afterward or at least rinse the mouth with water. (Children's medications that are sweetened for pallatabiliy can be a hidden source of sugar.)
3. Encourage regular, preventive dental health check-ups. Ideally, the child should see a dentist (or pedodontist) soon after the first teeth erupt, and no later than by 2½ years when primary dentition is complete. The recommended frequency of check-ups is usually twice yearly, but this depends on the individual child.
4. Discuss the role of fluoride in preventing dental caries.

UNIT VII

## PRODUCT REFERENCES AND TEACHING RESOURCES

Ross Laboratories
Sleeptight Order Department
1208 East Hudson St.
Columbus, OH 43211
1-800-662-6542
Offers the Sleeptight Infant Soother.

## REFERENCES

American Academy of Pediatrics, Committee on Nutrition: Fluoride supplementation, Pediatrics 77(5):758-761, 1986.

American Academy of Pediatrics Task Force on Circumcision: Report of the Task Force on circumcision, Pediatrics 84(4):388-391, 1989.

American Academy of Pediatrics Task Force on Pediatric AIDS: Pediatric guidelines for infection control of human immunodeficiency virus (acquired immunodeficiency virus) in hospitals, medical offices, schools and other settings, Pediatrics 82(5):801-807, 1988.

American Dental Association, Council on Dental Therapeutics: Accepted dental therapeutics, ed 40, Chicago, 1984, American Dental Association.

Austin AP et al: A survey of factors associated with diaper dermatitis in thirty-six pediatric practices, J Pediatr Health Care 2(6):295-299, 1988.

Benjamin L: Clinical correlates with diaper dermatitis, Pediatrician 14(suppl 1):21-26, 1987.

Bersani G and Carl W: Oral care for cancer patients, Am J Nurs 83(4):533-536, 1983.

Brown JL: Hair shampooing technique and pediatric vulvovaginitis (letter), Pediatrics 83(1):146, 1989.

Campbell RL: Clinical tests with improved disposable diapers, Pediatrician 14(suppl 1):34-38, 1987.

Campbell RL et al: Effects of diaper types on diaper dermatitis associated with diarrhea and antibiotic use in children in daycare centers, Pediatr Dermatol 5(2):83-87, 1988.

Cotton WH and Davidson PJ: Aspiration of baby powder, N Engl J Med 313(26):1662, 1985.

Council on Dental Therapeutics: Guidelines for the acceptance of fluoride-containing dentifrices, JADA 110(4):545-547, 1985.

Creative care unit: getting a grip on the situation, AJN 82(7):1115, 1982.

Davis L, McKemie FW, and McEnery PT: False crystalluria with superabsorbent disposable diapers, Am J Dis Child 142(6):586, 1988.

Driscoll WS et al: Prevalence of dental caries and dental fluorosis in areas with optimal and above-optimal water fluoride concentrations, JADA 107:42-47, 1983.

Feldman AL and Aretakis DA: Herpetic gingivostomatitis in children, Pediatr Nurs 12(2):111-113, 1986.

Gillies C: Infant colic: is there anything new? J Pediatr Health Care 1(6):305-312, 1987.
Hansen FH: Nursing care in the neonatal intensive care unit, JOGNN 11(1):17-20, 1982.
Hashimoto T: A comparison of the amount of dust produced by disposable and cloth diapers in incubators, Pediatrician 14(1):44-47, 1987.
Hathaway G et al: Clinical problem: mucositis, J Assoc Pediatr Oncol Nurs 3(3):23-34, 1986.
Henningsson A et al: Bathing or washing babies after birth? Lancet 19(26):1401-1403, 1981.
Hess CS et al: Fluoride: Too much or too little, Pediatr Nurs 10(6):397-403, 1984.
Hess CS et al: Fluoride and caries prevention, Child Nurs 4(2):1-4, 1986.
Hill EM et al: Sweetener content of common pediatric oral liquid medications, Am J Hosp Pharm 45(1):135-142, 1988.
Jackson MM et al: Why not treat all body substances as infectious? Am J Nurs 87(9):1137-1138, 1987.
Joyner M: Hair care in the black patient, J Pediatr Health Care 2(6):281-287, 1988.
Kronmiller JE and Nirschl RF: Preventive dentistry for children, Pediatr Nurs 11(6):446-449, 1985.
Krueger H and Osborn L: Effects of hygiene among the uncircumcised, J Fam Pract, 22(4):353-355, 1986.
Kuller JM, Lund C, and Tobin C: Improved skin care for premature infants, MCN 8(3):200-203, 1983.
Leyden J: Cornstarch, *Candida albicans,* and diaper rash, Pediatr Dermatol 1(4):322-325, 1984.
Loadman W et al: Reducing the symptoms of infant colic by introduction of a vibration/sound-based intervention, Pediatr Res 21(4):82A, 1987.
Martin RJ et al: Effect of supine and prone positions on arterial oxygen tension in the preterm infant, Pediatrics 63(4):528-531, 1979.
McCormick MA et al: Hazards associated with diaper changing, JAMA 248(17):2159-2160, 1982.
McDonald RE and Avery DR: Dentistry for the child and adolescent, ed 5, St Louis, 1987, The CV Mosby Co.
Merenstein GB and Gardner SL: Handbook of neonatal intensive care, ed 2, St Louis, 1989, The CV Mosby Co.
Miller AM and Norton BA: Skills for professional nursing practice, Norwalk, Conn, 1986, Appleton-Century-Crofts.
Muscari ME: Effective nursing strategies for adolescents with anorexia nervosa and bulimia nervosa, Pediatr Nurs 14(6):475-482, 1988.
Neifert M: Information from the experts: Dr. Neifert answers, Baby Talk, August, pp. 10-12, 1989.
Niehaus CS et al: Oral complications in children during cancer therapy, Cancer Nursing, 10(1):15-20, 1987.
Perry AG and Potter PA: Clinical nursing skills and techniques, ed 2, St Louis, 1990, The CV Mosby Co.
Perry AG and Potter PA: Fundamentals of nursing, ed 2, St Louis, 1989, The CV Mosby Co.
Rasmussen JE: Classification of diaper dermatitis: overview, Pediatrician 14(suppl 1):6-10, 1987.
Sasso SC: Erythromycin for eye prophylaxis, Am Matern Child Nurs J 9(6):417, 1984.
Starr RM and Gravitz RF: Pit and fissure sealants in the prevention of tooth decay, Pediatr Nurs 11(4):289-291, 1985.
Thomas KA: How the NICU environment sounds to a preterm infant, MCN 14(4):249-251, 1989.
Timely teaching for uncircumcised preschoolers, Am J Nurs 86(9):993, 1986.
Tomovitch T: Looking out for OTC hydrocortisone use, Patient Care 15:170-183, 1981.
Turick-Gibson T: Infant botulism, Pediatr Nurs 14(4):280-283, 1988.
Wagaman MJ et al: Improved oxygenation and lung compliance with prone positioning of neonates, J Pediatr 94(5):787-791, 1979.
Wagner TJ and Hindi-Alexander M: Hazards of baby powder, Pediatr Nurs 10(2):124-125, 1984.
Weibley, TT: Inside the incubator, MCN 14(2):96-100, 1989.
Weinstein LB et al: Increasing awareness of sugar ingestion among children, Pediatr Nurs 14(4):277-279, 1988.
Wells R and Trostle K: Creative hairwashing techniques for immobilized patients, Nursing 14(1):47-51, 1984.
Whaley LF and Wong DL: Essentials of pediatric nursing, ed 3, St Louis, 1989, The CV Mosby Co.
Whaley LF and Wong DL: Nursing care of infants and children, ed 4, St Louis, 1991, The CV Mosby Co.
Wiswell TE and Geschke DW: Risks from circumcision during the first month of life compared with those for uncircumcised boys, Pediatrics 83(6):1011-1015, 1989.
Wong DL and Whaley LF: Clinical manual of pediatric nursing, ed 3, St Louis, 1990, The CV Mosby Co.

# UNIT VIII Nutrition and Fluids

# SKILL 58 Selecting Age-related Foods

*Peggy J. Drapo*

Nutritional needs vary as children progress from infancy through childhood. The younger child needs and likes different amounts and types of foods than the older child. The child's feeding skills and physical condition must also be considered. While metabolic needs and personal preferences vary with growth periods, children must consume sufficient high quality protein, vitamins, minerals, and calories to provide for energy needs and growth. This skill focuses on information the nurse needs to provide a proper diet for the hospitalized child, as well as to provide anticipatory guidance to families for appropriate food selection throughout infancy and childhood.

**NURSING DIAGNOSES**

Altered nutrition: less than body requirements related to insufficient intake for metabolic needs; Altered nutrition: more than body requirements related to excessive intake for metabolic needs; Altered parenting related to lack of knowledge and/or resources to provide for child's nutritional needs; Altered growth and development related to nutritional deficiencies.

| Steps | Rationale |
|---|---|
| **Assessment** | |
| 1. Determine age and developmental status related to feeding skills, including fine and gross motor skills (see Table 61-1 on p. 393 for developmental sequences that affect feeding). | Food selection and feeding methods vary depending on child's age and motor/neurologic development. ***Special Considerations:*** *The feeding skills of developmentally disabled children may not match chronological age. (For the child with feeding difficulties related to developmental delay, see Skill 61.)* |
| 2. Assess nutritional status (see Skill 29). | Information related to food habits can indicate nutritional deficiencies (Eschelman, 1988) and guide food selection and teaching efforts. |
| a. Dietary intake, using assessment tools such as 24-hour diet recall, food frequency record, 3- or 7-day food diary. | ***Special Considerations:*** *Depth of assessment depends on present information needs, e.g., selecting nutritious meals for a hospitalized child, providing anticipatory guidance, or problem solving with a family.* |
| b. Family food preferences, including child's specific likes and dislikes; cultural, regional, and religious influences; and eating patterns. | Sensitivity to preferences and familiar food practices aids child's acceptance of the meal and helps to ensure that selected foods are consumed. Cultural and religious influences provide insights related to forbidden foods (e.g., pork for Jewish children) and frequently eaten foods (e.g., rice for Asian children, or beans and corn products for Mexican children) and usual mealtimes. ***Special Considerations:*** *Cultural factors may also play a part in the child's feeding skills. Individual families may vary in adherence to cultural practices (see Skill 41).* |
| c. Patterns of food purchasing and preparation, including adequacy of financial resources for obtaining food. | Financial resources may significantly influence ability to obtain food and follow dietary recommendations. |

| Steps | Rationale |
|---|---|

**TABLE 58-1** Dietary Treatments for Selected Genetic/Metabolic Disorders

| Condition | Cause | Signs/Symptoms | Treatment |
|---|---|---|---|
| 1. Lactose intolerance. | Lack of enzyme lactase or damage to site of lactase absorption. | Abdominal distension, cramps, diarrhea, and failure to thrive. | Lactose-free diet. Eliminate milk and milk products. Also bread, cake, cookies, etc. which use a milk base. For children, substitute formulas such as Prosobee, Soyalac, or Isomil. |
| 2. Sucrose intolerance. | Missing enzyme sucrase. | Diarrhea. | Eliminate all sugar, honey, and anything sweetened with sugar. Give sugar-free formulas, milk, meat, fish, eggs, vegetables, and cheese. Allow only one piece of fruit per day. |
| 3. Galactose/glucose malabsorption. | Missing enzyme to break down galactose. | Damage to kidney, brain, and eyes from high blood levels. Newborns develop jaundice, vomiting, convulsions, lethargy, bleeding difficulties, and blindness. | Dietary restriction such as for lactose except no galactose should be present in formulas. |
| 4. Fructose intolerance. | Missing enzyme aldolase. Fructose accumulates in liver. | Vomiting, diarrhea, abdominal pain, and failure to thrive. | Fructose-free diet (found in honey and fruit). Sorbitol products (found in "sugar-free" diabetic foods) metabolize to fructose and should be avoided. Avoid sucrose for same reason. Vitamin C and extra servings of vegetables should be given to replace the fruit in diets. |
| 5. Cystic fibrosis. | Autosomal recessive disorder associated with widespread dysfunction of exocrine system. | Thick, tenacious mucus secreted from glands causing obstruction or inefficiency of pancreatic enzymes. Causes poor absorption of protein, carbohydrates, and fats, flatulence, and foul-smelling stools. | Nutritionally adequate diet, especially protein, fat, and carbohydrates. Pancreatic enzyme replacement. |
| 6. Celiac disease. | Intolerance to gluten (the protein of wheat, rye, oats, and barley). | Chronic diarrhea, irritability, vomiting, abdominal distension, steatorrhea (fat in the stools), and failure to thrive. | Exclusion of gluten from diet. Supplements of Vitamin B group. May eat gluten-free products such as corn flour. |
| 7. Phenylketonuria (PKU). | Absence of enzyme that converts phenylalanine to tyrosine in the body. | Phenylalanine accumulates in the blood causing abnormal concentration in tissues; excessive concentration causes mental retardation. | Intake of low phenylalanine products such as Lofenalac with measured quantities of milk added. Older children have a vegetarian diet and protein substitutes, vitamins, and minerals. Frequent monitoring of blood serum levels. |

| Steps | Rationale |
|---|---|
| d. Child's physical growth (see Skill 28). | Growth measures provide a baseline for evaluation of adequacy of nutritional intake and assist in identifying significant deviation from norms. This data will directly impact both food selection and teaching. |
| 3. Review child's history for medical conditions requiring dietary restrictions or alterations, e.g., food allergies, phenylketonuria (PKU), or pregnancy (see Table 58-1 for selected genetic/metabolic disorders). | Conditions such as diabetes, cystic fibrosis, and PKU require dietary alterations as part of the medical regime. Disorders such as hypothyroidism may reduce the metabolic rate, altering caloric requirements. Other disorders, e.g., Prader-Willi Syndrome, may be the cause of overeating and eventual obesity (Greenswag, 1990). Nutritional requirements increase during pregnancy. Acute illness such as gastrointestinal disorder may require temporary alterations in the diet. |

| Steps | Rationale |
|---|---|
| 4. Determine if family has any specific concerns or questions related to child's intake, e.g., when to start cereals for an infant, or that a toddler is not eating an adequate variety of nutrients. | Identification of specific concerns can direct further assessment and teaching efforts. |

## Planning and Goal Setting

| Steps | Rationale |
|---|---|
| 1. Review nutritional needs for this child (see Table 58-2 for recommended daily intake). | A review of the child's nutritional needs allows evaluation of present intake and preparation for food selection and/or teaching. Nutrients to be analyzed include carbohydrates, proteins, fats, minerals, vitamins, fiber, and water. |
| 2. If teaching, review nutritional intake assessment and other assessment data for anticipatory guidance needs or for common or potential problems such as inadequate/excessive caloric intake, excess salt, fat, sweets, or nutritionless "junk" food. | Identification of potential or existing problems or areas for anticipatory guidance directs individualized teaching. |
| 3. Gather teaching materials, e.g., pamphlets or charts, if necessary. | Written materials and visual aids reinforce teaching. |
| 4. Develop individualized child and family goals:<br>▪ The child's nutritional intake is adequate for daily requirements.<br>▪ Appropriate foods are selected considering the child's stage of development and any existing health problems.<br>▪ The child/family exhibits adequate knowledge to provide for the child's nutritional needs. | |

## Implementation

| Steps | Rationale |
|---|---|
| 1. Develop an individualized food plan, selecting age-appropriate food, and/or discuss nutritional requirements and food selection with child/family (see Table 58-2 for amounts and selection alternatives). | Nutritional requirements should be adapted to individual preferences, needs, and health conditions. Long-term impact on dietary practices is accomplished only if the family and child have adequate nutritional knowledge. |
| ***0 to 3 months*** | |
| a. Provide breast milk or commercially prepared iron-fortified formula. Hold and cuddle infant during feeding. Do not prop bottles (see Skills 59 and 60). | Breast milk and formula are the only appropriate foods at this age. The American Academy of Pediatrics (1982) recommends breast milk as the ideal source of nutrition; an acceptable alternative is commercial iron-fortified formula. A young infant can easily choke and aspirate if formula bottles are propped.<br>***Special Considerations:*** *For the infant with a family history of allergy, breastfeeding is especially recommended to avoid triggering allergic reactions. Unmodified whole cow's milk is not recommended for the young infant, because the iron in cow's milk is poorly absorbed by the infant (James and Mott, 1988) and it is an inferior source of vitamin C; it also places the infant at risk for enteric blood loss and exposure to chemicals used by farmers as pesticides. Goat's milk is low in vitamins C and D, folic acid and iron. If using a cow's milk-based formula, suspect an allergy if rash (eczema), irritability, vomiting, or diarrhea presents.* |
| b. If exclusively breast-fed, if no water is used to prepare formula, or if water supply contains less that 0.3 ppm fluoride, provide supplemental fluoride of 0.25 mg per day (see Skill 56). | Breast milk and formula do not contain fluoride; if fluoride is not ingested by the infant (e.g., in concentrated or powdered formula mixed with fluoridated water), then supplementation is necessary before eruption of teeth to achieve maximum dental benefits (Hess et al, 1984). |
| c. For breast-fed infant, provide vitamin D supplement (400 IU/day) if infant has inadequate exposure to ultraviolet light, either because of lack of sunlight or dark skin color. | Available vitamin D may be insufficient in these situations. Adequate amounts are necessary for absorption of calcium and phosphorus for bone and teeth mineralization. Vitamin D deficiency may cause rickets. |
| d. Discourage the use of infant cereals to promote sleeping at night. | Macknin, Medendorp, and Maier (1989) found no relationship between sleeping through the night and introduction of rice cereal at 5 weeks versus 4 months of age.<br>***Special Considerations:*** *Feedings thickened with rice cereal are sometimes prescribed for reflux, although the benefits are unproven (see Skill 63).* |

***TABLE 58-2*** Recommended Daily Intake

| | Birth-3 months | 4-5 months | 6-12 months | 12-18 months |
|---|---|---|---|---|
| **CALORIC REQUIREMENTS** | | | | |
| Kilocalories | 115 kcal/kg/day. | 115 kcal/kg/day. | 105 kcal/kg/day. | 100 kcal/kg/day |
| **PROTEIN REQUIREMENTS** | | | | |
| Grams | 13 g/day. | 13 g/day. | 14 g/day. | 16 g/day. |
| **MILK GROUP** | **BREAST MILK OR IRON-FORTIFIED COMMERCIAL FORMULA:** | | | |
| ½ cup whole milk = ¾ oz cheese, ½ cup yogurt or pudding, 1 cup cottage cheese, ¾-1 cup ice cream | 2-4 oz every 2-4 hrs, gradually increased to 5-6 oz every 4-5 hrs. | 6-8 oz, 4-5 times daily. | 24-32 oz daily gradually decreased to 18-24 oz. | 3-4 servings of ½-¾ cup each. |
| **MEAT GROUP** | | | | |
| 1 oz meat = 1 egg, 1 oz cheese, 2 Tbs peanut butter, ¼ cup tuna, ½ cup cooked legumes | — | — | 2 servings of strained meats of 1-2 Tbs each. | 2 servings of 1-2 oz each. |
| **VEGETABLE, FRUIT GROUP** | — | — | 2 servings of 1-2 Tbs each. | 3-4 servings of 2-3 Tbs each. |
| Vitamin A sources: deep yellow and dark green fruits and vegetables | — | — | 1 serving every other day or | |
| Vitamin C sources: citrus fruit, melons, strawberries, broccoli, tomatoes, cabbage, vitamin C fortified juices | — | — | | At least 1 |
| **BREAD/CEREAL GROUP** | | | | |
| 1 slice bread = ¾ cup dry cereal, ½ cup cooked pasta, rice, or cereal, ½ hamburger bun, 1 small muffin or biscuit | — | Dry, iron-fortified infant cereal, 2 servings of approximately 2 Tbs each. | Dry, iron-fortified infant cereal, 2 servings of 2-4 Tbs each. Gradually add other products. | 4 servings of ½ slice bread each. Continue iron-fortified cereal for 2 or 4 servings daily. |

| Steps | Rationale |
|---|---|
| ***4 to 5 months*** | |
| a. Continue breast milk or formula. Continue vitamin/mineral supplements as for younger infant. | Breast milk or commercial iron-fortified formula should be the primary source of milk for the first year of life. ***Special Considerations:*** *For the lactating mother returning to work or for convenience, see the box on p. 388 in Skill 60.* |
| b. May begin dry, iron-fortified infant cereal, approximately 2 Tbs twice daily. Mix cereal with milk to consistency of thin paste and warm slightly. | Prenatal iron stores begin to diminish at 4 to 5 months; cereal provides a nutritious source of iron. |
| ▪ Start with rice cereal; other single grain types may be gradually added to diet. Introduce mixed grain cereal last. | Rice cereal is introduced first since it is usually easily digested and has a low allergenic potential. |
| ▪ Feed with a small, straight-handled spoon, placing it toward the back of the tongue. Expect much of the cereal to be pushed out by the tongue; scoop up and refeed. Avoid adding cereal to bottles or feeding with "bottle feeder." | The extrusion reflex is still present, making spoon feeding a slow process. However, giving cereal by bottle or "bottle feeder" deprives the infant of important feeding experiences for needed development of oral musculature; it can also contribute to overfeeding and/or choking. |

| 1½-3 years | 4-6 years | 7-10 years | Adolescents |
|---|---|---|---|
| 1300 kcal/day. | 1800 kcal/day. | 2100 kcal/day. | 11-14 yrs.: 2400 kcal/day.<br>15-18 yrs.: Males—3000 kcal/day.<br>Females—2100 kcal/day. |
| 16 g/day. | 24 g/day. | 28 g/day. | 11-14 yrs.: 45 g/day.<br>15-18 yrs.: Males—59 g/day.<br>Females—44 g/day. |
| 3-4 servings of ½-¾ cup each. | 3-4 servings of ¾ cup each. | 3-4 servings of 1 cup each. | 4 servings of 1 cup each. |
| 2 servings of 1-2 oz each. | 2 servings of 1-2 oz each. | 2 servings of 2-3 oz each. | 2 or more servings of 3-4 oz each. |
| 4 servings of 3-4 Tbs each.<br>at least three to four servings weekly.<br><br>serving daily. | 4 servings of ¼ cup each. | 4 servings of ¼-½ cup each. | 4 or more servings of ½ cup each. |
| 4 servings of ½ slice bread each. | 4 servings of 1 slice bread each. | 4 servings of 1-2 slices bread each. | 4 or more servings of 2 slices bread each. |

| Steps | Rationale |
|---|---|
| | ***Special Considerations:*** *The unnecessary addition of other solids before 6 months of age adds excess calories, imposes a heavy renal solute load, and increases water demands (James and Mott, 1988).* |

***6 to 8 months***

a. Continue breast milk or formula. Infant may be able to hold own bottle, but should still be held for feedings. Discourage allowing child to take a bottle to bed; if permitted, bottle should contain only water (see Skill 56).

Development of gross motor skills at this age usually includes being able to hold bottle and remove it from mouth when finished. However, holding and cuddling is still needed to meet emotional and socialization needs. Also, lying flat while sucking from a bottle allows milk to pool in the pharynx, providing a medium for bacterial growth. This bacteria may then enter the eustachian tube, predisposing the infant to middle ear infections. The pooled milk or juice also bathes teeth and gums with sugars during sleep, leading to "nursing bottle caries."

| Steps | Rationale |
|---|---|
| b. Provide dry, iron-fortified infant cereal: 2 servings of 2 to 4 Tbs/day. | For infants 6 to 12 months of age, the RDA for iron is 15 mg/day. Three to four tablespoons of dry infant cereal provides 7 mg of elemental iron, thus two servings per day will meet iron requirements. **Special Considerations:** *Avoid wet-pack infant cereals, which are lower in iron.* |
| c. May begin apple or other non-citrus fruit juices: 1 to 2 oz and increasing to 4 oz daily. Offer juices in a cup. | The infant is now able to approximate lips to a cup and form a seal. Encouraging drinking of juices from a cup may help to reduce development of "nursing bottle mouth" and promotes bottle weaning. |
| d. Begin strained fruits, vegetables, and meats, using a small, straight-handled spoon and placing food toward the back of the tongue. | Around 6 months, the infant is ready both physiologically and developmentally for solid foods. The digestive system is sufficiently developed to handle foreign proteins and to produce enzymes necessary for absorption and use of specific nutrients (James and Mott, 1988). The previous strong tongue thrust progresses into lateral movement by 6 months, allowing improved spoon feeding. Head and neck control is developed, allowing the infant to sit with support and turn head away to express disinterest in food. |
| e. Introduce only one new food per week. Avoid egg whites, wheat (gluten) products, cow's milk and milk products, citrus fruits and juices, tomatoes, strawberries, corn syrup solids, seafood (protein and iodine), spices, and chocolate in early feedings. | Isolating foods during introduction allows easier identification of any food intolerance or allergies. The listed foods to avoid are more likely to trigger allergic responses or be poorly tolerated. **Special Considerations:** *Signs of food allergy include rash (eczema), irritability, vomiting, or diarrhea.* |
| f. Commercially prepared baby foods may be used; avoid combination dinners and desserts. Baby food may also be prepared at home by steaming unseasoned food in a small amount of water, then pureeing in blender or food grinder/processor along with cooking liquids. Avoid canned foods, or home prepared beets, spinach, collard greens or turnips. See also the box on p. 380 in Skill 59. | Commercial baby foods are convenient and contain no added salt. Commercial combination dinners are a poor source of protein; dinners and desserts are high in carbohydrates and calories, and low in nutritional value. Home-prepared baby foods are more economical and relatively simple to prepare. All cooking liquid must be used to avoid loss of water-soluble vitamins. Canned foods are high in sodium and may be a source of lead from the container. Home-prepared beets, spinach, collard greens, and turnips may contain excessive nitrates (Austin, 1989), which increase the risk of methemoglobinemia in infants. |
| g. Introduce large finger foods, e.g., crackers, wafer cookies, and sliced bananas. | A beginning pincer grasp and coordination of hand-to-mouth movements allow manipulation of large finger foods. Few teeth and limited experience with solids make choking and aspiration a high risk. Foods easily softened by saliva help prevent this risk (James and Mott, 1988). |
| h. Avoid honey as a sweetener for food or on pacifiers. | Impure honey may cause infant botulism (Long, 1985). |
| ***9 to 12 months*** | |
| a. Continue breast milk or formula, but gradually reduce number of feedings, offering more liquids by cup. Continue to discourage taking a bottle to bed. | The infant is generally ready for weaning at about 1 year of age, if given the opportunity. **Special Considerations:** *Whole cow's milk may be given after 7 months of age if at least one third of the child's total caloric intake consists of a balanced mixture of supplemental foods (cereals, vegetables, etc.) to ensure adequate sources of vitamin C and iron (American Academy of Pediatrics, 1983).* |
| b. Continue iron-fortified infant cereals. | Infants continue to need significant amounts of iron from one or more sources during the first year. |
| c. Begin providing more textured foods such as finely chopped table foods, or commercial "junior foods." | With the eruption of teeth and development of oral feeding skills, the child is ready for textured foods to facilitate development of the oral musculature and provide sensory "chewing" experience. **Special Considerations:** *To promote development of self-feeding skills, give the child a separate spoon while feeding, and praise attempts to feed self.* |
| d. Introduce a three meals per day pattern of eating. | Milk is decreasing as the primary source of nutrition. Introduction of set mealtimes assists in socializing the infant to family life. **Special Considerations:** *A large hospital food tray may overwhelm a small child. Instead, place appropriate portions on a small plate.* |

| Steps | Rationale |
|---|---|
| e. Introduce small finger foods such as Cheerios, cooked vegetables, cheese cubes, hot dogs (sliced, quartered and with casing removed), peeled and diced apples or peaches. Avoid nuts, popcorn, raw vegetables (especially carrots), grapes, and hard candy. | Motor skills are becoming more refined, but choking is still a hazard, especially with hard foods that do not soften with saliva or round foods that may lodge in the trachea or esophagus. |
| f. Avoid high-fat foods such as gravy, bacon, and fried foods. | Fats are hard for the infant to digest, high in calories, and low in nutritional value. |
| ***Toddler*** | |
| a. Begin whole milk, and complete weaning from bottle. Limit milk intake to 16 to 24 oz daily. Discourage low-fat or skim milk until age 2. | A toddler still needs the fatty acids in whole milk for growth and development. Also, skim milk increases the renal solute load. Excessive milk intake makes the child less hungry for solid foods, leading to nutritional deficiencies. |
| b. Continue to offer iron-fortified infant cereals, two servings per day of approximately 1/4 cup (dry) each, along with other breads and cereals. | Dry iron-fortified infant cereals are recommended through the second year of life to meet iron requirements. |
| c. Gradually change to table food. Suitable foods include canned fruits, well-cooked vegetables, liverwurst, well-cooked ground meats, minced chicken liver, drained tuna, custards, and puddings. Continue to avoid excessive fat, salt, and sugar intake. Avoid spicy foods. Continue to avoid small hard or round foods. Expect a decreased appetite. | The growth rate slows during this period thus reducing calorie and protein needs. Spicy foods may be poorly tolerated and are often disliked by toddlers. Choking on food is still a high risk.<br>***Special Considerations:*** *Toddlers may be picky eaters with strong taste preferences. Appetite and food preferences tend to be sporadic with "food jags" being common. Toddlers also tend to dislike mixed foods such as stews and casseroles. Avoid making an issue of eating to diffuse power struggles but continue to offer a balanced diet. Also, avoid introducing new foods to the hospitalized child, unless a long-term stay is required (Dickey, 1987).* |
| d. Offer nutritious snacks between meals such as fruits, cheeses, crackers, and peanut butter. | The toddler's stomach capacity is small, making small, frequent meals desirable. If nutritious snacks are given, there is less need for concern if the child eats less at mealtime.<br>***Special Considerations:*** *Do not force a child to eat, and do not use food as a punishment or reward for behavior at any age.* |
| e. Encourage the child's use of a cup and spoon, but expect frequent spills. | Fine motor skills are improving, and independence is an important developmental task for the toddler. |
| ***Preschooler*** | |
| a. Provide diet from the four basic food groups. A general guideline for minimum serving size is 1 tablespoon for each year of age for each food served. | The preschooler needs a balanced diet that meets nutritional needs. Quality is generally more important than quantity because exact amounts of foods eaten will vary depending on the child's appetite.<br>***Special Considerations:*** *Table manners may become an issue. The 3- to 4-year-old child is not developmentally ready to sit quietly through a long meal. By 5 to 6 years of age the child should be better able to participate in mealtime socialization.* |
| b. Low-fat or skim milk may be introduced after 2 years of age. To meet caloric needs, three fat servings daily may be provided, e.g., 1 tsp butter or margarine, 1 slice bacon, 1 Tbs salad dressing. Discourage excessive fat intake. | Cholesterol intake is an important consideration even for young children. More than 10% of the children in the U.S. have elevated total blood cholesterol levels (Davidson et al, 1989). Avoiding excessive fat intake early prevents establishing a habit of high-fat intake.<br>***Special Considerations:*** *Bacon is considered a fat, not a meat serving.* |
| c. Sweets, chips, and other high fat/salt/sugar-low nutrient foods should be limited to 1 to 2 servings daily and offered only after basic diet requirements are met. | Excessive intake of these foods may cause reduced intake of more nutritious foods, leading to diet deficiencies and excess weight gain.<br>***Special Considerations:*** *Ice cream, puddings, and fruit cobblers have desirable nutrients, although sugar and fat content is high. Yogurt, raisins, and graham crackers may be satisfying to the child in place of sweet desserts.* |
| d. Continue fluoride supplements as recommended (see Skill 57). | Fluoride helps make the enamel more resistant to caries (Hess et al, 1984). |

| Steps | Rationale |
|---|---|
| ***School-age child*** | |
| a. Provide diet from the four basic food groups. Gradually increase portion size. | Caloric and protein requirements increase as the child grows. |
| b. Continue to avoid excessive intake of fats, desserts, and other "junk" foods. | ***Special Considerations:*** *Peer pressure becomes an increasingly important influence on food selection as the child becomes more independent from the parents. Good nutrition becomes a joint responsibility of both child and parent. This is an excellent age to teach children about healthy foods.* |
| ***Adolescent*** | |
| a. Provide balanced diet from the four basic food groups. Caloric requirements are increased, particularly for males. | Growth and maturation are occurring rapidly with significant body changes. Protein and iron needs are increased. Choice of foods is strongly influenced by peers. Diet and body image are closely related. ***Special Considerations:*** *The family should try to be flexible to the adolescent's personal choices about food (Dickey, 1987). Pregnant teens require added calories and nutrients. Vitamin A, calcium, iron, and total calories are common deficiencies for a pregnant teenager. Diet should be evaluated in early pregnancy, and diet counseling should be provided frequently.* |
| 2. If teaching, develop diet plan with family and child. Provide written materials and visual aids. | Involvement of family and child in development of a food plan promotes compliance. Written materials reinforce teaching. |
| 3. Provide resources and referral if finances are inadequate to obtain a nutritious diet. | Governmental programs, e.g., food stamps and the Special Supplemental Feeding Program for Women, Infants and Children (WIC), may assist low-income families in attaining an adequate diet. In addition, WIC provides nutrition education for all participants. |
| 4. Refer and/or collaborate with other health professionals, e.g., nutritionist, physician, psychologist, or speech pathologist, if the child has conditions requiring dietary alterations, restrictions, or counseling beyond the scope of nursing practice. | A nutritionist can provide more in-depth nutritional counseling. The physician will prescribe required medical regimes for conditions such as diabetes, PKU, celiac disease, or food allergies. A psychologist may assist the child/family with emotional problems such as failure to thrive, anorexia nervosa, bulimia, or obesity. A speech pathologist may assist children with delayed feeding skills related to oral motor problems such as cerebral palsy or cleft palate. |

| Evaluation Outcomes | Observational Guidelines |
|---|---|
| 1. Child's nutritional intake meets daily requirements. | Compare daily intake to recommended requirements in Table 58-2. Weigh daily/weekly, compare to baseline, previous weights, and/or growth charts. |
| 2. Foods are selected based on child's stage of growth and development, personal preferences, and any health problems requiring a special diet. | Note appropriateness of selected food compared to recommendations for age, and individual assessment factors. Note adherence to special diet regimen. Observe amount of selected food/diet consumed; question child (if possible) regarding selections not eaten. |
| 3. Child and family possess adequate knowledge and resources to provide for child's nutritional needs. | Child and/or family are able to discuss nutritional requirements of the child. Family is able to plan 3-day menu that is appropriate to child's age and meets recommendations for daily intake. If financial resources are inadequate, referral to appropriate agencies is made. |

## Documentation

Document the nutritional assessment. For food selection, note type of feeding or food the child received and toleration of feeding or meal. Specify amounts of food/liquids consumed. For teaching to child/family, document topics discussed, written materials provided, and evaluation of goal achievement, e.g., the family was able to plan an appropriate 3-day menu for the child. The individualized food plan is recorded.

### Child and Family Teaching

1. Discuss strategies to reduce fat intake. For example, use yogurt and cheeses that are low- or nonfat; ice milk, low-fat frozen yogurt, or frozen fruit juice bars instead of ice cream; bake or broil meats instead of frying; bake or steam vegetables; boil or poach eggs; use 2%, 1%, ½% or skim milk, gradually working to a lower content to facilitate transition; avoid snack foods and candy that are high in fat such as chips and chocolate bars, substituting lower fat snacks such as pretzels, popcorn, hard candies, and fresh fruits. Teach the family how to interpret fat content on food labels. Making changes gradually is easier, e.g., alternate serving ice cream with frozen low-fat yogurt until ice cream is only an occasional treat.
2. Discuss the value of exercise in controlling weight by increasing body metabolism. Very low-calorie diets are not recommended for children because the low intake can lead to muscle loss, not fat loss, and retard growth.
3. For the child who needs to increase caloric intake, e.g., child with a malabsorption syndrome, suggest nutritious foods and a balanced diet with increased total calories. Some examples include fruit pies, butter and jelly on toast, whole milk, ice cream, puddings, peanut butter with crackers, and fried chicken.
4. To restrict sodium intake, e.g., for children with renal or cardiovascular problems, or weight reducing programs, suggest the use of herbs instead of salt to flavor foods. One mixture is *Herb Shaker:* mix 2 tsp of garlic powder (not garlic salt) with ½ tsp of one of the following—curry, dry mustard, paprika, basil, marjoram, thyme, mace, onion powder, pepper, or sage. Teach families how to read for the sodium content on food labels; most processed foods have a high sodium content.

# *SKILL* 59 Feeding with a Bottle and Burping

*Lynda Lowe Odaffer*

The majority of parents in the United States will choose to feed their infants entirely by bottle, as a supplement to breastfeeding, or after weaning from the breast. The bottle-fed infant will require special considerations when ill. Nurses have a unique opportunity to teach the family about bottle feeding in special situations to increase the family's confidence, esteem, and attachment to the infant.

### NURSING DIAGNOSES

Altered nutrition: less than body requirements related to insufficient intake for metabolic needs; Altered nutrition: more than body requirements related to excessive intake for metabolic needs; Altered parenting related to lack of knowledge about infant satiety cues, preparation, storage and/or administration of bottle feedings.

| Steps | Rationale |
|---|---|
| **Assessment** | |
| 1. Assess infant's health history and present condition.<br>a. Age.<br>b. Physiologic and developmental status.<br>c. Previous feeding experience and problems.<br>d. Current feeding ability.<br>e. Scheduled treatments.<br>f. Procedure or medications.<br>g. Presence of family members. | Numerous factors influence feeding abilities and nutritional requirements. Early identification of special needs facilitates appropriate individualized care and prevents additional problems.<br>***Special Considerations:*** *With neonates, assess maternal drug use during labor and at birth, as drugs crossover to fetus and may temporarily affect neonatal behavioral status, interest in feeding, and coordination of sucking and swallowing.* |
| 2. Determine:<br>a. Type of formula.<br>b. Nipple preferred.<br>c. Frequency and amount of feedings.<br>d. Positioning for feeding.<br>e. Special equipment needed. | Knowledge of recommended formula and infant's usual feeding behavior ensures compatible product formulation, enhances feelings of familiarity, and minimizes stress during feeding, thus increasing formula intake.<br>***Special Considerations:*** *See Table 58-2 for usual feeding amount and frequency during infancy.* |

| Steps | Rationale |
|---|---|
| 3. Observe during feeding for:<br>a. Positioning of head above stomach.<br>b. Nipple on top of tongue.<br>c. Efforts to enhance sucking.<br>d. Response to satiation cues.<br>e. Burping and positioning on completion of feeding. | During hospitalization, the family's desire to feed their infant may vary depending on their fatigue level. Validating family's knowledge reveals areas to reinforce, modify, and add when teaching. |
| 4. Assess family's ability to purchase formula and supplies. | Identification of family's resources enables referrals to local financial assistance programs. |
| 5. Validate family's knowledge about preparing and storing formula and care of equipment (see Home Care Modifications). | Validation verifies family uses safe measures with formula feeding. |

### TIPS ON INFANT FOOD PURCHASING, PREPARATION, AND STORAGE

Inform parents that:

1. Reading food labels before purchasing will identify undesired ingredients (e.g., sugar, sodium, additives, preservatives, and/or allergenic substances).
2. Unopened jars of commercially prepared infant food can be stored indefinitely at room temperature.
3. When opening jar, listen for the popping sound of the seal to know that the food is safe to use.
4. If infant is fed directly from the jar, bacteria is introduced through the infant's saliva, which necessitates discarding unused portion at the end of a feeding. To minimize waste, pour the expected amount for a feeding into a bowl and feed infant. The remainder can be refrigerated and used up to 24 hours (Bobak and Jensen, 1987).
5. Commercially dried, prepared infant foods come in single portion servings that minimize waste of unused food. Dilute only if the label instructs.
6. When transporting food that needs to be refrigerated, take unopened jars of juice and food if possible, and open just before feeding, or keep food in an ice cooler (Whaley and Wong, 1991).

## Planning and Goal Setting

| Steps | Rationale |
|---|---|
| 1. Collect equipment and supplies:<br>a. Formula.<br>b. Bottle (check glass for cracks).<br>c. Disposable liner, if indicated.<br>d. Nipple (check for intactness and collapsibility).<br>e. A clean, soft cotton cloth for burping. | Collecting all supplies beforehand saves time and improves efficiency.<br>***Special Considerations:*** *When teaching family, supplement with audiovisual aids, e.g., films, pamphlets, flip charts, feeding equipment, and doll or infant to facilitate learning.* |
| 2. Arrange teaching around family convenience and feeding times. | Collaboration between family and health care team increases receptivity and goal attainment. |
| 3. Plan for an environment that is quiet, private, comfortable, and free of distractions. | A therapeutic setting enhances learning by increasing relaxation, comprehension, and retention of information. |
| 4. Develop individualized child and family goals:<br>▪ Infant's nutritional needs will be met.<br>▪ Family will demonstrate safe and correct techniques when formula feeding.<br>▪ Family concerns related to bottle feeding are promptly identified and managed. | |

## Implementation

| Steps | Rationale |
|---|---|
| 1. Recognize infant's hunger cues: awake state, smacking lips, rooting, bringing fingers to mouth, or vocalizing. | Infants feed more eagerly when in quiet alert state.<br>***Special Considerations:*** *Infants who are preterm or experience jaundice, infection, pain, fatigue, analgesia, or neurologic problems often require sensory stimulation for arousal: talking to, rubbing head, palms, soles, patting legs, unwrapping and/or sitting up in lap. Do not unwrap infants with labile temperatures.* |
| 2. Check bottle label for expiration date and formula type. | Giving incorrect formula may lead to adverse reactions or nutritional deficits. Outdated formula may be inadequate in vitamins and minerals. |
| 3. Shake bottle and screw on appropriate sterile nipple. | Shaking reconstitutes formula and nutrients. Using a sterile nipple minimizes microorganisms and pathogens infant will be exposed to during feeding. |

| Steps | Rationale |
|---|---|
| 4. Give formula at room temperature. Warm refrigerated formula by placing bottle in pan or large cup of warm water and periodically shaking. | Warming formula to room temperature may encourage infant to suck. Using hot water or a microwave can lead to hot spots in formula and burning. Overheating also destroys some vitamins and plastic bottle liners may develop leaks or split (Martell, 1987; Nemethy and Clore, 1990). |
| 5. Before feeding, hold bottle upside down to test formula temperature on inside of wrist or forearm and observe rate at which formula drips. | The wrist and forearm are more sensitive to temperature than fingers or hand. Formula released in steady drops facilitates ingestion.<br>***Special Considerations:*** *If bottle has to be shaken to release formula, more energy is required to feed. Formula flowing in a stream may lead to gulping, choking and/or swallowing air, which may compromise respiratory or gastrointestinal status.* |
| 6. Rather than propping bottle, cradle infant in arms with head slightly above stomach. | Holding infant close during feedings provides security and sensory stimulation, enhancing ingestion. Keeping head above stomach during feedings decreases choking, reflux, and minimizes fluids entering the eustachian tube, which may lead to otitis media (Whaley and Wong, 1991; Bobak and Jensen, 1987).<br>***Special Considerations:*** *Some infants begin rooting when held close, making it difficult to introduce the nipple. It may be necessary to hold infant away from body until infant latches onto nipple. Infants with poor suck-swallow coordination, esophageal reflux, or pyloric stenosis may need to be held more upright using gravity to enhance ingestion. Infants in intensive care, traction, or with a myelomeningocele may need to be fed in their incubator or crib. The infant's head can be elevated above the stomach by raising the head of the bed, placing blanket rolls under infant's head and chest, or placing an arm under neck and/or shoulders, or supporting head with hand and elbow on bed.* |
| 7. Rub nipple along lower lip and down chin. | Rubbing nipple around the oral area stimulates infant to open mouth and grasp nipple.<br>***Special Considerations:*** *Preterm infants may latch on and suck better when environment is quiet and dim.* |
| 8. Place nipple on top of tongue. | Placing nipple on top of tongue, against roof of mouth, enables adequate sucking and swallowing. |
| 9. Hold bottle at an angle so formula fills nipple neck. | Angling the bottle so that formula fills the nipple neck reduces air swallowing. |
| 10. Determine sucking pattern, interest, and status throughout feeding. | Early changes in feeding behavior, which are particularly significant in preterm or ill infants, may indicate developing problems such as infection, respiratory or cardiac distress, and/or changes in intracranial pressure (Whaley and Wong, 1991).<br>***Special Considerations:*** *Use a softer nipple or one with two holes (such as a preemie nipple) to enable tired, preterm, postsurgical, and congenital-heart infants to ingest milk more easily. Use a firm nipple with smaller holes to slow milk flow and reduce choking and regurgitating in infants with low muscle tone, esophageal reflux, and pyloric stenosis.* |
| 11. Attempt to burp infant after every ½ oz to 1 oz and at end of feeding. | Burping helps remove air swallowed during feeding and prevents abdominal distension and discomfort (Whaley and Wong, 1991). |
| a. Place a clean, soft cotton cloth under infant's chin. | Using a clean, soft cloth decreases brushing pathogens across mouth and is less irritating to skin when wet burps or reflux occurs. |
| b. Position infant in lap and support chin and trunk with one hand and arm (Fig. 59-1). | Sitting up in lap allows for continuous observation. Supporting chin and trunk facilitates burping (Bobak and Jensen, 1987). |
| c. Firmly and slowly rub or pat back from lower back upward along either side of spine. | Slowly and firmly rubbing or patting upward promotes release of swallowed air.<br>***Special Considerations:*** *To burp infants with myelomeningocele or a cast over their back, place infant in prone position and rub gently between the shoulders/scapulae or rock on a firm surface (Riordan, 1983). Infants with pyloric stenosis or esophageal reflux must be carefully handled and gently patted after every ½ oz or every 5 minutes during a feeding to prevent reflux or vomiting.* |

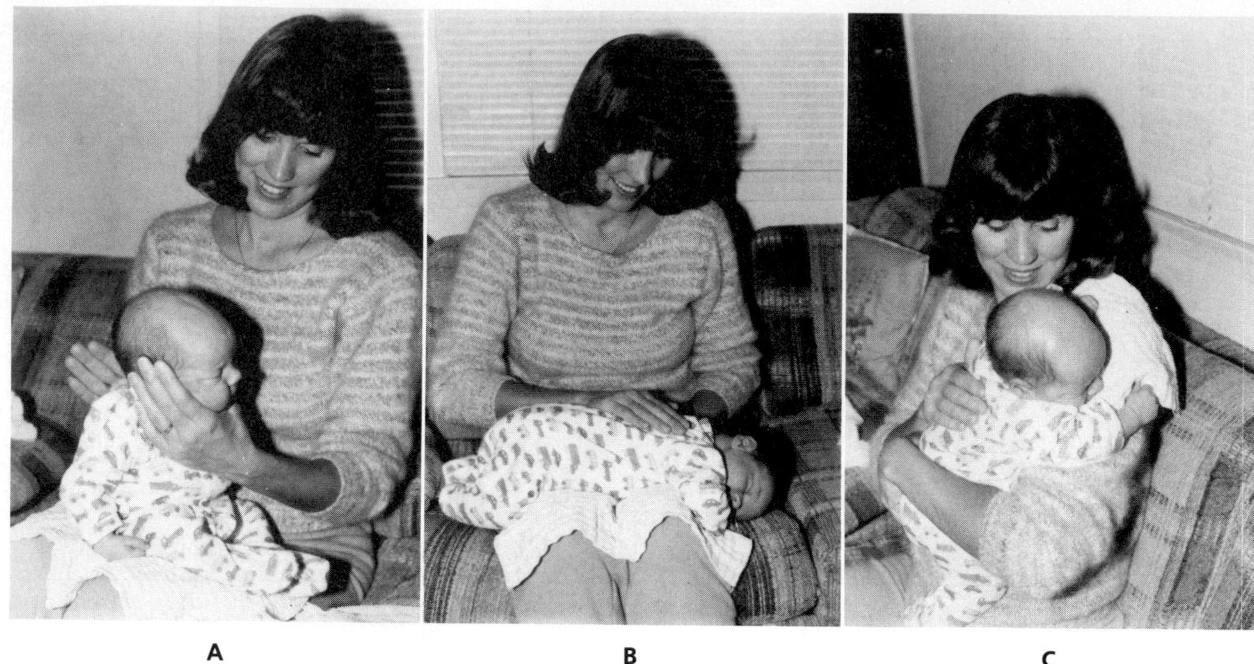

**FIG. 59-1** Positions for burping a baby. **A,** Upright. **B,** Across the lap. **C,** Shoulder position.
From Bobak I and Jensen M: Maternity and gynecologic care, ed 4, St Louis, 1989, The CV Mosby Company.

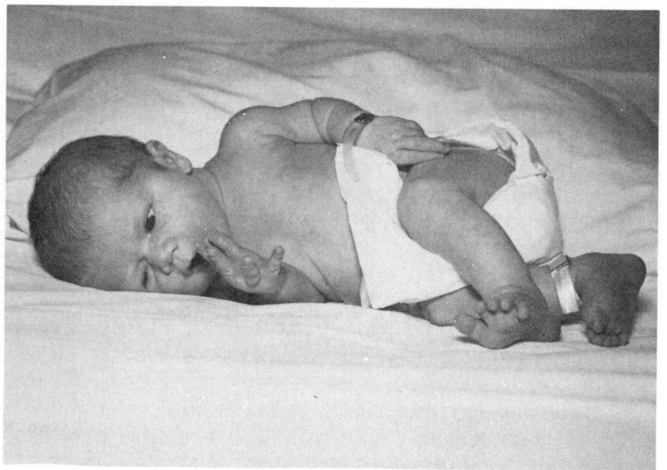

**FIG. 59-2** Right-side lying position after feeding.
From Whaley LF and Wong DL: Nursing care of infants and children, ed 4, St Louis, 1991, The CV Mosby Co.

| Steps | Rationale |
|---|---|
| 12. Respond to satiety cues (sucking slows or stops, infant refuses bottle after burping, falls asleep or appears peaceful if awake after feeding). | Acknowledging signs of satiety prevents infant from overfeeding and developing poor eating habits early in life (Whaley and Wong, 1991). |
| 13. Position on the right side with support behind back or place infant in prone position after feeding (Fig. 59-2). | These positions facilitate expelling swallowed air and help prevent regurgitation or aspiration of stomach contents (Whaley and Wong, 1991). |
| 14. Discard remaining formula at end of feeding. | Discarding excess formula prevents reuse and ingestion of rapidly multiplying bacteria that have entered the bottle during feeding (Whaley and Wong, 1991). |
| 15. Do not give bottle in bed at naptime or bedtime. | During sleep saliva decreases. Formula given over a few hours allows sucrose to bathe the teeth, causing caries to develop (McDermott and McCormack, 1986). |
| 16. Teach family techniques for bottle feeding. | Teaching family these techniques will increase their ability to feed the infant safely and increase their confidence. |

## Evaluation Outcomes

1. Infant's nutritional needs are met.
2. Family demonstrates safe, correct techniques when preparing, storing, giving formula, and caring for equipment.
3. Family's bottle feeding concerns are identified early and resolved.

## Observational Guidelines

Assess infant's health and behavior, review anthropometric measurements and/or lab data to determine nutritional status.

Observe a bottle feeding. Interview family about preparation, storage of formula, and caring for equipment.

Have family state concerns and resolutions.

## Documentation

Record on infant's chart: type of formula given, amount, time, infant's toleration of feeding, burps, positioning after feeding, and any adverse effects (choking, reflux, vomiting, decreased or lack of interest, suck dysfunctions). After teaching family, record specific information given, both verbally and in writing, and feeding supplies provided, validation of family's understanding (verbalization or return demonstration), points needing reinforcement, and referrals made (if any).

## Home Care Modifications

1. Ready-to-feed bottles and disposable nipples are not economical for frequent use at home. The family will usually prepare formula from liquid concentrate or powder in reusable bottles.
2. Wash all equipment in top rack of dishwasher, bottle sterilizer, or clean sink. When using a sink, use hot, soapy water and friction, and rinse in hot water to reduce microorganisms. Squeeze water through nipples during washing and rinsing. Air dry bottles and nipples on a clean towel.
3. Clean bottles and nipples for a full day's feedings for time and cost efficiency.
4. Before opening, wash top of formula cans with hot, soapy water, then rinse and dry to decrease pathogens.
5. Follow health professional's and manufacturer's recommendations when preparing formula.
   a. Use clean technique.
   b. If a clean water supply and refrigeration are not available or if infant's immune system is immature or deficient, the aseptic (sterile) technique should be used instead of the clean technique (Martell, 1987). See Bobak and Jensen (1987) for specific guidelines on sterilizing formula, bottles and nipples.
   c. Shake liquid formula to reconstitute nutrients.
   d. Use a clean can opener to open.
   e. Ready-to-feed formula should be given without dilution to ensure availability of nutrients and avoid dehydration or decreased weight gain. Measuring powder without packing it into a spoon prevents overconcentration, overfeeding, and high renal solute load (Bobak and Jensen, 1987).
   f. Measure and mix according to label instructions.
   g. Pour about ½ oz more into each bottle than what infant usually drinks.
   h. Place nipples pointing down into bottles with caps and collars on top. If using bottles with disposable liners, place bottle cover on top of nipple.
   i. If not using immediately, tightly cover bottles, refrigerate, and use within 24 hours or discard to decrease risk of introducing microorganisms, which cause gastrointestinal distress (Martell, 1987).
   j. Date, tightly cover, and promptly refrigerate opened cans of liquid formula. Use opened liquid formula within 48 hours and opened powdered formula within 1 month (Whaley and Wong, 1991).
6. Safely transport prepared formula:
   a. Ready-to-feed formula manufactured in sterile bottles can be stored at room temperature until the expiration date on label or bottle seal is broken.
   b. Prepared formula that is at room temperature should be used within one hour or discarded. For longer periods, the formula should be kept in a small cooler that maintains the same temperature as a refrigerator.

# SKILL 60 Supporting Breastfeeding in Special Situations

*Lynda Lowe Odaffer*

Professional literature has cited numerous advantages of breastfeeding for both mother and infant. The committee on Nutrition of the American Academy of Pediatrics (AAP) recommends that ideally breastmilk be the source of nutrition the first 4 to 6 months of life, and that either breastmilk or formula be the primary source of milk the first year of life. In recent years there has been an increasing number of mothers opting to breastfeed. Mothers of infants with special needs (illness or hospitalization) may face obstacles that hinder initiating or maintaining lactation to meet their infants' nutritional needs. Education, support, and reassurance from the nurse promotes successful breastfeeding (even in challenging situations), which meets the infant's nutritional needs, increases the mother's confidence in parenting, and strengthens maternal-infant attachment.

## NURSING DIAGNOSES

Altered nutrition: less than body requirements related to insufficient intake for metabolic needs; Ineffective breastfeeding related to infant prematurity, physical anomaly, or knowledge deficit; Altered infant growth and development related to nutritional deficiencies; Altered parenting related to breastfeeding difficulties; Pain related to nipple irritation or breast engorgement.

| Steps | Rationale |
|---|---|
| **Assessment** | |
| 1. Assess maternal health history and current status, e.g., breast surgeries or conditions (plugged ducts, mastitis, inverted, flat, dimpled, sore, blistered or cracked nipples, fibrocysts, scar tissue), perceptions of breast fullness before and after nursing, signs of milk let-down, current medications, previous breastfeeding experience(s), feelings concerning breastfeeding, emotional state (anxiety, frustration, anger, fatigue, self-esteem level, and confidence, and/or depression), and adequacy of support system (Neifert and Seacat, 1986). | Assessment of maternal health status reveals factors that can influence the success of breastfeeding. Anticipatory guidance and empathic support are then provided as indicated. Identifying psychosocial factors reveals the value mother has placed on breastfeeding, her knowledge level, usual coping skills, and availability and understanding of significant others who also affect confidence level and breastfeeding outcome (Kearney, 1988).<br>***Special Considerations:*** *A mother who is highly anxious, dependent, inflexible, or unresponsive to her infant is at high risk for breastfeeding problems and requires frequent reassurance and support (Kearney, 1988).* |
| 2. Assess infant's history and determine current health status, e.g., infant's special needs, current medications and treatment, age, growth rate, developmental level, feeding patterns, quality of suckling, duration of feedings, satiation cues, use of supplements, solid foods, pacifiers or thumbsucking, frequency and characteristics of voiding and stools (Neifert and Seacat, 1986). | Thorough assessment of infant allows identification of factors that may challenge breastfeeding and prompt management to prevent additional problems with breastfeeding/nutrition. |
| 3. Observe maternal and infant behaviors during a feeding including: | Observation validates techniques to reinforce, modify or add.<br>***Special Considerations:*** *Establish rapport with mother before observing because breastfeeding is an intimate experience. Using the approach of "Let's see how baby does . . . " decreases the pressure on mother's ability and facilitates relaxation.* |
| a. Responds to infant's early hunger cues (increased eye and body movements, smacking lips, rooting, or bringing fingers to mouth). | Infants nurse more readily with less negative pressure on the nipple, when in a quiet, alert state, and when exhibiting early hunger cues (L'Esperance and Frantz, 1985). |

| Steps | Rationale |
|---|---|
| b. Assumes proper support and positioning when putting infant to breast: | |
| ▪ Is in a comfortable position (with support for back and arms). | Comfort promotes relaxation and enhances milk let-down. |
| ▪ Supports breast underneath with hand and fingers. Thumb may be gently placed on top. | Supporting the breast moves areola forward helping infant latch on and keeps weight of breast off infant's chin, facilitating milk flow. Gentle placement of thumb on top of areola may prevent occlusion of a duct or misalignment of nipple. **Special Considerations:** *With a preterm or neurologically weak infant, mother will need to continue support throughout the feeding or the weight of the breast will push infant's mouth open.* |
| ▪ Turns infant to side, and stimulates wide opening of mouth by rubbing nipple over lower lip and down chin. | Close positioning and a wide open mouth (as if yawning) allows nipple and ½ to 1 inch of areola to be taken into mouth so that compression occurs over the collecting sinuses, maintaining nipple integrity, and enhancing milk let-down (Tibbetts and Cadwell, 1985; Danner, 1986). |
| ▪ Brings infant close (chest to chest contact), supporting head and body, centering nipple in mouth (Danner, 1986). | Bringing infant's head and body close, in a "c" fashion, prevents arching back, leading to faulty positions at breast (Walker, 1988). **Special Considerations:** *Preterm and infants with low muscle tone will open mouths wider when downward pressure is placed on chin. This pressure will need to be maintained during nursing until infant learns to keep mouth open wide enough to suckle properly (Neifert and Seacat, 1986).* |
| c. Proper positioning of infant's mouth for suckling: ▪ Infant has nipple and ½ to 1 inch of areola in mouth, lips are turned outward, tongue is cupped under nipple and over gums. ▪ Suckling is quiet and rhythmical, with cheeks only drawn in slightly (Danner, 1986). | Proper positioning during suckling increases let-down, stimulates milk production and maintains nipple integrity (Danner, 1986). **Special Considerations:** *To increase rhythmical suckling in infants with low muscle tone, hold infant close in a flexed position, using pillows to keep head and bottom at same level (McBride and Danner, 1987).* |
| d. Milk let-down occurs within a few minutes: a "pins and needles" feeling, tightening, tingling, or painlike sensation in breasts, milk leaking from other breast, uterine contractions, and/or relaxed feeling (Neifert and Seacat, 1986). | Let-down indicates that milk is available. **Special Considerations:** *Observing a slowing down or a more rhythmical swallowing pattern (nutritive suckling) is also a reliable indicator of milk let-down when a mother does not experience the more common sensations (McBride and Danner, 1987).* |
| e. Breaks suction by inserting tip of clean little finger into mouth between gums and pulling downward, before removing from breast. | Breaking suction maintains nipple integrity (Tibbetts and Cadwell, 1985). |
| f. Offers both breasts at each feeding. | Offering both breasts decreases risk of plugged ducts or infection and stimulates a more equal milk production (Dilts, 1985). |
| g. Attempts to burp infant before offering other breast and at end of nursing; positions infant prone or on right side with support behind back (see Skill 59). | Burping allows swallowed air to be expelled and helps prevent regurgitation, aspiration and abdominal distension (Whaley and Wong, 1991). |
| 4. Validate mother's knowledge about: | |
| a. Alternating "starting" each breast nursing. Wearing a safety pin or tying a piece of ribbon on bra can signal which breast was nursed last. | Alternating breasts stimulates a more equal milk production, since infants usually suckle more eagerly on the first breast. **Special Considerations:** *Temporary exceptions include sore or cracked nipples, plugged ducts, or a breast infection.* |
| b. Frequent nursing on infant's hunger cues (every 2 or 3 hours during day and at least once at night) until satiation. | Gastric emptying for young infants takes about 1½ hours (Lawrence, 1985). Frequent nursing facilitates milk let-down and milk production, increasing infant's intake and weight gain (L'Esperance and Frantz, 1985). **Special Considerations:** *Older infants, who are on solid foods, require less frequent nursing.* |
| c. Frequent rotating of positioning around areola (cradle [Fig. 60-1*A*], football or side-cradle [Fig. 60-1*D*], and side-lying [Fig. 60-1*B*]). | Rotating positions varies pressure exerted by jaws around areola, thus maintaining nipple integrity (L'Esperance and Frantz, 1985). **Special Considerations:** *Infants on oxygen by nasal cannula often nurse easier when in the football (side-cradle) position.* |

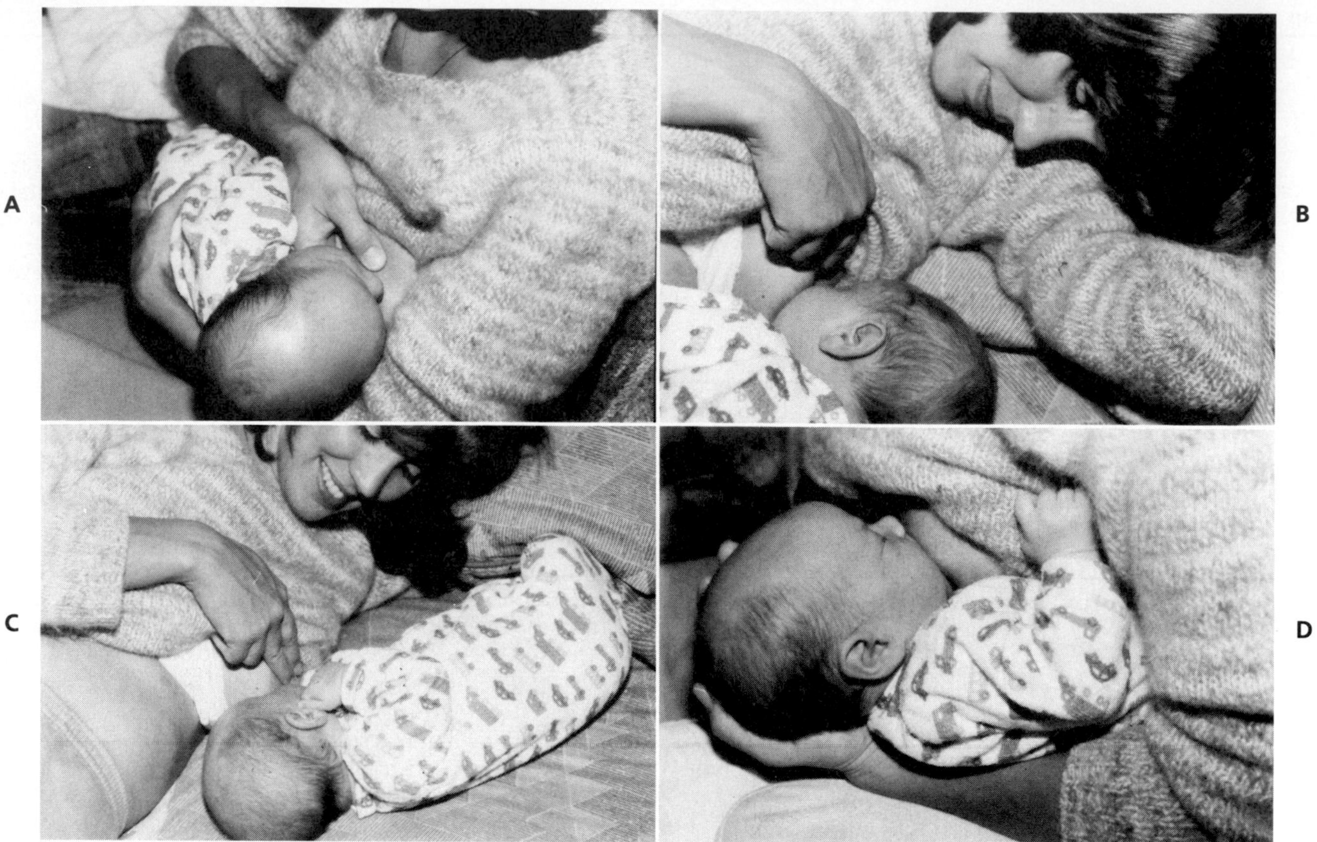


***FIG. 60-1*** Positioning the baby: series. **A,** Cradle hold. One arm and hand support baby; other hand supports breast (thumb above and fingers below). Breast is guided into baby's mouth. **B,** Side-lying position. Pillows support mother's head. Baby is turned toward mother. Mother depresses breast to facilitate baby's breathing. **C,** Variation on side-lying position. **D,** Football hold. Baby is held in one arm with hand supporting head.

From Bobak I and Jensen M: Maternity and gynecologic care, ed 4, St Louis, 1989, The CV Mosby Company.

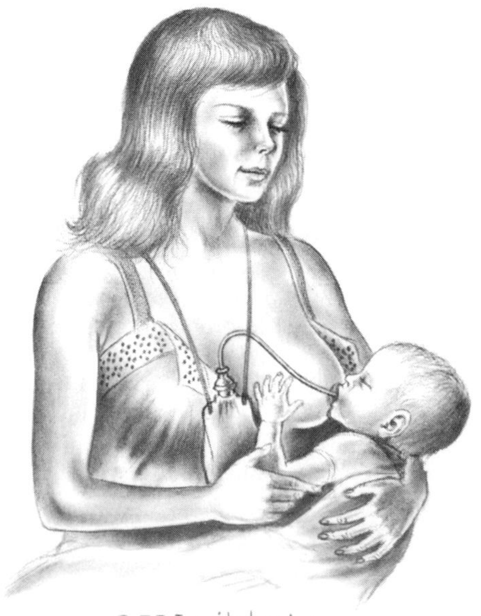


***FIG. 60-2*** Lact-Aid Nursing Trainer in use.

From Bobak I and Jensen M: Maternity and gynecologic care, ed 4, St Louis, 1989, The CV Mosby Company.

| Steps | Rationale |
|---|---|
| **Planning and Goal Setting** | |
| 1. Gather available teaching aids and pamphlets. | Learning is facilitated through use of audiovisual aids and written materials. ***Special Considerations:*** *Education level, previous experience with breastfeeding, feelings about breasts, the desire for privacy, and sensory capabilities (sight, hearing) need to be considered.* |
| 2. Arrange a time that is convenient for mother and does not conflict with scheduled care. | Consulting mother and other care givers beforehand increases receptivity and goal attainment. |
| 3. Create an environment conducive to learning and feeding, e.g., arrange for privacy and comfort. Use an unhurried approach. | Relaxation, concentration, and retention are enhanced in a setting that is free of distractions and unhurried. |
| 4. Develop individualized child and family goals including: ▪ Mother will demonstrate correct breastfeeding techniques. ▪ Infant's nutritional needs will be met. ▪ Difficulties related to breastfeeding will be resolved. | |
| **Implementation** 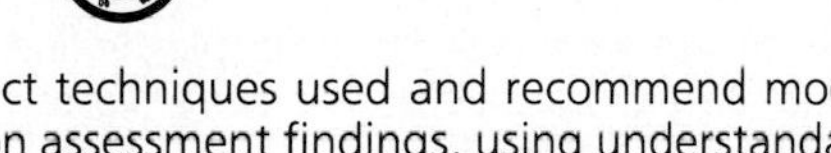 | |
| 1. Reinforce correct techniques used and recommend modifications based on assessment findings, using understandable terms. | Reinforcement enhances mother's confidence. Suggesting changes based on mother/infant data with rationale augments mother's compliance. |
| 2. Counsel mother about identified concerns or provide anticipatory guidance. Common problems include: | |
| a. Sleepy infant (preterm, hospitalized, acute illness, jaundice, pain, analgesic, or anesthetic). ▪ Recommend mother: | |
| (1) Talk to and unwrap infant, stroking/rubbing infant's face, arms, palms, legs, or soles for a few minutes. | Infants usually feed more completely and exert less negative pressure on the nipples when alert (L'Esperance and Frantz, 1985). |
| (2) Sit infant in her lap, supporting chin and cheeks in her hands. Stroke and talk to infant while infant is sitting up (Danner, 1986). (3) Establish eye contact with infant. (4) Change diaper or pat face or legs with a cool cloth before feeding or between breasts (Saunders, 1988). | ***Special Considerations:*** *Closely monitor preterm infants, those with infections and congenital heart problems, as they may become stressed under stimulation and demonstrate variations in color, vital signs, and activity (Walker, 1988). Some infants become so comfortable in mother's arms they fall asleep and will need intermittent restimulation.* |
| ▪ Validate that mother positions infant correctly at breast. | Proper positioning encourages infant to attend during nursing (Saunders, Carroll, and Johnson, 1988). |
| ▪ Recommend mother massage breasts and express a small amount onto nipple just before putting infant to breast. | Smelling and tasting milk entices infant to attend and suckle. |
| b. Infant has physiologic jaundice. ▪ Recommend mother: | |
| (1) Nurse infant until satiated every 1½ to 3 hours or 10 to 12 times every 24 hours. | Early and frequent nursings facilitate excretion of bilirubin in stools (DeCarvalho, Klaus, and Merkatz, 1982; Auerbach and Gartner, 1987). |
| (2) Avoid water or formula supplements. | Supplementing infant with water does not reduce serum bilirubin concentrations, and use of a rubber nipple may lead to nipple confusion, resulting in impaired breastfeeding (DeCarvalho, Hall, and Harvey, 1981; Nicoll, Ginsburg, and Tripp, 1982). |
| (3) Consider using a nursing supplementer (Fig. 60-2), e.g., Medela SNS Lact-Aid, or oral gavage tube to provide additional breastmilk or formula if infant has limited interest in feeding or a poor suckling response. | Using a nursing supplementer meets infant's nutritional needs without nipple confusion, reluctance to nurse, and maternal engorgement (Auerbach and Gartner, 1987). |
| c. Suckling variations: nipple confusion, weak, uncoordinated suck or flutter suck (as seen with preterm, neuromotor dysfunctions, congential heart defects, oral anatomic protrusion of tongue, micrognathia, cleft lip and/or palate). ▪ Recommend mother: | |
| (1) Avoid use of artificial nipples. | Avoiding use of artificial nipples prevents nipple confusion (Saunders, Carroll, and Johnson, 1988). |

## EXPRESSING AND STORING BREASTMILK

1. Explain principles for success:
   a. Begin within 12 to 24 hours of birth or cessation of infant's suckling to prevent stasis and bacterial growth (Forte, 1987).
   b. Express breastmilk at infant's usual feeding times during day, with spontaneous milk let-downs and once at night (if possible) to maintain or increase milk supply.
   c. Nipple stimulation from a pump is less efficient than infant suckling, and a smaller milk return is expected.
   d. Privacy, patience, relaxation, and persistence enhance milk let-down and supply.
2. Discuss criteria for selecting a pump (if one is desired).
   a. Expected frequency and duration of use. If daily use or more often consider a battery operated or electric model with single or double pumping units. Simultaneously pumping both breasts shortens time required, may increase prolactin levels, and frees hands (Neifert and Seacat, 1986).
   b. Adequate nipple fit and stimulation.
   c. All pump parts should be sterilizable.
   d. Portability—size, weight, attachments, batteries, or outlet required.
   e. Cost to rent or purchase (often covered by insurance when physician orders).
   f. Readily available—hospital, lactation consultant, or pharmacy (Walker, 1987).
3. Support and instruct about expressing, storing, defrosting, and transporting breastmilk and caring for equipment.
   a. Gather supplies (towel, pump, collecting container, tape, and pen).
   b. Prepare to express breastmilk:
      - Thoroughly wash hands with soap. Clean under and around nails to decrease risk of contaminating milk.
      - Provide privacy and encourage a comfortable position and relaxation. Some mothers are most successful pumping at infant's bedside with a screen around them (Walker, 1988).
      - Massage each breast for at least 1 minute, covering all quadrants, but avoiding nipples.
      - Begin hand expression by placing thumb and fingers just outside areola about 1 to 1½ inches back from nipple. Press in toward chest wall, and gently press thumb and fingers together. Be careful not to pinch or pull nipple out. Express 2 to 3 tsps, and discard to help flush contaminated milk away from superficial ducts (Meier and Wilks, 1987).
   c. Express breastmilk by either continuing with hand expression or using a pump:
      - Hand expression—Collect milk in sterile container. Using a hand expression funnel may decrease splashes and spills. Alternate breasts to facilitate multiple milk let-downs. Rotate hand position around breasts to reach all the ducts and to empty reservoirs, spending about 10 to 12 minutes per breast (Danner, 1986).
      - Pumping—Choose nipple adaptor that is snug on nipple yet allows nipple to slide in. Center nipple in opening to prevent nipple trauma. Lean forward and allow nipple and areola to comfortably move into flange. According to product instructions, pump for 5 minutes or until the spray of milk stops. Repeat pumping up to 15 minutes on each breast (Danner, 1986).
   d. Store breastmilk:
      - Immediately pour breastmilk into a sterile plastic container, bottle, or presterilized liner. Do not touch inside of container or lid. Seal lid, leaving about ½ inch at the top for the milk to expand as it freezes. Date with tape. If using plastic liners, place inside air-tight plastic bag to store (Forte, 1987).
      - Milk can be stored in the refrigerator and used for up to 24 hours. Milk can be stored for up to 2 weeks in a freezer within a refrigerator, for up to 3 months in back of a self-contained freezer in a refrigerator, and for up to 1 year in a deep freezer at 0° F (Forte, 1987).
      - Refrigerated milk can be added to frozen milk. The milk added must be less than the amount of frozen milk to prevent thawing of frozen milk (Danner, 1986).
   e. Promptly care for equipment. Wash supplies and pump parts with hot soap and water. Rinse with hot water and air dry on a clean towel. Sterilize pump parts once every 24 hours in top rack of dishwasher without other dishes or in a pan of boiling water on the stove. Check rubber gaskets when reassembling pump, as the heat may harden and/or shrink them.
   f. Defrost or thaw milk in a cup under cool then warmer water, gently shaking to maintain fat globules. Avoid using boiling water or a microwave to defrost milk, as heat destroys some of the protective cells and antibacterial properties, and may heat milk unevenly, causing hot spots that could burn infant's mouth. Defrosted milk can be stored in the refrigerator and used for up to 24 hours. Discard milk remaining in bottle at end of feeding (Danner, 1986).
   g. Transport breastmilk (both frozen and thawed) in a cooler with ice that will maintain milk at 4° C or lower to decrease bacterial multiplication. Refrigerate or freeze immediately on arrival.

| Steps | Rationale |
|---|---|
| (2) Frequently attempt to nurse when infant is in a quiet, alert state. | Infants are more likely to suckle at breast if not sleepy, crying, or fatigued. |
| (3) Establish milk let-down just before nursing. | Infant promptly receives milk with less effort, which encourages repeated suckling (Walker, 1988). |
| (4) Express a small amount of milk onto nipples just before nursing (Saunders, 1988). | Smelling and tasting the milk entices infant to latch on and suckle. |
| (5) Place one finger under infant's jaw and gently press upward intermittently. | Supporting infant's jaw encourages continued suckling. |
| (6) Acquire a breast pump that provides adequate nipple stimulation, and pump after each feeding until infant is able to correctly suckle an amount equivalent to a full feeding (see box at left). | Additional nipple stimulation will be required to build up or maintain an adequate milk supply. The milk obtained may be given to infant through a nursing supplementer (Neifert and Seacat, 1986). |
| (7) Consider using a nursing supplementer (Fig. 60-2) such as the SNS by Medela or Lact-Aid, oral gavage tube, eye dropper, or cup while feeding if the problem lasts more than 48 hours and infant's breastfeeding intake is inadequate (Neifert and Seacat, 1986) (see box at left). | |
| ▪ Instruct mother in the suck-training technique when an infant suckles incorrectly (e.g., back of tongue is pulled up, tongue on roof of mouth, or pushes nipple out). | |
| (1) Stroke infant's cheeks with fingertip toward lips; brush over lips several times; massage outside of lower and upper gums. | Stroking and massage minimizes the intrusiveness of the training technique. |
| (2) Insert finger with pad up, and gently rub back along hard and soft palate. | This initiates infant's sucking response. |
| (3) When infant starts to suck, press a finger downward and forward against the tongue. | Pressure helps infant bring tongue into correct position to nurse effectively. ***Special Considerations:*** *A nursing supplementer can be used to provide feeding during suck training.* |
| (4) Alternate rubbing infant's palate with downward and upward pressure on the tongue when infant needs pacification or before and during nursing (if infant reverts to negative suckling) until infant consistently uses proper suckling (Marmet and Shell, 1984). | Repetition creates a conditioned reflex (Marmet and Shell, 1984). ***Special Considerations:*** *Hold infant with a cleft lip close, pressing the breast into the cleft and placing a finger over the cleft to form a seal. Place infant upright in lap with head slightly tilted back, and use a cleft palate nipple, or place one finger on top of and one under areola during feeding. Infants with cleft palate and/or low muscle tone may suckle more if mother firmly pushes up and down under jaw (Riordan, 1983; Lawrence, 1985; Danner, 1986).* |
| d. Infant tires easily (preterm, low muscle tone, congenital heart, respiratory limitations, e.g., respiratory distress syndrome (RDS) or bronchopulmonary dysplasia (BPD), infection, anemia, postanesthesia, with analgesia). | |
| ▪ Recommend mother: | |
| (1) Nurse infant when in the quiet, alert state. | Infants nurse more eagerly when in this state. |
| (2) Establish milk let-down before nursing. | Ready milk let-down allows infant to obtain more milk with less effort (Walker, 1988). |
| (3) Position infant upright as much as possible during feeding, stabilizing the head. (The mother may need assistance in positioning.) | This position is less stressful to infant, avoids excess pressure on the diaphragm, and prevents infant from pulling away, which is fatiguing (Riordan, 1983). |
| (4) Provide jaw and chin support by moving thumb and forefinger forward to form a "u". Gently hold cheek and chin (Dancer hand position), or place forefinger under chin during nursing. | Providing jaw and/or chin support will keep the weight of breast from pressing on mouth and chin and will stabilize jaw, enhancing sucking with less energy expenditure (McBride and Danner, 1987). |
| (5) Modify sensory stimulation during feeding by keeping area quiet, dark, and warm and by patting, rocking, or talking only as infant tolerates. | Limiting stimulation avoids stressing infant's immature nervous system (Walker, 1988). |
| (6) End feeding when infant exhibits satiation cues or signs of stress occur. | Promptly responding to infant's behavior avoids stressing infant, distending stomach, and impeding respiratory function (Riordan, 1983). |
| ▪ Monitor infant's growth (weight and circumferences), frequency and duration of nursings, activity level, and nutritional status. | Frequent assessments allow early detection of inadequate weight gain, nutritional disruptions, and delayed development. |

| Steps | Rationale |
|---|---|
| e. Preference for nursing on one breast (mother has variation in one breast or nipple, or infant is uncomfortable, e.g., IV fluids infusing through scalp vein, fractured clavicle, surgical incision). | |
| ▪ Recommend mother: | |
| (1) Nurse infant on the preferred breast in the cradle position (Fig. 60-1*A*) until milk let-down occurs. | Limiting nursing on the preferred breast avoids satiating infant. |
| (2) Switch infant to football (side cradle) (Fig. 60-1*D*) hold, and offer other breast (Saunders, Carroll, and Johnson, 1988). | This position provides minimal stimulation or disturbance to infant. |
| (3) Nurse on preferred breast in the side-lying position (Fig. 60-1*B*) until milk let-down occurs, then roll over more on the same side, and offer the other breast without changing infant's position. | |
| (4) Nurse on the less preferred breast first if infant is sleepy or just waking up. | Infants will often accept this breast more readily if not fully awake or crying. |
| (5) Nurse in a dark, quiet room. | Decreased sensory stimulation enables infant to attend to nursing (Saunders, Carroll, and Johnson, 1988). |
| ▪ Reassure mother that usually this preference lasts only a few days (Saunders, Carroll, and Johnson, 1988). | Reassurance decreases maternal anxiety, which can affect milk let-down and infant's behavior. |
| f. Infant gulps or chokes with milk let-down (preterm, neuromuscular disorders, esophageal reflux). | |
| ▪ Recommend mother: | |
| (1) Nurse and/or pump on a regular basis. | Frequent nursing/pumping prevents breasts from becoming overly full with a strong milk let-down. |
| (2) Perform breast massage, and express a small amount just before nursing. | Massage and expression elongates nipple and softens areolae, helping infant latch on correctly. |
| (3) Position infant so that back of neck and throat are higher than the nipple, e.g., use an elevated football or cradle position leaning back so that breast is angled upward, or a side-lying position with towel under infant so that infant's face looks slightly down toward the nipple, or the Australian position (lying supine with infant laying across chest) (Danner, 1986). | These positions slow the flow of milk, preventing it from shooting to back of mouth, enabling infant to swallow more easily (Danner, 1986). |
| g. Infant regurgitates during or after feedings (pyloric stenosis, esophageal reflux, preterm). | |
| ▪ Recommend mother: | |
| (1) Position infant so throat and neck are higher than nipple during feeding. | This position slows release of milk from ducts (Danner, 1986). |
| (2) Frequently nurse infant (every 1½ to 2 hours) for a shorter time, gradually increasing the duration as infant tolerates (Riordan, 1983). | Frequent, shorter nursing prevents infant from getting overly hungry and distending stomach (Riordan, 1983). |
| (3) Gently rub infant's back instead of traditional burping before, between breasts, and after nursing. | Rubbing facilitates expulsion of swallowed air. |
| (4) Slowly and gently handle infant after nursing and place infant in prone position, with head above stomach (Riordan, 1983) (see Skill 63). | This position prevents stimulation of the sphincter(s) and avoids excess pressure on the abdomen. |
| ▪ Maintain a log of the time and duration of feedings, when infant regurgitates and amount, and voidings and stools. | Maintaining a log identifies potential or actual problems that may rapidly develop. |
| ▪ Assess infant's nutrition and hydration status at least every 8 hours (see Skill 64). | Dehydration and fluid and electrolyte imbalances can quickly develop in infants (Riordan, 1983). |
| ▪ Reassure mother that regurgitation is not related to her ability to nurse or to her milk and that breastmilk is beneficial for infant. | Reassurance helps restore mother's self-confidence and encourages continued breastfeeding (Riordan, 1983). |
| h. Infant with slow weight gain. | |
| ▪ Recommend mother: | |
| (1) Frequently nurse infant (every 1½ to 3 hours) around the clock. | Frequent suckling increases nipple stimulation and prolactin release, leading to increased milk production (Danner, 1986). |
| (2) Alternate between breasts every 5 minutes during feeding until satiated (switch nursing). | Frequent switching between breasts arouses infant and stimulates multiple milk let-down during feedings and release of hind milk (Neifert and Seacat, 1986). |
| (3) Avoid non-nutritive sucking on a pacifier or thumb and use of rubber nipples and shields (Neifert and Seacat, 1986). | Frequently putting infant to breast meets sucking needs. If possible avoid nipple shields because they limit nipple and areolar stimulation, may traumatize nipples, and can lead to nipple confusion (Riordan, 1983). |

| Steps | Rationale |
|---|---|
| ▪ When ordered, instruct and support mother in: | |
| (1) Supporting infant's suckling when indicated by providing head, jaw, or chin support or by inserting finger into infant's mouth (for a cleft palate). | Adequate suckling with nipple stimulation is the key to stimulating milk let-down and further milk production (Riordan, 1983). |
| (2) Using a nursing supplementer such as the SNS or a gavage tube to supplement with breastmilk or formula until infant's weight gain is adequate. | Using a SNS or gavage tube encourages infant to nurse in response to a steady flow of milk and avoids use of artificial nipples (Neifert and Seacat, 1986). |
| i. Maternal anxiety while breastfeeding/collecting milk. | |
| ▪ Reassure mother that anxiety is normal while learning, and keep her informed of infant's condition. | Maternal stress and fatigue escalate when infants are hospitalized and/or are acutely or chronically ill (Whaley and Wong, 1991). |
| ▪ Generously reinforce what mother is doing correctly regarding breastfeeding/collecting milk. | Reinforcement promotes maternal confidence enhancing relaxation and milk let-down. |
| ▪ Consult mother about relaxation techniques that might decrease her anxiety, then support her use of them. Examples include: Privacy while nursing/pumping; quiet; comfort; music; slow, deep breathing; active or passive relaxation of muscle groups; having a warm drink; or visualizing positive aspects of infant or nature scenes such as a waterfall or ocean. | Collaborating with mother allows individualized interventions and augments their effectiveness. Relaxation is individualized. ***Special Considerations:*** *When milk let-down is affected by maternal anxiety and tension, the following are also often effective: taking a shower; applying warm packs to breasts for 15 to 20 minutes or performing breast massage for 1 to 2 minutes on each breast before nursing/pumping (Danner, 1986). An oxytocin nasal spray that stimulates milk let-down can be obtained by prescription and if needed, used before and during nursing (Lawrence, 1985).* |
| j. Maternal sore nipples. | |
| ▪ Recommend mother: | |
| (1) Nurse frequently for shorter periods (5 to 8 minutes each breast), increasing nursing time gradually as soreness subsides. | Frequent, shorter nursing and rotating infant's position at breast minimizes stress on nipples and varies pressure points (L'Esperance and Frantz, 1985). |
| (2) Rotate infant's position at breast at each feeding (Danner, 1986). | |
| (3) Begin nursing on the least sore breast (Danner, 1986). | Infants tend to nurse more vigorously on the first breast (Danner, 1986). |
| ▪ Reassess infant's position during feeding and reposition as indicated. | Infant may have slipped down on nipple. Improper positioning traumatizes nipple, leading to pain (L'Esperance and Frantz, 1985). |
| ▪ Instruct and reinforce use of proper nipple care. | Correct nipple care facilitates healing and increases comfort. |
| (1) Allow colostrum to dry on nipples after feedings. | Colostrum is absorbed and may promote healing. |
| (2) After feeding, air dry nipples 10 to 15 minutes, or use a hair dryer for 30 seconds set on cool, held at arm's length. | Naturally drying nipples allows circulation and promotes nipple healing and integrity (L'Esperance and Frantz, 1985). |
| (3) Wear a dome-shaped breast shell/cup (with holes over entire surface) inside bra between feedings. | Breast shells/cups permit air to circulate around nipples and prevent clothing from rubbing and irritating nipples (L'Esperance and Frantz, 1985). |
| (4) Briefly apply a cold cotton cloth to nipples just before feeding. | Cold decreases pain sensations and facilitates nipple erection (Danner, 1986). |
| k. Maternal breast engorgement/plugged ducts. | |
| ▪ Recommend mother: | |
| (1) Nurse every 1½ to 3 hours around the clock on both breasts until infant is satiated (Danner, 1986). | Frequent nursing promotes milk release, prevents stasis, and augments resolution (Dilts, 1985). |
| (2) Take a shower or apply warm moist packs 15 to 20 minutes before nursing. | Warmth, breast massage, and expression helps open milk ducts, moves milk forward, softens areolae, and enhances milk let-down (Storr, 1988). |
| (3) Massage breasts, and stimulate milk let-down before nursing. | |
| (4) With a plugged duct, begin on affected breast, positioning infant with nose toward lump, intermittently and gently massaging breast. | This technique facilitates duct drainage, decreases risk of infection, and increases comfort (Danner, 1986). |
| (5) With engorgement, support breast underneath and gently compress areola as infant latches on. | Support helps infant to grasp nipple and position properly (Tibbetts and Cadwell, 1985). |
| (6) Express a small amount if breasts are still uncomfortable after nursing (Danner, 1986). | Expression enhances comfort and decreases stasis. |
| (7) Apply a cold cotton cloth to breasts for a few minutes after or between feedings (Danner, 1986). | Cold packs promote comfort by increasing vasoconstriction and decreasing vascularity (Danner, 1986). |
| ▪ Encourage wearing a fitted support bra when awake and avoid sleeping in prone position. | Supporting breast tissue increases comfort. Sleeping in prone position places pressure on breasts and may inhibit duct drainage (Danner, 1986). |
| 3. Provide follow-up counseling, or refer to other health professionals as indicated. | Follow-up counseling and referrals provide support and evaluation of outcomes. |

## Evaluation Outcomes

1. Mother verbalizes understanding of and uses techniques promoting successful breastfeeding.
2. Infant's nutritional needs are met as indicated by weight gain and developmental achievements.
3. Breastfeeding difficulties in special situations are identified early and resolved with continuation of breastfeeding.

## Observational Guidelines

Interview and observe mother's use of proper techniques during feeding.

Plot infant's growth on a growth chart, and observe for developmental achievements.

Interview mother about resolution of difficulties and observe mother/infant behaviors. Note continuation of breastfeeding.

## Documentation

Charting will include learning needs, specific information provided both verbally and in writing, supplies obtained (e.g., breast pump, breast shells, hand expression funnel, nursing supplementer), validation of mother's understanding through verbalizations and/or return demonstrations, areas to reinforce through follow-up counseling and referrals made.

# *SKILL* 61 Feeding the Hospitalized Child with Special Needs

*Peggy J. Drapo*

Estimates show that ¼ to ⅓ of hospitalized children have some type of nutrition or feeding problem. Feeding problems range from difficulties in sucking, swallowing, or chewing and are attributed to lack of energy, acute infective conditions, economic barriers, psychological factors, or some combination of these. In the case of a sick child, for whom the feeding or nutritional problem is temporary, some simple modifications and creativity may be all that is necessary. In contrast, for the child with a more chronic problem, a thorough assessment is needed to determine the cause of the feeding difficulty and to determine appropriate interventions. Nutrition is an essential component of nursing care because nutrition-related problems frequently occur among children with disabilities, and because adequate nutrition is important to the prevention, treatment, and habilitation of disabling conditions in children.

## NURSING DIAGNOSES

Altered nutrition: less than body requirements related to difficulty chewing/swallowing, loss of appetite, nausea/vomiting, chronic illness, or limited access to food; Altered growth and development related to inadequate nutritional intake or parental knowledge deficit about appropriate interventions for child with chronic illness; Self-care deficit: feeding related to developmental disability or neuromusculoskeletal impairment; Potential for aspiration related to impaired swallowing or inability to sit upright.

| Steps | Rationale |
|---|---|
| **Assessment** | |
| 1. Determine age and developmental level. | Age and developmental level provide guidelines for nutritional needs, preparation of food, and feeding abilities. |
| 2. Review feeding history from birth for previous feeding difficulties and present conditions that commonly influence feeding abilities such as food sensitivities, failure to thrive, cerebral palsy, multiple sclerosis, muscular dystrophy, Down syndrome, prematurity, or any other developmental or neuromuscular disability. | These special conditions will require individualized feeding plans.<br>***Special Considerations:*** *Parents may request assistance if problems occur with the child's diet. Be familiar with services offered in the hospital as well as referral resources in the community for discharge planning. In many of these disorders, dietary consultants are needed to assist in teaching parents the basic requirements and methods of substitution (Hinson, 1985).* |

| **Steps** | **Rationale** |
|---|---|
| 3. Interview family for usual dietary amounts and patterns (include allergies, likes and dislikes, and cultural patterns related to nutrition) and feeding interventions tried in the past. See Skill 29. | Some families are vegetarians or have religious taboos for certain types of meat or mixture of foods. Some genetic conditions cause increased intake, e.g., Prader-Willi syndrome. In cases of children with developmental disabilities, parents may have been previously instructed about various feeding positions that have been successful. |
| 4. Assess oral motor skills and feeding behaviors including suck, swallow, bite, and gag reflexes, lip control, tongue movement, muscle tone, and positioning. (See Tables 61-1 and 61-2 for assessment of normal and abnormal development.) | Identification of special needs or physical problems will facilitate an individualized care plan. Physical disorders can include problems with feeding involving the oral phase: tongue, teeth, labial, and buccal musculature. Smooth functioning in the oral phase is necessary to position food in mouth, manipulate food in mouth with tongue, chew bolus, recollect bolus for swallowing, and organize lingual peristalsis to propel bolus backward. Problems involving swallowing can occur in the pharyngeal or the esophageal phase. These problems may arise from oral or oropharyngeal cancers, laryngeal cancers, and neuromuscular disorders caused by neurologic lesions from trauma, stroke, infectious disease, congenital damage, and/or degenerative neuromuscular disease (Logemann, 1983). The ability to swallow saliva is one indication of ability to swallow fluids or foods (Eschelman, 1988). |
| 5. Review medical records for special dietary orders, diagnosis, treatments, or procedures that indicate feeding or swallowing problems. | Children with disabilities may have problems with muscle coordination that inhibit ability to reach or feed themselves. This may result in malnutrition. Children with disorders such as cerebral palsy may have growth rates below normal in height, weight, and bone structure. Information related to these disabilities will help in planning more realistic goals (Urban et al, 1983). |

***TABLE 61-1*** Assessment of Normal Developmental Sequences that Affect Feeding

| **Age** | **Sequence** | **Assessment Parameters/Comments** |
|---|---|---|
| Birth-3 mo | Rooting | Turns face and opens mouth in response to light touch to cheek. |
| | Suckling | Immature sucking motion in newborn. Lips do not close in a tight seal. |
| Birth-5 mo | Suck-swallow reflex | Sucking and then swallowing immediately as a reflexive pattern. |
| | Tongue protrusion (extrusion) | Innate response of infant to prevent foreign objects from entering mouth. |
| Birth-7 mo | Bite reflex | Involuntary and immediate biting when object introduced into the mouth. |
| Birth-lifetime | Gag reflex | Normal gagging action if stimulus applied to back of tongue. If child gags too easily, the condition is termed *hyper gag reflex*. If the child has had a persistent tube (NG) in place, he or she will have a *hypo gag reflex* and will not show a choking reflex. May aspirate easily. |
| 4-5 mo-lifetime | Lip closure | Brings lips together to form seal. Helps in removing food from spoon or drinking. Prevents drooling. |
| | Sucking | Oral activity that matures after suckling. Sucking activity must precede chewing. May drink from straw. |
| 6 mo-lifetime | Chewing or mastication | Vertical up and down motion to manipulate food. Rotary chewing (begins at 9 months) used in conjunction with vertical or circular motion of jaw. |
| 9 mo-lifetime | Tongue movements that are essential to eating: | |
| | 1. Retraction | Locating or moving tongue to back of mouth. This movement assists in manipulating food in preparation for swallowing. |
| | 2. Projection | Voluntary projection of tongue forward. |
| | 3. Lateralization | Side to side movement of tongue. |
| | 4. Elevation | Moving tongue upward toward roof of mouth. |
| | 5. Depression | Moving tongue downward toward floor of mouth. |
| | 6. Licks | Licks from spoon. |
| 6-8 mo-lifetime | Hand activity | Can hold a bottle. Picks up large finger foods. |
| 9-12 mo | | Feeds self with fingers. Can hold cup. |
| 12-15 mo | | Picks up cup. Can pick up smaller finger foods. |
| 16-19 mo | | Eats with spoon. |
| 20-23 mo | | Can take wrapper off candy. |
| 24-36 mo | | Begins to manipulate fork. |

**TABLE 61-2** Assessment of Abnormal Development Related to Feeding or Nutrition

| Structure or Function | Abnormal Finding | Description or Cause |
|---|---|---|
| Tongue | Thrust (past 6 mo) | Involuntary forward movement of tongue. |
| Gag Reflex | Hyperactive | Occurs when pressure is applied anywhere on the tongue. |
| | Hypoactive | Slow or complete lack when any area of tongue is stimulated. May be seen with Down syndrome or other conditions where child is hypotonic. |
| Saliva | Uncontrolled drooling | Attributed to poor lip closure, sluggish swallow, or lack of control of tongue or other oral muscles. |
| Gums | Hypertrophic | Caused by hyperplastic gingivitis or from drugs such as Dilantin. Overgrowth of gum tissue. Gingiva is firm and fibrous and covers more area of the teeth than usual. Tissue is insensitive. |
| Swallow | Hypoactive | Slow and sluggish. May result in choking, drooling. Nasogastric tubes depress voluntary swallow. |
| Jaw | Macrognathia | Large jaw, poor jaw and teeth alignment. |
| | Micrognathia | Small jaw, poor jaw and teeth alignment. |
| | Prognathism | Protruding jaw, poor jaw and teeth alignment. |
| Teeth | Macrodontia | Larger than normal teeth. |
| | Microdontia | Smaller than normal teeth. |
| | Anodontia | Absence (congenital) of all or part of teeth. |
| | Bruxate | Grinding teeth other than when eating. May cause wearing away of teeth. |
| Oral Mucosa | Anesthesia | Decreased sensitivity in oral area. |

| Steps | Rationale |
|---|---|
| 6. Assess family's understanding of basic nutritional facts and/or any barriers to nutrition such as economic, cultural, and/or religious beliefs. | Instruction will need to be based on the level of understanding of the child and/or the child's caretaker. For example, if the family does not have the nutritional background necessary to understand the four basic food groups and the body's nutritional requirements, then teaching should begin at that level. If the child's nutritional deficits are the result of economics, the intervention should first be directed toward securing resources. Dietary habits, language, values and beliefs, and family influence may all reflect cultural considerations that must be incorporated into education program planning (Anderson and McFarland, 1988). |

## Planning and Goal Setting

| Steps | Rationale |
|---|---|
| 1. Contact nutritionist, physical therapist, and/or physician for child's individualized feeding techniques if plan was previously developed. Inquire about special equipment that will be needed. | Children who have difficulty eating as a result of developmental delay or problems with reflexes or body tone require individualized feeding techniques. If the feeding difficulty is preexisting, a program may have been developed. Working with the physician, nutritionist, and physical therapist aids understanding of the underlying cause of feeding problems. ***Special Considerations:*** *Document on the care plan names and telephone numbers of team professionals and actions agreed on.* |
| 2. Wash hands. | Handwashing reduces transmission of microorganisms. Thorough cooking and other safety preparation methods will not help if food is contaminated after cooking (Boston Center, 1987). |
| 3. Gather necessary supplies: | Having supplies available facilitates a smooth and pleasant feeding time. |
| a. Formula/food (see Skill 58). | ***Special Considerations:*** *Constipation is always a problem for inactive children. Selecting too few fruits and vegetables and allowing too much milk will aggravate the problem. Do not use infant bottle feeders (see Step 3b). Preferences for sweet drinks and food are established early; serve sweets sparingly to promote acceptance of nutrient-rich foods.* |

***FIG. 61-1*** Cup with a cut out space.

| **Steps** | **Rationale** |
|---|---|
| b. Liquids and bottle/cup: begin transition to cup as soon as developmentally ready. Use a cup with cut out space for the nose (Fig. 61-1). | A child should not be bottle fed when developmentally ready to drink from a cup because continued bottle use inhibits development of muscles for speech and chewing. A cup with a cut out space for the nose allows the child to tip the cup and swallow fluid more easily.<br>***Special Considerations:*** *At 6 to 8 months the child is able to drink from a cup with assistance. By 9 to 12 months the child can drink independently from a cup if the child does not have a developmental disability or delay. Often children with special needs do not (or cannot) ask for fluids, therefore frequently offer fluids. Suitable fluids are water, juice, and milk.* |
| c. Use appropriately sized utensils, adaptive devices, and bib for the child (see Fig. 61-2 and the box below). | Appropriately sized utensils and adaptive devices contribute to the success of feeding. They should be selected to allow the child to participate as normally, efficiently, and safely as possible.<br>***Special Considerations:*** *Avoid plastic or uncoated metal spoons, especially if the child has a hyperactive bite reflex. Rubber coated spoons are more suitable.* |

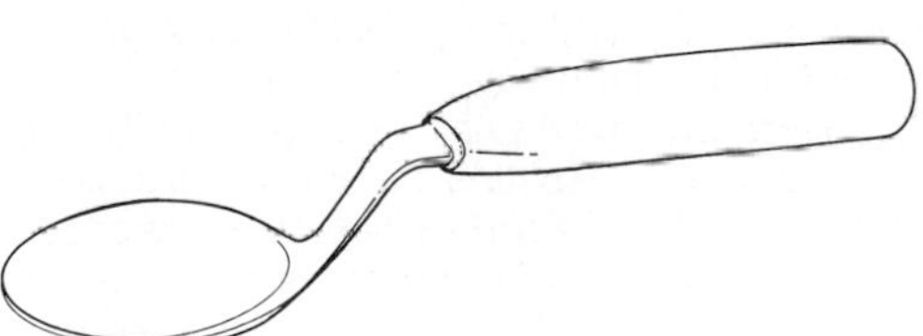

***FIG. 61-2*** Angled spoon.

### *COMMERCIALLY AVAILABLE SPECIAL UTENSILS*

Angled spoon—angled to right or left; used for children who have trouble with normal supination or pronation of the hand (Fig. 61-2).

Horizontal palm spoon or cuff device—used for children who have no grasp.

Swivel spoon—helps decrease spilling.

Extension utensils—used with child who has contractures and cannot flex or extend elbows.

Utensils with built-up handles—useful for children with weak grasps.

Dishes—scoop dish, plate guard, or bowl; assists children who have difficulty getting food onto spoon.

Dycen—a plastic rubbery material that will adhere to the table or tray, can be placed under the plate to keep the plate from sliding.

Weighted cups and glasses—weighted cups with a slit lid.

Flexible straws—enable children to drink from a cup that is stationary on table.

Homemade devices:

- In place of a horizontal palm spoon or a universal cuff, one can cut the handle of a Clorox jug and put the handle on the child's hand, and stick the spoon handle in the hollow of the jug handle.
- In place of Dycen, use wet paper towels or modeling clay.
- Cut plastic tubing that is used in fish aquariums into shorter pieces and use instead of expensive straws.
- Build up regular utensils with gauze, styrofoam, and tape for better grasping. Bicycle grips or rubber foam curlers can also be used on the utensil handles.

| Steps | Rationale |
|---|---|
| d. Positioning aids:<br>■ Chair, pillows, footrest for person feeding child.<br>■ Pillow to support child's back.<br>■ Rolled towel to place in back of child's head.<br>■ Table or counter to place child's back against for support.<br>■ Small table to place food and equipment on. | Since feeding is a lengthy process, supporting the child's weight and compensating for hypertonic or hypotonic musculature during this time is exhausting (Kosowski and Sopczyk, 1985). Using positioning aids to properly support the child promotes comfort for the person feeding.<br>***Special Considerations:*** *If special rehabilitative equipment is not available, infant seats, high chairs, and lounge chairs can be adapted. Use blankets, towels, or other suitable padding. Bean bag chairs, a small inner tube, or a child's life preserver are excellent. If necessary, use the child's bed with head elevated and knee gatched (Kosowski and Spoczyk, 1985).* |
| 4. Provide a quiet environment with minimal stimulation. | A quiet environment facilitates feeding. If the child retains a primitive startle reflex and hears a loud noise, the child will throw his or her head back and arms outward, losing control of utensils and food. When this happens the child may also fall if not secured or may aspirate a mouthful of food. |
| 5. Develop individualized child and family goals:<br>■ Child will receive adequate food and fluid intake for growth and development.<br>■ Child will be correctly positioned for feeding.<br>■ Child will be fed using correct technique.<br>■ Child feeds self appropriately for developmental age and ability.<br>■ Child experiences minimal fatigue and stress. | |

## Implementation

| Steps | Rationale |
|---|---|
| 1. Position child: | Proper positioning facilitates feeding and minimizes physical stress for the child. The feeding process requires significant energy for the child with feeding disabilities, attributable to the incoordination of sucking and swallowing and weak oral muscles. |
| a. For small babies, place on lap with arms around baby supporting shoulders, head, and neck (Fig. 61-3). Do not feed a child in a reclining position. | Children who are hypotonic require extra support. A reclining position may cause middle ear infections or aspiration and does not foster the development of feeding skills. |
| b. Older babies or children can be seated on a pillow on the feeder's lap, facing the feeder (Fig. 61-4). The feeder should be seated with feet on a small stool or box. Place pillows behind the child's back and lean the child against the edge of a table for support (feeder facing table; child and pillow with back to table edge). To help the child sit upright with head slightly forward, place a rolled towel behind the neck (McClannahan, 1983). | ***Special Considerations:*** *A small child's plastic inflated swimming ring may be used for seating the child in a support position. Hold the ring on its end and seat child on the edge of the ring with head and neck resting on the top part of the ring (Fig. 61-5). This frees the child's arms. A kitchen counter at home works well.* |
| c. When the child is old enough to feed in a chair, promote development of good posture by supporting from the ground up.<br>■ Support feet.<br>■ Place child back in chair to produce flexion of the hips and knees.<br>■ Support head at midline, tilted slightly forward. | Since feeding a child with developmental or other disabling conditions is sometimes a long procedure, comfort is imperative. A hospitalized child is even more prone to tiring easily. Supporting the child and positioning for comfort will reduce stress and facilitate safe feeding.<br>***Special Considerations:*** *If the child is hypertonic, as with cerebral palsy, avoid placing any pressure on the back of the head as this may cause a reflex action that pushes the head back and the child's feet and torso forward.* |
| 2. Spoon feed the child. General measures: | |
| a. Put only the right amount of food on the child's spoon. | Too much food on the spoon may cause the child to choke or gag. |
| b. Feed the child with head tilted slightly forward and supported at midline, but not back in a "bird feeding" position (Fig. 61-6). | The child might aspirate food with the head tilted back while feeding. Tilting the head back during eating will throw all swallowing mechanisms out of line and may contribute to permanent deformities. |
| c. If the lower lip is "floppy" (hypotonic) and food does not stay in the mouth, use the nondominant hand to feed and use the index finger on the dominant hand over the upper lip and the third finger under the lower lip. The ring finger is used to support the jaw. Assist the child in holding the lips closed until he or she is able to swallow. The child needs to do as much of the feeding process as possible. | Using the muscles will help the child to develop skills.<br>***Special Considerations:*** *The family should be encouraged to try new foods (based on therapist's advice) even though it takes longer to feed, and encourage the child's attempts at feeding.* |

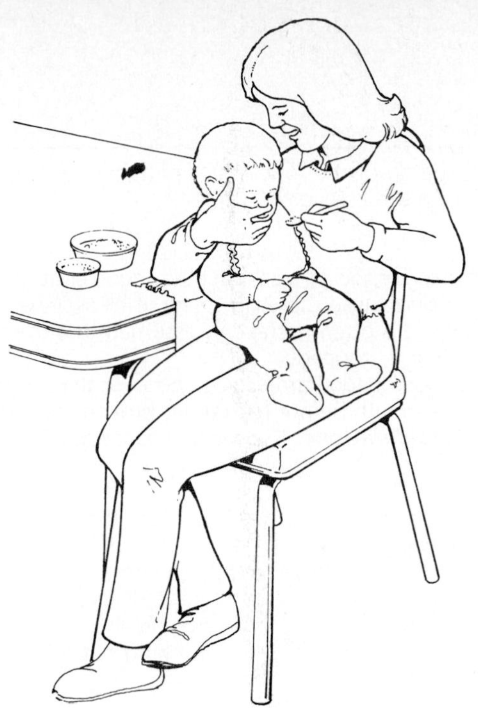

***FIG. 61-3*** Child is placed on lap with proper support during feeding.

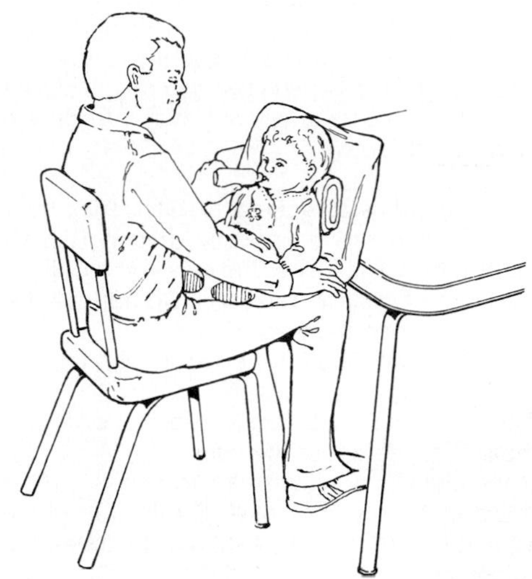

***FIG. 61-4*** Child is positioned facing feeder with pillows and towel behind back.

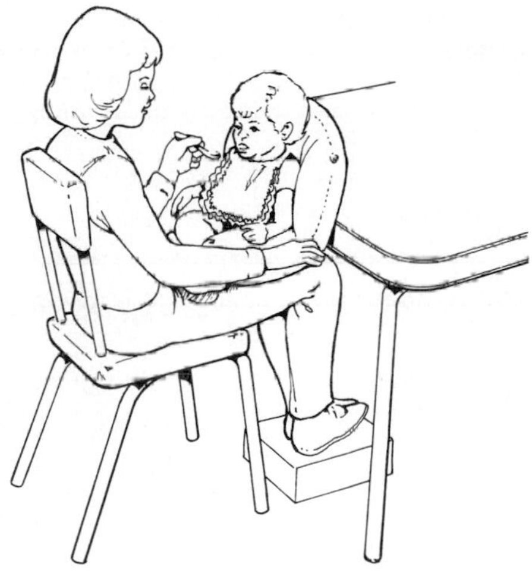

***FIG. 61-5*** A small inflatable inner tube may be used to provide support.

A

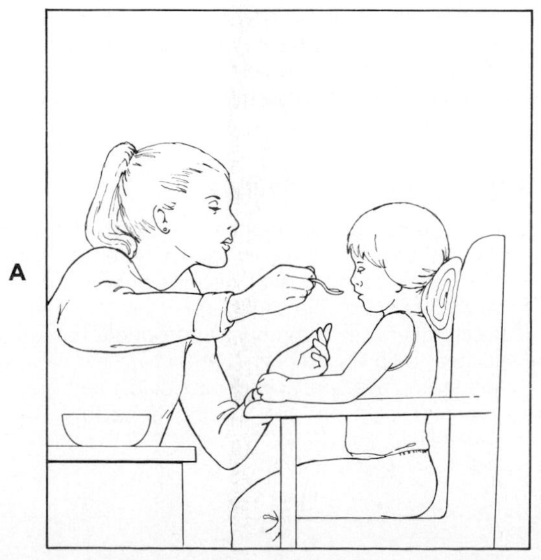

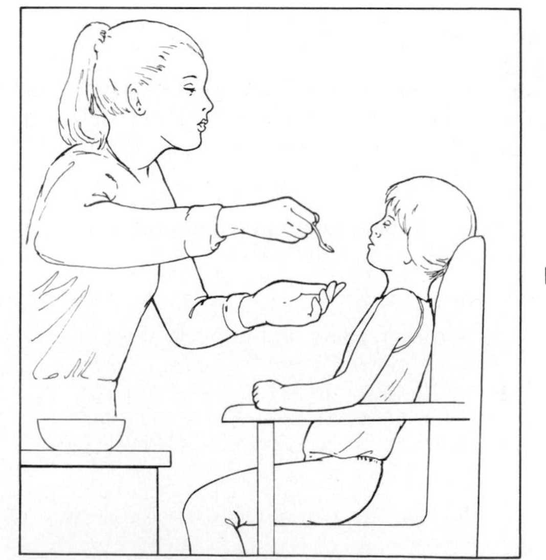

B

***FIG. 61-6*** **A,** Correct and **B,** Incorrect positions for feeding the child with special needs.

| Steps | Rationale |
|---|---|
| d. If the child has tongue thrust and pushes the food out of the mouth, do not touch the tip of the tongue with the spoon. Place the food well behind the tip of the tongue and press down firmly but gently. | Touching the tip of the tongue encourages a tongue thrust reaction with these children. |
| e. If the child has a hyperactive gag reflex, place the spoon forward on the tongue, and slowly introduce semi solids or textured foods. | Placing the spoon too far back on the tongue elicits a gag reflex. Gagging may cause the child to vomit or aspirate. When the child gags, it is often mistakenly assumed that the child is full and feeding is stopped. |
| f. If the child has a hyperactive bite reflex he or she will clamp down on the spoon when it is placed in the mouth. Massage below the ears and along the angle of the jaw to facilitate relaxation. Do not pull the spoon or try to pry open the jaw. | If the child clamps too hard on the spoon or the spoon is pulled out of the mouth before relaxation, broken teeth may result. ***Special Considerations:*** *Use rubber coated spoons for this type of disorder.* |
| g. Do not scrape food off the spoon with the child's teeth. | Lips should be used to remove food from the spoon to develop proper feeding patterns. |
| h. If the child is slow to chew, rub in a circular motion on the soft tissue under the chin. | This procedure stimulates the child to chew. |
| 3. Assist the child to drink with a cup. | |
| a. If the child does not have lip closure when drinking, assist by using the thumb under the lip and around the cup to ensure a better seal (Fig. 61-7). | This will help keep the fluid from running out of the mouth. |
| b. Tilt the cup to allow the child to suck the liquid into the mouth. | A cup with a cut out space for the nose allows the child to tip the cup and swallow the fluid more easily. |
| c. Wait for the child to swallow before adding more fluid. To facilitate the swallow reflex, gently press upward under the chin at the base of the tongue. An ice cube rubbed over the skin on the throat may facilitate swallowing (Eschelman, 1988). | Unless the child swallows the fluid given previously, he or she will choke or lose the fluid from the mouth when more fluid is introduced. ***Special Considerations:*** *Orenstein et al (1988) reported blowing a small puff of air into the face reliably elicited a swallowing reflex in infants under 11 months and children with severe neurologic disorders.* |

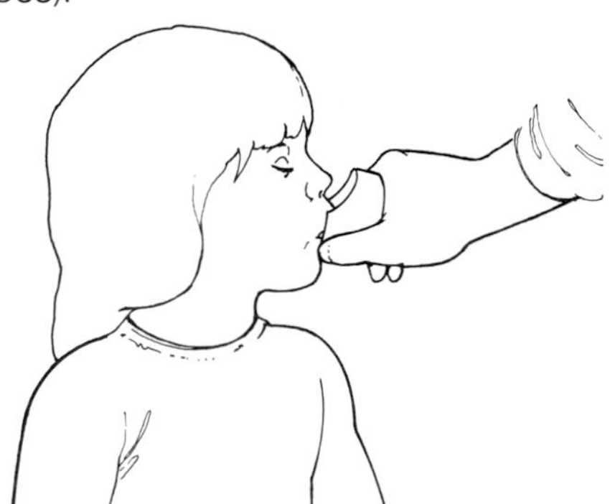

***FIG. 61-7*** Assisting the child with poor lip closure to drink.

| Steps | Rationale |
|---|---|
| 4. Do not wipe child's face. Blot it instead to wipe food and drink from the face. | Wiping the mouth of a child with a neurologic impairment may encourage reflexive opening of the mouth. |
| 5. Talk to the child, and encourage him or her to eat and drink. Keep environmental stimuli, e.g., soft music or dim lights at a relaxing level. | Reassurance and encouragement will decrease the child's anxiety. Meals should be unhurried and uninterrupted. Eye contact and conversation are reassuring. Music and dim lights work well to relax child (Kosowski and Sopczyk, 1985). |
| 6. Clean child's teeth or assist child to clean own teeth (see Skills 56 and 57). | Children who do not have good oral musculature may be prone to develop dental problems. |
| 7. Encourage family to express feelings related to child's feeding program. | Family participation is essential to a successful feeding program. |

| Evaluation Outcomes | Observational Guidelines |
|---|---|
| 1. Child is gaining weight and exhibits no dehydration or signs and symptoms of nutritional deficiency. | Use age standards for height and weight. Plot growth curves on these standardized forms to assess serial trends, recognizing that some children with disabilities will not be at the same level as peers of the same age. |
| 2. Caretakers use correct feeding and drinking techniques at all meals. | The caretaker uses techniques appropriate for conditions of child related to lip closure, stimulation to chew or swallow, blotting food from face, and appropriate placement of spoon in mouth. |
| 3. The child exhibits normal development of feeding behaviors for age or demonstrates progression from previous feeding behaviors. | Compare child's present feeding behaviors with previous assessment. |

| Steps | Rationale |
|---|---|
| 4. The child responds positively at mealtime and is not fatigued from feeding. | Child cooperates with feeding; intake is adequate for needs. Stimuli in the child's eating area are reduced. Child is alert and does not exhibit signs of fatigue after feeding. |
| 5. Family members express their concerns about the child's feeding. | Attitude and concerns of parents are verbalized. |

## Documentation

Document child's feeding behaviors. Record intake for each meal. When teaching the family, note techniques that have worked in the past for successful feeding. Any techniques taught to the family or discussed with them should be documented. Relate how validation of family's or child's feeding skills were assessed and the level of their understanding for teaching purposes, e.g., repeated the technique, asked pertinent questions, or discussed the rationale for care given. Document areas that may need to be repeated or reinforced with the family. Discuss referrals that were made for the child and the family and the rationale for making them after hospitalization. If the background of the child's condition or any part of the feeding program is researched, list references or attach copies of the article to the child's care plan or chart.

## Home Care Modifications

Referral to home health care, public health or school nurse, an outreach team, or an early childhood intervention program will be useful for the family. Occupational therapists can show parents how to make utensils out of ordinary household items. Some programs will loan special equipment to a family. (See resource list on p. 438 for some home care references.)

# *SKILL* 62 Feeding the Child with Cleft Lip/Cleft Palate

*Mary Breen*

Newborns with cleft lip and/or cleft palate present a feeding challenge to the medical professional. Every attempt should be made to provide a normal feeding experience for both the infant and parent. This involves assessing the oral structures, selecting the best feeding method, and giving instruction and guidance to the family. This skill focuses on feeding the child who has not yet had surgical correction for the defect. Postoperative feeding methods vary with the surgeon and institution (see the box on the following page).

## NURSING DIAGNOSES

Altered nutrition: less than body requirements related to insufficient intake for metabolic needs; Altered infant growth and development related to nutritional deficiencies; Altered parenting related to lack of knowledge about cleft lip/cleft palate infant feedings; Anxiety related to feeding difficulties of newborn with cleft lip/cleft palate.

| Steps | Rationale |
|---|---|
| **Assessment** | |
| 1. Assess type of cleft and degree of interference with feeding. | The type and degree of severity of the cleft will have an impact on feeding. Infants with cleft lip may have difficulty achieving lip closure around the nipple. Infants with cleft palate may have an ineffective suck. |
| 2. Determine if the infant will be bottle fed or breast-fed. | ***Special Considerations:*** *Breastfeeding the infant with cleft lip/palate is an emotional and often controversial subject. Infants with isolated cleft lip may breastfeed without problems—the mother's breast may mold to the defect. However, infants with a cleft of the palate may not be able to effectively obtain milk from the breast but may take pumped breastmilk from a bottle or Lact-Aid device. A Lact-Aid feeding device comprises a sterile plastic bag and a small capillary tube. The tube comes out of the bag filled with breastmilk and the opening is placed in the area of the mother's nipple. The baby sucks on the breast and tube at the same time to obtain milk.* |

### *FEEDING METHODS AFTER CLEFT LIP/PALATE REPAIR*

**TRADITIONAL (SYRINGE) VS. UNRESTRICTED**

Postoperative feeding protocols following cleft lip/palate repair vary with the institution. In the past, most surgeons did not allow postoperative feeding for 2 to 3 weeks, while methods such as the Brecht feeder, syringe, or cup feeding were recommended. Currently, these traditional methods are being discarded, and more physicians are allowing bottle or breast-feeding within 24 to 48 hours after surgery.

Elkins, Cohen, and Schafer (1988) compared two postoperative care protocols using a sample of 80 infants aged 2 to 13 months with unilateral or bilateral cleft lip and palate. Protocol A called for feeding with a tube and syringe for 7 days following cleft lip surgery and for 10 days following cleft palate repair. Protocol B called for bottle and nipple feeding on the first postoperative day for cleft lip repair and on the second postoperative day for cleft palate repair. With the exception of one partial lip dehiscence after cleft lip repair in an infant fed according to Protocol A, all infants healed primarily. Although weight measurements were not recorded, the investigators' overall impression was that the weight gain and nutritional status in Group B was better. Therefore their conclusion was that immediate unrestricted feeding following cleft lip and cleft palate repair is possible without fear of dehiscence or other complications and should be reinforced.

Another study (Weatherley-White et al, 1987) investigated the results of immediate breastfeeding following cleft lip repair. Sixty mothers were offered this choice; 16 chose to breastfeed their infants for a minimum of 6 weeks, while 22 started with breastfeeding but switched to a bottle within 6 weeks. No complications attributed to breastfeeding were observed. An improved rate of weight gain and shorter hospital stay was also described.

Since nurses are responsible for educating parents in postoperative care, they should be aware that feeding protocols vary and need to be informed concerning the postoperative feeding practices at their institution.

| Steps | Rationale |
|---|---|
| 3. Determine infant's weight. | A baseline weight will provide accurate growth evaluation. |

## Planning and Goal Setting

| Steps | Rationale |
|---|---|
| 1. Select from appropriate nipple and bottle choices. | Some babies with a cleft defect can use a regular bottle and nipple. However, in most cases, the equipment must be modified or special products used. ***Special Considerations:*** *Parents should be advised that each infant with a cleft defect is different and they should try several bottles and/or nipples before deciding on the best method.* |
| a. Nipples.<br>▪ Regular nipple with enlarged, cross cut opening.<br>▪ Nuk nipple.<br>▪ Soft preemie nipple with cross cut opening. | Cross cutting the nipple opening improves milk flow; premie nipples are soft and easily compressible. Nuk nipples may allow better lip closure if the cleft is extremely wide. |
| b. Bottles.<br>▪ Regular bottle.<br>▪ Soft squeeze bottle (Fig. 62-1). | The squeeze bottle assists the infant's own sucking mechanism and prevents excessive fatigue. ***Special Considerations:*** *As the infant practices sucking, he or she will develop the muscles that will be important for both eating and later speech development.* |
| 2. Gather supplies:<br>a. Bottle and nipple.<br>b. Prescribed formula.<br>c. Bulb syringe.<br>d. Burp cloth. | Having supplies ready prevents interruptions during feeding time. |
| 3. Allow 30 to 45 minutes in schedule for feedings. | Parents should be encouraged to view the longer feeding time as a chance to spend quality time with the infant and develop the parent-child relationship. |
| 4. Develop individualized child and family goals:<br>▪ Adequate intake for growth needs.<br>▪ Reasonable time for length of feedings.<br>▪ Family comfortable with feeding method. | |

| **Steps** | **Rationale** |
|---|---|

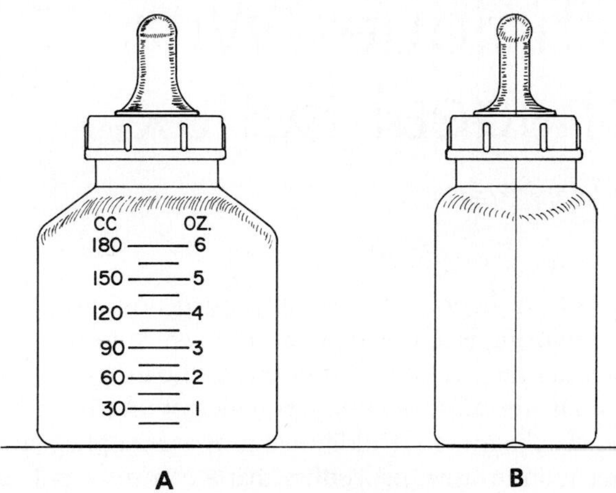


***FIG. 62-1*** A cleft lip/cleft palate nurser. **A,** Front view. **B,** Side view.

From Smith MJ, Goodman JA, and Ramsey NL: Child and family concepts of nursing practice, ed 2, St Louis, 1987, The CV Mosby Co.

## Implementation

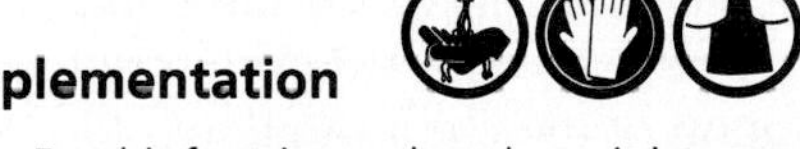

1. Feed infant in a relaxed, upright, or semi-reclining position.

   The upright position reduces the amount of nasal regurgitation.
   ***Special Considerations:*** *The family should be instructed in the use of the bulb syringe in case of regurgitation (see Skill 87).*

2. Place nipple in infant's mouth on the opposite side from cleft or where there is the greatest amount of palatal tissue available for compressing nipple.

   This placement facilitates infant's "stripping" or chewing action to get formula from bottle.
   ***Special Considerations:*** *Occasionally infants may develop areas of redness or irritation on the oral mucosa from the nipple, thus placement may need to be rotated to different sites.*

3. If using a squeeze bottle, gently squeeze the bottle before putting the nipple into the infant's mouth to estimate how much pressure is needed to get an even flow.

   Formula flowing too fast may cause the infant to choke, while a slow flow will lengthen feeding time.
   ***Special Considerations:*** *Parents should be cautioned against squeezing formula into the mouth when the infant is resting. This disturbs the natural suck/swallow pattern and could also cause the infant to choke.*

4. Burp infant after every ½ to 1 oz.

   Infant may swallow more air than usual, causing discomfort.
   ***Special Considerations:*** *Parents must be cautioned about removing the nipple too often. This may cause the infant to tire and become frustrated.*

5. Discuss feeding techniques with family, address concerns, and answer questions.

   Usually successful feeding is the most immediate need for the family with a newborn with cleft lip/palate. They may also have many questions regarding issues such as surgery, speech development, dental concerns, and explanations to other family members.
   ***Special Considerations:*** *Refer parents to a cleft palate team and/or parent support group for accurate information, support, comprehensive care, and treatment (if not already in contact with these resources).*

## Evaluation Outcomes

1. Reasonable feeding schedule is established with the infant taking required calories in 30 to 45 minutes.
2. Infant demonstrates adequate weight gain for age.
3. Family demonstrates confidence in feeding infant.

## Observational Guidelines

Ask parent to describe feeding schedule, length of feeding, and formula amount per feeding.
Weigh infant daily and plot changes on growth chart.
Observe family members feeding infant. Note relaxed posture and hold on child, eye contact, ability to cope with regurgitation, and infant's behavior.

## Documentation

Document type and amount of formula, length of feeding time, type of bottle/nipple successfully used, person feeding, and infant's behavior.

# SKILL 63 Feeding Techniques With Gastroesophageal Reflux

Donna Phillips Smith and Mary Breen

Gastroesophageal reflux (GER) results when the incompetent or relaxed sphincter between the esophagus and stomach allows acidic stomach contents to reflux or flow back up into the esophagus. The frequency of occurrence and severity of the resulting clinical symptoms varies considerably, from no noticeable effect to serious complications and even death. GER in early infancy is considered physiologically normal until about 6 weeks of age, although it often persists much longer. GER also commonly occurs in children with neurologic impairment (pathophysiologic GER) and failure-to-thrive cases (pathologic GER).

The infant's history of vomiting or regurgitation must be carefully evaluated. A detailed history, physical examination, and diagnostic testing are essential to confirm a diagnosis of GER. Several tests are available to aid in differential diagnosis and treatment. A barium swallow test is usually ordered first. It is fairly accurate in identifying GER, and it can also eliminate two other serious causes of vomiting: pyloric stenosis and bowel obstruction. Esophageal pH monitoring is a more specific test, which uses a probe to measure the pH of the lower end of the esophagus over a 24-hour period, detecting frequency of gastric contents in the esophagus. Two additional tests are esophageal manometry, an invasive procedure that measures esophageal pressures to evaluate esophageal sphincter tone, and radionuclide gastroesophagraphy, in which the child swallows a radionuclide that can be detected during reflux by radiographic visualization of the chest (Aquilina, 1987).

## NURSING DIAGNOSES

Altered nutrition: less than body requirements related to gastric reflux/vomiting due to incompetent or relaxed cardiac sphincter; Ineffective family coping related to inadequate information about gastroesophageal reflux disorder, feeding, and positioning techniques; Altered growth and development related to inadequate nutritional intake.

| Steps | Rationale |
|---|---|
| **Assessment** | |
| 1. Determine age and developmental level of the child. | Regurgitation or physiologic GER is considered normal in the first 6 weeks of life, although it is not uncommon for it to continue for many months. Reflux may also persist asymptomatically into adulthood.<br>***Special Considerations:*** *Physiologic GER is especially common in premature infants, possibly attributable to immature development.* |
| 2. Interview the family: | |
| ***Infant*** | |
| a. Determine type and method of feeding, preparation of formula, amount, and frequency of feedings. Also type of feeder: slow, gulps, or difficult to burp (Aquilina, 1987). | Reviewing the typical feeding routine may identify possible causes or factors contributing to reflux.<br>***Special Considerations:*** *Observe feeding technique if needed to validate or clarify information obtained.* |
| b. Determine vomiting patterns such as when it occurs (with burps, every feeding or one half the time, 2 hours after feeding, only in certain positions), if the vomiting is forceful, and if the child acts hungry after vomiting (Aquilina, 1987). | Reflux and vomiting patterns can provide additional information for diagnosis and treatment. Therapeutic management usually depends on the severity. For example, if reflux only occurs when placed in an infant seat after feedings, positioning may alleviate the symptoms.<br>***Special Considerations:*** *Forceful vomiting without a loss of appetite is characteristic of pyloric stenosis, a congenital condition requiring prompt surgical intervention.* |
| c. Ask if child is irritable after a feeding, has blood-tinged emesis or stool, or has inconsistent sleeping patterns. | These symptoms are associated with esophagitis, an irritation of the esophageal mucosa from the reflux of acidic gastric contents. The development of this complication of GER can result in heartburn, blood loss, and iron deficiency anemia. |

| Steps | Rationale |
|---|---|
| d. Assess associated pulmonary symptoms such as coughing, cyanosis, stridor, and apnea. | In addition to commonly known aspiration pneumonia, reflux of acidic gastric contents can trigger reflex bronchospasm, reflex laryngospasm (obstructive apnea, stridor), and reflex central apnea and bradycardia (Orenstein and Orenstein, 1988). GER is a well-known risk factor for apneic episodes in infants. |
| ***Older child*** | |
| a. Determine usual eating patterns including types and amounts of food and times. | Large meals can exacerbate existing reflux. Eating before bedtime allows reflux while in a recumbent position. |
| b. Determine patterns of symptoms such as vomiting, heartburn in relation to time of day and positioning (e.g., at night while sleeping). | Patterns of symptoms help guide diagnosis and treatment. Just as in infants, management usually depends on severity.<br>***Special Considerations:*** *Heartburn is a frequently reported symptom in older children, although it may go unrecognized in infants.* |
| c. If fed enterally, determine type and method of feeding (gastrostomy tube, nasal feeding tube), preparation of formula, amount and frequency of feedings (bolus or continuous). | The feeding management program for the child may need to be altered if reflux is identified. For example, bolus feedings may need to be smaller. Indwelling nasogastric tubes or gastrostomy tube placement may also cause or aggravate GER (Orenstein and Orenstein, 1988; Mollitt et al, 1985).<br>***Special Considerations:*** *A controversial issue in gastrostomy tube placement in children with neurologic damage is whether to perform a fundoplication at the same time. While some recommend it routinely, Ross et al (1988) found it most indicated with a child with central nervous system (CNS) insult causing cerebral injury, while children with more global damage (perinatal asphyxia or postterm progressive encephalopathy) were more likely to tolerate a gastrostomy tube alone.* |
| d. Assess for associated symptoms such as coughing at night and wheezing. | Prominent nocturnal asthma symptoms may result from reflex bronchospasm triggered by GER.<br>***Special Considerations:*** *Reflux may not even be suspected but should be considered in nocturnal asthma symptoms without an allergic basis that is resistant to medical management (Orenstein and Orenstein, 1988).* |
| 3. Review medical history for recurrent pneumonia, asthma, cystic fibrosis, bronchopulmonary dysplasia (BPD), food allergies, neurologic injury, neuromuscular or developmental delay such as cerebral palsy, and/or repaired tracheoesophageal fistula or esophageal atresia. | Respiratory disorders, symptoms and treatments can provoke reflux if they alter antireflux barriers such as increasing abdominal pressure (coughing, wheezing) and counteracting natural gravitational pull (chest physiotherapy, supine positioning) (Orenstein and Orenstein, 1988). Neurologic injury and neuromuscular or developmental delay are often associated with pathophysiologic GER (Aquilina, 1987) possibly because of supine positioning, increased abdominal pressure attributed to spasticity, and poor swallowing and gag reflex. Repaired esophageal malformations also tend to reflux, possibly from associated congenital factors (Orenstein and Orenstein, 1988). |
| 4. Assess for use of bronchodilators such as theophylline, caffeine, isoproterenol, metaproterenol, and carbuterol. Also assess for cigarette smoking by the child or family. | These medications relax the lower esophageal sphincter, allowing reflux. Theophylline increases gastric acid secretion. Smoking promotes esophageal sphincter relaxation; it is unknown if passive smoking has the same effects (Orenstein and Orenstein, 1988). |
| 5. Assess family and home environment. | The ability of the family to continue treatment at home must be evaluated, especially if failure-to-thrive is associated with GER. Contributing factors may indicate pathologic GER. |
| 6. Assess growth measurements and review growth curve if available. | Frequent vomiting or reflux may lead to weight loss or poor growth, possibly the first sign of an existing problem. Assessing present measurements provides a basis for evaluation. |
| 7. Perform a physical assessment, paying particular attention to child's behavior such as irritability or contentedness, respiratory rate, adventitious breath sounds, cyanosis or retractions, and symptoms of anemia (Aquilina, 1987) (see Skill 27). | A physical assessment assists in validating and/or clarifying the previous assessment data obtained to further assist in diagnosis and treatment. |

| Steps | Rationale |
|---|---|

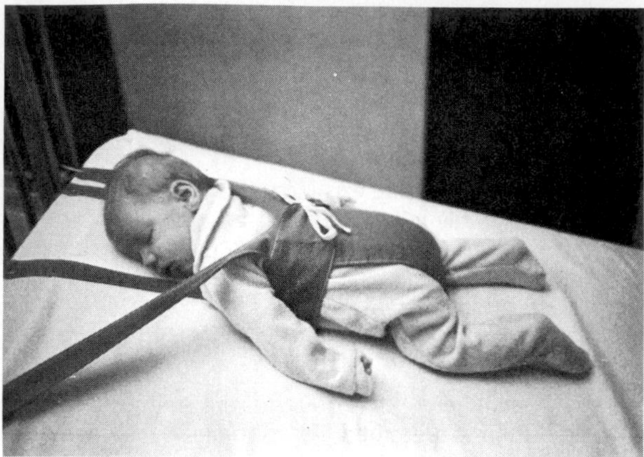

***FIG. 63-1*** Infant positioned in fabric harness.
From Orenstein SR and Whittington PF: Positioning for prevention of infant gastroesophageal reflux, J Pediatr 103, 534-537, 1983.

## Planning

1. Review physician's orders on feeding such as type, frequency, thickeners (if infant), and positioning requirements.

The physician determines the therapeutic plan. Some controversy exists on optimum therapeutic management, as well as variations in treatment, depending on severity.
***Special Considerations:*** *Pharmacologic agents for the treatment of GER are also controversial and may or may not be ordered.*

2. Gather necessary items such as positioning aids, formula, and thickeners.

***Special Considerations:*** *Positioning aids can include blanket and towel rolls, a fabric harness, an elevated board with a spindle, or commercial positioning bed (Fig. 63-1 and see Product References).*

3. Bathe and diaper child immediately before feedings. For the older ambulatory child, schedule the last meal of the day to be eaten at least 4 hours before bedtime.

Proper planning prevents delay of effective positioning for the infant after feeding. For the older child, timing meals properly allows for gastric emptying before bedtime.

4. Plan time to teach family about GER and the purposes and techniques of the selected therapy (see Skill 43).

Selecting a convenient time for teaching will facilitate learning.

5. Develop individualized child and family goals:
   - Child will exhibit decreased symptomatology of reflux.
   - Child and family will demonstrate adequate knowledge and use of techniques to minimize reflux.

## Implementation 
### *Infant*

1. Thicken formula or expressed breastmilk with rice cereal if ordered. The usual amount is one tablespoon to one ounce of formula (usually 2 to 4 ounces). Enlarge the nipple opening as necessary.

The traditional treatment is to provide a smaller feeding to prevent overdistension of the stomach and thickened to prevent reflux.
***Special Considerations:*** *Studies are conflicting as to the value of thickening the feeding. Bailey et al (1987) found no differences in radiologically detected reflux, but less episodes of emesis, less crying time, and more sleep time was demonstrated after the thickened as compared with the unthickened formula.*

2. Feed slowly in an upright position, burping at least every ½ ounce.

The upright position prevents reflux by use of gravity. Frequent burping prevents overdistension of the stomach, and large burps tend to allow formula to flow up at the same time.

3. After feeding, gently place in a prone position with head elevated 30° (see Fig. 63-1).

Orenstein et al, (1983) demonstrated that infants in the prone, head-elevated position had fewer episodes of reflux than in the traditionally used infant-carrier position, in which the slumped posture usually submerged the gastroesophageal junction, allowing reflux.
***Special Considerations:*** *A recent study found the prone, head-elevated position to be no better than flat prone in decreasing reflux (Orenstein, 1990).*

| Steps | Rationale |
|---|---|
| 4. Feed 2 to 4 ounces every 2 to 3 hours or as ordered. The amount and frequency may be gradually increased as the infant gets older. For the breast-fed infant, have the mother express some milk before feeding to prevent a sudden surge of milk and to prevent the infant from getting a larger feeding. Limit feeding to 10 to 15 minutes on each breast (Aquilina, 1987). | Reflux can occur when intragastric pressure exceeds sphincter pressure, therefore frequent, smaller amounts may prevent increased pressure. ***Special Considerations:*** *Orenstein and Orenstein (1988) questioned the use of frequent feedings, which increase the postprandial time, when most episodes occur. The prone position alone may achieve improvement in reflux episodes (Aquilina, 1987).* |
| 5. Maintain the prone, elevated position except for feeding, bathing, and diaper changes for 24 hours a day or as ordered. Maintain upright position as much as possible for these caretaking activities. | ***Special Considerations:*** *The positioning aid may need to be padded with sheepskin or eggcrate foam padding to protect the infant's knees and elbows (Whaley and Wong, 1989).* |
| 6. Provide developmental stimulation appropriate to degree of immobility (see Skill 15). | Continuous prone positioning minimizes opportunities for developmental stimulation, particularly as the child gets older and more mobile. ***Special Considerations:*** *The physician may allow the older infant to be positioned upright in a walker for short periods.* |
| ***Older Child*** | |
| 1. Provide smaller, more frequent meals during the day (solid and liquid gastric/enteral feedings). | Reflux can occur when intragastric pressure exceeds sphincter pressure; smaller meals help prevent increased abdominal pressure. |
| 2. Have ambulatory child sit upright or stand during the day and avoid semi-reclining positions. | Gravity helps prevent reflux. |
| 3. Have child fast at least 4 hours before bedtime. | Fasting allows gastric emptying, which makes nocturnal reflux less likely. |
| 4. Position prone if possible with the head of the bed elevated 30° for sleep. | The prone position is better than supine for recumbency with older children as well as infants. ***Special Considerations:*** *Although it is difficult to place the child on assisted ventilation in the elevated prone position for sleep, it can be beneficial (Orenstein and Orenstein, 1988).* |
| 5. Perform chest physiotherapy, which requires supine or head down positions several hours after a meal, and/or administer antacid (Orenstein and Orenstein, 1988). | Chest physiotherapy in these positions can induce reflux by gravity, and the usual accompanying coughing maneuvers increase abdominal pressure, aggravating the situation. |
| ***General Measures*** | |
| 1. Avoid tight diapering or tight, restrictive clothing. | Restrictive items around the abdomen will increase abdominal pressure, promoting reflux. |
| 2. Discuss the pathophysiology of GER, principles of the recommended treatments, and expected course with the family and child. | An understanding of the disorder and treatment modalities enhances cooperation and is essential to discharge planning. ***Special Considerations:*** *Physiologic GER usually lasts until about 8 months of age (Aquilina, 1987). Surgical correction (fundoplication), usually performed after 1 year of age, is reserved for pathophysiologic and pathologic cases with severe complications such as reflux-mediated respiratory disease, failure-to-thrive, and neurologically devastated children with reflux (Orenstein and Orenstein, 1988).* |
| 3. Provide emotional support for the family. Problem solve with them for anticipated areas of concern. | Home management of GER is time-consuming, exhausting, and stressful, especially for families of infants with round-the-clock feeding schedules, apnea monitoring, reluctance of other family members to hold or feed for fear of emesis or choking, and a need for sitters qualified to give CPR. |

| Evaluation Outcomes | Observational Guidelines |
|---|---|
| 1. Child exhibits reduced or lessened symptomatology of GER. | Review initial presenting symtoms of GER; compare with present status, e.g., frequency of emesis, weight loss or poor growth, episodes of apnea or aspiration, frequency of night coughing or bronchospasm, blood-tinged emesis. |
| 2. Family demonstrates adequate knowledge base of mechanism of GER, and principles of selected treatments. | Ask family to explain the disorder and how the treatments are effective in minimizing GER. |
| 3. Family demonstrates correct feeding and positioning techniques. | Observe family prepare a feeding, feed and burp, and position the child. |
| 4. Family develops strategies to promote development for the infant needing to remain prone 24 hours. | Ask family to discuss their plans to provide developmentally appropriate stimulation for the child positioned prone. |
| 5. Family demonstrates comfort with feeding schedule at home. | Ask family to discuss their plans to manage the frequent feeding schedule. |

### Documentation

Record the type and amount of formula and how prepared (thickener added, how much). Note how infant tolerates the feeding and indicate positioning used, as well as toleration of position. Document episodes of emesis as well as the amount and related symptoms. Describe any teaching conducted with child and family.

### Child and Family Teaching

1. The family will need to learn simple airway clearance methods such as using a bulb syringe and oral suctioning (see Skill 87).
2. Provide instruction on use of an apnea monitor if the child will be discharged with continuous monitoring. The family, including alternate caregivers for respite care, will also need to receive CPR training (see Skills 93 and 126).

### Home Care Modifications

1. Assist the family in the construction or purchase of a device that provides secure, 30 degree head-elevated prone positioning. Simple towel or blanket rolls are satisfactory for temporary situations such as diaper changing or baths, but a more stable device is needed for long-term positioning. The crib mattress can be elevated with blankets, blocks, or a cardboard box. A harness can be sewn from heavy duty, washable fabric. A padded, wooden board with a padded spindle securely attached can be constructed. A portable, adjustable commercial bed is also available (see Product Resources).
2. Car travel is a difficult problem because the car seat position predisposes to reflux (Clark, 1987). Suggest planning short trips at least 2 hours after a feeding. Suggest providing a pacifier while in the car seat, since sucking on the pacifier while seated in this position may reduce episodes of reflux (Orenstein, 1988). One federally approved car bed permits the prone position (see Skill 45).
3. Avoid "umbrella" type strollers that allow the small infant to slump forward, promoting reflux similar to the infant seat position.

# *SKILL* 64 Monitoring Hydration

*Krena Hunter White and Donna Phillips Smith*

Assessing and monitoring fluid balance is a significant part of nursing care with most hospitalized children and is often a concern in a number of mild childhood illnesses. Fluid balance is especially important in children because of major physiologic differences that increase the risk of imbalance. Children have a higher total body water percentage by weight, which gradually decreases by age: preterm infant, 80% to 85%; full-term infant, 75% to 80%; by age 3, 63%; and by age 12 and older, approximately 58% depending on amount of body fat (Whaley and Wong, 1991). The distribution of water between intracellular and extracellular (interstitial and intravascular) compartments also differs by age, with the majority of water located extracellularly in infants, gradually changing to intracellularly in the older child/adult. Despite this greater total water content, children are more vulnerable to imbalances because they must ingest and excrete (turnover) a greater volume per day (up to one half total body water compared with one sixth for adults) to excrete metabolic wastes produced with a metabolic rate twice that of adults. In addition, a child has a greater body surface area in relation to body weight than adults, which results in greater insensible water losses (undetected losses through the lungs and the skin). Functional renal immaturity significantly contributes to the risk of fluid imbalances, especially under age 2. A less efficient renal ability to concentrate or dilute urine or to retain or excrete sodium allows fluid deficit or overload and/or sodium imbalance to rapidly develop.

Fluid balance is a complex interaction of numerous physiologic principles, with many additional closely related concepts such as nutrition and acid-base balance. In addition to the complexities involved in fluid balance, an imbalance is usually a combination of several problems, and single disruptions are seldom seen. The scope of this skill is limited to presentation of a framework for clinical application of fundamental fluid balance concepts to allow meaningful observation, permit knowledgeable collaboration with the physician, and provide basic principles of therapy to guide both dependent and independent nursing practice. A brief review of the major forces, electrolytes, and hormones influencing fluid balance is presented in the box at right.

For a more complete review, to gain fundamental concepts, or for acid/base dynamics, consult an authoritative text on fluid and electrolytes.

### NURSING DIAGNOSES

Fluid volume deficit related to excessive fluid loss or failure of regulatory mechanism; Fluid volume excess related to excessive fluid/sodium intake or compromised regulatory mechanisms; Altered tissue perfusion related to hypovolemia or hypervolemia; Altered thought processes related to electrolyte imbalances and/or hypervolemia; Potential altered parenting related to lack of information about importance of child's fluid balance and goals of therapy.

## OVERVIEW OF FLUID BALANCE

### ELECTROLYTES

The major electrolytes significantly influencing fluid balance are sodium ($Na^+$) and potassium ($K^+$) (both cations), and chloride ($Cl^-$) (an anion). Sodium and chloride are primarily extracellular; potassium is the major intracellular cation. For chemical neutrality in a solution (including body fluids), anions and cations must balance, e.g., electrolytes in IV solutions are always in combination: sodium chloride, potassium chloride, sodium bicarbonate.

### FLUID MOVEMENT

In considering fluid balance, the forces that move fluid into and out of the vascular space include osmotic forces, oncotic pressures, hydrostatic pressures, and changes in capillary permeability (Hazinski, 1988). Of these, osmotic forces, as a result of serum osmolality (concentration of solution measured in mOsmols), most commonly influence movement. Sodium is the major cation determining serum osmolality. Since free water moves from an area of low osmolality to one of high osmolality (by osmotic draw), a low serum sodium causes fluid movement out of the intravascular space into interstitial tissues, and a high serum sodium (less common) causes water to move into the intravascular space. Glucose also contributes to serum osmolality, causing similar fluid shifts, especially with increased levels. While osmotic forces work at the vascular level, the other forces function at the capillary level (Hazinski, 1988). Plasma proteins exert oncotic pressure, which tends to hold fluid in the capillary vascular spaces; decreased plasma protein levels allow fluid to escape. Hydrostatic pressure generated by myocardial function helps maintain fluid balance in the vascular spaces. Myocardial dysfunction may lead to increased venous pressure and a net filtration of fluid into the interstitial tissues. Capillary permeability is the last factor opposing fluid filtration; the membrane is normally impermeable to plasma proteins. If capillary permeability increases, as it commonly does with sepsis, the proteins pass into the interstitial spaces, drawing fluid with them (Hazinski, 1988).

### HORMONAL INFLUENCES

The two major hormones that influence fluid balance are antidiuretic hormone (ADH), which is secreted by the posterior pituitary, and aldosterone, a mineral corticoid produced by the adrenal cortex. Release of ADH, normally triggered by an increase in serum osmolality, increases reabsorption of water in the renal tubules and collecting ducts, thus increasing vascular volume by decreasing urine output. The stimulus for aldosterone release is reduced renal blood flow. Aldosterone acts on the distal tubules to reabsorb sodium by excreting potassium in exchange; water is reabsorbed by association with the sodium. To a lesser extent, the glucocorticoids, which are also excreted by the adrenal cortex, cause sodium and water retention; this effect is mimicked by steroid medications.

| Steps | Rationale |
|---|---|
| **Assessment** | |
| 1. Determine age and developmental level. | Fluid balance concerns and requirements vary based on age; younger children are especially susceptible to rapid changes in status. Developmental level influences ability to cooperate and determines teaching needs. |
| 2. Review physician/practitioner orders. | Awareness of ordered therapies related to fluid balance such as fluid replacement/restriction and relevant medications guides assessment, monitoring, and intervention. |
| 3. Assess preexisting conditions, present status, and current therapies for factors influencing fluid balance (Table 64-1). | Awareness of the actual/potential affect of conditions and therapies on fluid balance allows appropriate monitoring and prompt intervention. |
| 4. Determine present weight and recent weight measures, if known, including date of measure. | Validated short-term weight changes provide the most reliable quantitative indication of fluid loss or gain. One kilogram of weight change represents one liter of fluid loss/gain (Hazinski, 1988). Also, fluid requirements and dosage calculations are usually based on weight. Rapid fluid loss or gain (<24 hours) is a factor in the severity of the imbalance. ***Special Considerations:*** *The neonate experiences a physiologic diuresis of total body water, especially the extracellular fluid (ECF), in the first 5 days of life, which results in a 5% to 10% weight loss (Rushton, 1988). Sequestered interstitial fluid, known as "third space" losses, results in intravascular volume deficit without weight loss.* |
| 5. Assess for physical signs of hydration status: | Clinical signs, in addition to weight changes, can be used to determine hydration status. |
| a. Infant only: anterior fontanel should be flat and soft. | A sunken, pulsatile fontanel indicates dehydration; tense bulging may be a sign of cerebral edema or increased intracranial pressure, especially in a quiet infant. |

**TABLE 64-1** Clinical Conditions Influencing Fluid Balance

| Clinical Situation/Examples | Primary Effects | Potential Clinical Imbalances | Comments |
|---|---|---|---|
| **FLUID VOLUME DEFICIT** | | | |
| **Water and electrolyte losses** | | | |
| Diarrhea, stoma drainage (ileostomy or colostomy) | Water and sodium losses | Hypovolemia, possibly hyponatremia, metabolic acidosis | Watery stools increase sodium losses |
| Vomiting, nasogastric suction, upper GI fistulas, gastrostomy | Water, $K^+$, $Cl^-$ and hydrogen ion losses | Hypovolemia, metabolic alkalosis | Pyloric stenosis typical of this imbalance |
| Hemorrhage, copious chest tube drainage | Water, sodium, albumin losses; decreased oncotic pressure | Inadequate intravascular volume, metabolic acidosis | Correct intravascular volume depletion with isotonic saline; may need packed red blood cells |
| **Water and electrolyte deficits** | | | |
| Decreased or absence of water and electrolyte intake (NPO, anorexia, inability to respond to thirst cues) | Inadequate replacement of normal losses; water deficit usually in excess of sodium deficit | Hypovolemia, hypernatremia | |
| **Water losses** | | | |
| Increased metabolic rate (fever, salicylate poisoning, radiant warmer, tachypnea) | Increased insensible water losses; increased osmolality | Hypernatremia, hypovolemia respiratory alkalosis | May have deceptively "normal" urinary output, but at expense of interstitial and intracellular fluids |
| Wound drainage | Mostly water losses, some electrolytes | Hypernatremia | |
| **Sodium losses** | | | |
| Cystic fibrosis | Excess sodium losses in sweat; decreased osmolality | Hyponatremia, intravascular volume depletion | |
| Renal salt-losing states (adrenal insufficiency, congenital adrenogenital hyperplasia) | Inability to retain/reabsorb sodium; decreased osmolality | Hyponatremia, intravascular volume depletion | |
| **Interstitial losses** | | | |
| Surgery, burns, major crush injuries, peritonitis, tissue ischemia/necrosis | Third space losses: movement of plasma, proteins, blood, or pus into tissues | Increased oncotic pressure of tissue draws fluid from intravascular space; intravascular volume depletion | Sequestered fluid returns to intravascular space 48-72 hours later |
| Sepsis | Increased capillary permeability; fluid loss at capillary bed | Intravascular volume depletion, pulmonary and systemic edema, ascites | Despite symptoms of fluid overload, e.g., pulmonary edema, needs fluid to maintain perfusion. Albumin solutions may be given as replacement fluids. Use fresh frozen plasma if clotting status is abnormal |
| Loss of plasma protein (burns, hemorrhage, nephrotic syndrome, inadequate protein intake) | Decreased oncotic pressure; fluid loss at capillary bed | Same as for sepsis | Same as for sepsis |
| **Hormonal alterations** | | | |
| Neurogenic diabetes insipidus (head injury, trauma, infection, brain tumor) | Hyposecretion of ADH | Uncontrolled diuresis; hypervolemia, hypernatremia, hyperchloremia | Exhibits symptoms of excessive thirst if conscious |
| Nephrogenic diabetes insipidus (congenital defect, renal failure, sickle cell disease, drug reactions) | Renal tubules unresponsive to ADH | Inability to concentrate urine; hypervolemia, hypernatremia, hyperchloremia | Exhibits symptoms of excessive thirst if conscious |
| **Drug therapy** | | | |
| Furosemide (Lasix), thiazides, bumetanide (Bumex), ethacrynic acid | Water and $K^+$ losses | Hypovolemia, hypokalemia | Hypokalemia may potentiate digitalis toxicity |
| Spironolactone (Aldactone) | Inhibits aldosterone activity; water excreted but $K^+$ spared | Hyperkalemia | Mild diuretic |

**TABLE 64-1** Clinical Conditions Influencing Fluid Balance—cont'd

| Clinical Situation/Examples | Primary Effects | Potential Clinical Imbalances | Comments |
|---|---|---|---|
| **FLUID VOLUME EXCESS** | | | |
| **Water intoxication** | | | |
| Excess free water intake (hypotonic IV administration, tap water enema, diluted formula, rapid dialysis, reflexive swallowing during water submersion, e.g., infant swimming lessons) | Dilution of serum sodium; decreased serum osmolality | Fluid shift into interstitial and intracellular spaces; cerebral edema | Greater risk if decreased ability to excrete excesses, e.g., infants, renal failure, inappropriate secretion of ADH |
| **Excess sodium/glucose** | | | |
| High solute intake (TPN, enteral feeds, or infant formula excessively concentrated); or high salt solution (undiluted broth, or accidental substitution of salt for sugar when preparing infant formula) | Excess sodium/solute load; increased serum osmolality; water reabsorption | Shift of fluid into intravascular; hypervolemia; dehydration of interstitial and intracellular spaces | Rapid shifts can rupture cerebral blood vessels, causing hemorrhage; adequate or increased urine output is a misleading indicator of hydration status |
| Diabetic ketoacidosis | Elevated glucose levels; increased serum osmolality | Increased or decreased intravascular volume; osmotic diuresis; dehydration of intracellular and interstitial spaces; hypokalemia | Rapid reduction in serum glucose (by giving IV insulin) can worsen cerebral edema |
| Renal failure | Sodium and fluid retention | Hypernatremia, hypervolemia, hyperkalemia | Severe imbalances may require emergency dialysis; may become hyponatremic from sodium restriction |
| Osmotic diuretics (Mannitol) | Increased serum osmolality; osmotic diuresis | Mild hypokalemia | Successive doses less effective; may eventually become hypovolemic |
| **Hormonal alterations** | | | |
| Stress (surgery, trauma, sepsis) | Increased release of aldosterone, ADH, and glucocorticoids; sodium and water retention | Hypervolemia, hypokalemia | Hormonal release part of general stress (adaptation) response to maintain systemic perfusion |
| Hyperaldosteronism | Hypersecretion of aldosterone; sodium retention | Hypernatremia, hypervolemia; hypokalemia | Potassium losses increase with increasing levels of aldosterone |
| Syndrome of inappropriate ADH secretion (SIADH): CNS disease/trauma, postoperative, pneumonia, mechanical ventilation, hydrocephalus, asphyxia in neonate, morphine & barbiturates | Increased ADH secretion; fluid retention | Hyponatremia; decreased serum osmolality | Although urine becomes concentrated (increased urine osmolality), treatment is fluid restriction |
| Cushing syndrome (adrenal), steroids | Increased glucocorticoids (from secretion or intake); sodium and water retention | Hypervolemia; hypokalemia | |
| **Myocardial dysfunction** | | | |
| Congestive failure | Decreased hydrostatic pressure and decreased perfusion; increased ADH and aldosterone secretion; sodium and water retention | Fluid loss from capillary bed into interstitial tissues, systemic and pulmonary edema; hypervolemia, dilutional hyponatremia | Potential for hypokalemia from diuretic therapy |

| Steps | Rationale |
|---|---|
| b. Eye globes and orbits should be firm. | Eyes may appear sunken, the globes may be soft, and periorbital skin may be drawn in severe dehydration. Fluid excess often shows up initially in loose tissue structures such as the periorbital area. |
| c. Conjunctivae and mucous membranes should be moist with salivary bubbles under the tongue. Tearing should be noted with crying (over 6 weeks of age). | Dryness of membranes and absence of salivation are indicators of dehydration; tearing may be absent.<br>***Special Considerations:*** *Mouth breathing can also cause dryness, but saliva should still be evident under the tongue if child is adequately hydrated. Dry, sticky mucous membranes are symptomatic of hypernatremia.* |
| d. When skin turgor of abdomen and inner thigh is pinched, skin should quickly recoil (within 1 second) on release. | With fluid volume deficit, the skin may remain raised (tented) for several seconds after release.<br>***Special Considerations:*** *Poor skin turgor may also be noted in malnutrition. Turgor may appear deceptively normal in an obese, dehydrated infant. Firm, "doughy" skin is characteristic of hypernatremia.* |
| e. Skin is firm and smooth; abdomen is soft and nondistended; hands and feet are not puffy; scrotum is not edematous. | Excess fluid can accumulate in interstitial tissues as generalized, localized, or dependent edema. |
| f. Breath sounds should be clear; respiratory effort should be minimal. | Fluid overload and/or increased capillary permeability with net fluid movement into interstitial tissue can result in pulmonary edema manifested by auscultation of rales or "wet" breath sounds, frothy pink sputum, tachypnea, and increased work of breathing. Tachypnea can also indicate metabolic acidosis.<br>***Special Considerations:*** *Pulmonary edema in the child on assisted ventilation may be noted by higher inspiratory pressure requirements, indicating decreasing lung compliance (Hazinski, 1988).* |
| g. Neck veins should have normal filling. If central monitoring is available, venous or right atrial pressure should be 0 to 5 mm Hg; pulmonary artery wedge or left atrial pressure should be 4 to 8 mm Hg. | Flat neck veins indicate decreased intravascular volume; distended neck veins or elevated central pressures indicate intravascular volume excess.<br>***Special Considerations:*** *Neck vein assessment is difficult in infants and young children because of their short, thick necks.* |
| h. Liver should not be palpable below the right costal margin. | Hepatomegaly may be indicative of excessive intravascular volume.<br>***Special Considerations:*** *In neonates, liver is normally palpable 1 cm below costal margin.* |
| 6. Assess for behavioral changes such as irritability, lethargy, confusion, seizures. Question the family about their observations. | Behavioral changes may accompany fluid shifts and electrolyte imbalances. Central nervous system cells are particularly vulnerable to fluid excess, resulting in behavioral changes such as confusion and seizures. Irritability may be exhibited with water intoxication, hypernatremia, or hypocalcemia. Tetany and seizures are also characteristic of hypocalcemia. |
| 7. Assess systemic perfusion: | Adequate intravascular volume and normal myocardial function are necessary for adequate systemic perfusion (Hazinski, 1988). |
| a. Capillary refill should be brisk (1 to 2 seconds), extremities should be warm, and peripheral pulses should be strong. | Sluggish capillary refill (>3 seconds), cool extremities (especially in the presence of fever), and weak peripheral pulses evidence poor peripheral perfusion.<br>***Special Considerations:*** *Hypothermia, especially in the neonate, may falsely prolong capillary refill (Adcock and Consolvo, 1989).* |
| b. Urine volume: minimum acceptable by weight: infants, 2 cc/kg/hr; child, 1 cc/kg/hr; and adolescent, 0.5 cc/kg/hr (Hazinski, 1988). | Adequate systemic perfusion is necessary for glomerular filtration to produce urine. Although the amount of urine produced can be influenced by other factors (e.g., renal function and hormone secretion), oliguria (decreased urine output) and anuria (absence of urine formation) are significant assessment factors related to fluid balance. |
| c. Urine specific gravity: Normal—1.005 to 1.020 | Decreased urine volume accompanied by an increased specific gravity may be an indicator of poor systemic perfusion (Hazinski, 1988). An increased urine volume with decreased specific gravity may signify water intoxication. |

| Steps | Rationale |
|---|---|
| | ***Special Considerations:*** *Neonates and infants minimally conserve or dilute urine, so specific gravity is a less useful measure. Suspect inappropriate ADH secretion when a decreased serum sodium and increased specific gravity occur (Adcock and Consolvo, 1989). A low specific gravity associated with dehydration suggests a defect in urinary concentrating mechanisms and intrinsic renal disease (Robson, 1987). Specific gravity may be falsely elevated by glucose or protein in the urine (Lattanzi, 1989).* |
| d. Skin color: consistent coloring and pink mucous membranes. | Pallor and grey or mottled color indicate poor systemic perfusion and development of metabolic acidosis from accumulation of wastes.<br>***Special Considerations:*** *Cherry-red lips are characteristic of hyperventilation from metabolic acidosis.* |
| e. Acid-base balance: pH, 7.35 to 7.45<br>$pCO_2$, 32 to 48<br>$HCO_3$, 21 to 28 mEq/liter | Metabolic acidosis (decreased pH, carbon dioxide, and bicarbonate) may indicate inadequate tissue perfusion (Hazinski, 1988).<br>***Special Considerations:*** *Normal values for the neonate and infant may vary. The neonate has a tendency to develop metabolic acidosis because of a high metabolic rate with acid formation.* |
| f. Vital signs: normal limits for age (see related skills). | Heart rate may increase in response to hypovolemia in an attempt to maintain systemic perfusion. However, blood pressure may remain normal since vasoconstriction also occurs to maintain perfusion. Hypotension is a late sign of hypovolemia and may signal a prearrest state. Tachypnea can signal metabolic acidosis or pulmonary edema. Hypertension may indicate intravascular volume excess.<br>***Special Considerations:*** *If ECG is monitored, dysrhythmias are symptomatic of hypokalemia. Classic changes of peaked T waves followed by a widened QRS complex signal a prearrest state in hyperkalemia.* |
| 8. Assess amount and character of recent intake and output (I & O): | Fluid and electrolyte needs are based on ongoing losses, both normal and abnormal (maintenance needs), and losses that occurred before replacement therapy began (deficit needs). Amount and type of I & O also assists in initial assessment of the child's hydration status. |
| a. Intake: amounts, type of food or liquids taken and retained, preparation methods, especially for formula or homemade electrolyte solutions. | Present body composition of fluid and electrolytes is influenced by losses and concomitant intake (Robson, 1987). Intake of excessive free water (plain or dextrose solution, diluted formula) could indicate fluid overload or hyponatremic dehydration when associated with diarrhea. High salt intake during diarrheal losses from broth, improperly prepared formula/electrolyte solution, or misuse of an oral rehydrating solution (ORS) for maintenance is associated with hypernatremic dehydration. |
| b. Urine and stool: amount of urine output, or if unknown, the number of times child has voided or number of wet diapers in past 24 hours; appearance of urine; and stool amount, consistency. | Approximate urinary output and concentration assist in hydration assessment and replacement needs. Less than three voids in 24 hours is considered oliguria. Negligible amounts of water are lost in normal stools, but liquid stools (more than 20 grams/kg/day) may account for significant fluid loss.<br>***Special Considerations:*** *The amount of sodium lost in stool increases with increasing water content, e.g., the more watery the stools, the greater the sodium loss and risk of hyponatremic dehydration.* |
| c. Insensible losses through respiration and evaporation through the skin. Perspiration (sweat) is not an insensible loss. | Insensible losses include electrolyte-free water loss and, under ordinary circumstances, account for one third of total maintenance volume (Lattanzi, 1989).<br>***Special Considerations:*** *Insensible losses are greatly reduced if the child is receiving humidified air such as with a mist tent, incubator, or ventilator; losses are increased with hyperthermia or tachypnea (Lattanzi, 1989).* |

***TABLE 64-2*** **Composition of Abnormal Body Fluid Losses**

| | Na | K | Cl |
|---|---|---|---|
| **Fluid** | | **mEq/L** | |
| Gastric | 20–80 | 5–20 | 100–150 |
| Small intestine | 100–140 | 5–15 | 90–130 |
| Bile | 120–140 | 5–15 | 80–120 |
| Ileostomy | 45–135 | 3–15 | 20–115 |
| Diarrhea | 10–90 | 10–80 | 10–110 |
| Sweat: | | | |
| Normal | 10–30 | 3–10 | 10–35 |
| Cystic fibrosis | 50–130 | 5–25 | 50–110 |
| Burns | 140 | 5 | 110 |

Adapted from Robson AM: Parenteral fluid therapy. In Behrman RE and Vaughn WE, editors: Nelson textbook of pediatrics, ed 13, Philadelphia, 1987, WB Saunders Co.

| **Steps** | **Rationale** |
|---|---|
| d. Abnormal losses such as sweat, vomitus, nasogastric suction, chest tube, and wound drainage (see Table 64-2). | Amount and electrolyte composition of abnormal losses must be considered in calculation of replacement therapy.<br>***Special Considerations:*** *Sodium chloride losses in sweat are generally minimal, except in children with cystic fibrosis (Robson, 1987).* |
| 9. Review lab data: | Laboratory data provides baseline information for monitoring progress and assists in determining the forces influencing fluid movement to guide therapy. |
| a. Serum sodium: normal—135 to 145 mEq/L. | Sodium is the major cation that determines serum osmolality. Serum sodium reflects the relative losses/gains of water to electrolytes.<br>***Special Considerations:*** *Sodium levels may be falsely low, with excess fluid in the intravascular space.* |
| b. Serum glucose: normal—60 to 105 mg/dL | Next to serum sodium, glucose is the second major force that determines serum osmolality. Hyperglycemia causes fluid to shift into the vascular space, which, in the presence of normal renal function, effects an osmotic diuresis, increasing urinary output. As this fluid shift depletes interstitial fluid reserves, the ultimate effect is dehydration. |
| c. Blood urea nitrogen (BUN): normal values—5 to 22 mg/dL and creatinine: normal—infant, 0.2 to 0.4 mg/dL; child, 0.3 to 0.7 mg/dL; adolescent, 0.5 to 1.0 mg/dL. | BUN and creatinine provide indirect data about glomerular filtration rate and extracellular fluid. The BUN is falsely elevated in dehydration and hemoconcentration of extracellular fluid; it is falsely low in overhydration and hemodilution.<br>***Special Considerations:*** *Values may not be reliable in first 24 hours of life (Rushton, 1988).* |
| d. Serum osmolality: normal value—272 to 290 mOsm/dL OR can be calculated: [2 × serum sodium] + [serum glucose ÷ 18] + [BUN ÷ 2.8] = _____ mOsm/dL (serum osmolality.<br>For example, for a serum sodium of 132, a serum glucose of 60, and a BUN of 30, the calculated osmolality is 278 mOsm/dL: (2 × 132) + (60 ÷ 18) + (30 ÷ 2.8) = (264) + (3.33) + (10.71) = 278.04 | Serum osmolality measures the proportion of solutes to water in the body. Serum osmolality is sensed by receptors in the hypothalamus to stimulate the thirst response and release ADH (Heitkemper and Bond, 1988).<br>***Special Considerations:*** *This formula does not reflect increased serum osmolality from administration of osmotic diuretics (Hazinski, 1988). If the BUN and glucose are normal, the calculated osmolality is approximately twice serum sodium value (Lattanzi, 1989).* |
| e. Total protein normal for neonate, 4.6 to 7.4 mg/dL; child, 6.2 to 8.0 mg/dL. | Oncotic pressure is exerted by plasma proteins. If plasma protein decreases, the oncotic pull of fluid back into the vascular space at the capillary level is hampered. Plasma protein can decrease from insufficient dietary intake or from abnormal losses such as with burns or nephrotic syndrome. |
| f. Serum potassium: normal values—3.5 to 5.5 mEq/L | Potassium levels at the beginning of therapy may be of limited usefulness because values can be falsely elevated from decreased renal function or acidosis, even when significant cellular deficiencies exist (Robson, 1987). However, a low serum potassium implies significant intracellular depletion (Adcock and Consolvo, 1989). |

| Steps | Rationale |
|---|---|
| | ***Special Considerations:*** *A hemolyzed blood specimen will result in falsely elevated potassium levels.* |
| g. Hematocrit: normal values—neonate, 48% to 69%; infant, 28% to 42%; child, 35% to 45%; adolescent, 36% to 49% (depending on sex). | Hemoconcentration (increase in hemoglobin, hematocrit, and plasma proteins) is often used as a gauge of dehydration, but a baseline measure is generally most useful to determine effectiveness of therapy in situations where there is not ongoing blood loss (Robson, 1987). |

## Planning and Goal Setting

| | |
|---|---|
| 1. Evaluate present fluid balance. | Fluid management in terms of maintenance/deficit therapy and monitoring concerns will be determined by present fluid balance. ***Special Considerations:*** *Although the physician usually determines type, amount and rate of IV fluids, it is appropriate nursing practice to be knowledgeable about factors affecting the decisions concerning fluid therapy.* |
| a. Fluid volume deficit: determine severity, preferably by weight loss or comparison with clinical signs (see Table 64-3); determine type by serum sodium levels, history, and clinical signs (see Table 64-4). | The severity of dehydration and type (isotonic, hypotonic or hypertonic) determines the amount, type, and rate of fluid needed for rehydration more than the underlying cause (Robson, 1987). ***Special Considerations:*** *To determine percentage of weight loss, divide amount of loss by the child's previous weight, e.g., if a 10 kg child loses 0.5 kg, this equals a 0.05 or 5% weight loss.* |

***TABLE 64-3*** **Degree of Dehydration***

| | Mild | Moderate | Severe |
|---|---|---|---|
| Weight loss | | | |
| Infant | 5% | 10% | 15% |
| Child | 3% | 6% | 9% |
| Skin color | Pale | Gray | Mottled |
| Skin turgor | Normal or decreased | Decreased | Tenting |
| Mucous membranes | Damp to dry | Very dry | Parched |
| Urine output | Decreased | Oliguria | Marked oliguria and azotemia |
| Blood pressure | Normal | Normal or lowered | Lowered |
| Heart rate | Normal or increased | Increased | Rapid and thready |
| Capillary filling | Brisk | Slow | >3 seconds |
| Behavior | Alert, thirsty | Irritable to lethargic | Marked sensorium changes |

*Classification applies to isotonic dehydration. With hypotonic dehydration, symptoms will appear more severe with less actual fluid loss. In hypertonic dehydration, symptoms may appear milder with greater fluid losses, because increased osmolality maintains intravascular volume.
Adapted from Whaley L and Wong D: Nursing care of infants and children, ed 4, 1991, St Louis, The CV Mosby Co.

***TABLE 64-4*** **Type of Dehydration**

| | Isotonic | Hypotonic | Hypertonic |
|---|---|---|---|
| Serum sodium | 130 to 150 mEq/L | <130 mEq/L* | >150 mEq/L* |
| Systemic perfusion | Decreased | Decreased | Normal or decreased |
| Skin texture | Poor turgor | Poor turgor | Firm, "doughy" |
| Mucous membranes | Dry | Dry | "Sticky" |
| Behavior | Depends on degree | Lethargic to comatose, may seize | Marked lethargy, irritable when stimulated, may seize |
| Prevalence of cases with diarrheal etiology | 70% | 10% | 20% |

*A low serum sodium level may be a result of dilution rather than a true sodium deficit, while an elevated serum sodium level is always a true excess.

| Steps | Rationale |
|---|---|
| b. Fluid volume overload: review history and clinical symptoms for potential causes such as excess free water intake, myocardial dysfunction, inappropriate ADH secretion. | Clinical presentation of fluid overload and involved mechanisms determine modifications in maintenance fluid requirements and other therapeutic measures, e.g., medications or sodium restriction. |
| c. Fluid volume balance: well-hydrated, no clinical signs of dehydration or fluid overload. | When fluid balance is appropriate, maintenance solutions (IV or PO) meet needs for a short time, e.g., while a child is awaiting surgery. |
| 2. Calculate maintenance fluid requirements based on one of three methods: metabolic rate, body weight, or body surface area. | Maintenance therapy replaces ongoing losses, both normal and abnormal, of fluid and electrolytes, to temporarily maintain an adequate fluid balance and allow excretion of the renal solute load (electrolytes and urea) (Ackerman, 1987).<br>***Special Considerations:*** *Maintenance solutions (IV or PO) always include fluid, electrolytes, and sufficient glucose to provide 20% of the child's caloric needs to minimize protein catabolism and prevent development of ketosis. Protein and calorie deficits will develop only if maintenance fluids are given for more than a few days (Lattanzi, 1989).* |
| a. Metabolic rate or body weight (Hazinski, 1988):<br><u>Kilogram wt.</u> — <u>24 hr. fluid needs</u><br>0 to 10 kg (>72 hr) — 100 ml/kg<br>11 to 20 kg — 1000 ml + 50 ml/kg for each kg over 10<br>21 to 30 kg — 1500 ml + 25 ml/kg for each kg over 20<br>31 to 40 kg — 1750 ml + 10 ml/kg for each kg over 30<br>Example: a 22 kg child's fluid requirements would be: 1500 + 50 = 1550 ml/24 hr. | Daily maintenance requirements are most accurate when based on metabolic rate; approximately 100 ml of fluid is needed for every 100 kcal expended. However, this method requires use of basal caloric output tables. A simpler, yet more acceptable method, is to use body weight as an indirect measure of caloric expenditure to allow fluid calculation.<br>***Special Considerations:*** *This method may overestimate a newborn's fluid requirements and underestimate the adolescent's (Hazinski, 1988). Since body fat does not contain water, use the 50th percentile ideal weight for the obese child to avoid overestimation of fluid requirements.* |
| b. Body surface area: Use Dubois or West surface nomogram to provide requirements of 1500 ml per $m^2$ body surface area.<br>Example: a child's fluid requirements with a body surface area ($m^2$) of 0.64 would be $1500 \times 0.64 = 960$ ml/24 hr. | This calculation method of fluid requirements is thought to provide an accurate estimation because heat production is proportional to body surface area (Hazinski, 1988).<br>***Special Considerations:*** *This method may underestimate fluid requirements in small infants and young children (Hazinski, 1988).* |
| 3. Modify maintenance fluid requirement calculations appropriate to conditions: | Maintenance requirements address only normal body fluid requirements and insensible losses. Adjustments must be made for activity variations, abnormal losses, disease states, or any condition in which increased or decreased losses of fluids/electrolytes occur (Robson, 1987). |
| a. Decreased requirements: renal failure, cardiac disease with failure, increased intracranial pressure, inappropriate (excessive) release of ADH (such as with meningitis), hypothermia, hypernatremia with fluid excess, hypothyroidism, unconscious or anesthetized, physiologic diuresis of neonate (first 3 to 5 days of life), and high humidity environment such as an incubator/ventilator. | Fluid administration must be below maintenance in conditions such as decreased metabolic needs, fluid retention, and decreased insensible losses, to prevent, minimize, or correct fluid overload. Excess fluid replacement in the neonate can prolong physiologic diuresis (Rushton, 1988).<br>***Special Considerations:*** *General guidelines: renal failure, limit replacement to insensible losses (300 ml/$m^2$ BSA) plus urine and any additional measured output; neonate 3 to 5 days age, 50 ml/kg/day; cardiac failure, two thirds maintenance; inappropriate ADH, one half to two thirds maintenance; and high humidity environment, decrease by one third.* |
| b. Increased requirements: hypermetabolic states (fever, salicylism, hyperthyroidism), chronic renal disease (concentrating and diluting ability lost), hyperventilation, diabetes insipidus, diaphoresis, cystic fibrosis, phototherapy or radiant warmer, abnormal losses of any body fluid, e.g., burns, nasogastric suction, diarrhea, and ostomy drainage. | Fluid requirements must be increased in situations of increased metabolic rate, increased insensible losses, abnormal losses, and impaired renal concentrating ability to prevent fluid deficits.<br>***Special Considerations:*** *General guidelines: add 10 ml/kg/degree >37° C; radiant warmer or phototherapy, increase by 25% to 50%; chronic renal, one and one half maintenance; and diabetes insipidus, up to 4 times maintenance (oral replacement safer than IV). Increased needs may be met by increasing volume of maintenance fluid or volume-for-volume replacement of abnormal losses with a solution of similar electrolyte composition to lost body fluid (Lattanzi, 1989).* |
| 4. Calculate deficit therapy requirements based on severity of dehydration and type. | Previously incurred losses must be replaced in addition to maintenance requirements for adequate rehydration. Deficits resulting from many different etiologies can be successfully treated in a similar manner based on severity and type of dehydration (Robson, 1987). |

| Steps | Rationale |
|---|---|
| a. Mild isotonic dehydration: up to 50 ml/kg evenly administered over next 24 hours. | The child with mild isotonic dehydration has lost approximately 5% of body weight or up to 50 ml/kg. |
| b. Moderate isotonic dehydration: replace up to 100 ml/kg over next 24 to 48 hours. | The child with moderate isotonic dehydration has lost approximately 5% to 10% of body weight or up to 100 ml/kg. |
| c. Severe isotonic dehydration: immediate fluid bolus of 20 ml/kg, then 150 ml/kg over next 24 to 48 hours. | The child with severe isotonic dehydration has lost approximately 10% to 15% of body weight or up to 150 ml/kg. Hypovolemic shock is present and requires immediate fluid resuscitation to restore systemic perfusion.<br>***Special Considerations:*** *Administration of blood or plasma volume expanders may be necessary initially to reverse shock.* |
| d. Hypotonic dehydration: use formula appropriate to degree of dehydration from above; replace 50% of fluid losses in first 8 hours of therapy, and remaining 50% during next 16 hours. | In hypotonic dehydration, losses are primarily from the intravascular space; rapid volume replacement restores systemic perfusion (Hazinski, 1988).<br>***Special Considerations:*** *Sodium replacement should be slow to prevent sudden fluid shifts into the intravascular space, unless symptoms of water intoxication are present such as seizures, then a 3% saline bolus may be necessary.* |
| e. Hypertonic dehydration: use fluid formula appropriate to degree of dehydration from above; replace 50% of losses during first 24 hours and 50% during next 24 hours. | In hypertonic dehydration, fluid has shifted from the cells to the intravascular space. Rapid fluid replacement can lead to a sudden fluid shift back into cellular spaces, causing cerebral edema and increased intracranial pressure. Also, since intravascular volume has been maintained at cellular expense, rapid volume expansion is usually unnecessary. |
| 5. Determine need for I & O monitoring: per facility policy, physician order, or for child at risk for fluid and electrolyte imbalance, e.g., receiving intravenous fluids, after major surgery, with thermal burns, renal disorder, congestive heart failure, sepsis, dehydration, diarrhea, vomiting, diabetes mellitus, oliguria, or diuretic or corticosteroid therapy (Whaley and Wong, 1991). | Monitoring I & O is always indicated when a child is at risk for fluid and electrolyte imbalance, regardless of facility policy or physician orders.<br>***Special Considerations:*** *Many facilities have a policy requiring routine I & O monitoring on all children.* |
| 6. Gather supplies to monitor I & O: reminder signs; bedside tally/flow sheet; scales for weighing diapers or urine collection device (urinal, urine collection bag, toilet seat container); and graduated metric containers appropriate to anticipated output amounts. | Visible reminders and easily available supplies for I & O monitoring assist in maintaining compliance. Appropriately sized metric containers allow accurate, easily calculated measures. The weight difference between a wet and dry diaper provides an indirect measure of urinary and liquid stool output.<br>***Special Considerations:*** *Use a scale that is accurate with small amounts, e.g., a dietary scale.* |
| 7. Obtain and/or select fluid and electrolyte solutions: | |
| a. Oral maintenance solutions such as Pedialyte and Lytren, containing approximately 3 mEq/100 ml sodium and 2 to 2.5 g/100 ml glucose (see Table 64-5). | Oral maintenance solutions contain recommended concentrations of fluids/electrolytes/carbohydrates to provide maintenance requirements after deficit therapy (oral or parenteral rehydration) or for child without evidence of dehydration (Ghishan, 1988). |
| b. Oral rehydration solutions (ORS), e.g., Gastrolyte, WHO solution, and Rehydralyte, containing 70 to 90 mEq/L sodium and 2 to 2.5 g/100 ml glucose (see Table 64-5). | ORS is a hypertonic solution recommended for deficit therapy only, generally given for a short time and followed by maintenance solutions.<br>***Special Considerations:*** *ORS is commonly used in underdeveloped countries for treatment of diarrhea, which is a leading cause of infant mortality. Its use is being advocated in the United States (Ghishan, 1988). Do not give ORS to an anuric child, since the solution contains potassium.* |
| c. Parenteral solutions (see Appendix D):<br>▪ Maintenance is usually 20 to 30 mEq sodium and chloride and 20 mEq potassium per liter, and 5% dextrose.<br>▪ Deficit solutions will vary. | Parenteral solutions may be used for maintenance or deficit therapy.<br>***Special Considerations:*** *Do not add potassium until renal function is demonstrated (1 to 2 voids). Replacement of potassium is often safely delayed until deficit therapy is underway, unless child is known to be hypokalemic or has had large potassium losses such as pyloric stenosis, diabetic ketoacidosis, or prolonged diarrhea (Robson, 1987).* |
| 8. Develop individualized goals of nursing care:<br>▪ Fluid balance will be improved/maintained.<br>▪ Complications of fluid therapy will be prevented or minimized.<br>▪ Child and family will demonstrate understanding of fluid therapy goals. | |

***TABLE 64-5*** **Composition of Oral Solutions**

**ORAL ELECTROLYTE SOLUTIONS**

| | Na† | K† | Cl | Other Anion | CHO (%) |
|---|---|---|---|---|---|
| WHO† solution | 90 | 20 | 80 | 30 | 2 |
| Gastrolyte | 90 | 20 | 80 | 30 | 2 |
| Pedialyte | 45 | 20 | 35 | 30 | 2.5 |
| Rehydralyte | 75 | 20 | 65 | 30 | 2.5 |
| Lytren | 50 | 25 | 45 | 30 | 2.0 |
| Infalyte | 50 | 20 | 40 | 30 | 2.0 |
| Gatorade | 23 | 3 | 17 | — | 5.9 |

**"CLEAR LIQUID" SOLUTIONS**

| | Na†* | K*† | CHO (%) |
|---|---|---|---|
| Pepsi-Cola | 1–2 | 0.1 | 10.9 |
| Coca-Cola | 1–2 | 0.1 | 10 |
| Ginger ale | 2 | 0.6 | 9.2 |
| Jell-O | 24–27 | 1.3 | 16 |
| Club soda | 12 | 0.6 | — |
| Root beer | 6 | 0.6 | 10.6 |
| Popsicles | 1–4 | 0.5 | 18 |

*Concentrations are mEq/L.
†WHO (World Health Organization)
From Ghishan FK: The transport of electrolytes in the gut and the use of rehydration solutions, Pediatr Clin North Am 35(1):35-50, 1988.

### *GUIDELINES FOR MEASURING INTAKE AND OUTPUT*

1. Use milliliters (ml) or cubic centimeters (cc) to record all measures. For conversion, one ounce equals 30 cc or ml; fluid weight in grams equals cc or ml. For example, 4 oz. formula equals 120 cc, and 60 grams of fluid equals 60 cc.
2. Oral Intake: include liquids taken with meals, medication administration, and liquids in solid state such as ice chips, ice cream and pudding. Determine breastfeeding milk intake by weighing infant immediately before and after feeding and converting difference in grams to ml or cc.
3. Gastric/Enteral Intake: include NG, GT, JT feedings, and flushes for feedings and medication administration.
4. Parenteral Intake: include all IV fluids, including blood and blood products, medication administration fluids and flushes. These are often overlooked yet significant to consider.
5. Urinary output: measure all urinary output. For the nontoilet-trained child who does not have an indwelling catheter, an adhesive collection bag with drainage tubing may be applied, or urine output may be estimated: weigh a dry diaper of the same material and size as the wet one, then weigh the wet diaper, and subtract the dry diaper weight; convert grams or ounces to cc (see step 1). For increased accuracy, record the dry weight of a diaper before placing it on the child, then reweigh the diaper after the infant has voided and determine the difference. Evaporative loss may occur if diaper weighing is delayed greater than 60 minutes, or if the diaper is left near radiant warmer or phototherapy lights (Williams & Kanarek, 1982; Hermansen & Buches, 1988). Superabsorbent diapers may actually gain weight in the absence of urinary output when used in warm, high humidity incubators (Hermansen & Buches, 1987).
6. Stool output: solid stools contain little fluid; generally the number and size of the stool is recorded. Liquid stools (including ostomies) may be measured/weighed in the same manner as urine output.
7. Abnormal output: include all measurable output, such as vomitus, nasogastric or other suction or gravity drainage (Jackson-Pratt drain, Hemovac, chest tube, externalized ventricular shunt). For accuracy in estimating wound drainage, weigh using the method described for diapers. For a critically ill child or premature infant, measure all blood drawn for laboratory studies for both I & O records and potential transfusion needs.

| Steps | Rationale |
|---|---|
| **Implementation** | |
| 1. Provide replacement fluids if indicated (deficit therapy). | Deficit therapy replaces previously incurred fluid and electrolyte losses. The first goal of therapy is to restore adequate intravascular volume and increase renal function. |
| a. Oral rehydration: give 50 ml/kg within 4 hours for mild dehydration; give 100 ml/kg within 6 hours for moderate dehydration. After ORS, allow plain water or breastfeeding ad lib to replace insensible losses. Continue breastfeeding or begin maintenance oral solutions. | Oral electrolyte solutions are increasingly being used for children with mild to moderate dehydration from diarrhea regardless of etiology (Bass and Walker, 1986; Ghishan, 1988; and Grill, 1989). The slow absorption from the GI tract minimizes adverse effects from excessive amounts of water or electrolytes. It also prevents trauma and potential complications of venipuncture, is more economical, and does not require hospitalization. |

| Steps | Rationale |
|---|---|
| | ***Special Considerations:*** *Vomiting may occur initially with ORS, but usually ceases, and treatment can continue.* |
| b. Parenteral rehydration: usually replaced over 24 to 48 hours. Initial administration rate may be higher, then decreased for duration of replacement. Maintenance requirements are usually administered concurrently. Potassium is usually added later when renal function is established, and may be replaced over 2 to 3 days. | Parenteral replacement of deficits is indicated for severe dehydration, shock, severe gastric distension, or inability to drink for any reason (Barness, 1986). Although a higher administration rate may be required initially to restore intravascular volume and adequate systemic perfusion, total replacement of losses is usually over a longer time. Adequate renal function is necessary to prevent hyperkalemia, which can lead to cardiac arrest. ***Special Considerations:*** *In hypernatremic dehydration, monitor serum sodium closely; a rapid drop may lead to cerebral edema and seizures (Hazinski, 1988).* |
| 2. Provide maintenance fluids. | Maintenance fluids replace ongoing losses, both normal and abnormal. ***Special Considerations:*** *Maintenance therapy (oral or parenteral) is appropriate for only a few days. If normal nutritional intake cannot be resumed, TPN or enteral feedings must be initiated (Robson, 1987).* |
| a. Oral: provide maintenance needs in calculated amounts, using acceptable maintenance solutions (see Table 64-5). Avoid liquids that are high in carbohydrates or have inappropriate electrolyte compositions, e.g., broth, flavored gelatins, carbonated beverages, glucose water. | Traditional "clear liquids" often have an inappropriate electrolyte composition to meet maintenance needs, and high carbohydrate levels can aggravate diarrhea (Ghishan, 1988). ***Special Considerations:*** *Reinstitution of oral liquids as soon as possible prevents deterioration and permits natural regulatory functioning of the gastrointestinal mucosa (Ghishan, 1988).* |
| b. Parenteral: administer at ordered maintenance rate. Replace abnormal losses as ordered, with maintenance solution or one similar in composition to body fluids lost (see Table 64-2). | ***Special Considerations:*** *If the child is taking and retaining fluids, the IV rate should be reduced so that the total PO and IV intake equals the calculated maintenance fluid requirements.* |
| 3. If fluids are being restricted: | Fluid restriction may be necessary as a preventive or therapeutic measure. |
| a. For oral intake, provide approximately 50% of total during the day; 35% to 40% during the evening; and 10% to 15% during the night. | ***Special Considerations:*** *This distribution should be individualized to the child's needs. For example, a young infant may need equal amounts for around-the-clock feedings.* |
| b. Assist in coping with fluid restriction: perform frequent mouth care; touch and cuddle frequently; provide infant with a pacifier; use distraction techniques such as games, crafts, activity. | In the absence of normal intake, mouth secretions tend to thicken and accumulate on the tongue, teeth, and mucous membranes. A slightly abrasive surface such as moistened gauze or sponge mouth swab may aid in removing accumulated secretions. |
| 4. Obtain body weight daily or more frequently, if indicated, and record. Use consistent technique and the same scale for each measurement. Make a written notation of any cause for weight variation that cannot be removed, e.g., a cast, chest tubes, or IV armboard (see Skill 28). | Weight changes in 24 hour periods reflect fluid gain or loss. Consistency is essential for accuracy, since weight changes from fluid may be small. ***Special Considerations:*** *Significant weight changes in 24 hours or less: infant, 50 gm; child, 200 gm; and adolescent, 500 gm (Hazinski, 1988).* |
| 5. Monitor I & O. | Accurate I & O records are essential to calculate fluid replacement needs and evaluate response to medications and treatments. |
| a. Explain to child and family the need and importance of monitoring I & O. Enlist the older child's participation and praise efforts. | An understanding of the importance of fluid balance in children will facilitate cooperation and compliance, since much of the information that should be recorded may occur during self-care or family caretaking activities, e.g., a diaper change. Participation contributes to the older child's sense of control and responsibility in own health care. |
| b. Measure and record all oral, enteral, parenteral intake and all measurable output, including normal and abnormal losses. Report significant imbalances (see the box at left). | Each source of intake and output must be considered for accurate monitoring of fluid balance. |
| 6. Perform ongoing assessment of hydration status. (Follow guidelines in Assessment, step 5.) | Many factors influence planning of fluid needs, therefore it is essential to systematically evaluate response to therapy, as unpredicted responses are common, and fluid calculations may need to be revised. ***Special Considerations:*** *"Third space" losses into interstitial fluid initially causing hypovolemia may be mobilized back into the intravascular space in 24 to 48 hours, leading to intravascular volume excess if fluid replacement is not decreased (Rushton, 1988).* |

| Steps | Rationale |
|---|---|
| 7. Perform ongoing assessment of systemic perfusion. (Follow guidelines in Assessment, step 6.) | Changes in intravascular status are likely in fluid therapy; ongoing assessment will detect any fluid shifts that may hamper systemic perfusion. |
| 8. Monitor neurologic status: level of consciousness, orientation, behavior, pupil size and response, and ability to follow commands. | Neurologic status should improve with fluid therapy; lack of improvement or deterioration in status should be reported promptly to allow reevaluation of therapy. ***Special Considerations:*** *In hypernatremic dehydration, seizures may occur during rehydration therapy particularly if the serum sodium level decreases too rapidly; a slow decline (not more than 10 mEq/L/24 hr) will minimize this risk (Robson, 1987).* |
| 9. Monitor serial lab measures. (Follow guidelines in Assessment, step 9.) | Serial lab measures can help determine effectiveness of therapy. |

| Evaluation Outcomes | Observational Guidelines |
|---|---|
| 1. Fluid balance status is improved or maintained. | Monitor hydration status, systemic perfusion, body weights, laboratory results, neurologic status, and I & O records. Compare with baseline or previous assessment. Compare calculated maintenance/deficit needs with intake records. |
| 2. Complications of fluid therapy are prevented or minimized. | Clinical status does not deteriorate as a result of therapy, e.g., development of cerebral edema from hypotonic fluids, seizures from precipitous drop in serum sodium, hypernatremia from inappropriate use of oral rehydration solutions, or hyperkalemia from adding potassium when renal function is inadequate. Any detrimental change in status is detected early, allowing prompt intervention. |
| 3. Child and family demonstrate an understanding of fluid therapy goals. | Ask child and family to explain goals of therapy; child and family actively participate in collecting intake and output information; other information relative to fluid status, e.g., behavioral changes, are promptly reported. |

### Documentation

Record complete baseline fluid balance assessment, continue appropriate documentation of child's behavior and ongoing monitoring of fluid balance. Document all measures such as body weights and urine specific gravities. Document appropriate fluid therapy, intake and output records, development of any complications related to therapy, and actions taken.

### Child and Family Teaching

1. Discuss potential for water intoxication during swimming lessons for infants. The infant may swallow large amounts of water during repeated submersion, leading to fluid overload or dilutional hyponatremia (Whaley and Wong, 1991).
2. Caution family to avoid high salt fluids (e.g., broth) and excess free water intake to replace vomiting/diarrhea losses.
3. Teach family to recognize signs of dehydration requiring attention of a health care professional.

# *SKILL* 65 Inserting and Maintaining a Gastric or Jejunal Tube

*Mary C. Oberc*

Tubes can be inserted into the stomach or jejunum of the child via the mouth or nose. The purposes for tube placement include: (1) to relieve distension by removing fluid and gas from the upper gastrointestinal tract (decompression); (2) to instill nutritional feedings, fluids, or medications directly into gastrointestinal tract; (3) to irrigate or lavage; (4) to remove gastric samples for diagnostic testing; and (5) to alleviate nausea or vomiting. Correct tube placement minimizes trauma to the child and family and ensures safety.

## NURSING DIAGNOSES

Altered nutrition: less than body requirements related to inadequate caloric intake; Potential fluid volume deficit related to loss of fluid due to vomiting or gastric decompression; Anxiety related to unmet informational needs about purpose and procedure for oral, nasal, or jejunal tube placement; Pain related to insertion/removal of oral, nasal, or jejunal tube.

| Steps | Rationale |
|---|---|
| **Assessment** | |
| 1. Assess purpose of tube placement. Check physician's order for type and purpose of tube (see box below and Fig. 65-1). | Knowing the purpose of tube insertion is helpful in selecting appropriate tube and equipment. Proper selection helps to decrease cost and trauma to the child and family. ***Special Considerations:*** *Only tubes made with radiopaque material should be used because these permit visualization by radiography (Hughes and Buescher, 1980).* |
| 2. Assess child's age, weight, and size. | Age, weight, and size help determine size of tube to be used. Equipment size should be proportional to child (Table 65-1). ***Special Considerations:*** *Oral insertion is preferred for premature infants (Pikl, 1981). Oral insertion may also be indicated in older infants and children who have structural defects of the nasal passage such as choanal atresia. Chronological age may not correlate with the tube size needed. For example, if a child is 3 years old but only weighs 5 kilograms, then a smaller size tube may be indicated. In such cases determine the age and correlate weight to select appropriate tube.* |
| 3. Determine patency of each nostril.<br>a. With an infant or small child, briefly occlude child's nostril with fingertip; place another finger tip under open nostril, and feel the passage of air. Repeat with opposite nostril.<br>b. With an older child, ask him or her to breathe through one nostril while the other is occluded. Repeat with opposite nostril. | Trauma is minimized when patency of nares is determined before attempting insertion. ***Special Considerations:*** *Sometimes one naris is smaller than the other. To facilitate passage of the tube for the first time, the tube should be placed through the larger nostril (Persons, 1987). To facilitate passage of the tube through nares with congested turbinates or inflamed mucosa, obtain order to instill .25% Neo-synephrine nose drops to decrease the swelling (Hughes and Buescher, 1980).* |

### *TYPES OF TUBES*

1. *Polyvinyl chloride (PVC):* The PVC tube can be used for intermittent or continuous feeding, gastric drainage, or irrigation or lavage. The tube is firm to provide stability during insertion but flexible to maneuver the curves of the child's nasal passage. Sizes are 5, 8, 10, and 12 French; lengths are 15 in, 36 in, or 42 in. This tube is most commonly used for feeding children and is referred to as a "feeding tube." The tube can remain in place for several days or be removed and reinserted with each feeding. In small infants, it may also be used for straight gastric drainage. Straight drainage involves allowing the tube to drain by gravity rather than applying suction. Mucosal damage may result from suction used for decompression because the tube is not vented. To facilitate drainage or irrigation, insert at least an 8 French tube. Smaller lumen tubes can produce greater resistance.
2. *Levine:* The Levine tube is used for irrigation, instillation, and withdrawal of fluids on a short term basis. It is an unweighted, single-lumen, firm polyvinyl tube without air vents. Sizes include 10, 12, and 14 French. The firmness of the tube may make insertion more difficult. Mucosal damage may result when the tube is attached to suction because it has no venting system. Aspiration of small amounts of gastric fluid for sample or culture does not produce mucosal damage.
3. *Salem-Sump:* The Salem-Sump tube is an unweighted, radiopaque, double lumen, clear plastic tube suitable for irrigation, decompression, monitoring, and instillation of fluids. The small blue air vent, if patent, prevents the nasogastric tube from adhering to the gastric mucosa (Persons, 1987). The tube is frequently used for postoperative gastric drainage and is usually attached to a suction apparatus.
4. *Silicone or polyurethane:* The silicone tube is a soft, pliable, weighted, small-bore, single-lumen feeding tube (e.g., Enteriflex, Nutriflex, Keofeed) used for long-term, intermittent, or continuous nasogastric or nasojejunal feedings. The tubes are available with a stainless steel or plastic stylet to stiffen the tube during insertion. A size 5 French (15 or 36 inches long) may be used for a premature infant. A size 8 French tube (36 or 43 inches long) is suitable for most infants and children. The silicone tube does not require regular replacement because it is less irritating to the gastric mucosa than polyvinyl tubes. It may be reused once it has been inspected for holes and rinsed with warm water. It is especially useful for comatose children, trauma victims, and children with low platelet counts (Sporing, 1984; Persons, 1987). Use of these small-bore feeding tubes reduces complications such as pharyngitis, otitis media, and incompetence of the lower esophageal sphincter (Wesley, 1988).

**Steps** | **Rationale**

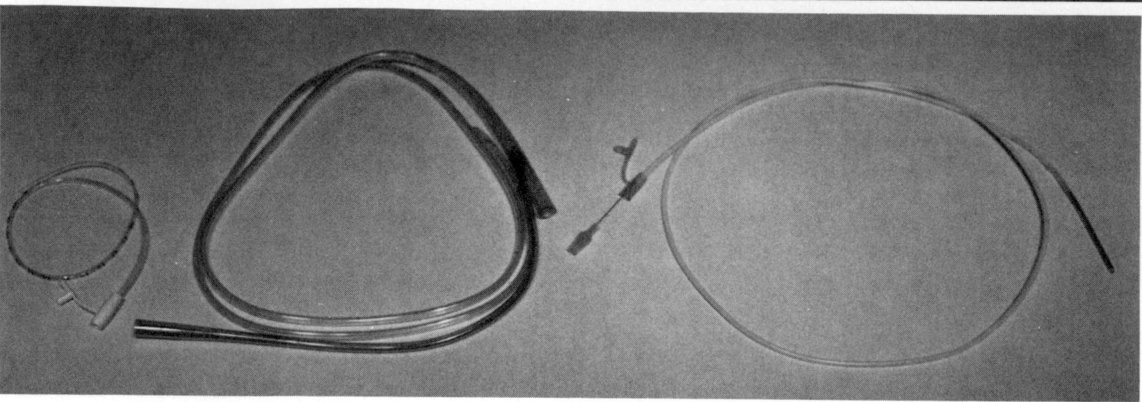

***FIG. 65-1*** Types of tubes: a polyvinylchloride tube, the Salem-Sump tube (with air vent), and a weighted silicone tube.

4. Assess child's and family's needs and concerns about the procedure.
   a. Previous experience with tube insertion.
   b. Ability to follow instructions.
   c. Fears and anxieties.
   d. Need for restraint.

Assessing child and family needs and concerns allows proper preparation for the procedure. Restraint may be needed for the child's safety and comfort.

***Special Considerations:*** *A tube insertion can be frightening for a parent to watch and for the child to experience. Parents familiar with the procedure may have helpful suggestions to facilitate tube insertion. An agitated child may require restraint. It is usually more effective and less traumatic to gain cooperation of the child. An older child who has had frequent experiences with tube insertion may prefer to insert the tube himself or herself (Hughes and Buescher, 1980).*

5. Assess possible precautions or contraindications for the procedure such as:
   a. Gastroesophageal surgery or trauma.
   b. Fracture of the face or nose.
   c. Recent nasopharyngeal or corrective surgery.
   d. Structural defects.
   e. Basal skull fracture.
   f. Deviated septum.
   g. Endotracheal tube (Persons, 1987).

Insertion of a tube through a recent surgical repair or fracture could injure or perforate newly formed tissue. Structural defects could interfere with normal passage of the tube. Inserting a nasogastric tube into a child with a basal skull fracture places the child at risk for passage of the tube into the cranium. The presence of an endotracheal tube tends to guide the feeding tube into the trachea (Persons, 1987).

***Special Considerations:*** *If contraindications are present, the physician may use fluoroscopy to help with tube placement. If the child dislodges a tube inserted during a surgical repair, notify the physician before attempting reinsertion.*

## Planning and Goal Setting

1. Gather supplies.

### *Infant*

   a. Select or obtain the ordered tube (see Table 65-1 and the box on p. 419).
   b. 5 cc or 12 cc syringe.
   c. Rolled blanket or towel, cloth diaper, or burping pad.

Collecting supplies in advance yields increased safety and efficiency.

***Special Considerations:*** *For Levine, Salem-Sump, and silicone tubes, a catheter tip or cone-shaped Asepto syringe is needed for aspiration. Polyvinyl chloride tubes use a regular tip syringe.*

***TABLE 65-1*** Suggested Sizes for Vented Tubes

| Age Group | Tube Size |
|---|---|
| Infants | 5 to 8 Fr |
| Toddlers | 8 to 10 Fr |
| Preschool | 10 to 12 Fr |
| School age | 12 Fr |
| Adolescent | 14 Fr |

To prevent a fistula of the septum, insert a smaller size tube into children intubated nasally.

| Steps | Rationale |
|---|---|
| d. ¼-inch or ½-inch hypoallergenic tape. | |
| e. Stethoscope. | |
| f. Medicine cup half filled with water. | |
| g. Water-soluble lubricant (for nasal insertion only). | |
| h. Pacifier. | |
| i. Suction apparatus (if ordered). | |
| j. Specimen container or basin. | A basin or container is needed to collect gastric contents. |
| k. Catheter tip syringe (also referred to as Asepto, Toomey, or irrigating syringe). | |
| l. Clamp (optional). | A clamp may be used to close the tube after insertion. |
| ***Older child*** | |
| a. All of the above except pacifier, cloth diaper, rolled blanket. | |
| b. Emesis basin. | |
| c. Glass of water with drinking straw. | |
| d. Safety pin. | |
| e. 50 cc syringe. | |
| f. Towel. | |
| g. Facial tissues. | Eyes may water during the procedure. |
| 2. Recruit an assistant if necessary. | An assistant may be needed for restraining purposes (see Skill 51). |
| 3. Prepare the child and family for the procedure (see Skill 1). Discuss possible discomfort and sensation of gagging during the procedure. Suggest the use of a hand signal to indicate if the child cannot breath or needs a break (Persons, 1987). | Proper preparation and teaching will help decrease child and family's fear of the unknown. **Special Considerations:** *For a child subjected to repeated tube insertions, allow child to poke a demonstration doll's nose as often as needed, remaining close for emotional support (see Skill 16).* |
| 4. Develop individualized child and family goals:<br>▪ Child will have a patent and functional tube inserted.<br>▪ Child will experience minimal discomfort during tube insertion.<br>▪ Child will receive therapeutic effect intended by the tube insertion (decompression, nutrition).<br>▪ Family and child will experience minimal anxiety as a result of the tube insertion. | |

## Implementation

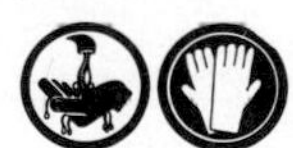

| Steps | Rationale |
|---|---|
| 1. Before performing the procedure, explain each step to the family and child. | Knowing what will happen next often reduces fears and anxieties. **Special Considerations:** *Even with infants, talk throughout the procedure because the sound and intonation of the human voice will often soothe and relax them.* |
| 2. Position the child. | |
| a. Elevate the head of the bed. Place infant on his or her right side or back on the elevated portion of the bed. Restrain as indicated.<br>b. Alternate methods of simulating elevation:<br>▪ Infant: use a folded blanket under head and shoulders or place infant in semi-sitting infant seat.<br>▪ Older child: ask the child to sit in a bed set at a high Fowler's position; support head and shoulders with a pillow. | Elevating the head of the bed allows gravity and easier swallowing to facilitate passage of the tube. For nasojejunal insertion, placement on the right side promotes drainage of stomach contents into the small intestine. Placing the child in a comfortable position promotes relaxation. **Special Considerations:** *If the infant is positioned on his or her side, support the back with rolled blanket or towel.* |
| 3. Arrange assembled equipment.<br>a. Open packages.<br>b. Cut three pieces of tape approximately 3 inches long. Hang them within easy reach on the night stand or bed rail. | Organization and preparation improves efficiency, decreases trauma to the child, and prevents needless repetition of procedure. **Special Considerations:** *Width and length of tape pieces will vary with size of the child. Only use enough to secure the tube. Avoid over-taping.* |
| 4. Place a towel or cloth diaper over the child's chest and shoulders. For an infant, place a portion of the cloth near mouth to absorb possible emesis. For an older child, place an emesis basin in his or her hands or within easy reach. | Vomiting may occur when the tube stimulates the gag reflex. **Special Considerations:** *For a premature or small infant, a cloth diaper or burping pad may be more appropriate than a towel.* |
| 5. Measure length of tube to be inserted. Place a piece of tape on the tube to mark the final length needed. | Measuring the tube length facilitates proper placement and prevents possible aspiration that can occur if the tube is incorrectly positioned in the esophagus. |

### CALCULATING PLACEMENT (OR INSERTION) LENGTH OF FEEDING TUBE

A reliable formula for calculating placement (or insertion) length of a feeding tube has not been determined. Ziemer and Carroll (1978) noted that using the conventional method of measurement, tip of the nose to ear lobe to xiphoid process, was often found to be too short because gastric contents could not be aspirated. They proposed a measurement from the tip of the nose to the ear lobe to a point midway between the xiphoid process and the umbilicus. It was reported that with this method, the tube was properly positioned in the body of the stomach at autopsy. However, Weibley et al (1987) performed an experimental study comparing Ziemer and Carroll's method with a variation of the conventional method to determine which resulted in the most accurate placement in the stomach of the premature infant. X-ray was used for verification. Method "A" began at the right corner of the infant's nostril or mouth, extended to the right ear lobe, and then extended to the termination of the xiphoid process. A strip of adhesive tape was wrapped 2 cm beyond the measured point, and the tube was inserted to the tape marker. In method "B," the tube was placed at the right corner of the right nostril or mouth, extended to the right ear lobe, and then to a point midway between the xiphoid and umbilicus. Results indicated that both methods "A" and "B" produced incorrect measurements. Method "A" yielded 55.6% incorrect placements; method "B" yielded 39.9% incorrect placements. Weibley concluded that other measurement methods should be explored.

| Steps | Rationale |
|---|---|
| *Nasogastric:* place the tip of the tube at the tip of the child's nose. Extend the tube to the child's ear lobe and then downward to a point midway between the xiphoid process and umbilicus (Ziemer and Carroll, 1978). Measurement may also be done in reverse, starting at a point midway between the umbilicus and xiphoid process (Wong and Whaley, 1990) (see box above). | ***Special Considerations:*** *If the measured distance for the tube insertion is within 1 or 2 inches of the total length of the tube, then use a longer tube to improve manipulation. Polyvinyl chloride tubes have dots on the side of the tube that may be used as a marker instead of tape. For a silicone feeding tube, measurement begins with the ports at the bottom of the tube and not the weighted tip.* |
| *Nasojejunal:* proceed with nasogastric insertion measurement, and then add 10 to 15 cm (4 to 6 in) beyond the point midway between the xiphoid process and the umbilicus. | This measurement approximates the distance from the nose into the jejunum.<br>***Special Considerations:*** *Occasionally the tube may need to be advanced a few centimeters further to obtain verification of placement by aspiration of jejunal contents.* |
| *Orogastric:* begin measurement at the corner of the mouth; extend the tube to the child's ear lobe and then downward to a point midway between the xiphoid process and the umbilicus. | |
| 6. Prepare the tube. | |
| a. Wrap approximately 15 cm (6 in) of the tube around the index finger to give the tube a natural curve. | A curved tube will pass more easily through the curved structures of the nasopharynx. |
| b. If the tube is too stiff, soak it in a basin of warm water until it is more pliable. | An excessively stiff tube may injure the nasal passage, while a very soft tube is difficult to insert. |
| c. If the tube is too soft, soak it in a basin of cold water until it is firmer. | ***Special Considerations:*** *Levine tubes are very firm and may require both wrapping and soaking. Gastric perforation is possible with forceful insertion of a stiff tube (Hughes and Buescher, 1980). Esophageal perforation has been reported in low birth weight infants following gavage feeding (Clarke, 1980).* |
| d. For a silicone feeding tube only: | |
| ▪ Remove the guide wire from the tube; spread water-soluble lubricant over the entire wire. | Lubricating the wire ensures easy removal of the wire once the tube is in place.<br>***Special Considerations:*** *Some feeding tubes with stylets are coated with a water-activated substance that facilitates stylet placement. Inject water through the feeding tube instead of lubricating the stylet before placement. Follow manufacturer's directions.* |
| ▪ Replace the wire inside the tube; avoid passing the wire through the feeding ports at the bottom of the tube. | Properly reinserting the wire prevents possible excoriation or perforation of the gastrointestinal tract by the exposed distal end of the wire. |
| 7. Lubricate the tube. | Lubrication facilitates passage of the tube through the nasopharynx. |
| a. *Nasogastric, nasojejunal:* lubricate 1 to 2 inches of the end of the tube with water-soluble lubricant or water. | ***Special Considerations:*** *Hydrocarbon aspiration pneumonia could result if an oil-based lubricant such as petroleum jelly is used. Some facilities prefer to lubricate the tube only with water. Refer to procedure manual.* |

| Steps | Rationale |
|---|---|
| b. *Orogastric:* no lubrication is necessary. | |
| c. *Silicone feeding tube:* lubricate the weighted tip with water-soluble lubricant. | |
| 8. Stabilize the child's head. | |
| a. Infant, side-lying position: place the palm of the non-dominant hand along side of the child's face without hyperextending the neck. | An infant is less likely to aspirate in a side-lying position. Hyperextension of the infant's neck can occlude the airway. |
| b. Infant, supine position: encircle mandible with an extended thumb and forefinger. | ***Special Considerations:*** *If an infant in the supine position begins to vomit, turn the head to the side to prevent aspiration.* |
| c. Older child: elicit cooperation by asking him or her to hyperextend the neck, keep the head still, breathe through the mouth, and swallow when instructed. | Hyperextending the neck relaxes the child and provides a better angle for tube insertion. |
| 9. Insert the tube with the dominant hand. | |
| *Nasogastric:* | |
| a. Insert tube into the selected nostril with the curved end facing downward, and advance along the base of the nose, directing straight back toward the occiput. | Following the curves of the nasal passage facilitates tube insertion and decreases trauma. Insertion at a downward slant decreases trauma to nasal mucosa by avoiding the nasal turbinates. |
| b. If resistance is met after advancing 2 to 3 cm (1 in) into the naris, slightly rotate the tube or have the child inspire. Wait for the feeling of release, and then thread the tube further into the naris. Do not poke or force the tube through the resistance. | ***Special Considerations:*** *For young children, rolling the tube clockwise between the thumb and fingers as the tube is advanced forward facilitates placement. A previously cooperative child or an active infant (premature or full-term) may grab and pull out the tube because of extreme discomfort.* |
| c. Continue to thread the tube to the posterior nasopharynx. In synchrony with child's swallowing reflex, advance the tube to the desired length. | Swallowing closes the epiglottis and facilitates passage of the tube into the esophagus. |
| ▪ Infants: encourage swallowing with use of a pacifier or blowing a small puff of air in the infant's face, eliciting the Santmyer swallow reflex. If gagging occurs during advancement, slightly withdraw the tube, and advance after gagging subsides. | A puff of air reliably elicits a reflexive swallow in developmentally normal infants and in older children with severe neurologic disorders (Orenstein et al, 1988). Stimulation of the posterior pharynx may inadvertently stimulate the vagus nerve, resulting in gagging. ***Special Considerations:*** *Moderate hyperflexion of infant's neck may facilitate esophageal placement. Extreme hyperflexion may occlude the airway.* |
| ▪ Older child: once the tube has passed the posterior naris, ask the child to flex neck forward. Give the child a glass of water with a straw, instructing to repeatedly swallow small sips of water. While the child is swallowing, advance the tube to the desired length. If gagging occurs, withdraw the tube slightly, allowing child to regain composure and take a few deep breaths. | Since the esophagus is situated behind the trachea, the tube is more easily inserted when the child's head is hyperflexed. Swallowing enhances peristalsis, and the water lubricates the tissue. This enables the tube to glide more easily into the stomach. ***Special Considerations:*** *Rotating a curved-tip tube 180 degrees after it passes through the posterior naris also may prevent the tube from entering the trachea, facilitating placement. Sips of water should only be offered to children who are conscious, able to follow commands, and are allowed fluids. If no fluids are allowed, instruct the child to perform a Valsalva maneuver, which will close the epiglottis and eliminate the need for swallowing during the insertion (Hughes and Buescher, 1980).* |
| d. Check the back of the child's throat for a coiled tube. If this occurs, withdraw the tube and reinsert. | A coiled tube at the back of the throat indicates improper placement. ***Special Considerations:*** *Tubes with small diameters such as size 5 French or less are especially prone to coiling because of their flexibility.* |
| e. Observe for signs of vagal stimulation while passing the tube past the gag reflex area: decreased pulse, gasping, apnea, coughing, gagging, and/or vomiting. If these symptoms occur, withdraw the tube and wait for the child's condition to stabilize before proceeding. | Vagal stimulation can cause cardiac depression, bronchial constriction, coughing, gagging, and vomiting. |
| f. Observe for indications that tube placement is in the trachea or bronchus: excessive coughing, choking, cyanosis, and/or absence of sound. If this occurs, retract the tube to the nasopharynx, and reinsert after the child is breathing more easily. | Presence of the tube in the trachea or bronchus occludes the airway and is potentially hazardous. ***Special Considerations:*** *Accidental placement in the trachea may not be as apparent with smaller diameter tubes. A cough may not be present if the child's cough reflex is suppressed or absent.* |

| Steps | Rationale |
|---|---|
| *Nasojejunal:* | |
| a. Follow procedure for nasogastric tube insertion.<br>b. Once the tube is in the stomach, advance the tube through the pylorus to the designated mark on the tube. | ***Special Considerations:*** *Resistance may be encountered when advancing the tube through the pylorus. The tube may coil in the stomach instead of advancing through the pylorus. See step 11, checking tube placement.* |
| *Orogastric:* | |
| a. Open the mouth.<br>▪ Infants and toddlers: grasp mandible at the chin, and gently pull down; or squeeze both cheeks toward the midline (Fig. 65-2); or pinch nose between thumb and forefinger; or demonstrate an open mouth and say "ahh."<br>▪ Older child: Ask the child to say "ahh", or give specific directions to open mouth. | Infants are nose breathers. Occluding the nose results in mouth breathing.<br>***Special Considerations:*** *If the child has teeth, oral insertion may be contraindicated because the child may bite the tube in half and aspirate it. If no other route is available, place a firm airway in the mouth to prevent biting.* |
| b. While the mouth is open, quickly advance the tube to the back of the throat. Approach from the side of the tongue. If the child gags, slightly withdraw the tube.<br>c. In synchrony with swallowing reflex (see above), advance the tube to the desired length. | Following the curves of the oropharynx facilitates tube insertion and decreases trauma. |
| 10. Temporarily secure the tube to check position. | The tube can become displaced if not secured, causing the placement check to be in error. |
| *Nasogastric, nasojejunal:* | |
| a. Cross both sides of the marking tape over the tube, and press the adhesive side of the tape onto the skin between the bottom of the nose and the top of the lips (Fig. 65-3). | |
| *Orogastric:* | |
| a. Temporarily tape tube to the cheek. Use cross over method. | |
| *Silicone feeding tube:* | |
| a. Remove the guide wire.<br>▪ Use nondominant hand to hold the tube in place.<br>▪ Use the dominant hand to disconnect the plastic end of the guide wire from the feeding tube.<br>▪ Straighten the tube, and remove the guide wire.<br>b. Secure the tube the same as nasogastric tube. | The guide wire is intended for insertion only, as it occludes the tube's lumen. |

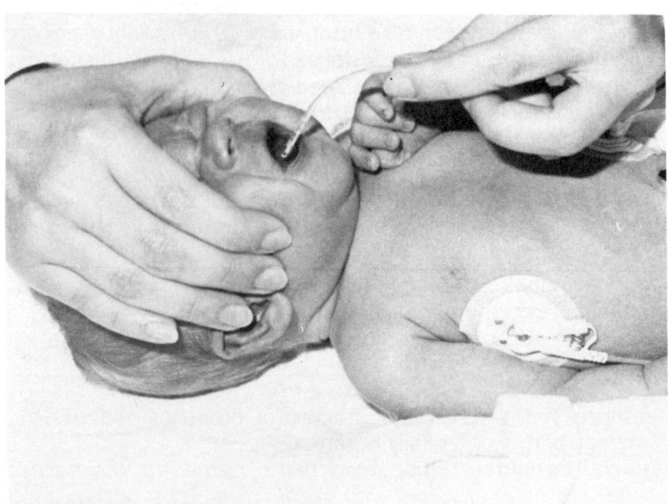

***FIG. 65-2*** Insertion of tube for gavage feeding.

From Whaley LF and Wong DL: Essentials of pediatric nursing, ed 3, 1989, St Louis, The CV Mosby Co.

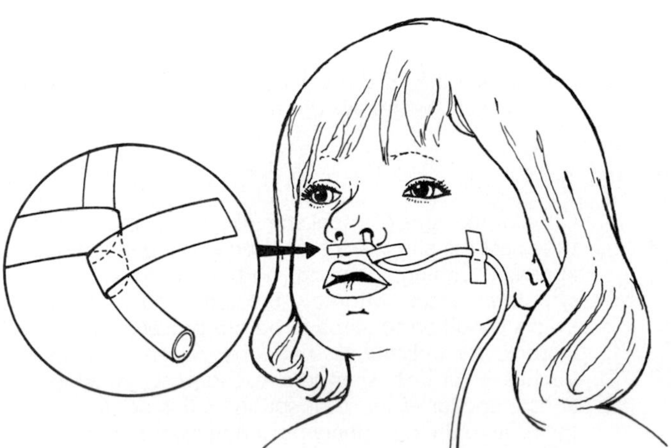

***FIG. 65-3*** Position of the tube is secured by cross over method.

| Steps | Rationale |
|---|---|
| 11. Check tube to verify gastrointestinal, not tracheal, placement. Use all three methods for each insertion. | Proper and safe functioning of the tube requires proper placement. Reliability of commonly recommended measures to test placement is unproven (Metheny et al, 1988).<br>**Special Considerations:** *Incorrect placement can have serious or fatal complications.* |
| a. Place free end of tube in a cup of water and observe for a stream of bubbles when the child exhales. | Bubbling in the water during exhalation indicates placement of the tube in the lungs. |
| b. Attach a syringe filled with 0.5 to 5 cc of air to the distal end of the tube.<br>▪ *Nasogastric, orogastric:* place a stethoscope over the stomach directly below the left costal margin or left upper abdomen. Rapidly inject the air into the stomach while simultaneously auscultating for a burp, gurgling, or whooshing sound. Aspirate air inserted. | When air is injected into a body cavity, a gurgling or burping sound indicates proper placement.<br>**Special Considerations:** *Use minimal air to prevent gastric distension. The amount of air injected is determined by the size of the child: 0.5 cc in premature or very small infants to 5 cc in larger children. This method can be misleading because a bolus of air can be auscultated over the stomach when the tube is still in the esophagus within 1 cm of the cardiac sphincter (Ziemer, 1978), or when one opening of the tube is in the stomach and another is in the esophagus (Metheny, 1986). Danger of aspiration exists if one or more of the lower openings is in the esophagus (Weibley, 1987).* |
| ▪ *Nasojejunal:* place a stethoscope over the right lower quadrant of the abdomen. Rapidly inject the air into the jejunum while simultaneously auscultating for a "swishing" sound. Aspirate air inserted. | The jejunum is located in the right lower quadrant of the abdomen. When air is injected, a "swishing" sound indicates proper placement.<br>**Special Considerations:** *Use above guidelines as to amounts of air to inject.* |
| c. Aspirate cavity fluids by applying gentle negative pressure with the syringe attached to the tube. | |
| ▪ *Nasogastric, orogastric:* aspirate approximately 1 cc of stomach fluids. If green bile stained fluid is obtained, withdraw the tube approximately 2.5 to 5 cm (1 to 2 inches), and aspirate again. | Aspiration of stomach contents indicates presence of the tube in the stomach. Green bile stained fluid suggests duodenal placement. Bolus feedings into the duodenum can cause an iatrogenic dumping syndrome: nausea, vomiting, warmth, sweating, increased pulse, empty feeling in upper abdomen, light headedness, or vertigo (Hanson, 1980).<br>**Special Considerations:** *Absence of fluid is not necessarily evidence of improper placement. The stomach may be empty, or the tube may not be in contact with stomach contents. If unable to aspirate stomach contents, turn the child on the left side to pool gastric contents, and aspirate again (Persons, 1987). If still unable to aspirate stomach contents, slightly advance the tube (approximately 1 cm) and reattempt aspiration.* |
| ▪ *Nasojejunal:* aspirate approximately 1 cc of jejunal fluid. Jejunal fluid will have a golden yellow color; pH will be 6 or above. If unable to aspirate jejunal fluid, wait 1½ hours. During this time keep the child on the right side with the tube vented to air. After 1½ hours, aspirate again. If no fluid is obtained, reinsert tube or consult with physician. | Aspiration of jejunal fluid indicates presence of the tube in the jejunum.<br>**Special Considerations:** *An x-ray or fluoroscopy, the most reliable methods of verifying jejunal tube placement, may be indicated. Continuous feedings at 1 cc or more per hour may be ordered to stimulate peristalsis. The tube should advance through the pylorus within 24 hours. Because the silicone tube is soft, it is prone to collapsing. If this occurs, inject 5 cc of sterile water and gently aspirate the same amount.* |
| d. Return aspirate to the cavity (stomach or jejunum) from which it was withdrawn. | Returning aspirate prevents electrolyte imbalance. |
| 12. Once proper placement is determined, completely secure the tube in place. | A securely taped tube decreases tube displacement, risk of aspiration, and allows for freedom of head movement.<br>**Special Considerations:** *Taping alone is usually sufficient. Excessive taping does not hold the tube more securely in place. Some sources recommend the use of a protective dressing wipe (such as skin prep). Avoid using tincture of benzoin to secure the tape. It can be irritating to the skin, and sometimes small pieces of skin can be pulled off when the tape is removed. A small piece of stoma adhesive, used to secure ostomy bags, can be placed on the skin, then the tape can be secured to it. This is especially helpful to protect the skin when repeated taping is necessary (Stoiko, 1989).* |

| Steps | Rationale |
|---|---|
| 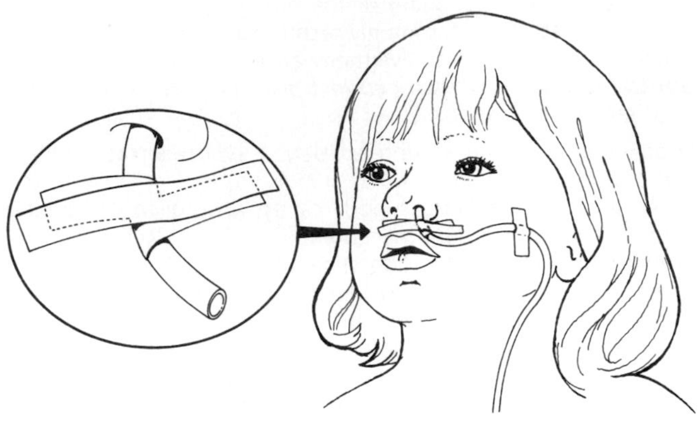 | ***FIG. 65-4*** An additional adhesive strip, placed over the crossover tape, is molded around the tube. |
| *Nasogastric, nasojejunal:* | |
| a. Over the piece of crossed tape under the nose, place an additional piece of tape, molding it around the tube (Fig. 65-4). | |
| b. Extend the tube to the side of the face, and tape the tube flat (avoiding distortion) as it leaves the naris (Fig. 65-4). | Prolonged pressure on the external nares from improper taping can lead to irritation and tissue damage. Avoid taping to the forehead because the tape will exert an upward pull on the naris. |
| c. For heavier tubes use tape tab, and safety pin the tube to the child's gown. | Securing tube to the gown helps support the weight of the tube and prevents it from pulling or dangling.<br>***Special Considerations:*** *For an infant or toddler, the polyvinyl chloride tube can be placed over the shoulder and taped to a T-shirt or gown.* |
| *Orogastric:* | |
| a. Over the piece of tape used to temporarily secure the tube to the cheek, place another piece of tape, and mold it around the tube.<br>b. If the tube is to be indwelling, mold another piece of tape around the tube approximately 2 to 3 inches away from the initial taping site, and attach to face. | ***Special Considerations:*** *Some facility policies do not recommend taping for intermittent gavage feedings because of possible damage to the skin. If this practice is followed, hold the tube firmly in place where it enters the mouth or nose. Also be aware that aspiration can result from tube dislodgement when taping is omitted.* |
| 13. Comfort the child.<br>a. Infant: pick up and hold or stroke head.<br>b. Older child: caress or hug. Thank for cooperation. Praise efforts at swallowing. | Praising and comforting reassures child that he or she is loved and accepted.<br>***Special Considerations:*** *Confirm that the procedure is uncomfortable. If the child vomits, reassure that adults sometimes do also.* |
| 14. If gastric decompression is ordered, attach the gastric tube to low, intermittent suction or straight gravity drainage. Use the lowest suction setting that effectively decompresses the stomach. | Intermittent suction is preferred in children because continuous suction can cause irritation to the gastric mucosa and may cause gastrointestinal bleeding (Hazinski, 1984). Intermittent suction can be obtained by using either a regulatory pump, e.g., Gomco, or a central source, e.g., wall suction. |
| *Intermittent suction:* | |
| a. Attach air vented tube to intermittent suction apparatus (e.g., central wall suction or portable device such as Gomco), using the largest lumen of the gastric tube. Use a low setting of 30 to 40 mm Hg. | Air venting is necessary to minimize mucosal damage from the vacuum created by the suction.<br>***Special Considerations:*** *An air vent may not be effective in preventing mucosal damage (Van Way, 1987).* |
| b. Secure the air vent pigtail of tube above the level of child's stomach. | A siphon effect may cause gastric fluid to drain into air vent when it hangs below level of stomach. |
| c. If suction is sluggish:<br>▪ Irrigate air vent with 5 to 20 cc of air or saline followed by air. | The air vent may be occluded with water-soluble lubricant or gastric contents from insertion. Irrigation will clear obstruction, return patency, and help prevent mucosal damage. |
| ▪ Irrigate primary lumen with 5 to 20 cc of normal saline every 2 hours or as ordered. | Loss of sodium ions during intermittent suctioning make normal saline the preferred solution for irrigating. Occlusion of the tube may result in gastric distension and vomiting. |

| Steps | Rationale |
|---|---|
| *Straight gravity drainage:* | |
| a. Place tube opening into a receptacle and secure in place. | The receptacle will be used to collect and measure the gastric drainage. ***Special Considerations:*** *Some possible containers are urine specimen or drainage bag, specimen cup with hole cut in lid, or a preweighed disposable diaper.* |
| b. Place collection receptacle below the child's stomach level. | Placing the tube opening below the stomach level is necessary to siphon off gastric drainage and air. |
| 15. For gravity or suction drainage, keep accurate and frequent measurements of intake and output, noting amount and characteristics of drainage. Replace gastric drainage with appropriate intravenous fluids milliliter for milliliter per physician's order (Hazinski, 1984). | Loss of large amounts of gastric secretion can result in dehydration and electrolyte imbalance. ***Special Considerations:*** *An increase in gastric secretions or a change to bilious color may be indicative of a bowel obstruction. The presence of blood may indicate gastric wall irritation or trauma. Unreplaced loss of hydrogen and potassium ions can result in metabolic alkalosis and hypokalemia.* |
| 16. Maintain the tube. | |
| a. Change the tube as needed. | |
| ▪ Polyvinyl chloride tube: Nasogastric, orogastric—change at least every 3 days unless contraindicated, e.g., surgically placed or difficult insertion. Nasojejunal—change at least every 5 days. ▪ Salem-Sump, Levine: Check with physician. | The tip of the polyvinyl chloride tube hardens and can perforate the stomach if it remains in the stomach for extended periods. Other complications that may develop from prolonged use are acute otitis media, sinusitis, stomatitis, parotiditis, and epistaxis (Hughes and Buescher, 1980). ***Special Considerations:*** *Refer to facility procedure manual for recommended frequency of tube change.* |
| ▪ Silicone feeding tube: Does not require changing. | ***Special Considerations:*** *Because of the difficulty with reinsertion, the silicone feeding tube should be maintained in place if any possibility exists that feeding may be resumed.* |
| b. Alternate nares when reinserting a tube. | Use of only one naris can result in deviated septum or tissue necrosis. |
| c. Change the adhesive tape as needed. | |
| d. Irrigate tube as needed unless contraindicated. ▪ Nasogastric or orogastric, see step 14c. ▪ Silicone feeding tube: Flush with 1 to 10 ml of tap or sterile water after each feeding or medication administration. Otherwise, flush once every 8 hours. | Regular irrigation helps maintain patency of tube. ***Special Considerations:*** *Some facilities require a physician's order for irrigations. Follow any irrigation of a vented tube with an injection of air through the air vent pigtail.* |
| 17. Provide daily oral and nasal care. a. Clean the nostril and tube with moistened cotton-tip applicators. b. Apply water-soluble lubricant to the nostril if it appears dry or encrusted. c. Inspect the nostril for discharge and irritation. d. Give frequent oral care (see Skills 56 and 57). | Mouth breathing and inability to drink may cause mucous membranes to become dry. The presence of the tube can be irritating to nasal tissues. ***Special Considerations:*** *A commercially made pacifier will help meet the infant's need to suck while not allowed oral feedings (Whaley and Wong, 1991).* |
| 18. Remove the tube when ordered by a physician or after intermittent feedings such as with orogastric tube. | |
| a. Remove tape securing tube to skin and unpin from gown. | |
| b. Kink the tube. | Kinking the tube prevents possible aspiration of contents present in the tube at the time it is withdrawn. |
| c. Have a towel held at the nose to grab the tube. | Grabbing the tube with a towel prevents soiling child's clothing and bedding with possible gastric contents. |
| d. Rapidly and steadily pull the tube out. | |
| e. Give oral and nasal care after removal. | |

| Evaluation Outcomes | Observational Guidelines |
|---|---|
| 1. Child has a patent and functional nasogastric or orogastric tube. | Stomach contents are aspirated with a syringe. A "burping" sound is auscultated in the left upper quadrant of the abdomen when air is injected through the tube. No bubbling is observed. |
| 2. Child has a patent and functional nasojejunal tube. | Jejunal contents are aspirated with a syringe. A "swishing" sound is auscultated in the right lower quadrant of the abdomen when air is injected through the tube. |
| 3. Child experiences minimal discomfort during tube insertion or removal. | Facial expressions are observed for signs of pain or gagging. Note if bleeding from nose or mouth occurs, caused by irritation from tube insertion. |

| Steps | Rationale |
|---|---|
| 4. Child experiences therapeutic effect of tube insertion as indicated for nutritional support, decompression, irrigation or lavage, or obtaining specimens. | Note improvement or relief according to intended therapeutic benefit compared with baseline assessment. |
| 5. Child and family experience minimal anxiety from tube insertion or removal. | Observe facial and body expressions for anger or fear. Note cooperation of child and family members. Listen to comments from child and family. |

## Documentation

Record type of tube, route, placement, check results, date and time of insertion and removal, child and family teaching, child's tolerance and reaction to the procedure, family's reaction to the procedure, and techniques that enhanced tube insertion. Record amount, type, and consistency of aspirate or fluid drained. Record any irrigation solution instilled if not aspirated. Record accurate intake and output and notification of physician of any significant changes in drainage. Record use of suction, type and pressure, gravity drainage, and child's response to decompression.

## Home Care Modifications

1. Tubes and syringes can be cleaned by soaking them in hydrogen peroxide to remove old mucus and dried formula. Long pipe cleaners and bottle brushes may be used in cleaning inner lumens. Tubes and syringes can then be washed in warm soapy water and rinsed with tap water. Attach the feeding tubes to a coat hanger with a spring clothes pin and hang them vertically on a shower rod to allow air drying. When tubes and syringes are dry they can be stored in a sealable plastic bag, clean glass jar, or plastic container.
2. Silicone tubes are rinsed in warm water without additional cleansing agents. Avoid inadvertently puncturing the tube with sharp objects such as safety pins.
3. Teach caregivers how to restrain child in the home setting if the child is not cooperative during the procedure.
4. Teach several caregivers in the family how to perform the procedure in case the primary caregiver becomes ill or incapacitated.
5. Refer to *Clinical Manual of Pediatric Nursing* (Wong and Whaley, 1990) for a home care instruction sheet that may be photocopied and distributed to families.

# *SKILL* 66 Administering Tube Feedings

*Jane Deacon and Patricia Beachy*

Children who are unable to take nourishment orally are often fed by way of a tube inserted orally or nasally to the stomach (gastric gavage), or duodenum/jejunum (enteral gavage), or by a device inserted through an abdominal incision into the stomach (gastrostomy) or jejunum (jejunostomy). Feedings may be intermittent or continuous, short-term or long-term, by gravity or by infusion pump. Astute nursing assessment and care is essential for safe administration of feedings and prevention of harm to the child.

## NURSING DIAGNOSES

Altered health maintenance related to lack of knowledge about care and administration of tube feedings; Potential for aspiration related to gastric reflux due to bolus tube feedings, feeding position, or delayed gastric emptying; Altered nutrition: less than body requirements related to inadequate caloric intake; Altered nutrition: more than body requirements related to excessive caloric intake.

| Steps | Rationale |
|---|---|
| **Assessment** | |
| 1. Determine the child's age and weight. | The type of food and fluid a child receives is determined primarily by age (Paarlberg and Balint, 1985). The amount is determined by weight. An initial weight also provides baseline information for evaluating effectiveness of a nutritional program. |
| 2. Check physician's order for: | Tube feedings must be ordered by a physician. |
| a. Type of formula. | ***Special Considerations:*** *Commercially-prepared or insititutionally-prepared formulas are available.* |

| Steps | Rationale |
|---|---|
| b. Amount of formula. | |
| c. Delivery rate. | |
| d. Frequency of feedings. | Feedings may be either continuous or intermittent. Gastric feedings are given most often intermittently as a bolus, while jejunal feedings tend to be continuous. |
| e. Amount and type of flush. | Tubes are flushed to complete feeding and to clear tubing to prevent obstruction of tip. |
| f. Information about whether tube should be vented or clamped after feeding, and if so, length of time. | |
| 3. Assess type of tube being used to administer feeding (see Skill 65). | The type of tube dictates additional assessment and intervention. It may also influence appropriate formula consistency and amount of flush needed. ***Special Considerations:*** *Enteral feeding tubes and gastrostomy devices remain indwelling between feedings. Nasogastric or orogastric tubes may be indwelling or removed after each feeding.* |
| 4. Review the child's history and record for information regarding: | Awareness of pertinent information related to feedings can facilitate safe administration. |
| a. Tolerance of previous feeding, e.g., gagging, vomiting. | |
| b. Allergies to foods such as eggs or milk. | Formulas commonly contain milk, sugar, eggs, and oil. Assessing allergies prevents local or systemic allergic responses. |
| c. Current clinical condition. | A deterioration in clinical condition may contraindicate proceeding with feeding. |
| 5. Assess gastrointestinal function of child especially: | |
| a. Abdominal girth. | Abdominal distension may be a contraindication to feeding since it may lead to emesis and possible aspiration of stomach contents. It also elevates the diaphragm, decreasing the functional residual capacity (FRC), which increases intrapulmonary right to left shunting. In infants and children with abnormal or compressed lung function, this can cause significant hypoxemia and apnea (Mize, Teitell, and Cunningham, 1984). |
| b. Bowel sounds. | Active bowel sounds indicate intestinal peristalsis. |
| c. Residual gastric volume (see Implementation step 3). | Residual volume is an indication of feeding tolerance. |
| d. Type of stools. | Some children occasionally develop osmotic diarrhea with bolus feedings. ***Special Considerations:*** *Children on tube feedings may develop diarrhea from an underlying problem such as malnutrition or as a result of other therapy such as antibiotic drugs, rather than from the tube feeding itself (Anderson, 1986).* |

## Planning and Goal Setting

| Steps | Rationale |
|---|---|
| 1. Schedule times for administering intermittent feedings to approximate the child's usual meal times (Paarlberg and Balint, 1985). | Normalizing feeding schedules mimics normal digestive function, which facilitates reinstitution of oral feedings. |
| 2. Determine whether scheduled by mouth (PO) medications can be given with the scheduled feeding. Flush tube with small amount of water before and after medication administration. | Administration of medications during the feeding will decrease the number of procedures for the child and improve nursing care and efficiency (Foster et al, 1989). Flushing tube before and after reduces risk of tube occlusion. ***Special Considerations:*** *Improperly administering medication with feedings is a common cause of tube occlusion. Viscous drugs may require dilution to avoid plugging the tube. Tablets must be finely crushed and completely dissolved. Administration of some medications with food or milk is contraindicated, whether PO or through a tube. Check with pharmacy or drug literature to determine appropriateness of administering drugs with feedings.* |
| 3. Prepare the child and family for the procedure. | Preparing the child and family reduces anxiety related to the procedure and enhances cooperation and identification of potential problems. |
| 4. Gather and prepare supplies and equipment. | Gathering needed items enhances the efficiency of performing the procedure. |
| a. Stethoscope, catheter-tip syringe.<br>b. Water at room temperature in a pour container.<br>c. Formula at room temperature in a pour container. | A stethoscope and syringe are used to assess proper tube placement. Water is used to flush the tube after the feeding is completed. Feedings are usually given at room temperature unless otherwise ordered. Heated feedings may irritate the mucous membranes and cold feedings may cause vasoconstriction and cramping. |

| Steps | Rationale |
|---|---|
| d. Pacifier (neonates and infants). | Pacifiers are used for non-nutritive sucking in infants. |
| e. Emesis basin. | ***Special Considerations:*** *Only pacifiers with a safe one-piece design must be used to prevent the possibility of aspiration.* |
| f. Feeding container: Catheter-tip (Toomey) syringe, 35 or 60 cc size to accommodate feeding OR standard feeding container or bottle with attached drip chamber, tubing, and flow regulator clamp.<br>g. Enteral/IV pump (optional). | ***Special Considerations:*** *Syringes and bags should be rinsed after intermittent feedings and changed every 24 hours for intermittent and continuous feeds. Infusion pumps designed for enteral feedings regulate the exact volume to be delivered. Infusion pumps may be used if child is on continuous infusion; feeding is being administered over several hours; a small-bore gastric tube is being used; or gravity flow is insufficient to instill the feeding. Follow manufacturer's directions for pump use. Some types have minimum flow rates that may be too fast for neonates. An IV pump may be used when increments of 1 ml/hour or less are desired (Mize, Teitell, and Cunningham, 1984).* |
| h. Methylene blue (1%): 1 cc for each 500 cc of formula (optional). | Methylene blue may be used to color enteral feedings to determine if pulmonary aspiration of feeding occurs. |
| i. For gastrostomy buttons only:<br>▪ Adaptor.<br>▪ Feeding tube: continuous or bolus.<br>▪ Decompression tube. | |
| 5. If applicable, prepare the feeding container:<br>a. Add methylene blue dye to formula in pour container (optional). | |
| b. Add no more than 6 hours worth of formula (McGee, 1987). | Because the formula will be open at room temperature, it is subject to bacterial growth. |
| c. Prime the attached tubing with formula. | Priming the tubing prevents a bolus of air from entering stomach. |
| 6. Arrange for continuous supervision or restrain child if necessary (see Skill 51). | Children must be cooperative during a feeding to avoid disconnection of tubing. Even neonates can grasp and dislodge the feeding tube. |
| 7. Develop individualized child and family goals, including:<br>▪ Child's nutritional and fluid intake will remain adequate.<br>▪ Child will experience minimal or no discomfort or complications from procedure. | |

## Implementation

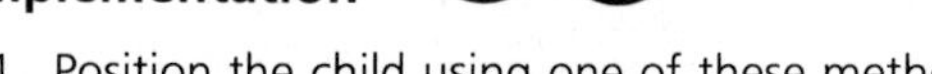

| Steps | Rationale |
|---|---|
| 1. Position the child using one of these methods:<br>a. Elevate head of bed with child or infant lying on back or on right side OR<br>b. Have adult hold infant or child on lap with head and chest elevated OR<br>c. With bed flat, position infant or child on right side with a folded blanket under the head and shoulders for infants and pillow for children.<br>d. Place older child in a Fowler's position in bed or normal sitting position in a chair. Provide for privacy. | Proper positioning enhances child's comfort and safety. Elevating the child's head and chest enhances gravity flow of feeding and reduces reflux through the lower esophageal sphincter (LES) (Perez, 1984).<br>***Special Considerations:*** *Reflux through the LES is sometimes associated with emesis and bradycardia. Discomfort during or after feeding in the absence of emesis may also be indicative of reflux.* |
| e. Place infant in an infant seat. | ***Special Considerations:*** *Infant seats are contraindicated for a child with gastroesophageal reflux (GER), as the position may increase reflux (see Skill 63).* |
| 2. Check nasal or orally inserted tubes for proper placement (see Skill 65). | Incorrect placement may result in administering feeding into the trachea, resulting in serious or fatal complications.<br>***Special Considerations:*** *Checking nasogastric placement by pH of stomach aspirate has been shown to be a reliable method (Metheny et al, 1989).* |
| 3. Check for residual from previous feedings, before each intermittent feeding or every 2 to 4 hours. Check tube for patency.<br>*For all except gastrostomy devices:*<br>a. Attach syringe to tube and gently aspirate gastric contents. | Aspiration of residual contents indicates correct placement, patency, and feeding tolerance.<br>***Special Considerations:*** *Absence of aspirate does not necessarily indicate tube misplacement. The stomach may be empty or the tube may not be in contact with stomach contents (Whaley and Wong, 1991).* |
| b. Note amount and character of the fluid aspirated. | ***Special Considerations:*** *If aspirate amount is greater than 10% to 20% of the previous feed on an intermittent feeding schedule report to the physician. Check physician's parameters or facility policy for amount of residual necessary to withhold feeding.* |

| **Steps** | **Rationale** |
|---|---|
| *Gastrostomy devices:* | |
| a. Do not aspirate (Perry, Johnson, and Trump, 1983; Whaley and Wong, 1991). | Suction created by aspiration may irritate the lining of the stomach wall and cause bleeding or perforation. |
| b. Attach syringe with water to end of tube and slowly inject; note any resistance. | Resistance may indicate tube/device occlusion. ***Special Considerations:*** *See Home Care Modifications for techniques used to clear tubes/devices.* |
| c. If occluded, follow facility policy or consult enterostomal therapist. | |
| d. If stomach distended before a feeding, check residual on a gastrostomy by suspending an empty syringe attached to tube and observing backflow of stomach contents. | |
| e. For a button GT, insert decompression tube. If formula comes out, wait one hour and repeat. | The one-way valve of the button prevents aspiration of gastric contents. |
| 4. Reinstill aspirate. | Partially digested formula contains electrolytes and enzymes that if lost in large quantities can cause an electrolyte imbalance (Perez, 1984). ***Special Considerations:*** *Aspirate of non-digestible material (e.g., mucus, old blood, curdled formula) may be discarded (Foster, Hunsberger, and Anderson, 1989).* |
| 5. Subtract residual amount obtained from prescribed amount of feeding according to orders/facility policy. Example: if prescribed feeding is 25 cc and aspirate is 5 cc, the aspirate returned, plus 20 cc of feeding, totals 25 cc. | Deducting residual amount avoids overdistending the stomach. |
| 6. Administer feeding: | |
| *Intermittent bolus:* | |
| a. Clamp or pinch off proximal end of tube, and attach the syringe barrel to the tube. For gastrostomy buttons, attach the adaptor and feeding catheter to the syringe. | Pinching or clamping off the tube prevents excess air from entering the stomach and causing distension. |
| b. Pour the formula into the barrel of the syringe. Prime feeding catheter, if using button. Adhere to handwashing protocol, and avoid touching inside of delivery system containers (Anderson, 1986). | Filling the feeding catheter prevents large amounts of air from entering the stomach and causing distension (Huth and O'Brien, 1987). Contamination of formula may occur when formula is poured into delivery system. |
| c. For gastrostomy button, open the safety plug and attach adaptor and feeding catheter to button (see Fig. 66-1). | |
| d. Unclamp the tube and allow the feeding to flow in slowly by gravity. If necessary, start flow of formula by either gently pushing 2 to 3 cc with plunger, then removing plunger, or by milking/stripping tube. | Forceful feeding with a plunger may result in gastric distension with esophageal reflux, thus increasing the risk of aspiration (Perry, Johnson, and Trump, 1983). |
| e. Adjust the height of the syringe above the stomach level approximately 6 inches or at a level that administers feeding over 15 to 30 minutes (Fig. 66-2). Do not exceed rate of flow greater than 5 cc every 5 to 10 minutes in premature and very small infants and 10 cc/minute in older infants and children (Wink, 1983; Whaley and Wong, 1991). | Gravity flow rate is determined by the diameter of the tubing and the height of the reservoir containing the feeding. The greater the height of the syringe, the faster the flow rate. Rapid feeding causes "dumping syndrome"—the sudden distension of the jejunum by hypertonic foods and liquids. This results in a rapid shift of body fluids from the vascular system into the intestines to dilute the contents. |
| f. Observe for signs of dumping syndrome: nausea, vomiting, diarrhea, cramps, pallor, sweating, heart palpitations, increased pulse rate and fainting after a feeding. | Identifying symptoms of dumping syndrome allows adjustments in the amount and frequency of the feedings. |
| g. If necessary, refill the syringe before it empties. | Refilling the syringe before it empties prevents air from entering stomach. |
| *Continuous feedings:* | |
| a. Hang the prepared container with attached clamped tubing from an infusion pole or pump. | |
| b. Attach the primed tubing to the feeding tube, unclamp feeding tube, and either regulate the drip by adjusting the clamp or set the pump rate. | |
| 7. Talk to the infant or child, and use facial expressions to encourage the infant or child to attend (DeBear, 1986). Hold or cuddle infant if permitted. Spend time reading to child during feeding (Whaley and Wong, 1991). Allow infant to suck on pacifier during feeding. | Talking and positive facial expressions help the infant and child associate feeding times with pleasant sensations and become accustomed to the social nature of feeding. Nonnutritive sucking has been shown to increase weight gain and decrease crying (Anderson, 1986). It also allows the infant to associate the oral experience of sucking with the feeling of satiation. ***Special Considerations:*** *A hole can be cut in top of nipple and the orogastric tube passed through it to stimulate sucking.* |

| Steps | Rationale |
|---|---|

A 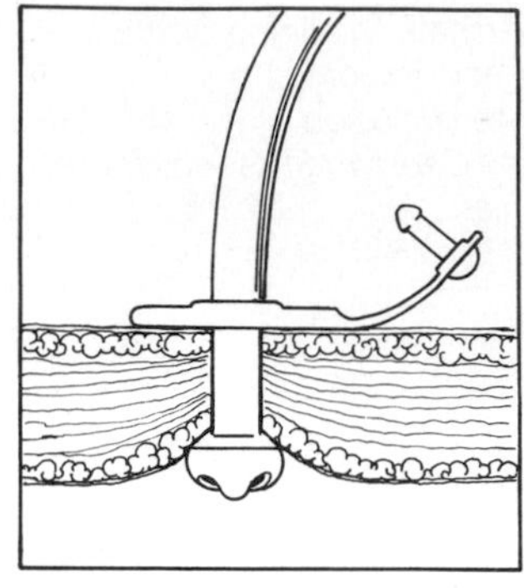 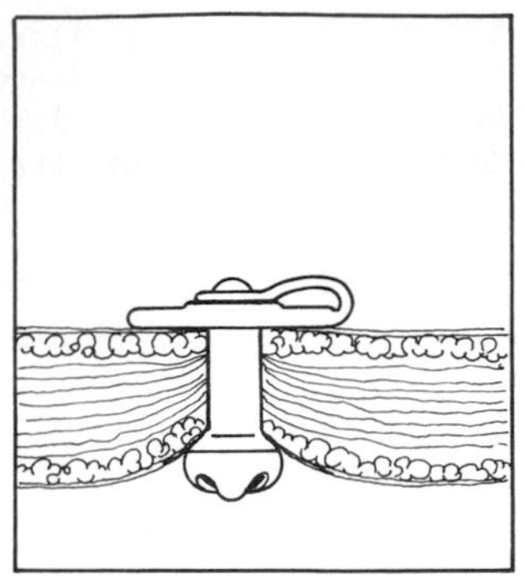 B

*FIG. 66-1* Gastrostomy button. **A,** With feeding catheter attached. **B,** With safety plug closed.

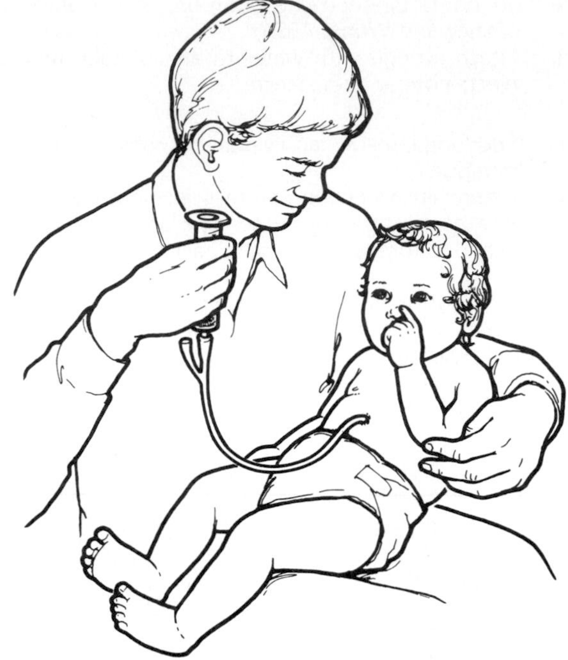

*FIG. 66-2* The height of the syringe is adjusted above the stomach level.

From Wong D and Whaley L: Clinical manual of pedicatric nursing, ed 3, 1990, St Louis, The CV Mosby Co.

8. As the last of the feeding empties from neck of syringe or drip chamber, pour in specified amount of flush. For the syringe method, use 1 to 2 cc for small bore tubes or 5 to 10 cc for other types. For a container/bottle, add enough flush to clear tubing.

Flushing the tube rinses feeding out of tube or button tip and prevents occlusion. Adding water before syringe is empty prevents instilling air into stomach.
***Special Considerations:*** *For child on fluid restriction, carefully adhere to amount and type of flush prescribed.*

9. Discontinue intermittent feeding:
   a. Pinch or clamp tube before removing syringe or tubing.

Clamping prevents reflux of the feeding.

   b. Clamp or cap indwelling tubes. Remove feeding catheter and adaptor from button, and snap safety plug in place (see box at right).

***Special Considerations:*** *If the antireflux valve of the button is functioning correctly, no formula or food should leak.*

   c. If tube is to be vented, suspend attached empty syringe barrel above stomach level. Venting is needed if the child has significant abdominal distension, appears to be trying to vomit, or if ordered.

Suspending the empty syringe above the stomach allows decompression into the syringe, thus preventing emesis and possible aspiration of stomach contents.
***Special Considerations:*** *The tube should be vented for 30 minutes if a child has had a Nissen fundoplication (Paarlberg and Balint, 1985).*

   d. If the tube is to be removed after feeding, pinch tube firmly and withdraw quickly.

Pinching prevents escape of fluid into the trachea as the tube is withdrawn.

10. If child's condition permits, bubble (burp) the child, especially infants, after feeding.

Air may enter the stomach during tube feedings and necessitates removal by either burping or venting.
***Special Considerations:*** *With a gastrostomy button, air can be removed by inserting decompression tube into unplugged button. This releases air by opening valve.*

11. Position infant or child on right side or on abdomen with head of bed elevated 30° for at least 1 hour after feeding.

Proper positioning minimizes the possibility of regurgitation and aspiration. A right lateral position facilitates movement of feeding from stomach into small intestines. The prone position minimizes reflux.

12. Observe child closely for toleration of feeding by performing ongoing gastrointestinal assessments.

Observing child closely for evidence of discomfort or intolerance facilitates prompt adjustments in flow rate, concentration, or quantity of feeding.

13. If equipment is to be reused, wash with soap and water and rinse thoroughly. Change equipment every 24 hours or according to facility policy.

Washing equipment and replacing it every 24 hours reduces risk of bacterial contamination.

### *Maintaining a Gastrostomy Tube/Skin-Level Gastrostomy*

A gastrostomy is performed to provide an alternative to oral feedings, either as a temporary or long term measure. Gastrostomy tube feedings have several advantages over nasogastric tube methods: they provide better decompression of the stomach; they allow obligate nose breathing; and, after initial placement, they are considerably more comfortable (Perry, Johnson, and Trump, 1983).

There are three main types of gastrostomies performed on infants and children (Gauderer, 1989):

1. Formation of a serosa-lined channel from the anterior gastric wall around an indwelling catheter (Stamm or Witzel type).
2. Formation of a permanent tunnel from full-thickness gastric wall to the skin surface with a catheter introduced intermittently for feeding (Depage or Janeway type).
3. Percutaneous endoscopic gastrostomy (PEG) in which the catheter holds the gastric and abdominal walls in apposition.

Gastrostomy tubes exist in a variety of types. Commonly used indwelling catheters are the Malecot and the Pezzar, with expanded tips to keep the tubes from easily dislodging, and balloon types such as the Foley, MIC, and Flow-Thru tubes with an inflatable balloon at the tip to prevent dislodgement. When a permanent tunnel gastrostomy is formed, straight or Foley catheters are often used for intermittent feedings.

Skin level devices include the Button or the Gastroport. The button type is a small, flexible silicone rubber device that has a mushroom-shaped tip at the intragastric end and two small retention flaps at the cutaneous end. The intragastric end of the shaft has a one-way anti-reflux valve to prevent leakage of the stomach contents. It also includes a snap-on safety plug that serves as an additional barrier. Skin level devices require a well established gastrostomy site, come in a limited number of sizes, and are more expensive than the conventional gastrostomy tube. Although care is simplified for the skin level device, there is the possibility that the valve may become clogged. The skin level devices are more cosmetically pleasing and carry a decreased incidence of skin breakdown and a diminished risk of migration and subsequent obstruction (Huth and O'Brien, 1987). An increased risk of gas bloat syndrome exists if a Nissen fundoplication has been performed, therefore button use is not recommended (CHLA, 1988).

Astute nursing care is required to ensure that the skin and stoma site remain clean and free of infection and that the gastrostomy feeding device is safely maintained. Inspect the stoma and peristomal skin daily, just before cleaning, to assess any abnormal findings (e.g., leakage around the tube, redness extending more than ½ to 1 cm beyond the site, pus, copious discharge, bleeding, and skin breakdown). Clean the peristomal skin with mild soap and water, with half-strength hydrogen peroxide, or as ordered. Care may be required one to two times daily, depending on the skin's condition. Secure a gastrostomy tube to the abdomen, either by taping it or by sliding it through a sterile disposable nipple. Access to the tube by the child may be prevented by taping or pinning a diaper or abdominal binder over the abdomen. Care must be taken to clean around the stoma, extending out approximately one inch, and to rotate all gastrostomy devices (especially skin level gastrostomies) to prevent adherence of granulation tissue. If a skin level device is used, it must be cleaned daily with a cotton-tip applicator and tap water. Allow the area to dry thoroughly, then apply a skin protectant, if needed. Provide regular monitoring, observing for signs that the gastrostomy tube/device needs replacement (e.g., catheter stretched or split, catheter balloon deflated, irreversible tube occlusion, anti-reflux valve malfunction, yeast-infested tube or button, tube length in excess of baseline postinsertion measurement).

| Steps | Rationale |
|---|---|
| **Evaluation Outcomes** | **Observational Guidelines** |
| 1. Child's nutritional and fluid intake remains adequate. | Weight measurements exhibit evidence of appropriate gain. Mucous membranes remain moist and intact. Skin turgor is good. Electrolyte and glucose levels are within normal range. Intake and outputs remain within normal limits. |
| 2. Child experiences minimal or no gastrointestinal complications from procedure. | Bowel sounds remain normal. No evidence of diarrhea, constipation, or dumping syndrome. No abdominal distension or firmness occurs. No vomiting or aspiration occurs. |
| 3. Child experiences minimal or no discomfort from procedure. | Child states a feeling of comfort during and after feeding. Child does not exhibit nonverbal signs of discomfort, e.g., agitation, irritability, crying, facial grimaces. |
| 4. Child and family experience feeding as a positive social, physical, and emotional event. | Child appears relaxed and at ease during the feeding. Older child interacts during feeding. Family remains present and at ease during feeding. Child and family express no distress regarding the feedings. Child and family cooperate with procedure. |

## Documentation

Record date and time of feeding. Document amount, color, consistency, and disposition of aspirate (e.g., re-fed or discarded). Note type and amount of formula given, as well as amount and type of irrigant. Record child's tolerance and response to feeding, noting any signs of complications, e.g., emesis, distension, and/or diarrhea. Document disposition of the tube after feeding, e.g., vented or clamped.

### Home Care Modifications

1. Wash equipment daily with warm soapy water, rinse thoroughly, and air dry. A bottle brush may be helpful, or a pipecleaner may be used to clean tubing. Rinse tubing and syringe after each feeding. Sealable plastic bags or clean plastic containers may be used to store syringes when they are completely dry.
2. If inside of tubing or syringe becomes coated with milky residue, clean them with a solution of one part vinegar to two parts water, then wash as above.
3. Include child in mealtime socialization to maintain and nurture normal interpersonal and family relationships (McGee, 1987).
4. Various treatments have been reported in the literature for tube occlusions. Carbonated beverages, cranberry juice, meat tenderizers, fresh pineapple juice (papain), and pancreatic enzymes have been used to open blocked tubes. Check with health care professional before employing a specific treatment. Careful flushing with water before and after medications will minimize occlusion (Gebus, 1990).
5. Tubes may be suspended in a variety of ways. Caregiver may pin the syringe to their shirt at shoulder height when holding an infant for feeding or suspend syringe from a pole such as a floor lamp (Paarlberg and Balint, 1985). Encourage family to adapt home environment to meet their needs.
6. A pillow or foam wedge can be used to elevate head and chest of child.
7. More than one caregiver should be familiar with feeding procedure.
8. Family will need to know the size of the button to purchase properly fitting tubing and/or replacement button. If giving continuous feeding, they will need continuous feed tubing rather than bolus tubing.
9. Tubing and supplies can be obtained from pharmacies that stock ostomy supplies or hospital supply companies.

# *SKILL* 67 Administering Total Parenteral Nutrition

*Elizabeth A. Marks and Karen T. Graves*

Total Parenteral Nutrition (TPN, hyperalimentation) is the intravenous infusion of protein (amino acids), carbohydrates (dextrose), fat (lipid), and additives (vitamins, minerals, electrolytes, trace elements). It can be delivered through central or peripheral veins.

TPN is indicated when nutritional needs of the child cannot be met through gastrointestinal digestion and absorption. In children, nutritional support must be adequate for growth and development in addition to anabolic needs. Since children have a higher metabolic rate per unit of body weight than adults, they require greater fluid and caloric intake per kilogram (Hazinski, 1984). The added stress of an acute illness or increased metabolic demands that often occur in chronic conditions (e.g., cystic fibrosis) further increases nutritional needs in children. Since children usually have limited body stores of essential nutrients, provision of nutritional support is vital (Testerman, 1989). Parenteral nutrition for infants and children is a supportive rather than a curative therapy. No standard has been set for length of therapy.

Peripheral vein TPN is used in children when the need for parenteral nutrition is short term (5 to 7 days), the child's nutritional status is good, and venous access is available. For example, peripheral TPN may be used effectively following uncomplicated gastrointestinal surgery when 3 to 5 days of bowel rest are required.

Central vein TPN is appropriate when parenteral nutrition is needed for longer than 7 days, or when the child is malnourished. Central TPN can provide the higher calories required for "catch up" growth. Central venous access is required for long term TPN.

TPN requires a multidisciplinary approach to achieve success. Nursing provides a vital part of that care with careful delivery and monitoring of TPN to prevent and minimize complications.

### NURSING DIAGNOSES

Altered nutrition: less than body requirements related to inadequate caloric intake; Potential for infection related to invasive peripheral/central venous catheter; Potential for injury related to adverse effects and/or extravasation of TPN solutions.

| Steps | Rationale |
|---|---|
| **Assessment** | |
| 1. Assess nutritional status and physical growth measures, including head circumference if the child is under 3 years of age (see Skills 28 and 29). | Baseline measurements provide comparison information for monitoring child's response to TPN. Weight measurement is necessary for determining caloric needs and dosages of TPN components. All areas of normal growth are monitored, including the rapid brain growth that occurs in children less than 3 years of age. **Special Considerations:** *Skin fold thickness measurements may be obtained by a dietician or skilled practitioner.* |
| 2. Assess baseline vital signs and activity level. | Baseline information provides comparative data necessary for ongoing monitoring. Changes in vital signs and activity may be indicative of complications such as infection or metabolic changes. |
| 3. Determine age and developmental level. | This information helps determine child's ability to cooperate with procedure and necessary safety precautions. |
| 4. Assess hydration and electrolyte status (see Skill 64). | Fluid and electrolyte status should be stabilized before beginning TPN. Children requiring fluid resuscitation may need frequent solution and rate changes. Since amino acid dextrose solutions must be delivered at a constant rate (based on glucose tolerance and calorie needs), these solutions are not suitable for use when fluid boluses or deficit replacement is necessary (Kerner, 1983). |
| 5. Determine venous access route: | The route of administration affects further planning and interventions. |
| a. Central. | Central venous access allows delivery of sufficient nutrients to support anabolism and growth. |
| b. Peripheral. | Peripheral venous administration limits the osmolarity of the glucose concentration. **Special Considerations:** *Concentrations greater than 10% dextrose/2% amino acids or 5% dextrose/4% amino acids are not recommended for peripheral TPN (CHLA, 1988). TPN can cause venous sclerosis, thrombosis, phlebitis, or burns and tissue sloughing if the solution infiltrates into surrounding tissues (Testerman, 1989).* |
| 6. Review indications for TPN. Review physician's orders for solution, rate, and initial and routine laboratory studies. | Understanding the purpose of TPN for this child aids in monitoring response to therapy. Reviewing orders ensures administration of correct solution over appropriate time period and that laboratory results are available when needed to evaluate/change TPN. **Special Considerations:** *TPN may be changed daily based on clinical status.* |
| 7. Determine if contraindications exist to fat emulsion administration: elevated serum triglyceride level (>250 mg/dL, 150 mg/dL in neonates); active bleeding present; or neonate with elevated serum unconjugated bilirubin (>5 mg/dL) (CHLA, 1989). | Preexisting elevated triglyceride level hinders monitoring for fat overload. Fat emulsion is not recommended for neonates with appreciable jaundice because it may increase the risk of kernicterus (Synderman, 1985). |
| **Planning and Goal Setting** | |
| 1. Prepare child and family for procedure, including the rationale for treatment and methods to avoid accidentally dislodging tubing. | Preparing the child and family promotes their understanding and may enhance their cooperation. |
| 2. Gather and prepare equipment and supplies: | |
| a. Infusion pump. | Regulation of the infusion is necessary for accurate and safe delivery, particularly in small children. |
| b. IV tubing, preferably with Luer-Lok connections. | Luer-Lok connections protect the integrity of the system. |
| c. 0.22 micron in-line filter. | Amino acid dextrose solutions require filtering because of the multiple additives used that increase the risk of particulate matter and microprecipitation of some solutes. **Special Considerations:** *Because of the size of fat molecules, fat emulsion should not be filtered (Kerner, 1983).* |
| d. Amino acid dextrose solution as ordered. | **Special Considerations:** *Percentages of dextrose and amino acid are ordered separately, based on calorie and protein needs per kilogram. Preparation of an amino acid dextrose solution under a laminar flow hood is recommended to prevent contamination.* |

| Steps | Rationale |
|---|---|
| e. Y-connector extension tubing. | A Y-connector placed distal to the filter allows concurrent delivery of fat emulsion with amino acid dextrose solution.<br>***Special Considerations:*** *Fat emulsion is compatible with amino acid dextrose solution. Use of stopcocks poses a contamination risk.* |
| f. Fat emulsion, 10% or 20%. | Fat emulsion is prepared from predominantly unsaturated fatty acids to provide essential fatty acids.<br>***Special Considerations:*** *Minimum fat requirement must be 4% to 7% of total calories to avoid essential fatty acid deficiency (Kerner, 1983). Do not shake fat emulsion bottle since this disrupts physical stability of microscopic fat globules (Perry and Potter, 1990).* |
| g. Items for infant oral stimulation, e.g., pacifier, Nuk toothbrush, soft rubber toys, infant spoons, textured cloth. | ***Special Considerations:*** *Textured cloth may be used for tactile stimulation of cheeks, lips, and torso (Orr and Allen, 1986).* |
| 3. Remove ordered amino acid dextrose solution from refrigerator and allow to warm to room temperature. | Infusing cold solutions can decrease body temperature, cause venospasm and pain. |
| 4. Verify solution with physician's order. | Verifying the solution ensures infusion of ordered solution.<br>***Special Considerations:*** *Dextrose concentration may be increased gradually (2.5% to 5% daily) to allow the child to accommodate increasing glucose load.* |
| 5. Develop individualized goals for child:<br>▪ Nutritional status will be maintained or improved.<br>▪ Development of oral-motor skills will be maintained.<br>▪ Complications of infection and metabolic disturbances from administration of TPN will be prevented or minimized. | |

## Implementation

| Steps | Rationale |
|---|---|
| 1. Using aseptic technique:<br>a. Connect tubing, filter and Y-set.<br>b. Connect tubing to solution. | Aseptic technique reduces risk of contamination. |
| c. Prime tubing with solution.<br>d. If administering lipid concurrently, attach container to tubing, purge tubing of air, and connect to Y-site below filter. | Priming purges air from the tube to prevent air embolism.<br>***Special Considerations:*** *Lipid may be admixed with the amino acid dextrose solution (3-in-1 mixture). A larger micron filter is required for 3-in-1 mixture to allow passage of fat molecules.* |
| e. Tape connection sites. | Securing connections prevents accidental disconnection. |
| 2. Insert tubing into infusion pump and set flow rate. | Flow rate is determined by physician's order and must be maintained at prescribed level.<br>***Special Considerations:*** *If solution is not infused in allotted time, do not increase infusion flow rate to "catch up" because this may lead to hyperglycemia.* |
| 3. After verifying patency of venous access, aseptically connect tubing and solution to established infusion site, and begin infusion (see Skills 108 and 111). | Verifying patency is necessary to avoid infusing solution into tissues and causing tissue necrosis and sloughing. |
| 4. Check peripheral insertion site hourly for signs of infiltration. | Frequent site checks ensure early detection and prompt intervention for complications such as extravasation. |
| 5. Monitor vital signs and activity level every 4 hours. Notify physician of fever or abnormal vital signs (see Skills 30, 31, 32 and 33). | Monitoring vital signs and activity level allows for early detection and intervention of complications. For example, an elevated temperature may be an early indicator of catheter-related sepsis.<br>***Special Considerations:*** *IV lipid use is occasionally associated with acute chills, fever, and local allergic skin reactions during the first 12 hours after infusion begins (Mize and Teitell, 1984).* |
| 6. Monitor urine or blood glucose levels every 8 hours (see Skill 120). | Monitoring urine or blood glucose provides a method to assess child's response to the increased glucose load.<br>***Special Considerations:*** *Glucose intolerance may be an early sign of sepsis. Glycosuria may also be the result of stress, certain chemotherapeutic drugs, or renal damage (Kennedy-Caldwell and Guenter, 1988). Occasionally, insulin is necessary to counteract hyperglycemia when reduction of infusion rate is not possible or effective (Mize and Teitell, 1984).* |
| 7. Monitor intake and output (see Skill 64). | Monitoring intake and output allows for determination of fluid balance and replacement. |

| Steps | Rationale |
|---|---|
| 8. Monitor and plot growth parameters (see Skill 28).<br>a. Weight (daily).<br>b. Height (under age 3 years, every 2 weeks; over 3 years, monthly).<br>c. Head circumference (same as height).<br>d. Skin fold thickness (weekly to monthly). | Monitoring growth parameters facilitates evaluating effectiveness of therapy and may signal fluid imbalances if significant gains/losses occur in short periods of time. |
| 9. Obtain laboratory tests as ordered and monitor results, e.g., serum electrolytes, blood glucose and blood urea nitrogen. | Metabolic complications are among the most common complications to occur. Laboratory tests make early detection and correction possible. |
| 10. Using aseptic technique, change solutions, tubings and filter every 24 hours. | Both amino acid dextrose solutions and fat emulsions are favorable media for bacterial growth (Kennedy-Caldwell and Guenter, 1988). |
| 11. Change the dressing and provide site care every 48 to 72 hours or more frequently if soiled or loose (see Skills 98 and 110). | Changing the dressing reduces the risk of infection and allows detection of problems at the site. |
| 12. Do not use TPN line to simultaneously: | Addition of other parenteral products to the TPN line is contraindicated unless flow is interrupted and tubing is completely flushed before and after addition. |
| a. Administer blood products. | Blood products are incompatible with TPN. |
| b. Administer incompatible antibiotics or other medications. | ***Special Considerations:*** *Verify medication compatibility with pharmacist.* |
| c. Obtain blood samples.<br>d. Measure central venous pressure. | Admixture of TPN with the blood sample may affect results. |
| 13. Simulate normal feeding interactions as closely as possible if child is NPO. Provide tactile stimulation, oral exploration, oral feedings, and pacifiers (Orr and Allen, 1986). | Providing optimal oral experiences to infants receiving long-term TPN promotes better feeding skills and decreases the transition time from parenteral to oral feedings. Some infants are hypersensitive to touch and progressive tactile stimulation may desensitize them. Introducing small volumes of oral feedings as early as possible and using pacifiers for nonnutritive sucking can promote the development of oral musculature. |
| 14. If discontinuing, cycling, or interrupting amino acid dextrose infusion: | Cycling an infusion consolidates delivery over 8 to 16 hours at night thus allowing child's participation in normal activities during day without the inconvenience of continous infusion. |
| a. Taper infusion rate 1 hour before discontinuing. For example: if the rate is 100 ml/hour, decrease the rate to 50 ml/hour for 30 minutes then 25 ml/hour for 30 minutes. | Tapering the rate allows the child's insulin production to adjust to the decrease in glucose intake. |
| b. If the child is NPO and disruption is abrupt, start a peripheral IV line and observe for signs and symptoms of hypoglycemia. Check blood glucose level 30 minutes after discontinuance. | Sudden cessation of amino acid dextrose solution may result in a hypoglycemic response since insulin production remains elevated. |
| c. Flush central venous access device after discontinuing TPN (see Skill 110). | |

| Evaluation Outcomes | Observational Guidelines |
|---|---|
| 1. Child's nutritional status is maintained or improved. | Rate of growth is appropriate for age. Compare current nutritional assessment with baseline. |
| 2. Normal oral-motor skills are maintained. | Oral feedings take place with minimal difficulty during or after completion of therapy. |
| 3. Metabolic-related or catheter-related complications are prevented or minimized. | Metabolic studies remain within normal limits. Vital signs remain stable and within normal limits. No evidence of infection at infusion site. No evidence of septicemia. No evidence of embolism. No evidence of vein sclerosing, phlebitis, tissue necrosis at peripheral infusion site. |

## Documentation

Record the date and time TPN and fat emulsion were initiated and completed. Note the concentration and flow rate of solutions. Document the child's growth measurements daily or weekly. Record intake and output measurements and urine or glucose measurement every 8 hours. Note vital sign measurements every 4 hours. Indicate child's activity level. Document condition or insertion site, care given, status of infusion, and date and time of dressing and/or tubing change. Note oral stimulation exercises performed. Document adverse clinical manifestations and nursing interventions taken, e.g., notification of physician.

## Home Care Modifications

1. Teach the family oral stimulation activities to perform with child. Refer to article by Orr and Allen, 1986, for specific exercises.
2. To allow child participation in normal daily activities, home TPN is given over 8 to 16 hours at night. Consolidation of delivery hours is done gradually, usually by 1 hour per day. To allow the child's rate of insulin production to adjust, taper the rate during final hour of infusion.
3. Daily glucose testing should be done in the home.
4. Amino acid dextrose solutions are stable with refrigeration for 2 to 4 weeks. Parenteral vitamins and certain medications must be added daily, before the bag is used.
5. Continue to include child in family mealtime socialization even if oral intake is not permitted. With infants not receiving oral feedings, maintain regular schedule of cuddling, rocking, and talking while the infant sucks on pacifier to stimulate feeding times (Berry and Jorgensen, 1988).
6. Infusion of large volumes of fluid at night may result in bed-wetting. Preparation of the child and family for this possibility is important. The use of bedpans, nighttime diapers, urinals, or bedside commodes may be helpful (Berry and Jorgensen, 1988).

UNIT VIII

## PRODUCT REFERENCES AND TEACHING RESOURCES

### Books

Bennett V: Feeding young children with cleft lip and palate, 1986. Contact:
Minnesota Dietetic Association
1821 University Avenue West
Suite S-280
St. Paul, MN 55104

Jones ML: Home care for the chronically ill or disabled child, New York, 1985, Harper & Row, Publishers Inc.

McClannahan C: Feeding and caring for infants with special needs, 1983. Contact:
Aota Products
1383 Piccard Drive
Rockville, MD 20850-4375

Perske R et al: Mealtimes for persons with severe handicaps, Baltimore, 1986, Paul H Brooks.

Wong D and Whaley L: Clinical manual of pediatric nursing, ed 3, St Louis, 1990, The CV Mosby Co.
Home care instructions for gavage and gastrostomy feeding.

### Products

Bard Interventional Products
C.R. Bard, Inc
5 Federal Street, Box 5069
Billerica, MA 01822
1-800-826-BARD
Offers the following:
Gastrostomy Button
Button Sizes: 18 Fr, 24 Fr, 28 Fr
Feeding Tubes: Continuous or Bolus, 18 Fr, 24 Fr, 28 Fr

Childbirth Graphics, Ltd.
1210 Culver Road
Rochester, NY 14609-5454
(716) 482-7940
Offers the following material by Sarah Danner and Edward Cerutti:
Breastfeeding: an illustrated introduction—Hardcover flip chart and slides available, both with teaching notes.
Nursing your premature baby (8 pages)
Nursing your baby with a cleft palate or cleft lip (16 pages)
Nursing your baby with Down's Syndrome (12 pages)
Nursing your neurologically impaired baby (8 pages)
Expressing breastmilk (12 pages)

Cozcon
24 Norwich Avenue
Colchester, CT 06415
1-800-221-5882
Offers Cozcon Reflux Bed.

Health Education Associates, Inc.
8 Jan Sebastian Way, Unit 13
Sandwich, MA 02563
(508) 888-8044
Offers the following pamphlets:
Teens can breastfeed
Breastfeeding your twins
Breastfeeding problems can be avoided
When your baby needs your milk: collecting milk for a baby who cannot nurse.
Wall chart—(17 × 22 inches) How to use a breast pump also available.

La Leche League International
PO Box 1209
Franklin Park, IL 60131-8209
(312) 455-7730
The Lactation Consultant Series offers the following articles by Kathleen Auerbach:
Back to the breast: retraining infant suckling patterns, (Unit 15), No. 288-15 (20 pages)
Breastfeeding techniques and devices (unit 17) No. 288-17 (14 pages)
Breastfeeding aids/products
Pumps: Medela (manual-electric)
Gentle Expressions
Loyd-B
Medela supplemental nutrition system—No. 416
Breast shell kit—No. 422
Breast shields—No. 402
Hand expression funnel—No. 423
Breastfeeding audio cassette and booklet: Breastfeeding your baby by Dr. William Sears, et al., 1988

Mead Johnson Laboratories
Nutritional Division
Evansville, IN 47721
Disposable Cleft Lip/Palate Nurser: Mead Johnson 6 oz squeezable bottle with crosscut nipple.

### Organizations

American Cleft Palate Educational Foundation
1218 Grandview Avenue
University of Pittsburgh
Pittsburgh, PA 15211
24-hour hotline 1-800-24-CLEFT
This organization assists patients, families, and the public in learning about cleft defects. The hotline provides information and referral sources for cleft palate teams and parent support groups.

Food and Nutrition Information Center
National Agricultural Library
Room 304
Beltsville, MD 20705
(301)344-3719

Serves the information needs of professionals interested in nutrition education. Acquires and lends books, journal articles, and audiovisual materials.

National Dairy Council
Food Nutrition Board
2101 Constitution Ave, NW
Washington, DC 20037

Provides teaching materials and information for schools and other health care professionals.

## REFERENCES


Ackerman AD: Fluid therapy. In Hoekelman RA, editor: Primary pediatric care, St Louis, 1987, The CV Mosby Co.

Adcock EW and Consolvo CA: Fluid and electrolyte management. In Merenstein GB and Gardner SL, editors: Handbook of neonatal intensive care, ed 2, St Louis, 1989, The CV Mosby Co.

American Academy of Pediatrics: Policy statement based on task force report: the promotion of breast feeding, Pediatrics 69(5):654-661, 1982.

American Academy of Pediatrics, Committee on Nutrition: The use of whole cow's milk in infancy, Pediatrics 72(2):253-355, 1983.

American Academy of Pediatrics, Committee on Nutrition: Pediatric nutrition handbook, ed 2, Elk Grove Village, Ill, 1985, American Academy of Pediatrics.

Anderson B: Tube feeding: Is diarrhea inevitable? Am J Nurs 86(6):704-706, 1986.

Anderson E and McFarland J: Community as client: application of the nursing process, Philadelphia, 1988, JB Lippincott Co.

Anderson G: Pacifiers: The positive side, MCN, 11(2):122-124, 1986.

Aquilina S: Gastroesophageal reflux, problem or nuisance? J Pediatr Health Care 1(5):233-239, 1987.

Auerbach K and Gartner L: Breastfeeding and human milk: their association with jaundice in the neonate, Clin Perinatol 14(1):89, 1987.

Austin C: Dietary assessment and management of the infant. In Simko MD, Cowell C, and Hreha MS, editors: Practical nutrition: a quick reference for the health care practitioner, Rockville, 1989, Aspen Publishers.

Bailey D et al: Lack of efficacy of thickened feeding as treatment for gastroesophageal reflux, J Pediatr 110(2):187-189, 1987.

Balluff M: Nutritional needs of an infant or child with a cleft lip or palate, Ear Nose Throat J 65:44-47, 1986.

Barness LA: Fluid and electrolyte therapy. In Gellis SS and Kagan BM, editors: Current pediatric therapy, ed 12, Philadelphia, 1986, WB Saunders Co.

Bass DM and Walker WA: Acute and chronic nonspecific diarrhea syndromes. In Gellis SS and Kagan BM, editors: Current pediatric therapy, ed 12, Philadelphia, 1986, WB Saunders Co.

Berry RK and Jorgensen S: Growing with home parenteral nutrition: adjusting to family life and child development, Pediatr Nurs, 14(1):43-45, 1988.

Bobak I and Jensen M: Essentials of maternity nursing, 2 ed, St Louis, 1987, The CV Mosby Co.

Boston Center for Study of Responsive Law: Eating clean: consumer guide book, Washington, DC, 1987, Boston Center for Study of Responsive Law.

Children's Hospital of Los Angeles (CHLA) Nutritional Support Team: Gastrostomy care, Nursing procedure manual, Los Angeles, 1988, CHLA.

Children's Hospital of Los Angeles (CHLA) Nutrition Support Team: Total parenteral nutrition manual, Los Angeles, 1989, CHLA.

Clark M: Car seats and gastroesophageal reflux (letter), J Pediatr 111(4):634, 1987.

Clark TA et al: Esophageal perforations in premature infants and comments on the diagnosis, Am J Dis Child 134:367-368, 1980.

Danner S: Expressing breastmilk: expressing, pumping, and storing your breastmilk, 1986, Rochester, NY, Childbirth Graphics.

Danner S and Cerutti E: Breastfeeding: an illustrated introduction, Rochester, NY, 1986, Childbirth Graphics.

Davidson DM et al: School-based blood cholesterol screening, J Pediatr Health Care 3(1):3-8, 1989.

DeBear K: Sham feeding: Another kind of nourishment, Am J Nurs 86(10):1142-1143, 1986.

DeCarvalho M, Hall M, and Harvey D: Effects of water supplementation on physiological jaundice in breastfed babies, Arch Dis Child 56:568, 1981.

DeCarvalho M, Klaus M, and Merkatz R: Frequency of breastfeeding and serum bilirubin concentration, Am J Dis Child 136:737, 1982.

Dickey S: A guide to the nursing of children, Baltimore, 1987, Williams & Wilkins.

Dilts C: Nursing management of mastitis due to breastfeeding, JOGNN, 14(4):286, 1985.

Elkins S, Cohen M, and Schafer M: Immediate unrestricted feeding following cleft lip and palate repair, paper presented at the American Cleft Palate Association Meeting, 1988.

Eschelman MM: Introduction to nutrition diet therapy, 1988, Philadelphia, JB Lippincott Co.

Farnan S: Nutrition and feeding of children with cleft lip palate, Nutr News 3(2):1-4, 1988.

Forte A, Mayberry L, and Ferketich S: Breastmilk collection and storage practices among mothers of hospitalized neonates, J Perinatol 7(1):35, 1987.

Foster R, Hunsberger M, and Anderson J: Nursing strategies: altered digestive function, Family centered nursing care of children, Philadelphia, 1989, WB Saunders Co.

Gallagher L and Kriedler M: Nursing and health, Norwalk, Conn, 1987, Appleton & Lange.

Gauderer M: Techniques for pediatric gastrostomies. Paper presented at the 13th Clinical Congress, American Society of Parenteral and Enteral Nutrition, Gastrostomies in Pediatrics: indications and practical aspects, Miami Beach, Fla, Feb 1989.

Gebus V: Pitfalls in "access" management. Paper presented at the 14th Clinical Congress, American Society for Parenteral and Enteral Nutrition on Optimum Nutrition of Children with Intestinal Disorders, San Antonio, Texas, January 1990.

Ghishan FK: The transport of electrolytes in the gut and the use of oral rehydration solution, Pediatr Clin North Am 35(1):35-50, 1988.

Grady E: Breastfeeding the baby with a cleft of the soft palate, Clin Pediatr 16(11):978-981, 1977.

Greenswag LR: A community outreach program for individuals with Prader-Willi Syndrome, J Pediatr Health Care 4(1):32-38, 1990.

Grill B: Oral rehydration, food allergy, and specialized nutrition, Current Opinion in Pediatr 1:384-393, 1989.

Hanson R: New approach to measuring adult nasogastric tubes for insertion, Am J Nurs 80:1334-1335, 1980.

Hazinski MF: Understanding fluid balance in the seriously ill child, Ped Nurs, 14(3):231-236.

Hazinski M: Nursing care of the critically ill child, St Louis, 1984, The CV Mosby Co.

Heitkemper MM and Bond E: Fluid and electrolytes: Assessment and interventions, J Enterostomal Ther 15(1):18-23, 1988.

Hermansen MC and Buches M: Super diapers and premature infants, Pediatrics 79(6):1056, 1987.

Hermansen MC and Buches M: Urine output determination from superabsorbent and regular diapers under radiant heat, Pediatrics 81(3):428-431, 1988.

Hess CS et al: Fluoride: too much or too little, Pediatr Nurs 10(6):397-403, 1984.

Hinson F: Handbook of pediatric nursing, 1985, Baltimore, Williams & Wilkins.

Hughes WT and Buescher ES: Pediatric procedures, ed 2, Philadelphia, 1980, WB Saunders Co.

Hunsberger M: Promoting healthy dietary practices. In Foster R, Hunsberger M, and Anderson J, editors: Family centered nursing care of children, Philadelphia, 1989, WB Saunders Co.

Huth M and O'Brien M: The gastrostomy feeding button, Pediatr Nurs, 13(4):241-245, 1987.

James S and Mott S: Child health nursing, Reading, Mass, 1988, Addison-Wesley Publishing Co.

Kearney M: Identifying psychosocial obstacles to breastfeeding success, JOGNN 17(2):98-105, 1988.

Keating S and Kelman G: Home health care nursing, Philadelphia, 1988, JB Lippincott Co.

Kennedy-Caldwell C and Guenter P: Nutrition support nursing: core curriculum, ed 2, Maryland, 1988, American Society for Parenteral and Enteral Nutrition.

Kerner J: Manual of pediatric parenteral nutrition, New York, 1983, John Wiley & Sons Inc.

Kosowski M and Sopczyk D: Feeding hospitalized children with developmental disabilities, MCN 10:190-194, 1985.

Lattanzi WE: Simplifying the approach to fluid therapy, Contemp Ped, 6(2):72-88, 1989.

Lawrence R: Breastfeeding: a guide for the medical profession, ed 2, St Louis, 1985, The CV Mosby Co.

Lederer J et al: Care planning pocket guide, ed 3, Fort Collins, Colo, 1990, Addison-Wesley Nursing.

L'Esperance F and Frantz K: Time limitation for breastfeeding, JOGNN 14(2):115, 1985.

Logemann J: Evaluation and treatment of swallowing disorders, San Diego, 1983, Collet-Hill Press.

Long SS: Epidemiologic study of infant botulism in Pennsylvania: report of the Infant Botulism Study Group, Pediatrics 75(5):928-934, 1985.

Macknin ML, Medendorp SV, and Maier MC: Infant sleep and bedtime cereal, Am J Dis Child 143(9):1066-1068, 1989.

Marmet C and Shell E: Training neonates to suck correctly, MCN 9:401-407, 1984.

Martell I: Teaching about bottle feeding, Childbirth Educator, pp 34-36; 42-43, fall 1987.

McBride M and Danner S: Sucking disorders in neurologically impaired infants: assessment and facilitation of breastfeeding, Clin Perinatol 14(1):109, 1987.

McClannahan C: Feeding and caring for infants and children with special needs, St Paul, 1983, Department of Health, Services for Children with Handicaps and Section of Health Education.

McDermott R and McCormack K: Nursing caries syndrome: Implications for children's health care professionals, Child Health Care 15(1):49-54, 1986.

McGee L: Feeding gastrostomy, part II: nursing care, J Enterostomal Ther 14(5):201-211, 1987.

Meier P and Wilks S: The bacteria in expressed mother's milk, MCN 12: 420, 1987.

Metheny NA, Eisenberg P, and Spies M: Aspiration pneumonia in patients fed through nasoenteral tubes, Heart and Lung 15:256-261, 1986.

Metheny NA et al: Measures to test placement of nasogastric and nasointestinal feeding tubes: a review, Nurs Res 37(6):324-329, 1988.

Mize C, Teitell B, and Cunningham C: Total enteral nutrition: special feeding techniques and formula selection: In Levin D, Morris F, and Moore G, editors: A practical guide to pediatric intensive care, ed 2, St Louis, 1984, The CV Mosby Co.

Mollitt D, Golladay E, and Siebert J: Symptomatic gastroesophageal reflux following gastrostomy for neurologically impaired patients, Pediatrics 75(6):1124-1126, 1985.

National Center for Education in Maternal Child Health: Reaching out: a directory of national organizations related to maternal and child health, Washington, DC, March 1989.

Neifert M and Seacat J: A guide to successful breastfeeding, Contemp Pediatr 3:109, 1986.

Nemethy M and Clore ER: Microwave heating of infant formula and breastmilk, J Pediatr Health Care 4(3):131-135, 1990.

Nicoll A, Ginsburg R, and Tripp J: Supplementary feeding and jaundice in newborns, Acta Pediatr Scand 71:759, 1982.

Orenstein S: Personal communication, Jan 28, 1990.

Orenstein S: Effect of nonnutritive sucking on infant gastroesophageal reflux, Pediatr Res 24(1):38-40, 1988.

Orenstein S and Orenstein D: Gastroesophageal reflux and respiratory disease in children, J Pediatr 112(6):847-858, 1988.

Orenstein S and Whitington P: Positioning for the prevention of infant gastroesophageal reflux, J Pediatr 103(4):535-536, 1983.

Orenstein S, Magill H, and Brooks P: Thickening of infant feedings for therapy of gastroesophageal reflux, J Pediatr 110(2):181-186, 1987.

Orenstein S et al: The Santmyer swallow: a new and useful infant reflex, Lancet 1(8581):345-346, 1988.

Orr M and Allen S: Optimal oral experiences for infants on long-term total parenteral nutrition, Nutrition in Clinical Practice 1(6):288-295, 1986.

Paarlberg J and Balint J: Gastrostomy tubes: practical guidelines for home care, J Pediatr Nurs, 11:99-102, 1985.

Perez R: Care of the child with a gastrostomy tube: Common and practical concerns, Issues Compr Pediatr Nurs, 7:107-119, 1984.

Perry A and Potter P: Clinical nursing skills and techniques, ed 2, St Louis, 1990, The CV Mosby Co.

Perry S, Johnson S, and Trump D: Gastrostomy and the neonate, Am J Nurs 83(7):1030-1033, 1983.

Persons CB: Critical care procedures and protocols: a nursing process approach, Philadelphia, 1987, JB Lippincott Co.

Peterson M: Esophageal pH monitoring, J Pediatr Nurs 1(5):354-357, 1986.

Pikl BH: Massachusetts General Hospital manual of pediatric nursing practice, Boston, 1981, Little, Brown and Co, Inc.

Pipes PL: Nutrition in infancy and childhood, ed 4, St Louis, 1989, The CV Mosby Co.

Riordan J: A practical guide to breastfeeding, St Louis, 1983, The CV Mosby Co.

Robson AM: Parenteral fluid therapy. In Behrman RE and Vaughan WE, editors: Nelson textbook of pediatrics, ed 13, Philadelphia, 1987, WB Saunders.

Ross M et al: The importance of acid reflux patterns in neurologically damaged children detected by four-channel esophageal pH monitoring, J Pediatr Surg 23(6):573-576, 1988.

Rushton CH: The surgical neonate: principles of nursing management, Pediatr Nurs, 14(2):141-151, 1988.

Saunders S, Carroll J, and Johnson C: Breastfeeding: a problem-solving manual, New York, 1988, Essential Medical Information Systems, Inc.

Sporing EM, Walton MK, and Cady CE: Pediatric nursing policies, procedures, and personnel, Oradell, NJ, 1984, Medical Economics Books.

Stoiko M: Personal communication, Sept 8, 1989.

Storr G: Prevention of nipple tenderness and breast engorgement in the postpartal period, JOGNN 17(3):203-209, 1988.

Synderman S: Total parenteral alimentation. In Zimmerman S and Gildea J: Critical care pediatrics, Philadelphia, 1985, WB Saunders Co.

Testerman E: Current trends in pediatric total parenteral nutrition, J Intravenous Nurs 12(3):152-162, 1989.

Tibbetts E and Cadwell K: Protocol for in-hospital breastfeeding teaching, part 1, Sandwich, Mass, 1985, Health Education Associates.

Urban H et al: Meeting the needs of the multiply handicapped, New York, 1983, United Cerebral Palsy Association of Western New York.

Van Way CW III: Prevention of suction-induced gastric mucosal damage in dogs, Crit Care Med 15:774-777, 1987.

Walker M: How to evaluate breast pumps, MCN 12:270-276, 1987.

Walker M: The challenge of breastfeeding the preterm baby, Childbirth Educator, 7(3):18, 1988.

Walsh J, Persons C, and Wieck L: Manual of home health care nursing, Philadelphia, 1987, JB Lippincott Co.

Weatherley-White R et al: Early repair and breastfeeding for infants with cleft lip, Plast Reconstr Surg 79(6):879-887, 1987.

Weibley TT et al: Gavage tube insertion in the premature patient, MCN 12:24-27, 1987.

Wesley JR: Special access to the intestinal tract, Enteral feeding: scientific basis and clinical application, Report of the 94th Ross conference on pediatric research, Columbus, Ohio, 1988, Ross Laboratories.

Whaley L and Wong D: Essentials of pediatric nursing, ed 3, St Louis, 1989, The CV Mosby Co.

Whaley L and Wong D: Nursing care of infants and children, ed 4, St Louis, 1991, The CV Mosby Co.

White J and Owsley V: Helping families cope with milk, wheat, and soy allergies, MCN 8:423-428, 1983.

Williams PR and Kanarek KS: Urine evaporative loss and effects on specific gravity and osmolality, J Pediatr, 100:626-628, 1982.

Wink D: The physical and emotional care of infants with gastrostomy tubes, Issues Compr Pediatr Nurs 6:195-203, 1983.

Wong D and Whaley L: Clinical manual of pediatric nursing, ed 3, St Louis, 1990, The CV Mosby Co.

Ziemer M and Carroll JS: Infant gavage reconsidered, Am J Nurs 78:1543-1544, 1978.

# UNIT IX Elimination

## SKILL 68 Inserting an Indwelling or Intermittent Urinary Catheter

*Karen S. Farr*

Bladder catheterization involves passing a tube of latex, silastic, or polyethylene (polyvinyl chloride) through the urethra into the urinary bladder. Intermittent or continuous drainage of urine is thereby provided in the child who is unable to control bladder emptying (e.g., the child in a coma or the child with neurogenic bladder secondary to disease, congenital anomaly, or injury of the spinal cord). Placement of a catheter, with continuous measurement of urinary output, may also be indicated for strict monitoring of fluid balance in the seriously ill child. Catheterization of the pediatric patient requires special consideration of anatomical and cognitive factors unique to children.

### NURSING DIAGNOSES

Altered patterns of urinary elimination related to neuromuscular impairment; Urinary retention related to neuromuscular disorders, obstruction, anesthesia, or medication side effects; Incontinence (functional or total) related to sensory, cognitive, or mobility deficits or neurological dysfunction.

| Steps | Rationale |
|---|---|
| **Assessment** | |
| 1. Assess child for age, size, and developmental level. | The age and size of the child influence selection of catheter size. The child's level of awareness and understanding affect the approach to explaining the procedure and enlisting cooperation.<br>***Special Considerations:*** *In children a size 8-10 French catheter is usually appropriate. For the small infant, however, a size 5 French feeding tube may be used in lieu of a catheter. Older children and adolescents may require up to a size 14 French catheter.* |
| 2. Assess family's level of understanding of the need for catheterization and the procedure involved. | Enhanced parental understanding enables provision of necessary support to their child, and eases anxiety. |
| 3. Review child's record for medical history, allergies, physician order, reason for catheterization, and time and amount of last void. | Child's history reveals factors influencing ability to void and need for catheterization (e.g., urinary tract infection, surgery, neurogenic bladder). Some children are sensitive to the iodine used in preparations such as Betadine. Bladder catheterization is not without risk and should be clearly indicated (Epstein, 1985). A physician order is required. |
| **Planning and Goal Setting** | |
| 1. Gather all necessary supplies.<br>a. Obtain pre-packaged sterile catheterization tray<br>OR<br>b. Assemble a tray including:<br>▪ Sterile gloves.<br>▪ Two to three sterile drapes, including one fenestrated.<br>▪ Antiseptic solution for cleansing (e.g., povidone-iodine).<br>▪ Cotton balls or large swabs.<br>▪ Sterile water-soluble lubricant. | Strict adherence to aseptic technique precludes interrupting the procedure to retrieve needed items (Burkitt and Randall, 1987). Lack of distractions also enhances ability to communicate with and comfort child. |
| ▪ Two catheters of appropriate size. | Having an extra catheter ready will save time if the first one becomes contaminated. |

| Steps | Rationale |
|---|---|
| ▪ Syringe filled with sterile normal saline to inflate balloon on indwelling catheter.<br>▪ Sterile urine specimen container.<br>▪ Receptacle for urine.<br>▪ Drainage bag and connecting tubing if catheter is to remain indwelling.<br>▪ Safety pin, elastic band, and tape for securing an indwelling catheter to the child's bed and leg. | ***Special Considerations:*** *The amount of saline needed for balloon inflation will be specified on the port of an indwelling catheter.* |
| c. Waterproof padding to protect bed, adequate light source (e.g., overhead examination light or gooseneck lamp) and wastebasket. | |
| d. Disposable gloves, warm water in a basin, soap, washcloth, towel. | Preliminary perineal care may be necessary to remove blood, stool, or diaper creams and powders. Introduced with the catheter, these agents may cause urinary tract infection. |
| 2. Determine whether the procedure would best be performed in the child's room or in a treatment room. | A child's bed should be maintained as a "safe place" (e.g., from invasive procedures) as much as possible. Evaluation of the child's coping skills, consideration of previous/pending painful procedures ordered, and ability to provide privacy will influence the decision. |
| 3. Explain the reason for the catheterization and the procedure to be performed. Use clear, simple terms and simplified pictures in keeping with the child's developmental level. Provide honest explanations with a positive tone of voice (see Skill 1). | Knowledge of what to expect reduces anxiety and enhances cooperation.<br>***Special Considerations:*** *Too much detail will heighten anxiety in the young child. Preschoolers are especially fearful of invasive procedures (Whaley and Wong, 1989).* |
| 4. If restraint of the child is necessary, have an assistant present from the initiation of the procedure through completion. | Movement during passage of the catheter can result in urethral trauma and subsequent development of strictures (Burkitt and Randall, 1987).<br>***Special Considerations:*** *Do not ask parents to restrain the child. This can create feelings of considerable anxiety in parents and mistrust in children. It is preferable to have parents distract or comfort child.* |
| 5. Develop individualized child and family goals:<br>▪ Unobstructed drainage of urine will occur and/or be maintained.<br>▪ Child will be free of catheter-induced complications. | |

## Implementation

| Steps | Rationale |
|---|---|
| 1. Assemble equipment on overbed table (do not open sterile supplies at this point). | |
| 2. Lower crib siderail completely or raise bed to comfortable working height if performing procedure in child's room. | Occupational back injuries are reduced by use of correct body mechanics. |
| 3. Provide privacy for child. | Even if the child is too young to be concerned, parents invariably appreciate efforts to preserve their child's dignity. |
| 4. Protect bedding with waterproof pad placed under child. | |
| 5. Position child: | |
| a. For the *female* unable to assist, an assistant can hold the child's legs flexed at hips and knees while she lies supine. | ***Special Considerations:*** *If a female child cannot lie supine, position side lying with the upper leg drawn up in a knee-chest position.* |
| b. *Males* are assisted in maintaining a supine position. | |
| 6. Wash perineal area with soap and water, rinse thoroughly, and dry. | Removal of diaper creams, powders, etc. is necessary in order to reduce risk of chemical inflammation of the bladder and urethra, which predisposes child to development of a urinary tract infection (UTI). |
| 7. If an indwelling catheter is to be used, suspend drainage bag from bed frame and thread tubing up between siderails and side of bed to facilitate immediate hookup once catheter is inserted and secured. Do not remove protective cap from end of drainage tubing until time of hookup. | Maintenance of a sterile system is essential for patient safety.<br>***Special Considerations:*** *Assure that tubing will not be pulled when siderails are lowered.* |
| 8. Adjust light source to provide optimum visualization of meatus. | The female meatus is difficult to visualize, and adequate lighting is essential (Burkitt and Randall, 1987). |
| 9. Open catheter kit/tray, maintaining sterile field. | |
| 10. Put on sterile gloves, organize supplies and test balloon on indwelling catheter for integrity by inflating with indicated amount of sterile normal saline from the syringe, then completely withdrawing fluid (do not discard). | Pretesting the balloon avoids need for recatheterization because of equipment malfunction. |

| Steps | Rationale |
|---|---|
| 11. Drape child: Place solid drape on bed, slipping one end just underneath buttocks, using caution not to contaminate gloves. Place fenestrated drape over perineum with slit exposing labia or over penis. | ***Special Considerations:*** *It may not be feasible to maintain placement of fenestrated drape on a struggling child. It may be preferable to omit this drape rather than risk contamination of the field.* |
| 12. Prepare urethral meatus. | |
| a. *Female:* Gently spread labia with nondominant hand in order to visualize meatus, maintaining this position throughout catheterization (Fig. 68-1). This hand is now considered contaminated. With antiseptic-soaked swabs or cotton balls, use a downward stroke and wipe inner labial folds, then meatus. Discard swab/cotton ball after *each* stroke. | Contamination will occur if labia are allowed to return to closed position during the procedure. Reduction of surface microorganisms minimizes risk of their introduction into the bladder with passage of the catheter. ***Special Considerations:*** *The meatus may be difficult to visualize. It may appear as a small dimple or may be concealed in the anterior wall of the vagina.* |
| b. *Male:* With nondominant hand, hold penis just proximal to glans, retracting foreskin if child is uncircumcised, and maintain position throughout catheterization (Fig. 68-2). This hand is now considered contaminated. Using antiseptic-soaked swabs/cotton balls, wipe meatus in a circular motion from center to periphery. Discard swab/cotton ball after *each* stroke. | Contamination will occur if penis is allowed to drop or foreskin returns to normal position. Reduction of surface microorganisms minimizes risk of introduction into the bladder with passage of the catheter. |
| 13. Pick up catheter with dominant hand or forceps, 2 to 4 inches from the tip, and lubricate the catheter. Place distal end of catheter in sterile urine receptacle. | |
| 14. Insert catheter: | ***Special Considerations:*** *Never force catheter. Ask the older child to bear down in order to relax the external sphincter. A slight change in the angle of the penis or rotation of the catheter may facilitate insertion if resistance is encountered.* |
| a. *Female:* Aiming slightly upward, insert catheter tip gently through meatus 1 to 2 inches or until urine appears, then advance another ½ to 1 inch. | |
| b. *Male:* Using light tension, hold penis at a 90° angle from body and gently insert catheter tip 2 to 3 inches or until urine appears, then advance another ½ to 1 inch. | |

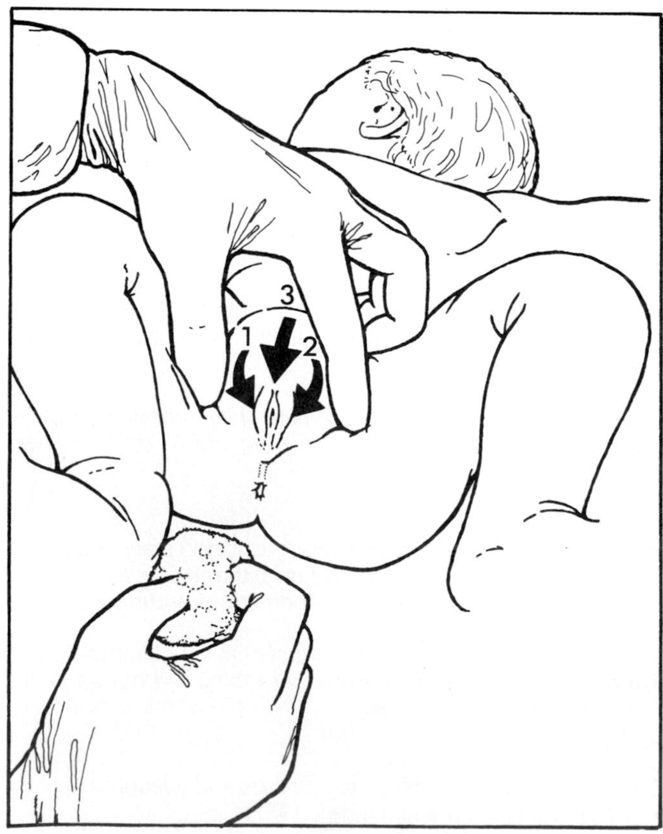


***FIG. 68-1*** Order of cleansing of female perineum before catheterization.

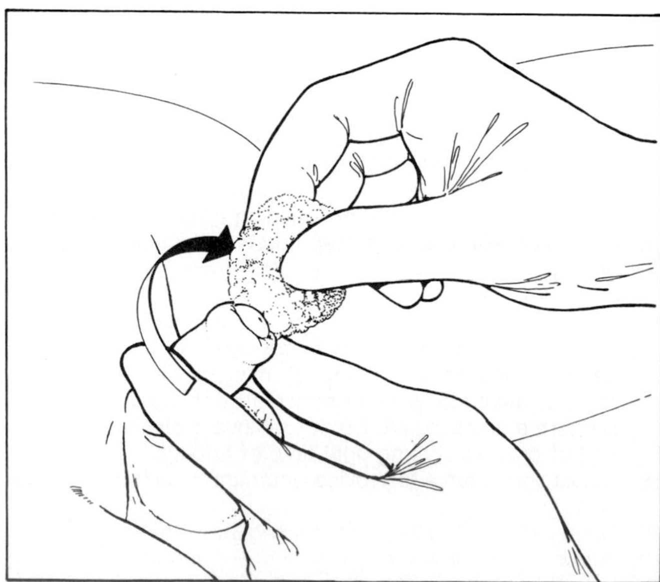

***FIG. 68-2*** Meatus is wiped with a circular motion.

| Steps | Rationale |
|---|---|
| 15. Collect urine specimen, if ordered, then provide for complete emptying of bladder into separate receptacle. | ***Special Considerations:*** *Traditional practice dictates that no more than 1000 ml of urine should be allowed to drain at one time as there is a risk for shock. In a small study of adults, Bristoll et al (1989) reported no adverse effects when complete bladder emptying in amounts up to 1950 ml was allowed.* |
| 16. a. Remove intermittent catheter slowly and smoothly, pinching lumen | ***Special Considerations:*** *Ask child with flaccid bladder to bear down gently, if able, or raise head of bed slightly to facilitate complete drainage, reducing risk of infection associated with residual urine.* |
| OR | |
| b. Inflate balloon of indwelling catheter, being careful not to overinflate balloon, and observing child for evidence of pain with inflation. If pain behaviors are noted, deflate balloon completely, slightly advance catheter, and reinflate. | Exhibiting pain behaviors can indicate that balloon is in urethra. ***Special Considerations:*** *Infants and very young children should be observed for change in cry and facial expression as evidence of pain.* |
| 17. Secure indwelling catheter to child's inner thigh or lower abdomen (for males) with tape, allowing enough slack to prevent any tension on catheter with extension of leg (Figs. 68-3 and 68-4). | Tension on catheter can result in urethral trauma. Taping the catheter to the abdomen on the male prevents pressure on the penile-scrotal angle. |
| 18. Connect indwelling catheter to closed drainage system, ensuring that collection bag is below level of bladder and that tubing is free of kinks (Ruge, 1987). | Maintaining patent tubing with adequate gravity drainage prevents reflux of urine into the bladder, which increases the risk of catheter-related UTI. |
| 19. Clip or pin drainage tubing to bottom sheet on bed (see Fig. 68-4). | This frequently neglected maneuver helps minimize tension on the catheter. ***Special Considerations:*** *If pin is used, tape it closed to protect against accidental opening and injury to the patient.* |
| 20. If necessary, provide for restraint of child's hands in order to protect against urethral trauma caused by pulling on catheter (see Skill 51). | ***Special Considerations:*** *Plan regular check of color, sensation, movement and temperature in hands, and periodic release of restraints to prevent circulatory impairment and provide psychological and physical comfort for child. Consider removal of restraints if child has adjusted to presence of catheter and parent is present to monitor child.* |
| 21. Praise child for any cooperation offered and/or comfort child with a hug. | ***Special Considerations:*** *If child's condition permits, assist parents in holding child after procedure, using care to preserve integrity of the catheter system.* |

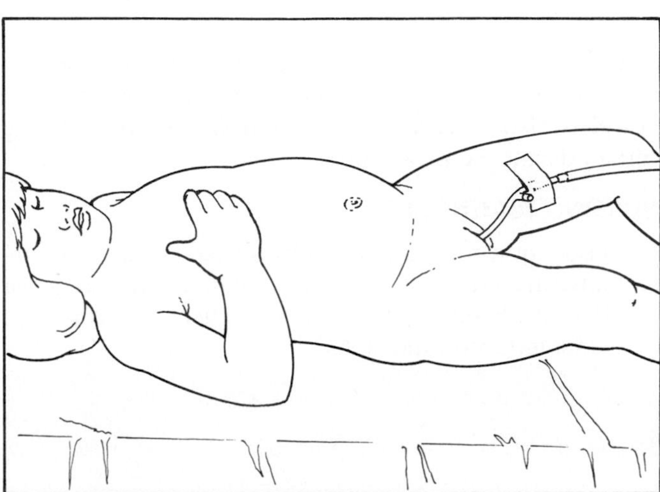

***FIG. 68-3*** Catheter is taped to child's inner thigh.

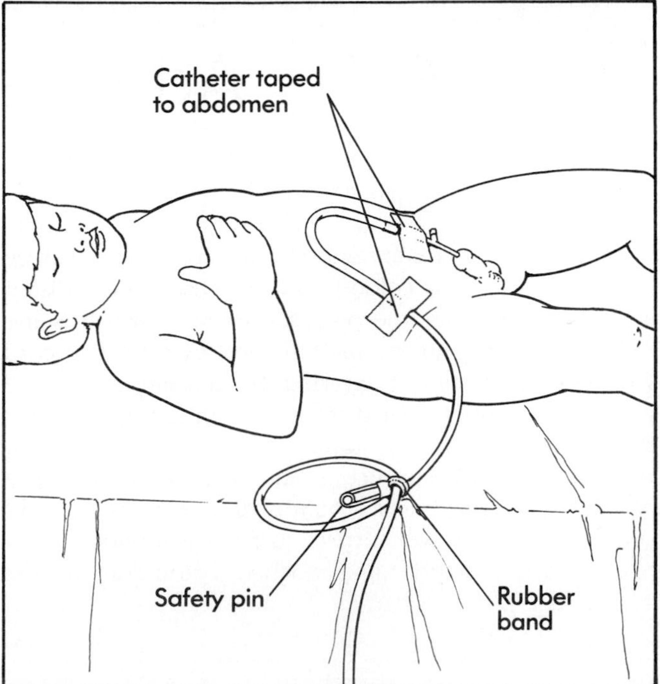


***FIG. 68-4*** Catheter taped to abdomen of male child.

## Evaluation Outcomes

1. Urinary retention/bladder distension is relieved.
2. Urine flow is unobstructed.
3. Child does not develop catheter-associated UTI.

## Documentation

Chart catheter type and size used, volume of fluid used for inflating balloon, urine appearance and volume, and collection of any specimen. Also chart child's response to the procedure and any necessary action taken to protect catheter. Include date and time.

## Home Care Modifications

1. Discuss equipment maintenance for intermittent catheterization: catheter is washed with soap and water, rinsed, and allowed to dry or placed in appropriate disinfectant solution. Remainder of supplies are kept together in a clean, dry place.
2. Discuss positioning of child on toilet for intermittent catheterization. A girl performing self-catheterization may find a mirror helpful for location of meatus. Unless mirror is free standing, assistance may be required and caution should be encouraged with the use of glass in the bathroom.
3. Following hypospadius repair, a child may be discharged to home with an indwelling catheter for a week or more. An anti-reflux leg drainage bag can be used to facilitate mobility. The bag attaches securely to the leg with straps and can be easily emptied periodically (Sugar and Firlit, 1988).

## Observational Guidelines

Palpate bladder to detect evidence of urine retention and note volume of urine obtained with catheterization.
Observe collecting system regularly for quality and volume of urine present, noting any clumps, sediment, or diminished flow. Check for patency of tubing every 1 to 2 hours.
Monitor for development of fever, vomiting, bladder tenderness, cloudy or foul smelling urine, irritability, or lethargy.

# *SKILL* 69 Administering an Enema

*Karen S. Farr*

Under normal circumstances, transference of feces occurs from the pelvic colon into the rectum. Rectal distension then stimulates the defecation reflex, which is mediated by centers in the medulla and sacral spinal cord. Deficient nerve supply, ignoring the defecation reflex repeatedly, and fiber-poor diet are among factors impeding this normal process. With administration of an enema, fluid is introduced into the rectum and sigmoid colon to precipitate peristalsis, hence stooling. An enema may also be ordered before bowel surgery to reduce numbers of intestinal flora (bacteria) and evacuate colon contents that could cause postoperative infection with their escape into the peritoneum during surgery. A thoroughly cleansed bowel is also essential to optimum visualization during certain diagnostic procedures.

### NURSING DIAGNOSES

Constipation related to neuromuscular impairment, immobility, inadequate fluid and/or fiber intake, stress or medications; Potential fluid volume deficit/excess related to enema-induced fluid shifts.

| Steps | Rationale |
|---|---|

## Assessment

1. Assess child for age, size, and developmental level.

Age and size influence type and volume of solution used and choice of rectal tube size. The child's level of awareness and understanding affect the approach to explaining the procedure and enlisting cooperation.

***Special Considerations:*** *In the neonate, the sigmoid colon makes a right angle to itself at a depth of 3 cm (Merenstein and Gardner, 1989) making rectal perforation a high risk with insertion of stiff tubing for an enema.*

2. Assess child's abdomen for bowel sounds, distension, pain, rigidity, or guarding.

Absence of bowel sounds, or presence of pain, rigidity, or guarding may indicate appendicitis, bowel perforation, or peritonitis. An enema is contraindicated in these conditions.

3. Review child's record for purpose of enema, current conditions affecting fluid/electrolyte balance, and recent vital signs. Verify physician order.

Reason for enema and current status of hydration influence the degree to which cleansing must be carried out, as well as the type and volume of solution used. Changes in vital signs can indicate enema-induced fluid shifts. A physician order is necessary to administer an enema in an inpatient setting.

***Special Considerations:*** *Administration of inappropriate electrolyte concentrations and/or volumes can be lethal in children (Nurses Drug Alert, 1987). Serum sodium, potassium, and phosphorus can be elevated, and serum calcium and arterial pH can be lowered, resulting in cardiac arrest and death. Children with preexisting fluid/electrolyte disturbance are particularly at risk. Plain tap water should* never *be used in children.*

4. Assess family's level of understanding regarding reason for enema.

Enhanced parental understanding enables parents to provide the necessary support to their child. Assessment may also reveal a teaching opportunity, since regular bowel movements are often a source of concern for parents.

## Planning and Goal Setting

1. Gather all supplies:
   a. Prepackaged enema kit (e.g., Pediatric Fleet).
   b. Supplies for isotonic or medicated enema:
      - Administration bag.
      - Connecting tubing.
      - Rectal tube of correct size for child.

***Special Considerations:*** *A size 10 to 12 French rectal tube may be used for infants and toddlers, with graduation up to size 22 French for adolescents.*

      - Correct type and volume of solution (as ordered by physician).

Many sources feel the only safe type of cleansing enema for infants and young children is the isotonic saline enema because of the potential dangers of fluid and electrolyte disturbances with other formulations (Behrman and Vaughan, 1987; Martin et al, 1987).

***Special Considerations:*** *An isotonic solution is made by the addition of one (1) measuring teaspoon table salt to 500 ml. (1 pint) of tap water. Neomycin is often used in preoperative enemas. Maximum recommended volumes are:*

| | |
|---|---|
| Infant | 120 to 240 ml |
| Small child | 240 to 360 ml |
| Large child | 360 to 480 ml |
| Adolescent | 480 to 720 ml (Whaley and Wong, 1989) |

      - Bath thermometer to assure proper temperature of solution.

Solution under 40.5° C can precipitate abdominal cramping and expulsion of solution. Solution over 43° C can burn the mucosal lining of the intestine.

      - Waterproof padding to protect bed.

***Special Considerations:*** *For the child in a spica cast, plastic wrap may be tucked around cast edges.*

      - Water soluble lubricant.
      - Bedpan, bedside commode or provision for safe and easy access to bathroom.
      - Disposable gloves.

Gloving reduces risk of transmission of microorganisms.

      - Basin of warm water, soap, washcloth and towel, and toilet tissue.

The child will need to be cleansed after evacuation of bowel.

      - IV stand.

An IV stand may be used to suspend bag of solution.

***Special Considerations:*** *Do not elevate bag higher than 12 to 18 inches above the anus to prevent forceful influx of solution and resulting discomfort (Perry and Potter, 1990).*

| Steps | Rationale |
|---|---|
| 2. Warm solution including prepackaged enema solutions to 41° to 42° C. | ***Special Considerations:*** *Solution may be placed (in its container) in a warm water bath or it can be heated very briefly in a microwave oven. Temperature* must *be checked with a thermometer.* |
| 3. Explain the reason for the enema and the procedure to be performed. Use clear, simple terms and simplified pictures appropriate to child's developmental level (see Skill 1). Also explain correlation of retention time with efficacy of enema. | Knowledge of what to expect greatly reduces anxiety and enhances cooperation.<br>***Special Considerations:*** *Too much detail will heighten anxiety in the young child. Preschoolers are especially fearful of invasive procedures.* |
| 4. Gather age-appropriate books and toys to provide diversion during retention time. Consult with child life specialist if available. | Child may have greater success in retaining enema for optimum time and in obtaining the best results if attention is distracted while waiting. |
| 5. Develop individualized child and family goals:<br>▪ Child's bowel will be adequately cleansed of stool.<br>▪ Child will experience minimal discomfort.<br>▪ Child's fluid/electrolyte loss will be minimized. | |

## Implementation

| Steps | Rationale |
|---|---|
| 1. Assemble equipment on bedside table, including prewarmed solution. | |
| 2. Lower crib siderail completely or raise bed to comfortable working height. | Occupational back injuries are reduced by use of correct body mechanics. |
| 3. Provide for privacy. | Even if the child is too young to be concerned, parents invariably appreciate efforts to preserve their child's dignity. |
| 4. Protect bedding with waterproof pads. | |
| 5. Obtain assistance for restraint of child as needed. | ***Special Considerations:*** *Avoid asking parent to restrain child. Encourage the parent to provide comfort and distraction.* |
| 6. Position child: Infants and small children may be maintained in the dorsal recumbent (supine) position with knees flexed. Older children may be assisted into Sim's position (on left side with right knee flexed). | Flexion of the knees promotes relaxation of abdominal muscles, reducing discomfort.<br>***Special Considerations:*** *Infants may be supported by resting head and torso on a pillow or folded bath blanket, and by resting buttocks over the padded edge of a bedpan (a towel may be used for padding) (Fig. 69-1).* |
| 7. Administer enema as ordered by physician:<br>a. Non-prepackaged enema:<br>▪ Clamp tubing shut. | Solution will escape when added to container unless tubing is clamped. |
| ▪ Add prewarmed isotonic saline or medicated solution to bag. | |
| ▪ Purge air from tubing and tip; reclamp tubing. | Purging prevents the introduction of air into colon. |
| ▪ Lubricate tip of tube well with water-soluble lubricant. | Lubrication reduces the risk of mucosal injury. |
| ▪ Separate buttocks with nondominant hand to visualize anus. | |
| ▪ Gently insert tip of tube into rectum (infant 1"-1½"; child: 2"-3"), while maintaining firm hold on tube (Fig. 69-2). | A firm grasp on tubing prevents accidental deep penetration and possible injury or slipping out.<br>***Special Considerations:*** *Never force tubing because it may puncture intestinal mucosa and result in serious injury or fatality.* |
| ▪ Allow solution to infuse slowly (approximately 100 cc/minute) and control the rate by raising or lowering the bag. Do not elevate bag higher than 12-18 inches above anus. | ***Special Considerations:*** *If child complains of cramping, stop infusion briefly, then resume. Lower bag slightly to slow rate and to minimize discomfort. Adequate pressure for infusion may be achieved by elevating the bag as little as 4 inches above anus in some cases (e.g., infants) (Wong and Whaley, 1990). Be alert to nonverbal cues of pain in infants and toddlers. These children may already be crying simply from being restrained, so be attentive to a change in cry, facial expression, and overall intensity in their response to the procedure.* |
| ▪ Clamp tubing as last solution infuses. | Clamping tubing prevents air from entering rectum following solution. |
| b. Pre-packaged enema:<br>▪ Remove cap from tip and apply additional lubricant if necessary. | Lubrication reduces risk of mucosal injury. |

| Steps | Rationale |
|---|---|

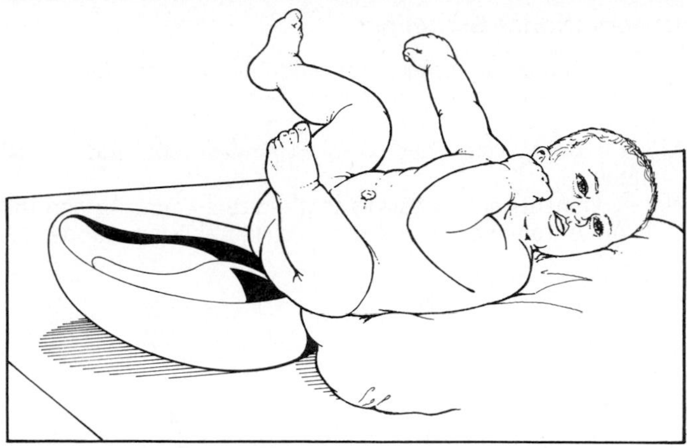

***FIG. 69-1*** Infant positioned over bedpan.

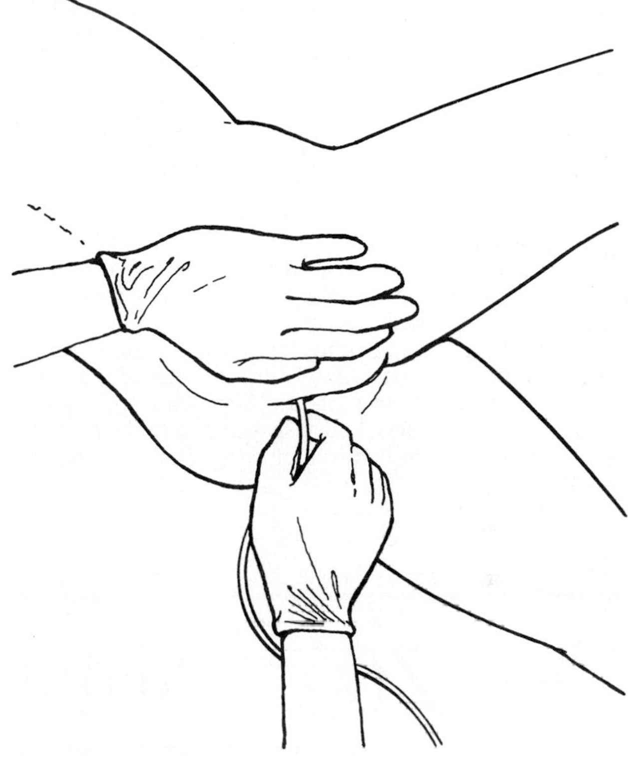

***FIG. 69-2*** Maintaining a firm hold on tube, gently insert into child's rectum.

- Separate buttocks with nondominant hand to visualize anus.
- Gently insert tip of tube into rectum (infant: 1″-1½″, child: 2″-3″).
- Slowly squeeze bottle until all of solution is emptied into rectum. As bottle empties fold it over (as with a toothpaste tube) to force liquid into the tip.

8. Gently withdraw tube and wipe child with toilet tissue.

Lubricant often collects on the anal area.

9. Encourage child to remain quietly in bed for as long as possible. Reinforce teaching about retention/efficacy if child is developmentally able to understand.

Length of retention time influences effectiveness of the enema. For maximum effect, solution should be retained for 10-20 minutes.

***Special Considerations:*** *Infants and young children will need to have buttocks held together because sphincter control is immature. Age appropriate puppets, stories, or board games may be employed as diversionary activities.*

10. Assist child onto bedpan, to commode/potty seat, or to bathroom.

A sense of urgency, coupled with inadequate sphincter control/leaking solution, places young children at increased risk for slips and falls when they get out of bed.

11. Observe evacuated contents of solution and feces.

Observing evacuate confirms efficacy of enema.

12. Assist older child with cleansing or thoroughly wash infant or young child with soap and water, using disposable gloves.

Enzymes in feces are skin irritants. Universal Blood and Body Fluid Precautions call for use of gloves (see Skill 50.)

13. Dispose of all single-use equipment in proper trash receptacle.
14. Praise child for any cooperation offered or comfort him or her with a hug.
15. Observe child for alteration in mental state, muscle tone, heart rate and rhythm, respiratory rate and pattern, and blood pressure after procedure. Also note urine output. Notify physician promptly should any signs of fluid/electrolyte disturbance develop.

Children are at an increased risk of significant fluid and electrolyte shifts, with potentially life-threatening results, from the administration of enemas.

| Steps | Rationale |
|---|---|
| **Evaluation Outcomes** | **Observational Guidelines** |
| 1. Bowel is adequately cleansed appropriate to reason for enema (e.g., fecal retention vs preoperative/prediagnostic preparation). | Observe evacuated contents for amount and characteristics of stool and amount of solution returned. |
| 2. Fluid/electrolyte losses are minimized. | Monitor child's vital signs, weight, urine output, and mental status. |
| 3. Child expresses minimal discomfort during procedure. | Note comments and behaviors that indicate cramping and the length of retention time. Observe child's ability to cooperate. |

## Documentation

Chart volume and type of solution, temperature of solution, and size of rectal tube used. Also chart the child's response to the procedure (e.g., if all solution ordered was actually administered, complaints of pain, and length of retention) and characteristics of evacuated contents. Document any signs and symptoms that indicate an adverse response to the procedure. Note if the child remained free of signs of adverse response.

# SKILL 70 Maintaining an Ostomy

*Karen S. Farr*

Diversion of feces or urine is required when normal pathways of elimination are temporarily or permanently inhibited. Hirschsprung's disease (aganglionic megacolon), intussusception, necrotizing enterocolitis, meconium ileus, ulcerative colitis, Crohn's disease, and imperforate anus are some conditions that require the formation of a colostomy or ileostomy. Location of the ostomy will dictate consistency of effluent (drainage), with ostomies along the ileum and ascending colon draining liquid stool. Descending colon and sigmoid colostomies will drain stool similar to a normal bowel movement. Obstructive uropathy, primary congenital anomalies such as extrophy of the bladder, and occasionally neurogenic bladder disease are indications for urinary diversion. Ureters may be brought out through the abdominal wall or anastomosed into a segment of bowel (e.g., ileal conduit). Nursing care of the child with an ostomy must extend beyond the attention to physical needs to incorporate a high level of sensitivity to the child's feelings about body image and self-worth, as well as to the parents' feelings of grief, fear, anger, and guilt.

## NURSING DIAGNOSES

Body image disturbance related to structural and functional changes in elimination due to ostomy; Potential altered health maintenance related to lack of knowledge about ostomy care; Impaired skin integrity related to effluent leaking, adhesive sensitivity, frequent appliance changes, or restrictive clothing; Anticipatory grieving related to perceived potential loss of bowel/urinary control.

| Steps | Rationale |
|---|---|
| **Assessment** | |
| 1. Determine child's age and developmental level. | The child's level of awareness and understanding influence the approach of explaining the procedure and enlisting cooperation. |
| 2. Assess family for level of understanding and stage of emotional adjustment regarding their child's ostomy and coping skills. | The birth of an imperfect infant or the development of illness that requires an ostomy in a child can be a devastating experience for parents and can create feelings of failure, guilt, and grief. Until these feelings are recognized and the appropriate support provided for parents, they will be unable to assimilate new information and care for their child. Parental attitudes are also critically important to assist their child to develop a positive body image and healthy self-care skills. |
| a. Review nursing care plan and nurses' notes for information previously gathered. | |
| b. Explore issues with open-ended questions (see Skill 12). | |

| Steps | Rationale |
|---|---|
| 3. Review child's record for medical history, type and location of ostomy (see operative report), allergies, physician orders, and history of frequency of appliance changes. | The patient history will reveal the condition that necessitates the formation of the ostomy and will reveal whether the diversion is temporary or permanent. Location of the ostomy influences the type of drainage expected. Composition/consistency of drainage, along with allergies, may affect selection of appliance and skin barrier (e.g., the ileum has more digestive enzymes; therefore, ostomies in this portion of bowel require more aggressive skin protection). Familiarity with the operative procedure performed is also necessary to anticipate complications. A physician's order is necessary to obtain reimbursement for supplies and home care referrals. |

## Planning and Goal Setting:

| Steps | Rationale |
|---|---|
| 1. Gather all necessary supplies. | Interrupting ostomy care to retrieve needed items creates a chaotic atmosphere. The unique needs of ostomates and families in regaining control over their body function call for an orderly, matter-of-fact approach to management. |
| a. Ostomy care using no appliance:<br>▪ Disposable gloves | Infants and toddlers may or may not wear an appliance (pouch); double diapering may be used instead. However, enzymes in stool or high urine pH can quickly macerate peristomal skin (Broadwell, 1987). Rubbing of the stoma by the diaper may cause abrasions and bleeding. Chronic blood loss can be significant in small babies, resulting in anemia (Webster, 1985). |
| ▪ Washcloth, towel, basin of warm water, mild/nonoily soap if needed (e.g., Ivory). | Thoroughly cleansed and dried peristomal skin, protected by a barrier, is resistant to breakdown by ostomy drainage. Soap can alter the natural acidic pH of skin, and it is not routinely used for peristomal skin cleansing. |
| ▪ Skin sealant (optional) (e.g., Bard Protective Barrier Film, Skin Prep by United Medical, or Hollister's Skin Gel). | A skin sealant (a liquid barrier that leaves a protective film) helps to prevent breakdown from occurring when skin is stripped as the old barrier is removed. |
| ▪ Skin barrier (e.g., Stomahesive wafers, powder or paste [ConvaTec], Comfeel Hollister Premium Wafers, Pericare or Unisalve ointments with karaya powder, Convatec Little Ones Sur-Fit Flexible Wafers, Dansac Supersquare and Bard ReliaSeal).<br>▪ Petroleum gauze.<br>▪ Disposable diaper.<br>▪ Diaper pins, tape or Montgomery straps. | ***Special Considerations:*** *Because urine often disintegrates pectin, a nonpectin based barrier may be preferable for the urostomate, e.g., ReliaSeal (Erickson, 1987).* |
| b. Ostomy care using an appliance:<br>▪ Disposable gloves. | |
| ▪ Washcloth, towel, basin of warm water, mild/nonoily soap (e.g., Ivory, Purpose [Johnson & Johnson], or Neutrogena [nonemollient formula]). | Skin must be gently (but thoroughly) cleansed and dried to promote secure appliance adhesion and prevent breakdown. |
| ▪ Skin sealant (see step a above). | Swabbing with skin sealant, especially at base of stoma before application of barrier, will help protect skin from mechanical stripping with next change. |
| ▪ Skin barrier (see step a above). | Skin barrier protects peristomal skin from maceration by effluent or urine. Since pouch opening must be cut $\frac{1}{16}$-$\frac{1}{8}$ inch larger than stoma, stoma paste can be applied around base of stoma to prevent seepage of effluent under barrier edge. |
| ▪ Ostomy pouch with clamp.<br>▪ Squeeze bottle or 60 cc syringe with 6 to 12 inch rubber tubing attached and container of warm water for irrigation of pouch between changes. | ***Special Considerations:*** *Pediatric pouches are made in a variety of sizes and styles, including those designed for premature infants and one or two-piece designs (Fig. 70-1). Pouches are also available with barriers especially designed for extra sensitive skin and urostomates. Antireflux valves prevent urine backflow.* |
| ▪ Gauze squares. | Gauze can be held against stoma (*not* inserted) to absorb fluids/drainage during barrier application.<br>***Special Considerations:*** *A tampon may also be used for this purpose.* |
| c. Irrigation of stoma. | Irrigation of a stoma is done only by a physician's order, and it is usually in preparation for surgery or diagnostic procedures. |
| ▪ Irrigating cone. | Use of an irrigating cone eliminates the risk of intestinal perforation associated with catheters (Yahle, 1976). This method also prevents backflow of solution. |

| Steps | Rationale |
|---|---|

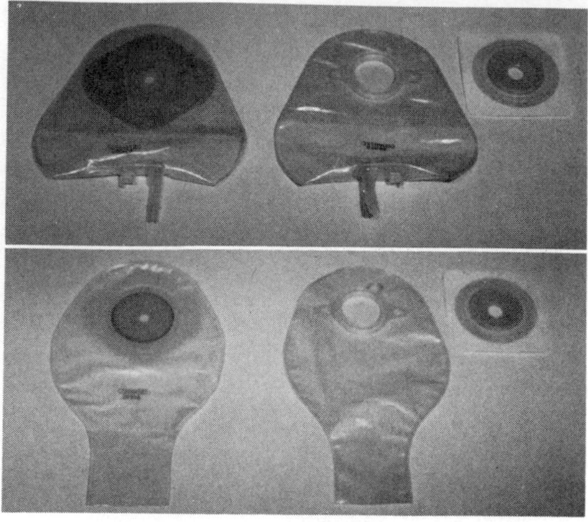

*FIG. 70-1* **A,** One- and two-piece urostomy bags. **B,** One- and two-piece colostomy bags.

- Colostomy irrigating set.
- Water soluble lubricant.
- Bath thermometer.
- Warmed irrigating solution (approx. 42° C) of correct volume/type as specified by physician's order.
- Washcloth, towel, basin of warm water, mild/nonoily soap if needed (e.g., Ivory, Purpose [Johnson & Johnson], Neutrogena [non-emollient formula]).
- Collecting basin or bedpan for drainage.

Lubricant reduces risk of stomal/intestinal trauma.

Solution cooler than 40.5° C can precipitate cramping and premature expulsion of solution. Solution warmer than 43° C can burn intestinal mucosa. Administration of inappropriate electrolyte concentrations and/or volumes can be lethal in children: serum sodium, potassium, and phosphorus can be elevated, serum calcium and arterial pH lowered, resulting in cardiac arrest and death. Children with pre-existing fluid/electrolyte disturbances are particularly at risk (Nurses Drug Alert, 1987).

***Special considerations:*** *Never use plain tap water or adult premixed formulas in children. Some recommended volumes are:*

| | |
|---|---|
| *Infant:* | *120 to 240 cc* |
| *Child 2-4 years:* | *240 to 360 cc* |
| *Child 4-10 years:* | *360 to 480 cc* |
| *Child 11+ years:* | *480 to 720 cc (Whaley and Wong, 1989)* |

2. Determine optimum time for pouch changes, if possible.

Pouches/faceplates are changed when leaking occurs and are routinely changed at least two to three times per week to permit thorough cleansing and evaluating of peristomal skin and checking for undetected leaks.

***Special Considerations:*** *For home care, assure parents that appliance changes are not emergency situations. It is preferable to comfort and calm the child first if he or she is agitated and crying. This reduces parental stress and anxiety that predispose to hurried and faulty application, leaks, and the need for yet another change.*

3. Explain the procedure to be performed using simplified diagrams, pictures, and product samples (see Skill 1):
   a. Begin teaching preoperatively, if possible.
   b. Individualize pacing of instruction.
   c. Use correct anatomical terms (e.g., no nicknames for the stoma) and approach the family tactfully with a matter-of-fact attitude.
   d. Repeat explanation frequently in the early postoperative period.

Teaching about ostomies requires sensitivity. Strong feelings regarding altered body image may affect immediate interest and participation on the part of the child or family. It often takes time for the child and the family to simply be able to look at the ostomy, so individualized pacing is essential. Repeated explanations are usually needed because the assimilation of new information is inhibited during times of great stress.

***Special Considerations:*** *Introduce parents/older children to another family that is successfully managing a similar appliance, if possible.*

4. Develop individualized client/family goals:
   - Free flow of urine (or evacuation of stool) will be maintained.
   - Healthy stoma and peristomal skin integrity will be maintained.
   - Child/family will be able to independently change the appliance and to maintain healthy peristomal skin and stoma.
   - Child/family will progress through stages of psychological adjustment to stoma.

| Steps | Rationale |
|---|---|
| **Implementation**  | |
| 1. Provide for child's privacy. | Even if the child is too young to be concerned, parents invariably appreciate efforts to preserve their child's dignity. |
| 2. Arrange all equipment on bedside table. | Organization promotes a calm, orderly approach and sets the tone for child and family to maintain or regain control. |
| 3. Enlist assistance, as needed, for restraint. | Assistance may be necessary to maintain child's position during care. Parents should not be asked to restrain the child, particularly in the early postoperative period. Very young children often cry as a response to being restrained, but parents may interpret their crying as an expression of pain instead. ***Special Considerations:*** *Enlist parents in entertaining/distracting their child at this point to initiate/reinforce a positive response to the procedure. Also, parents are better able to concentrate on learning about the procedure if they are not involved in restraining their child.* |
| 4. Place child in supine position in crib or bed for diaper or pouch changes or for pouch irrigation. Stoma irrigation should be done in a treatment room. | Supine position facilitates thorough cleansing, accurate assessment, and secure barrier/pouch adhesion. Stoma irrigations, which are usually perceived as a negative experience by children, should be carried out in a treatment room, thereby retaining the bed as a "safe place." |
| 5. Ostomy care using no appliance: | |
| a. Put on gloves (and cover gown if indicated). Explain gloving to parents. | Universal Blood and Body Fluid Precautions call for use of gloves to minimize risk of transmission of infectious disease (e.g., HIV, hepatitis). Explaining this precaution to the family helps them to understand that it is not an aversion to effluent or the stoma. |
| b. If appropriate, remove diaper(s) and place in trash or laundry receptacle. | Diapers are usually used on infants and toddlers only. ***Special Considerations:*** *Talking/cooing to the infant, as with any diaper change, promotes a positive response to stoma care and positive role modeling for the parents as well.* |
| c. Remove peristomal skin barrier. | ***Special Considerations:*** *If a wafer-type barrier was used, peel gently from edges toward center. Check skin-side for eroded finger-like areas that indicate seepage of ostomy drainage because of poor adhesion of barrier. If an ointment or paste was used, completely remove all layers once a day to allow thorough assessment of peristomal skin. Only the top layer needs to be removed for other diaper changes after the immediate postoperative period.* |
| d. Wash skin thoroughly using warm water and pat dry. Use a mild, nonoily soap only if necessary. | Cleansing permits accurate assessment and promotes optimal skin condition for reapplication of barrier. |
| e. Assess stoma for color, integrity, size, and elevation. The well-perfused stoma should be deep pink to cherry red. The stoma may initially be edematous from surgical manipulation, but it should decrease in size over the next 3 to 6 weeks. The stoma should be elevated from skin level. Postoperative stomal bleeding should be minimal, although there may be scant bleeding with washing. | A bluish or black color signals poor circulation (as in volvulus, prolapse, adhesions) to the intestinal segment that creates the stoma. Pallor may indicate decreased oxygen-carrying capacity of blood due to anemia. Persistent edema may be caused by a too tight barrier/appliance. If scar tissue develops around the stoma, it can become retracted (pulled in) or flush with surrounding skin surface, which makes protecting the peristomal skin difficult. Stomal abrasions that result from contact with crystals precipitated from alkaline urine or rubbing by diapers or dressings increases the risk of infection or necrosis (Broadwell, 1987; Watson et al, 1976). ***Special Considerations:*** *Parents often fear that the stoma is painful because it is red. Anticipate this concern, even if it is not voiced, and explain that the stoma is normally not painful.* |
| f. Assess peristomal skin (including any peristomal sutures). Peristomal skin should look like the skin over the rest of the child's abdomen. | Maceration can occur when effluent or urine seeps under the skin barrier. Peristomal skin is most commonly infected by *C. albicans* (yeast); a bright red, papular rash with satellite lesions, which progresses to scaling and crusting (Broadwell, 1987). A sensitivity to the adhesive is suspected if erythema/rash exactly match size and shape of the adhesive disc or other adhesive material used (Chezem, 1976). Frequent stripping of adhesives/barriers from skin is a common reason for trauma. A reevaluation of the system in use may be indicated if this occurs (Broadwell, 1987). Suture lines close to the stoma are at risk |

| Steps | Rationale |
|---|---|
| | of dehiscence and infection due to mechanical trauma and contact with drainage. |
| g. Assess drainage from stoma for amount, consistency, and odor in relation to type/location of the diversion. Minimal drainage can be expected from an ileostomy or colostomy immediately post-op (48 to 96 hours) due to NPO status and effects of anesthesia. Urinary drainage should occur immediately post-op. Functional ileostomy drainage is usually dark green, liquid, and odorless. As adaptation/partial water absorption occurs and solid foods are introduced, consistency should become mushy and a musty odor should develop. Colostomy drainage will more closely resemble normal stool in color, consistency, odor, and gas content. Initially, urine will be pink (first 48 hours), but should be amber by the third postoperative day. Some mucus will be present with ileal conduits, giving urine a cloudy appearance. | Familiarity with the surgical procedure performed is essential in evaluating the appropriateness of drainage and detecting signs of dysfunction or obstruction. Abundant, watery effluent from a colostomy indicates dysfunction and can rapidly result in hyponatremia, dehydration, and metabolic acidosis. Excessive mucus may indicate a UTI secondary to inflammation of bowel mucosa (Petillo, 1987). |
| h. Wipe peristomal skin with skin sealant, if desired. | Sealant leaves a protective film, which reduces the risk of mechanical trauma. The resulting "tacky" skin surface also promotes snug, even, barrier adhesion.<br>***Special Considerations:*** *Sealant must be thoroughly dry before attempts are made to apply barrier. Sealants can sting and burn denuded skin. Pain associated with stoma care can cause strong, negative feelings, including fear in very young children.* |
| i. Apply protective barrier.<br>▪ Wafer: Use template provided with product to assure that the hole cut will not constrict stoma, yet completely cover all peristomal skin. Cut a hole 1/16-1/8 inch larger than stoma. If stoma is irregular, place transparent film over stoma and trace outline with a marking pen. Use this as a template, being careful not to reverse tracing when cutting barrier.<br>▪ Paste/Powder: Apply a thick, even coat on peristomal skin right up to the stoma's edge, covering approximately a 3" radius. | Barrier protects peristomal skin from breakdown by effluent or urine.<br>***Special Considerations:*** *Skin must be meticulously clean and dry before application of a barrier. Gauze may be used to blot drainage as it occurs during the assessment of skin and stoma and barrier application. Barrier must be replaced whenever it is no longer intact, and it should be carefully inspected with each diaper change. When pastes or powders are used, they should be applied thickly and only the top layer should be removed with each diaper change. Replace top layer with fresh barrier. Making a mixture of paste and karaya powder can increase skin protection. Wash off all barrier daily to allow a thorough assessment of peristomal skin.* |
| j. Place a folded cloth diaper over stoma, securing it with regular diaper, tape, pins, or Montgomery straps. | ***Special Considerations:*** *A small square of petroleum gauze placed directly over the stoma before application of the diaper may help reduce stomal abrasions and bleeding. If pins are used to secure diaper, tape them closed to prevent accidental opening and injury.* |
| k. Discard disposable diapers, gloves, and soiled linen in appropriate receptacles and wash hands. | |
| l. Praise child for any assistance or cooperation offered. | |
| 6. Ostomy care using an appliance: Proceed as in steps 5a and 5b, then: | ***Special Considerations:*** *Encourage child's participation whenever possible.* |
| a. Remove pouch and barrier as a single unit, peeling gently from periphery to center, and discard in appropriate trash receptacle. | This method facilitates ease of removal.<br>***Special Considerations:*** *If wafer-type barrier was used, check skin-side for signs of erosion that indicate seepage of ostomy drainage because of poor adhesion of wafer.* |
| Proceed as in steps 5d to 5g, then:<br>b. Apply one or two-piece unit:<br>▪ Using template, cut hole in barrier no greater than 1/16-1/18 inch larger than stoma. Stoma paste may be carefully applied in this narrow space. | ***Special Considerations:*** *Be sure that skin has remained thoroughly clean and dry before attempting to apply unit or adhesion will be lost. Do not allow paste to extend underneath wafer. Wiping peristomal skin with skin sealant immediately before unit application will enhance adhesion (allow several seconds for sealant to dry). Wrinkles or gaps under a wafer will allow seepage of effluent, loss of adhesion, and skin breakdown.* |
| ▪ If using two-piece unit, attach pouch to barrier.<br>▪ Center hole over stoma and press entire unit carefully from stoma base to periphery of barrier, assuring a smooth wrinkle-free contact with skin.<br>▪ Apply clamp or elastic band to end of bag. | Two-piece units usually have a flange or collar on both barrier and pouch. Be sure these are properly snapped and securely together to prevent leakage of ostomy drainage.<br>***Special Considerations:*** *Instruct parents that rapid physical growth during baby's first year, accompanied by stomal growth, necessitates frequent checks with template for proper fit.* |

| Steps | Rationale |
|---|---|
| c. Assist child with dressing in nonconstrictive clothing. | Clothing without tight waistbands reduces risk of stomal abrasion and dislodging of pouch.<br>***Special Considerations:*** *One piece playsuits work well with infants and toddlers. They eliminate constriction and prevent disturbing the appliance. A cloth pouch cover in bright colors or juvenile prints can be purchased or sewn to conceal pouch contents for aesthetic appeal to older children and parents.* |
| 7. Irrigation of colostomy pouch between changes of unit: | ***Special Considerations:*** *Pouch irrigation may be carried out with emptying of drainage or as child/family preference indicates.* |
| a. Provide for patient privacy. | Even if the child is too young to be concerned, parents invariably appreciate efforts to preserve their child's dignity. |
| b. Arrange all supplies on bedside table. | Organization promotes a calm, orderly approach, setting the tone for patient and family to gain control. |
| c. Remove closure from end of pouch.<br>d. GENTLY express drainage into collection receptacle and observe characteristics/amount (see Implementation step 5g). | ***Special Considerations:*** *Empty pouch when one third full of gas or drainage to prevent overdistension and leaks.* |
| e. Using squeeze bottle or 60 cc syringe of warm water, thoroughly wash out pouch, allowing to drain in collection receptacle. | ***Special Considerations:*** *Attaching a 6"-12" length of flexible rubber tubing to the syringe is helpful in irrigating narrow spaces along the top of the pouch and around the stoma in small babies. Use of stiff tubing may traumatize stoma. Infants may experience significant drop in body temperature and subsequent cold stress with undressing and use of room temperature water. Therefore, keep infant's upper body covered and do not prolong procedure. Premature and sick infants may need to have the procedure carried out under a radiant warmer.* |
| f. Assess condition of stoma (see Implementation, step 5e).<br>g. Assure that barrier is still secure. Inspect pouch for leaks at juncture with barrier and tears elsewhere. | |
| h. Before clip is applied, dry outside with toilet tissue. Also use tissue as a wick to dry lower 2 inches of inside of pouch. | Drying helps prevent odor formation.<br>***Special Considerations:*** *Odor formation may also be reduced by rinsing inner pouch with dilute mouthwash, taking care to avoid stoma during the initial postoperative period.* |
| i. Gently press pouch flat to expel air, and reapply clamp or elastic band to end.<br>j. Assist child with any additional cleansing needed from procedure.<br>k. Assist child with dressing in nonconstrictive clothing. (See 6c above.) | |
| l. Give child praise and encouragement for any cooperation or assistance offered during procedure. | ***Special Considerations:*** *Reassure parents that it will not harm stoma to hold child close and give hugs.* |
| 8. Irrigation of colostomy stoma (usually confined to preoperative or prediagnostic study use in children). | Routine irrigation for control of colostomy is not done in children. They are seldom independent in self-care, their ostomies are often temporary, and they are at increased risk for fluid/electrolyte disturbances secondary to irrigation, as with enemas (Connors, 1987). |
| a. Provide for child's privacy.<br>b. Assemble all equipment on treatment room table, including prewarmed solution of volume and type as ordered by physician. | |
| c. Attach cone to irrigating set and lubricate well. | Lubrication reduces risk of mucosal injury.<br>***Special Considerations:*** *A rubber baby bottle nipple, with enlarged hole, may be used in lieu of a cone.* |
| d. Purge air from set, including cone. | This step prevents introduction of air into intestines. |
| e. Enlist the assistance of a coworker to provide any necessary restraint of child. | |
| f. Position child. | ***Special Considerations:*** *Infant without a pouch may rest on a folded bathblanket or pillow alongside a bedpan or may be supported on a bedpan with padded edges. Child with a pouch may lie supine with the end of pouch draped into bedpan.* |
| g. Gently insert cone approximately ½"-1" into stoma in direction of ascending intestine, and allow solution to flow in slowly (no faster than 100 cc/minute). | Rapid influx of solution can precipitate cramping and premature expulsion of contents.<br>***Special Considerations:*** *Insert enough of cone to prevent leakage of solution during procedure.* |

| Steps | Rationale |
|---|---|
| h. Remove cone and allow ostomy to drain into bedpan. | |
| i. Evaluate volume and characteristics of return. | |
| j. Proceed with ostomy care as decribed in steps 5, 6, or 7 as appropriate. | |
| k. Observe child closely for signs of fluid/electrolyte disturbance (see Skill 64). | |
| 9. Observe child and parents for psychological response to procedures and for readiness to participate in self-care. | Inadequately addressed issues of child/parent grief, anger, and fear seriously hamper regaining control and maintaining a positive body image. ***Special Considerations:*** *Be alert to facial expressions and body language that may indicate an aversion to ostomy.* |
| 10. Provide on-going teaching and reinforcement of instructions. | Learning promotes independence. |
| 11. Encourage return demonstrations and evaluate child/parent skills. | |

| Evaluation Outcomes | Observational Guidelines |
|---|---|
| 1. Peristomal skin is free of maceration and rash. | Observe skin for integrity. Note its similarity to rest of child's abdominal skin. |
| 2. Stoma is healthy and functional. | Observe stoma regularly for evidence of stricture and excoriation. Note edema, elevation, color, and bleeding. |
| 3. Postoperative complications are minimized by early recognition and management. | Evaluate ostomy regularly for evidence of dysfunction, obstruction, and circulatory impairment. Note characteristics of effluent and appropriateness to type/location of ostomy. Promptly report any abnormal findings to physician. |
| 4. Child/parents are able to participate in care such as assessment of stoma, skin care, and appliance changes/irrigation. | Observe parent's demonstration of these skills. If child is old enough, observe his or her ability to assist with care. |
| 5. Child will have positive self-image restored/maintained. | Observe child's nonverbal cues during ostomy care, ability to enter into play with other children, and interaction with family. |

## Documentation

Chart condition of stoma and peristomal skin, amount and characteristics of ostomy drainage, whether appliance changed or simply flushed, type of barrier used. For stoma irrigation: chart type, volume and temperature of solution used, amount and characteristics of return and patient tolerance of procedure. Document pertinent verbal and nonverbal cues for patient and/or family that indicate degree of acceptance and subsequent ability to provide self-care.

UNIT IX

## PRODUCT REFERENCES AND TEACHING RESOURCES

### Books

Wong D and Whaley L: Clinical manual of pediatric nursing, ed 3, St Louis, 1990, The CV Mosby Co.
Home care instructions: Performing clean intermittent self-catheterization; Caring for the child with a colostomy.

### Products

Convatec—A Squibb Company
CN 5254
Princeton, NJ 08543-5254
Offers "Little Ones" Pediatric Ostomy Product Line.

### Organizations

The United Ostomy Association
2001 W. Beverly Blvd
Los Angeles, CA 90057
Booklet—Chris has an ostomy

## REFERENCES


Adams D and Selekof J: Children with ostomies: comprehensive care planning, Pediatr Nurs 12(6):429-433, 1986.

Behrman RE and Vaughan WE, editors: Nelson textbook of pediatrics, ed 13, Philadelphia, 1987, WB Saunders Co.

Boarini J: Principles of stoma care for infants, J Enterostomal Ther 16(1):21-25, 1989.

Bolinger B: The adolescent patient, In Broadwell D and Jackson B, editors: Principles of ostomy care, St Louis, 1982, The CV Mosby Co.

Bristoll SL et al: The mythical danger of rapid urinary drainage, Am J Nurs, 89(3):344-345, 1989.

Broadwell D: Peristomal skin integrity, Nurs Clin North Am 22(2):321-332, 1987.

Burkitt D and Randall J: Catheterisation: urethral trauma, Nurs Times 83(43):59-63, 1987.

Burkitt D and Randall J: Safe procedures, Nurs Times 83(43):65-66, 1987.

Chezem J: Urinary diversion, Nurs Clin North Am 11(3):445-456, 1976.

Connors M: Colostomy care, Ostomy Quarterly 24(2):6-7, 1987.

Deegen S: Intermittent catheterisation for children, Nurs Times 81(14):72-74, April, 1985.

Epstein S: Cost effective application of the Centers for Disease Control guideline for prevention of catheter-associated urinary tract infections. Reprinted from the Twelfth Annual Educational Conference of Association for Practitioners in Infection Control, Cincinnati, Ohio, May 13-17, 1985.

Erickson P: The art of pouching, Nurs Clin North Am 22(2):311-320, 1987.

Hutchinson S and Shipes E: The psychosocial care of children with stomas: a primer for home and school, Springfield, Ill, 1981, Charles C Thomas.

Jeter K: The pediatric patient: ostomy surgery in growing children. In Broadwell D and Jackson B, editors: Principles of ostomy care, St Louis, 1982, The CV Mosby Co.

Martin et al: Fatal poisoning from sodium phosphate enema: case report and experimental study, JAMA 257:2190-2192, 1987.

Merenstein GB and Gardner SL: Handbook of neonatal intensive care, ed 2, St Louis, 1989, The CV Mosby Co.

Metheny N et al: Effectiveness of pH measurements in predicting feeding tube placement, Nurs Res 38(5):280-285, 1989.

Motta G: Life-span changes: implications for ostomy care, Nurs Clin North Am, 22(2):333-339, 1987.

Nurses Drug Alert, Infant death from enemas, Am J Nurs 87(9):1194-1195, 1987.

Perry AG and Potter PA: Clinical nursing skills and techniques, ed 2, St Louis, 1990, The CV Mosby Co.

Petillo M: The patient with a urinary stoma: nursing management and education, Nurs Clin North Am 22(2):263-279, 1987.

Rideout B: The patient with an ileostomy: nursing management and education, Nurs Clin North Am 22(2):253-262, 1987.

Ruge D: Catheter-related UTIs: what's the best way to treat them? Nursing 17(12):50-51, 1987.

Sugar EC and Firlit CF: Urinary prophylaxis and postoperative care of children at home with an indwelling catheter after hypospadius repair, Urology 32(5):418-420, 1988.

Watson P et al: Comprehensive care of the ileostomy patient, Nurs Clin North Am 11(3):427-444, 1976.

Webster P: Special babies, Community Outlook 7(19):21-22, 1985.

Whaley L and Wong D: Essentials of pediatric nursing, ed 3, St Louis, 1989, The CV Mosby Co.

Wong D and Whaley L: Clinical manual of pediatric nursing, ed 3, St Louis, 1990, The CV Mosby Co.

Yahle M: An ostomy information clinic, Nurs Clin North Am 11(3):28-31, 1976.

# UNIT X Mobility and Immobility

# SKILL 71 Assisting Ambulation with Crutches

*Frances Lynn McCullough*

Ambulating with crutches is initially viewed by many children as a fun and exciting experience. They often do not understand the reason for crutches and the consequences of improper use. They also do not realize the extent to which the crutches will limit their activities. The use of crutches may be temporary or permanent depending upon the physical impairment creating the need for crutches.

Although instructing a child in the use of crutches, including the fitting, is generally the responsibility of the physical therapist, nurses must be able to reinforce this teaching and be knowledgeable enough to assist and supervise the child in ambulation. There are also situations when a physical therapist is not available.

## NURSING DIAGNOSES

Potential for injury related to altered mobility, improper ambulation assistance devices, or environmental hazards; Potential for self-care deficit (bathing, dressing, toileting) related to impaired physical mobility and loss of independence; Activity intolerance related to pain and fatigue.

| Steps | Rationale |
|---|---|
| **Assessment** | |
| 1. Obtain health history data that may affect ambulation:<br>a. Age/developmental level including physical maturation/gross motor skills.<br>b. Other health problems or conditions, such as paralysis, contractures, and developmental delay. | This data is necessary to plan appropriate interventions.<br>***Special Considerations:*** *Children under the age of 6 years or with other physical or mental handicaps usually require a walker because they cannot manipulate crutches.* |
| 2. Review physician's order for type of crutch-gait to be used e.g., non-weightbearing, partial weightbearing, touchdown weightbearing, four-point, and time to be initiated. | Proper use of crutches and ordered crutch-gait is necessary to prevent loss of surgical correction, loss of fracture reduction, delayed healing, and increased pain. Appropriate crutch-gait is important for children with permanent physical limitations so that they can ambulate safely and with the most efficient gait possible. Ambulation and crutch-gait training are initiated only when ordered by the physician. The type of crutch-gait will depend on child's stability, weightbearing allowed on affected extremity, and goal of crutch-gait (Whaley and Wong, 1991). |
| 3. Assess type of crutches to be used: | Selection is determined by individual needs. |
| a. Axillary. | This is the most commonly used type when crutches are needed for a short period of time. |
| b. Forearm (Lofstrand). | This type is usually used by individuals with permanent handicaps. |
| c. Platform or trough. | This type is used when an upper extremity is involved and weight cannot be taken through hand and wrist but needs to be distributed through the forearm. |
| 4. Review the child's present diagnosis, purpose of crutches, and amount of weightbearing allowed. | These factors will aid in understanding why the crutch-gait ordered was selected and in planning interventions. |

| Steps | Rationale |
|---|---|
| 5. Assess length of immobilization. | The longer the child has been immobilized, the more prone he or she will be to postural hypotension, and endurance and strength will be decreased.<br>***Special Considerations:*** *Exercises to strengthen arms and shoulders while still on bedrest are important if immobilization has been prolonged.* |
| 6. Assess child/family's understanding of need for crutches and crutch-gait ordered. | Knowledge of reason for crutches assists in teaching and gaining cooperation. |

## Planning and Goal Setting

| Steps | Rationale |
|---|---|
| 1. Discuss with family/child the goals of crutch ambulation, crutch device to be used, and type of crutch-gait. | When the goals are understood, better cooperation is obtained and anxiety is decreased.<br>***Special Considerations:*** *Often children who are to be full or partial weight bearing on the affected extremity are reluctant to do so fearing pain or injury. However, it has been shown that in select instances, weightbearing is beneficial and promotes bone healing (Latta and Sarmiento, 1981; Ogden, 1982; Trickey, 1982).* |
| 2. Measure for appropriate axillary crutch size:<br>(As this is the most commonly used type, its use will be the focus of the following discussion.)<br>a. Place child in standing position. If unable to stand, place supine.<br>b. Measure from 1 to 2 inches below axilla to 6 to 10 inches out from sole of foot. | Appropriately sized crutches promote proper posture and weight bearing. Correctly sized crutches prevent pressure on the brachial plexus in the axilla, increase ease in walking, and decrease falls.<br>***Special Considerations:*** *Preoperative fitting and instruction will ease postoperative course for children undergoing elective procedures.* |
| 3. Obtain equipment/supplies<br>a. Crutches.<br>b. Rubber crutch tips.<br>c. Safety belt.<br>d. Proper clothing and shoes. | Collecting supplies improves organization, decreases child/family's anxiety, and optimizes time with child/family.<br>***Special Considerations:*** *Ask the family to bring the child's usual walking shoes or nonskid house shoes. Avoid long, full robes and gowns that could trip the child.* |
| 4. Plan the best time for ambulation with child/family. | Planning enhances a positive outcome and experience for the child. Including the child and family increases their cooperation and allows them to participate in care.<br>***Special Considerations:*** *Time selected should be when child is rested and when pain is manageable. It should not interfere with other therapies, routines, or meals. The presence of a family member may increase the child's cooperation and feeling of security.* |
| 5. Administer analgesic if indicated, with the peak effect timed to coincide with ambulation. | A decrease in pain will increase cooperation with ambulation.<br>***Special Considerations:*** *Analgesic should not cause excessive sedation or dizziness. If it does, ambulation will need to be delayed or a different analgesic used.* |
| 6. Determine location for ambulation to take place and distance to be ambulated. Clear the area of obstacles such as chairs, tables, waste baskets, and throw rugs. An extra wide pathway will be needed. | Planning allows the child to know what is expected. Selection of an area with few obstacles and little traffic promotes safe ambulation.<br>***Special Considerations:*** *Places to rest should be easily accessible. If child knows resting is allowed, his or her anxiety will be reduced.* |
| 7. Develop individualized child/family goals:<br>▪ Child will demonstrate proper crutch-gait ambulation, sitting and rising, and stair-climbing.<br>▪ Child/family will verbalize proper crutch-gait technique and safety considerations for crutchwalking. | |

## Implementation

| Steps | Rationale |
|---|---|
| 1. Adjust crutches according to measurements and secure rubber tips. | Rubber tips are necessary to prevent crutches from sliding on slippery surfaces. |
| 2. With bed at its lowest position, assist child to a sitting position. | |
| 3. Assist child to put on chosen clothing and footwear. | Allowing a child to dress self as much as possible fosters independence and allows him or her to participate in care. |

| Steps | Rationale |
|---|---|
| 4. Secure safety belt around child's waist. | Use of safety belt is essential to provide a secure hold on the child and to prevent falls. |
| 5. Assist child to stand and allow him or her to feel secure without dizziness. Support child so that only a permitted amount of weightbearing occurs until crutches are aligned. | Postural hypotension is possible with each position change. Allowing child to gain equilibrium provides security and prevents falls.<br>***Special Considerations:*** *Two people should always be present for the first crutch-walking attempt in case the child becomes dizzy or loses his or her balance.* |
| 6. Align crutches. Assume tripod position. Crutches should be slightly to the side and approximately 10 inches in front of the child (Fig. 71-1). | This allows for a wide base of support and for weight to be borne through the crutches. |
| 7. Verify that crutches are the proper length. Adjust handpiece of axillary crutches so that elbow is flexed no more than 30 degrees. | |
| 8. Instruct child to bear weight on hands and not axilla. | Bearing weight on the axilla results in pressure on the brachial plexus. |
| 9. If possible, demonstrate gait to child. | Different individuals learn best different ways. Younger children and children with learning difficulties often learn best visually. |
| 10. Assist child to ambulate using ordered crutch-gait. | |
| a. Non-Weightbearing (3-point): Crutches and involved leg are moved forward together. Weight is taken on the palms and wrists while the uninvolved leg follows (Fig. 71-2). | Non-weightbearing on an extremity is used when extremity cannot tolerate any weight due to the degree of the injury or instability after surgery. The uninvolved leg bears all the body weight alternately with the crutches. |
| b. Partial Weightbearing (2-point): Involved leg shares weight with palms and wrists (Fig. 71-2). | This gait is used when extremity is stable enough to bear some weight but not the full weight. |
| c. 4-Point Gait: Three points are in contact with the floor at all times. Sequence is right crutch, left foot, left crutch, right foot (Fig. 71-2). | This gait is used when both extremities are involved.<br>***Special Considerations:*** *This is a very slow gait. It must be stressed to the child not to rush or be tempted to alter the gait pattern to move more rapidly.* |
| d. Swing-through and swing-to: Both crutches are moved forward, and the body is lifted and swung to or beyond the crutches (Fig. 71-2). | This gait is used when both lower extremities are paralyzed and braced.<br>***Special Considerations:*** *This is a rapid but less stable gait and is usually reserved for individuals with permanent handicaps.* |
| 11. Assist child with sitting and standing while using crutches.<br>a. Sitting in chair.<br>▪ Position with back to chair.<br>▪ Transfer both crutches to the hand on the involved side.<br>▪ Grasp the armrest with the other hand and lower body into chair (Fig. 71-3). | ***Special Considerations:*** *Choose a firm chair with armrests suitable to the child's size; the child's feet should be able to touch ground. The chair should be placed firmly against the wall or other stationary object to prevent sliding.* |

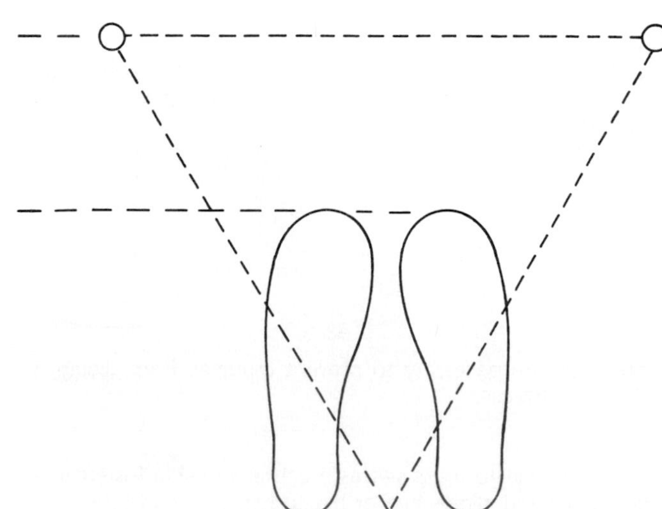

***FIG. 71-1*** Tripod position.

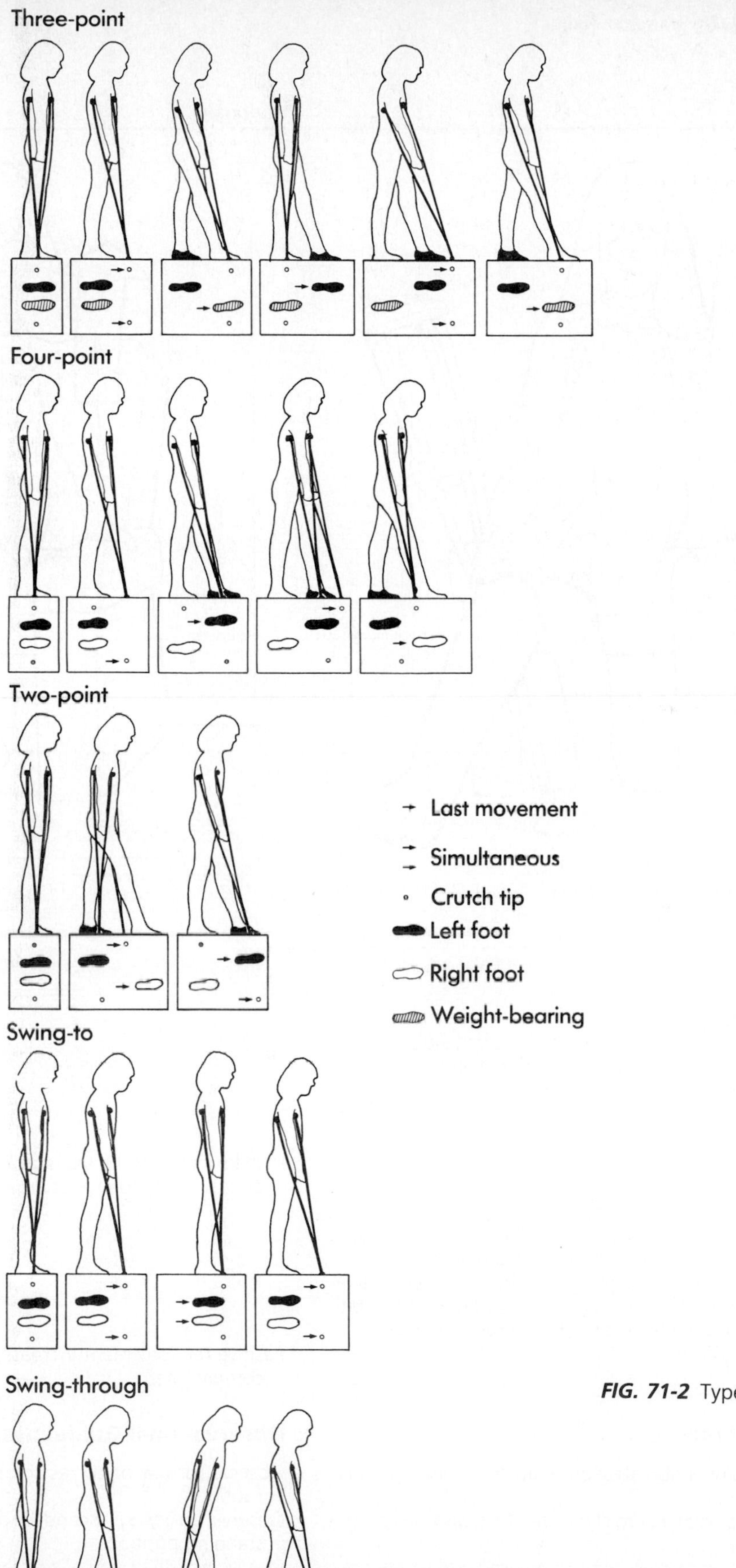


***FIG. 71-2*** Types of crutch gaits.

| Steps | Rationale |
|---|---|

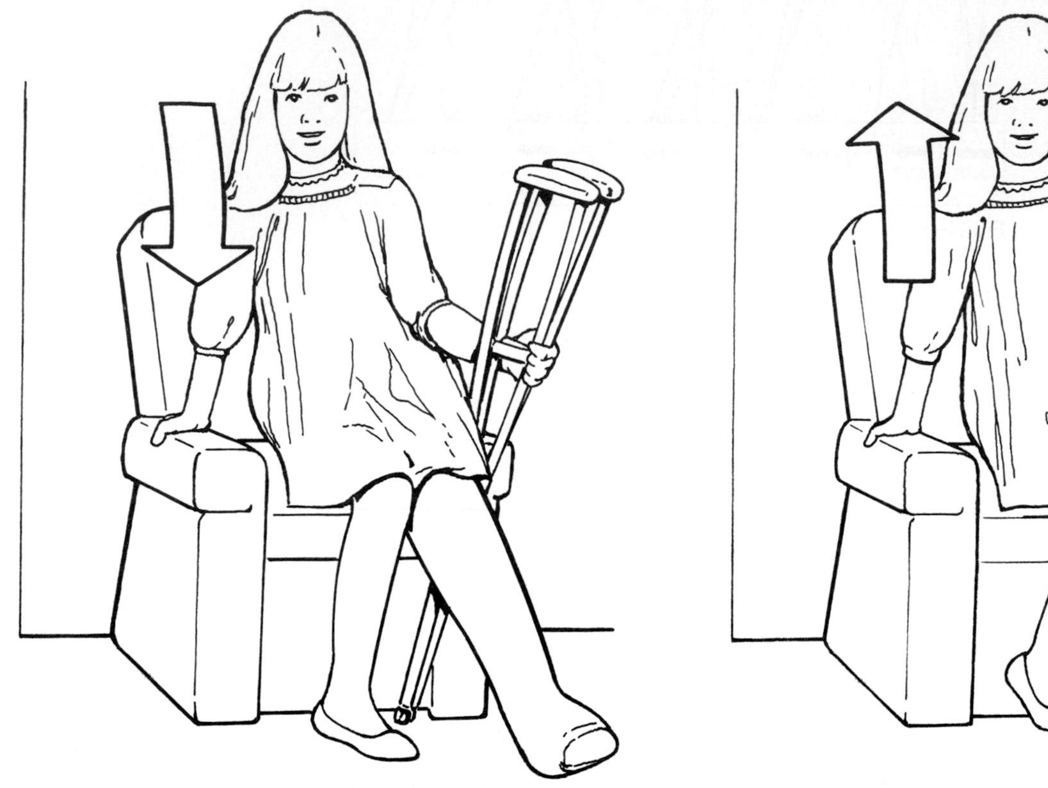

***FIG. 71-3*** Correct positioning and placement of crutches for sitting.

***FIG. 71-4*** Crutches provide support when rising from chair.

b. Rising from chair.
   - Move to edge of chair.
   - Grasp crutches in hand on the involved side.
   - Place uninvolved leg slightly under chair.
   - Grasp armrest with other hand and push to stand (Fig. 71-4.)
   - Reposition crutches.

12. Assist child with stair-climbing. Begin in tripod position with weight on crutches.
    a. Ascending: Place uninvolved leg on step and shift weight to it. Then place crutches on step, bring involved leg up onto step, shift weight, and repeat sequence.
    b. Descending: With weight on uninvolved leg, lower crutches and involved leg down a step first, follow with uninvolved leg, shift weight and repeat sequence.

    *Rationale:* If child must handle stairs at home or at school, this skill must be learned before discharge.

13. Praise child for efforts.

    *Rationale:* Positive reinforcement increases cooperation and feelings of accomplishment.

## Evaluation Outcomes

1. Child successfully ambulates on crutches using the prescribed crutch-gait.
2. Child demonstrates ability to climb stairs, sit, and stand from a sitting position.
3. Family and child understand gait to be used and safety principles related to use of crutches.

## Observational Guidelines

Observe for use of correct crutch-gait, posture, and safety precautions.

Observe ability to ascend and descend stairs, sit, and rise to standing position.

Family and child verbalize steps in prescribed gait and safety principles and demonstrate these before discharge from hospital.

## Documentation

Record type of crutch-gait used, type of crutch device, fit of crutches, and child's tolerance while ambulating with crutches. Note child's ability to use crutches on flat surfaces, ascend/descend stairs, sit, and rise to standing position. Document the family's understanding of crutch-gait and safety principles, as well as any additional teaching performed.

## Home Care Modifications

Instruct family in making the home environment safe for ambulation with crutches, maintaining crutches, and applying principles of crutch ambulation. Tell them to:

1. Check crutch tips for wear. Most drugstores carry crutch tips.
2. Remove throw rugs, toys, and electric cords from child's path.
3. Clean any spills immediately to prevent slips.
4. Keep small children and pets from underfoot.
5. Rearrange furniture if necessary to have room to safely maneuver with crutches.
6. If the child's bedroom is on a second floor, consider making a sleeping area on the first floor for easier escape in case of fire.

# *SKILL* 72 Applying a Spinal Orthosis

*Frances Lynn McCullough*

A number of spinal conditions require the use of a spinal orthosis (brace). An orthosis is often used for 6 to 9 months after spinal surgery until healing is complete. If the orthosis is being used for postoperative immobilization, it should be worn at all times during ambulation to prevent disruption of spinal instrumentation and allow healing to occur. A spinal orthosis may also be used for immobilizing spinal fractures, and as nonoperative treatment for spinal disorders such as scoliosis.

## NURSING DIAGNOSES

Impaired physical mobility related to presence of spinal orthosis; Impaired health maintenance related to lack of knowledge about application, removal and restrictions of brace; Potential for impaired skin integrity related to mechanical irritation of brace; Potential for injury related to restricted mobility with brace; Body image disturbance related to use of spinal orthosis.

| Steps | Rationale |
|---|---|
| **Assessment** | |
| 1. Assess child and family's understanding of need and use for body brace and feelings regarding it. | Most children are very apprehensive about wearing a brace and about their first ambulation. Allowing them to express their feelings and understanding of brace wear provides an opportunity to correct any misinformation. |
| 2. Assess other factors affecting use of the brace:<br>a. Physical condition.<br>b. Age/developmental level.<br>c. Purpose of brace.<br>d. Type of brace.<br>e. Wearing schedule. | Knowledge of these factors is necessary to develop an individualized plan of care for the child and family.<br>***Special Considerations:*** *The physician usually specifies the type of brace and the wearing schedule.* |
| 3. Assess skin for preexisting areas of irritation or preexisting conditions that make the skin more prone to breakdown. | Conditions such as paraplegia, decreased sensation, or little subcutaneous tissue over bony prominences make the skin more prone to breakdown.<br>***Special Considerations:*** *Children with insensate skin may need brace modifications such as special linings to protect the skin.* |

| Steps | Rationale |
|---|---|
| **Planning and Goal Setting** | |
| 1. Plan time with child/family for when the brace will be fitted and teaching performed. | By planning in advance, the child and family are prepared to learn about the brace and its use, allowing more effective discharge planning. |
| 2. Ask family to obtain a close-fitting, cotton T-shirt to be worn under the brace. | A T-shirt is worn to decrease skin irritation. It should be close-fitting because wrinkles will be irritating under the brace. Cotton is best because it will better absorb perspiration. ***Special Considerations:*** *The T-shirt should be long enough to cover all skin under the brace. Most children prefer the sleeveless "tank top" style. If the family has not provided a T-shirt, a stockinette can be used in its place.* |
| 3. Ask family to bring nonskid footwear. | |
| 4. Obtain spinal orthosis (Fig. 72-1). | ***Special Considerations:*** *The two types of braces are the univalve, a one-piece shell with a front and back, hinged at the side; and a bivalve, a two-piece shell that fastens together. These are usually custom ordered from a company that specializes in orthotics.* |
| 5. Refer to Planning and Goal Setting steps 4 to 6 in Skill 71, p. 459. | |
| 6. Develop individualized child/family goals:<br>▪ Child/family will verbalize understanding of purpose and uses of brace.<br>▪ Child/family will demonstrate application and removal of brace.<br>▪ Skin integrity will be maintained under brace.<br>▪ Child will safely ambulate in brace. | |
| **Implementation** | |
| 1. Discuss how the brace will be applied, the sensations that may be experienced (e.g., tightness, feeling of inability to breathe, dizziness when sitting/standing for the first time), and the wearing schedule. Usual schedule for initial adjustment includes:<br>a. Postoperative immobilization or spinal fracture immobilization: 24 hours daily. May be removed for shower daily with physician's order.<br>b. Nonoperative use: 23 out of 24 hours daily or as prescribed by physician. | This assists in reducing fear of the unknown and enhances child/family cooperation. |
| 2. Allow to hold and examine brace if desired. | Becoming familiar with the brace decreases anxiety. ***Special Considerations:*** *Talking to another child who has worn a brace can be helpful in reducing anxiety.* |
| 3. Place T-shirt on child. | A T-shirt should be worn at all times under the brace to prevent skin breakdown. ***Special Considerations:*** *If the child has had elective surgery, it is helpful to inform the family in advance of this need.* |
| 4. Logroll child to the side, keeping his or her shoulders and pelvis in the same plane without twisting (see Skill 74). | Logrolling avoids a twisting motion that stresses the spine and could cause further injury or dislodge spinal instrumentation. ***Special Considerations:*** *Children who have had spinal fractures or spinal surgery should always be logrolled.* |
| 5. Slide the brace or posterior shell of the bivalved brace under the child as far as possible with iliac crest pads aligned over the anterior iliac crests (see Fig. 72-2). | For proper fit, the crest pads for the brace must rest on the anterior iliac crests of the child. |
| 6. While stabilizing brace in place, logroll child to supine position. | |
| 7. Check position of brace.<br>a. Iliac crest pads of brace must be well down on the anterior iliac crests of child.<br>b. For univalve brace, check that brace is centered over spine and buckle tightly (Fig. 72-3).<br>c. For bivalve brace, check that posterior shell is centered over spine, apply the anterior shell, and buckle tightly (Figs. 72-4 and 72-5). | The brace must be positioned correctly and fit tightly to provide proper immobilization and minimize discomfort and irritation. ***Special Considerations:*** *Pulling on the T-shirt from top and bottom can help remove wrinkles and prevent pinching of the skin while the brace is being tightened.* |
| 8. Logroll to other side if necessary to position brace properly. | |
| 9. Assess child's tolerance of brace. | ***Special Considerations:*** *Children often complain of being unable to breathe when adapting to the brace. Explain the need for tightness and assure them that this sensation will pass.* |

A

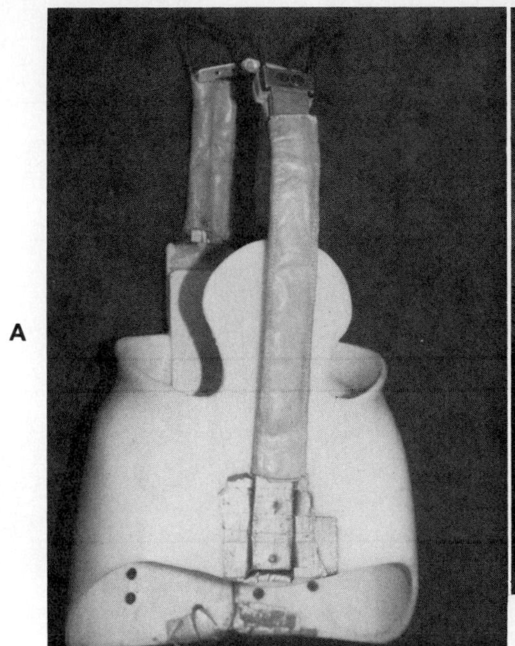

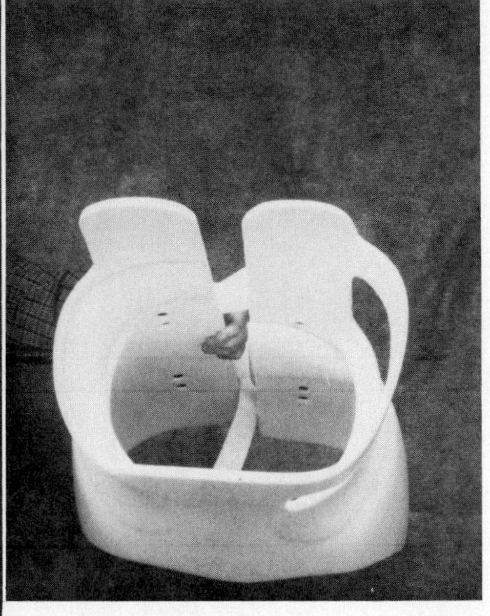

B

C

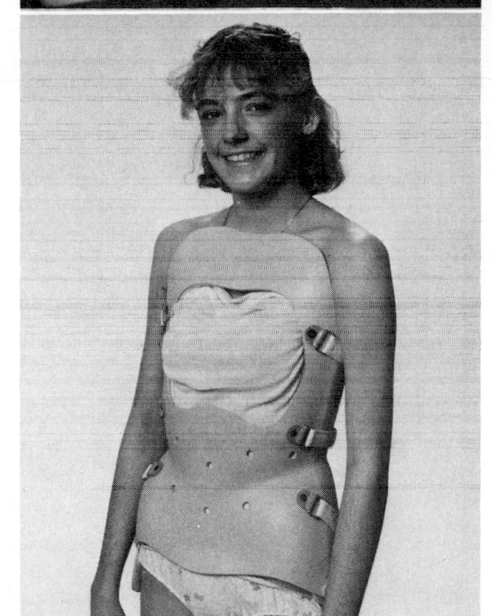

***FIG. 72-1*** Types of orthoses: **A,** The Milwaukee brace. **B,** A low profile (Boston) univalve brace. **C,** Anterior view of a bivalve brace.

(**C** from Smith M, Goodman J, and Ramsey N: Child and family: Concepts of nursing practice, ed 2, St Louis, 1987, The CV Mosby Co).

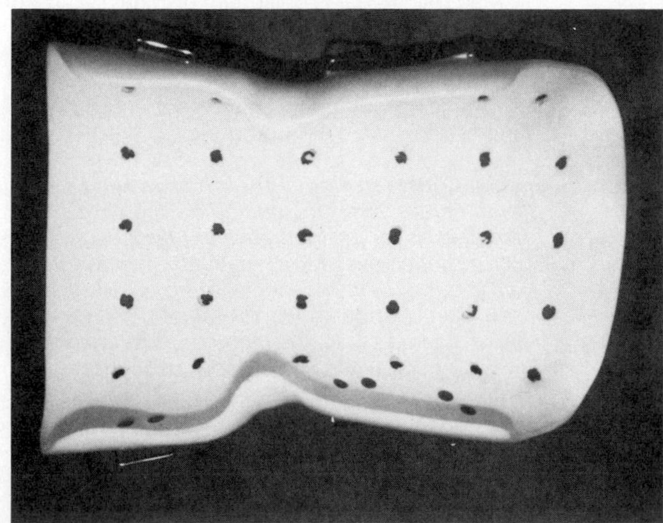

***FIG. 72-2*** Posterior shell of bivalve brace.

| Steps | Rationale |
| --- | --- |

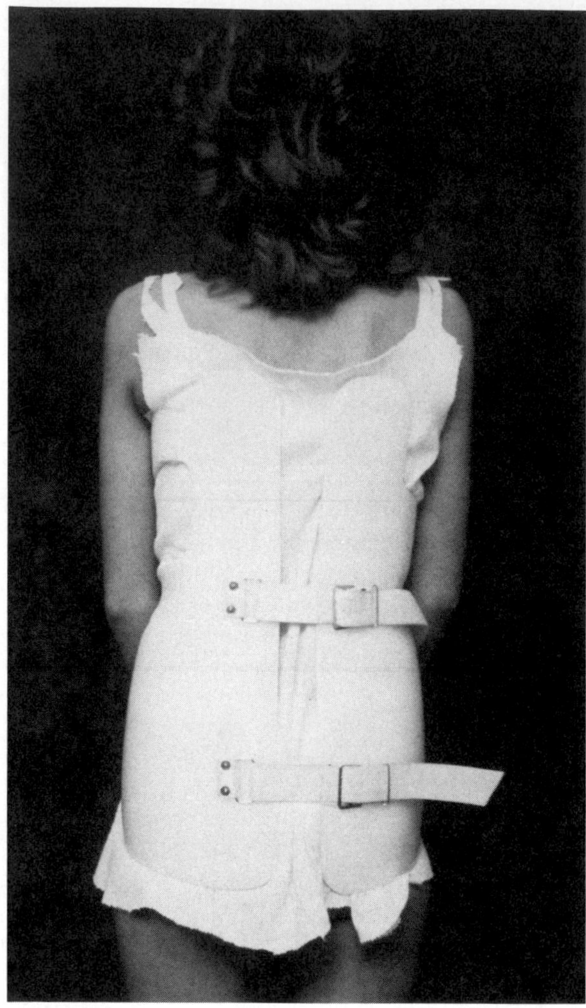

***FIG. 72-3*** Univalve brace is centered over spine and buckled securely.

***FIG. 72-4*** Anterior shell is attached to side of bivalve.

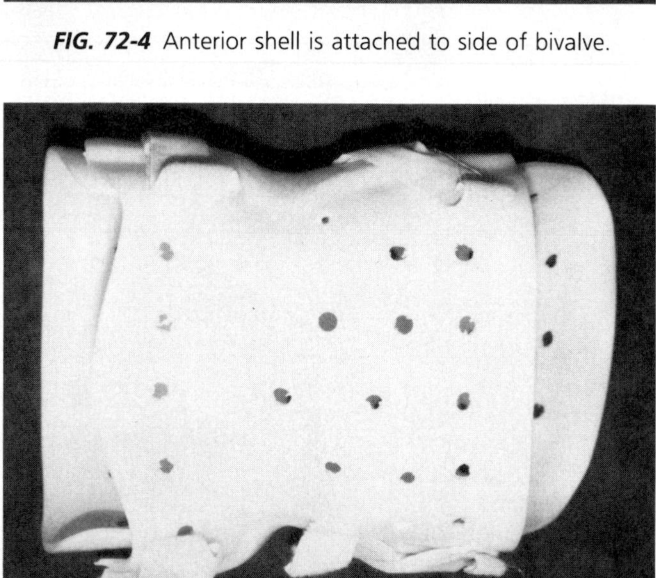

***FIG. 72-5*** Anterior and posterior shells buckled.

| Steps | Rationale |
| --- | --- |
| 10. Assist child to a standing position and allow him or her to become steady before proceeding. | Postural hypotension is possible with each position change. Allowing child to gain equilibrium provides security and prevents falls. |
| 11. Encourage a normal walking posture with the child looking ahead and not at his or her feet. | Walking in a slumped position inhibits breathing and causes earlier fatigue. |
| 12. During ambulation, observe gait (steady/unsteady, limp, ataxia, amount of assistance needed), tolerance, and signs of fatigue, pain, or discomfort. | Observation will determine nature of subsequent ambulations and assist in evaluating progress. |
| 13. After ambulation, assist the child to a chair or return him or her to bed. Remove brace if the child is at maximum tolerance or if this is the first time the brace has been worn. The child should be supine and logrolled to remove brace. | ***Special Considerations:*** *The initial wearing schedule to adapt to the brace varies depending on the child's tolerance and if the brace is for postoperative or nonoperative immobilization. For postoperative status, gradually increase the wearing time while out of bed, then increase up to full-scheduled time in a few days. Nonoperative tolerance develops more gradually, increasing up to full wearing schedule in about 2 weeks.* |
| 14. Inspect skin after brace removal. | Skin tolerance is important to assess immediately after wearing the brace to identify areas that will be prone to breakdown or require brace modifications. |

| Steps | Rationale |
|---|---|
| | ***Special Considerations:*** *Expect some redness, particularly over iliac crests. Redness should disappear within 30 minutes. If it does not, decrease the amount of time that brace is worn the next time, and/or assess whether the brace needs to be modified.* |
| 15. Rub reddened areas with alcohol. | Reddened areas are those receiving the most pressure and are those areas the most susceptible to breakdown. Applications of alcohol will help toughen the skin. ***Special Considerations:*** *If the child objects to the smell of alcohol, witch hazel or an astringent high in alcohol may be substituted.* |
| 16. Provide positive reinforcement for the child's efforts during brace application, ambulation, and brace removal. | Positive reinforcement is important to increase the child's self-esteem and sense of accomplishment. |
| 17. On future applications, allow the family to apply the brace with supervision. | Allowing the family to perform the care before discharge provides an opportunity to assess their understanding and ability, and it increases their confidence in their ability to care for child at home. |

| Evaluation Outcomes | Observational Guidelines |
|---|---|
| 1. Child/family verbalize understanding of need for wearing brace. | Ask family to list the purposes of brace. |
| 2. Child/family verbalize correct schedule to wear the brace. | Ask child/family to outline correct wearing schedule. |
| 3. Child/family demonstrate application and removal of the brace. | Observe application and removal of brace including the use of T-shirt, correct placement, correct tightness, and correct inspection of the skin after brace removal. |
| 4. Child tolerates ambulation in brace. | Observe distance ambulated, gait, signs of discomfort, verbalizations of discomfort, fatigue, and pain. |
| 5. Child experiences no skin breakdown from brace. | Observe skin for redness or breakdown under brace. |

## Documentation

Record type and fit of brace. Note the length of time that the brace is worn by the child and the child's level of tolerance. Indicate the skin condition before and after the brace is worn. Document the child/family's understanding of care and any teaching performed.

## Home Care Modifications

1. Although skin breakdown is usually less of a problem the longer the brace is worn, the child/family must be taught to continue skin care throughout the course of brace wear to prevent problems from occurring. Continued observation of the skin is necessary because growth of the child and changes in weight can alter the fit of the brace, which necessitates modifications.
2. The child/family should be instructed to call if the fit of the brace changes for any reason. It is not unusual for the brace to need modifications 2 to 3 weeks after the initial fitting because of the compression of soft-tissue and the resolution of any abdominal distension following surgery. Reiterate to the family that the brace must fit tightly to be effective.
3. For use when adjusting to the brace in the immediate post-operative period, loose-fitting tops and pants with elastic waists (e.g., sweatsuits) are ideal. After the child is sufficiently recovered from surgery, various styles of clothing can be tried. Encourage the child/family to try different brands because they will be cut in different ways. Generally, sizes will increase one or two sizes above what is normally worn to accommodate the brace.
4. The use of a "reacher," which can be obtained through the occupational therapy department of most hospitals, may be helpful until the child becomes confident in squatting in the brace to retrieve dropped articles or articles stored near the floor. Motion takes place at the hips rather than the waist.
5. Avoid tub baths; getting in and out of the tub places too much stress on the spine. With the physician's permission, the brace may be removed for a shower. Very specific instructions should be given. All items needed should be assembled ahead of time. The brace should be removed as the very last step and reapplied in the standing position as soon as the shower is complete. Complete tightening of the brace can be performed in the supine position after the brace is put on while standing. The child should be instructed to move as if the brace were still on (e.g., no bending, twisting, etc.).
6. Activity restrictions vary tremendously from one child to another depending upon what is being treated, the type of surgery performed, the instrumentation used, or if the brace is for nonoperative treatment. In general, activities after surgery are restricted to exclude all sports, roller skating, ice skating, and running activities for 4 to 6 months. It usually takes 6 months for the fusion mass to become solid, after which restrictions can be lifted. A daily walk of increasing distance is begun immediately after discharge. Return to school with no physical education activities is usually permitted 2 to 3 weeks after discharge from the hospital. After 6 to 8 weeks, driving can be resumed. There is no restriction on riding as a passenger in a car, provided seatbelts/shoulder straps are used. If a brace is being used as a nonoperative treatment for scoliosis, no activity restrictions may be placed on the child. It is up to the physician to set specific restrictions.

# SKILL 73 Transferring and Transporting the Nonambulatory Child

*Frances Lynn McCullough*

There are a number of reasons why a child may be nonambulatory. These reasons include age, illness requiring activity limitations, fractures, traction, casting, spinal surgery or injury, and postoperative status. The infant who is nonambulatory because he or she is too young to walk requires different techniques of transport than the child immobilized in traction. There are more choices of transport vehicles for children than for adults.

## NURSING DIAGNOSES

Potential for injury related to lack of knowledge about transportation of the immobilized child; Impaired physical mobility related to pain, neuromusculoskeletal impairment or developmental level.

| Steps | Rationale |
|---|---|
| **Assessment** | |
| 1. Determine child's age, developmental level, and cognitive level. | Knowledge of these factors facilitates planning for an efficient and safe transfer. |
| 2. Assess current physical/medical condition; reason for immobilization; goal of transfer/transport. | Awareness of the child's physical condition, limitations, etc., guides selection of a safe method of transfer and transport. |
| 3. Determine if physician has ordered transfer and/or transport method. | Children restricted to bedrest or in traction should have a physician's order that permits transfer or transport for a specific purpose. |
| 4. Determine method of transfer and transport best suited to situation. Possible methods include bed, crib, stretcher, wheelchair, wagon, stroller, and other mobilization devices. | ***Special Considerations:*** *Infant/child should not be transported off the unit for tests, etc., in one's arms for both safety and legal reasons. The carrier could trip and fall, injuring the child and placing the institution in a liability situation.* |
| 5. Assess presence of IV lines, oxygen, catheters, nasogastric tubes, etc. | The presence of these necessitates special handling that requires advanced planning.<br>***Special Considerations:*** *Portable ventilators can be used to provide mobility for the ventilator-dependent child.* |
| **Planning and Goal Setting** | |
| 1. Gather and inspect equipment:<br>a. Wagons with raised sides.<br>b. Stretchers with siderails and safety belts.<br>c. Wheelchairs and strollers with safety belts.<br>d. Pillows, blankets, towel rolls, etc., for positioning and comfort. | Gathering equipment in advance enhances safety and efficiency. |
| 2. Obtain personnel to assist if needed. | It may be necessary to have adequate assistance to protect the nurse and the child from injury. |
| 3. Prepare child/family for anticipated procedure. Describe the method of transfer and reassure the child of adequate support of his or her body. | Including the child/family encourages their cooperation and helps reduce anxiety. Older children and those with a heavy cast may be especially afraid of being dropped.<br>***Special Considerations:*** *Administering pain medication prior to the transfer/transport of child who is experiencing pain with movement may enhance the child's tolerance of the procedure.* |
| 4. Develop a nursing goal of care:<br>▪ To transfer and transport child safely. | |

| Steps | Rationale |
|---|---|

## Implementation

### *Infant/toddler*

1. Methods of transfer:
   a. Horizontal carry.
      - Comfortably position child's head in bend of own elbow. Maintain child's head and back in alignment by supporting with own forearm, firmly grasping thigh and buttocks with hand (Fig. 73-1*A*).
      - Free hand may be used for other activities or may be placed under child's back for cuddling and comforting.
      - Align face to same parallel plane with child's face (*en face* position).

   b. Football carry.
      - Comfortably position child's head in the palm of the hand, supporting the back on own forearm with child's buttocks securely held between the elbow and body (Fig. 73-1*B*).

   c. Shoulder carry.
      - Carefully move the child into an upright position, supporting his or her weight with one hand or forearm under the buttock (Fig. 73-1*C*).
      - Support the child against own chest by holding the newborn's head and neck or the older infant's back.

The football carry is suitable only for small infants. The horizontal carry is suitable for an infant, and the shoulder carry is suitable for infants and toddlers.

2. Methods of transport:
   a. Parent's arms.

Children are more secure and less anxious in their parents' arms.
***Special Considerations:*** *Check with the facility's policy regarding allowing parents to carry a child to diagnostic departments or surgery.*

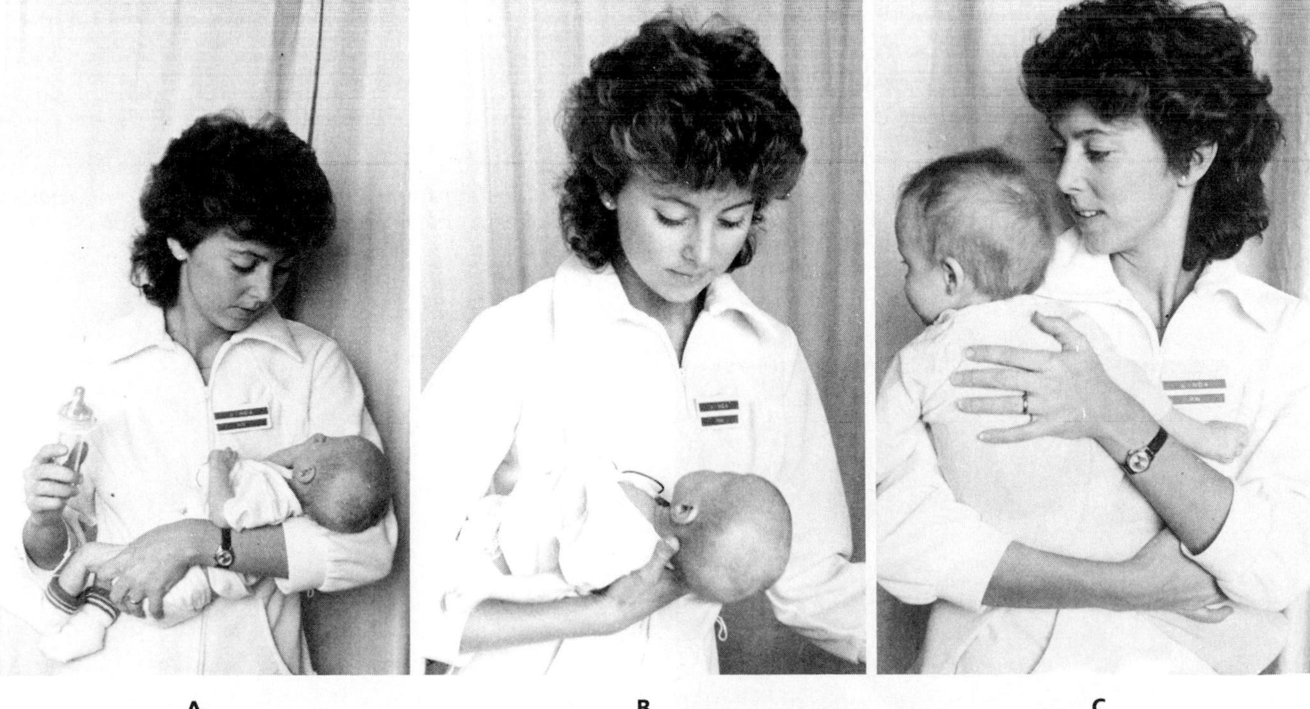

A B C

***FIG. 73-1*** **A,** The horizontal carry protects against sudden infant movement. **B,** Use of the football carry to transport the infant. **C,** The shoulder carry allows close head-to-head contact.
From Whaley LF and Wong DL: Nursing care of infants and children, ed 3, 1987, St Louis, The CV Mosby Co.

| Steps | Rationale |
|---|---|
| b. With parent in wheelchair. | Sitting in a parent's lap in a wheelchair is comforting for the child and guards against the possibility of the parent tripping or falling. |
| c. Wagon or stroller, stretcher, bassinet, or other mobilization devices. | These methods are safe for transporting the child, provided seatbelts and/or siderails are used. ***Special Considerations:*** *Strollers should have a strap between the legs to prevent the child from sliding down in the stroller. Never leave a child unsupervised in a transport device.* |
| d. Crib with siderails up and child not standing. | A standing child could fall, bump on the crib sides, and be injured. |

***Child***

| Steps | Rationale |
|---|---|
| 1. Methods of transfer/transport: a. Transfer of small child. ▪ Place child in sitting position. ▪ Place one arm around shoulders and under arms. ▪ Place one arm under knees. ▪ Lift to appropriate seating or vehicle for transport. | ***Special Considerations:*** *Maintain good body mechanics during transfers to prevent injury.* |
| ▪ Fasten safety belts and restrain as needed. | ***Special Considerations:*** *If a wheelchair is not equipped with a safety belt, a jacket or vest restraint may be used.* |
| b. Transfer of older child. ▪ Place child in sitting position. ▪ One person stands behind child and places his or her arms under child's arms and across child's chest. ▪ Second person stands in front of child and places hands under child's knees/thighs. ▪ Lift and transfer child simultaneously. ▪ Elevate extremity, if needed. ▪ Fasten safety belt and restrain as needed. | Having assistance prevents injury to both the nurse and child. ***Special Considerations:*** *The child with an injured or casted extremity may require two people even if the child is small. One person supports the child while the second supports the extremity.* |
| c. Alternate transfer method to chair. ▪ Place chair/wheelchair at bedside. ▪ Assist child to stand at bedside with weight-bearing as ordered. ▪ Support child and assist to pivot until back is to chair. ▪ Assist to sit. ▪ Elevate extremity if needed. ▪ Fasten safety belt and restrain as needed. | ***Special Considerations:*** *This method is suitable for the child able to bear weight.* |
| d. Transfer from bed to stretcher. ▪ Place stretcher and bed side by side at same height with all wheels locked. | |
| ▪ Place child in supine position, if allowed. ▪ If movement is not restricted, child may move himself or herself from bed to stretcher with assistance. | ***Special Considerations:*** *If supine position is contraindicated, place in comfortable prone or side-lying position.* |

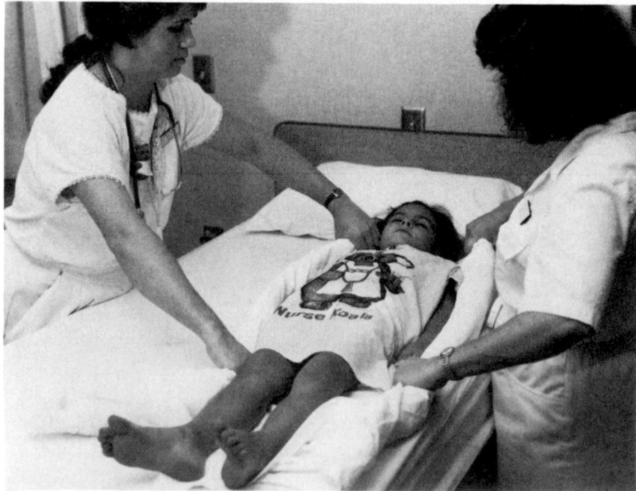


***FIG. 73-2*** Transfer of a small child using a drawsheet.

| Steps | Rationale |
|---|---|
| ▪ If movement is restricted, as after spinal surgery, use drawsheet and two or more people. One person should be positioned at head and one at pelvis, with additional people as needed, depending on the size of child, to move the body by keeping the shoulder and the pelvis in same plane at all times. Move child to edge of bed and then to stretcher (Fig. 73-2). | A child who has had spinal surgery must be transferred keeping the shoulders and pelvis in the same plane at all times without twisting. This prevents injury to the spine and prevents the disruption of spinal instrumentation. After spinal injury or spinal surgery, transfers should be kept to a minimum. |
| ▪ Check body alignment. | |
| ▪ Fasten safety belt and restrain as needed; place covering on child and raise siderails. | |
| e. Transfer in spica cast. | ***Special Considerations:*** *Do not use the crosswise bar on a spica cast to lift or move the child. It is only intended for stabilization and could separate from the cast. If a Bradford frame is used, transport options will be limited to bed, wagon, or stretcher.* |
| ▪ Transfer to transport vehicle (wagon, reclining wheelchair, or stretcher) using a two-person transfer (see Implementation step 1b). The method of transport will depend on the child and position casted (Fig. 73-3). | |
| ▪ Drape child properly to provide warmth and modesty. | |
| ▪ Support casted area as needed with pillows. | |
| ▪ Restrain as needed. | |
| f. Transfer/transport of child in traction: | |
| ▪ If the purpose of traction is to rest a joint or gain motion, it can generally be interrupted for short periods of time without a physician's order. Transport can then be made by a stretcher, wheelchair, or as specified by the physician. | |
| ▪ If the purpose of traction is fracture reduction and immobilization, do not interrupt the traction for transfer/transport. With a physician's order, however, the child can often be transported in the bed with the traction. | Interruption of fracture reduction traction may result in loss of bone alignment, soft tissue damage, and pain for the child. ***Special Considerations:*** *Fracture reduction and immobilization are accomplished with skin or skeletal traction.* |
| ▪ If transporting the child by bed, move slowly and carefully to protect ropes and weights from excessive motion. | Excessive motion can cause pain as well as disrupt fracture alignment or postoperative position. ***Special Considerations:*** *Keep transfers of the child in traction to a minimum.* |

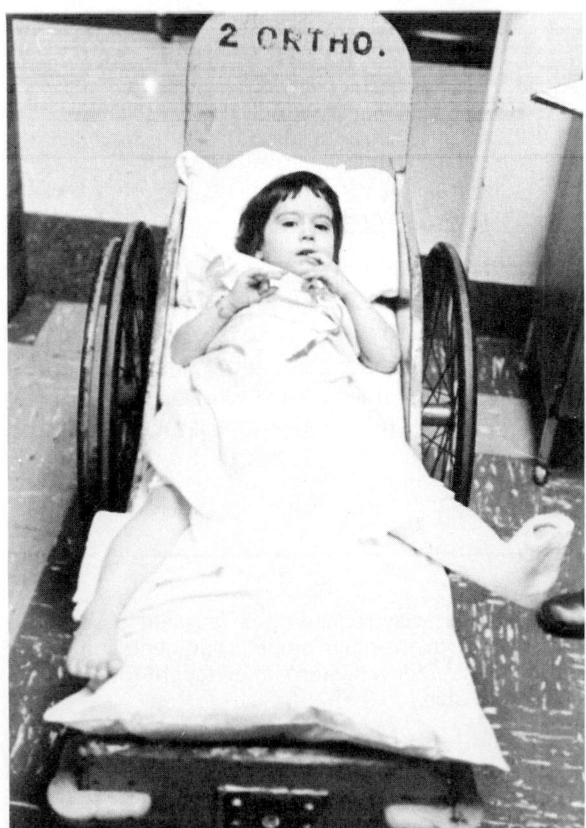


***FIG. 73-3*** A child with a hip spica cast can be placed in a cart to permit movement outside the bedroom.

From Smith M, Goodman J, and Ramsey N: Child and family: concepts of nursing practice, ed 2, New York, 1987, McGraw-Hill, Inc.

### Evaluation Outcomes

1. Child is safely transferred and transported.
2. Child experiences minimal pain and anxiety.

### Observational Guidelines

Note that transfer and transport to intended destination occurred without injury.

Ask child to rate pain experience, if able. For a younger child, note verbal cries and ability to be comforted. Note restlessness, expressions of anxiety.

### Documentation

List method of transfer, method of transport, time, destination, child's tolerance of procedure, and parental teaching.

### Child and Family Teaching

1. Discuss auto safety and use of car seat adaptations before discharge (Shesser, 1985) (see Skill 45).

### Home Care Modifications

1. It is important to determine the best method of transport (wagon, stroller, standard wheelchair, child-size wheelchair, reclining wheelchair, etc.) before discharge so that the family can provide this at home after having an opportunity to practice in the hospital.
2. The use of a mechanics creeper can give immobilized small children, especially those in a spica cast, a measure of independent mobility. The creeper should be large enough to not be overbalanced by the weight of the child and to support the child. Family may want to construct a larger version for their child (Hilt and Schmidt, 1975).

# *SKILL* 74 Positioning the Child in Bed

*Frances Lynn McCullough*

For the child in a cast, in traction, recovering from surgery, or unable to move himself or herself for any reason, positioning is important to obtain the optimum benefit and to prevent complications of immobilization such as skin irritation, constipation, contractures, respiratory congestion, or edema. For the child who is unable to verbalize his or her discomfort or to change his or her own position, keen observation is needed.

### NURSING DIAGNOSES

Impaired physical mobility related to cast, traction, surgery, pain, or developmental level; Potential for impaired skin integrity related to presence of cast, traction, or physical immobility; Potential for injury related to improper positioning; Potential for disuse syndrome related to neuromuscular impairment, prescribed immobility in bed or pain.

| Steps | Rationale |
|---|---|
| **Assessment** | |
| 1. Assess age and developmental level of child. | Younger children may require more frequent observation and repositioning to maintain proper alignment and to prevent complications. Older children can be taught to maintain alignment when able. |
| 2. Review physician's orders for positioning specifications. | |
| 3. Assess physical condition and factors contributing to positioning needs, including preexisting conditions such as impaired sensation, paralysis, obesity, emaciation, and/or contractures. | Physical condition and factors such as recent spinal surgery or injury, traction, casting, skin ulcers, respiratory infection, potential for excessive secretions/reflux/vomiting, and the child's ability to assist will help determine interventions needed to maintain proper positioning. |

| Steps | Rationale |
|---|---|
| 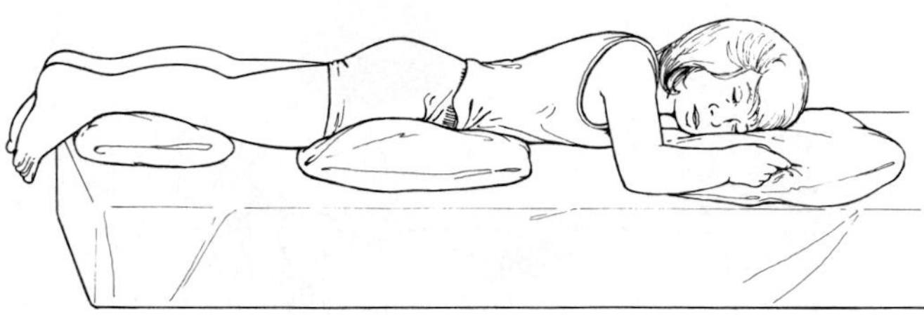 *FIG. 74-3* Child lying in prone position. | 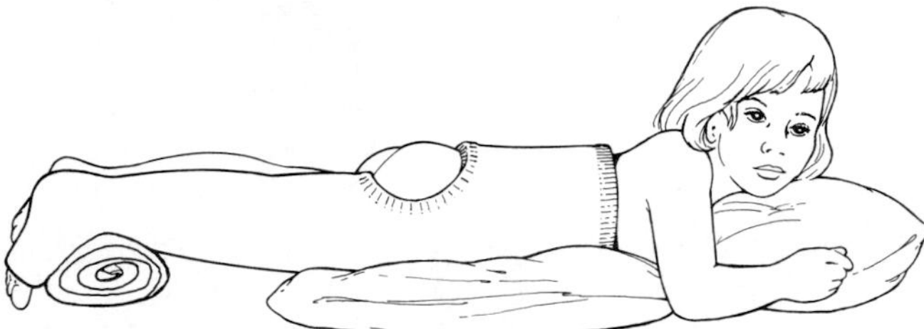 *FIG. 74-4* Prone position for child in hip spica cast. |
| | ***Special Considerations:*** *This position is contraindicated in child with respiratory distress, abdominal surgery, joint contractures, and/or cervical injury. For the child with a tracheostomy, positioning prone is difficult but sometimes done to prevent reflux (see Skill 63). A child who has undergone spinal surgery should not be placed in prone position without a physician's order.* |
| ▪ Move child's body toward the side and foot of bed prior to turning prone. | Moving the child to the side allows proper body placement in the center of the bed after the turn. Moving the child down allows feet to freely hang over end of mattress after turning. ***Special Considerations:*** *May use small pillow to elevate feet if knee extension is not required.* |
| ▪ Turn prone with arms at the side of the body. | Positioning the arms at the side prevents them from falling under the chest during the turn and putting uncomfortable stress on the shoulder joint. ***Special Considerations:*** *If there is an injured extremity, always turn the child with the uninjured extremity down on the bed because it will take the body weight during the turn. If the child has a cast that is still damp, handle it with the palms of the hands only, not the fingertips. This prevents pressure areas as the cast dries.* |
| ▪ After turning, turn face toward one side. Position arms with upper arm at 90 degrees from the shoulder and elbow flexed 90 degrees or greater for comfort. | ***Special Considerations:*** *Alternate side to which head is turned.* |
| ▪ Use flat pillow under head and shoulders, if desired. | A flat pillow avoids shoulder rounding and prevents hyperextension of neck. ***Special Considerations:*** *To encourage the development of the neck muscles in the prone position, especially in developmentally delayed children, elevate the chest on a pillow and place a toy in the child's line of vision (Steele, 1988).* |
| ▪ Place small pillow/towel roll under abdomen/pubic area. | This support decreases lordosis and pressure on genitalia. It also promotes chest expansion. ***Special Considerations:*** *Child in spica cast will need a pillow under his or her shoulders, chest, and abdomen to maintain alignment and keep trunk level (Fig. 74-4).* |
| ▪ Place small pillow/towel roll under ankles and lower legs. | This prevents hyperextension of knees. |
| ▪ Allow feet to hang freely over end of mattress or elevate feet with small pillow or towel roll. | This avoids excessive plantar flexion and hip rotation and prevents injuries to toes. |
| d. Side-lying (Lateral). | Properly positioned, side-lying is a position of comfort. It allows increased respiratory expansion and facilitates drainage of secretions or emesis. |
| ▪ Place pillow under head. | A pillow keeps head level with spine. |
| ▪ Pull hips posteriorly toward edge of bed. Tuck pillow or rolled blanket or commercial aid lengthwise along back and tuck in snugly. | This provides support to trunk. |
| ▪ Bring top leg forward and flex to rest on two pillows. | Using two pillows avoids dependent edema and internal hip rotation. |

| Steps | Rationale |
|---|---|

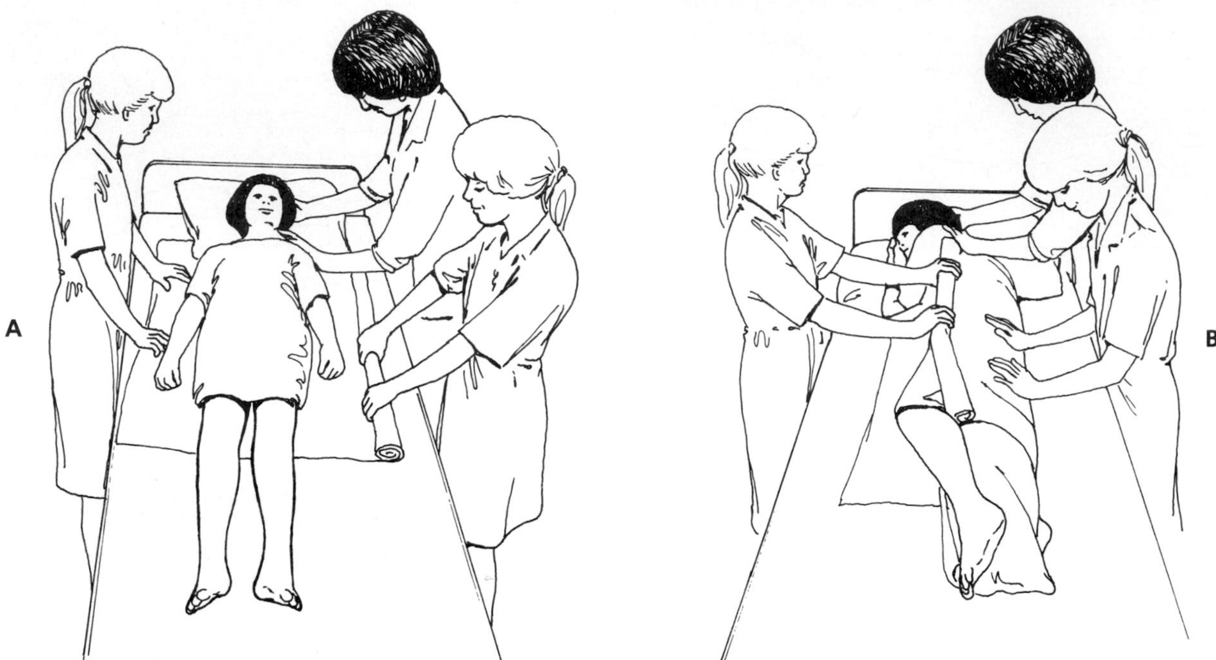


*FIG. 74-5* **A,** Head, neck, shoulders and pelvis are supported during turn. **B,** Turning as a single unit avoids disruption of body alignment.

| Steps | Rationale |
|---|---|
| ▪ Flex bottom leg slightly or keep straight for comfort. | |
| ▪ Pull lower shoulder forward. | This provides balance and prevents undue pressure on the shoulder joint. |
| ▪ Flex bottom arm and place hand under or beside pillow at head. | This prevents hyperextension of elbow joint. |
| ▪ Support top arm on one or two pillows; keep them level with the shoulder. | Support prevents dependent edema and internal rotation of the shoulder. |
| e. Sim's (Semi-prone). | Sim's is useful if prone position is uncomfortable or is not tolerated.<br>***Special Considerations:*** *This position is also more secure for children who are difficult to maintain in a side-lying position.* |
| ▪ Place in side-lying position. | |
| ▪ Flex hip and knee of top leg and rest knee and foot on bed. | Flexed leg serves as support keeping gluteal and abdominal area off bed. |
| ▪ Raise arm on top with shoulder and elbow at 90 degrees and forearm parallel with head. | |
| ▪ Move dependent shoulder slightly posterior. | |
| ▪ Dependent arm is placed at side behind back. | |
| ▪ Allow to turn toward abdomen. | |
| ▪ Use pillow to support abdomen, if needed. | ***Special Considerations:*** *Other pillows usually not required.* |
| f. Logrolling; head, neck, spine, pelvis turned as a unit without twisting (Fig. 74-5). | Prevents stress on spine after spinal injury or surgery.<br>***Special Considerations:*** *Requires one to three people depending on size of child. A drawsheet is helpful.* |
| ▪ Place pillow between legs to keep them slightly apart and parallel. Fold arms across chest. | A slight separation of the legs prevents back strain. Folding the arms across the chest prevents them from falling under the body during turning and disrupting alignment. |
| ▪ Support head, neck, shoulders, and pelvis, and turn as a single unit. | |
| ▪ Place pillows as previously described to maintain supine or side-lying position. | ***Special Considerations:*** *Sim's position is contraindicated after spinal injury or surgery.* |
| ▪ Flex hips and knees slightly, keeping legs parallel. | |
| 2. Use restraints if needed to maintain position (see Skill 51). | ***Special Considerations:*** *Use the minimum that will accomplish the goal. Emphasize that the restraint is a reminder to maintain position and not a punishment.* |

| Steps | Rationale |
|---|---|
| 3. Praise child for cooperation during positioning and for maintaining position. | Praise increases cooperation, compliance, and child's self-esteem. |
| 4. Inspect skin with each position change for redness that does not fade in 30 minutes, or breakdown and abrasion. | Skin observation allows detection of irritation/potential breakdown early so more frequent turning, different position, or other appropriate interventions can be made. ***Special Considerations:*** *Various aids such as sheepskin, foam mattresses, alternating pressure mattresses, heel and elbow protectors are available to aid in the prevention of skin breakdown in higher risk children.* |

| Evaluation Outcomes | Observational Guidelines |
|---|---|
| 1. Proper positioning is maintained at all times. | Note maintenance of proper alignment, use of variety of positions, and contraindicated positions not used. |
| 2. Skin integrity is maintained. | Observe skin for redness, irritation, and breakdown after each position change. Compare to assessment of skin condition. Note the use of a variety of positions and the frequency of changes. |
| 3. Child/family understand basic principles and reasons for positioning. | Child/family verbalize reason for positioning and basic principles. Observe child maintaining proper alignment and family cooperation. |
| 4. Child is positioned comfortably. | Note absence of irritability and restlessness in younger children. Ask older child if position is comfortable. Note ability to rest or sleep in various positions. |

### Documentation

Record position utilized, time positioned, and child's tolerance of position. Note skin condition, as well as the presence of traction, cast, special positioning aids, and/or restraints. Document child/family knowledge about positioning and any teaching performed.

### Home Care Modifications

For a complete review of positioning needs and aids for the disabled child at home, refer family to: Jones ML: Home care for the chronically ill or disabled child: A manual and source book for parents and professionals, New York, 1985, Harper & Row.

# *SKILL* 75 Applying Skin Traction to an Extremity

*Frances Lynn McCullough*

Skin traction can be used to attain fracture alignment, to reduce muscle spasms, to stretch tendons and muscles, to rest and hold the extremity, and to prevent further injury. Skin traction is used when traction is needed for a short period of time and when a large amount of weight is unnecessary. The skin can tolerate only small amounts of weight (5 to 10 lb) depending on body size. The most common types are Buck, Russell, and Bryant traction. In children, both lower extremities are often placed in traction rather than only the one involved extremity. This assists in maintaining proper body alignment in bed. Lower extremity traction may be extended to the top of the thigh rather than to below the knee to assist in traction maintenance and to distribute the force over a larger surface area.

The exact procedure for application of skin traction will vary according to individual institutions and physicians. This skill discusses basic concepts for skin traction application. In many institutions, only personnel with specific training or the physician are allowed to apply skin traction.

## NURSING DIAGNOSES

Potential for disuse syndrome related to physical immobilization (skin traction); Fear/anxiety related to hospitalization, traction and separation from family; Diversional activity deficit related to lengthy treatment (skin traction).

| Steps | Rationale |
|---|---|

## Assessment

1. Assess child's age and developmental level.

A knowledge of the child's level of development is necessary to plan age appropriate interventions and explanations.

2. Assess child/family's understanding of traction and its purposes.

An understanding by the child/family helps to gain their cooperation.

***Special Considerations:*** *If possible, have the child/family visit another child in traction.*

3. Perform baseline neurovascular assessment of extremity (see Skill 77).

It is important to know if any deficits or abnormal conditions exist so that these will not be attributed to the traction.

4. Assess skin integrity thoroughly before application of traction.

Any areas of irritation or breakdown (e.g., abrasions, lacerations, insect bites, bruising) should be noted before traction application so that they will not be attributed to the traction and special care may be taken to prevent further breakdown.

5. Review medical history and current physical status for other conditions that may have implications for the use of traction and immobility, such as developmental delay, paralysis, impaired sensation, scarring from surgeries or trauma, poor nutritional status, and/or skin allergy to benzoin.

An awareness of preexisting conditions that may have implications for the application and maintenance of skin traction guides nursing care planning and implementation.

## Planning and Goal Setting

1. Review physician's order for the type of skin traction, the weight to be used, the goal of traction, and the duration.
   a. Types of Skin Traction.
      - Buck extension (Fig. 75-1) is usually applied to both lower extremities in an extended position. It is frequently used for correcting contracture or bone deformities, such as Perthes disease, or congenital hip dislocation.
      - Russell (Fig. 75-2) is applied to one lower extremity with a padded sling under the knee to immobilize the hip and knee in a flexed position. Used for femoral fracture.
      - Bryant (Fig. 75-3) is applied bilaterally to the lower extremities, flexing them at a 90° angle to the body. Its use is limited to children under 2 years of age and less than 12 to 14 kg. Used primarily for femoral fractures, it carries a high risk of postural hypertension and other circulatory impairment problems.
      - Dunlop (Fig. 75-4) is applied to an upper extremity with a fracture of the humerus. The arm is suspended horizontally with a 90 degree flexion at the elbow. This type is less commonly used as it is difficult to maintain good alignment in children.

***Special Considerations:*** *Skin traction used for reasons other than fracture reduction can be removed and reapplied as needed. To remove traction from a fractured extremity requires a physician's order. Manual traction must be maintained at all times on the fractured extremity.*

2. Gather equipment (adhesive traction strips, stockinette, cotton cast padding, Benzoin spray, elastic bandages, traction rope, pulleys, bars, spreader bars, and weights).

Collecting supplies in advance improves organization, decreases child/family anxiety, and optimizes time with child/family.

***Special Considerations:*** *The exact equipment will depend upon type of traction to be used, age and size of child, and facility's policy.*

3. Discuss procedure with child/family.

This reduces anxiety and increases cooperation.

4. Develop individualized child/family goals:
   - Traction will be maintained.
   - Skin integrity will be maintained.
   - Neurovascular status of extremity(s) will be unimpaired by traction.
   - Child/family will understand the reason for traction.

## Implementation

1. Wash extremity with soap and water and dry thoroughly.

Washing removes surface bacteria/debris that may contribute to skin breakdown. Traction also adheres better to clean, completely dry skin.

***Special Considerations:*** *Do not use oils or lotions that will make the skin softer and more prone to breakdown and may interfere with adherence of traction to skin. Do not shave skin without specific physician's order.*

**Steps** | **Rationale**

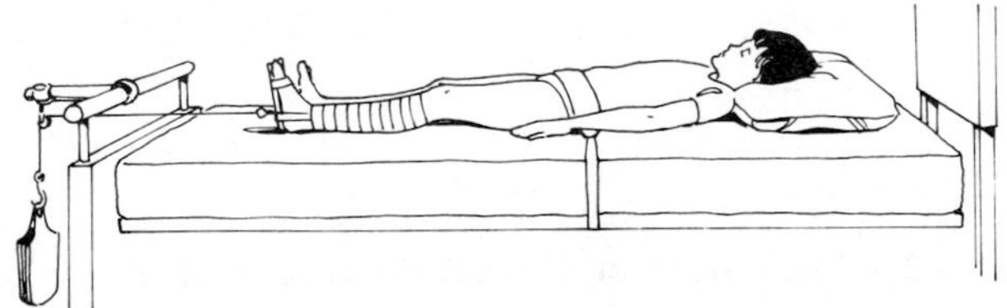

***FIG. 75-1*** Buck extension traction.

From Hilt NE and Schmitt EW: Pediatric orthopedic nursing, St Louis, 1975, The CV Mosby Co.

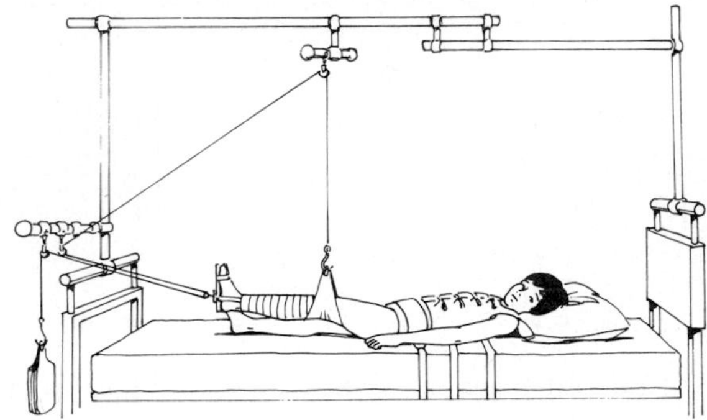

***FIG. 75-2*** Russell traction.

From Hilt NE and Schmitt EW: Pediatric orthopedic nursing, St Louis, 1975, The CV Mosby Co.

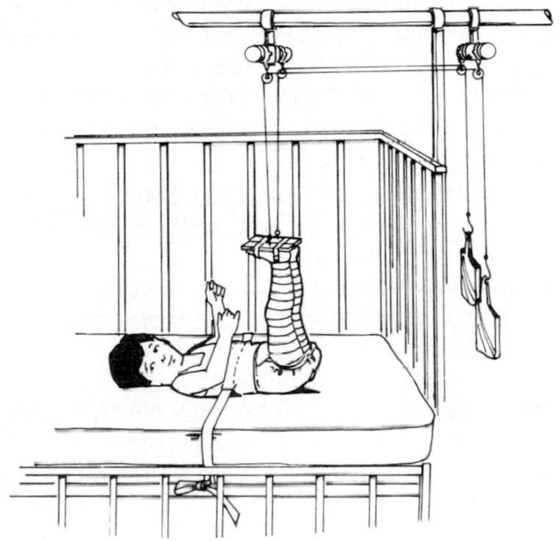

***FIG. 75-3*** Bryant traction.

From Hilt NE and Schmitt EW: Pediatric orthopedic nursing, St Louis, 1975, The CV Mosby Co.

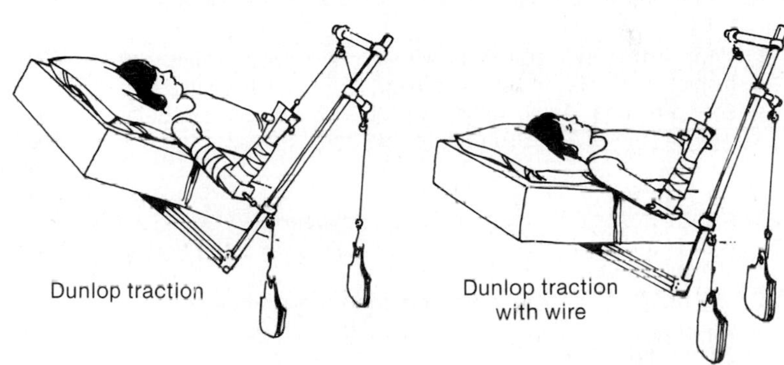


***FIG. 75-4*** Dunlop traction.

From Hilt NE and Schmitt EW: Pediatric orthopedic nursing, St Louis, 1975, The CV Mosby Co.

2. Cut a piece of stockinette approximately 3 to 4 inches longer than the extremity that is wide enough to fit easily over extremity but narrow enough to fit smoothly without wrinkles.

Stockinette is used to protect the skin.

***Special Considerations:*** *Some facilities' procedures require the use of cotton cast padding instead of a stockinette, or no leg covering to be used.*

3. Roll the cut stockinette into a "doughnut" (as a sock is rolled before putting on foot) before application.

Rolled stockinette is easier to apply quickly and smoothly without wrinkles.

4. Spray skin thoroughly with Benzoin and allow it to dry until it feels "tacky" and not wet.

Benzoin provides adhesive to hold the traction in place and to protect the skin.

***Special Considerations:*** *Protect the child from Benzoin fumes by spraying away from the head and by shielding the face. Protect bed linens by placing towel or pad under extremity while spraying Benzoin. Allergic contact dermatitis to tincture of benzoin compound has been reported (James, White, and Yanklowitz, 1984; Rademaker and Kirby, 1987). The benefits of its use in better adherence of skin traction must be weighed against potential skin disruption. Determine physician preferences.*

5. Unroll stockinette over extremity removing all wrinkles. Leave fingers/toes exposed.

Wrinkles cause discomfort and increased pressure that can lead to breakdown.

***Special Considerations:*** *A strip of cotton cast padding or stockinette can be applied over the malleoli bilaterally or the styloid process for protection.*

**Steps** | **Rationale**

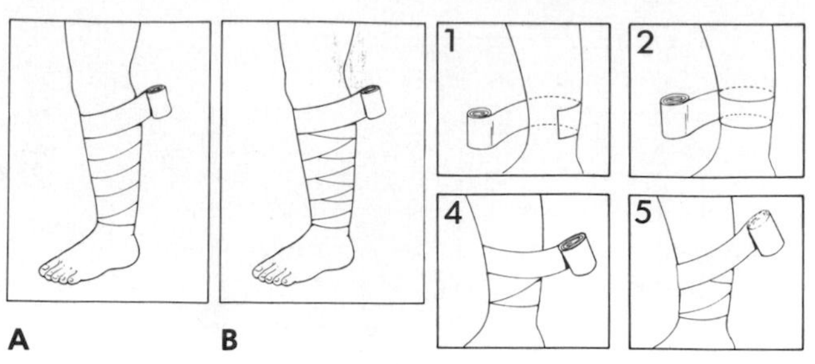


***FIG. 75-5*** Elastic bandage is wrapped in **A,** a circular or **B,** a figure-eight pattern. The figure-eight wrap (detailed in steps 1 through 5) is more secure and stays in place longer.

6. Measure extremity for length and width of traction strips.

***Special Considerations:*** *Strips should be longer than the extremity to accommodate the spreader bar. Strips should be as wide as possible without overlapping to distribute the forces over as much skin surface as possible.*

7. Measure to malleoli of ankle or styloid process of wrist and remove adhesive backing only to this point.

By not adhering to the bony prominences, the risk of skin breakdown is decreased. This also provides a way to determine if the traction is slipping and needs to be reapplied.

8. Apply adhesive traction strips over stockinette to both sides of the extremity allowing room for the spreader bar or footplate.

***Special Considerations:*** *If nonadhesive strips are used, they will need to be held in place while elastic bandage is secured. (See step 9.)*

9. Wrap extremity distal to proximal in a circular or figure 8 fashion with elastic bandage (Fig. 75-5). Secure ends with adhesive tape. Avoid wrapping too tightly over the fibular head to prevent pressure to the peroneal nerve.

Wrapping distal to proximal promotes vascular return and decreases edema. Adhesive tape is used rather than metal clips because the clips are a safety hazard.

***Special Considerations:*** *A figure 8 is a more secure method of wrapping and stays in place longer. More than one elastic bandage may be necessary.*

10. Attach to spreader bar/footplate and weights.
11. Assess traction equipment immediately after setup and at least every two hours thereafter:
    a. Weights are proper amount and hanging freely.
    b. Ropes are not frayed and are aligned in pulley.
    c. Knots are securely tied.
    d. Spreader bar/footplates do not touch siderails or footboard and are not exerting pressure on foot.

Traction that is improperly setup or maintained will not accomplish its purpose and can cause neurovascular compromise. It must be checked frequently because the child's movement will change the position of the traction.

12. Position child in bed for proper alignment in traction and reassess frequently.
    a. In Bryant traction (see Fig. 75-3):
       - Hips in 90 degree flexion.
       - Hips directly under pulleys.
       - Buttocks should be lifted off mattress just enough to slip hand between buttocks and mattress.
       - Child must remain flat on back and not turn on side or abdomen.

Children are very active and their position must be constantly reassessed and repositioned as necessary. If correct positioning is not maintained, the traction will not be as effective.

    b. In Russell, Buck, and Dunlop traction (see Fig. 75-1, 75-2, and 75-4):
       - Position in center of width of bed except for Dunlop traction for which the body should be positioned to the edge of the bed on the affected side.

***Special Considerations:*** *Attaching a toy or balloon or wrapping the siderail with tape at the point that the child should be in bed will allow the child and family to maintain his or her position without restraints and helps the family to participate in his or her care.*

       - Position aligned with pulleys.
       - Position lengthwise in center and toward the head of the bed. The head of the bed may be elevated 30 degrees with Russell traction.

The risk of footplate/spreader bar resting against the foot of the bed and/or weights resting on the floor is increased if the child is positioned toward the foot of the bed.

***Special Considerations:*** *With the physician's permission, sandbags under the hips may prevent the child from sliding down in bed. "Shock blocks" should not be used because they restrict movement of the bed in an emergency.*

13. Restrain child as needed.

Proper alignment is essential in order to derive full benefit from the traction and to ensure safety of child.

***Special Considerations:*** *Do not restrain unless absolutely necessary. Use a minimum of restraints that will accomplish the goal. Jacket or vest restraints work well with traction. Emphasize that the restraint is a reminder to maintain position and is not a punishment (see Skill 51).*

| **Steps** | **Rationale** |
|---|---|
| 14. Praise the child frequently for cooperating during application and maintenance of traction. | |
| 15. Perform neurovascular assessment 30 minutes after application and reapplication and at least every 4 hours thereafter (see Skill 77). | Neurovascular status must be reassessed frequently and after rewrapping to ensure traction is not applied too tightly or that the injury is not producing neurovascular compromise. ***Special Considerations:*** *Neurovascular assessment is especially important for the child in Bryant traction. Bilateral 90 degree hip flexion increases the risk of neurovascular compromise, and the child is too young to verbalize complaints other than by crying.* |
| 16. Assess child's tolerance to traction. If there are complaints related to the traction (tightness, burning, itching, rash, blistering) or a child is irritable and/or crying with no reason evident, the traction should be removed and the skin inspected. | Permanent nerve, vascular and muscle damage can occur within 4 to 6 hours from compartment syndrome if the pressure is not relieved. Skin breakdown can occur in an even shorter period of time. |
| 17. Provide age-appropriate activities to prevent boredom and assist in meeting developmental tasks (see Skill 15). | Children require mobility to reach out for new experiences that will aid them in developing and attaining new skills. If this mobility is decreased, activities must be brought to them to accomplish the same goal. ***Special Considerations:*** *If traction is for reasons other than fracture reduction, the bed can frequently be moved to the playroom with the physician's permission. Toys, pictures, balloons, paper chains, etc., can be hung from the traction frame without impairing the traction apparatus itself. The family may bring favorite toys from home to give the child added security.* |
| 18. Remove elastic bandage and rewrap every 8 hours. | Rewrapping the elastic bandage aids in correct maintenance of the traction and provides an opportunity to inspect the condition of traction wrapping underneath the bandage. |
| 19. Remove all traction, inspect skin, and reapply every 24 to 48 hours, as needed, or as individual institution policy dictates. | ***Special Considerations:*** *The exception is for the fractured extremity which requires a physician's order to remove and reapply. Manual traction must be maintained at all times on the fractured extremity. Do not wash extremity to remove Benzoin if used. Do not use lotions or oils prior to reapplication.* |

| **Evaluation Outcomes** | **Observational Guidelines** |
|---|---|
| 1. Skin traction is properly applied and maintained. | Observe for: body alignment; type of traction; extremity involved; amount of weight; and condition of traction equipment (e.g., ropes are not frayed, knots intact, ropes aligned in pulleys, weights hanging freely). |
| 2. Skin integrity is maintained. | Note if behaviors of skin breakdown occur, e.g., itching, irritability, excessive crying. Inspect skin for redness, rash, blisters, and/or areas of breakdown. |
| 3. Neurovascular status is not impaired by traction. | Observe neurovascular status through ongoing neurovascular assessment (see Skill 77). Note signs of discomfort caused by traction, e.g., irritability, crying, and pulling at traction. |
| 4. Child/family demonstrate understanding of the reasons and goals of traction. | Ask child/family to describe reason and purpose of traction. Note their cooperation with and attempts to maintain traction. |

## Documentation

Record the type of traction, the amount of weight used, and the extremity involved. Note the time the traction was applied and/or reapplied. Document findings from the neurovascular assessment including time performed, frequency of removal of traction to inspect skin, condition of skin, and treatment of any observed skin irritation or breakdown. Note the child's tolerance of traction and whether or not restraints were used. Document notification of the physician in the event of changes in neurovascular status, skin breakdown, or intolerance of traction. Indicate any child/family teaching performed.

# SKILL 76 Monitoring Skeletal Traction to an Extremity

*Bonnie Uthoff Dolson*

Skeletal traction is used when bone realignment is not possible with skin traction or cast immobilization. Steinmann pins or Kirschner wires are inserted into the bone and the continuous pull of traction is exerted on the bone instead of the skin and tissue. Fractures of the humerus and femur are frequently treated with this type of traction. Astute nursing assessment and care of the child in skeletal traction is essential to prevent neurovascular impairment of the extremity, infection of skeletal pin sites, and the physiological and psychological problems of immobility.

## NURSING DIAGNOSES

Potential for disuse syndrome related to physical immobilization (skeletal traction); Potential for infection related to traumatized tissue at skeletal pin sites; Fear/anxiety related to hospitalization, traction, and separation from family; Self-care deficit, bathing/hygiene, feeding, and toileting related to musculoskeletal impairment; Diversional activity deficit related to lengthy treatment.

| Steps | Rationale |
|---|---|
| **Assessment** | |
| 1. Assess traction apparatus:<br>a. Weights hang free, e.g., do not touch bed or floor.<br>b. Correct amount of weight is applied.<br>c. Ropes are intact and taut. | Correct use of traction, weights and pulleys provides effective traction for proper bone alignment and subsequent bone union and callus formation. Any disruption or impairment of traction can cause improper fracture alignment and delayed bone union.<br>***Special Considerations:*** *Traction set up, amount of weight, and weight changes are ordered by physician.* |
| d. Rope knots are securely tied and taped. | Securing knots prevents slipping or untying. |
| e. Ropes run freely through pulleys.<br>f. Ropes are free from bed linens, toys.<br>g. Proper direction of pull is applied on traction/wires. | Toys used to provide diversional activity may impair use of ropes and pulleys.<br>***Special Considerations:*** *Toys, art work, posters should be put on wall or frame of traction and not placed on or near ropes and pulley pathways.* |
| h. Skeletal pins/wires are covered with corks or protective caps. | Covering pins/wires prevents accidental trauma to child, family, or health care personnel.<br>***Special Considerations:*** *Corks/caps should be secured with tape in young children to prevent removal and possible aspiration.* |
| i. Pin screws are tight in holder, which attaches traction to pin. | Secure attachment prevents slippage and improper traction pull and alignment. |
| 2. Assess child's position and alignment in traction (see Figs. 76-1, 76-2, and 75-4 for proper alignment diagrams). | Supine positioning is required for extremity in skeletal traction. Incorrect positioning prevents proper fracture alignment for healing. Fear, anxiety, and curiosity about traction may cause increased movement and misalignment.<br>***Special Considerations:*** *Restlessness or irritability may be signs of pain or discomfort in children. Restraining vests or sandbags may be used if position maintenance is difficult to achieve.* |
| 3. Assess pin/wire sites for signs of infection: redness, purulent drainage, odor, pain, tenderness, warmth, swelling. | Exposed ends remain in contact with external environment and have increased risk for contamination. Superficial pin site infections may lead to osteomyelitis.<br>***Special Considerations:*** *Serosanguineous drainage or erythema may be expected for one to two days after insertion (Celeste, Folcik, and Dumas, 1984). Continuation of drainage or other signs of infection require prompt physician notification.* |

**Steps** | **Rationale**

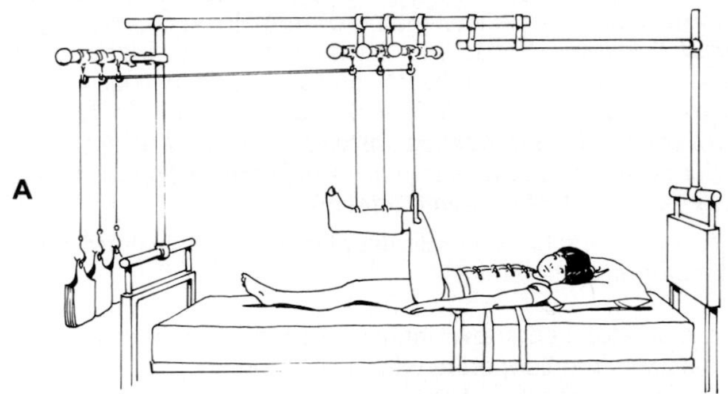


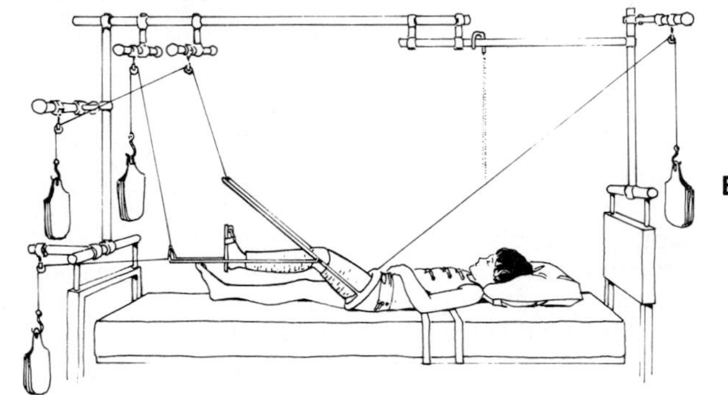


***FIG. 76-1*** Types of skeletal traction. **A,** 90°–90° traction. **B,** Balance suspension with Thomas ring splint and Pearson attachment.

From Whaley LF and Wong DL: Nursing care of infants and children, ed 4, St Louis, 1991, The CV Mosby Co.

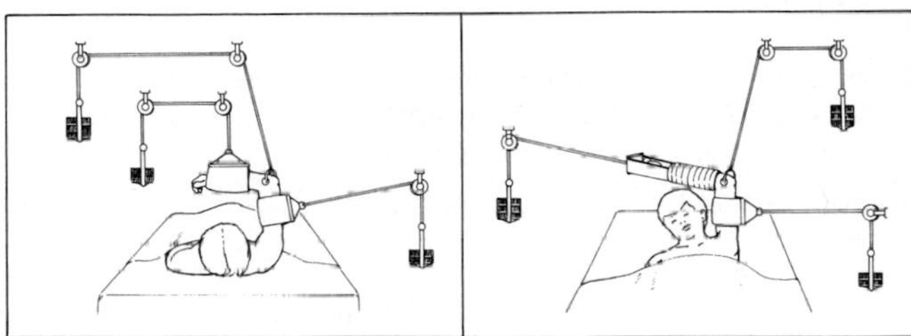

***FIG. 76-2*** Overhead skeletal traction.

4. Assess pin/wire sites for slippage: pulling or puckering of skin.

Excessive motion around insertion site may cause increased tissue damage and drainage.

5. Assess neurovascular status of extremity (see Skill 77).

Tissue hypoxia can cause irreversible damage to extremity within six to eight hours (McCullough and Evans, 1985).

***Special Considerations:*** *Notify physician immediately of changes in neurovascular status. Neurovascular assessment and documentation has significant legal implications since damage caused by impaired blood flow or nerve compression can be permanent.*

6. Assess alignment and condition of casts, splints, or wraps used with traction.

Adjunctive immobilization with casts or splints is frequently used. These may cause pressure areas or neurovascular impairment.

***Special Considerations:*** *90°-90° traction uses a boot cast on lower leg and foot to provide support and proper traction alignment. Balanced suspension traction for fractured femur uses a Thomas ring splint with a Pearson attachment. Overhead skeletal traction to the humerus uses a sling or skin traction to support the forearm (see Fig. 76-2).*

7. Assess skin integrity for pressure or friction area.

Children are prone to pressure sores from supine positioning and friction from movement on bed linens. The type of traction also indicates specific sites subject to pressure.

***Special Considerations:*** *Potential pressure sites—90°-90° traction: Popliteal area at cast edge. Balance suspension: heel, Achilles tendon, and calf where supported on Pearson attachment; and groin and gluteal fold where ring of Thomas splint rests. Dunlop traction: posterior aspect of shoulder and scapula. Overhead traction to humerus: inner wrist, antecubital fossa.*

| Steps | Rationale |
|---|---|
| 8. Assess child's and family's understanding of traction's purpose. | Anxiety and confusion most commonly occur because of lack of information or misunderstanding of terminology. **Special Considerations:** *Use open-ended questions to elicit ideas/concerns, e.g., "Why do you have a cast on your foot?" "How will this traction help your leg get better?" "Tell me why your child has traction instead of a cast." A frequent misunderstanding relates to purpose of boot cast on uninjured lower leg in 90°-90° degree traction.* |
| 9. Obtain health history data from family/child that may affect assessment of extremity, fracture healing, or increased risk for problems of immobility. | An accurate health history facilitates planning individualized nursing care for child/family. |
| a. Age and developmental level of child. | Age and developmental level influences child's fears and ability to understand and cooperate with assessment. |
| b. Cause of injury. | Traction/cast application frequently follows motor vehicle accidents or falls with concomitant head injuries and impaired consciousness. **Special Considerations:** *The child with multiple fractures, especially in long bones (e.g., the femur), is susceptible to fat emboli from the injured marrow.* |
| c. Previous health problems. | Preexisting conditions can influence assessment, fracture healing, and risk for problems of immobility. **Special Considerations:** *Conditions commonly affecting neurovascular status before current trauma or surgery: congenital heart disease, myelomeningocele, muscular dystrophy. Conditions commonly influencing fracture healing: diabetes mellitus, anemia, chronic renal failure, hemophilia. Conditions increasing risk for problems of immobility: bronchial asthma, cystic fibrosis, psoriasis, atopic dermatitis.* |

## Planning and Goal Setting

| Steps | Rationale |
|---|---|
| 1. Plan to perform assessment in organized manner. | Organization promotes complete identification of potential/actual problems. **Special Considerations:** *Frequencies other than every 4 hours will be determined by the child's status, the physician's order, or the hospital policy (see Implementation, step 9).* |
| 2. Adapt assessment and care to child's developmental level including consideration of major fears and concerns. | Consideration of developmental level facilitates accurate and valid assessment, decreases child's fear, and increases cooperation. **Special Considerations:** *See Skill 11 for major fears/concerns of each age group.* |
| 3. Plan care with child/family. | Collaborative planning of care with child and family fosters their sense of control and enhances their cooperation in the plan of care. |
| 4. Develop individualized child/family goals:<br>▪ Proper traction alignment and positioning will be maintained.<br>▪ Adequate peripheral circulation and sensory and motor function of affected extremity will be maintained.<br>▪ Pin/wire sites will be intact.<br>▪ Pain will be decreased.<br>▪ Skin integrity will be maintained.<br>▪ Child/family will understand need for traction.<br>▪ Child/family will participate in activities of daily living. | |

## Implementation

| Steps | Rationale |
|---|---|
| 1. Explain traction apparatus to child and family. Include:<br>a. How traction and adjunctive splints/cast work.<br>b. Correct alignment/positioning.<br>c. Use of overhead trapeze (if applicable). | Explanations help to decrease fear and anxiety and facilitate positive coping mechanisms. Understanding is vital since duration of traction is usually 2 to 6 weeks. **Special Considerations:** *Adapt explanations to child's developmental level. Diagrams, pictures, and demonstrations with dolls or toys help the child to visualize explanations.* |

| Steps | Rationale |
|---|---|
| 2. Explain what nursing care will be required and how child/family can assist with care (see Child and Family Teaching Section). | Inclusion of child/family enables them to understand and participate in care and allows control over the situation. It also facilitates adaptation to hospitalization and develops coping mechanisms. Encouraging the child to perform age-appropriate self-care activities as permitted by traction promotes independence and positive self-concept.<br>***Special Considerations:*** *Families often feel their role is taken over by health professionals. Plan collaboratively with families to provide care and play.* |
| 3. Encourage child/family to ask questions and verbalize fears/concerns. | Children often have misconceptions about the reason for hospitalization and treatment. Encouraging a discussion of feelings enables correction of misconceptions.<br>***Special Considerations:*** *See Skill 12.* |
| 4. Encourage families to spend time away from the child. | Family anxiety can be "contagious" and can influence the child's anxiety. Fatigue may decrease the family's objectivity. Older children are also not accustomed to continuous parental presence. Family may share concerns if they are given time away from the child's room.<br>***Special Considerations:*** *Reassure the family about how the child's needs will be met in their absence. Families may need help in identifying times to leave (e.g., during bath and child life activity times) or other persons to stay with child (e.g., grandparents and friends).* |
| 5. Accept the child's reaction to skeletal traction and immobilization. | Acceptance of child's reaction helps him or her to deal with stressful situation and develop positive coping mechanisms.<br>***Special Considerations:*** *Demanding behavior may occur because of the child's loss of control. Limit setting should be done by health professionals and by the family to provide the child with a sense of security. Assist the family to accept and deal constructively with the child's behavior.* |
| 6. Maintain proper alignment of child in traction (see Figs. 76-1 and 76-2):<br>a. Child in center of bed.<br>b. Extremity aligned with traction pull on pins/wires.<br>c. Proper degree of extremity flexion. | Proper traction alignment promotes correct fracture healing. Improper alignment and/or weight application decreases effectiveness and prolongs duration of traction.<br>***Special Considerations:*** *Skeletal traction is never released by the nurse. Weights should not be lifted or removed when moving the child into proper alignment (Osborne and DiGiacomo, 1987). Overhead trapeze allows child with lower extremity fracture to assist with movement and positioning thus fostering self-care and independence.* |
| 7. Praise the child's efforts to maintain traction alignment, perform self-care activities, and demonstrate socially acceptable behavior. | Positive reinforcement gives the child a sense of accomplishment and encourages cooperation/participation in their own care.<br>***Special Considerations:*** *Use of positive reinforcers such as playing with stickers, playing a game, and earning points for a prize/treat provides motivation to continue positive behavior. It is important to use reinforcers that are motivators for this particular child.* |
| 8. Implement measures to decrease risk of skin breakdown:<br>a. Place sheepskin, egg crate mattress, or alternating pressure mattress under back and hips. | Skeletal traction requires continuous supine positioning, which places the child at increased risk for pressure areas. Special padding and mattresses decrease pressure/friction over bony prominences. |
| b. Wash exposed skin with mild soap, rinse, and dry thoroughly. Perform at least twice daily. | Skin care removes perspiration and debris that cause skin irritation and provides an opportunity to inspect skin and assess it for irritation or pressure areas. |
| c. Gently massage pressure points at least every 8 hours. | Massaging stimulates circulation and decreases venous stasis.<br>***Special Considerations:*** *Reddened areas over pressure points should fade with repositioning and relief of pressure on the soft tissue. The effectiveness of massaging reddened soft tissue areas is controversial.* |
| d. Check under child for crumbs, small objects, toys, and wrinkles. | Hidden small items and wrinkles can cause skin irritation and potential pressure sores.<br>***Special Considerations:*** *Use of overhead trapeze for child with leg fracture allows the child to pull self up for back care and skin inspection. It also helps the child to maintain some degree of independence.* |

| Steps | Rationale |
|---|---|
| 9. Perform neurovascular assessment every 1 hour for 24 hours; then every 4 hours for duration of traction, or more often if necessary (see Skill 77). | Frequent assessment allows early detection of impaired circulation or sensory/motor function and prevents potential permanent damage.<br>***Special Considerations:*** *Failure to detect, report, and take corrective action with neurovascular impairment has significant legal implications.* |
| 10. Cleanse and dress pin/wire sites, if ordered, using sterile technique. | If site care is ordered, sterile technique is used to prevent superficial infection and osteomyelitis.<br>***Special Considerations:*** *Pin site care may be ordered by physician or established by hospital policy and standards of care. Pin site care is controversial (Sproles, 1985).* |
| 11. Monitor bowel and bladder elimination. | Immobility causes urinary stasis and decreased bowel elimination. Using a bedpan or urinal is awkward and embarrassing for child, so constipation and enuresis are common. |
| a. Determine what words child uses to indicate his or her needs. | Young children do not understand void and defecate. Children frequently use unique words to communicate their need to eliminate. |
| b. Encourage oral fluids and high fiber foods, e.g., fresh fruits and whole grains. | Water absorption by fiber softens and increases volume of stool, causing bowel to contract and empty. |
| c. Discuss favorite fluid and food preferences with child/family. | Providing fluid and foods that the child likes will increase intake and will provide child with control.<br>***Special Considerations:*** *Regression of toilet skills is common for toddlers and preschoolers because of the stress of hospitalization. Reassure family that regression is normal and not to correct or punish child. Pain medications or oral iron supplements may be the cause of constipation.* |
| 12. Monitor for signs and symptoms of blood, air or fat embolus: classic signs of shock, chest pain, dyspnea, and petechial hemorrhages of the chest and shoulders. | Post injury bleeding and clotting and fat deposits in the fractured bone marrow may produce an embolus that travels to the heart, lungs, or brain, causing life-threatening vascular obstruction and ischemia (Whaley and Wong, 1991).<br>***Special Considerations:*** *Fat embolus is generally the most common, usually occurring within the first 24 hours after injury.* |
| 13. Provide age-appropriate diversional activities. | Activities divert attention, decrease boredom, and facilitate cooperation with nursing care. Activities should be selected according to child's likes/dislikes and developmental level and needs.<br>***Special Considerations:*** *Encourage the family to bring favorite toys, crafts, and books. Visits by siblings/peers, telephone calls, and letters help the child to keep contact with those who are important to him or her.* |

| Evaluation Outcomes | Observational Guidelines |
|---|---|
| 1. Proper traction alignment and positioning is maintained. | Observe type of traction applied to involved extremity; extremity aligned with traction pull on pin/wire; proper degree of extremity flexion; amount of weight; child's position in bed; presence and condition of adjunctive splints/casts. |
| 2. Toes/fingers are warm and pink with brisk capillary refill, palpable pulses, decreased pain, and intact motor and sensory function to involved extremity. | Observe skin temperature, skin color, and capillary refill time. Palpate pulses for presence, strength, and equality. Observe for sensation in response to touch by report, by movement, or by changes in behavior or facial expression. Observe for active movement and performance of passive movement without increasing pain. If pain occurs note what movement induces pain (e.g., extension, flexion). |
| 3. Pin sites are intact without signs of bleeding, infection, or slippage. | Observe medial and lateral pin sites for bleeding, redness, purulent drainage, odor, pain, tenderness, warmth, and swelling. Observe for skin pulling or puckering. |
| 4. Child experiences decreased, minimal or no pain. | Determine amount and frequency of pain medication required. Assess level of pain and child's response to pain. |
| 5. Skin integrity remains intact. | Inspect all body skin for excessive dryness, redness, blisters, abraded or open areas over bony prominences, and potential sites related to specific traction types. |
| 6. Child and/or family verbalizes reason for traction. | Ask child/family to verbalize their understanding of reason for traction and how it works. |
| 7. Child and/or family participates in care activities. | Observe child's/family's participation in care (e.g., feeding, bathing, play). |

### Documentation

Record the type of traction and intactness, the extremity involved, the presence of a cast or splint used adjunctively, and the amount of weight used. Note the child's position and traction alignment. Indicate the condition of the pin/wire site (e.g., drainage, pain, redness, tenderness) and any care administered to the site. Note the neurovascular status of the involved extremity including color, temperature, pulse, pain, sensation, and movement. Document the condition of skin integrity, especially potential pressure areas and the use of preventive measures. Record the child/family's participation in care activities as well as any patient teaching conducted including content taught and child/family's ability to verbalize information or demonstrate skill. Specify problems identified and actions taken.

### Child and Family Teaching

1. Discuss the purpose and frequency of neurovascular assessment to the extremity.
2. Discuss modifications of daily hygiene such as bathing, shampooing, and oral care.
3. Discuss clothing modifications.
   a. If upper extremity in traction:
      - Modify shirt/top: Open shoulder seam of top, and open top of sleeve or cut off. Use snaps or velcro strips to fasten top at shoulder.

   b. If lower extremity in traction:
      - Modify gym-type shorts: Open side seam. Use snaps or velcro strips to fasten shorts on side.

# *SKILL 77* Monitoring Neurovascular Status for the Child in Traction or a Cast

*Bonnie Uthoff Dolson*

Neurovascular assessment of the child's extremity following an injury and immobilization with traction or casting is a primary nursing responsibility. Neurovascular assessment covers four areas: circulation, sensation, movement, and pain. This assessment is commonly referred to as the 5 P's: pulse, pallor, paresthesia, paralysis, and pain. Early detection of circulatory impairment and sensory and/or motor changes is vital because tissue hypoxia can cause irreversible damage within 6 to 8 hours. The use of developmental concepts helps the health professional to obtain an accurate and valid assessment of the child's neurovascular status.

### NURSING DIAGNOSES

Impaired tissue integrity related to circulatory and neuromuscular impairment; Altered (peripheral) tissue perfusion related to interruption of venous flow; Potential for impaired skin integrity related to physical immobilization (cast/traction); Altered health maintenance related to lack of information about neurovascular assessment following cast/traction application.

| Steps | Rationale |
|---|---|
| **Assessment** | |
| 1. Obtain baseline data of extremity's neurovascular status before cast and/or traction application if possible. | Determination of normal or previous status of extremity provides basis for comparing data and identifying actual or potential problems.<br>***Special Considerations:*** *Neurovascular assessment and documentation of status has significant legal implications because damage caused by blood vessel or nerve compression can be permanent. Early detection of neurovascular alterations can prevent or reduce the risk of permanent damage.* |
| 2. Obtain health history data from family/child that may affect neurovascular assessment of extremity: | Obtaining an accurate health history facilitates planning individualized nursing care for child/family. |

**Steps** / **Rationale**

a. Age and developmental level of child.

Age and developmental level influence child's fears and ability to understand and cooperate with assessment.

b. Cause of injury.

Traction/cast application frequently follows motor vehicle accidents or falls with concomitant head injuries and impaired consciousness.

c. Previous health problems.

Preexisting conditions may have impaired neurovascular status prior to current trauma or surgery (e.g., congenital heart disease, myelomeningocele, muscular dystrophy, diabetes mellitus, thrombophlebitis).

***Special Considerations:*** *Fractures in very young children are frequently the result of physical abuse; therefore, careful and accurate history taking is vital. Inconsistent information or injuries inconsistent with stated cause of fracture must be reported to appropriate agency personnel (see Skill 7).*

3. Assess neurovascular status following application of cast and/or traction:
   a. Every hour for 24 hours.
   b. Then every 4 hours for duration of therapy; unless ordered otherwise (see Implementation steps 2 to 5).

Frequent assessment facilitates early detection of blood vessel or nerve compression and can prevent possible permanent damage. Tissue hypoxia can cause irreversible damage to extremity within 6 to 8 hours (McCullough and Evans, 1985).

## Planning and Goal Setting

1. Plan to perform neurovascular assessment in an organized manner.

Organization promotes complete assessment and identification of actual/potential problems.

***Special Considerations:*** *Using a checklist will promote a complete assessment.*

2. Adapt assessment to child's developmental level.

Developmental considerations facilitate accurate and valid assessment of the child's status and decrease fear and anxiety.

***Special Considerations:*** *Knowledge of the child's major fears/concerns related to developmental level allows understanding of child's behavior.*

3. Develop individualized child/family goals:
   - Adequate peripheral circulation, sensory function, and motor function of affected extremity will be maintained.
   - Pain will be decreased.
   - Child/family will understand need for assessment.
   - Family will be able to perform neurovascular assessment upon discharge.

## Implementation

1. Explain purpose of neurovascular assessment to child and/or family.

Explanations help decrease fear of the "unknown" and increase the child's and family's use of available coping mechanisms. Decreasing family anxiety also increases the child's cooperation.

***Special Considerations:*** *Fear of strangers often inhibits the child's cooperation. Use simple comparisons with older children, e.g., say, "Your brain and nerves are like telephone lines. They call up the muscles and tell them to move."*

2. Check circulation of involved extremity.

Assessment of skin color indicates blood supply and tissue oxygenation.

a. Observe color of exposed skin using good overhead lighting. (Do not use a flashlight.)

Pink indicates adequate blood flow. Pale/white indicates decreased arterial blood flow. Dusky/cyanotic indicates venous stasis. Good overhead lighting provides optimal inspection of extremity. Flashlights or bedside lights may produce shadows or untrue colors.

***Special Considerations:*** *Describe color as: pink, pale, dusky, or cyanotic. Inform family why room light is essential, even at night, to decrease anger and frustration.*

b. Assess capillary refill: depress nail until nailbed becomes pale; quickly release pressure and observe rate of color return.

Rate of capillary blood return indicates status of arterial blood flow to extremity. Refill should take less than 3 seconds. Refill greater than 3 seconds indicates obstructed blood flow. Comparison of uninvolved extremities may help to validate a slow response.

| Steps | Rationale |
|---|---|
| | ***Special Considerations:*** *Describe refill as: rapid/brisk: less than 3 seconds; or slow/sluggish: greater than 3 seconds. Remove nail polish to visualize nailbed.* |
| c. Touch involved extremity to assess skin warmth. | Warm skin indicates adequate perfusion. Coolness indicates decreased blood circulation. If cool or cold, compare with uninvolved extremity to validate assessment.<br>***Special Considerations:*** *Skin temperature is the least reliable sign of circulation. Cold external room temperatures may cause peripheral vasoconstriction, cyanosis, and cool-to-touch skin. Describe as: warm, hot, cool, or cold.* |
| d. Palpate distal peripheral pulses on involved extremity (Fig. 77-1):<br>Upper: brachial, ulnar, and radial.<br>Lower: femoral, popliteal, posterior tibial, and dorsalis pedis. | Presence of pulses indicates adequate arterial blood flow to extremity. Pulselessness is a *late* sign of impaired circulation. Permanent tissue damage will have occurred by time pulse is absent.<br>***Special Considerations:*** *Describe as: present/absent, strong/weak, or equal/unequal. Marking pulse site with an "X" or face drawing ensures consistent accuracy of assessment. An ultrasonic flow detector or doppler should be used if pulse is difficult to assess. Cast location may inhibit assessment of all pulses. Document if pulse is not accessible because of cast/dressing.* |

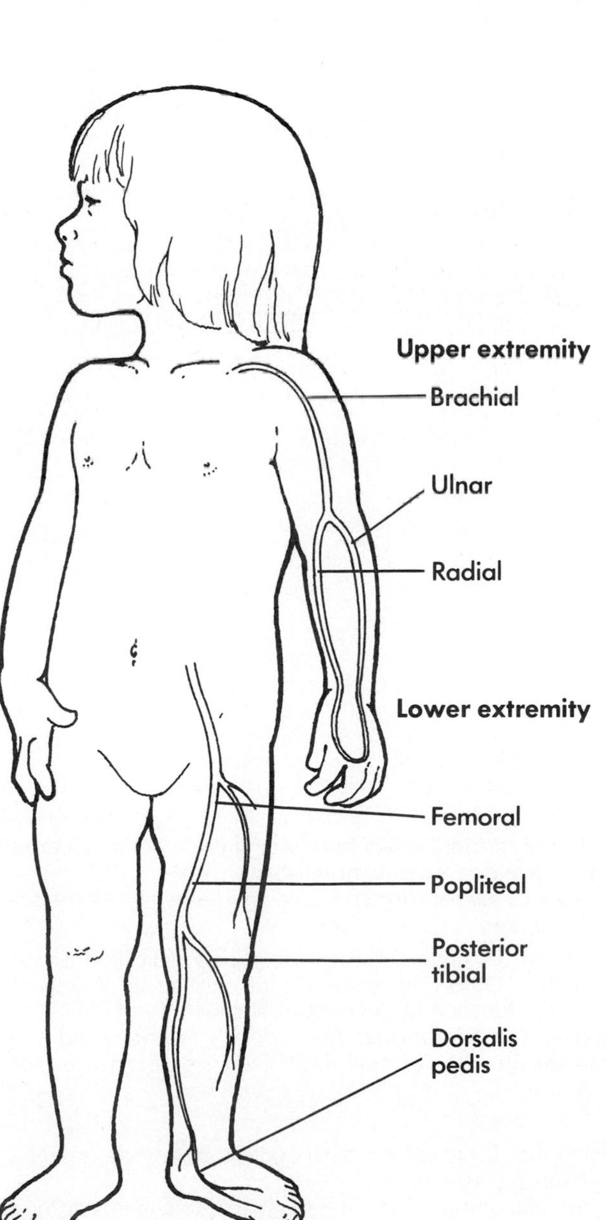


***FIG. 77-1*** Neurovascular assessment of circulation.

| Steps | Rationale |
|---|---|
| e. Assess for edema by inserting fingertips under cast edge. | Presence of edema increases risk of blood vessel and nerve compression. **Special Considerations:** *Elevation of casted extremity above the level of the heart will prevent or decrease edema. Describe as: Absent/present; number of fingerwidths/centimeters between cast edge and surface of exposed extremity.* |
| 3. Test sensory function according to extremity involved (see Fig. 77-2): Upper: Ulnar nerve, Radial nerve, Median nerve. Lower: Peroneal nerve, Tibial nerve. | Sensory changes are the most reliable signs of nerve compression. Sensation should be assessed in each finger/toe because one nerve does not innervate the entire extremity. **Special Considerations:** *Sensation is the most difficult aspect to accurately assess in children due to their limited vocabulary, lack of experience, and need for cooperation.* |

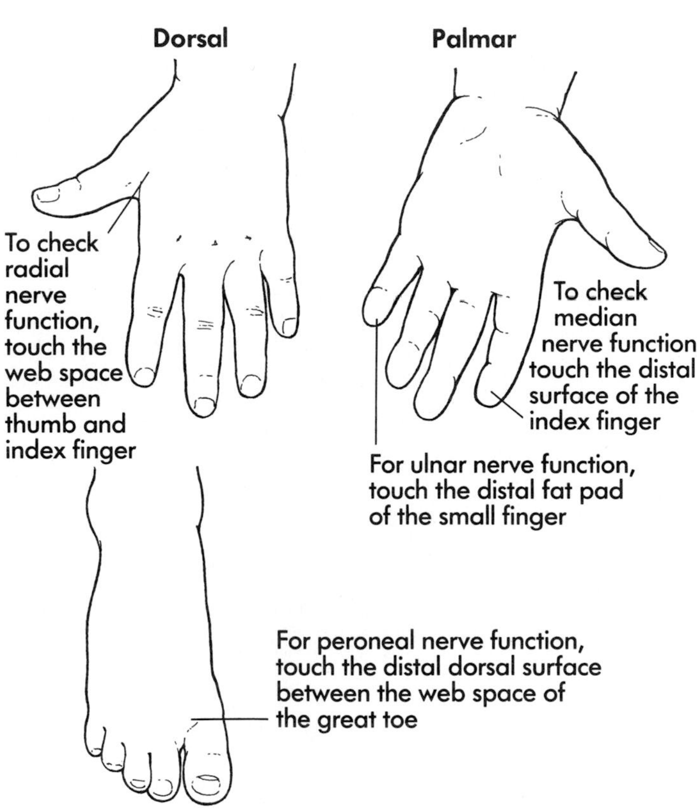


***FIG. 77-2*** Assessment of sensory function.

| Steps | Rationale |
|---|---|
| *Infants and toddlers:* | |
| a. Use toys or ask parents to help distract attention away from extremity being tested. | Distraction prevents child from seeing examiner touch extremity and increases assessment reliability. **Special Considerations:** *Including the family decreases the child's fear.* |
| b. Lightly touch or tickle each finger or toe. Observe for movement and changes in behavior or facial expressions. | Movement of fingers/toes gives a gross indication of sensory function. Observing behavior is the only means of determining sensory function in the nonverbal child. **Special Considerations:** *The toddler's favorite word is "No", so asking "Do you feel this?" will not obtain a reliable response.* |
| *Preschoolers and older:* | |
| a. Have child cover eyes with his or her hands, stuffed animal, or bed linens. | Child's inability to see examiner and extremity increases reliability of sensory assessment. |
| b. Alternate touching with nontouching until each finger/toe is tested. | Alternation of touch helps detect reliable statements by the child. **Special Considerations:** *Using pins for pricking skin is frightening for children. Use pen cap tip or point of pen. Use pin only if sensation is questionable.* |

| Steps | Rationale |
|---|---|
| c. Tell child to say when touch is felt and what part is touched (e.g., big toe). | Having child identify touch increases accuracy of sensory assessment. Children preschool age and older know names of body parts and can say them.<br>***Special Considerations:*** *Avoid saying "Do you feel this?". Child may give inaccurate yes/no answers.* |
| d. Have child describe how fingers/toes feel. | A child's limited vocabulary and experiences inhibit understanding words like "numb" or "tingling." Asking "yes" or "no" questions limits accurate assessment. Descriptions of unusual feelings may be the first signs of sensory impairment.<br>***Special Considerations:*** *Child may use words such as "heavy," "asleep," "funny" or "hurts" (e.g., "My hand feels heavy," "My foot is asleep," or "My arm feels funny").* |
| 4. Test motor function according to extremity involved: Observe flexion, extension, abduction, and adduction (Fig. 77-3):<br>Upper: Radial nerve, Median nerve, Ulnar nerve.<br>Lower: Peroneal nerve, Tibial nerve. | Changes in motor abilities indicate nerve compression. Different nerves initiate the movements of flexion, extension, abduction, and adduction.<br>***Special Considerations:*** *Movement can be difficult to assess because children fear pain from moving or being moved. If pain occurs, note what movement induces pain (e.g., extension).* |

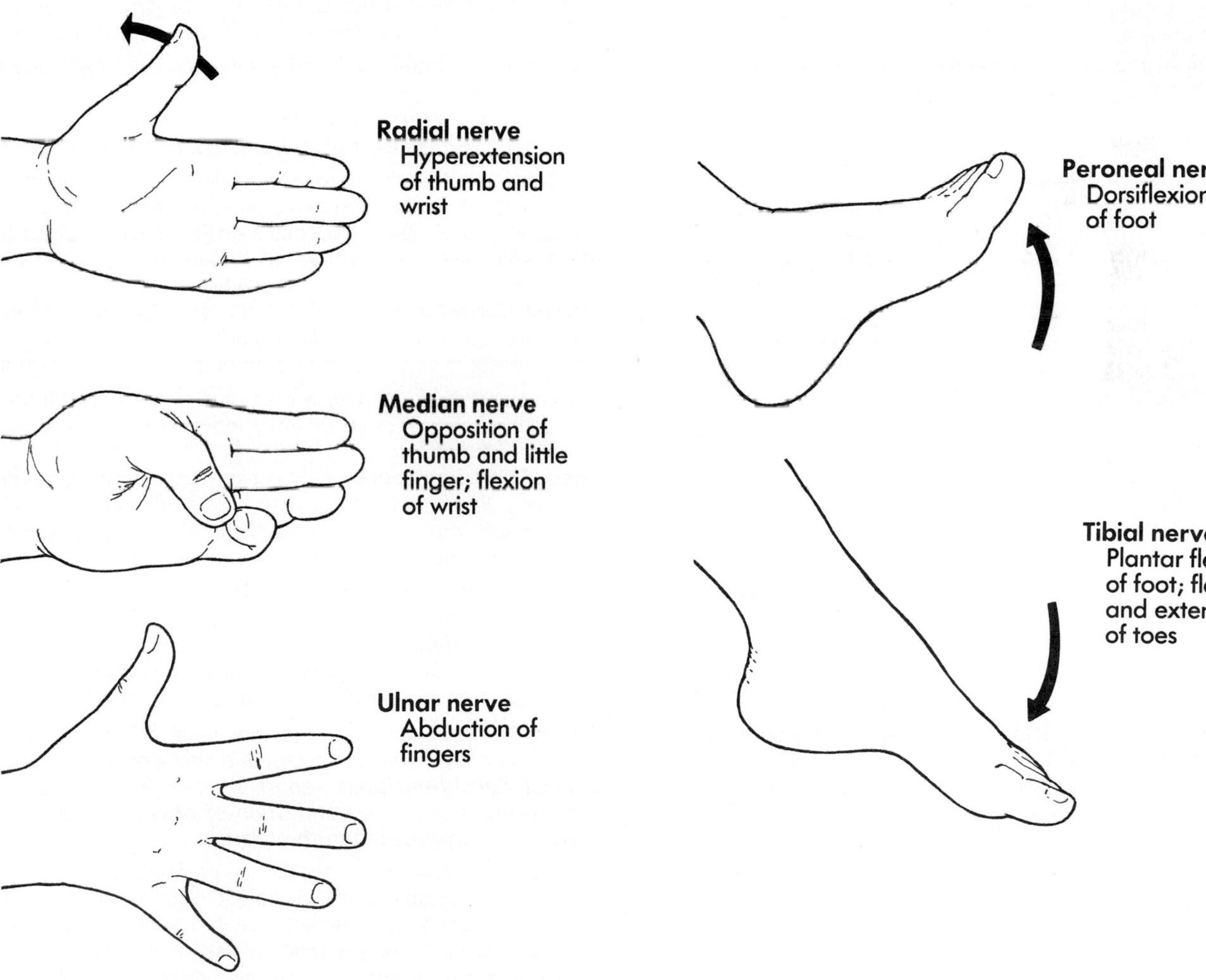


***FIG. 77-3*** Nerve testing for motor function.

| Steps | Rationale |
|---|---|
| *Infants and toddlers:* | |
| a. Observe movement during activity or play with family. | Spontaneous movement may occur during play with family when a child is relaxed and not afraid. |
| b. Place favorite toy within reach and observe child's ability or attempt to grasp or touch. | Play is a natural part of a child's daily routine and provides a nonthreatening method to observe extremity movement. ***Special Considerations:*** *Ask family to bring child's favorite toys. Toys can be used for testing and as security objects.* |
| c. Passively move exposed digits of extremity. | Passive range of motion should not produce pain. Pain indicates nerve compression and/or tissue hypoxia. ***Special Considerations:*** *Games like "This little piggy" can be used. Do this part of motor assessment last. It is the most threatening and may cause pain if there is nerve impairment or severe injury. Traumatic severing or crushing extremity injuries may initially require restricted motion; therefore, verify with the physician the amount of motion permitted.* |
| *Preschooler and older:* | |
| a. Make testing a game. | Playing games provides an activity children enjoy and provides a nonthreatening method of assessment. ***Special Considerations:*** *Games like "Simon says spread your fingers!" "Follow the leader," or "Show me five" can be used.* |
| b. Show and tell child what movement to perform (see Fig. 77-3.) | Child may not understand verbal directions but can copy body movements. ***Special Considerations:*** *Demonstration also works well when language barriers exist (e.g., deafness, non-English speaking).* |
| c. Tell child to wiggle fingers/toes. | Assessing only the ability to wiggle digits gives incomplete assessment data regarding nerve innervation, but it does initiate rapport and establish the child's ability to follow directions. |
| d. Passively move exposed digits of extremity. | Active and passive movement of extremity must be tested to ensure intactness of nerve innervation. ***Special Considerations:*** *Traumatic severing or crushing extremity injuries may initially require restricted motion; therefore, verify with physician the amount of motion permitted.* |
| 5. Determine presence of pain (see Skill 52). | Movement should not cause excessive pain or discomfort. Increased pain or discomfort may indicate impaired circulation or nerve function. ***Special Considerations:*** *Pain is expected following trauma or surgery. Pain should lessen with time and medication. All pain complaints must be evaluated. Fear, anxiety, and absence of family may increase child's perception of pain.* |
| 6. Praise child's efforts to cooperate with neurovascular assessment. | Positive reinforcement gives the child a sense of accomplishment and encourages continued participation. ***Special Considerations:*** *Praise all attempts at cooperation. Using stickers, playing a game, or awarding points for a special privilege provides motivation and rewards child's behavior.* |
| 7. Record assessment data in chart using nurse's notes or neurovascular flowsheet. | Recording assessment data provides legal documentation verifying neurovascular assessment and status of child's condition. ***Special Considerations:*** *Report all changes to physician immediately. Document notification of physician and any interventions implemented in the chart.* |
| 8. Teach family to perform neurovascular assessment on involved extremity. | Neurovascular assessment should be performed for duration of extremity immobilization to detect signs of blood vessel or nerve compression. Teaching family members during child's initial treatment allows time to ask questions and perform assessment proficiently before discharge. Teaching also promotes confidence and accurate assessment following discharge. |

## Evaluation Outcomes

1. Toes/fingers remain warm and pink with brisk capillary refill and palpable pulses.
2. Sensory function of involved extremity remains intact.
3. Motor function of extremity is exhibited by flexion, extension, abduction, and adduction.
4. Child experiences decreased, minimal, or no pain.
5. Child/family verbalizes reason for neurovascular assessment.
6. Family demonstrates proper neurovascular assessment of child's extremity prior to discharge.

## Observational Guidelines

Observe skin temperature, skin color, and capillary refill time. Palpate pulses for presence, strength, and equality.

Observe for sensation in response to touch by report, movement, changes in behavior, or facial expression.

Observe for active movement and perform passive movement without increasing pain. If pain occurs, note what movement induces pain (e.g., extension).

Determine amount and frequency of pain medication required. Assess level of pain.

Ask child/family to verbalize their understanding of the purpose for neurovascular assessment.

Observe family's ability to correctly perform assessment on involved extremity, identify potential problems, and verbalize frequency of assessment at home and when and whom to contact if problems/questions arise.

## Documentation

Document the following: color of extremity; capillary refill time; temperature of skin; pulses, pulse site and use of doppler. Note presence of edema, elevation of extremity, use of ice/cold applications; sensation, describe in child's own words; movement, active and passive; and pain, describe in child's own words. Document child/parent teaching, content taught, ability to verbalize information or demonstrate skill; and identification of problems and action taken, changes in neurovascular status, notification of physician, and interventions implemented.

UNIT X

## PRODUCT REFERENCES AND TEACHING RESOURCES

Wong D and Whaley L: Clinical manual of pediatric nursing, ed 3, St Louis, 1990, The CV Mosby Co.
Home care instruction: caring for the child in a cast.

## REFERENCES

Baker CM and Wong DL: Q.U.E.S.T.: a process of pain assessment in children, Orthop Nurs 6(1):11-19, 1987.

Benz J: The adolescent in a spica cast, Orthop Nurs 5(3):22-23, 1986.

Boos M: A program of home traction for congenital dislocation of the hip, Orthop Nurs 1(2):11-16, 1982.

Carpenito LJ: Nursing diagnosis: application to clinical practice, Philadelphia, 1983, JB Lippincott Co.

Celeste SM, Folcik MA, and Dumas KM: Identifying a standard for pin care site using the quality assurance, Orthop Nurs 3(4):17-24, 1984.

Creighton H: Law every nurse should know, ed 5, Philadelphia, 1986, WB Saunders Co.

Cuddy C: Caring for the child in a spica cast: a parent's perspective, Orthop Nurs 5(3):17-21, 1986.

Donahoo C and Dimon J: Orthopedic nursing, Boston, 1977, Little, Brown & Co.

Ellis JA: Using pain scales to prevent undermedication, MCN 13(3):180-182, 1988.

Farrell J: Illustrated guide to orthopedic nursing, ed 3, Philadelphia, 1986, JB Lippincott Co.

Feller N et al: A multidisciplinary approach to developing safe transportation for children with special needs, Orthop Nurs 5(5):25-27, 1986.

Hilt N and Cogburn S: Manual of orthopedic nursing, St Louis, 1980, The CV Mosby Co.

Hilt N and Schmidt E: Pediatric orthopedic nursing, St Louis, 1975, The CV Mosby Co.

James W, White S, and Yanklowitz B: Allergic contact dermatitis to compound tincture of benzoin, J Am Acad Dermatol 11(5, part 1):847-850, 1984.

Karn MA and Ragiel CA: The psychological effects of immobilization on the pediatric orthopaedic patient, Orthop Nurs 5(6):12-16, 1986.

Keefer B and Levine A: Total contact for immobilization of thoracolumbar fracture, Orthop Nurs 4(6):36-42, 1985.

Kozier B and Erb G: Techniques in clinical nursing, ed 2, Reading, Mass, 1987, Addison-Wesley Publishing Co.

Latta L and Sarmiento A: Mechanical behavior of tibial fractures. In Moore TM, editor: American Academy of Orthopedic Surgeons: symposium on trauma to the leg and its sequela, St Louis, 1981, The CV Mosby Co.

Leifer G: Principles and techniques in pediatric nursing, ed 4, Philadelphia, 1982, WB Saunders Co.

Lewis SM and Collier IC: Medical-surgical nursing: assessment and management of clinical problems, New York, 1987, McGraw-Hill Inc.

McCullough FL and Evans LM: Assessment of neurovascular status in children, Orthop Nurs 4(4):19-25, 1985.

Nelson N and Beckel J, editors: Nursing care plans for the pediatric patient, St Louis, 1987, The CV Mosby Co.

Norton B and Miller A: Skills for professional nursing practice, Norwalk, Conn, 1986, Appleton-Century-Crofts.

O'Brien SW and Konsler GK: Alleviating children's postoperative pain, MCN 13(3):183-186, 1988.

Ogden JA: Skeletal injury in the child, Philadelphia, 1982, Lea and Febiger.

Osborne LJ and DiGiacomo I: Traction: a review with nursing diagnoses and interventions, Orthop Nurs 6(4):13-18, 1987.

Palmer M and Wyness MA: Positioning and handling: important considerations in the care of the severely head injured patient, J Neurosci Nurs 20(1):42-49, 1988.

Pikl B, editor: Massachusetts General Hospital manual of pediatric nursing practice, Boston, 1981, Little, Brown & Co.

Rademaker M and Kirby J: Contact dermatitis to a skin adhesive, Contact Dermatitis, 6(5):297-298, 1987.

Rockwood CA Jr, Wilkins KE and King RE: Fractures in children, vol 3, Philadelphia, 1984, JB Lippincott Co.

Shesser L: Car seat modification for children under treatment for congenital hip dislocations, Orthop Nurs 4(6):11-13, 1985.

Smith M: Setting up portable Bryant traction, Orthop Nurs 1(2):18-20, 1982.

Smith M: Transport traction, Orthop Nurs 1(5):28-31, 1982.

Sporing E, Walton M, and Cady C: The Children's Hospital of Philadelphia manual of pediatric nursing policies, procedures, and personnel, Oradell, NJ, 1984, Medical Economics Books.

Sproles KJ: Nursing care of skeletal pins: a closer look, Orthop Nurs 4(1):11-19, 1985.

Steele S: Young children with meningomyelocele, with special reference to handling, positioning, and child-adult play interactions, Issues Compr Pediatr Nurs 11(4):213-225, 1988.

Swearingen P, editor: Photo-Atlas of nursing procedures, Reading, Mass, 1984, Addison-Wesley Publishing Co.

Taylor JW and Ballenger S: Neurological dysfunctions and nursing intervention, New York, 1980, McGraw-Hill Book Co.

Trickey EL: Injuries of the leg. In Wilson JN, editor: Watson-Jones fractures and joint injuries, vol 2, ed 6, New York, 1982, Churchill Livingstone.

Villalon D and Smith M: At home with traction, Pediatr Nurs 8:15-16, 1982.

Whaley L and Wong D: Nursing care of infants and children, ed 4, St Louis, 1991, The CV Mosby Co.

Whitson B and McFarlane J: The pediatric nursing skills manual, New York, 1980, John Wiley & Sons Inc.

Wieck L, King E, and Dyer M: Illustrated manual of nursing techniques, Philadelphia, 1986, JB Lippincott Co.

Wong D and Whaley L: Clinical manual of pediatric nursing, ed 3, St Louis, 1990, The CV Mosby Co.

# UNIT XI Skin Therapy

## SKILL 78 Cleansing and Dressing a Burn Wound

*Roberta S. Wilson*

Burns result in a variety of physical and psychosocial changes for a child that also influence the family. Child and family response may be affected by the extent and location of the burn. Physical care in the form of wound management is only one aspect of burn care; short- and long-term psychosocial needs provide additional challenges to health care providers working with the child, family and community where the child lives.

Cleansing burn wounds promotes wound healing by preventing infection. The efficacy of topical antimicrobial agents is dependent on a wound surface clean of debris and sources of infection. Application of dressings aids in further debridement of wounds by dislodging eschar when dressings are removed. Moreover, dressings provide a barrier that protects the wound and new epithelium.

### NURSING DIAGNOSES

Impaired skin or tissue integrity related to thermal trauma; Pain related to nerve ending injury and/or treatment procedures; Anxiety related to unmet informational needs about cleansing and dressing burn wound; Potential for infection related to interruption of primary defenses (skin/tissue); Potential alteration in body temperature related to hydrotherapy treatments or infection; Potential ineffective thermoregulation related to 20% to 25% or more loss of skin.

| Steps | Rationale |
|---|---|
| **Assessment** | |
| 1. Assess condition of the wound at each dressing change: | Frequent wound assessment permits early detection of signs of infection and other complications, which may convert a partial-thickness burn to full-thickness. |
| a. Color of the burn wound and surrounding tissue. | Tissue surrounding the burn wound should be clean and of usual skin color. Signs of infection are: redness of the skin extending beyond the burn, a bluish-green exudate, black discoloration of burn wound or surrounding skin, vesicles or blisters present on skin. |
| b. Drainage. | Burn wounds normally drain serous fluid; however, an increase in amount or a change in the consistency or color of drainage may indicate infection. |
| c. Odor. | An infected burn wound may produce a pungent, foul, or sweet smelling odor. |
| d. Granulation tissue (pink to red, moist and shiny) and/or epithelial tissue (pale pink to white spikes). | Granulation tissue develops in areas of full-thickness injury and requires coverage with a skin graft to achieve closure of the burn wound; it develops approximately 14 to 21 days after injury. Epithelial tissue appears in healing areas of partial thickness injury approximately 5 to 7 days after injury when the wound is free of eschar and infection. Epithelial tissue forms new dermis and epidermis. |
| e. Necrotic tissue. | Tissue necrosis is a sign of severe infection and may be the first visual indication of burn wound sepsis. Areas of tissue necrosis may also develop in nonburn tissue in burn sepsis. Tissue necrosis develops as large numbers of bacteria invade tissue and can be visible as patches of dark blue to black. |

| Steps | Rationale |
|---|---|
| 2. Assess age and developmental level of the child (see Skill 25). | Knowledge of developmental level allows appropriate teaching and evaluation of coping skills. Age and developmental level influence ability to cope with burn injury, pain, anxiety, burn care procedures, and separation from family and friends. |
| 3. Assess amount and severity of pain associated with burn care procedures (see Skill 52). | Injury to nerve endings results in pain, which may be intensified by exposure to air and burn care procedures; fear and anxiety increase perception of pain. |
| 4. Assess for changes in thermoregulation by monitoring child's temperature and other vital signs. | Loss of greater than 20% to 25% of the skin results in alteration of core body thermoregulation, which continues for several weeks after burn wound closure. Nursing interventions to conserve and maintain core body temperature at approximately 38° C, and to prevent shivering that massively increases metabolic demands, are essential to decrease physiologic stress and promote recovery. |
| 5. Assess changes in fluid and electrolyte balance (see Skill 64). | Changes in fluid and electrolyte balance may result from treatments and cleansing of the burn wound, and from the type of dressing or topical antimicrobial agent being used (Carjaval and Parks, 1988). |
| 6. Assess for additional signs and symptoms of burn wound sepsis, including: absence of bowel sounds, vomiting, changes in blood studies, changes in vital signs, psychological disorientation, or positive tissue/blood cultures. | Assessing for early signs and symptoms of sepsis allows prompt detection and intervention. Burn wound sepsis is a major cause of death in the burned child. |
| 7. Assess for allergies to cleansing solutions, e.g., povidone-iodine, sulfa-based antimicrobial creams, analgesics. | Assessing allergies affects the selection of medications and solutions used to prevent adverse effects. |

## Planning and Goal Setting

| Steps | Rationale |
|---|---|
| 1. Gather supplies:<br>a. For cleansing and dressings:<br>▪ Sterile gloves and gown.<br>▪ Hair cover and face mask.<br>▪ Sterile scissors.<br>b. For cleansing only:<br>▪ Gauze pads, fluff-squares, or washcloths.<br>▪ Clean linen.<br>▪ Sterile thumb forceps. | Supplies needed depend on method of cleansing and type of dressing to be applied. Gathering supplies before beginning the procedure assists in organization and keeps time of exposure of the burn to a minimum, thereby decreasing heat loss, fluid loss, metabolic stress, and discomfort for the child. |
| c. Additional supplies for hydrotherapy:<br>▪ Cleansing solution such as povidone-iodine solutions according to facility policy or physician preference. | ***Special Considerations:*** *Methods, equipment, and supplies to clean and debride burn wounds vary considerably among facilities. Hydrotherapy tubs are not available or used at all facilities. If used, a detergent germicide is needed to clean the tub before and after use.* |
| d. Additional supplies for bedside cleansing:<br>▪ Sterile basin with warmed povidone-iodine solution or other detergent.<br>▪ Sterile basin with warmed water or normal saline solution. | Wound cleansing can be effective at child's bedside. The decision of type of cleansing used is based on the physician's order. |
| e. Additional supplies for dressing application:<br>▪ Antimicrobial cream and/or biologic membrane.<br>▪ Sterile fine-mesh, rolled gauze, Kerlix, or kling.<br>▪ Stretch gauze, netting, elastic wraps, or Kerlix (optional). | ***Special Considerations:*** *Stretch netting is an expensive supply.* |
| 2. Plan for pain control methods. Administer medication timed appropriately to deliver peak effect during painful aspect of procedure (see Skill 52). | Adequate management of pain is necessary to reduce the discomfort caused by the burn and treatment therapies.<br>***Special Considerations:*** *Pain resulting from burn injuries and performance of burn care procedures may not be completely alleviated; however, it may be decreased with appropriate pain management.* |
| 3. Control environmental temperature of the hydrotherapy and dressing room with central heat, radiant heating shields, or heat lamps. Maintain environmental room temperature between 28° and 33°C (82.4° to 91.4° F). Avoid overheating or underheating (Whaley and Wong, 1991) (see Skill 83). | Controlling environmental temperature minimizes the child's metabolic expenditure, maximizes comfort, and facilitates maintenance of normal body temperature. |
| 4. Prepare hydrotherapy area if using:<br>a. Clean hydrotherapy tank, tub, or shower. | Cleansing the hydrotherapy area minimizes exposure of the burn wound to infectious agents.<br>***Special Considerations:*** *Follow appropriate hospital policies and procedures for the cleansing and disinfection of this area and equipment.* |

| Steps | Rationale |
|---|---|
| b. Fill tub with an appropriate amount of water. Maintain water temperature between 98° to 100.4° F. | The use of warm water in hydrotherapy helps to prevent heat loss from the burn wound. |
| c. Add selected ingredients and/or detergents to the cleansing solution. | |
| 5. Establish a sterile field with debridement and dressing supplies. | Aseptic technique is imperative to limit bacteria on the burn wound that can lead to infection and/or sepsis. |
| 6. Develop individualized goals of nursing care:<br>▪ Promote healing by preventing burn wound infection.<br>▪ Prevent additional complications of burn wounds such as fluid and electrolyte imbalance and ineffective thermoregulation.<br>▪ Minimize pain and anxiety. | |

## Implementation

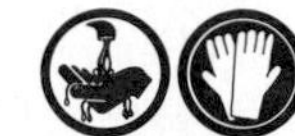

| Steps | Rationale |
|---|---|
| 1. Explain the procedure to the child prior to performing each step (see Skill 1). | Preparing the child may reduce anxiety and improve cooperation with the procedure. |
| 2. Remove old dressing: | |
| a. Put on mask, hair cover, sterile gown, and nonsterile gloves. | Mask should be worn when a burn wound is exposed. |
| b. Using clean technique, slit outer layers of the dressing with blunt end scissors. | Clean technique is sufficient to remove outer layers of old dressing using infection control precautions. |
| c. Turn or lay open the outer layers of dressing down to the fine-mesh gauze strips. | |
| d. Using sterile technique, unwrap the layer of fine-mesh gauze strips. | Sterile technique is used when exposing the burn wound. |
| e. Place all removed dressings in a biologic approved waste receptacle. | Biologic disposal of contaminated dressings reduces sources of infection. |
| 3. Clean the wound by one of the following methods: | |
| *Hydrotherapy:* | |
| a. After placing child in the water, turn agitators on for 5 to 10 minutes using gentle agitation or water pressure. | Water agitation assists with removal of topical antimicrobial creams and cleansing of the skin and burn wound. This procedure also increases peripheral blood flow to the burned areas, and permits easier range of motion exercises.<br>***Special Considerations:*** *Never leave a child unattended in the tub.* |
| b. Using the sterile fluff gauze squares and prescribed cleansing solution, gently wash all burn and surrounding areas. | Washing with gauze helps remove loose tissue and eschar.<br>***Special Considerations:*** *A school-age child or adolescent can assist with this step.* |
| c. Within 20 minutes, remove child from bath and place on clean sheets or towels. | Limiting immersion time prevents excess fluid and electrolyte loss from wound. |
| d. Gently pat burn areas dry. | Patting the burn areas dry is less painful than rubbing and limits damage to new epithelial tissue. |
| *Bedside cleansing:* | |
| a. Place gauze squares, fluffs, or washcloth in sterile basin with warm water and designated cleansing solution. | Warmed solutions minimize loss of body heat. |
| b. With gentle firm pressure, wash burn areas moving from center of wound to outer edge. | It is important that all areas be completely washed of accumulated creams and exudate to reduce bacteria. |
| c. Rinse all areas with warm solution if indicated. | Certain agents are irritating to tissues and must be rinsed. For example, povidone-iodine solutions harden eschar and may increase serum iodine to toxic levels. Hibiclens, however, is not rinsed since it may increase effectiveness of Silvadene. |
| d. Pat areas dry. | |
| e. Using scissors and thumb forceps, remove any loose tissue or eschar present on the wound. | Since loose tissue or eschar provides a medium for bacterial growth, removal is necessary. Extensive debridement should be avoided to prevent loss of blood and damage to new epithelial tissue under the eschar. |
| f. Place the child on clean sheets or towels. | |
| 4. Apply dressings using the following method: | |
| a. Change into sterile gloves. | Using the same gloves used for cleansing may transfer bacteria to dressings. |
| b. Apply topical antimicrobial cream or biologic membrane as ordered by the physician (Table 78-1). | |
| ▪ If using fine-mesh gauze impregnated with antimicrobial cream, apply overlapping strips to the burn areas. | A small amount of overlap for each strip maintains total coverage and allows for movement or edema. |

**TABLE 78-1** Comparison of Common Topical Preparations for Burn Wound Care

| Agent | Dressing Features | Advantages | Disadvantages |
|---|---|---|---|
| Silver nitrate, 0.5% ($AgNO_3$) | Occlusive<br>Impedes joint movement<br>Dressings changed twice daily | Reduces evaporative losses<br>Does not interfere with wound healing<br>Nonallergenic<br>Inexpensive<br>Effective against major burn flora, including *Pseudomonas* and *Staphylococcus* | Cannot allow dressings to become dry; requires frequent soaking (at least every 2 hours)<br>Difficult to use, stains all contacts black<br>Does not penetrate eschar; therefore, should be applied before bacterial growth occurs<br>Ineffective on established burn wound infections<br>Hypotonicity pulls electrolytes from wound, causing depletion of sodium, chloride, potassium, and magnesium, necessitating continuous monitoring and replacement<br>Little effect on *Klebsiella* and *Aerobacter* groups |
| Mafenide acetate (Sulfamylon), 10% | Usually exposure<br>Occasionally with dressings<br>Reapplied twice daily | Diffuses rapidly into burn wound and underlying tissues<br>Rapidly excreted<br>Easily applied<br>Penetrates through eschar and deeply into burn wound; therefore, effective against many gram positive and gram negative organisms including *Pseudomonas* and *Clostridium*<br>Topical of choice for electrical injury | Severe acidodis caused by inhibition of carbonic anhydrase in kidney<br>Hypersensitivity reaction in many children (sulfa-based)<br>Causes severe pain for approximately 20 minutes after application<br>Inhibits wound healing |
| Silver sulfadiazine (Silvadene), 1% (AgSD) | Occlusive or open<br>Motion of joints maintained<br>Applied 1 to 3 times daily | Nontoxic<br>Combines advantages of silver nitrate and mafenide acetate<br>Painless<br>Easy to apply<br>Absorbs slowly<br>Effective against gram positive and gram negative bacteria | Does not penetrate eschar as well as mafenide acetate<br>May cause neutropenia<br>Limited effectiveness against yeast |
| Povidone-iodine (Betadine) ointment | Exposure, modified or occlusive<br>Impedes joint movement | Effective against a broad spectrum of organisms including yeast | Elevation of protein-bound iodine causing CNS depression<br>Use associated with considerable pain<br>Causes eschar to "tan" and become very stiff, making debridement, movement and evaluation of burn wound difficult<br>May cause iodine toxicity |

Adapted from Whaley LF and Wong DL: Nursing care of infants and children, ed 4, 1991, St Louis, The CV Mosby Co.

| Steps | Rationale |
|---|---|
| ▪ If using direct application of topical antimicrobial cream from a container, use nondominant gloved hand to remove cream from container and drop into dominant hand. Then use dominant gloved hand to apply a thin layer over the entire burn area. | This method is employed to avoid contamination of cream in the container. |
| c. Wrap finger and toe digits individually. | Individual wrapping allows greater range of motion and prevents burned surfaces from adhering. |
| d. If using antimicrobial cream, apply one layer of dressing in overlapping strips to cover the burn area. | |
| e. Apply one or more layers of sterile fluff gauze rolls as continuous wrap over the dressing layer. | Continuous wrapping secures the dressing strips in place. ***Special Considerations:*** *When wrapping extremities, wrap distal to proximal to prevent edema and venous congestion. Excessive wrapping may limit range of motion.* |
| f. Apply stretch gauze, netting, elastic wrap or Kerlix over the entire dressing (optional) (Fig. 78-1). | The additional covering allows greater mobility for the child by keeping the eschar soft and pliable to promote active range of motion. |

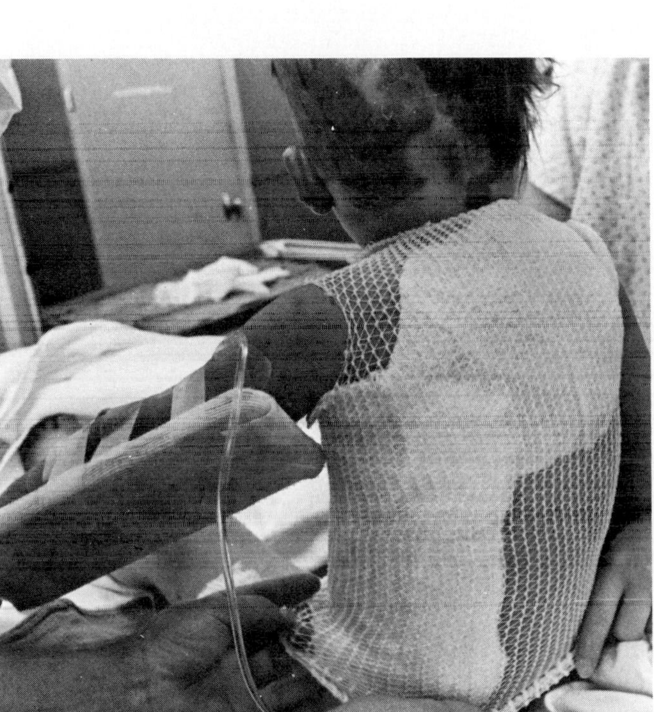

***FIG. 78-1*** Burn wound covered with gauze dressings and secured with tubular elastic netting.

From Whaley L and Wong D: Nursing care of infants and children, ed 4, 1991, St Louis, The CV Mosby Co.

| Steps | Rationale |
|---|---|
| 5. Monitor vital signs before and after procedures, particularly body temperature to determine extent of heat loss. See Skills 30, 31, 32, 33, and 83. | Close monitoring of vital signs permits early detection of hypothermia. ***Special Considerations:*** *Heat loss from hydrotherapy, wound cleansing, and application of dressings may not manifest for 2 to 4 hours after procedures.* |

| Evaluation Outcomes | Observational Guidelines |
|---|---|
| 1. Burn wound is free of infection and forms granulation or epithelial tissue. | Observe for purulent drainage or wound margin cellulitis, changes in odor or color. Review wound culture results. |
| 2. Pain is minimized during procedures. | Note type and frequency of analgesics administered. Note indicators of pain, both verbal and nonverbal, and behavior before, during, and after procedures. Note child's response to analgesia and other pain control interventions. |
| 3. Anxiety is reduced through use of appropriate coping skills during procedure. | Observe the child's coping techniques during procedures. |
| 4. Additional complications from burn wound are prevented. | Vital signs remain within normal limits. Electrolytes remain within normal range. Hydration is adequate. Signs and symptoms of burn wound sepsis are absent. |

## Documentation

Document appearance of the wound and surrounding tissue at each dressing change or procedure performed; application of topical preparation or biologic membrane; location and type of dressing applied; length of the procedure and the child's tolerance of the procedure; notification of the physician of changes in the burn wound and/or signs and symptoms of impending complications and the interventions implemented; analgesic given before the procedure being performed and child's response to analgesic; coping techniques implemented and child's response to the technique; and vital signs before and after the procedures and every 4 hours or as needed.

# *SKILL 79* Caring for Skin Grafts and Donor Sites

*Roberta S. Wilson*

The purpose of permanent skin grafting is to close a burn wound and restore integumentary function. Grafted skin initially receives nourishment by osmotic interchange with the recipient bed until a blood supply is established, usually 48 to 72 hours post-graft. The recipient area produces fibrin that attaches the graft, permitting wound healing to occur. Leukocytes and fibroblasts infiltrate the fibrin and capillary beds of granulation tissue spread through the fibrin. Within 3 days, vascularization of the graft occurs. After 2 weeks, the graft is attached to the base by connective tissue (Whaley and Wong, 1991).

Meticulous care of skin grafts fosters maximum functional and cosmetic results. Grafts may be managed by several methods. This skill addresses open and closed methods. Open, exposed grafts are left uncovered and open to air; closed grafts are covered by multiple layers of wet dressings.

Harvesting skin grafts produces a superficial partial thickness injury at the donor site. Prevention of infection in donor sites decreases conversion to a deeper wound that might also require grafting.

## NURSING DIAGNOSES

Potential for infection related to interruption of primary defenses (skin/tissue); Impaired physical mobility related to imposed restrictions to protect graft and donor sites; Pain related to exposure of donor site nerve endings to air and care procedures; Body image disturbance related to changes in physical appearance due to extent of burn, dressings, number of donor sites, scar formation, and peer/family acceptance.

| Steps | Rationale |
|---|---|
| **Assessment** | |
| 1. Determine child's age and developmental level. | Nursing interventions and interactions are based in part on the age and developmental level of the child. Age and development also influence the child's ability to participate in care. |
| 2. Assess condition of graft site, donor site, or dressings postoperatively and hourly for first 24 hours and then every 4 hours, noting drainage, odor, and color. | Assessment of skin graft site, donor site, and dressings helps detect and prevent postoperative complications. ***Special Considerations:*** *Most skin grafts are wrapped in wet bulky dressings for 48 to 72 hours postoperatively. Serosanguinous drainage may occur through the dressing; however, fresh bleeding should not occur. A large amount of drainage, the presence of a strong odor, and/or yellowish-white or green drainage indicates infection. If the skin graft is exposed or open, inspect graft more frequently. If a semipermeable membrane is used at the donor site, it may need to be removed by the physician if purulent drainage develops.* |
| 3. Assess pain related to graft and donor site (see Skill 52): | Assessment of pain indicates need for pain management measures and provides a basis for evaluation of effectiveness. |
| a. Skin graft site. | The area of skin graft placement usually does not cause discomfort because it is a closed wound. |
| b. Donor site. | The donor site is usually painful because it is equivalent to a healing partial thickness burn injury. |

| Steps | Rationale |
|---|---|
| | ***Special Considerations:*** *Drying the donor site with heat lamps or maintaining the site with a closed or semipermeable membrane dressing decreases the pain caused by exposure of nerve endings to air.* |
| 4. Assess child's alteration in body image. | Alteration in body image occurs at the time of the burn injury; acceptance of alteration in body image is necessary for optimal recovery. ***Special Considerations:*** *Change in appearance should be addressed in preoperative teaching and through the course of healing and recovery.* |

## Planning and Goal Setting

| Steps | Rationale |
|---|---|
| 1. Gather supplies. | Gathering supplies enhances the efficiency of care provided. |
| a. Skin graft care: ▪ Sterile cotton-tipped applicators. ▪ Cleansing solution. ▪ Lubricating ointment or lotion. ▪ Sterile 18 gauge needle. ▪ Sterile suture or staple removal set. ▪ Sterile scissors. ▪ Sterile thumb forceps. | The physician usually orders the cleansing solution and lubricating lotion to be used. |
| b. Additional items (closed graft care): ▪ Sterile fine-mesh gauze. ▪ Sterile bulky dressing. ▪ Stretch gauze, netting, elastic wraps, or Kerlix. | |
| c. Donor site care: *Fine-mesh gauze method:* ▪ Heat lamp. ▪ Sterile scissors. ▪ Lubricating lotion. *Semipermeable or biologic membrane:* ▪ Sterile bulky dressing. ▪ Sterile 18 gauge needle. ▪ Sterile cotton-tipped applicators. ▪ Lubricating lotion. | Supplies depend on type of donor site covering, and treatment as closed or open. |
| 2. Plan for pain relief measures (see Skill 52). | Adequate management of pain is necessary to reduce discomfort caused by the burn and burn therapies. Additional pain may result from adherence of dressings to skin. |
| 3. Plan for sedation or restraint if necessary to maintain immobilization of graft area (see Skill 51). | Excess movement may result in shearing and dislodgement of graft. |
| 4. Establish individualized goals of nursing care: ▪ Promote healing by preventing burn wound infection and protecting the graft from trauma. ▪ Minimize pain and reduce anxiety. | |

## Implementation

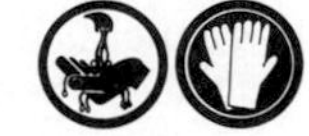

| Steps | Rationale |
|---|---|
| 1. Explain procedure to the child before performing each step (see Skill 1). Permit child as many choices as possible during the graft and donor site care and encourage active participation. | Age-appropriate explanations enhance the child's understanding and cooperation with the procedure. Apprehension is a major factor contributing to child's discomfort. Children are more cooperative and demonstrate less anxiety and depression when they are allowed to actively participate in their care. |
| 2. Protect graft and donor sites: | Facilitating a "take" of the graft, and preventing conversion of the donor site to a full-thickness injury are priority goals of nursing care. |
| a. Immobilize area of skin graft for 3 to 5 days using bulky dressings, splints, sedation, age-appropriate restraints, etc. | Immobilization is essential to prevent skin graft loss secondary to rubbing or shearing. |
| b. Keep child from scratching or picking at wound by providing distractions, explaining reasons to older children or applying restraints to the younger child. | Scratching or picking at wound could damage tissues or result in graft loss. |
| 3. If graft site is located on an extremity, maintain in extension. Reposition immobilized extremity frequently. | Extension positioning decreases risk of contracture formation. Immobilization of grafted extremities may result in stiffness and discomfort of joints. |

| Steps | Rationale |
|---|---|
| 4. Provide open graft care, using aseptic technique and infection control measures. | Following aseptic technique and infection control measures aids in preventing contamination of graft area and self-exposure to serous/blood body fluid. |
| a. Set up a sterile field at bedside. | Open graft care is performed at the bedside. |
| b. Moisten cotton-tipped applicators with cleansing solution. | Moistened applicators cleanse drainage and crust from the graft without dislodging it. |
| c. Gently roll the applicator from the center of the graft to the outer edge. Grafts should be rolled every 2 hours for the first 24 hours after application and then every 4 hours for 48 hours. | Rolling the graft in this manner removes fluid which collects under the graft, thus promoting graft adherence to underlying granulation tissue. The first 72 hours after grafting is the time during which grafts are adhering to underlying granulation tissue and graft take occurs. |
| d. When the edges of the graft become adherent, gently pierce any bleb or blister present on the graft with an 18 gauge needle and roll the fluid toward the opening in the blister. | It is important to maintain the adherent areas of the graft at all times. Opening the blister and draining the fluid does not disturb parts of the graft which have already adhered. |
| e. Apply lubricating ointment very lightly on graft using a cotton-tipped applicator. | A layer of lubricating ointment helps to prevent drying of the graft. |
| f. Remove sutures and/or staples between 3 to 7 days postgrafting or per physician's order. | The graft generally adheres in 3 days and the sutures/staples are no longer needed. Sutures or staples left in after 7 days may become a source of infection. |
| g. Trim excess graft from healed graft area with scissors and thumb forceps. Excess graft may have a dry paper-like shriveled appearance with dark edges. Areas of graft loss may appear as white to yellow blister-like areas with dark edges. | Excess graft or areas of graft loss must be trimmed from the graft as they become a source of infection and can prevent total graft incorporation into dermis. |
| 5. Provide closed graft care, using aseptic technique: a. Establish a sterile field. | Whenever the skin graft dressing is changed, aseptic technique must be maintained to prevent contamination. ***Special Considerations:*** *Dressings on closed grafts are usually changed starting on the third to fifth day after grafting, and daily thereafter.* |
| b. Remove graft dressing by slitting the outer layers of the dressing with blunt end scissors down to the layer of fine-mesh gauze directly over the graft. | ***Special Considerations:*** *Take care when removing the outer dressing to not disturb the graft.* |
| c. Remove the fine-mesh gauze, wetting with sterile saline or water if needed. | The mesh gauze must be easily removed to prevent dislodging the graft. |
| d. Remove the fluid from beneath the graft as in Steps 4c and 4d, then wash the graft gently with sterile cleansing solution and sterile gauze. | Washing cleans the surface of the graft. |
| e. Cover the graft with fine-mesh gauze dressing. | |
| f. Apply bulky dressing over the fine-mesh gauze. Moisten dressing every 4 hours or per physician order with normal saline or antimicrobial solution. | A large bulky dressing protects a new graft from damage due to rubbing, bumping or shearing. ***Special Considerations:*** *Moist dressings are usually covered with a dry, absorbent gauze. Plastic wrappings should not be used because they build up heat and moisture, which may cause skin maceration (Whaley and Wong, 1991).* |
| g. Apply elastic wrap, stretch gauze or netting over the entire dressing. | A pressure dressing prevents epithelial breakdown, stimulates circulation, and enhances mobility (Whaley and Wong, 1991). |
| 6. For donor site care using fine-mesh gauze exposure: a. Follow same procedure as for closed graft care (see steps 5a and 5b). | The donor site is covered with fine-mesh gauze and left exposed until dressing falls off. Dressings are not changed on donor sites to prevent tearing delicate, new epithelium (Whaley and Wong, 1991). |
| b. If ordered, apply heat lamp to donor site for 15 to 20 minutes:<br>250 watt: Place 3 to 4 feet from site.<br>60 watt: Place 18 to 24 inches from site.<br>Repeat every 2 hours until fine-mesh gauze is dry. | |
| c. Trim the fine-mesh gauze as it peels from the donor site using blunt end scissors. | The fine-mesh gauze will lift from the donor site as the site heals over 7 to 10 days. |
| d. Soak the donor site daily (during bath if desired) after 5 days. | Soaking helps loosen the fine-mesh gauze and aids in its removal between 7 and 10 days after harvest of the donor skin. |
| e. Apply lubricating lotion to the healed donor site. | Lubricating lotion decreases dryness of donor site until the skin is able to secrete oil. |
| 7. For donor site care with a semipermeable or biologic membrane: | |
| a. If wrapped, remove outer dressing as with fine-mesh gauze procedure. | ***Special Considerations:*** *Most institutions do not wrap membrane coverings except for a few hours postoperatively.* |

| Steps | Rationale |
|---|---|
| b. Drain areas of accumulated fluid using same technique as in step 4d. | Large amounts of fluid accumulation under the membrane may break the seal at the edges, lifting the membrane from the donor site. |
| c. Remove the membrane when the donor site is healed (approximately 7 to 10 days after harvesting) by soaking the area in the bath tub. | The membrane peels off easily when the donor site is healed. |
| d. Apply lubricating lotion to the donor site. | |
| 8. Measure vital signs every 4 hours. | Close monitoring of vital signs may provide early detection of infection. |
| 9. Assist child in building self-esteem and positive self-image (Whaley and Wong, 1991):<br>a. Explore feelings about physical appearance.<br>b. Discuss feelings about returning to home and family, school and friends.<br>c. Provide reinforcement of positive aspects of appearance and capabilities.<br>d. Point out evidence of healing.<br>e. Discuss methods for improving appearance, e.g., wigs, clothing, make-up. | Children's perceptions of their appearance have a strong impact on their body image and self-esteem. Emotional scars may be as damaging as physical scars.<br>***Special Considerations:*** *The extent of body image change depends on condition of the child, extent of the burn, location and number of donor sites, the appearance of the graft site and extent of scar formation, and parental acceptance.* |

| Evaluation Outcomes | Observational Guidelines |
|---|---|
| 1. Skin grafts and donor sites are free of infection and show evidence of healing. | Skin grafts and donor sites are clean, without signs of infection, and have minimal or no bacterial growth on the culture results. Grafts are dry, soft, and incorporated into the body tissue. Donor site skin is dry and of usual color. Vital signs remain within normal limits. |
| 2. The child experiences minimal pain associated with donor site care procedures. | Pain assessment demonstrates effectiveness of pain reduction measures. |
| 3. The child and family appropriately cope with alteration in body image as a result of the burn injury, grafts, and donor sites. | Observe the child's and family's reaction to changes in skin color, texture, and appearance of the burn injury, grafts, and donor sites. Monitor the child and the family interaction and verbalization of their concerns of the changes in body image. |

### Documentation

Note appearance of skin grafts and donor sites at every dressing change/procedure. Document notification of the physician of changes in skin grafts or donor sites and interventions implemented. Record analgesics given and child's response. Record vital signs. Note child and family's response to alteration in body image.

# *SKILL* **80** Controlling Pruritus

*Donna Phillips Smith and Noreen Heer Nicol*

Pruritus, or itching, is a symptom rather than a disease. Pruritus presents a particular challenge to the nurse because of its common occurrence and the major effect it frequently has on the quality of the suffering child's life. The urge to scratch may be mild and self-limiting, or it may be intense and lead to severely excoriated lesions, infection, and scarring. Pruritus can be a secondary symptom of conditions ranging from dry skin to carcinoma. Systemic diseases that often have associated itching include chickenpox, chronic renal failure, hepatitis, and cancer. Itching is the most common symptom of diseases affecting the skin primarily. Common pediatric dermatologic disorders in which pruritus plays a major role include scabies, insect bites, atopic and contact dermatitis, miliaria, fungal infections, poison ivy, and drug reactions. Appropriate management of the itching child requires an understanding of the itch sensation, an exhaustive search for the underlying cause, and a knowledge of the appropriate therapeutic modalities.

## NURSING DIAGNOSES

Impaired skin integrity related to excoriated lesions and pruritis; Potential for infection related to traumatized tissue; Body image disturbance related to perceived skin imperfections; Pain related to pruritus.

| Steps | Rationale |
|---|---|
| **Assessment** | |
| 1. Review current medical record for age, general health status, immunizations, and physician orders for medications and treatments. | An overview of general status and physician-ordered therapy provides a basis for planning care. |
| 2. Examine the skin for a primary skin lesion that is the direct result of the disease process. | Characteristic cutaneous lesions are often present that provide the diagnosis of one of multiple pruritic dermatoses, such as scabies, atopic or contact dermatitis, or chickenpox. However, the primary lesion is often difficult to find because of secondary changes such as excoriation and lichenification (thickened skin from chronic scratching or rubbing). |
| 3. Examine the skin for secondary changes such as scratch marks, pigment alterations, infection, scarring, and lichenification. | The extent and severity of excoriations indicate the degree of the child's itching and discomfort. The distribution and characteristics may identify external factors (e.g., fiberglass, airborne distribution), specific diseases (e.g., atopic dermatitis), or infestations (e.g., scabies). |
| 4. Examine the skin for dryness, redness, and scaling. Also inspect the condition of the nails. | Xerosis (dry skin) is a common cause or contributing factor of pruritus, which can be relieved by adequate topical hydration and therapy. Xerosis may be exacerbated by low humidity, high altitude, dry cold wind, central heating, and frequent washing with soap and hot water. Ragged and unclean edges of fingernails can contribute to skin breakdown and infection. |
| 5. Assess the nature of the itching:<br>a. Generalized or localized.<br>b. Provoking and relieving factors.<br>c. Character.<br>d. Severity.<br>e. Mode of onset and course.<br>f. Past treatment and effectiveness. | Generalized itching with no rash or identifiable primary lesion may indicate serious systemic disease, e.g., cancer, liver or renal failure, or diabetes (Madden, 1986). Itching associated with cancer (most frequently Hodgkin's) is seldom mild and usually not localized (Dangel, 1986).<br>Itching from exposure to aeroallergens or foods may point to atopy. Itching after a hot bath may point to aquagenic or cholinergic pruritus. Failure to obtain relief from usual symptomatic measures may indicate severity or inability to identify the mediator involved. The pathophysiology of pruritus is not well understood; however, histamine released from skin mast cells is believed to be the most important mediator. |
| 6. Determine if psychosocial factors are present that are contributing to or manifesting as pruritus. | Emotional stress, anxiety, fear, anger, and depression may be major exacerbating factors of pruritus. Pruritus triggered by psychologic factors requires the same symptomatic treatment; however, psychosocial referral is an essential component of therapy. |
| 7. Assess for exposure to any new agents including: current medications (systemic, topical, and OTC), parasites, infectious organisms, chemotherapy, or radiation therapy. | Pruritus can be caused by drug reaction, infectious process, chemotherapy, and radiation therapy. Also, children's skin is usually more easily irritated than is adult skin. Itching with or without a rash can indicate a drug reaction. Itching can also be a sign of infection in the immunosuppressed child. |
| 8. Assess for environmental conditions that may contribute to or cause pruritus. | Extremely high humidity may produce sweat retention. Heat increases cutaneous blood flow and may enhance itching. Tight or overabundant clothing, especially of wool or certain synthetics, can produce irritation. Exposure to irritants such as fiberglass can induce severe pruritus. |
| 9. Determine child's ability to cooperate with therapies and avoid scratching. | Age, developmental and cognitive level, self-control, and motivation influence cooperation. Younger children may require more protective measures. Older children may be more motivated to avoid scarring out of peer acceptance concerns. |
| **Planning and Goal Setting** | |
| 1. Plan therapy collaboratively with child and/or family based on assessment. | Collaborative planning will increase cooperation and success with therapy. Also an individualized approach is essential because of the subjective nature of pruritus. |
| 2. Assemble needed supplies according to therapy(ies) selected (see Implementation section). | Ready access to supplies allows efficient and safe treatments (e.g., emollients must be applied while skin is damp, so they should be obtained before the bath). |
| 3. Develop individualized child and family goals:<br>▪ Skin breakdown is minimized.<br>▪ Infection is prevented.<br>▪ Comfort is promoted. | |

| Steps | Rationale |
|---|---|

## Implementation 

1. Explain to the child and family:
   a. The itching symptom as it relates to etiology, if possible.
   b. The mechanism of the "itch-scratch-itch" cycle (scratching leads to the enhanced sensation of itching).
   c. The principles of the selected therapies.
   d. The factors that are known to exacerbate pruritis and ways to avoid them.

   Understanding the physiologic or psychologic process and principles of itching and its treatment helps increase cooperation.

2. Use general measures.
   a. Keep finger and toenails cut short and filed smooth.

      Small children are likely to scratch with both fingernails and toenails. Short, smooth nails prevent damage to the skin when scratching.

   b. Wash child's hands and scrub under nails frequently.

      Hands and nails should be kept clean to help prevent infecting nonintact skin during scratching.
      ***Special Considerations:*** *A nail brush should be kept at the sink to facilitate cleaning under nails.*

   c. Cover the child's body and extremities with one piece long-sleeved and legged clothing. Infant gowns with hand covers are also useful. If necessary, loosely tape or safety pin mittens or socks over hands and feet.

      Covering the child's body with clothing will minimize the child's ability to scratch. Covering nails will decrease skin damage when scratching.
      ***Special Considerations:*** *The skin should be kept covered only as much as is needed to prevent scratching. Covering and restraints may only frustrate the child and intensify the urge to scratch. Care must also be taken to avoid overdressing and overheating the child.*

   d. Plan care to provide adequate rest time.

      Being tired and irritable usually intensifies the urge to scratch.
      ***Special Considerations:*** *See Implementation step 5 on p. 508.*

   e. Use distraction, play therapy with hands, imagery, and relaxation techniques.

      Another activity allows for diversion of the child's attention.
      ***Special Considerations:*** *Hands-on activities such as modeling clay are ideal (see Skills 16 and 17).*

3. Avoid environmental irritants.
   a. Provide a consistent cool room temperature approximately 68° to 75° F. Also avoid vigorous exercise.

      Heat, presumably through vasodilation and increased cutaneous blood flow, promotes itching.
      ***Special Considerations:*** *Some families may need financial assistance to obtain a fan or air conditioner for the home if this plays a key role.*

   b. Wash all linens, clothing, and undergarments in a mild laundry soap, avoiding fabric softeners and making certain the laundry is thoroughly rinsed free of any residual detergents.

      Pruritus is often precipitated by exposure to the irritant effect of certain components of detergents and fabric softeners (Krowchuk, 1987). The actual laundry detergent that is used is not the key, but rather that all soap is rinsed out.
      ***Special Considerations:*** *Use of an extra rinse cycle or running the items through another wash cycle without soap is often very beneficial.*

   c. Provide lightweight cotton or cotton-blend clothing for the child to wear, especially next to the skin. Avoid overdressing, wool or rough surface fabrics, and tight-fitting garments with restrictive waists and cuffs. In hot weather, avoid synthetic fabrics.

      Light cotton or cotton-blend clothing that is loosely woven allows air circulation and minimizes perspiration, which intensifies itching. Synthetic fabrics, which poorly aerate, increase perspiration.

   d. Use flannel, or old soft sheets laundered as in 3b.

      The child may rub against harsh sheets to scratch, excoriating the skin.

4. Use topical therapy.
   a. Provide baths, immediately followed by an appropriate topical emollient to ensure well-hydrated intact skin. Bathe the child at bedtime when possible.

      Bathing is sometimes discouraged because of its alleged drying effect. Drying is usually the result, however, of failure to apply appropriate topicals to the skin immediately after bathing. The use of a drying soap may also compound the problem. Proper selection of soap and application of the appropriate topical immediately afterward make baths beneficial. Bathing at bedtime may help to promote sleep.

      - Use tepid water (32° to 38° C or 90° to 100° F).

        Hot water causes vasodilation that increases pruritus.

      - Soak in the bath for 15 to 20 minutes. Immediately upon leaving the bath, pat dry and apply emollient or prescribed topical. For tips on applying topical medications, see the box on the following page.

        Soaking 15 to 20 minutes allows the stratum corneum to become saturated with water. Applying an emollient or some occlusive within 2 to 4 minutes of leaving the bath is critical to prevent evaporation of water from the hydrated epidermis. Vigorously rubbing the skin removes more water from the skin and increases vasodilation.

### TIPS ON APPLYING TOPICAL MEDICATIONS

1. Always apply the Five Rights of Medication Administration (see Skill 101).
2. Topical medications are prepared in creams, lotions, pastes, gels, ointments, powders or aerosol base forms, which will affect factors such as occlusive ability, acceptibility to the child/family, and application considerations.
3. The skin is a poor protective barrier for infants of less than 28 weeks gestation; absorption of topical agents may be similar to oral administration (Rutter, 1987).
4. Wash the area of the skin where the medication will be applied if needed to inspect the skin. Also, the new application will be poorly absorbed if applied to skin over previous applications, exudate, crusts, or other debris. Skin inspection is necessary to identify inflamed or denuded skin, which may be a contraindication to use of topical medication.
5. Well-hydrated skin enhances topical drug absorption, therefore application after a bath or soaks is an effective strategy.
6. To check for sensitivity to a topical medication, an open-patch or occluded test application may be ordered on a small area of skin.
7. Verify topical medication concentration carefully to avoid a dosage error. For example, a 1.0% concentration is 10 times that of the same medication with a 0.1% concentration. Many topical agents are available in varying strengths.
8. Sterile gloves or a sterile applicator must be used when applying medication to an open lesion or wound. Nonsterile gloves provide a barrier to undesired exposure to or absorption of medication, although their use may hinder ability to assess the skin. Another consideration is that using gloves may convey nonacceptance of the child's skin appearance.
9. Withdraw medication from a container with an applicator (tongue blade, cotton tip swab, gauze sponge), using a fresh applicator each time to avoid contaminating the remaining medication.
10. To soften or warm topical medication to make application easier rub between the palms of the hands. When applying powder, shake first into hand, then apply to the child's skin to avoid puffs of dust that might be inhaled.

Courtesy Nix KS, Tulsa, Okla.

| **Steps** | **Rationale** |
|---|---|
| ▪ Use superfatted soaps (e.g., Dove, Basis), or soaps for sensitive skin (e.g., Neutrogena, Aveeno, Purpose) or omit soap. | These soaps and cleansers are generally less alkaline and less drying to the skin.<br>***Special Considerations:*** *Bubble bath products are drying and irritating and should be avoided. Provide bath toys and sponge shapes for water play instead of bubbles.* |
| ▪ Adding a colloidal oatmeal treatment (Aveeno) or ½ cup of baking soda to bath water may be beneficial (Rajatanavin, Withers, and Bernhard, 1987). | These traditionally recommended products may be soothing, although their value is unproven.<br>***Special Considerations:*** *Continue product additions to the bath water only if they seem to help the itching; otherwise, they are of no value and may be an added expense. The addition of cornstarch to the bath is not recommended, as it can exacerbate an existing candidial infection (see Home Care Modifications for oatmeal bath).* |
| ▪ Avoid adding mineral oils and bath oils to the bath water. | Adding oil at the beginning of the bath prevents adequate skin cleansing and water absorption. In the pruritic patient who has obvious xerosis, adding it at the end of the bath is not sufficiently occlusive to prevent evaporation of water from the hydrated epidermis and may interfere with the occlusive ability of more appropriate topicals. |
| b. Apply an emollient preparation that may or may not contain menthol (0.25%), camphor (0.25% to 0.50%) or phenol (1%). Use emollients two to three times per day, particularly immediately after a bath or shower. | Creams and ointments seal in water and thereby hydrate skin. Camphor and menthol produce a cooling effect; phenol has a numbing effect to decrease itching. Although the use of phenol is controversial, it is considered safe in low concentrations (Kahn, 1988).<br>***Special Considerations:*** *Lotions such as Lubriderm, Moisturel, Curel, DML, and Vaseline Dermatology Formula have an advantage because they can be applied to a large surface area in a reasonably short time and are cosmetically appealing to children and parents. Creams and lotions may cause an allergic response because of ingredients in the base such as preservatives, stabilizers, and fragrances rather than the drug itself. Plain mineral oil, petroleum jelly, or vegetable shortening may be recommended (Bernhard, 1987). The particular emollient selected mostly depends on patient preference and whether or not it is acceptable as a compounding base if there are to be additives.* |

## *WET DRESSINGS AND SOAKS*

Wet dressings, when properly applied, can be more effective and considerably safer in relieving an exudative process than the most potent topical steroid (Dobson and Abele, 1985). Wet dressings increase moisture and thus hydrate the skin. As the solution evaporates, the resulting heat loss cools the skin and results in vasoconstriction of surface blood vessels, reducing erythema. Also, the cooling process often has an antipruritic effect. Debridement is enhanced by both soaks and wet dressings by gently softening crusts, scabs, and scale. Soaks generally use the same solutions as wet dressings and are employed when young children are not able to cooperate with the dressings.

1. Commonly used solutions include:
   a. Normal saline—used for clean wounds; no bacteriocidal properties.
   b. Aluminum acetate (Burow's solution)—used for cleansing and disinfecting oozing, crusting lesions; mild astringent effect. Dilute one DomeBoro tablet in one pint (1 : 20 mix) or one quart (1 : 40 mix) of water (Dobson and Abele, 1985).
   c. Potassium permanganate (1 : 8000 dilution)—used for gram positive bacterial infections.
   d. Acetic acid or white vinegar 0.25% (1 : 12 dilution)—used for gram negative infections, particularly *Pseudomonas* (Dobson and Abele, 1985; Smith, 1985).
2. The room should be warmer than usual to prevent chilling from rapid evaporation of the solutions and from convection heat loss caused by drafts.
3. For soaks, fill basin, tub, or Ziploc bag with solution. If solution is to be warm, check temperature to ensure it does not exceed 32° to 38°C (90° to 100°F). Use lower temperatures for younger children. If using a basin, pad the edges with towels for comfort. If using a Ziploc bag, some leakage may occur, but children find this method entertaining (Perelson and Seyler, 1985). The usual duration of a soak is 15 to 20 minutes. If the water cools and fresh, warm solution must be added, do not add it while the child is soaking to avoid burn injury. To encourage cooperation, scatter poker chips, marbles, or brightly colored objects that will sink to the bottom of the container and have the child retrieve them; give them dishes to wash or a baby doll to "bathe"; challenge them to hold a floating object below the surface; or punch holes in a plastic cup, fill it with solution and hold it up to "rain" on the child (also see box on p. 75). Always maintain constant supervision when a child is near water.
4. For wet dressings, place dressing material (e.g., bolt gauze; Kerlix; Dermpak gauze gloves; or freshly laundered diapers, washcloths, towels, pillowcases, undershirts, long-sleeved pajamas, long underwear, or tube socks) into clean basin and thoroughly moisten with appropriate solution. Gently squeeze excess moisture from the dressings; excessive moisture may cause skin maceration. Wrap the dressing material firmly and smoothly over the affected skin, but avoid excessive tightness, which may restrict circulation or movement. On the head, leave openings for eyes, mouth, and nose. Cover hands and feet with wet tube socks or gauze; individual wrapping of digits may be overly restrictive and uncomfortable. Wrap elbows and knees in a bent position to maintain mobility. For extremities and the trunk, soaked pajamas, underwear, or towels are convenient. If chilling is a serious risk, cover no more than one third of the body at a time (Whaley and Wong, 1991). Immediately cover the wet dressings with a dry, nonocclusive covering to permit a slow evaporation and cooling process, and prevent maceration. Dry coverings may be the same materials used for wet dressings, or tubular bandages (Stockinette) or elastic wrap (Ace) may be used (Fig. 80-1). If the dry coverings need to be secured, use gauze ties; avoid tape, which can be occlusive and may be irritating to the skin.
5. When wet dressings begin to dry and must be reapplied (e.g., continuous treatment is ordered), always prepare fresh solution, remove dressings and repeat procedure in step 4. Old solutions may become concentrated from evaporation, and could be harmful if poured or squirted on dressings wrapped on the child (Whaley and Wong, 1991).
6. Topical medications may be ordered for concurrent use with wet dressings or for immediate application after dressings are removed. Medications and emollients are more effective if applied to well-hydrated skin.
7. When using waterproof padding to protect bedding, never place plastic directly next to the child's skin because it may cause skin maceration.
8. Always discard contaminated dressings in a moisture-resistant trash bag.

Courtesy Kemper JL, Casper, Wy.

| Steps | Rationale |
|---|---|
| c. Apply wet wraps to the skin immediately after soaking and applying topicals to achieve additional relief and drug absorption (see box above). | Use of wet wraps immediately after soaking and applying topicals to the skin increases absorption of the topicals and decreases itching. The wraps cool the skin as the water gradually evaporates. This gradual cooling has an anti-inflammatory effect and reduces itching.<br>***Special Considerations:*** *An ice pack may be useful for an area of localized itching such as an insect bite.* |
| d. Avoid the use of topical antihistamines and caine-type anesthetics. | Topically applied antihistamines and anesthetics are relatively ineffective and are best avoided because they can be potent allergic sensitizers (Tonnesen, 1988). This is especially true if these products are used on inflamed skin. |

| Steps | Rationale |
|---|---|

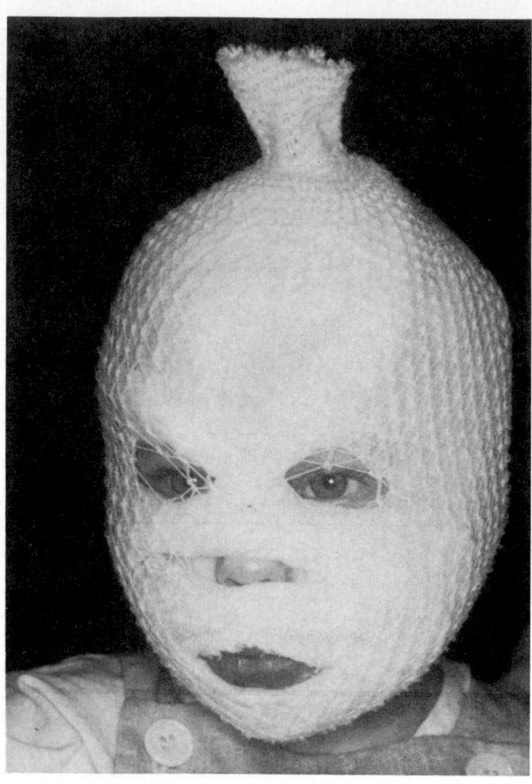

***FIG. 80-1*** Tubular bandage is applied over the head with openings for eyes, nose, and mouth.

From Nicol N: Atopic dermatitis: the (wet) wrap-up, Am J Nurs 87(12):1560-1563, 1987.

| Steps | Rationale |
|---|---|
| e. Avoid the use of diphenhydramine-containing calamine lotion. | The use of diphenhydramine topically can be very sensitizing.<br>***Special Considerations:*** *The value of calamine is unproven; however, it could be tried in children with chickenpox or insect bites and discontinued if not helpful.* |
| f. Avoid the use of topical corticosteroids unless ordered by the physician for specific therapy. For special considerations on the use of topical steroids, see the box on the following page. | Topical corticosteroids should not be used unless a specific steroid-responsive dermatosis is diagnosed (Bernhard, 1987). Topical steroids have many potential side effects including skin atrophy, acneiform eruptions, folliculitis, miliaria, striae, dermatitis, and itching. |
| 5. Use systemic medications | |
| a. Administer antihistamines (e.g., hydroxyzine, diphenhydramine, chlorpheniramine) on a regular schedule or as indicated for itching caused by histamine release and for sedation. | Histamine is the most commonly known itch mediator; however, since it is not the only mediator, it is clear why antihistamines are not always markedly effective. They often provide relief because of their sedative effect; however, patients eventually develop tolerance with prolonged use. Regularly scheduled administration is more effective than intermittent (Rubenstein, 1987).<br>***Special Considerations:*** *Care must be taken to avoid unnecessary sedation in children, especially during productive daytime activities. Time administration to coincide with rest periods and bedtime for maximum benefit. The physician may order a higher than usual recommended dosage to control itching, titrating against the effect of drowsiness (Krowchuk, 1987). Toxic blood levels have been reported when combining oral and topical diphenhydramine-containing preparations (Schunk and Svendsen, 1988).* |
| b. Administer sedatives (e.g., chloral hydrate) as indicated at bedtime to allow adequate rest. | If nighttime scratching is severe and continues in spite of adequate antihistamines and other topical therapy, use a sedative to offer temporary relief and allow adequate rest. Children who are uncomfortable and restless while trying to sleep can potentially do a great deal of damage to their skin by scratching (Nicol and Clark, 1988). |

### *SPECIAL CONSIDERATIONS WITH TOPICAL STEROIDS*

Steroid preparations are among the most common topical drugs used. They are available in varying strengths, from over-the-counter to stronger prescription-only preparations. Because topical steroids have a high potential for misuse, the following guidelines offer considerations for their safest and most effective use.

1. Steroids modify the inflammatory reaction in the skin. Their action is considered suppressive, not curative. Therefore topical steroids may mask signs of infection and actually promote growth of bacteria, fungi, and viruses.
2. The lowest potency that is effective should be used as a general rule. Avoid high-potency preparations especially on the face, diaper area, or genitals because gradual thinning of the skin, hyperpigmentation, and/or delayed healing may occur. In addition, natural or diaper occlusion of these and other intertriginous areas increases absorption.
3. Steroids in ointment form tend to be longer lasting and more potent because of occlusive effect but are often less acceptable than creams and lotions to the child/family. For the scalp and areas where hair growth is thick, sprays and lotions are easier to use.
4. Since topical steroids are better absorbed by hydrated skin, apply immediately after a bath or soaks.
5. Apply only a thin layer, rubbing into the skin thoroughly. Excess application does not increase penetration.
6. Occlusive dressings (e.g., plastic wrap) may significantly enhance penetration (as much as tenfold with some steroids) (Lester, 1984). The dressings may be most useful at night. Consider the increased risk for side effects, if using with occlusion.
7. Intermittent rather than continuous use of topical steroids often results in a better skin response, and poses less risk for side effects. More frequent than twice a day application is usually no more effective and greatly increases the cost of therapy.
8. Monitor for side effects indicating systemic absorption, especially with use over large areas of skin, prolonged use, inflamed or denuded skin, or high potency steroids. Such effects include adrenal suppression, slow growth, and Cushing syndrome. Especially in infants, the greater ratio of surface area to body weight means a larger area of skin for absorption, increasing the risk of systemic effects. Also consider that diapers or plastic pants provide continuous occlusion when the topical agent is applied to that area.

| **Steps** | **Rationale** |
|---|---|
| c. Avoid the administration of oral or systemic corticosteroids. | Systemic corticosteroids have no role in the management of the child with pruritus of unknown origin (Bernhard, 1987). |
| 6. Provide emotional support to child and family for the guilt feelings and controlling behaviors associated with scratching, for the stress associated with the etiologic cause of the pruritus, and for the often unsightly appearance of the child and rejection by others. Provide a referral of the child and/or family for therapy as appropriate. | The provision for the referral of the child and/or family for therapy or counseling in severe cases is essential. Emotional stress, anxiety, fear, anger, and depression can exacerbate pruritus and make the child less tolerant of the itching.<br>***Special Considerations:*** *In addition to the more conventional psychosocial interventions, unconventional therapies such as biofeedback, acupuncture, and transcutaneous nerve stimulation ultimately may become clinical adjuncts in the treatment of chronic idiopathic pruritus (Tonnesen, 1988).* |

| ## Evaluation Outcomes | ## Observational Guidelines |
|---|---|
| 1. Skin remains intact and any previous areas of breakdown are healing. | Observe intact skin for areas of redness and irritation, and inspect old lesions for evidence of granulation. |
| 2. Skin lesions show no evidence of secondary infection, the child is afebrile. | Examine skin lesions for redness or purulent drainage; measure the child's temperature. |
| 3. The child scratches minimally, engages in normal activities, and sleeps well. | Observe the child's behavior, activities, and sleeping patterns. |

## Documentation

Record measures and therapies implemented, success with each, child's response to therapies, skin condition, complications encountered, and child/family teaching.

### Home Care Modifications

1. Most often, therapies for pruritus are implemented in the home by the family. The therapies can be quite stressful, frustrating, and overwhelming to them. Use meaningful terminology, e.g., 1 cup solution mixed in 20 cups water, rather then the term "parts." Carefully review the procedure with them, ask for return demonstration, and provide them with written instructions and a phone number for questions or problems.
2. Assist the family in identifying cloth items that could be used for wet dressings and containers that could serve for soaks. Help them devise distracting activities and protective restraints to prevent scratching.
3. Develop a written schedule of medications and treatments to help them organize therapy.
4. To give an oatmeal bath at home: Add 2 cups oatmeal to 2 cups of boiling water. Boil for 5 minutes, stirring constantly. Pour the cooked cereal into a mesh or gauze bag. Fill a bathtub one-half full (or less, depending on the child's age) of tepid water, and swirl the bag through the water for several minutes, turning the water opalescent. Bathe the child using the bag to gently scrub crusts and debris, if desired (Phipps, 1983). Always remain with the child during the bath.

# SKILL 81 Providing Neonatal Phototherapy

*Sharon M. Glass*

The application of high-intensity fluorescent light to unshielded skin has been shown to reduce indirect serum bilirubin by photoisomerization. Light absorbed by the tissue converts unconjugated bilirubin to photobilirubin that can move from the tissue to the blood by diffusion. Photobilirubin can then be transported to the liver for biliary excretion into the duodenum and removed with feces without requiring conjugation by the liver (Maisels, 1987). Although phototherapy prevents rising bilirubin levels, it does not alter the underlying cause of jaundice. While phototherapy is usually performed in the hospital, in specific circumstances it can be safely and effectively accomplished in the home setting.

## NURSING DIAGNOSES

Potential for injury related to hyperbilirubinemia, enterohepatic recirculation of bilirubin, temperature instability, dehydration, and conjunctivitis; Parental anxiety related to unmet informational needs about a newborn with jaundice; Parental fatigue related to caring for a newborn receiving home phototherapy.

| Steps | Rationale |
|---|---|
| **Assessment** | |
| 1. Assess prenatal and perinatal factors that predispose to the development of neonatal jaundice:<br>a. Rh, ABO incompatibility.<br>b. Hydrops fetalis.<br>c. Cord bilirubin >5 mg/dl.<br>d. Prematurity.<br>e. Asphyxia.<br>f. Hypothermia.<br>g. Hypoglycemia.<br>h. Acidemia.<br>i. Hypoxemia.<br>j. Polycythemia.<br>k. Enclosed hemorrhage.<br>l. Congenital viral infection.<br>m. Hemolysis.<br>n. Hypothyroidism. | Bilirubin is normally cleared by the placenta in utero. Total bilirubin at birth is <3 mg% unless an abnormal hemolytic process is present. Conjugation of bilirubin depends on rate of hemolysis, liver maturity, and number of albumin-binding sites. Asphyxia decreases the ability of bilirubin to bind to albumin. Hypoxemia and acidosis impair the capacity of albumin to hold bilirubin. Hypothermia and hypoglycemia release free fatty acids that compete with bilirubin for albumin-binding sites. Congenital infections affect the liver's ability to process bilirubin. Sepsis and hemolytic disease cause an increased rate of red cell hemolysis. Polycythemia and enclosed hemorrhages result in an increased rate of red cell lysis with release of bilirubin (Maisels, 1987). |
| 2. Assess cultural factors<br>a. Hyperbilirubinemia is more prevalent in children of Chinese, Japanese, Greek, Korean, and American Indian extraction. | Serum bilirubin concentrations in Oriental and American Indian children may be double those of other populations. Glucose-6-phosphate dehydrogenase (G-6-PD) deficiency is more common in Oriental and Greek infants and can cause prolonged jaundice (Maisels, 1987). |

| Steps | Rationale |
|---|---|
| 3. Assess infant for jaundice: | |
| a. Assess in daylight. | Natural daylight allows better assessment of true skin color. |
| b. Blanch skin over bony prominence. | Blanching causes yellow staining to be more prominent. |
| c. Observe sclera, oral mucosa.<br>d. Observe palms, soles of feet, and hard palate in dark-skinned infants. | ***Special Considerations:*** *Yellow staining of skin is more difficult to assess in dark-skinned infants. Jaundice can be detected by observing yellow staining of sclera, posterior portion of the hard palate, palms, and soles of feet (Committee on Practice, 1986). Transcutaneous bilimetry is a noninvasive method of screening jaundice (see box below).* |
| 4. Assess behavior for neurologic signs of kernicterus:<br>a. Hypotonia.<br>b. Diminished reflexes.<br>c. Lethargy.<br>d. Seizures.<br>e. Opisthotonos.<br>f. High-pitched cry. | High concentrations of unconjugated bilirubin can be neurotoxic. Deposition of unconjugated bilirubin in the basal ganglia of the brain, called kernicterus, will cause abnormal neurologic signs. The increased risk of kernicterus at total bilirubin levels <20 mg% in term infants and <10 mg% in sick preterm newborns has been associated with asphyxia, respiratory distress, acidosis, sepsis, hypothermia, and low serum albumin levels (Streeter, 1986). |
| **Planning and Goal Setting** | |
| 1. Gather supplies: phototherapy unit with Plexiglas shield, photometer, bili mask, eye patches, and heat source such as an incubator or radiant warmer (Fig. 81-1). | A Plexiglas shield will minimize undesirable ultraviolet light exposure and protect infant from bulb breakage (Fanaroff and Martin, 1987). |
| 2. Prepare family by explaining equipment, eye covering, positioning, nudity, and frequency of bilirubin testing. | Preparation of the family will foster understanding and help reduce anxiety.<br>***Special Considerations:*** *Explain that eye covering is usually not distressing to the infant who has been accustomed to darkness while in utero.* |
| 3. Develop individualized goals of nursing care:<br>▪ Identify jaundice and refer for therapy.<br>▪ Promote effective and safe phototherapy.<br>▪ Provide emotional support to family and infant.<br>▪ Prevent potential complications of phototherapy. | |

### *TRANSCUTANEOUS BILIMETRY*

Transcutaneous bilimetry is a noninvasive method of screening neonatal jaundice by application of a bilirubinometer to the infant's skin. It is ideal for home screening because the usual peak of bilirubin levels with physiologic jaundice occurs at approximately 72 hours of age, which is often after discharge. The bilirubinometer illuminates the skin using a fiberoptic light source that measures the intensity of the yellow color of the skin. It is only a screening device to identify infants who require further investigation of serum bilirubin levels.

1. The obtained measure may be inaccurate if the equilibrium between skin bilirubin and serum levels is shifted such as with phototherapy use, changes in serum albumin concentration, or if exchange transfusion is performed (Goldman, Penalver, and Penaranda, 1982).
2. Supplies needed include a bilirubinometer (see Product References on p. 518) and alcohol wipes. Determine adequate functioning of the meter by activating the power switch and depressing the reset button. This step charges the photo circuit and illuminates the "ready" light in 5 to 10 seconds if the batteries are charged (Yamanouchi, Yamauchi, and Igarashi, 1980).
3. Calibrate the meter by constructing regression curves for each racial and gestational age group to be examined (follow manufacturer instructions). This curve is necessary because the meter generates a numerical index value that is not equal to, but correlates with the serum bilirubin concentration (Cassady, 1983).
4. Determine agency protocol for "action level," the numerical value above which the infant will be referred for serum bilirubin testing.
5. Clean the fiber optic probe with alcohol.
6. Activate the power switch and depress the reset button (see step 2).
7. Apply the fiber optic probe to the infant's skin surface over a bony prominence (forehead, sternum) with enough pressure to blanch the skin. An audible click will be heard from the machine (Maisels and Conrad, 1982).
8. Read the numerical index value, usually displayed on the digital readout within 5 seconds.
9. Compare the value to agency action level. Follow agency protocol as needed for repeated measurements every 8 hours or refer for serum bilirubin levels.

| Steps | Rationale |
|---|---|

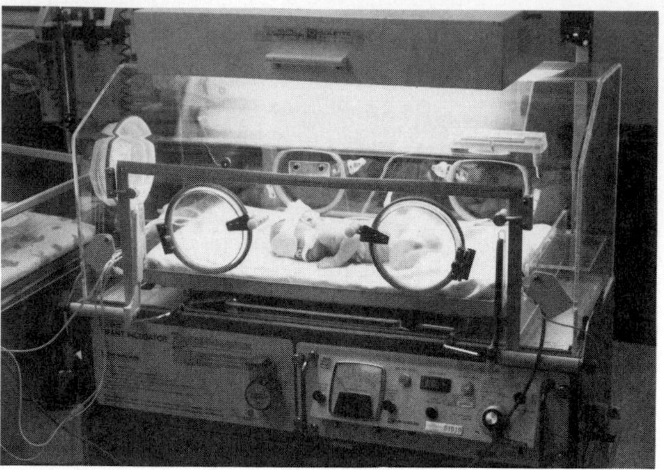

***FIG. 81-1*** Child receiving phototherapy in incubator.

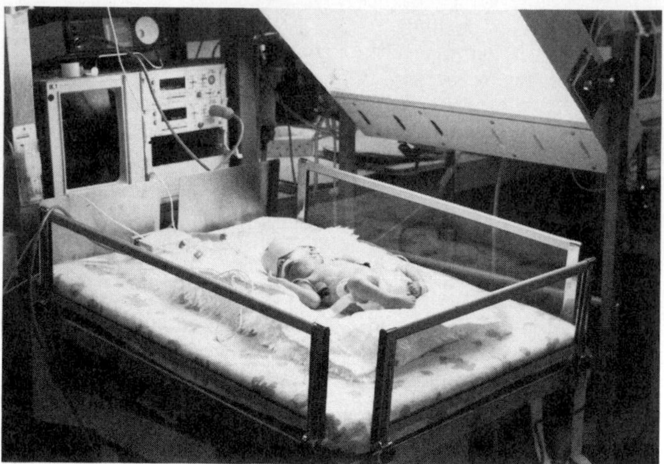

***FIG. 81-2*** Patches protect infant's eyes from high-intensity light.

## Implementation

1. Ensure proper functioning of all lights. Aperture should be adjusted to allow for maximum field exposure.

Properly functioning phototherapy lights will prevent injury and ineffective therapy.

***Special Considerations:*** *Fluorescent bulbs may be daylight, cool light, blue, or special blue. Light range for maximal absorption by bilirubin is 400 to 500 nanometers. Blue or special blue lamps are considered most effective, but they may interfere with the detection of cyanosis and cause eye strain on the part of the staff (Fetus and Newborn Committee, 1986).*

2. Shield infant's eyes:
   a. Cover eyes with soft, absorbent patches.
   b. Ensure lids are closed before applying patches.

Opaque eye coverings prevent possible retinal damage due to high-intensity light (Maisels, 1982).

   c. Position mask over eye patches and fasten securely (Fig. 81-2).

Eye covering must be secured to prevent slipping that can result in occlusion of the nasal airway or exposure of the eyes to potentially harmful light (Maisels, 1982).

   d. Change patches and check eyes every 4 hours for signs of drainage, irritation, or infection. (See also step 6.)

Conjunctivitis and corneal abrasions may be caused by irritation from eye patches (Fetus and Newborn Committee, 1986).

3. Position infant undressed and undiapered under lights.

Effectiveness of phototherapy is directly related to the degree of surface area exposed (Fanaroff and Martin, 1987).

   a. Change position frequently (every 2 hours).

Position changes ensure adequate irradiance of all skin areas.

   b. Position prone at least 2 hours after each feeding.

Prone positioning reduces the risk of aspiration if reflux or vomiting occurs (Streeter, 1986).

   c. Shield testes when positioned supine.

In vitro studies have shown breaks in DNA chains and decreased cell survival when cells were exposed to light similar to that used in phototherapy (Fetus and Newborn Committee, 1986).

***Special Considerations:*** *Soft surgical masks with ties can be used as bikini diapers to shield testes.*

4. Maintain intact skin:
   a. Change linen and diapering material as soon as soiled.
   b. Cleanse diaper area with sterile water and cotton balls.

***Special Considerations:*** *Soft surgical masks may also be used to minimize linen changes if the infant has frequent loose stools. Avoid lotions and oils on the skin.*

5. Ensure proper level of irradiance:
   a. Position lights to deliver ordered microwatt range.
   b. Check microwatt delivery every 8 hours.

The irradiance level at the skin will determine the effectiveness of the phototherapy. A photometer will measure irradiance in microwatts per square centimeter per nanometer. An irradiance level of at least 4 microwatts is necessary for effective phototherapy. The therapeutic response increases with increasing dose until a saturation point is reached at approximately 10 to 12 microwatts (Maisels, 1982).

| Steps | Rationale |
|---|---|
| 6. Remove infant from lights and remove eye patches for feedings and short family visits. Encourage family to visit during feeding time. | Removing light and patches provides visual and sensory stimulation. Parental-infant cuddling and interaction help minimize the effects of separation. **Special Considerations:** *In most instances, phototherapy can be interrupted for short periods of routine care without affecting its overall efficacy (Fetus and Newborn Committee, 1986).* |
| 7. Provide adequate fluid intake: a. Encourage feedings every 3 to 4 hours. | Additional fluid intake is needed to compensate for increased insensible water loss through the skin and loose stools. Increased bilirubin excretion results in loose stools and increased urine output. Inadequate fluid intake will result in dehydration (Maisels, 1987). |
| b. Administer intravenous fluids as ordered. | **Special Considerations:** *Intravenous fluids may be used in the presence of dehydration or other complications.* |
| 8. Monitor: a. Temperature of infant and incubator every 2 hours. | Hypothermia and hyperthermia can be complications of phototherapy. Phototherapy lights provide additional radiant heat. Maintaining skin temperature at 36.5° C by servocontrol minimizes increased insensible water loss and prevents overheating (Fetus and Newborn Committee, 1986). **Special Considerations:** *Infants are often placed under radiant heat or in servocontrolled incubators for optimal thermoregulation.* |
| b. Intake and output, weight, and skin turgor. | Output, weight, and skin turgor are the most sensitive measurements for hydration status. **Special Considerations:** *Specific gravity measurements may indicate state of hydration in healthy term infants, but they can be falsely elevated in preterm infants with proteinuria or glycosuria (Avery, 1987).* |
| c. Neurologic status for signs of kernicterus. | Deposition of unconjugated bilirubin in the basal areas of the brain will cause abnormal neurologic signs. |
| d. Bilirubin levels: turn phototherapy lights off momentarily for blood sampling. | Phototherapy irradiance of blood samples may result in falsely lowered bilirubin values. |
| 9. Observe for side effects of phototherapy: a. Loose, watery stools. | Increased amounts of unconjugated bilirubin in the intestine as a result of phototherapy may induce secretory diarrhea (Fetus and Newborn Committee, 1986). |
| b. Skin color changes. | Use of phototherapy with an elevated direct serum bilirubin level or liver disease may result in a temporary bronzing of the skin (Streeter, 1986). |
| 10. Provide family support: a. Explain reason for jaundice and usual course of therapy. b. Explain procedures, positioning, and expected side effects. c. Encourage family to express feelings about interruption of family-infant relationship. | Families will have many fears concerning their infant's disease and the proposed treatment. Thorough explanations of the infant's problem, the benefits and risks of phototherapy, and the precautions that will be taken can reassure the family and gain their support. |

| Evaluation Outcomes | Observational Guidelines |
|---|---|
| 1. Jaundice is identified. | Observe for yellow staining of skin, sclera, and mucous membranes. |
| 2. Phototherapy is effectively and safely maintained. | Monitor microwatt delivery; note use of eye patches and testes shields. Monitor lab reports. |
| 3. Bilirubin levels are decreased. | Compare bilirubin levels to prephototherapy levels. |
| 4. Dehydration, eye injury, and temperature instability are prevented. | Observe for poor skin turgor, depressed fontanelles, sunken eyes, decreased urine output, weight loss, electrolyte changes, eye drainage or erythema of conjunctiva. Monitor temperature. |
| 5. Neurologic injury is prevented or signs are detected early and appropriate interventions initiated. | Observe for irritability, hypotonia, lethargy, poor suck reflex, opisthotonic posturing, and seizures. |
| 6. Family demonstrates an understanding of infant's disease process and rationale for phototherapy treatment. | Interview family regarding their understanding of their infant's disease and the expected outcome of phototherapy. |
| 7. Family verbalizes feelings and concerns. | Family asks questions and expresses feelings. |
| 8. The effects of parent-infant separation are prevented or minimized. | Infant is out of incubator or radiant warmer with patches removed every 3 to 4 hours for feeding and interaction. Eye contact, cuddling, and other bonding behaviors are exhibited. |

### Documentation

Documentation should include time of onset of jaundice with signs and symptoms identified. When phototherapy is initiated, documentation should include time of initiation, type and number of phototherapy lamps used, measured level of microwatt irradiance, application of eye patches and mask, and explanations to the family including their reactions regarding the disease process and therapeutic interventions. Every 8 hours, documentation should include microwatt level; changing of eye patches and any evidence of eye drainage; irritation or infection; position changes; intake and output; temperature and specific actions required to maintain temperature; efforts to provide comforting and sensory stimulation; and any abnormal neurologic signs or other phototherapy side effects.

# SKILL 82 Treating Head Lice Infestation

*Donna Phillips Smith*

The diagnosis of head lice (pediculosis capitis) requires administering a pediculicidal product and/or manual removal of nits (eggs). Pediculicides, with varying degrees of effectiveness, are available both over the counter and by prescription. Proper administration is essential to ensure effective treatment and to prevent serious side effects from the chemicals. Educating the child and family will help prevent reinfestation.

### NURSING DIAGNOSES

Impaired skin integrity related to parasite infection; Potential for injury related to improper administration of pediculicides; Anxiety related to unmet informational needs regarding prevention and treatment of pediculosis.

| Steps | Rationale |
|---|---|
| **Assessment** | |
| 1. Determine the severity of the infestation. | ***Special Considerations:*** *The primary symptom is itching (see Child and Family Teaching section).* |
| a. Presence of adult lice or nits only. | Adult lice are fast moving and difficult to spot. Usually just nits are seen.<br>***Special Considerations:*** *The prolonged killing time of lindane may cause the child distress if adult lice are found (Table 82-1).* |
| b. Extensive cuts, scratches, or excoriated areas on head or neck. | Potential for systemic absorption of pediculicide exists. Consult with physician prior to treatment. |
| 2. Determine the child's age. | Pediculicides are contraindicated in infants because of high potential for toxicity. Nits must be manually removed on infants (generally under 2 years of age). |
| 3. Assess for sensitivity to ragweed or chrysanthemum. | Pyrethrins and permethrin are derived from these plants and are contraindicated for those sensitive to them. If sensitivity is detected, use other preparation (see Table 82-1). |
| 4. Assess for infestation among contacts: | |
| a. Inspect other family members for nits. | Over half of infested children have one or more infested family members.<br>***Special Considerations:*** *Consider cost and compliance factors when several members require treatment. Do not treat persons who show no signs of infestation. Only permethrin has a limited preventative effect (see Table 82-1).* |
| b. Determine school/child care attendance. | Infestations are common in schools and child care facilities.<br>***Special Considerations:*** *Notify the facility of case identification so they may inspect for other cases and take environmental measures. Encourage the family to contact others, such as playmates and sitters who have been in close contact recently.* |

**TABLE 82-1** Product Information For Lice Shampoos

| Product/Brand | Application | Effectiveness/Considerations |
|---|---|---|
| Lindane<br>Kwell (Prescription) (Reed & Carnick) | Shampoo | Killing-time of active lice following treatment reported as 3 hours and 12 minutes; 30% of eggs survived and hatched (Meinking et al, 1986). Lice-free 2 weeks following treatment reported as 43% (Taplin et al, 1986) and 76% (Bowerman et al, 1987). High potential for toxicity and misuse (Lindane, 1986). Retreat only if necessary due to systemic absorption. Prolonged killing time reported as distressing due to hyperactivity and twitching of lice (Meinking et al, 1986). |
| Pyrethrins with piperonyl butoxide* | Shampoo | |
| RID (OTC) (Pfizer) | | Killing time of active lice reported as 10.5 minutes; 26% of eggs survived and hatched (Meinking et al, 1986). Manufacturer recommends second application in 7 to 10 days. |
| A-200 Pyrinate (OTC) (Norcliff Thayer) | | Killing time of active lice reported as 22.5 minutes; 23% of eggs survived and hatched (Meinking et al, 1986). Manufacturer recommends second application in 7 to 10 days. Recent formulation change increased active ingredient to same strength as other pyrethrin products. |
| R & C Liquid (OTC) (Reed & Carnick) | | Killing time of active lice reported as 18.6 minutes; 25% of eggs survived and hatched (Meinking et al, 1986). Second application recommended in 7 to 10 days. |
| Permethrin<br>Nix (OTC) (Burroughs-Wellcome) | Rinse | Lice-free 2 weeks following single treatment reported as 97% (Taplin et al, 1986) and 98% (Bowerman et al, 1987). Unlike other products, helps prevent reinfestation as it retains insecticidal activity up to 2 weeks. |

*Other pyrethrins available OTC include Pronto (Commerce) and Triple X (Carter).

| Steps | Rationale |
|---|---|
| 5. Determine the child/family's knowledge regarding transmission and prevention measures. | Child/family may have inadequate or incorrect knowledge that could increase the risk of reinfestation or result in harmful practices.<br>***Special Considerations:*** *Education is essential to prevent reinfestation. Home remedies, such as using kerosene or gasoline, are potentially dangerous and should be discouraged. Educational materials written in Spanish are available from manufacturers.* |
| 6. Explore the child/family's anxiety regarding infestation. | Panic and embarrassment are common feelings; the child may be ridiculed by others.<br>***Special Considerations:*** *Infestation is not related to social class or personal hygiene despite traditional stigma.* |

## Planning and Goal Setting

| Steps | Rationale |
|---|---|
| 1. Select and obtain a pediculicide. Read the directions thoroughly, free from distraction. Obtain a nit comb. | Products vary considerably in recommended method and length of application. Directions must be followed carefully to ensure effective treatment.<br>***Special Considerations:*** *Several factors to consider when selecting the product include safety, effectiveness, cost, and anticipated compliance with nit removal and retreatment. (See Table 82-1.)* |
| 2. Select a location for the treatment that will allow the child to lie face up with the head leaning back into a sink, basin, or wash tray (see box on shampooing tips in Skill 55). | Treatment should not be done in the shower or bathtub to reduce exposure of body areas and risk of chemical conjunctivitis. The supine position poses the least risk for eye and body exposure to the chemicals.<br>***Special Considerations:*** *An older child may lean over a sink with a dry towel securely protecting the eyes if there is no other suitable location. A plastic drape around the child's shoulders provides further protection.* |

| Steps | Rationale |
|---|---|
| 3. Do not administer the treatment immediately following a warm bath or shower. | Vasodilation from steam increases skin absorption of chemicals. |
| 4. Gather towels, drape, gloves, clean-up supplies, and shampoo (if pre-shampoo required). | Gloves should be worn by the person administering the treatment to prevent exposure to the chemicals and infestation to themselves. ***Special Considerations:*** *Pregnant or breastfeeding women should consult their obstetrician before administering or being treated with a pediculicide.* |
| 5. Plan an activity to occupy the time period that the product must remain on the hair. Most application times are approximately ten minutes. Select an activity appropriate to the child's age (see Skill 15). | |
| 6. Develop individualized child and family goals: ▪ Child will receive safe and effective treatment for head lice. ▪ Child and family will be knowledgeable of measures to prevent reinfestation of self and others. | |

## Implementation 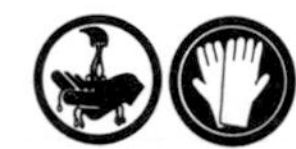

| Steps | Rationale |
|---|---|
| 1. Remove upper clothing except for a T-shirt or hospital gown if desired. Secure a plastic drape around the child's shoulders. | All linens and clothing will need to be washed following treatment, including those of the person administering the treatment. |
| 2. Position the child supine with the head leaning back into a sink or basin. Use rolled towels under the neck and shoulders for support. Give the child a towel or washcloth to cover the eyes. Make the child as comfortable as possible. Ensure safety from falls. Instruct the child to keep the eyelids closed. If the product does get in the eyes, flush with tepid water for 15 minutes. | The supine position and the dry towel will prevent the product from dripping into the eyes. |
| 3. Apply pediculicide as directed in instructions, leaving the product on the child the recommended length of time. | Proper application for the recommended length of time is necessary for maximum effectiveness. ***Special Considerations:*** *Some products are shampoos, some are rinses applied after a shampoo, and some are applied to dry hair, thus instructions must be carefully read.* |
| 4. To soften nit attachment, suggestions include vinegar rinses, wrapping the hair in a towel, or wearing a shower cap for 15 minutes (Reeves, 1987). | The adult louse secretes a glue-like substance that binds the nits to the hair shaft. ***Special Considerations:*** *Although vinegar rinses are a common practice, there is no research to document the effectiveness (Clore, 1989).* |
| 5. Towel dry or allow the hair to air dry. | Nit removal is easier with dry or slightly damp hair. ***Special Considerations:*** *Permethrin contains alcohol, so a hair dryer is not recommended. Heat can also decrease the effectiveness of the medication.* |
| 6. For nit removal, have the child sit up in a chair. Use a towel or sheet to cover the shoulders. | The covering over the shoulders catches the nits as they are removed. ***Special Considerations:*** *Lay a towel under the head of the immobilized child in bed to remove nits. With younger children, it is helpful for an assistant to hold them and provide distraction. A protective covering such as a gown should be worn.* |
| 7. Separate the hair into sections, working with one small section at a time. Start at the top of the head working down. | A systematic approach will minimize the chance of missing nits. Starting at the top of the head prevents nits from falling onto already combed sections (Clore, 1989). ***Special Considerations:*** *If a child has long hair and numerous nits, have the child and family consider cutting the hair shorter to make nit removal easier. It is unnecessary to shave the head, as it could subject the child to ridicule, and length of hair has no relation to infestation rates (McLaury, 1983).* |
| 8. Remove all visible nits with the extra fine tooth comb usually provided with the product. a. Comb from the scalp to end of hair shaft. If hair collects on the comb, tissue off and discard in toilet or in a sealed bag. | Products rarely kill all of the nits. Those surviving will hatch into active lice in 7 to 10 days if not manually removed. ***Special Considerations:*** *If the child is younger or has numerous nits, more than one removal session may be required.* |

| Steps | Rationale |
|---|---|
| b. The nits may also be removed using tweezers or grasping the nit between two fingernails and pulling it the length of the hair shaft. Also backcombing from the end of the hair to the scalp may be effective (Reeves, 1987). | Nit removal decreases the need for a second treatment and increases the effectiveness of the weaker products (About nits, 1986). Also, lindane-resistant lice have been reported in the Far East, the Netherlands, and Great Britain.<br>***Special Considerations:*** *The National Pediculosis Association (see Product References and Teaching Resources section) recommends a* No Nit *policy for day-care centers and schools, meaning that when sent home for treatment, a child must be inspected upon return for nit removal. If more than one or two nits are seen, the child is not allowed to reenter. This policy will document that treatment has occurred, and it serves to prevent further transmission.* |
| 9. To clean up:<br>a. Change the child's clothes.<br>b. Machine wash in hot water (140° F) and dry for 20 minutes in a hot dryer all linens and clothing worn during the procedure.<br>c. Soak comb in pediculicide product for 1 hour.<br>d. Clean the sink area.<br>e. Vacuum carpets. | Following recommended environmental measures will help prevent reinfestation or infestation of others.<br>***Special Considerations:*** *The following are some additional environmental measures for the home. All washable clothing and linens that have been in contact with the infested child in the 3 previous days should be washed as directed earlier. If no washer or dryer is available, boil the washables and iron them for ten minutes on the highest safe setting. Nonwashable items such as coats, hats, and stuffed toys can be dry cleaned, or put in a hot dryer for 20 minutes, or sealed in a plastic bag for 14 days. Soak all combs, brushes, headbands (etc.) as directed above. Vacuum mattresses, carpets, rugs, and upholstered furniture. Discourage the use of environmental lice sprays, as they are a potential hazard to humans and pets (Atkinson et al, 1986).* |
| 10. Discuss measures needed to eliminate lice and nits in the home with family (see step 9). | Adult lice can survive in the environment 48 hours; nits can survive up to 12 days. |
| 11. Discuss with child and family how lice are transmitted, and emphasize the need to avoid sharing personal items. | Knowledge of transmission allows avoidance of risk situations. |
| 12. Recheck the child daily for 7 days for lice or nits. Retreat at the end of this time if pediculicide instructions recommend or if evidence of infestation remains. | Treatment and nit removal may not be 100% effective. A second treatment is recommended by many product manufacturers. Even if not recommended, a second treatment is necessary if there is evidence of new nits or newly hatched lice.<br>***Special Considerations:*** *Teach the family to do the recheck and/or treatment at home if not performed by them initially, and a discharge is planned. Caution the family to avoid frequent and harsh shampooing in an effort to prevent future infestation. It can lead to an irritated and itchy scalp, which may be misinterpreted as evidence of reinfestation by the family.* |

| Evaluation Outcomes | Observational Guidelines |
|---|---|
| 1. No active lice or viable nits are present in child's hair following treatment. | After shampooing and drying child's hair, separate hair and inspect for adult lice, or pearly white nits firmly adhering to hair shaft. Hatched or nonviable nit cases are translucent in color. |
| 2. Retreatment occurs in seven days if recommended by pediculicide product or if active lice or viable nits present. | Schedule retreatment date and interview family to determine if recheck and/or retreatment occurred. |
| 3. The family performs the recommended environmental measures at home. | Interview family as to actions taken at home to prevent lice transmission. |
| 4. The child and family verbalize situations to prevent lice transmission. | Have the child and family list common situations of lice transmission (e.g., sharing combs, brushes, barrettes, hats, and coats). |

## Documentation

Document when treatment occurred, which product was used, and the nit removal performed. If reactions occurred from skin or eye contact, record measures taken. Document child and family teaching including when recheck and/or retreatment should occur if to be done by family. Notify school or day-care center that child may return.

## Child and Family Teaching

1. *Facts of transmission.* Lice are transmitted by direct contact, generally with personal items of an infested person. Lice cannot jump or fly, but can crawl quickly between items, such as coats piled together. Household pets do not carry or transmit lice. Contrary to popular belief, cleanliness and frequent shampooing do not prevent transmission. Black children seldom become infested. Girls have a higher infestation rate than boys, although length of hair is not a factor. Infestation occurs in all socioeconomic groups.

   Common sources of transmission include combs, brushes, barrettes, hair bows, headbands, hats, coats, scarves, caps, pillows, bedding, and stuffed toys recently used by an infested person. Other easy sources of transmission include seating on public transportation, in theaters, at slumber parties, and sharing lockers at school.
2. *Identifying an infestation.* Frequent scratching of the head by the child is the most noticeable symptom but may be absent. As the adult louse moves quickly and is usually not seen, family members should look for the nits to confirm reinfestation or the need for a second treatment. The best time to inspect is after washing and drying the child's hair when dandruff and hair casts are minimal. The nits are tiny, pearly white specks usually found one per hair shaft. They adhere firmly to the hair shaft, and cannot be flicked away as can dandruff and hair casts. They are also most commonly found on hairs behind the ears and at the nape of the neck. Although they are generally found ¼ inch from the scalp, evidence shows that viable nits may be found further along the shaft, especially in warmer climates (Taplin and Meinking, 1987). Hatched or nonviable nit cases are translucent in color.
3. *Prevention measures for schools and child care.* Children should have individual cubbies to store personal items. Coats should be hung on hooks with adequate spacing, not piled together. Children should have individual cribs, cots, sleeping mats, and nap toys. Rugs, carpets, and upholstered furniture should be vacuumed frequently. Dress-up centers pose a serious risk. The school should schedule regular nit checks throughout the year in a discreet manner to prevent embarrassment of individual children.

## UNIT XI
## PRODUCT REFERENCES AND TEACHING RESOURCES
### Products

Air-Shields Vicker
330 Jacksonville Road
Hatboro, PA 19040
1-800-523-2404
Offers Minolta Air Shields Jaundice Meter.

Burroughs Wellcome Co (Nix)
3030 Cornwallis Road
Research Triangle Park, NC 27709
1-800-FOR-LICE

Norcliff Thayer Inc (A-200 Pyrinate)
For educational materials:
PO Box 3842
Stanford, CT 06905
1-800-922-LICE
(203) 329-A-200 (call collect from within Connecticut)

Walt Disney Educational Media Company
500 South Buena Vista St.
Burbank, CA 91521
Offers a video for children—"Advice on Lice."

### Organizations

The National Pediculosis Association (NPA)
PO Box 149
Newton, MA 02101
(617) 449-6487
"The Latest Greatest Coloring Book about Lice" is available for children.

## REFERENCES


About nits, Progress 2(3):2, 1986.

American Academy of Pediatrics, Committee on Fetus and Newborn: Home phototherapy, Pediatrics 76(1):136-137, 1985.

Atkinson L et al: Internal and external parasites, Pediatrics: Nursing Update 1(23):1-7, 1986.

Avery GB: Neonatology: pathophysiology and management of the newborn, Philadelphia, 1987, JB Lippincott Co.

Bernhard JD: Clinical aspects of pruritus. In Fitzpatrick TB et al, editors: Dermatology in general medicine, ed 3, New York, 1987, McGraw-Hill Inc.

Bernstein N and Robson M, editors: Comprehensive approaches to the burned person, New Hyde Park, New York, 1983, Medical Examination Publishing Co.

Bowerman JD et al: Comparative study of permethrin 1% creme rinse and lindane shampoo for the treatment of head lice, Pediatr Infect Dis J 6(3):252-255, 1987.

Brucker MC and MacMullen NJ: Neonatal jaundice in the home: assessment with a noninvasive device, JOGNN 16(5):355-358, 1987.

Carvajal H and Parks D, editors: Burns in children: Pediatric burn management, Chicago, 1988, Year Book Medical Publishers.

Cassady G: Transcutaneous monitoring in the newborn, J Pediatr 103(6):837-848, 1983.

Clore E: Prioderm and permethrin: product update, Progress 1(2):1, 1985.

Clore E: Dispelling the common myths about pediculosis, J Pediatr Health Care 3(1):28-33, 1989.

Committee on Practice of NAACOG: OGN nursing practice resource: phototherapy and nursing care of the newborn with hyperbilirubinemia, Washington, DC, 1986, NAACOG.

Dangel R: Pruritus and cancer, Oncol Nurs Forum, 13(1):17-21, 1986.

Dobson R and Abele D: The practice of dermatology, Philadelphia, 1985, Harper and Row.

Fanaroff AA and Martin RJ, editors: Neonatal-perinatal medicine, diseases of the fetus and infant, St Louis, 1987, The CV Mosby Co.

Fetus and Newborn Committee, Canadian Paediatric Society: use of phototherapy for neonatal hyperbilirubinemia, Can Med Assoc J, 134:1237-1245, 1986.

Goldman SL, Penalver A, and Penaranda R: Jaundice meter: evaluation of new guidelines, J Pediatr 101(2):253-256, 1982.

Hawkins K: Wet dressings, Crit Care Update 9(11):24-26, 1982.

Hummel R: Clinical burn therapy: A management and prevention guide: Littleton, Mass, 1982, PSG Publishing Co.

Kahn G: Principles of treatment. In Schachner L and Hansen R, editors: Pediatric dermatology, vol 1, New York, 1988, Churchill Livingstone.

Kravitz M: Thermal injuries. In Cardona V et al, editors: Trauma nursing from resuscitation through rehabilitation, Philadelphia, 1988, WB Saunders Co.

Krowchuk DP: Practical aspects of the diagnosis and management of atopic dermatitis, Pediatr Ann 16(1):57-66, 1987.

Lester RS: Topical formulary for the pediatrician, Pediatr Clin North Am 30(4):749-765, 1983.

Lindane: Isn't it time to say no? Progress 2(3):1, 1986.

Madden E: Starting from scratch, Am J Nurs 86(7):846-847, 1986.

Maisels MJ and Conrad S: Transcutaneous bilirubin measurements in full-term infants, Pediatrics 70(3):464-467, 1982.

Maisels MJ: Jaundice in the newborn, Pediatr Rev 3:305-319, 1982.

Maisels MJ: Neonatal jaundice. In Avery GB, editor: Neonatology: pathophysiology, and management of the newborn, Philadelphia, 1987, JB Lippincott Co.

McLaury P: Head lice: pediatric social disease, Am J Nurs 83(9):1300-1303, 1983.

Meinking T et al: Comparative efficacy of treatments for pediculosis capitis infestations, Arch Dermatol 122:267-271, 1986.

Millar S, Sampson L and Soukup M: AACN procedure manual for critical care, Philadelphia, 1985, WB Saunders Co.

Nicol NH: Atopic dermatitis: The wet wrap up, Am J Nurs 87(12):1560-1563, 1987.

Nicol NH and Clark RAF: Atopic dermatitis. In Provost TT and Farmer ER, editors: Current therapy in dermatology-2, Philadelphia, 1988, BC Decker, Inc, The CV Mosby Co.

Perelson A and Seyler M: First aid: soaking an injured finger or toe, Emerg Med Clin North Am 16:158, 1985.

Phipps W, Long B, and Woods N: Medical-surgical nursing, ed 2, St Louis, 1983, The CV Mosby Co.

Rajatanavin N, Withers A, and Bernhard J: Baking soda and pruritis (letter), Lancet 2(8565):977, 1987.

Reeves JR: Head lice and scabies in children, Pediatr Infect Dis J 6(6):598-600, 1987.

Rubenstein R: Pruritus: a new look at an old problem, J Fam Pract 24(6):625-629, 1987.

Rutter N: Drug absorption through the skin: a mixed blessing, Arch Dis Child 62:220-221, 1987.

Sanford-Driscoll M: Pharmacotherapy of head lice in children: an update, J Pediatr Health Care 1(5):284-287, 1987.

Schunk JE and Svendsen D: Diphenhydramine toxicity from combined oral and topical use, Am J Dis Child 142(10):1020-1021, 1988.

Senter SB: Use of topical steroids in children, Pediatr Nurs 14(4):337-340, 1988.

Slater L and Brewer M: Home versus hospital phototherapy for term infants with hyperbilirubinemia: A comparative study, Pediatrics 73(4):515-519, 1984.

Smith S: Clinical nursing skills, Los Altos, Calif, 1985, National Nursing Review.

Streeter NS: High-risk neonatal care, Rockville, MD, 1986, Aspen Publishers.

Taplin D and Meinking T: Head lice infestation: biology, diagnosis, management, Research Triangle Park, NC, 1987, Burroughs Wellcome.

Taplin D et al: Permethrin 1% creme rinse for the treatment of Pediculus humanis var capitis infestation, Pediatr Dermatol 3:344-348, 1986.

Tomlinson G, Helfaer M, and Wiedermann B: Diphenhydramine toxicity mimicking varicella encephalitis (brief report), Pediatr Infect Dis J 6(2):220-221, 1987.

Tonnesen MG: Pruritus. In Provost TT and Farmer ER, editors: Current therapy in dermatology: 2, Philadelphia, 1988, BC Decker Inc, The CV Mosby Co.

Whaley L and Wong D: Nursing care of infants and children, ed 4, St Louis, 1991, The CV Mosby Co.

Yamanouchi J, Yamauchi Y, and Igarashi I: Transcutaneous bilirubinometry: preliminary studies of noninvasive transcutaneous bilirubin meter in the Okayama National Hospital, Pediatrics 65(2):195-202, 1980.

# UNIT XII Temperature Regulation

# SKILL 83 Managing Hypothermia

*Sandra L. Gardner*

Heat balance is a function of heat production (metabolic activity of the body), heat loss, and the heat supplied from external sources. Hypothermia, a result of heat loss being greater than heat production, is defined as a decrease in core temperature to ≤35°C (95°F). Children are at increased risk for hypothermia because of larger body surface area from which to lose heat and their lesser developed temperature regulation system. The younger the child, the more rapid the cooling.

Preventing further heat loss and allowing the body to rewarm without supplying external or internal heat sources is known as spontaneous rewarming. Active rewarming entails addition of internal or external heat to return body temperature (Lloyd, 1986). This skill contains guidelines appropriate for all neonates, full-term, preterm and ill, as well as older infants and children who are hypothermic as a result of environmental exposure, such as cold water submersion or frostbite.

## NURSING DIAGNOSES

Hypothermia related to environmental exposure, trauma/illness, or extremes of age; Potential for trauma related to contact with intense cold; Impaired tissue integrity related to temperature extremes (cold); Anxiety related to unmet informational needs about therapeutic interventions for hypothermia and separation from family.

| Steps | Rationale |
|---|---|
| **Assessment** | |
| 1. Obtain health history data from child/family and medical record that may affect assessment of risk for increase in heat loss or decrease in heat production. | An accurate health history enables recognizing infants/children at increased risk for hypothermia, facilitates planning individualized nursing care, and facilitates preventing complications. |
| a. Age and developmental level of child: *Preterms/neonates:* ▪ Gestational age. | Preterm, term, or postterm small for gestational age (SGA) infants are at the greatest risk for developing hypothermia due to (Merenstein, Gardner, and Blake, 1989): 1. A higher surface area-to-body mass ratio that results in a high surface area from which to lose heat. Flexion development decreases exposed surface from which heat is lost. Since preterm infants lack flexion development, primarily lying in extension, they expose a greater surface area to the environment. 2. Decreased subcutaneous tissue (insulation), brown fat, and glycogen stores. 3. Immature CNS (preterm) that results in a muted and immature response to cold stress; chronic hypoxia (SGA) depresses CNS and impairs response to cold stress. 4. Frequent interventions and procedures that increase their stress and the possibility of exposure to cold. |
| *Infant/older child:* ▪ Chronological age and developmental level. | Older children flex their extremities to their trunk when cold stressed, thus decrease surface area exposed to cold. Age and developmental level influence child's ability to understand and cooperate with assessment. |

| **Steps** | **Rationale** |
|---|---|
| b. Factors that increase heat loss: | |
| ▪ Impaired CNS temperature regulation: prematurity; CNS depressants (analgesics, anesthetics, alcohol, tranquilizers); trauma; shock; head injury; water intoxication; asphyxia and infection. | An immature, depressed, injured, or infected CNS mutes the hypothalamic response to temperature changes. |
| ▪ Decreased insulation: prematurity; low birth weight or SGA; infants; thinness; males; inadequate clothing. | Any of these factors are associated with less subcutaneous fat/body insulation that allows greater heat loss. |
| ▪ Increased vasodilation: fetal alcohol syndrome; alcohol ingestion; medications (antihypertensives; methylxanthines—theophylline, aminophylline; cardiac drugs—reserpine, apresoline; anesthetics). | Increased blood flow to the periphery increases peripheral heat loss. |
| ▪ Overactivity: exhaustion; panic. | Aimless activity wastes energy and increases heat loss. |
| ▪ Exposure: a "too cool" or cold environmental temperature (delivery or operating room; winter night; exchange transfusion with cold blood); wind; moisture (immersion in cold water, sweating). | Not only exposure to a cool temperature, but wind chill and moisture also increase heat loss. Two thirds of evaporative heat loss occurs on the skin; water draws heat away from the body 26 times faster than air current. |
| c. Factors that decrease heat production: | |
| ▪ Increased predisposition to frostbite: genetic; regional; prior exposure to cold; cigarette smoking (Wilkerson, Bangs, and Hayward, 1986). | Black-skinned people shiver at lower temperatures; their fingers cool faster in water; they reach a lower temperature before they start warming, and they do not rewarm as much. White-skinned people with Type O blood are more prone to frostbite. Those born in the south are four times more likely than northerners to become frostbitten. Those at higher altitudes are exposed to colder temperatures, experience more hypoxia, and are less able to rewarm themselves. Smoking causes vasoconstriction that decreases blood flow to periphery and predisposes to frostbite. |
| ▪ Illness: hypothyroidism; congenital heart disease; diabetes; CNS disorders (e.g., sepsis, stroke) or depression (e.g., anesthetics, barbiturates and phenothiazines); renal failure and uremia. | Hypothalmic dysfunction or depression mutes the CNS response to cold stress. Poor peripheral perfusion, hypoxia, decreased basal metabolic rate and activity, and increased caloric expenditure of organs in failure decrease heat production. |
| ▪ Inactivity: sleep; paralysis (spina bifida, spinal cord injury, muscular dystrophy); general anesthesia. | Muscle activity increases heat production. |
| ▪ Decreased ability to shiver: neonates; shock; head injury; alcohol intake; general anesthesia. | An immature, depressed, or injured CNS mutes the shivering response to cold stress and the ability to produce heat. |
| ▪ Decreased nutrient availability to generate heat: malnutrition (protein-calorie); dehydration; prematurity; low birth weight or SGA infants; hypoglycemia; decreased caloric intake (NPO; nausea and vomiting; gastric suction). | Fuel/substrate is necessary to generate heat. |
| 2. Assess temperature using appropriate method for measuring body temperature (based on age, developmental stage, anatomy and physiology). | Measuring body temperature provides baseline temperature data, guides the type and evaluates the effectiveness of interventions (see Skill 30).<br>***Special Considerations:*** *Consider the time of day the temperature is obtained. Humans have cyclic variations in bodily functions, including temperature, in a 24-hour period. These daily fluctuations are innately controlled by the brain's "biologic clock." Diurnal variations in core temperature range from .7° to 2.1°C; the lowest core temperature is between 4 to 5 AM and the highest between 7 to 9 PM (Lloyd, 1986).* |
| 3. Assess temperature for evidence of cold stress. | In an environment that is less than thermal neutral, cold stress begins as skin temperature decreases because of vasoconstriction (Fig. 83-1). Cold stress initiates nonshivering thermogenesis in neonates (norepinephrine is released, brown fat is metabolized, and heat is produced). These thermogenic processes require oxygen and glucose, and they result in hypoxia, acidosis, and hypoglycemia (Merenstein, Gardner, and Blake, 1989). |
| 4. Assess for signs/symptoms of hypothermia: | |
| a. Preterms/neonates (Merenstein, Gardner, and Blake, 1989): | |
| ▪ Skin feels cold to touch (hands, feet, trunk). | Cool skin is an early vasoconstrictive response to cold stress or the result of a decrease in core temperature. |
| ▪ Poor feeding: poor sucking, decreased intake, increased gastric residual, apathy toward feedings, abdominal distension or vomiting. | Poor feeding is common in infants with thermal instability due to CNS depression. |

**Steps** | **Rationale**

- Other behavioral changes: increase/decrease in spontaneous activity, hypotonia, weak cry, irritability/lethargy, difficult to arouse.

***Special Considerations:*** *Neonatal behavioral changes in hypothermia are subtle and may mimic other problems (e.g., sepsis, hypoglycemia).*

- Color changes:
  (1) Pallor.

Vasoconstriction decreases heat loss from skin.

  (2) Cyanosis: central (lips, mucous membranes, circumoral or orbital), peripheral (acrocyanosis of hands and feet).

A small drop in temperature results in a marked increase in oxygen consumption that may produce cyanosis.

  (3) Bright red skin color.

Bright red coloring is present after the failure of oxyhemoglobin dissociation at low temperatures.

- Autonomic changes: respiratory (tachypnea, slow rate, apnea), bradycardia.

Hypothermia is a frequent cause of apnea and bradycardia in the premature infant.

b. Infant/older child (Boswick et al, 1986; Lloyd, 1986):

- Mild hypothermia: core temperature between 32.2° to 34.4°C (90° to 94°F); conscious but stumbling, disorientation, incoordination and slurred speech; amnesia; shivering; ashen gray skin, bradycardia, decreased blood pressure.

Heat production is increased by increased muscle metabolism and tone. This leads eventually to shivering, which may double or triple oxygen consumption in an attempt to produce heat.

- Moderate hypothermia: core temperature between 26.6° and 32.2°C (80°-90°F); bradycardia, dysrhythmia, decreased blood pressure; decreased respiratory rate and cough reflex; decreased urinary output.
- Severe hypothermia: core temperature between 21.1° to 26.6°C (70° to 80°F); hypotension, shock; cardiac arrest <25°C; respirations difficult to discern because of extremely slow rate; apnea <24°C; deep coma, cold and stiff (appearance of death), fixed and dilated pupils; metabolic acidosis, hyperglycemia.

At core body temperatures below 32° C the excitation phase of heat production gives way to a slowing of organ system function (Robinson and Seward, 1986):

*Cardiovascular*—Blood pressure, heart rate and cardiac output fall at temperatures <32°C. Dysrhythmias (atrial/ventricular) and conduction delays (bradycardia) occur at core temperatures <30°C. Pulse and blood pressure may be difficult to determine. The bradycardia may be profound enough to resemble asystole (yet rate increases with rewarming). As core temperature drops <26°C, the risk of spontaneous ventricular fibrillation increases. Physical manipulation may also precipitate dysrhythmia.

*Pulmonary*—Hypoventilation results in a respiratory acidosis.

*CNS*—Below 32°C a decreasing level of consciousness (confusion and incoordination) gives way to unconsciousness.

*Metabolic*—The metabolic requirements of all tissues are decreased with severe hypothermia. Shivering and poor tissue oxygenation produce a metabolic acidosis that further impairs organ function. Acidosis and hypothermia cause a left shift in the oxyhemoglobin dissociation curve, thus impairing oxygen release at the tissue level. A hyperglycemic response (proportional to the depth of the hypothermia) is common.

*Local cold injury*—Perfusion changes such as hemoconcentration and sludging precipitate thrombus formation. As tissue temperature approaches the freezing point of water, ice crystallization occurs within the frostbitten tissues.

*Renal*—Ability to concentrate urine is impaired, resulting in a diuresis. Acute tubular necrosis may occur secondary to renal hypoperfusion and myoglobinuria.

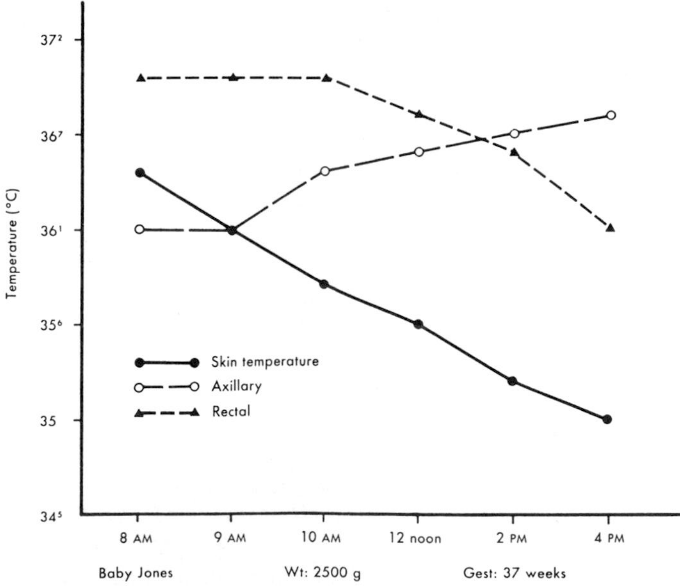


***FIG. 83-1*** Temperature measurement at various sites during cold stress.

From Merenstein GB and Gardner SL: Handbook of neonatal intensive care, ed 2, St Louis, 1989, The CV Mosby Co.

5. Assess skin integrity of frostbitten areas if applicable, especially fingers, hands, toes, feet, ears, and nose.
   a. First symptoms (Wilkerson et al, 1986):

Assessing for frostbite (localized cold injury characterized by freezing and ice crystal formation in the tissues) will determine what further interventions will be needed after core temperature has been raised.

- Pain.

As tissue freezing progresses, the pain subsides.

- Color—pale→purple.

Purple tissue represents circulatory stasis and sludging, a sign of severe tissue damage.

- Texture—firm, hard tissue.

| Steps | Rationale |
|---|---|
| b. Superficial injury:<br>▪ Hyperthermia (vascular congestion resulting in reddened skin areas); burning sensation. | Hyperemic discoloration represents increased blood flow; crust formation occurs and superficial skin is lost. A burning sensation occurs when circulation is reestablished to affected areas. |
| c. Second degree injury:<br>▪ Blister formation; paresthesia (tingling, numbness). | Blisters develop on tissue within hours or days of rewarming. Blisters that contain clear fluid and extend to the tips of the digits represent tissue that will survive. Blisters containing bloody fluid and not extending to the end of the digits overlay tissue that will not survive. |
| d. Full thickness injury:<br>▪ Eschar formation; anesthesia. | Tissue injury occurs as a result of water extraction from within the tissue cell and from the obstruction of blood supply to the tissues.<br>***Special Considerations:*** *Within a week or more after injury, a thick, gray, dark green or black eschar (like a third degree burn) develops. Black mummified eschar loses sensation and will either fall off or be amputated as the subcutaneous tissues become gangrenous.* |
| 6. Assess child/family's understanding of cold stress/hypothermic insult. | A lack of information, explanation, or misunderstanding of terminology will contribute to anxiety, fear, and confusion. |

## Planning and Goal Setting

| Steps | Rationale |
|---|---|
| 1. Plan frequency of assessment of body temperature (Merenstein, Gardner, and Blake, 1989):<br>a. Every 1 to 2 hours in low birth weight (preterms and SGA's) and sick neonates.<br>b. Every 2 to 3 hours after birth, during neonatal transition from intra to extrauterine life.<br>c. Every 3 to 4 hours in healthy, term neonates.<br>d. Every 30 to 60 minutes during rewarming of a cold-stressed neonate/infant/child.<br>e. Every 2 to 3 hours after rewarming period, if child is stable. | Frequent body temperature assessments establish baseline data, guide efficacy of interventions and determine need for more vigorous methods of rewarming. |
| 2. Plan frequency of assessment of vital signs in hypothermic infant/child:<br>a. Hourly vital signs during initial rewarming.<br>b. Every 2 to 3 hours after rewarming period, if child is stable. | Close monitoring of vital signs is necessary to evaluate the infant/child's general condition and response to interventions. |
| 3. Plan care collaboratively with child/family. | Collaborative planning encourages cooperation of child/family in care. |
| 4. Develop individualized child/family goals:<br>▪ Heat imbalance and its sequelae will be prevented.<br>▪ Complications of hypothermia and rewarming will be prevented or minimized.<br>▪ Pain will be decreased.<br>▪ Skin integrity will be maintained.<br>▪ Child/family will understand need/methods for rewarming.<br>▪ Child/family will participate in rewarming and prevention of recurrent cold stress and complications. | |

## Implementation

| Steps | Rationale |
|---|---|
| 1. Maintain neutral thermal environment for neonates (Merenstein, Gardner, and Blake, 1989). See Table 83-1 for neutral thermal environmental temperatures for newborns. | Neutral Thermal Environment (NTE) is the environmental temperature that enables a neonate's body temperature to remain normal with minimal metabolic effort and therefore minimal oxygen consumption.<br>***Special Considerations:*** *Neutral thermal environmental range:*<br>*32.5° ± 1.4°C (90.5° ± 2.6°F) for larger babies.*<br>*35.4° ± 0.5°C (95.7° ± .9°F) for smaller babies (Merenstein, Gardner, and Blake, 1989).* |

**TABLE 83-1** Neutral Thermal Environmental Temperatures

| AGE AND WEIGHT | STARTING TEMPERATURE (°C) | RANGE OF TEMPERATURE (°C) |
|---|---|---|
| 0-6 hours | | |
| 1501-2500 g | 33.4 | 32.8-33.8 |
| Over 2500 g (and >36 weeks) | 33.9 | 32.0-33.8 |
| 6-12 hours | | |
| 1501-2500 g | 33.1 | 32.2-33.8 |
| Over 2500 g (and >36 weeks) | 32.8 | 31.4-33.8 |
| 12-24 hours | | |
| 1501-2500 g | 32.8 | 31.8-33.8 |
| Over 2500 g (and >36 weeks) | 32.4 | 31.0-33.7 |
| 24-36 hours | | |
| 1501-2500 g | 32.6 | 31.6-33.6 |
| Over 2500 g (and >36 weeks) | 32.1 | 30.7-33.5 |
| 36-48 hours | | |
| 1501-2500 g | 32.5 | 31.4-33.5 |
| Over 2500 g (and >36 weeks) | 31.9 | 30.5-33.3 |
| 48-72 hours | | |
| 1501-2500 g | 32.3 | 31.2-33.4 |
| Over 2500 g (and >36 weeks) | 31.7 | 30.1-33.2 |
| 72-96 hours | | |
| 1501-2500 g | 32.2 | 31.1-33.2 |
| Over 2500 g (and >36 weeks) | 31.3 | 29.8-32.8 |
| 4-12 days | | |
| 1501-2500 g | 32.1 | 31.0-33.2 |
| Over 2500 g (and >36 weeks) | | |
| 4-5 days | 31.0 | 29.5-32.6 |
| 5-6 days | 30.9 | 29.4-32.3 |
| 6-8 days | 30.6 | 29.0-32.2 |
| 8-10 days | 30.3 | 29.0-31.8 |
| 10-12 days | 30.1 | 29.0-31.4 |

Adapted from: American Academy of Pediatrics and American College of Obstetricians and Gynecologists: Guidelines for perinatal care, ed 2, Evanston, Ill, 1988, American Academy of Pediatrics and American College of Obstetricians and Gynecologists.

| Steps | Rationale |
|---|---|
| a. Use a servocontrolled device.<br>▪ Attach the skin probe with tape to the upper right abdominal quadrant.<br>▪ If a radiant heater is used, cover the probe with a deflecting metal or foam pad. | Servocontrolled devices are used to automatically adjust heat output so the infant's skin temperature is maintained at a preset level. |
| ▪ Set the servo mechanism to the desired skin temperature (between 36° to 36.5°C/96.8° to 97.7°F). | The neutral thermal skin temperature is the skin temperature at which oxygen consumption is minimal. The range of thermal neutrality is narrow and there is a critical temperature below this range where oxygen consumption increases in an attempt to maintain temperature.<br>***Special Considerations:*** *Factors such as ambient air temperature, humidity, air velocity, and the temperature of objects in direct contact with the infant or surfaces involved in heat exchange should all be considered as part of the environment. Newer incubators also enable air temperature to be servocontrolled so that heat output fluctuates to maintain a set air temperature within the incubator. Interpretation of hypo/hyperthermia in the servocontrolled neonate may* not *be obvious since temperature is automatically maintained at the preset level.* |
| b. Use a nonservocontrolled or manual heating device. | Although manual heating devices are available, their use is not optimal because a decrease in skin temperature is not automatically detected, therefore more heat is not generated to warm the infant. |

| **Steps** | **Rationale** |
|---|---|
| ▪ Set the warming device at the neutral thermal environmental temperature desired (see Table 83-1). | Setting the warming device at neutral thermal environmental temperature and adjusting it manually to maintain the desired skin temperature will avoid cold stressing or overheating the baby.<br>***Special Considerations:*** *For example, an infant weighing 2 kg who is 2 days old should be placed in a prewarmed (32.5° C/90.5° F) incubator. Approximately 1°C/1.8°F should be added to this operative temperature when the room temperature is <27°C/80.6°F and a single-walled incubator is being used (Merenstein, Gardner, and Blake, 1989).* |
| 2. Block avenues of heat loss and apply external heat sources (Merenstein, Gardner, and Blake, 1989). | The risks of cold stress are minimized by blocking avenues of heat loss (Merenstein, Gardner, and Blake, 1989). Heat exchange from warmer to cooler objects takes place between the body surface and the environment as a function of the physical properties of radiation, evaporation, conduction, and convection. |
| *For the neonate:*<br>a. Avoid evaporative heat loss:<br>▪ Keep baby dry by removing wet clothes and linens and replacing with dry warmed clothes, blankets and bed linens, as often as necessary. | Evaporation causes heat loss from the mucosa of the respiratory tract and from skin. |
| ▪ Keep hair/head dry and wrap/cover head with dry towel or hat. | The head is one fourth (25%) of the neonate's body surface so covering the head decreases heat loss from a large surface area. |
| b. Decrease radiant heat loss and increase radiant warmth. | Radiation is the transfer of heat from skin to cooler surrounding surfaces that are *not* in contact with the skin. It is the largest avenue of heat loss in the neonate as he or she radiates heat to the incubator wall, which then radiates heat to surrounding cooler objects. |
| ▪ Use a heat shield or inner wall of a double-walled incubator that is warmed by the heated ambient air inside the incubator. | The temperature gradient between the infant and this interposed surface is much less than the difference between the infant and the cooler, outer incubator wall, thus the radiant heat lost by the infant is less. |
| ▪ Keep incubators away from cooler surfaces (e.g., windows, air conditioner ducts). | |
| ▪ Keep ambient room temperature between at least 22.2° to 24.4°C/72° to 76°F. | Proper room temperature minimizes both radiant and convective heat losses. |
| ▪ Use a radiant warmer that is preset to a control point (36.5°C) neonatal skin temperature. A radiant warmer provides easy access to an infant requiring frequent intervention. | Radiant warmers maintain temperature by pumping a large amount of infrared light energy into the infant's skin (Merenstein, Gardner, and Blake, 1989).<br>***Special Considerations:*** *Wide swings in heat balance will occur if hands, head, drapes, and blankets block the heat source from the infant's skin. Infants in radiant warmers tend to have an increased insensible water loss, oxygen consumption, and cardiac output over infants in incubators (the clinical significance of this is unknown) (Merenstein, Gardner, and Blake, 1989).* |
| ▪ Use rapid rewarming (set servocontrol at 37°C) for more severe hypothermia. | ***Special Considerations:*** *Rapid rewarming may be hazardous to the already compromised, cold stressed infant and is associated with apnea. It should only be implemented in an intensive care setting with continuous cardiorespiratory monitoring and attention to metabolic derangements of cold stress. Rapid rewarming is associated with decreased mortality in severely hypothermic infants (Kaplan and Eidelman, 1984; Sofer et al, 1986).* |
| ▪ Drape a blanket of plastic wrap (e.g., Saran Wrap) above but not touching the infant and over the sides of the warmer. | Plastic wrap enables radiant heat to reach the infant's skin while decreasing evaporative, convective and radiant heat losses.<br>***Special Considerations:*** Do not use *a Plexiglas heat shield over the infant in a radiant warmer or blankets, clothes, and insulating materials (e.g., foil, bubble wrap) that prevent radiant heat from contacting the infant's skin.* |
| c. Minimize conductive heat loss and increase conductive warmth. | Conductive heat loss occurs when heat is transferred directly from a warmer surface in contact with a cooler surface. |

| Steps | Rationale |
|---|---|
| ▪ Warm all objects to be in contact with the neonate's skin: examiner's hands, stethoscope, scales, x-ray plates, treatment tables, diapers/bed linen. | |
| ▪ Place the healthy newborn skin-to-skin with the mother and wrap both in a warm blanket. | Mother's body warmth is conducted to the skin of her infant and helps keep the baby warm. |
| ▪ Place heated pads that do not exceed 40°C in incubator or on radiant warmer.<br>(1) Cover heat pad with blanket or sheet.<br>(2) Place infant on covering and *not* directly onto heated pad. | ***Special Considerations:*** *Hot water bottles should* not *be used with neonates because of the risk of thermal burns. A regulatable pad that is* not *in direct contact with the skin is safer.* |
| ▪ Warm food and fluids (oral, intravenous, blood).<br>(1) Use blood/IV fluid warmers.<br>(2) Warm fluids to 40° to 42°C. | Warming fluids is a method of core rewarming. The majority of hypothermic children are dehydrated, hypovolemic, and need fluids.<br>***Special Considerations:*** *Intravenous fluids are the best method for core rewarming. Warmed oral fluids may trigger dysrhythmia in a cold heart.* |
| d. Minimize convective heat loss and increase convective warmth. | Convective heat loss results from air currents on the skin surface. The actual amount of heat loss depends on the velocity of air flow and the air temperature.<br>***Special Considerations:*** *Convective loss inside an incubator is minimal because the velocity is low and the air temperature is relatively high.* |
| ▪ Slowly rewarm infant by maintaining incubator ambient temperature 1 to 1.5°C/2 to 2.6°F above infant's skin temperature and increase every 2 to 3 hours until the temperature is within neutral thermal range. | Slow rewarming is preferred if the hypothermia is mild since oxygen consumption is minimal when the difference between skin and ambient air temperature is <1.5°C/2° to 2.6°F (Merenstein, Gardner, and Blake, 1989). |
| ▪ Decrease drafts over infant's body surface by:<br>(1) Minimizing unnecessary opening of incubator portholes.<br>(2) Organizing care.<br>(3) Placing open (radiant) warmers away from drafts.<br>(4) Not blowing air/oxygen directly into infant's face (point line away from face/head). | |
| ▪ Heat airway gases to 31° to 34°C/88° to 94°F. | Heating prevents cold stress and increased oxygen consumption that results from a cold flow on neonate's face/head. |
| (1) Measure the temperature of the heated gas at the delivery site (not as it leaves the nebulizer).<br>(2) Warm endotracheal tube gases to 35° to 36.6°C/95° to 97°F. | Cooling of the gas occurs in the tubing (Hagedorn, Gardner, and Abman, 1989). |
| ▪ Swaddle neonate in warmed blankets, put on clothing, wrap in insulating materials (bubble wrap or foil). | Swaddling decreases heat losses from radiation, evaporation, and convection.<br>***Special Considerations:*** *Visualizing the swaddled infant is more difficult. Infant must be warm* prior *to wrapping in insulating materials because these retain body warmth rather than generate heat.* |
| *For the infant/older child in mild hypothermia:*<br>a. Avoid evaporative heat loss. | Avoiding evaporation blocks heat loss. |
| ▪ Remove wet clothes.<br>▪ Dry off, including head and hair.<br>▪ Place in dry warm clothes or blankets; cover head. | These measures decrease evaporative heat loss from wet clothes, skin, and large surface areas (e.g., a child's head). |
| b. Minimize radiant and convective heat loss by placing in warm environment. | By placing in a warm environment, the child will passively warm himself or herself. |
| c. Increase conductive heat gain.<br>▪ Warm oral fluids. | Oral fluids have no effect on elevating core temperature but may make child "feel better."<br>***Special Considerations:*** *Warmed oral fluids may warm blood perfusing the brain, signaling that the child is "too hot" and may result in vasodilation (child feels warm and loses heat from skin). Block avenues of heat loss before giving warmed oral fluids (see step a above).* |

| **Steps** | **Rationale** |
|---|---|
| d. Provide external heat sources. | ***Special Considerations:*** *Great care must be exercised in the use of topical heat in any immobilized, anesthetized, unconscious person, or infant/child because of the increased potential for thermal injury resulting from their inability to feel pain of heat or inability to escape heat. The threshold at which heat causes pain is 43° to 45°C/109° to 113°F (Feldman et al, 1985).* |
| ▪ Hot water bath/shower: water <45°C (113°F) for infants/older children.<br>▪ Rewarming blanket (a circulating water blanket) at 37°C (98.6°F). | ***Special Considerations:*** *Hot water bottles, hot packs, and heating pads should not exceed 45°C/113°F (Feldman et al, 1985). Water that is warmer than 54°C/130°F increases the risk of full thickness thermal burns of the skin.* |
| ▪ Hot water bottles, hot packs, heating pads: first, wrap them in dry towel/cloth; then apply to areas with least insulation (e.g., inguinal area, axilla and sides of chest, neck-carotid/jugular area). | A layer of dry material between the skin and the warm surface will help protect the skin by providing insulation from direct contact. Since major heat loss occurs from the least insulated areas, application of external warmth facilitates raising core body temperature. |
| *For infant/child with moderate to severe hypothermia:*<br>a. Minimize evaporative/convective heat losses.<br>▪ Heat and humidify airway gases (40° to 42°C/104° to 108°F). | ***Special Considerations:*** *Heated, humidified gases decrease evaporative losses as well as convective loss from a cool flow. Warmed air/oxygen delivered directly to the airway by endotracheal tube is more effective than mask delivery. However, intubation and alkalosis of manual ventilation are potential triggers of ventricular fibrillation.* |
| b. Increase conductive heat gain.<br>▪ Administer warmed IV fluids (40°C/104°F). | Warm IV fluids increase core temperature. The fluids also expand the circulating blood volume, which elevates blood pressure, improves flow and oxygenation to the heart, and decreases the risk of rewarming shock and ventricular fibrillation. |
| c. Assist physician with central rewarming techniques (Lloyd, 1986). | ***Special Considerations:*** *Central rewarming is used only in extreme situations (e.g., cold water immersion, outdoor exposure).* |
| ▪ Extracorporeal blood warming:<br>(1) Cardiopulmonary bypass.<br>(2) Hemodialysis at 37°C. | This technique directly perfuses the heart with warmed blood that reduces cardiac irritability and the risk of ventricular fibrillation and cardiac arrest.<br>***Special Considerations:*** *Disadvantages include the availability of equipment and trained personnel and the risks of hemolysis, infection, and bleeding.* |
| ▪ Irrigation of body cavities:<br>(1) Gastric lavage with warmed solution (40.5° to 42.5°C). | Gastric lavage supplies heat to the core (like peritoneal dialysis) but without penetrating the skin. |
| (2) Peritoneal dialysis with warmed fluid (40.5° to 42.5°C). | Peritoneal dialysis conducts heat to the heart through the diaphragm and by warming the blood in the inferior vena cava. Abdominal cavity and organs are directly heated by the warmed fluid. |
| (3) Mediastinal irrigation with 40°C saline solution. | Mediastinal irrigation is an efficient means of transferring heat directly to the heart.<br>***Special Considerations:*** *This technique requires a thoracotomy and a high level skilled staff. It also carries the risk of infection.* |
| d. Minimize child's movements and handle gently. | At core temperatures <29.4°C/85°F, positional changes that may jar the heart (e.g., chest percussion, intubation, or rough handling) may trigger fibrillation and arrest. Sudden movement of extremities pumps cold, hypoxic and acidotic blood with a high potassium level into an already cold, compromised heart which is suddenly hit with colder blood containing cardiac irritants. Ventricular fibrillation results.<br>***Special Considerations:*** *The mortality rate in mild to severe hypothermia is 50% to 80%, because of ventricular fibrillation (Boswick et al, 1986; Lloyd, 1986; Robinson and Seward, 1986; Wilkerson et al, 1986).* |

| Steps | Rationale |
|---|---|
| 3. Provide continuous cardiorespiratory monitoring with high/low alarms set (see Skill 100). | Cardiorespiratory monitoring enables detection of cardiac dysrhythmias as well as apnea. |
| 4. Administer cardiopulmonary resuscitation (CPR) if needed. Use special precautions in administering CPR to a hypothermic person: | The cold heart is very irritable and ventricular fibrillation may be precipitated by chest massage, intubation, vein cannulation, and patient transfer/positioning. |
| a. Handle gently, using only the most necessary measures. | |
| b. Administer oxygen. | Hypothermic children are also hypoxic. Hypothermia protects the brain and other organs from hypoxia/anoxia by decreasing basal metabolic rate and oxygen utilization. |
| c. Initiate CPR if no pulse or respirations are discernible (see Skill 126). | A pulse of 5 to 10 bpm is adequate to sustain life in a hypothermic person.<br>***Special Considerations:*** *"No one should be considered cold and dead until he has been warm and dead" (Wilkerson et al, 1986). Children with core temperatures as low as 23°C (68°F) have survived with full CNS recovery (Robinson and Seward, 1986).* |
| ▪ Bag and mask preferred over intubation. | Risk of fibrillation increases with intubation. |
| ▪ If intubation is required, pre-oxygenate. | |
| ▪ Chest compressions. | Chest compressions are needed for asystole/ventricular fibrillation. |
| ▪ Defibrillation. | Defibrillation is often not effective at temperature $<$30°C because the sodium pump of the heart is disabled by such low temperatures so that the electrical shock of defibrillation is not transmitted to the conduction system of the heart. |
| ▪ Drug therapy. | ***Special Considerations:*** *Drug therapy is ineffective in hypothermic children until the core temperature is at least 30°C. Use of drugs during hypothermia may lead to drug toxicity on rewarming.* |
| 5. Monitor for signs/symptoms of systemic complications of hypothermia. | The hypothermic neonate/infant/child's response to rewarming may be hampered by the development of systemic complications of hypothermia. |
| a. Metabolic derangements: | |
| ▪ Hypoglycemia. | Hypoglycemia results from an increased use of carbohydrate stores in an effort to maintain core temperature. |
| (1) Test blood with reagent strip and/or obtain serum glucose level every hour until infant is stable.<br>(2) Observe for signs and symptoms: tremors and jitteriness, respiratory difficulty and apnea, lethargy or irritability, seizures, and poor feeding. | |
| ▪ Hyperglycemia.<br>(1) Test blood with reagent strip and/or obtain serum glucose levels every hour until stable.<br>(2) Measure urinary output and test for glycosuria. | Insulin is usually not used in treatment because the pancreas will resume insulin secretion when it is rewarmed.<br>***Special Considerations:*** *Either hypoglycemia or hyperglycemia occurs in infants and children in response to hypothermia.* |
| ▪ Hyperkalemia.<br>(1) Draw blood for electrolytes.<br>(2) Monitor additives in IV fluids. | The child is often hyperkalemic when cold, then hypokalemic when rewarmed. |
| ▪ Hypoxia and metabolic acidosis.<br>(1) Interpret arterial blood gas values.<br>(2) Observe continuous pulse oximetry and administer oxygen and assisted ventilation as needed. | Hypothermia causes pulmonary vasoconstriction in the neonate that further perpetuates the hypoxia-acidosis cycle. |
| ▪ Elevated blood urea nitrogen (BUN).<br>(1) Interpret BUN lab value.<br>(2) Measure intake and output hourly.<br>(3) Test urine for blood, protein, pH and sugar. Measure specific gravity (see Skill 117). | Decreased renal blood flow predisposes the child to acute tubular necrosis and diuresis, because of an inability to concentrate urine. Measurement of intake and output facilitates fluid management to prevent fluid overload and/or dehydration. |
| ▪ Hyperbilirubinemia.<br>(1) Observe for jaundice discoloration in a head to toe progression.<br>(2) Interpret serum bilirubin values. | Hypothermia alters the blood-brain barrier that increases risk of kernicterus at lower serum bilirubin levels. |
| b. Hypotension.<br>▪ Observe vital signs, including blood pressure every 30 to 60 minutes during acute rewarming. | Hypotension may occur secondary to peripheral vasodilation associated with rapid rewarming. |

| **Steps** | **Rationale** |
|---|---|
| c. Seizures.<br>▪ Observe for signs/symptoms of seizure behavior which may be subtle in the neonate (i.e., tremors, jitteriness, opisthotonos, hypo/hypertonia, chewing or boxing motions, apnea, staring facial expression). | Seizures in the neonate are the result of ischemic brain insult from low blood flow following peripheral vasodilation. In the infant/child, seizures result from cerebral edema secondary to ischemia of brain. |
| d. Apnea.<br>▪ Observe respiratory patterns.<br>▪ Provide continuous cardiorespiratory monitoring with alarms. | Apnea may be the result of hypoxia or an unknown central nervous system mechanism. |
| e. Dehydration.<br>▪ Observe urinary output, amount and color; test for specific gravity, protein, blood, pH, and sugar hourly.<br>▪ Evaluate skin turgor, mucous membrane moisture, arterial blood pressure, activity level, and body weight. | Dehydration after hypothermia is caused by increased insensible water loss of 3- to 4-fold during rewarming. |
| f. Pneumonia.<br>▪ Observe respiratory effort: rate, rhythm, and use of accessory muscles.<br>▪ Auscultate breath sounds. | Pneumonia is the most common complication after rewarming. |
| 6. Implement techniques for rewarming local tissue injury (frostbite) (Wilkerson et al, 1986). | ***Special Considerations:*** *Do not treat frostbite until core temperature is responding to rewarming efforts. Rewarming (of extremities) should not be attempted if danger of tissue refreezing exists (e.g., during evacuation attempts) because more extensive damage to tissues will occur.* |
| a. Remove wet or constrictive clothing. | Removing wet, constrictive clothing decreases evaporative heat loss and increases blood flow to the extremities. |
| b. Wrap affected areas with warm, dry material (e.g., blankets). | |
| c. Do *not* rub affected areas or expose them to dry heat. | Temperature of dry heat sources cannot be controlled as easily as a warm water bath. Rubbing, for example, applies warmth unevenly to the area. |
| d. For rapid rewarming, immerse affected parts in warm water (40° to 42° C/104° to 108° F) for 20 to 30 minutes, until tissues are soft and pliable or until a flush returns to the most distal tip of the thawed part. | Warm water thaws frozen tissue and helps to improve peripheral circulation. Slow rewarming will increase tissue loss. |
| ▪ Maintain constant water temperature by adding warm water to bath.<br>▪ *Do not* heat water container.<br>▪ Remove extremity when adding water.<br>▪ Stir water thoroughly and check temperature before returning extremity to water. | Warmer temperature increases tissue damage. |
| ▪ Suspend frozen part to avoid touching sides/bottom of water container. | Suspending immersed body part avoids injury from bumping sides of container surfaces.<br>***Special Considerations:*** *Do not rub with snow or immerse in cold water because it will aggravate vasoconstriction and circulatory sludging. Areas that do not flush indicate a lack of return of blood flow and will probably not survive.* |
| e. Administer pain medications during rewarming (see Skill 52). | As rewarming occurs, the child will regain sensation and frostbitten tissue may be extremely painful. When tissues are thawed and perfused, pain decreases.<br>***Special Considerations:*** *Aspirin may not only relieve pain, but improve circulation by its prostaglandin-inhibiting action and its alteration of bleeding/clotting time.* |
| f. Protect injured tissue after rewarming.<br>▪ Keep child warm. | |
| ▪ Elevate injured part. | Elevation helps to decrease edema. |
| ▪ Pad between frostbitten fingers and toes with sterile gauze or cotton. | Preventing contact between injured tissue protects it from further trauma/irritation. |
| ▪ Keep bed linens off frostbitten, thawed tissue with a bed frame. | Blister formation occurs after rewarming; keeping blisters intact decreases secondary infection. |
| ▪ Encourage active extremity movement. | Active movement increases blood flow to extremities.<br>***Special Considerations:*** *The child sets his or her own limits of mobility when pain is elicited with movement.* |
| 7. Provide information, reassurance and emotional support to family and child, such as explaining the importance of keeping child warm and why child may resist covers and clothes. | Information about equipment, condition, and therapies for family/child assists in mastery and elicits cooperation and collaboration. |

**Steps** | **Rationale**

***Special Considerations:*** *Sometimes a hypothermic child will resist being covered, a phenomenon called paradoxical undressing, which is the result of a drop in core temperature that confuses the thermal regulating mechanism and gives the victim a false sense of being too warm (Sivaloganathan, 1986).*

## Evaluation Outcomes / Observational Guidelines

1. Proper body temperature is maintained.

   Measure temperature at recommended intervals for age and condition and plot on temperature chart. Maintain temperature at:
   *Neonate:*
   telethermometer with the skin probe between 36° to 36.5° C/ 96.8° to 97.7°F and axillary between 36.5° to 37.5°C/97.7° to 99.5°F.
   *Infant/older child:*
   rectal probe 36.6° to 37.5°C/97.8° to 99.5°F; axillary between 36.5° to 37.5°C/97.7° to 99.5°F.

2. Signs and symptoms of hypothermia are reversed.

   Observe reversal in state of consciousness: deep coma to confusion and incoordination to conscious to able to speak. Fixed, dilated pupils become reactive. Observe reversal in cardiopulmonary symptoms: decrease in cardiac dysrhythmias, slow heart rate and respiratory rate to increased heart and respiratory rates.

3. Localized areas (toes, feet, fingers, hands) regain adequate circulation, intact sensory and motor function.

   Observe skin color, blisters, and temperature. Localized areas are warm and pink with brisk capillary refill. Observe for active movement and reports of and/or behavioral and facial expressions of pain. If pain occurs, note the movements that induce it.

4. Child experiences decreased, minimal, or no pain.

   Assess level of pain and child's response to pain.
   Determine amount, frequency, and route of pain medication required, as well as the response to pain medication.

5. Skin integrity remains intact.

   Inspect skin areas actively involved in rewarming for redness, blisters, abraded, or open areas.

6. Child/family understand reason for hospitalization and treatments.

   Ask child/family to verbalize their understanding of reason for development of hypothermia and need for hospitalization.

7. Child/family participates in self-care activities.

   Observe child's/family's participation in care (e.g., feeding, bathing, play).

## Documentation

Record temperature values:

a. Neonate—skin, axillary, environmental, control.
b. Infant older than 3 months/child—axillary, rectal. Note signs and symptoms of hypothermia, rewarming interventions, and responses to those interventions. Document skin integrity of frostbitten areas and of areas directly involved in rewarming efforts. Indicate pain experienced by child, comfort measures and pain medications administered, and the child's responses. Note child/family's participation in self-care activities and any child/family teaching conducted, including content, ability of child/family to understand/repeat information and demonstrate skill. Identify any additional problems and actions taken.

# *SKILL 84* Managing an Elevated Temperature

*Anne Scott*

An elevated body temperature measurement may result from fever or hyperthermia. Fever is defined as core body temperature greater than 38° C (100.4° F) as a result of an organized response by the body to an insult or disease (Burstin, 1985). Hyperthermia is defined as a core body temperature greater than 38° C (Morriss, 1984) in spite of the body's attempts to lower it. Mild degrees of fever or hyperthermia may not warrant intervention, depending on the underlying cause. Causes of elevated temperature include infection and thermoregulatory failure (Morriss, 1984).

Fever is a result of an increase in the hypothalamic setpoint in response to an infectious agent. This resetting of the hypothalamic thermostat results in increased heat production. Controversy exists concerning treatment of fevers caused by infection. Many authors argue that fever is nature's defense against illness and fevers below 104°-106° F should usually be left untreated. (Cunha et al, 1984; Fruthaler, 1985; Griffin, 1986; Gurevich, 1985). Most authorities agree that children can tolerate fevers up to 107.6° F without permanent damage. Irreversible brain damage has been reported with body temperatures above 42° C (108° F) (Burstin, 1985). Fever aids in fighting infectious agents by triggering the release of interleukin 1, which deprives the infectious agents of needed zinc and iron (Griffin, 1986; Fruthaler, 1985). Thus, to treat a fever may be detrimental to the body's natural defense mechanisms (Reeves-Swift, 1990). Comfort would be the primary reason for treating fever in an otherwise healthy child (Fruthaler, 1985). For the critically ill infant or child with compromised cardiopulmonary or neurologic status, fever may have serious consequences and should be treated aggressively (Burstin, 1985; Morriss, 1984).

Elevated temperatures caused by thermoregulatory failure can occur as a result of: (a) hypermetabolic states such as malignant hyperthermia resulting in excessive heat production; (b) disordered hypothalamic function such as with CNS injury or infection; (c) defective heat loss or elevated environmental temperature such as heat exhaustion or heat stroke. In these situations, the body temperature exceeds the hypothalamic setpoint although the setpoint may be normal.

This skill focuses on the most common causes of elevated temperatures in children, that of infection and impaired heat dissipation. Severe hyperthermia caused by abnormal heat production (e.g., malignant hyperthermia) will not be addressed because it requires specific medical management.

## NURSING DIAGNOSES

Hyperthermia related to infection, exposure to a hot environment, dehydration, or medication side effects; Parental anxiety related to unmet informational needs about fever and treatment modalities; Potential impaired tissue integrity related to cool/cold treatment measures.

| Steps | Rationale |
|---|---|
| **Assessment** | |
| 1. Assess body temperature, pulse, respirations and blood pressure (see Skills 30, 31, 32 and 33). | Establishing a child's baseline vital signs is important to evaluate elevated temperatures.<br>***Special Considerations:*** *For every 1° F elevation in temperature, heart rate increases 10 beats/minute and respiratory rate increases 2 breaths/minute. Systemic blood pressure may decrease as a result of peripheral vasodilation caused by fever. With heat stroke, initial sweating and water loss lead to decreased blood volume and then peripheral vasoconstriction (Burstin, 1985).* |
| 2. Consider the probable cause of the elevated temperature by reviewing the history, performing a physical assessment (see Skill 27) and collaborating with other health professionals. | The method or need to reduce temperature depends upon the underlying cause.<br>***Special Considerations:*** *Viral infection is the cause of 80% to 90% of childhood fever (Fruthaler, 1985).* |
| 3. Review history for risk factors: | Certain conditions warrant more aggressive treatment of temperature elevations. |

| Steps | Rationale |
|---|---|
| a. Febrile seizures. | Fever is known to lower the seizure threshold although the seizures are usually a result of the disease process rather than the fever (Fruthaler, 1985).<br>***Special Considerations:*** *Only 4% of children have seizures associated with high temperatures.* |
| b. Diabetes. | An elevated temperature can rapidly cause a child with diabetes to become acidotic because of an increased metabolic rate. |
| c. Recent medications. | A medication reaction may cause an elevated temperature. Anticholinergic drugs decrease sweating and affect the child's ability to dissipate heat. |
| d. Cardiac disorders. | Vasoconstriction of pulmonary arterioles and systemic hypotension from peripheral vasodilation caused by a temperature elevation can increase intrapulmonary and/or intracardiac shunting (Burstin, 1985). |
| e. Pulmonary disorders. | Fever shifts the oxyhemoglobin dissociation curve to the right (Burstin, 1985). A generalized hypermetabolic state caused by high fever may initially result in hyperventilation causing alkalosis and tetany (Morriss, 1984). |
| f. Neurologic disorders. | Fever increases intracranial pressure, metabolic and oxygen requirements of the brain thus aggravating existing neurologic deficits (Burstin, 1985). |
| g. Prematurity. | Premature infants younger than 32 weeks gestation are at particular risk when overheated since they are unable to sweat and dissipate heat. Hyperthermia may result in apnea. |
| h. Cystic fibrosis, ectodermal dysplasia, familial dysautonomia, and fluid deprivation. | Children with these conditions are predisposed to heat stroke (decreased heat dissipation caused by high ambient temperature) (Burstin, 1985). |
| 4. Observe for signs of dehydration (see Skill 64). | Dehydration is a frequent result of an elevated temperature because of excessive fluid losses via skin and lungs. Insensible fluid losses increase by 10% for every 1° C increase in temperature (Morriss, 1984). |
| 5. Assess family's knowledge and concerns about elevated temperatures. | Family beliefs and concerns will clarify their perspective to guide teaching and collaborative efforts.<br>***Special Considerations:*** *See the box on the following page for further information.* |

## Planning and Goal Setting

| Steps | Rationale |
|---|---|
| 1. Gather equipment:<br>a. Temperature measuring device, e.g., glass thermometer, electronic thermometer. | |
| *Environmental cooling:*<br>a. Fan with protective cage surrounding blades. | Protective cage is necessary for safety reasons. |
| *Sponge bath:*<br>a. Basin.<br>b. 5 washcloths.<br>c. 3 towels.<br>d. Bath blanket. | |
| *Hypothermia blanket:*<br>a. Hypothermia control unit.<br>b. Hypothermia coiled blanket.<br>c. Fluid for control unit.<br>d. 12 towels (3 for each extremity).<br>e. Adhesive tape.<br>f. Bath blanket. | |
| *Antipyretics:*<br>a. Acetaminophen, aspirin or ibuprofen as ordered. | Aspirin and acetaminophen are the preferred drugs for fever management (Table 84-1).<br>***Special Considerations:*** *Aspirin should not be given to children with chickenpox or flu symptoms because of the reported association with Reye syndrome (Fruthaler, 1985; Hurwitz et al, 1985). Ibuprofen is not recommended for children under 12 years of age (Whaley and Wong, 1991).* |

## *PARENTAL KNOWLEDGE AND TREATMENT OF FEVER*

Kilmon (1987) reported a descriptive study using a convenience sample of 100 parents of children aged 2 months to 5 years 10 months. The purpose of the study was to obtain information about parental knowledge and practices related to treatment of their children's fevers. Results included: 21% to 32% of the parents treated their children for fever when the children's body temperatures were actually within the normal range; 99% indicated the use of antipyretic medications. Of these, only 35.7% gave the correct dose; 38.7% gave a dose that was too low (from 10% to 75% of the correct dose); 12.2% gave a dose that was too high by 133% to 200%. When asked where they sought information about the correct dosage, 72.2% said they relied on the product package, 14.4% named a health care provider, 6.2% relied on a relative or friend, and 7.2% said they knew from "experience." Half of the parents indicated that they sponged their child for a fever. Only 18% of these parents used tepid water; 36% used potentially toxic alcohol or an alcohol/water mixture, 36% used cold water, and 10% did not specify what they used.

The implications for nurses are many. Parents need guidance and instruction in the proper home management of fever. Of utmost importance is teaching when to treat a fever, the proper medication dosage, and the proper solution and indications for sponging a child. Nurses can easily accomplish this task in both hospitals and well-child clinics, especially during immunization visits.

***TABLE 84-1*** Recommended Dosages of Acetaminophen for Each Age/Weight Child*

| Age | 3 Mo | 4-11 Mo | 12-23 Mo | 2-3 Yr | 4-5 Yr | 6-8 Yr | 9-10 Yr | 11-12 Yr |
|---|---|---|---|---|---|---|---|---|
| Weight (lb) | | 12-17 | 18-23 | 24-35 | 36-45 | 44-64 | 66-76 | 77 |
| Dose (mg) | | 80 | 120 | 160 | 240 | 320 | 400 | 480 |
| **TYPE OF MEDICINE** | | | | | | | | |
| *Liquids* | | | | | | | | |
| Drops (1 dropper = 80 mg/0.8 ml) | | 1 | 1½ | 2 | 3 | 4 | 5 | |
| Elixir/syrup 160 mg/5 ml (1 tsp) | | ½ tsp | ¾ tsp | 1 tsp | 1½ tsp | 2 tsp | 2½ tsp | 3 tsp |
| *Tablets* | | | | | | | | |
| Chewable tablets (80 mg/tablet) | | | 1½ | 2 | 3 | 4 | 5 | 6 |
| Swallowable tablets (160 mg/tablet) | | | | | | 2 | 2½ | 3 |

Acetaminophen brand names:

| Liquids | Tablets |
|---|---|
| Panadol | Chewable Anacin 3 |
| Tylenol | Chewable Tylenol |
| Tempra | St. Joseph Aspirin Free Chewable |
| | Junior Strength Tylenol |

*Give the dose that is recommended for the child's weight if his weight is higher or lower than the weight listed for his age.
Modified from Whaley L and Wong D: Clinical manual of pediatric nursing, ed 3, 1990, St Louis, The CV Mosby Co.

| Steps | Rationale |
|---|---|
| 2. Develop individualized child and family goals:<br>▪ Discomfort will be minimized.<br>▪ Child will be adequately hydrated.<br>▪ Skin integrity will remain intact.<br>▪ Family will demonstrate an understanding of fever and recommended treatment.<br>▪ Family anxiety will be reduced. | |
| **Implementation** 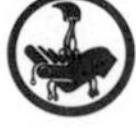 | |
| 1. Explain procedure to child and family (see Skill 1). | |
| 2. Monitor temperature and treat as indicated (see Skill 30). | Treatment is dependent on the underlying cause of the temperature elevation and the degree of risk to the child.<br>***Special Considerations:*** *Treatment may consist of environmental measures, antipyretics, or both.* |
| 3. Maintain a neutral thermal environment for neonates (see Skill 83). | Neutral thermal environment enables a neonate's body temperature to remain normal with minimal metabolic effort and therefore, minimal oxygen consumption (Merenstein, Gardner, and Blake, 1989). |

| Steps | Rationale |
|---|---|
| ***Hyperthermia (environmental) measures*** | |
| 1. Eliminate external heat sources. | By removing external heat sources the body is able to release heat and lower its temperature. |
| a. Expose skin to air, removing blankets or excess clothing. | A common cause of hyperthermia is overdressing infants and young children. |
| b. Reduce environmental temperature. | ***Special Considerations:*** *Infants in servocontrolled heating devices must be carefully monitored for accidental dislodgement of skin probe, which can cause a sudden increase in the device's heat production. Infants left in locked cars for short periods of time in the summer may suffer heat stroke. The associated mortality in children younger than 1 year of age is very high (Burstin, 1985).* |
| 2. Increase air circulation by providing child with a fanning device directed over child's body surface, opening windows, etc. | Increased air movement increases convective heat loss. Infants and young children have a large surface area-to-volume ratio and thus lose more heat to the environment through convection and evaporation than adults (Hazinski, 1984). |
| 3. Immerse or sponge child with tepid water. | Tepid water on the skin helps reduce core temperature. Cooled blood from the skin surface is conducted to inner organs and tissues and warm blood is circulated to the skin surface to be cooled and recirculated. Surface blood vessels dilate as the body attempts to dissipate heat to the environment and facilitate the cooling process (Whaley and Wong, 1991). ***Special Considerations:*** *Sponging is beneficial only with elevated temperatures resulting from hyperthermia in which the physical removal of heat is required, e.g., high environmental temperature or a child's inability to perspire (Newman, 1985).* |
| a. Fill basin or tub with water 1° to 2°F lower than body temperature. | Tepid water lowers the temperature gradually to avoid triggering heat producing mechanisms (e.g., shivering) caused by rapid cooling. ***Special Considerations:*** *Do not use ice water, vigorous sponging, or alcohol to lower body temperature. These cause rapid cooling and chilling, elevating the temperature even further due to shivering. Alcohol sponging may cause peripheral vasoconstriction and CNS depression secondary to inhaling alcohol fumes (Morriss, 1984).* |
| b. Remove gown from child while keeping covered with bath blanket or sheet. | A light sheet or bath blanket preserves modesty and prevents chilling. |
| c. Using washcloths and towels soaked in tepid water, gently sponge child for 20 to 30 minutes unless shivering or chilling occurs, at which time sponging should stop immediately. | ***Special Considerations:*** *A floating toy or other water toys can provide distraction during the bath. Never leave child unattended in the tub.* |
| d. Pat skin dry and dress child in lightweight gown, allowing child to rest. Repeat vital sign measurements 30 minutes after completion. | |
| 4. Use a cooling (hypothermia) blanket with servocontrol or manual control set between 32° and 35° C (Morriss, 1984). | A child at high risk of vital organ compromise may benefit by the use of a cooling blanket. ***Special Considerations:*** *Major concerns in the use of a hypothermia blanket are shivering, frostbite, and skin breakdown.* |
| a. Prepare unit and set parameters according to manufacturer's instructions and physician's orders. | Unit operation may vary. |
| b. Wrap 3 towels around each arm from the elbow to beyond the hands. Fold up the ends of the towels, forming a large mitten, and wrap tape loosely around the towels on the arm. Repeat the procedure with the legs. | Wrapping prevents shivering, which increases cell metabolism and body temperature and counters the purpose of the intervention. The tape is applied loosely to avoid obstructing circulation. ***Special Considerations:*** *Avoid use of pins because accidental puncture of blanket can result in fluid leakage from the coils or cables.* |
| c. Place an absorbent sheet or blanket between skin and cooling blanket. Check bath blanket, gown, or sheet frequently and change when wet. | Keeping child completely dry prevents frostbite. Dampness conducts cold. Frostbite welts may occur if any form of dampness (e.g., perspiration, antiseptic ointments, Vaseline, urine) gets between the skin and the cooling blanket. Freezing can occur if moisture accumulates on cooling blanket. |

| Steps | Rationale |
|---|---|
| d. Remove any kinks or folds in the cooling blanket or bath blanket. | Kinks or folds can cause uneven circulation of fluid in the cooling blanket, causing hot and cold spots. |
| e. Observe for signs of frostbite welts (see Skill 83). | Rapid cooling may cause frostbite. |
| f. Pad bony prominences and avoid use of gowns with metal snaps/closures. | Bony prominences and metal closures are potential sites of increased pressure. Metal snaps and closures may also conduct heat or cold to the skin. |
| g. Gently reposition child every hour. Avoid shearing forces on the skin (Jones, 1984). | Repositioning prevents skin breakdown. Vasoconstriction caused by cooling process decreases circulation to the skin, increasing the risk of skin breakdown. |
| h. Monitor vital signs, neurologic status, skin color, and capillary refill every 15 minutes until desired body temperature is reached and stabilized; every 1 hour thereafter (Persons, 1987). | Lowering body temperature can result in depression of vital functions. |
| ***Fever reduction measures*** | |
| 1. If fever is a response to infectious agent:<br>a. If child is not high risk and with physician's order, do not treat except for comfort. Keep child lightly covered based on child's preference. | Fevers caused by infectious agents are physiologically beneficial because of the chemical changes they produce that inhibit microbial survival. Fever patterns may provide diagnostic information and are an excellent indicator of how the child is responding to antibiotic therapy (Griffin, 1986). |
| b. If child is high risk, uncomfortable, or if the physician orders, give antipyretic drug and/or use environmental measures. | More aggressive therapy is needed if child has existing risk factors. Antipyretics lower the hypothalamic setpoint thus lowering heat production.<br>***Special Considerations:*** *Antipyretics have not been shown to reduce the risk of febrile seizures (Ellenburg et al, 1986; Consensus Statement, 1980). Sponging may temporarily lower the body temperature but does not lower the setpoint. Sponging as a mode of temperature reduction when elevation is in response to an infectious process does not lower the temperature significantly nor contribute to the child's comfort (Newman, 1985).* |
| ***General measures*** | |
| 1. Provide adequate hydration intravenously or orally as per order. Measure strict intake and output (see Skill 64). | Hydration is necessary to replace fluid loss that occurs with an elevated temperature.<br>***Special Considerations:*** *Radiant warmers greatly increase an infant's insensible water loss. This loss must be considered when calculating fluid requirements.* |
| 2. Promote rest periods during which the child is not disturbed by visitors or interventions. | Rest periods reduce energy expenditure thereby reducing stress on vital body organs during febrile periods. |
| 3. Discuss common myths and basic pathophysiology of elevated temperatures with the child and family, focusing on the type that child has. Allow time for questions and verbalization of concerns. | Understanding the purposes of treatments for temperature elevation helps allay fears, increases cooperation, and fosters trust. |

| Evaluation Outcomes | Observational Guidelines |
|---|---|
| 1. Child's discomfort is minimized. | Ask child how he or she feels. Observe muscle tension, especially in the face. Observe degree of playfulness when appropriate toys are provided. Observe child's response to fatigue. During sleep, note body movements, muscle tension, and duration of sleep. |
| 2. Child is adequately hydrated. | Observe for signs of adequate fluid balance, e.g., brisk capillary refill, adequate urine output, good skin turgor. |
| 3. Skin integrity remains intact. | Inspect skin areas actively involved in cooling process for redness, frostbite welts, abraded or open areas. |
| 4. Family demonstrates understanding of etiology of elevated temperature if known. | Ask family to describe the cause of child's temperature elevation and the body mechanisms involved. |
| 5. The family experiences minimal anxiety. | Observe the family's ability to talk easily and openly, and to maintain eye contact. |
| 6. The family is supportive and compliant with treatment measures. | Ask the family if they agree to the recommended treatment of elevated temperature. Observe their nonverbal agreement or disagreement by how they assist and support in the care given to their child. |

## Documentation

Document vital signs, sensorium, appearance of comfort or discomfort, hydration status, skin integrity, anxiety behaviors in family before and after teaching, presence or absence of chills/shivering, presence or absence of sweating, measures taken to decrease temperature and effectiveness of measures.

## Home Care Modifications

1. Instruct families not to overdress their infant or child in hot weather or leave infant/child in locked car. This may lead to hyperthermia, dehydration, and possibly death.
2. Instruct parents on guidelines for when to seek professional health care for child with fever as well as safe and effective measures to reduce fever (Whaley and Wong, 1991).
3. Instruct parents on how to take a child's temperature and read the thermometer accurately. Review normal measurements with them (see Skill 30).
4. Parents should understand the choices for antipyretics, know to avoid aspirin for chickenpox or other viral illness, the proper time intervals between doses, the proper dose (see Table 84-1), and the most accurate method of measurement. Determine the type of antipyretic being used in the home before discussing dosages.
5. Teach indications for a sponge bath. Caution against the use of ice or alcohol.

UNIT XII

**PRODUCT REFERENCES AND TEACHING RESOURCES**
**Books**

Wong DL and Whaley LF: Clinical manual of pediatric nursing, ed 3, St Louis, 1990, The CV Mosby Co.
Home care instructions: Measuring your child's temperature; Giving medications to children.

**REFERENCES**

American Academy of Pediatrics and American College of Obstetricians and Gynecologists: Guidelines for perinatal care, ed 2, Evanston, Ill, 1988, American Academy of Pediatrics and American College of Obstetricians and Gynecologists.

Boswick JA, Martyn JW, and Schultz AL: Hypothermia: not just a winter problem, Patient Care 20(18):84-116, 1986.

Burstin H: Temperature regulation. In Zimmerman S and Gildea J, editors: Critical care pediatrics, Philadelphia, 1985, WB Saunders Co.

Consensus statement: Febrile seizures: long-term management of children with fever-associated seizures, Pediatrics 66(6):1009-1012, 1980.

Cunha B et al: Implications of fever in the critical care setting, Heart and Lung 13(5):460-465, 1984.

Dunne KP and Matthews TG: Hypothermia and sudden infant death syndrome, Arch Dis Child 63:438-440, 1988.

Ellenberg J, Hirtz D, and Nelson K: Do seizures in children cause intellectual deterioration? New Engl J Med 314(17):1085-1088, 1986.

Feldman KW, Morray JP, and Schaller RT: Thermal injury caused by hot pack application in hypothermic children, Am J Emerg Med 3(1):38-41, 1985.

Fruthaler G: Fever in children: phobia vs facts, Hospital Practice 20(11A):49-53, 1985.

Griffin J: Fever: when to leave it alone, Nursing 16(2):58-61, 1986.

Gurevich I: Fever: when to worry about it, RN, 48:14-17, 1985.

Hagedorn MI, Gardner SL, and Abman SH: Respiratory diseases. In Merenstein GB and Gardner SL, editors: Handbook of neonatal intensive care, ed 2, St Louis, 1989, The CV Mosby Co.

Hazinski MF: Nursing care of the critically ill child, St Louis, 1984, The CV Mosby Co.

Hurwitz E et al: Public health service study on Reye's syndrome and medications, N Engl J Med, 313(14):849-857, 1985.

Jones S: The use and misuse of hypothermia blankets, RN 47:55, 1984.

Kaplan M and Eidelman AI: Improved prognosis in severely hypothermic newborn infants treated by rapid rewarming, J Pediatr 105(3):470-474, 1984.

Kilmon C: Parents' knowledge and practices related to fever management, J Pediatr Health Care, 1(4):173-179, 1987.

Klaus MH and Fanaroff AA: Care of the high-risk neonate, ed 3, Philadelphia, 1986, WB Saunders Co.

Lloyd EL: Hypothermia and cold stress, Rockville, Md, 1986, Aspen Systems Corp.

Merenstein GB, Gardner SL, and Blake WW: Heat balance. In Merenstein GB and Gardner SL, editors: Handbook of neonatal intensive care, ed 2, St Louis, 1989, The CV Mosby Co.

Morriss F: Abnormalities in temperature regulation. In Levin D, Morriss F, and Moore G, editors: A practical guide to pediatric intensive care, St Louis, 1984, The CV Mosby Co.

Newman J: Evaluation of sponging to reduce body temperature in febrile children, Can Med Assoc J 132:641-642, 1985.

Persons C: Critical care procedures and protocols: a nursing process approach, Philadelphia, 1987, JB Lippincott Co.

Reeves-Swift R: Rational management of a child's acute fever, MCN 15(2):82-85, 1990.

Robinson M and Seward PN: Environmental hypothermia in children, Pediatr Emerg Care 2(4):254-257, 1986.

Sofer S et al: Improved outcome of hypothermic infants, Pediatr Emerg Care 2(4):211-214, 1986

Sivaloganathan S: Paradoxical undressing and hypothermia, Med Sci Law 26(3):225-229, 1986.

Whaley LF and Wong DL: Nursing care of infants and children, ed 4, St Louis, 1991, The CV Mosby Co.

Wilkerson JA, Bangs CC, and Hayward JS, editors: Hypothermia, frostbite and other cold injuries, Seattle, 1986, The Mountaineers.

# UNIT XIII Neurologic Management

# SKILL 85 Implementing Seizure Precautions

*Pamela K. Christensen and Deborah S. Lammert*

Children with seizure disorders may have a sudden loss of consciousness, loss of muscle tone, or forceful muscle contractions accompanying the seizure that may cause injury to themselves. A child who is known to have convulsive episodes or who is under observation for seizures requires special precautions. The extent of these measures depends on the type and frequency of the seizure (Whaley and Wong, 1991). Promoting the safety of the child is the primary goal of nursing care.

## NURSING DIAGNOSES

Potential for ineffective airway clearance related to tonic-clonic activity of facial and mandible muscles; Potential for aspiration related to pooling of oral secretions and inability to control gastric secretions; Potential for injury (tissue) related to tonic-clonic movements of extremities or hypoxia due to tonic-clonic activity of thoracic muscles; Anxiety related to unmet informational needs about seizure disorders and required safety precautions.

| Steps | Rationale |
|---|---|
| **Assessment** | |
| 1. Review child's current health and neurologic status including:<br>a. Level of consciousness.<br>b. Motor functioning.<br>c. Cerebellar functioning.<br>d. Behavior. | Knowledge of the child's current status including functioning abilities is essential in establishing baseline data. Also, the child may have other related or unrelated conditions that would have implications (e.g., febrile status or diabetes). |
| 2. Assess child's developmental level:<br>a. Mental age.<br>b. Chronologic age.<br>c. Ability to cooperate with procedure. | The child may have neurologic deficits affecting his or her mental age and ability to cooperate with procedures. |
| 3. Assess history for previous seizure activity or potential risk factors:<br>a. Previous type, intensity, progression, duration, "triggering factors," preconvulsive warning signs, and medications.<br>b. Potential: recent head injury (cerebral edema, hemorrhage); central nervous system infections (intracranial, meningeal); metabolic alterations; space occupying lesions (cysts, tumors); anoxia; toxins (drugs, bacterial, lead); febrile; omitted doses of anticonvulsants; post-neurosurgical status. | Information concerning previous history has implications for interventions. The implementation of safety measures as a precautionary activity will enhance the promptness and appropriateness of treatment for the child should a seizure occur. Some seizure types present minimal risk for injury that should also be reflected in care planning.<br>***Special Considerations:*** *Preconvulsive warning signs may include visual auras of varying colors or shades, auditory changes such as "ringing in the ear" or sounds becoming more distant or muffled, and vision changes such as blurring or diplopia. Triggering factors may include fatigue, pain, specific photo stimuli (e.g., rapid and rhythmically flickering lights or images; direct, bright light) (Hazinski, 1984) emotional stress, and loud or buzzing noises.* |

| Steps | Rationale |
|---|---|
| 4. Assess safety of environmental conditions:<br>a. Bed or crib with side rails.<br>b. Floor covering.<br>c. Toys.<br>d. Furniture arrangement.<br>e. Physical space. | Certain aspects in the environment may need to be changed to prevent injury from a seizure. |
| 5. Assess the child's and family's level of anxiety and understanding concerning child's disorder and its ramifications. | Seizure disorders generate a high level of anxiety in family members, which interferes with understanding and compliance. Determining present level of understanding and meaning of disorder provides a baseline for effective teaching and initiating supportive measures.<br>***Special Considerations:*** *Seizures can elicit feelings of fear, misunderstanding, and helplessness in the child, family, and in health professionals unfamiliar with seizure disorders (Mott, Fazekas, and James, 1985).* |

## Planning and Goal Setting

| Steps | Rationale |
|---|---|
| 1. Gather supplies: | Gathering supplies promotes efficiency in the health care setting.<br>***Special Considerations:*** *The need for airway, suction and oxygen equipment at the bedside depends on the frequency and severity of the child's seizures. Because of additional cost and/or potential anxiety, equipment need only be readily accessible unless a bedside need is determined. Collaborate with the practitioner and/or follow facility protocol.* |
| a. Appropriate size airway. | Protection of airway by artificial means may be required during seizure activity.<br>***Special Considerations:*** *The use of a bite block or padded tongue blade is controversial. If one is used, it should never be forcefully placed because it may injure the teeth. With a generalized seizure and the onset of the first major muscle contraction, the child will clench teeth and bite the tongue. Thereafter, the placement of a solid object into the child's mouth is pointless and may cause aspiration of broken teeth (Friedman, 1988).* |
| b. Oropharyngeal suction equipment. | Child may require suctioning of oropharynx during or after seizure activity due to pooling of secretions and/or inability to control oral secretions. Emesis may also occur. Removal of these materials by suctioning may help to prevent pulmonary aspiration. |
| c. Oxygen apparatus, source and face mask. | Oxygen will be readily available for administration if needed for respiratory impairment during severe or prolonged seizure activity. |
| d. Waterproof mattress or sheet. | Child may be incontinent during a seizure. |
| e. Padding for bedrails.<br>▪ Bath towels.<br>▪ Bath blankets.<br>▪ Commercial pads. | Rail padding protects the child from striking any body part on a hard or pointed surface.<br>***Special Considerations:*** *There are commercially available pads for bedrails.* |
| f. Sign at bedside stating "seizure precautions" (optional). | Communication with other staff members alerts them to the potential for seizure activity and indicates the need for precautionary measures.<br>***Special Considerations:*** *Posting a sign at the bedside may be embarrassing to the child, affecting self-image. The potential harm of a sign must be weighed against the benefit. Institutional policy may dictate whether such a sign must be posted.* |
| 2. Arrange for a room/bed with adequate visualization for caregivers. | Observation of seizure activity and prompt intervention promotes safety for the child experiencing a seizure. |
| 3. Develop individualized nursing goals of care:<br>▪ To prevent injury and promote safety in the event of a seizure.<br>▪ To reduce the risk of seizure activity occurring.<br>▪ To increase child's and family's understanding of seizure disorder and reduce anxiety related to same. | |

| **Steps** | **Rationale** |
|---|---|
| **Implementation** | |
| 1. Explain the precautions to the child and family. Address any concerns they may express. | Explanations and instructions to the child and family increase their knowledge base and enhance compliance with the required precautions. |
| 2. Place airway at head of bed or in a readily accessible location. | The oral airway needs to be readily available should the child's airway become compromised. The oral airway should be out of the reach of the child. |
| 3. Assemble suction and oxygen equipment and verify functioning. Keep in readily accessible location (see Special Considerations, Planning and Goal Setting step 1, p. 538.) | During a seizure, oral secretions or blood from mouth may need to be suctioned to prevent aspiration. Oxygen administration is indicated when respiratory effort is difficult or impaired in any way. |
| 4. Prepare bed:<br>a. Use a waterproof mattress or pad in linen change. | The bed should be protected from an incontinent episode that may occur during or following a seizure.<br>***Special Considerations:*** *A waterproof pad may be a potential source of embarrassment to the older child.* |
| b. Adjust siderails to full upright position when child is in bed. | Keeping siderails up prevents injury that may occur if a child would fall from bed during a seizure. |
| c. Keep bed in low position. | A bed in low position reduces the risk of injury should a child fall from the bed during a seizure. |
| d. Pad bed/cribrails and headboard with several thicknesses of folded bath blankets, or use special foam siderail pads. Secure to rails so that all hard surfaces or pointed edges are covered. | Strong muscle contractions may cause the child to jerk causing injury from striking the bedrails. |
| 5. Post "seizure precautions" sign at bedside if indicated. | (See Special Considerations, Planning and Goal Setting step 1f, p. 538.) |
| 6. Establish a safe physical environment (see Skill 49). | Establishing a physically safe environment reduces risk of injury during seizure activity. |
| a. Remove sharp objects, blunt toys, and other solid items from the bed or crib during periods when the child is unsupervised. | Removing objects when unsupervised protects the child from injury caused by involuntary striking of a hard object during a seizure. |
| b. Avoid use of oral glass thermometers. | If the child has a generalized seizure during temperature measurement, forceful teeth clenching would break the glass, possibly injuring the child. |
| c. Remove excess furniture, keeping the floor arrangement open. | During a generalized seizure, the child may fall to the floor. |
| d. Ensure that the child is wearing nonrestrictive clothing. | Nonrestrictive clothing prevents restriction of respirations by tight clothing or banding of cloth items during the uncontrolled movements characteristic of a seizure. |
| e. Restrict from shower bathing if indicated by assessment information. For a tub bath, pad the tub with towels or a bath blanket, and remain in constant attendance. | Injury from a fall during seizure activity while in the shower could occur.<br>***Special Considerations:*** *Review assessment information, collaborate with practitioner, and/or refer to institutional policy to determine safety of allowing showering.* |
| 7. Reduce environmental triggering factors if an assessed problem in this child. | A child with a seizure disorder may be photosensitive and require dim lights. Bright, direct blinking lights, and video games can precipitate seizures in some children (Dahlquist, Mellinger, and Klass, 1983). |
| 8. Explain to child and family how to summon assistance from nursing staff. Demonstrate use of call light, and instruct in the need to call for supervision and assistance if child must be out of bed or crib. | Child/family may alert nursing staff to impending or actual seizure activity allowing prompt observation and interventions. Seizure precautions and supervision must be continued when the child is out of the protected bed or crib. |
| 9. Administer routine and nonroutine prescribed doses of anticonvulsant medications. Observe for effects and side effects. Monitor serum levels of medication and assist in maintaining therapeutic blood levels (see Unit XVI). | The maintenance of therapeutic blood levels of anticonvulsant medications creates an elevated seizure threshold and decreases the likelihood of seizure activity. A child's reactions and tolerance to anticonvulsant medications provides data regarding the effectiveness of the specific medication for the particular child. |
| 10. Implement additional safety measures for children with frequent grand mal seizures or poorly controlled seizure disorders:<br>a. When ambulatory, use a soft protective helmet.<br>b. Observe closely at mealtime.<br>c. When in wheelchair or chair, secure child with soft safety straps or sheets around the trunk and hip areas. | Providing safety measures for the child allows an appropriate activity level otherwise not possible. |

| Evaluation Outcomes | Observational Guidelines |
|---|---|
| 1. The child remains free of injury and preventable complications of seizure activity. | Observe for any injury or complications following seizure activity, e.g. breaks in skin integrity, swelling of soft tissue, improper alignment or decreased movement of an extremity, complaint of pain or headache not present before seizure, aspiration of secretions, emesis, or gastric contents. |
| 2. The child exhibits a reduction in or absence of seizure activity. | Observe frequency of seizure activity. Observe child's responses to environmental stimuli and medications. |
| 3. Child and family demonstrate an increase in understanding and a decrease in anxiety regarding seizure disorder and precautions taken. | Ask child/family to verbalize their understanding of the purpose of seizure precautions. Observe family's ability to correctly demonstrate the initiation/maintenance of seizure precautions during the child's hospitalization. Ask family to verbalize their feelings and concerns. |

## Documentation

Record indicators that place the child at high risk for seizure activity. Document the baseline neurologic assessment of the child. Note the institution and maintenance of precautionary measures, (e.g., padded siderails, oral airway at bedside, etc.). Document any seizure activity or pre-seizure activity noted, the child's postictal state, anticonvulsants administered and child's responses to medication. Record any child/parent teaching of seizure precautions during hospitalization and post-discharge. Note content taught, ability to verbalize information and/or demonstrate skill, written information given to parents. Identify any problems or abnormalities and actions taken to modify or correct the problems.

## Child and Family Teaching

1. Explain to the family the effects and side effects of prescribed anticonvulsant medications. Emphasize the importance of regular dosing and accurate measurements as well as follow-up medical visits and serum determinations of anticonvulsant medications for optimal therapeutic effects. Provide the child's primary caregiver at home with a written copy of medication generic and trade names, dosages, times of administration, and side effects. Provide written copy of schedule for follow-up outpatient visits.
2. Instruct family members and visitors in appropriate actions during a seizure, such as remaining with the child and turning the child to the side to prevent aspiration. Warn them *not* to attempt to insert an object into the child's mouth during a seizure.

## Home Care Modifications

1. Lightweight protective helmet or faceguard may be appropriate to prevent head and facial injuries for children with daily seizures. Siderails may be required at home for night-time safety of child. Provide family with information of stores carrying these items, such as baby/child furniture stores for siderails and bicycle shops for soft, fitted helmet.
2. The child should carry a card or wear a Medic Alert bracelet with pertinent information about his or her condition.
3. The child should have a regular schedule to avoid excess stress and fatigue that can precipitate seizure activity.
4. The child with daily or frequent seizures should avoid engaging in activities in which he or she might be injured, such as climbing, swimming or handling sharp objects (Whaley and Wong, 1991).
5. The child who has infrequent seizures or who is relatively free of seizures should have few restrictions on activities. Normal healthy activities are encouraged, and participation in competitive sports is determined on an individual basis. Contact sports such as football, karate, or wrestling should be avoided. Basketball, baseball, and tennis are preferable (Whaley and Wong, 1991).
6. The well-controlled epileptic child can ride a bicycle or swim when accompanied by a companion.
7. Inform teachers and school nurses of child's condition and therapy so that they can assist in ensuring regular dosing of medication and any special care child might need.

# SKILL 86 Assisting with Ventricular Puncture or Shunt Tap and Maintaining a Ventriculostomy

*Mary C. Baron*

A ventricular puncture is a procedure performed by a physician for a variety of indications, but most commonly to drain off excess cerebrospinal fluid that may be causing increased intracranial pressure. In children, this procedure is often associated with hydrocephalus. The circumstances under which the procedure is performed may be life-threatening, diagnostic, or palliative prior to surgery. Ventriculostomy drainage is a temporary measure and is used in conjunction with other methods of treatment.

Either a needle with a stylet or a catheter with a stylet is introduced through the scalp or burr hole into the anterior horn of the lateral ventricle in the nondominant hemisphere. In infants, if the anterior fontanel or coronal suture is sufficiently open (up to 15 months of age), the puncture may be performed through these routes. In older children, a trephine opening (burr hole) is necessary.

When a catheter is used, (i.e., for ventriculostomy), it is sutured into place and connected to a drainage system, leveled by the neurosurgeon. This procedure is usually done in a treatment room and requires skillful restraint of the child. The complications that can result from the procedure include infection and trauma to the brain tissue or blood vessels along the course of the needle.

Sometimes it is necessary after the acute phase to internalize the system to a ventriculoperitoneal shunt. If the child is unable to effectively circulate cerebrospinal fluid due to damage from trauma, tumor, or congenital conditions, the shunt provides primary drainage of cerebrospinal fluid from the ventricles to an extracranial location, usually the peritoneum. The shunt system is usually a permanent device and requires revisions as the child grows or complications occur (see Child and Family Teaching section). Shunt systems consist of a ventricular catheter, a reservoir, a unidirectional flow valve, and a distal catheter.

## NURSING DIAGNOSES

Anxiety related to perceived threat to body integrity or unmet informational needs about ventricular procedure; Potential fluid volume deficit related to loss of cerebrospinal fluid through indwelling ventricular catheter; Potential for infection related to presence of ventricular catheter; Potential for injury related to inadequate restraint while ventriculostomy in place.

| Steps | Rationale |
|---|---|
| **Assessment** | |
| 1. Assess child's neurologic and vital sign status, especially:<br>a. Response to voice.<br>b. Ability to follow commands.<br>c. Response to painful stimuli.<br>d. Respirations, pulse, blood pressure, and temperature.<br>e. Pupillary response to light.<br>f. Lethargy/irritability. | The child's neurologic and vital sign status prior to the procedure will determine the urgency of performing the procedure and will provide a baseline for post procedure neurologic assessment.<br>***Special Considerations:*** *A slow, irregular heart rate and widened pulse pressure indicate an elevation of intracranial pressure.* |
| 2. Determine child's age and development level. | Age and developmental level determine the child's ability to understand and cooperate with the procedure. |
| 3. Determine indications for ventriculostomy placement/shunt tap (e.g., diagnostic as with malfunction; palliative or life-threatening as with increased intracranial pressure due to trauma, tumor, bleeding, acute hydrocephalus, or cerebral edema). | The reason for the tap influences how quickly it must be performed, as well as whether tubing will be connected for continuous or intermittent drainage. |
| 4. Review physician's orders and chart for the following information: | Continuous versus intermittent drainage is usually determined by the physician. Informed consent is necessary because of the invasive nature of the procedure. |

| Steps | Rationale |
|---|---|
| a. If ventricular drainage is to be maintained following puncture.<br>b. Presence of signed consent form, if required by the facility (see Skill 8). | ***Special Considerations:*** *If drainage is to be intermittent, an intracranial pressure monitoring device must be utilized with specific parameters set up for fluid drainage. In many cases of increased intracranial pressure (especially acute rather than chronic), unless the child can be taken to surgery immediately for intervention, drainage will be maintained.* |
| 5. Review medical history for related factors such as seizures, head injury, shunt malfunction, and symptoms. | The child's medical history will provide important information as to predisposing factors and events that led to the illness or injury.<br>***Special Considerations:*** *In the case of trauma, it is important to note if the child had any loss of consciousness or seizure activity.* |
| 6. Assess child's/family's understanding of procedure, rationale, and potential complications. | The family's and child's understanding of the procedure and its ramifications influences their compliance with the procedure. |

## Planning and Goal Setting

| Steps | Rationale |
|---|---|
| 1. Prepare the child and family for the procedure (see Skill 1). | Preparing the child and family for the procedure reduces fear and anxiety and enhances feelings of control and trust.<br>***Special Considerations:*** *The family and child (depending on developmental level) should be informed that the procedure does not damage brain tissue and that restraint may be necessary for the child's safety.* |
| 2. Recruit assistant(s) for restraining, if necessary. | Adequate staff to securely restrain the child and to assist the physician is needed to maintain strict asepsis and to ensure safe performance of procedure.<br>***Special Considerations:*** *The family should not be recruited to restrain for painful procedures because this may damage the trust relationship with their child.* |
| 3. Implement seizure precautions if assessment data indicates this is warranted (see Skill 85). | Seizures may be precipitated by increases in intracranial pressure or fever. A preexisting seizure disorder is common with some conditions associated with this procedure. |
| 4. Assemble supplies needed, preferably in a treatment room. | Gathering supplies in advance enhances the safety and efficiency of the procedure. A treatment room provides adequate lighting, privacy, and accessibility to the child. It also maintains the hospital bed as a "safe" environment. |
| a. Ventricular puncture and shunt tap:<br>▪ Hair clippers and/or straight-edged razor or safety razor (determine physician preference). | A straight-edged razor is more effective than a safety razor for closeness of shave. However, it is less safe and may produce micronicks that can lead to infection. A straight-edged razor should only be used by someone with high level skill. |
| ▪ Appropriate bactericidal solution. | A strong bactericide decreases contamination of the wound with organisms on the skin.<br>***Special Considerations:*** *Verify that child is not allergic to selected bactericide.* |
| ▪ Alcohol. | Alcohol is used after cleaning with bactericidal solution to enhance visibility of the area as well as remove soap residue. |
| ▪ Sterile gauze 4 × 4's. | Gauze is used for friction in sterile cleaning to remove microorganisms and as a dressing when the procedure is complete. |
| ▪ Sterile drapes. | The area is draped after shaving and prepped to maintain sterility. |
| ▪ Sterile gloves and masks. | Gloves and masks help prevent contamination of the exposed area. |
| ▪ 3 to 5 sterile culture tubes, if the tap is diagnostic. | If diagnostic, cerebrospinal fluid will be analyzed for culture, gram stain, and cell count. |
| ▪ Restraints, if needed. | It is crucial that the child remain still during the procedure to avoid injury. |
| ▪ Manometer. | Manometer may be used to assess intracranial pressure by measuring opening pressure of cerebrospinal fluid. |
| b. Additional items for ventricular puncture:<br>▪ Twist drill if burr hole is necessary. | Twist drill is needed to make an opening into the skull if fontanel and sutures are closed. |

| Steps | Rationale |
|---|---|
| ▪ Scalpel. | Scalpel is used to make a small skin incision before the trephine. |
| ▪ Local anesthetic—1% or 2% xylocaine with sterile syringes and needles for administration. | Xylocaine will anesthetize the scalp over the site. |
| ▪ Catheter with stylet. | ***Special Considerations:*** *A lumbar puncture needle or special ventricular catheter may be used.* |
| ▪ Cotton balls with collodion. | After the catheter is removed, these items are used to seal the puncture site. |
| c. Additional items for shunt tap: | |
| ▪ 23 or 25 gauge butterfly needle. | A small puncture hole will seal easier in the shunt reservoir and a butterfly needle is flexible for easy positioning. |
| ▪ Sterile adhesive bandage. | Because the shunt reservoir is self-sealing, only an adhesive bandage is necessary after the needle is removed. |
| d. Additional items for ventriculostomy/external ventricular drain. Add the following to the above items to convert a shunt tap or ventricular puncture: | Circumstances such as infection or increased intracranial pressure may necessitate an external drainage system. |
| ▪ Suture silk. | Sutures are necessary to hold the needle or catheter in place. |
| ▪ Tape and tincture of benzoin. | Tape and benzoin help secure the dressing around the catheter. ***Special Considerations:*** *Tincture of benzoin has been reported to cause allergic contact dermatitis (James, White, and Yanklowitz, 1984).* |
| ▪ Clear transparent film dressing. | Transparent film allows visualization of the needle in the reservoir at all times. |
| ▪ Sterile drainage system consisting of tubing, collection container, drip chamber and pressure monitoring devices, if desired. | A closed, sterile system prevents infection. |
| ▪ Leveling instrument: usually a meter stick similar to a carpenter's level with a bubble in a glass tube. | The leveling instrument is used to determine the height at which to secure the system. ***Special Considerations:*** *The physician determines the head elevation level.* |
| 5. Use strict aseptic technique in preparing equipment. | Strict asepsis is necessary because brain tissue and cerebrospinal fluid are exposed. Cerebrospinal fluid, because of its glucose content, provides a favorable environment for bacterial growth (Hickey, 1986). ***Special Considerations:*** *Have extra supplies readily available in the event of contamination.* |
| 6. Develop individualized child/family goals: ▪ The child/family will experience minimal pain and anxiety during and after the procedure. ▪ Complications during and following the procedure will be prevented or minimized. | |

## Implementation

***Ventricular puncture or shunt tap***

| Steps | Rationale |
|---|---|
| 1. Administer short-acting sedative, if ordered. | Potent long-acting sedatives may interfere with accurate neurologic assessment. ***Special Considerations:*** *In an emergency situation, there may not be sufficient time to allow a sedative to achieve its full effect. If short-acting sedatives are administered, provide cardiac-respiratory monitoring and/or pulse oximetry and have oxygen, mask, and manual resuscitation bag available in case of respiratory depression.* |
| 2. Apply body restraints if needed with child in supine position (e.g., mummy, papoose, posey) (see Skill 51). | Unless the child is totally unresponsive, even to deep pain, secure restraint is necessary. Insufficient restraint may interfere with the sterility and safety of the procedure. |
| 3. Mask and glove aseptically, and ensure that everyone in the room is adequately prepared. | Masks must be worn by everyone in the room, and gloves by the staff directly involved in the procedure. This decreases the chance of infection. |
| 4. Prep site to be utilized on child's head (or assist physician in doing so): a. Apply restraints. b. Remove hair. c. Cleanse skin with bactericide. d. Cleanse skin with alcohol. e. Dry site with sterile gauze. | Restraints should be applied before preparing the site to prevent contamination of the area or injury to the child. The site is cleansed to decrease the amount of bacteria at the site as much as possible. |

| Steps | Rationale |
|---|---|
| 5. Position self or assistant at child's side, close to the head but not blocking physician's access to site. Apply firm restraint to head by placing hands on either side of head and elbows stabilized on treatment table, while being careful not to apply pressure over ears (Fig. 86-1). Maintain this position throughout procedure, avoiding contamination of the sterile field. | Stability of the head is vital in preventing injury to the scalp or brain tissue from the drill and/or needle that may be caused by sudden movement. **_Special Considerations:_** *If one person must maintain restraint throughout procedure, an additional person will be needed to assist physician.* |
| 6. Assist with the procedure as needed by physician. Additional nursing responsibilities include: a. Frequent assessment of child. b. Comforting child as needed. c. Maintaining asepsis. d. Obtaining and opening new supplies as needed. | The physician's responsibility is performing the procedure as quickly and safely as possible. |
| 7. Dispatch any lab specimens obtained. a. Label specimens accurately. b. Complete necessary requisitions. c. Arrange for transport to lab. | The cerebrospinal fluid specimens should be sent for analysis as soon as possible to obtain valid results. |
| 8. Comfort the child after procedure is completed. | Providing comfort helps the child to reestablish trust. Careful postprocedural monitoring may prevent or minimize complications of infection, increased intracranial pressure, or cerebrospinal fluid leakage. Deteriorating clinical status may indicate improper catheter placement. Gradual as well as sudden changes in level of consciousness can be clinically significant. |
| 9. Monitor child closely (every 15 to 30 minutes) postprocedure until awake and stable, then routinely (every 2 to 4 hours): a. Neurologic assessment. b. Vital signs and skin color. c. Drainage on dressing. d. Cerebrospinal fluid drainage in bag if on continuous drainage. | |
| ***Maintaining ventriculostomy/external ventrlcular drainage*** | |
| 1. Maintain collection container and head elevation level designated by physician (Fig. 86-2). | If the level of the container is too low, cerebrospinal fluid will drain off too quickly, causing subdural bleeding, or even brainstem herniation (Hickey, 1986). However, if the level of the container is too high, lack of drainage will result in increased intracranial pressure, which may also subsequently lead to herniation (Bonta and Blichfeldt, 1984). **_Special Considerations:_** *Neither the level of the child's head nor the container level may be changed without first clamping the system.* |
| 2. Restrain the child as necessary, using jacket, wrist, and elbow restraints (see Skill 51). | The child must be securely restrained to prevent injury caused by changing the level of the head. **_Special Considerations:_** *Often the elbows must be restrained also to prevent the child from pulling out the catheter if he or she slides down in bed.* |

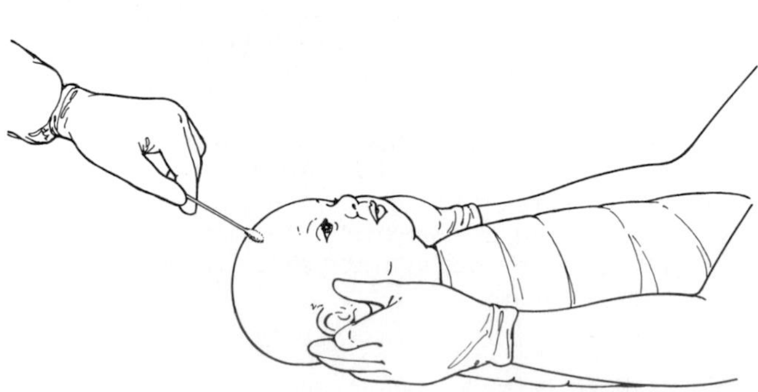

***FIG. 86-1*** Stability of the head is vital throughout the procedure.

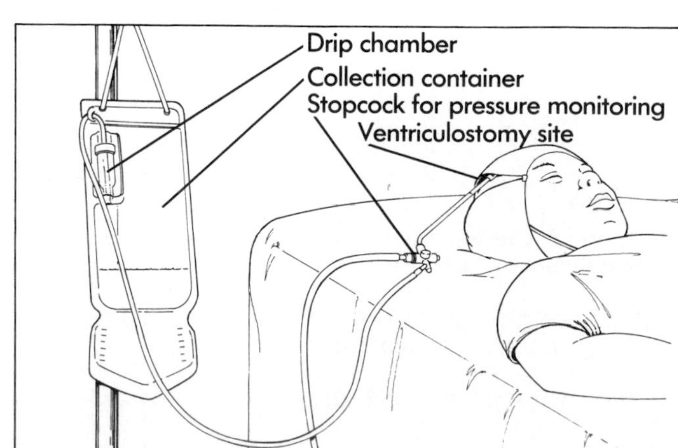


***FIG. 86-2*** Ventriculostomy drainage requires maintenance of proper head elevation and collection container levels.

| Steps | Rationale |
|---|---|
| 3. Provide diversional activities which are appropriate for age (see Skill 15). | Diversional activities enhance the child's compliance with restriction in movement. ***Special Considerations:*** *If possible, have the collection container leveled by physician to a wheelchair or go-cart so the child may be mobile.* |
| 4. Assess dressing frequently for intactness and drainage, reinforcing as necessary. | A wet dressing provides an ideal medium for bacterial growth, which may lead to infection. However, drainage from the catheter site and incision frequently occurs despite careful suturing (Hickey, 1986). ***Special Considerations:*** *Dressing changes to catheter site are usually performed only by a physician.* |
| 5. Observe for fluctuation of cerebrospinal fluid and patency of the system at least every hour. If absent:<br>a. Check tubing for kinks or clamps.<br>b. Notify physician if unable to locate an external source of the problem.<br>c. Perform more frequent neurologic assessments until problem is resolved. | Failure to see fluctuation of cerebrospinal fluid in the drip chamber could indicate that the tubing is kinked or clamped or that the catheter is obstructed. The catheter may become clogged with blood, thick proteinaceous cerebrospinal fluid, or tissue. This heightens risk for increased intracranial pressure. ***Special Considerations:*** *If the tubing becomes disconnected, it should not be reconnected, but clamped close to the catheter. A new system should be connected using aseptic technique after cleaning the old connector site with alcohol. Ideally, the entire system should be changed, including the catheter or needle.* |
| 6. Perform neurologic checks at least every 4 hours, more often if warranted. In children under 2 years of age, measure head circumference daily. | Frequent and accurate neurologic assessment will allow early detection of complications. In a child whose cranial sutures are open, the fontanel may expand before the child becomes symptomatic. |
| 7. Monitor intake and output every shift, as well as serum electrolyte values per physician's order. Record the amount of cerebrospinal fluid drained as part of the child's output totals. | Cerebrospinal fluid contains sodium, so children losing cerebrospinal fluid to external drainage may become hyponatremic. ***Special Considerations:*** *The physician will often order the drainage amount to be partially or fully replaced with intravenous or oral normal saline.* |
| 8. Administer antibiotic therapy and monitor drug levels as ordered. | Intravenous antibiotics are often ordered prophylactically or for identified cases of infection, due to the serious consequences. Peak and trough serum levels of certain antibiotics may be ordered to ensure maximum effectiveness and minimal side effects. |
| 9. Encourage the family to be involved in the child's care as much as possible. | The presence of a ventriculostomy is very intimidating to most families, and reassurance is needed so that they can continue to be involved in their child's care. ***Special Considerations:*** *Holding the child or changing the child's position requires nursing assistance and possibly a physician's order.* |

| Evaluation Outcomes | Observational Guidelines |
|---|---|
| 1. The child is cooperative and exhibits minimal anxiety during and following the procedure. | Observe the child's reactions during the procedure, statements of discomfort, and reactions to staff after the procedure. Also observe the child's willingness to get involved in diversional activities when given the opportunity. Easy distractibility and cooperation with restrictions demonstrates decreased anxiety. |
| 2. The child does not experience complications from increased intracranial pressure. | Observe and assess the child's level of consciousness, head circumference if appropriate, vital signs, and behavioral changes. Determine whether behavioral changes are due to decreased neurologic status or fear and anxiety. Compare to assessment findings. |
| 3. The child is well hydrated and normonatremic. | Observe for signs of dehydration: decreased urine output, high urine specific gravity, dry mucous membranes, and poor skin turgor. Review sodium levels and note replacement when needed. |
| 4. The child remains free from injury from ventriculostomy placement. | Observe child frequently, note secure restraints when utilized. Note family cooperation with restraints. Ventriculostomy remains securely in place for the duration of treatment. |
| 5. The child remains free from infection. | Observe for fever spikes, monitor results of serial cerebrospinal fluid cultures, and note site appearance under dressing. |

## Documentation

Chart procedure, physician performing procedure, date and time performed, and child's toleration of procedure. Note level of system. Record amount and character of cerebrospinal fluid drained during procedure and per shift as well as cumulative 24 hour totals. Document sedatives administered—including amount, route, time given, and child's response. Indicate specimens sent to lab. Note child's neurologic status. Document whether restraint was needed. Provide an hourly record of patency of system. Note any child/family teaching done.

## Child and Family Teaching

When the child has a ventriculoperitoneal shunt:

1. Discuss basic purpose and circulation of cerebrospinal fluid.
2. Explain and draw a diagram of the shunt system.
3. Discuss signs and symptoms of most common complications of shunts:
   a. Infection: Fever (generally, a consistent elevation); headache; redness and/or swelling along shunt tract; nuchal rigidity; nausea/vomiting.
   b. Malfunction/obstruction: Headache; high-pitched cry in infants; vomiting without nausea, often projectile; lethargy; irritability; poor feeding; full, tense fontanel in infants; Sunsetting eyes in infants; eye deviations, visual disturbances, or pupil changes.
4. Instruct family to notify primary health care provider if shunt problems are suspected.
5. Discuss activity restrictions based upon child's age, developmental level, and physician's recommendations.
6. Reassure the family that normal activity will not interfere with the shunt's functioning.

UNIT XIII

## PRODUCT REFERENCES AND TEACHING RESOURCES

### Organizations

Epilepsy Foundation of America
4351 Garden City Drive
Landover, MD 20785
(301) 459-3700

Guardians of Hydrocephalus Reasearch Foundation
2618 Avenue Z
Brooklyn, NY 11235
(718) 743-GHRF
Offers: An Introduction to Hydrocephalus.

## REFERENCES


American Nurses' Association and American Association of Neuroscience Nurses: Neuroscience nursing practice, Kansas City, 1985, American Nurses' Association.

Bonta S and Blichfeldt M: What to watch for if your patient has a ventriculostomy, RN, 47(12):63-73, 1984.

Conway-Rutkowski BL: Neurological and neurosurgical nursing, ed 8, St Louis, 1982, The CV Mosby Co.

Dahlquist N, Mellinger J, and Klass D: Hazard of video games in patients with light-sensitive epilepsy, JAMA 249:776-777, 1983.

Friedman D: Seizures: coping with the unpredictable, Nursing 18(2):52-59, 1988.

Hazinski M: Nursing care of the critically ill child, St Louis, 1984, The CV Mosby Co.

Hickey J: The clinical practice of neurological and neurosurgical nursing, ed 2, Philadelphia, 1986, JB Lippincott Co.

James W, White S, and Yanklowitz B: Allergic contact dermatitis to compound tincture of benzoin, J Am Acad Dermatol 11(5):847-850, 1984.

Mott S, Fazekas N, and James S: Nursing care of children and families: a holistic approach, Menlo Park, Calif, 1985, Addison-Wesley Publishing Co.

Roberts J and Hedges J: Clinical procedures in emergency medicine, Philadelphia, 1985, WB Saunders Co.

Whaley LF and Wong DL: Nursing care of infants and children ed 4, St Louis, 1991, CV Mosby Co.

# UNIT XIV Oxygenation and Ventilation

## SKILL 87 Clearing an Oral or Nasal Airway

*Mary C. Oberc*

Suctioning is an important element in the maintenance of a patent airway in children. Because their respiratory tract structures have small lumen size, air passages are more easily blocked by the presence of excessive mucus, foreign particles, and swelling of mucous membranes. When a child is unable to remove the obstruction without help, oral and/or nasal suctioning is performed to facilitate airway clearance. Oral or nasal suctioning involves placing a suction device into the mouth or nose to remove obstructive material. Proper selection and use of various suction devices can decrease mucous membrane damage and maintain airway patency.

### NURSING DIAGNOSES

Ineffective airway clearance related to tracheobronchial secretions or obstruction; Ineffective breathing pattern related to tracheobronchial obstruction; Altered oral mucous membrane related to trauma from oropharyngeal/nasotracheal suctioning.

| Steps | Rationale |
|---|---|
| **Assessment** | |
| 1. Assess respiratory status.<br>a. Skin color.<br>b. Respiratory effort.<br>c. Diaphragmatic movement, lung expansion, and use of accessory muscles.<br>d. Breath sounds.<br>e. Abnormal sounds.<br>f. Signs of early stage respiratory distress.<br>g. Cardinal signs of respiratory failure. | Assessment of respiratory status helps determine course of action and provides a baseline for comparison after the intervention.<br>***Special Considerations:*** *Signs that may indicate need for suctioning include pallor; restlessness or anxiety; increased pulse, respiration, and temperature; dyspnea; bubbling (copious amounts of thin secretions); rattling (thick, tenacious secretions); drooling; mouth breathing; nasal flaring; grunting; gasping; retractions; cyanosis; and erythema (flushed face). An infant's restlessness or anxiety may be exhibited by an anxious look in the eyes or constant fidgeting. Older children may constantly seek attention with no explanation, toss and turn in bed, or finger a blanket edge.* |
| 2. Examine mouth, anterior nares, and nasopharyngeal tract for evidence of obstruction. | Assessment of anatomic airway structures facilitates proper intervention and prevents further trauma.<br>***Special Considerations:*** *Possible contraindications for insertion of a nasal catheter include fracture of face or nose, structural defect, basal skull fracture, or corrective surgery on nose. Insertion of a tube into a child with a basal skull fracture places the child at risk for placement of the tube into the cranium. Placing a suction device into the back of the oropharynx is contraindicated in child with croup or epiglottitis unless intubated (Hazinski, 1984).* |
| 3. Assess type of obstruction.<br>a. Amount, color, and consistency of mucus or vomitus.<br>b. Hard, foreign body, e.g., hard candy, hot dog. | Assessment of type of obstruction facilitates proper selection of suction device and determines type of intervention required. |

| Steps | Rationale |
|---|---|
| | ***Special Considerations:*** *Suctioning is only indicated when secretions are audible in airway, when there are signs of airway obstruction, or signs of oxygen deficit (Sporing, Walton, and Cady, 1984).* |
| 4. Assess size of child.<br>a. Age.<br>b. Weight.<br>c. Size of nasal passages. | Use of equipment proportional to child decreases physical and psychologic trauma.<br>***Special Considerations:*** *Size of suction catheter is based on weight rather than age of the child (JAMA, 1986). For example, if a child is 3 years old but only weighs 5 kg, a smaller size catheter is indicated. In such cases, determine the age for which the weight correlates to select appropriate tube (Table 87-1).* |
| 5. Assess the mental and emotional status of child and family.<br>a. Knowledge about procedure.<br>b. Fears and anxieties.<br>c. Need for restraint.<br>d. Disorientation.<br>e. Ability to comprehend. | Baseline knowledge about the child and family's understanding allows individualized care and proper preparation for the procedure.<br>***Special Considerations:*** *The child and family may not have a clear understanding about the procedure and its purpose despite previous suctioning. To facilitate the procedure, restraint may be needed for the child's safety and comfort. For an agitated infant or small child, "mummying" is effective.* |

## Planning and Goal Setting

| Steps | Rationale |
|---|---|
| 1. Gather supplies:<br>a. Box of tissues.<br>b. Vacuum apparatus.<br>c. Connecting tubing.<br>m. Oxygen on stand-by.<br>e. 100 ml of sterile saline or sterile water for nasal or oropharyngeal suctioning.<br>f. 100 ml of water (sterile or tap) for oropharyngeal suctioning only.<br>g. Sterile gloves or one sterile glove and one nonsterile glove.<br>h. Sterile basin for nasal or oropharyngeal suctioning.<br>i. Nonsterile basin for oral pharyngeal suctioning only.<br>j. Proper type and size device (Fig. 87-1).<br>▪ Oral: bulb syringe, saliva ejector, Yankauer tip, straight suction catheter.<br>▪ Nasal: bulb syringe, straight suction catheter.<br>k. Water-soluble lubricant for nasal suctioning.<br>l. Sterile suction kit if available; in addition, assemble above listed items not noted in kit contents.<br>m. Clean cloth to wrap bulb syringe after use. | Collecting supplies in advance yields increased efficiency and safety.<br>***Special Considerations:*** *Bulb syringe (ear bulb syringe) and straight suction catheters can be used for both oral and nasal suctioning. Saliva ejector and Yankauer tip can only be used for oral suctioning. Both saliva ejector and Yankauer tip are referred to as tonsil tip suction. All four types come in various sizes and can be effectively used on both infants and children, although the bulb syringe is used most with infants. Saliva ejectors, Yankauer tips, and straight suction catheters require connecting tubing and vacuum apparatus. The saliva ejector is slightly flexible and has numerous openings for collecting secretions and vomitus. The tip may be bitten off or may accidentally fall off in the child's mouth. The Yankauer tip is made of hard, nonflexible plastic and has fewer openings. The rigid plastic may cause trauma in an active child unless the child's head is stabilized. The rigidity of the Yankauer tip allows it to be more easily directed and prevents it from coiling in the back of the mouth.* |

***TABLE 87-1*** **Catheter Sizes for Nasopharyngeal and Oropharyngeal Suctioning of Nonintubated Patient**

| Age | Size of Catheter (French) |
|---|---|
| Newborn | 5 to 6½ |
| 6 months | 8 |
| 1 year | 8 to 10 |
| 2 years | 10 |
| 5 years | 12 |
| 10 years or older | 12 to 14 |

Adapted from Hazinski MF: Nursing care of the critically ill child, St Louis, 1984, The CV Mosby Co.

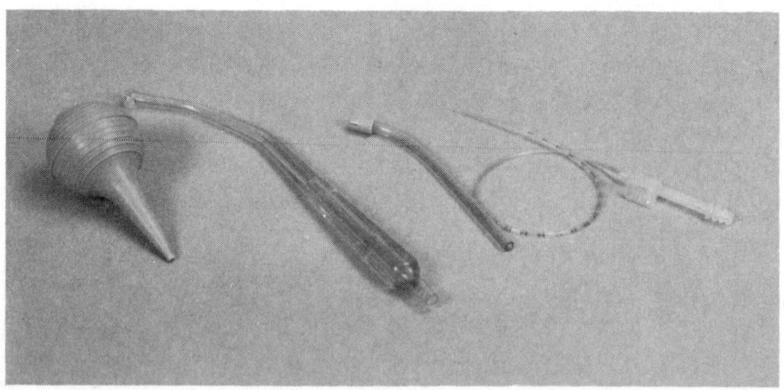

***FIG. 87-1*** Devices used for oral and/or nasal airway clearing. Shown from left to right: bulb syringe, Yankauer tip, saliva ejector, and straight suction catheter.

| **Steps** | **Rationale** |
|---|---|
| 2. Set up vacuum apparatus and tubing at bedside if needed. | A vacuum source is required to remove excess secretions and vomitus from the mouth with tonsil tip devices and straight suction catheters. |
| 3. Prepare child and family for procedure (see Skill 1).<br>a. Explain purpose of suction.<br>b. Discuss discomfort and loud noise of suction apparatus.<br>c. Respond to fears and concerns. | Proper preparation and teaching will help to decrease fear and enhance cooperation.<br>***Special Considerations:*** *For a small child, demonstrate how the machine operates by suctioning some water from a cup. Reassure the child that the machine is only suctioning excess fluid from the mouth or nose and not body contents. Use play therapy for children requiring frequent suctioning to promote understanding and decrease anger and frustration. In an emergency, simply state, "I need to suction the child."* |
| 4. Obtain an assistant if necessary to perform the procedure:<br>a. Noncooperative child.<br>b. Unstable child who may become bradycardic or require oxygen to be directed on airway during procedure. | Having an assistant may be necessary to ensure the child's safety.<br>***Special Considerations:*** *If no assistance is available, gather equipment necessary for proper restraint as needed. Mummy, papoose board, football hold, and clove hitch restraints are useful. See Skill 51.* |
| 5. Develop individualized goals of nursing care:<br>▪ Provide a patent airway.<br>▪ Prevent trauma (physical and psychologic).<br>▪ Decrease fear and anxiety of child and family. | |

## Implementation

| | |
|---|---|
| 1. Position child properly for effective access to suctioning: | Correct positioning provides easier access to and more effective removal of secretions. |
| a. Positioning for bulb syringe suctioning.<br>▪ Use football hold (see Skill 73).<br>▪ "Mummy" the child and place on nurse's lap (see Skill 51).<br>▪ Cradle child in nondominant arm. Place the child's arm closest to self behind own back. Hold the child's free arm with the arm cradling the child (Perry and Potter, 1990).<br>▪ While infant is lying in bed, clasp the infant's hands together with own nondominant hand. | Restraining the child's arms allows a safer and more efficient procedure. |
| b. Positioning for bulb syringe, nasal, or oropharyngeal suctioning:<br>▪ Elevate child's upper torso 45 degrees or place in semi-Fowler's or Sim's position if not contraindicated. | An elevation of 45 degrees allows for maximum movement of diaphragm, which promotes deep breathing and effective coughing (Fuchs, 1984).<br>***Special Considerations:*** *Do not elevate head of bed for premature infants or infants suspected of having intracranial hemorrhage. Keep the head level with the body to prevent increasing intracranial pressure and possible bleeding as a result of gravity (Jensen and Bobak, 1985).* |
| ▪ Restraint methods for infant or small child.<br>(1) Place child on back or side. Position own upper body lightly across the child, wedging child's chest and arms between own body and upper arm (Perry and Potter, 1990). | Strategically applied pressure provides restraint. |
| (2) "Mummy" the child (see Skill 51). | ***Special Considerations:*** *When suctioning a toddler in a mummy restraint, position the feet away from self. Preferably, the bodies of the child and nurse should be perpendicular to one another (Fig. 87-2). This prevents the child from kicking or launching himself off the bed, which could occur with a side-lying position.* |
| (3) Ask an assistant to restrain the child's arms and hands. | |
| ▪ For an older child, find a comfortable position for both the child and nurse. | A comfortable position promotes the child's comfort and prevents back strain in the nurse (Perry and Potter, 1990). |
| ▪ Stabilize the head by using three fingers (little, ring, and index) and palm of the nondominant hand. | Stabilizing the head prevents trauma, which could be caused by sudden movement of the head. |

| Steps | Rationale |
|---|---|

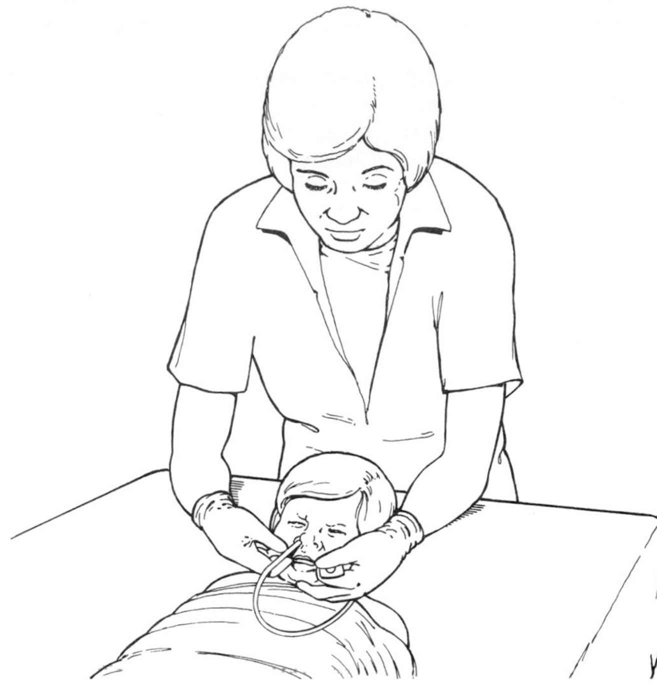

*FIG. 87-2* Child in mummy restraint during nasal suctioning.

| Steps | Rationale |
|---|---|
| 2. Use of bulb syringe. | |
| a. Grasp the bulb syringe by placing index and forefinger around the snout near the bulbous end. Place the thumb over the center of the bulb. | |
| b. Compress the bulb before inserting it into the naris. To compress the bulb, push the thumb toward the index and forefinger, (Fig. 87-3). | Removal of air inside the bulb decreases the possibility of secretions being forced further down the respiratory tract. Compression of the bulb creates a vacuum needed for the suction effect. |
| c. Suction the nose first. Place the tip of the bulb syringe snugly into one naris. Gradually release the pressure on the bulb by lifting the thumb. | The nose is suctioned first because the mouth is considered more contaminated. Effectively suctioning the nares requires a snug fit between the surface of the bulb syringe and nares. Gradual release of pressure prevents tissue trauma, yet removes secretions.<br>***Special Considerations:*** *Always suction the nares first except at the moment of birth when the mouth should be suctioned first. Most infants are nose breathers, therefore patency of nares is essential.* |
| d. When the bulb is reinflated remove it from the naris, and expel contents into a tissue. | Emptying the bulb removes aspirated contents that could be blown back into the airway. |
| e. Recompress the bulb, and reinsert into the other naris. | Recompression restores the vacuum needed for suction. |
| f. Repeat steps c through e until the nose is clear. | Suctioning nose until clear restores airway patency.<br>***Special Considerations:*** *Air as well as secretions are removed with suctioning, therefore reassess respiratory status between suction attempts.* |
| g. Recompress the bulb and insert the tip inside the mouth between cheeks and gums. Gradually release the pressure on the bulb. Discard secretions as above. | Secretions in the mouth could occlude the airway if not removed. |
| h. Repeat procedure on both sides of mouth until clear. | Suctioning until clear restores airway patency.<br>***Special Considerations:*** *Suctioning is complete when the cry is clear and no excessive secretions are noted in the nose and mouth.* |
| i. After use, wrap the bulb syringe in a clean cloth and place in an easily accessed location. | Consistent placement after each use will make it easier to find.<br>***Special Considerations:*** *Some manufacturers' inserts recommend only single use of the bulb syringe. Once contaminated mucus is trapped inside the bulb syringe, pathogens continue to survive even after the syringe is cleaned with soap and water or the mucus dries. A recent study noted that replacing the bulb syringe every 24 hours may suffice to limit colonization of the bulb syringe (Patel et al, 1988).* |

| **Steps** | **Rationale** |
|---|---|

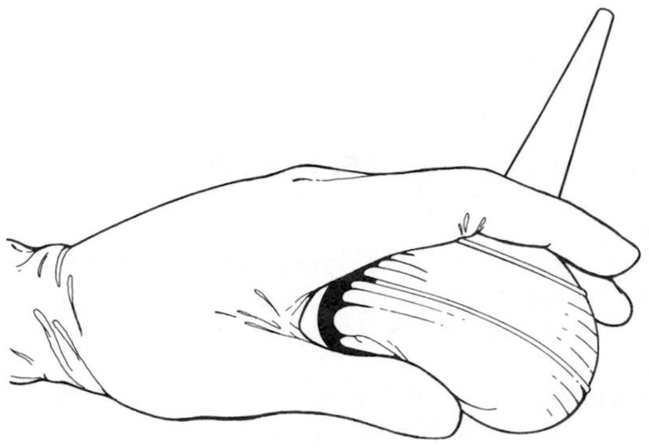

***FIG. 87-3*** Use of bulb syringe for nasal suctioning.

3. Use of tonsil tip devices (Yankauer tip and saliva ejector).
   a. Pour approximately 100 ml of water into a paper cup or basin (sterile or nonsterile). Sources of water can include:
      - Bottle of sterile water.
      - Fresh tap water from sink faucet.

A clean source of fluid is needed to flush the device. Clean technique can be used because the mouth is not a sterile cavity.
***Special Considerations:*** *Gram negative bacteria multiply rapidly in solutions and equipment used for respiratory care. To minimize growth, the water bottle should be discarded every 8 to 12 hours. It should also be labeled with date and time of opening (Rhoades, Adcock, and Jovanovich, 1980). Sterile saline can be substituted for the sterile water.*

   b. Turn on vacuum apparatus.

Adequate suction pressure is needed to remove secretions.

   c. Check suction pressure by kinking the connecting tube between the thumb and forefinger. Note the amount of pressure (mm Hg or cm of $H_2O$) registered on the gauge, and adjust to the correct pressure (see Table 87-2) (Hoffman and Maszkiewicz, 1987; Perry and Potter, 1990).

Excessive negative pressure may cause edema and trauma to mucous membranes, bradycardia, laryngospasm, and cardiac dysrhythmia. When the tube is occluded, the gauge registers the maximum suction pressure that the system is exerting. The gauge indicates only partial pressure without occlusion (Hoffman and Maszkiewicz, 1987).
***Special Considerations:*** *Hospital policies may vary on the amount of negative pressure that may be used. Check the agency's manual.*

***TABLE 87-2*** Recommended Pressures for Airway Suctioning

| | Wall Suction (mm Hg) | Portable Suction (mm Hg) | Negative Pressure (cm of water) |
|---|---|---|---|
| Infants | 60-100 | 3-5 | 60-90 |
| Children | 100-120 | 5-10 | 90-110 |
| Older child | — | — | 110-150 |
| Adult | 120-150 | 7-15 | — |

Data from Blodgett D: Manual of respiratory care procedures, Philadelphia, 1980, JB Lippincott Co; and Hazinski MF: Nursing care of the critically ill child, St Louis, 1984, The CV Mosby Co.

   d. Put on a pair of nonsterile gloves.

Wearing gloves decreases risk of contamination with body secretions.

   e. Open the suction tip package, and attach the tapered end of the tip to the connecting tube.

Connecting the parts prepares the apparatus for suctioning.
***Special Considerations:*** *If a sputum specimen is needed and the child is unable to expectorate spontaneously, connect a mucus trap device between the suction catheter and the suction tubing. A specimen will be collected during suctioning. This method will also work with endotracheal or tracheostomy suctioning.*

   f. Suction water to moisten the tip, and determine patency and equipment function.

Properly working equipment increases efficiency and safety.
***Special Considerations:*** *Some tonsil tip devices are equipped with a finger control opening. If present, place the thumb of the hand holding the device over the finger control opening to achieve suction. Devices without a finger control opening provide continuous suction.*

| Steps | Rationale |
|---|---|
| g. Insert the tip into the mouth along the base of the tongue. If a child resists opening the mouth, try the following:<br>▪ Infants and toddlers: grasp mandible at the chin, and gently pull down; squeeze both cheeks toward the midline; demonstrate an open mouth.<br>▪ Older child: ask child to say "ahh," give specific directions to open mouth. | Inserting the tip along the base of the tongue decreases the possibility of triggering a laryngospasm.<br>***Special Considerations:*** *If a finger control opening is present, remove thumb from the opening and insert the device into the mouth. Then apply suction after the device is in position. Avoid placing fingers in child's mouth as child may bite.* |
| h. Suction for approximately 3 to 4 seconds (Whaley and Wong, 1989).<br>▪ Place thumb over finger control opening if present.<br>▪ Move the device throughout the mouth. | Continual movement of the device decreases mucosal damage caused by suction on tissues. Suctioning for longer than 3 to 4 seconds obstructs the airway (American Heart Association, 1988).<br>***Special Considerations:*** *Although this recommendation is specific to tracheal suctioning, the same principles could apply. No research is available on oral or nasopharyngeal suctioning. To keep track of time, hold breath during suctioning or slowly count to four (Birdsall, 1985; Perry and Potter, 1990).* |
| i. Remove device and observe for:<br>▪ Bradycardia.<br>▪ Apnea.<br>▪ Cyanosis.<br>▪ Laryngospasm.<br>▪ Vomitus.<br>▪ Excess secretions. | Movement of the device inside the mouth, especially at the back of the throat, may inadvertently stimulate the vagus nerve. Vagal stimulation can cause cardiac depression, bronchial tree constriction, coughing, gagging, and vomiting. Also, air as well as secretions are removed with suctioning, therefore reassess respiratory status between suction attempts.<br>***Special Considerations:*** *Administer oxygen as indicated.* |
| j. Repeat steps g through i until the mouth is clear of vomitus or excess secretions. | Suctioning until clear restores airway patency.<br>***Special Considerations:*** *Encouraging the child to cough between suction attempts will help to move secretions from the lower airway into the mouth where they can be more easily removed. The child may need a slight respite to catch his breath between suction attempts. Allow 30 to 60 seconds unless concern for aspiration indicates aggressive suctioning. If device becomes clogged with thick secretions, aspirate water through it until clog is removed.* |
| 4. Use of straight suction catheter for nasopharyngeal or oropharyngeal suctioning.<br>a. Follow step 1b of Implementation section. | |
| b. To adjust suction gauge to correct pressure see steps 3b and c in Implementation. | Higher suction pressures do not remove more secretions (Shekleton and Nield, 1987; Kuzenski, 1978).<br>***Special Considerations:*** *The literature varies on the maximum amount of suction pressure to be used. See Table 87-2 or consult hospital procedure manual.* |
| c. Maintaining sterile technique, assemble catheter kit contents.<br>▪ Open catheter package and water-soluble lubricant packet if needed. | Sterile technique reduces the risk of introducing microorganisms into the respiratory tract, which could result in nosocomial infection.<br>***Special Considerations:*** *Suction catheter kits vary in contents. Most provide the catheter, one or two sterile gloves, and a container for the sterile saline.* |
| ▪ Put sterile glove on dominant hand. | Because the dominant hand touches the catheter, a sterile glove is used to prevent infection. |
| ▪ Using the sterile gloved hand, lift the kit's container for saline and place on bedside table. | |
| ▪ Use ungloved hand to pour sterile normal saline into container. | Saline lubricates the catheter, tests its patency, and clears catheter and tubing of secretions.<br>***Special Considerations:*** *Sterile water may be substituted for normal saline.* |
| ▪ If water-soluble lubricant is to be used, squeeze the desired amount onto the sterile surface of the package with the ungloved hand. | Water-soluble lubricant prevents risk of hydrocarbon aspiration pneumonia, which could occur with oil-based lubricant.<br>***Special Considerations:*** *Facility policies on recommended lubrication vary.* |
| ▪ Grasp the inner package containing the catheter near the tapered port with the sterile gloved hand.<br>▪ With the ungloved hand connect tubing onto tapered port of catheter. Return inner package to sterile field. | |

| Steps | Rationale |
|---|---|
| ▪ Glove the ungloved hand. This will be the clean hand. | Because the clean hand does not touch sterile equipment, a sterile glove is not needed. However, using a glove protects from contact with body secretions and possible infections such as herpetic whitlow and HIV (Birdsall, 1985). |
| ▪ Grasp connecting tube and finger control opening with clean hand. Remove catheter from inner package, coiling catheter in the palm of the sterile gloved hand. | Catheters have a tendency to spring out in various directions when covering is removed, increasing risk of contamination. |
| ▪ Recheck suction pressure:<br>(1) Bend or pinch catheter with sterile gloved hand to occlude lumen.<br>(2) Place thumb of clean hand over finger control opening.<br>(3) Adjust gauge with clean hand if needed. | Excessive negative pressure may cause edema and trauma to mucous membranes, bradycardia, laryngospasm, and cardiac dysrhythmia. When the tube is occluded, the gauge registers the maximum suction pressure that the system is exerting. |
| d. Check patency of catheter and lubricate.<br>▪ Place tip of catheter in sterile normal saline. Aspirate a small amount of saline into catheter. This also lubricates the catheter tip. If water-soluble lubricant is preferred roll the tip of the catheter in lubricant on sterile field. | Checking patency ensures the equipment is properly functioning before entering the nares. Lubrication facilitates passage of catheter through the nasal passage.<br>***Special Considerations:*** *Do not use uncapped or undated sterile saline, because it may be colonized with gram negative organisms. Saline should be labeled with the date and time of opening and discarded every 8 to 12 hours (Rhoades, Adcock, and Jovanovich, 1980).* |
| e. Administer oxygen as needed. | Since duration of suctioning has been shown to be related to development of hypoxia, administer oxygen to minimize depletion of oxygen supply (Shekleton and Nield, 1987).<br>***Special Considerations:*** *Studies conducted on preoxygenation were done in relation to nasotracheal or endotracheal suctioning, not nasopharyngeal. Use of oxygen should depend on child's clinical status and facility policy (Shekleton and Nield, 1987).* |
| f. Insert catheter into one nostril. Thread the catheter along the base of the nasal passage. Little resistance should be met. However, resistance may be encountered 2 to 3 cm into the naris. Touching the nasal membrane with the tip of the catheter, slightly rotating the catheter, or having the child inspire usually removes the resistance. Wait for the feeling of release and then thread the catheter further into the nostril. Do not poke or force the catheter through the resistance. | Correct insertion is required to prevent trauma to mucous membranes or perforation of closed structures by forceful advancement of catheter. Nasopharyngeal suctioning should be done before oropharyngeal suctioning to prevent transfer of oral microorganisms to the nasal passages.<br>***Special Considerations:*** *Congenital anomalies that could be perforated include choanal and esophageal atresia (Jensen and Bobak, 1985). If the catheter keeps advancing more than expected, and no resistance is encountered, the child may have swallowed the catheter, and it is in the esophagus.* |
| g. Advance catheter to the nasopharynx using a slightly downward slant. Recommended length of catheter insertion is:<br>▪ Infants and small children: 4 to 8 cm.<br>▪ Older children: 8 to 12 cm (Perry and Potter, 1990). | Distance for catheter insertion is measured from the tip of the nose to the base of the ear lobe. Insertion at a downward slant decreases trauma to nasal mucosa by avoiding the nasal turbinates (Perry and Potter, 1990).<br>***Special Considerations:*** *Gagging and coughing may indicate that the catheter has advanced beyond the nasopharynx. A tube in the trachea yields a cough. A tube in the esophagus yields a gag (Jensen and Bobak, 1985). If the child has been fed recently, be especially careful not to advance the catheter past the nasopharynx, because of the potential for vomiting and aspiration (Jensen and Bobak, 1985).* |
| h. Slightly withdraw the catheter and apply suction, not exceeding 3 to 4 seconds.<br>▪ Place thumb of clean hand over finger control opening.<br>▪ Slowly withdraw the catheter from the nostril while rotating the catheter between the thumb and forefinger of the sterile gloved hand.<br>▪ Suction only when the catheter is being withdrawn. Each suction attempt should not exceed 3 to 4 seconds. | Rotation decreases mucosal damage caused by tissue being drawn up into the catheter. Not exceeding 3 to 4 seconds of suctioning helps to avoid hypoxia and danger of bradycardia. Using the thumb and forefinger to rotate the catheter is sufficient and less tiring than twirling the arm and wrist.<br>***Special Considerations:*** *The 3 to 4 second recommendation is specific to tracheal suctioning (American Heart Association, 1988). No research is available on oral or nasopharyngeal suctioning. Occasionally the catheter may become clogged with thick mucus. Place tip of catheter in saline container, and aspirate to remove the clog.* |
| i. Repeat with each nostril, allowing 30 to 60 seconds between suction attempts. | ***Special Considerations:*** *See step 3j. When suctioning the child, observe facial expression for signs of respiratory distress or need for a break.* |

| Steps | Rationale |
|---|---|
| j. Repeat steps f through i until nasopharnx is clear of excess secretions. | |
| k. Suction the oropharynx. Follow Implementation steps 3f through j. | ***Special Considerations:*** *Small children may attempt to bite the end of the catheter, so observe catheter when it is withdrawn.* |
| l. Disconnect catheter from connecting tube. Remove the glove holding the catheter by pulling it off inside out so that the catheter remains coiled inside the glove (Fig. 87-4). Remove other glove, and dispose of properly. | Single use of suction catheter in hospital setting decreases risk of nosocomial infection. ***Special Considerations:*** *Suctioning is complete when the airway sounds clear and respirations return to baseline status.* |
| 5. For suctioning procedures using vacuum apparatus, rinse the connecting tubing until clear by suctioning saline or water through it. Turn off the vacuum apparatus. | Rinsing clears the connecting tubing for future use and decreases the probability of transmitting microorganisms. ***Special Considerations:*** *Frequency of changing device, tubing, and sterile water varies according to hospital policy. Usual recommendation is to change straight suction catheter and tonsil tip devices after each use; change sterile saline or water bottle every 8 to 12 hours; change connecting tubing and suction cannister between patients (Simmons and Wong, 1983).* |

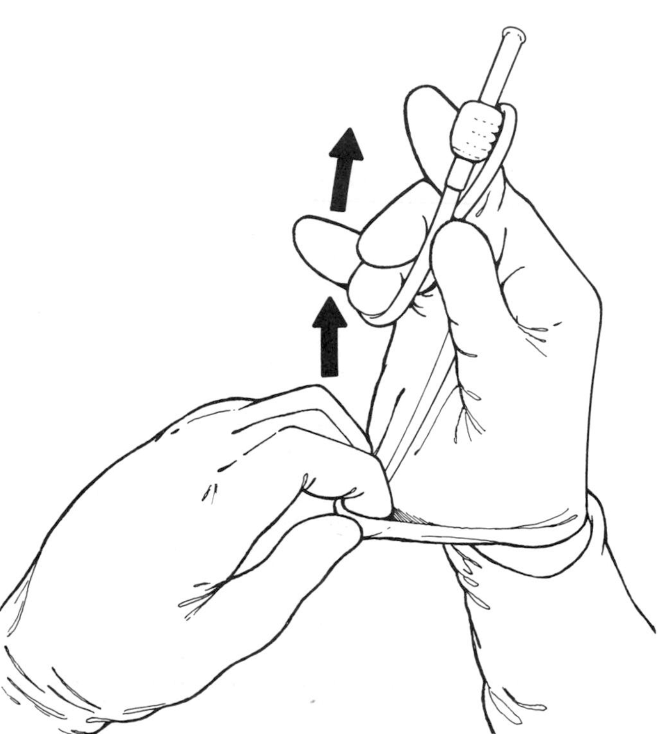

***FIG. 87-4*** Glove is removed so that catheter remains coiled inside.

| Steps | Rationale |
|---|---|
| 6. Following all suction procedures, hold infant and caress or hug child when finished. Praise child for cooperation. | Verbal and physical reinforcements reassure and calm child. |
| 7. Provide comfort for child. | |
| a. Cleanse face and nares if needed with tissue or wash cloth. | Removal of foreign substances from the skin prevents skin breakdown. |
| b. Provide oral care after emesis (see Skills 56 and 57). ▪ Infant/toddler/comatose patient: use swab moistened in normal saline. ▪ Older children: offer mouth rinse. | Providing oral hygiene enhances comfort of child. Gastric acid in emesis can erode tooth enamel if not removed. |
| c. Position appropriately. | ***Special Considerations:*** *The Sim's position promotes safe drainage of respiratory secretions, especially for unconscious or semi-alert child.* |
| 8. Dispose of device, contaminated saline or water, and paper cup. | Appropriate disposal of soiled equipment decreases spread of microorganisms. ***Special Considerations:*** *For tonsil tip suction only: if a basin was used, wash in warm, soapy water, dry, and replace at bedside.* |

| Evaluation Outcomes | Observational Guidelines |
|---|---|
| 1. The child's airway is cleared, allowing adequate oxygenation. | Listen near the child's mouth and nose for "bubbling" and "rattling" sounds. Observe nose and mouth for excessive mucus or vomitus. Reassess respiratory status. |
| 2. Trauma to the airway mucosa is prevented or minimized. | Observe for bright red blood or mucosa/tissue being drawn into suction catheter during suctioning procedure. Observe for bleeding in the mouth and nares. |

### Evaluation Outcomes—cont'd

3. The child experiences minimal discomfort or psychologic trauma.
4. The child and family demonstrate understanding of the necessity for suctioning.
5. The child and family experience decreased fear and anxiety from improved respiratory status.

### Observational Guidelines—cont'd

Observe child's cooperation with procedure, verbal or behavioral expression of discomfort, ability to be comforted after procedure.

Observe family's facial expression, listen for comments of understanding.

With infant or small child, observe for less anxious look in the eyes and decreased fidgeting. For an older child there are verbal expressions of feeling better, decreased tossing and turning in bed. Parents express feelings of relief at sight of improved color and increased ease of child's respirations.

### Documentation

Record type of suction apparatus used; amount, color, odor, consistency of secretions obtained; change in respiratory status; child's toleration of the procedure; episodes of apnea, bradycardia, cyanosis with description of measure taken; child/family teaching such as instructing in use of suction.

### Home Care Modifications

1. Cleansing the bulb syringe—if mucus secretions are crusted on, hydrogen peroxide can be used to loosen them before boiling the syringe. Boil the water-filled syringe daily for 10 minutes before reuse (Patel et al, 1988).
2. The family can rent or purchase a portable suction machine.
3. Oropharyngeal and nasopharyngeal suctioning can be done as clean procedures at home. Use good handwashing and nonsterile gloves for suctioning. Tap water in a new paper cup can be used to rinse the catheter. Use fresh water and a new paper cup for each procedure (Pfaff and Terri, 1980).
4. Steps for cleansing suction catheters at home are as follows: (a) presoak the catheters and tubing in a hydrogen peroxide solution to loosen mucus (1 cup hydrogen peroxide to 3 cups water); (b) wash in soap and water; use long pipe cleaners and small bottle brushes to clean lumens; (c) thoroughly rinse with tap water; a syringe may be used to force water through the catheter; (d) disinfect with white vinegar solution in an enamel or glass pot (1 cup vinegar to 3 cups water). Vinegar reacts with aluminum or plastic by leaching those substances into the solution. White vinegar is used because of its antiseptic properties. Boiling is not recommended because it causes the catheter to disintegrate. Soak the catheters for 15 to 20 minutes. The length of time is accepted practice but has not been thoroughly researched; (e) using a clean spring clothespin, hang catheters from a wire coat hanger in the shower and allow to dry; and (f) store in a plastic zip-lock bag or clean glass jar (Pfaff and Terri, 1980).

# *SKILL* 88 Suctioning an Endotracheal or Tracheostomy Airway

*Debbie R. Berry*

A child with an endotracheal or tracheostomy tube requires suctioning to help keep the airway patent and clear of secretions. The amount of suctioning needed for any child depends on the nature of the child's pulmonary problem. It may vary from every 15 minutes to every 2 hours. Suctioning is invasive and unpleasant for the conscious child. The nature of the artificial airway forces the glottis to remain open, and the child is unable to effectively cough.

## NURSING DIAGNOSES

Ineffective airway clearance related to excessive or thick secretions, ineffective coughing, or intubated trachea; Impaired gas exchange related to altered oxygen supply; Anxiety related to change in breathing pattern, suctioning procedure, or protective restraints.

| Steps | Rationale |
|---|---|

## Assessment

1. Assess child's respiratory status for indicators that secretions are accumulating in the respiratory tract: bubbling, rattling, decreased breath sounds, coarse expiratory rales, tachypnea, or dyspnea (see Skill 27).

Assessing respiratory status will provide supportive information regarding whether a need for suctioning exists.
***Special Considerations:*** *A rise in peak pressure with mechanical ventilation may also indicate a need for suctioning (Knipper, 1984).*

2. Assess child for signs of hypoxia or anoxia: increased pulse rate, cyanosis or pallor, restlessness, irritability, decrease in oxygen saturation measurements, respiratory effort.

Hypoxia/anoxia can be caused by accumulation of secretions or mucus plugs and can be remedied by suctioning.
***Special Considerations:*** *Suction only when there is evidence of pooled secretions or indications of mucus plugs. Unnecessary or careless suctioning can result in mucosal damage and stimulate increased mucus production (Hazinski, 1984).*

3. Assess whether child is receiving supplemental oxygen or mechanical assistance.

Suctioning removes oxygen from the airways and may produce hypoxia. Accessibility to supplemental oxygen is necessary.

4. Review child's chart for information such as: physician's orders regarding suctioning, frequency of suctioning, tolerance of procedure, type of secretions last suctioned, or any contraindications to suctioning.

This information provides baseline data useful in identifying changes in child's respiratory status.
***Special Considerations:*** *Suctioning a child with increased intracranial pressure may cause pressure to further increase. If necessary, suctioning should be used judiciously and be preceded by hyperventilation with 100% oxygen (Whaley and Wong, 1991).*

5. Assess child's ability to cooperate with procedure, and determine if assistance or restraint will be necessary.

The child will need to be cooperative or restrained to safely perform procedure.

## Planning and Goal Setting

1. Gather supplies:

Having supplies ready improves the efficiency and safety of the procedure.

   a. Suction collection bottle.
   b. Connecting tubing.
   c. Vacuum source with regulator.
   d. Appropriate size sterile suction catheter—with or without thumb port (Table 88-1).

Using the proper size suction catheter prevents hypoxia and tissue damage while allowing adequate secretion removal.

   e. Y-connector if catheter does not have thumb port.

Y-connector is used to join the catheter to the suction tubing. One arm of the Y is used to control the suction.

   f. Pair of sterile gloves.

***Special Considerations:*** *Only the dominant hand needs to have a sterile glove; the nondominant hand is used for clean tasks, and a nonsterile glove may be used.*

   g. Disposable sterile container.

***TABLE 88-1*** Suction Catheter Size in Relation to Size of Tracheostomy Tube

| Age | Tracheostomy (Internal Diameter in mm) | Suction Catheter (in French Sizes) |
|---|---|---|
| Premature | 4-5 | 5½-6 |
| Newborn | 4-5 | 6-8 |
| 6 months | 5.5 | 6-8 |
| 18 months | 6.0 | 8-10 |
| 24 months | 6-7 | 10 |
| 2 to 4 years | 6-7 | 10-12 |
| 4 to 7 years | 7.0 | 12 |
| 7 to 10 years | 8.0 | 12-14 |
| 10 to 12 years | 9.0 | 14 |

Adapted from Hazinski MF: Nursing care of the critically ill child, St Louis, 1984, The CV Mosby Co.

### *EFFECTS OF SALINE INSTILLATION*

Instillation of normal saline into the airways to facilitate removal of secretion during suctioning is often done as part of the routine suctioning procedure. However, mucus is not miscible in saline and is not actually thinned or liquified as commonly thought. Benefits in secretion removal may be due to a lavage effect or stimulation of cough by the saline (Demers and Saklad, 1973).

Recommendations regarding the amount of saline to be instilled may vary considerably. Suggested amounts for children range from 0.5 to 3.0 cc (Hazinski, 1984), while amounts for adults range from 2 to 10 cc (Burton, Gee, and Hodgkin, 1984). A study by Bostick and Wendelgass (1987) of 45 adults who had open heart surgery looked at instillation of saline during suctioning and presuctioning and postsuctioning oxygen tension values. They found a greater decrease in postsuctioning oxygen tension (as compared with presuctioning oxygen tension) in patients who had 5 cc saline instilled vs. those with no saline instilled and also in those who had 10 cc saline instilled vs. those who had 5 cc saline instilled.

| **Steps** | **Rationale** |
|---|---|
| h. Sterile water or saline solution. | Sterile solution is used to flush and lubricate the catheter. |
| i. Stethoscope. | The stethoscope is used immediately after each suctioning episode to auscultate the lungs. |
| j. Ampule or syringe (without a needle) of sterile bacteriostatic free saline: use 0.5 ml for infants and 1 to 3 ml for older children (Hazinski, 1984). | Sterile saline is often used to lavage the airway, making secretions easier to remove.<br>***Special Considerations:*** *Tracheal lavage may be ordered by physician or may exist as an institutional policy. The use of lavage is considered controversial (Hazinski, 1984) (see the box on previous page).* |
| k. Oxygen source and equipment. | Hyperoxygenation before suctioning reduces postsuctioning decreases in arterial oxygen tension ($PaO_2$). |
| l. Manual resuscitation bag with pressure manometer or mechanical ventilator. | Manual hyperventilation is often required before suctioning. The use of a pressure manometer helps ensure that high inspiratory pressures are avoided (Hazinski, 1984). |
| m. Tracheostomy adaptor. | The adaptor is attached to the resuscitation bag, allowing for a proper size fit into the tracheostomy or endotracheal tube. |
| 2. If necessary, recruit an assistant or apply restraints. | Some form of restraint may be needed to ensure that sterility and safety are maintained throughout the procedure.<br>***Special Considerations:*** *Some institutional policies require that endotracheal suctioning be performed by two people.* |
| 3. Explain procedure and possible sensations to child and family (see Skill 1). | Explaining the procedure to the child and family can reduce fear and anxiety.<br>***Special Considerations:*** *Explain that the child may experience a choking sensation when the suction catheter passes through the artificial airway into the trachea.* |
| 4. Develop individualized child/family goals, including:<br>▪ Patent airway will be maintained.<br>▪ Gas exchange will be improved.<br>▪ Child/family will experience minimal anxiety related to procedure. | |

## Implementation

| **Steps** | **Rationale** |
|---|---|
| 1. Assemble supplies on bedside table with easy access to child. | Supplies should be available and within easy reach when suctioning to improve efficiency and safety. |
| 2. Turn on suction, check suction source, regulator, and suction bottle for proper functioning. Loosen lid on sterile water or saline bottle. | Checking and preparing equipment before "gloving" is necessary to maintain sterile technique during procedure.<br>***Special Considerations:*** *High suction pressures may cause trauma to airway tissue (Whaley and Wong, 1991) (see Table 87-2 on p. 551).* |
| 3. Using sterile technique:<br>a. Open suction kit package. | Sterile technique is used to prevent direct contamination of lower airways because inserting a suction catheter through an endotracheal or tracheostomy tube bypasses the upper airway's defenses against infection (Tafuro and Ristuccia, 1984). |
| b. Spread wrapper on bedside table. | Inside of package wrapper will serve as sterile field. |
| c. Put on gloves: maintain dominant hand as sterile; nondominant hand may be used for clean tasks. | ***Special Considerations:*** *Gloving both hands when suctioning lessens the risk of herpetic whitlow and HIV infection (Soule, 1983).* |
| d. Set up disposable sterile container with sterile hand; pour sterile water or saline solution into container with nonsterile hand. | Sterile water or saline will be used to flush catheter between suctioning passes. |
| e. Connect suction catheter to connecting tubing by grasping suction catheter in dominant sterile hand and connecting tubing in nondominant nonsterile hand. | |
| 4. Check suction pressure by suctioning a small amount of sterile solution through the suction catheter. | This lubricates the catheter and ensures that the equipment is working properly. Lubricating eases insertion, reduces tissue trauma, and prevents secretions from adhering to catheter lumen. |
| 5. Hyperventilate the child:<br>a. Using nonsterile hand, set oxygen at 100%. | Suctioning removes both secretions and oxygen from the airways. Hyperventilating with high oxygen concentrations increases alveolar oxygenation.<br>***Special Considerations:*** *If a plug is suspected in a larger airway, or copious secretions are present, suction before hyperventilating to avoid forcing the plug or secretions downward into distal airway.* |

| Steps | Rationale |
|---|---|
| b. If using manual resuscitation bag, attach the adaptor of the bag to the tracheostomy or endotracheal tube. | This method provides the ability to instantly start and stop the increased oxygen concentration. The disadvantages are the need for extra equipment and the required disconnection from the ventilator (Riegel and Forshee, 1985).<br>***Special Considerations:*** *Because excessive inflation pressure can cause barotrauma and pneumothoraces, inflating pressures of less than 30 cm of water are generally used in the intubated child (Hazinski, 1984).* |
| c. If child is able to breathe spontaneously, compress the resuscitator bag or the ventilator sigh button in synchrony as child inspires for 8 to 10 breaths. If apneic, deliver breaths about every 3 seconds. | The sigh setting on the ventilator will hyperinflate the child. An advantage of this method is the ability to control inspired volume and inspiratory pressure without extra equipment. Disadvantages include: the inability to instantly start and stop the increased oxygen concentration because most ventilators require a predetermined amount of time to increase the oxygen concentrations; and the possibility of forgetting to lower the oxygen concentration once suctioning is completed (Pierce and Piazza, 1987). |
| d. Observe the rise and fall of the child's chest with each ventilation. | Observing chest excursion ensures adequacy of ventilation. |
| e. Observe for possible gastric distension with continued use of bag. | Gastric distension can interfere with chest expansion and ventilation. |
| f. If distension occurs and is persistent, notify physician for possible nasogastric tube insertion (see Skill 65). | Insertion of a nasogastric tube can alleviate gastric distension caused by air being forced into stomach during hyperventilation. |
| 6. Disconnect child from oxygen source or ventilator and introduce catheter into artificial airway no further than 1 cm beyond the length of the tube. Do not advance until resistance is met (see the box below and Fig. 88-1). | Tissue damage can occur when suction catheter impacts airway tissue while being advanced (Kleiber, Krutzfield, and Rose, 1988). Deep suctioning results in significantly more tracheobronchial pathology than a shallow, premeasured technique (Bailey et al, 1988).<br>***Special Considerations:*** *Do not apply suction while catheter is being inserted. If resistance is met, withdraw catheter 1 to 2 cm before applying suction.* |

### *DEEP VERSUS SHALLOW SUCTION TECHNIQUE*

The traditional practice of inserting the suction catheter until resistance is met when suctioning may result in tracheal mucosa damage. A study done using anesthetized, intubated kittens compared four suction procedures. Animals in group 1 had the suction catheters inserted at a predetermined distance and withdrawn without the application of suction. In group 2, a catheter was inserted as in group 1 and withdrawn with suction applied at 75 mm Hg. In group 3, a catheter was advanced until resistance was met and withdrawn. Group 4 had the catheter advanced until resistance was met and withdrawn with suction applied at 75 mm Hg. Histologic examinations of animals in groups 1 and 2 revealed normal tracheal tissue. Nine of ten animals in groups 3 and 4 had multifocal areas of denuded epithelium and varying degrees of inflammation (Kleiber, Krutzfield, and Rose, 1988).

Another study by Bailey et al (1988) compared deep suctioning using a shallow, premeasured technique on anesthetized, intubated rabbits, yielding similar results. Increased tracheal mucosal necrosis and inflammation, greater loss of cilia, and increased mucus production were found with the deep suctioning technique. A mail survey of neonatal intensive care unit (NICU) physicians throughout the country was also conducted (Bailey et al, 1988) to assess the extent to which the deep suctioning technique was still being used. Of the 405 (43%) NICU physicians who responded, 82% reported frequent or exclusive use of the deep technique for routine suctioning.

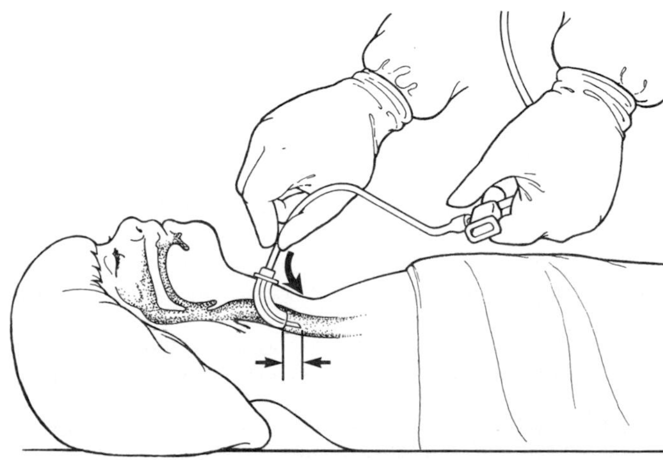

***FIG. 88-1*** The suction catheter is inserted into artificial airway.

| Steps | Rationale |
|---|---|
| 7. While obstructing suction port with thumb of nondominant hand, intermittently rotate suction catheter between thumb and forefinger of dominant hand as it is being withdrawn. Suction time should be as brief as possible, never longer than 5 to 10 seconds (Hazinski, 1984). Tracheostomy suctioning should not require more than 3 to 4 seconds since the length of the artificial airway is shorter than with an endotracheal tube (Chameides, 1988). | Rotating the catheter helps prevent invagination of airway tissue into openings on the suction catheter tip. Suctioning time is restricted to minimize oxygen loss. |
| 8. Monitor child's response to the procedure, including heart rate and rhythm, blood pressure, skin color, and oxygen saturation by pulse oximetry if available (see Skill 91). | Duration of suctioning has been shown to be related to the development of hypoxemia (Baun and Flones, 1984). Tachycardia is a sign of hypoxemia. Prolonged suctioning or repeated insertion of the suction catheter may produce vagal stimulation, which can cause profound bradycardia (Persons, 1987).<br>***Special Considerations:*** *Suctioning should be terminated immediately if child becomes bradycardic, hypotensive, cyanotic, mottled or develops pallor. The child should then be manually ventilated until stable (Hazinski, 1984).* |
| 9. Repeat suctioning until airways are cleared or child shows adverse signs as noted in Step 8. | |
| a. Allow at least 60 seconds between suctioning passes. | Sixty seconds or longer is required before oxygen tension returns to baseline values (Baun and Flones, 1984). |
| b. Hyperoxygenate and hyperventilate child before each suction pass. | Reoxygenating prevents hypoxia. |
| c. Rinse catheter with sterile solution between suction passes, observing amount, consistency, color, and odor of secretions obtained. | Rinsing keeps catheter and tubing patent. Observing secretions provides helpful information for assessing child's status. |
| 10. If secretions are thick and tenacious, instill appropriate amount of sterile saline solution into artificial airway just before hyperventilation. | Instilling saline may facilitate secretion removal through a lavage effect. (See the box on p. 556.) |
| 11. Use catheter to suction oropharynx and nasal passages after tracheal suctioning is completed (see Skill 87). | Failure to remove upper airway secretions can result in epiglottitis or pharyngitis (Perry and Potter, 1990).<br>***Special Considerations:*** *Never reuse catheter for (sterile technique) tracheal suctioning after (clean technique) oropharynx and nasal passage suctioning.* |
| 12. Manually ventilate child immediately after completing procedure. | Manually ventilating the child minimizes possible microatelectasis and reverses hypoxia or hypercapnia, which may have developed as a result of suctioning. |
| 13. Turn off the suction, and disconnect the catheter from the tubing. | |
| 14. Wrap used suction catheter around the fingers of sterile hand, and pull glove off over the catheter (see Fig. 87-4). Discard in proper waste container. | Proper disposal of contaminated catheters helps prevent nosocomial infections. |
| 15. Discard container with saline. | A container of saline for multiple use is discouraged; it serves as a reservoir for organisms from secretions aspirated through the tube (Whaley and Wong, 1991). |
| 16. Auscultate chest with stethoscope for breath sounds and equality of air movement, while observing for symmetrical chest movement. | Lungs should be carefully auscultated for ventilation adequacy and presence of congestion. Adventitious breath sounds should decrease with removal of secretions from airways. Asymmetrical movements may indicate migration of the endotracheal tube into a main stem bronchus.<br>***Special Considerations:*** *Be alert to the possibility of the endotracheal tube migrating into a main stem bronchus with manual ventilation (Hazinski, 1984).* |
| 17. Place the child in a position that is comfortable, safe, and facilitates breathing. | Proper positioning can enhance air exchange and promote comfort. |
| 18. Return oxygen concentration on ventilator to the prescribed maintenance amount. | Delivering higher concentrations of oxygen than needed for prolonged periods may have detrimental effects such as ciliary paralysis, interstitial thickening, and fibrotic changes of the retina in premature infants (retinopathy of prematurity) (Whaley and Wong, 1991). |
| 19. Replenish supplies so that suction is ready to be used again. | Because suctioning is often quickly needed, it is vital to leave the equipment ready for immediate use. |

| Evaluation Outcomes | Observational Guidelines |
|---|---|
| 1. The airway is cleared of excess secretions. | Auscultate breath sounds and compare with presuctioning assessment. Note amount of secretions removed in suction catheter during procedure. |
| 2. Oxygenation is improved. | Monitor heart rate, respiratory rate and effort, blood pressure, color of skin, and oxygen saturation by oximetry. Compare with presuctioning assessment. |
| 3. Hypoxemia is prevented or minimized during suctioning. | Monitor heart rate, oxygen saturation, and skin color changes during procedure. |
| 4. Trauma to airway tissues is prevented during suctioning. | Observe for blood-tinged aspirate, monitor suction pressures, note catheter rotation during suctioning. |
| 5. Discomfort to the child is minimized during suctioning. | Observe child's behavior and facial expressions during suctioning. Note if child is excessively fatigued afterward. |

### Documentation

Record time of suctioning and route suctioned; give description of secretions, including amount, consistency, color, and odor; amount of sterile saline instilled; child's tolerance of procedure; respiratory status before and after procedure.

### Home Care Modifications

1. In some cases, clean (and not sterile) technique suctioning may be used when caring for a child with a tracheostomy at home. A clean and disinfected catheter should be used each time. See Home Care Modifications in Skill 87. Home care instruction sheets on suctioning a tracheostomy are available in the *Clinical Manual of Pediatric Nursing* (Wong and Whaley, 1990).

# *SKILL* 89 Performing Chest Physiotherapy

*Bobbie J. Mackay*

Chest physiotherapy (CPT) is a therapeutic intervention applied to help natural airway clearance mechanisms (cough and ciliary cleansing mechanisms) reduce or prevent blockage of airways by thick, tenacious mucus. Bronchial (postural) drainage combines manual maneuvers such as percussion, vibration, and gravity to facilitate drainage and expectoration of lung and bronchial secretions. It is a means of moving mucus from the small airways to the larger central airways so that they may be coughed up or removed by suctioning. The area to be drained determines the position that the child is to assume.

## NURSING DIAGNOSES

Ineffective airway clearance related to inability to cough effectively, tracheobronchial secretions, or lack of family information about purpose and procedures for chest physiotherapy; Ineffective breathing pattern related to decreased lung expansion, immobility or musculoskeletal impairment.

| Steps | Rationale |
|---|---|
| **Assessment** | |
| 1. Identify physical indications for CPT:<br>a. Impairment of airway clearance.<br>▪ Weak, ineffective cough.<br>▪ Rapid, shallow respirations.<br>▪ Crackles. | Certain physical conditions predispose children to impaired airway clearance. These include impaired neuromuscular function, cough, mucociliary transport, or airways; a postoperative status or immobilization; and those with artificial airways or atelectasis. CPT with percussion and vibration can prevent or reduce associated complications. |
| b. Abnormal breath sounds.<br>▪ Wheezing.<br>▪ Crackles.<br>▪ Egophony (a nasal quality to speech that occurs when the voice sounds are transmitted through consolidated lung tissue). | Abnormal breath sounds indicate pathology often related to lung congestion and loose airway secretions. Egophony indicates consolidation of secretions in the lungs.<br>***Special Considerations:*** *CPT is not indicated in the initial phase of asthma.* |

| Steps | Rationale |
|---|---|
| c. Thick, tenacious, foul-smelling, and discolored secretions that are difficult to mobilize. Note the quantity, color, consistency, and odor of sputum. | The degree and location of lung congestion, if localized, will determine the postures used and areas to which chest physiotherapy is directed. Areas to be drained can be detected through auscultation of abnormal lung sounds, indicating loose secretions in the airways. For children with diffuse disease, treatments may need to be repeated over all lung areas several times per day (Irwin and Tecklin, 1985). |
| d. Breathing pattern.<br>■ Respiratory rate and depth.<br>■ Use of accessory muscles.<br>■ Chest wall movement. | Rapid, shallow breathing is a sign of serious chronic obstructive lung disease, asthma, or hypoxemia. |
| 2. Identify possible contraindications for CPT:<br>a. Conditions that preclude use of Trendelenburg position:<br>■ Increased intracranial pressure.<br>■ Bronchospasm.<br>■ Severe dyspnea.<br>■ Hypertension.<br>■ Hypoxemia, decreased arterial oxygen tension.<br>■ Lung hemorrhage or rupture.<br>■ Certain surgical procedures such as neurosurgery.<br>■ Traction.<br>■ Decreased cardiac output. | In children with severe respiratory insufficiency, movement of secretions into large airways can precipitate or potentiate bronchospasm, dyspnea, and hypoxemia.<br>***Special Considerations:*** *The physician should be notified if conditions develop that are contraindications for CPT.* |
| b. Conditions that preclude use of percussion or vibration:<br>■ Hemoptysis.<br>■ Pneumothorax.<br>■ Pulmonary emboli.<br>■ Areas of pain, tenderness, or swelling on shoulders, chest, or back.<br>■ Easily fractured bones, e.g., osteogenesis imperfecta.<br>■ Chest pain. | CPT can potentiate these conditions and should be discontinued until child's condition improves.<br>***Special Considerations:*** *Physician should be notified if symptoms of these conditions appear.* |
| 3. Determine child's age, developmental level, ability to understand procedure, and ability to cooperate. Assess diversional activities child might enjoy during CPT. | A child's age, developmental level, ability to understand, and ability to cooperate affect the achievement of effective treatments.<br>***Special Considerations:*** *Young children often fight the confinement of treatments. School-age children may exercise more self-control. They are likely to use diversional activities to help them pass the time. Treatment time serves as a prime time to develop a closer relationship with the child, discuss school activities, feelings, or concerns. School-age children are likely to respond to diversional activities such as watching television, listening to music or a radio program. Teenagers resent interference with their activities and goals and often are noncompliant.* |
| 4. Determine parents' understanding of and ability to perform CPT at home. Assess:<br>a. Health beliefs and behaviors that might interfere with parents' willingness to comply with therapy recommendations.<br>b. Perceived need for CPT.<br>c. Barriers to learning.<br>d. Willingness to learn. | Assessment allows for appropriate discharge planning. Home CPT is indicated in children with chronic lung conditions such as cystic fibrosis, bronchiectasis, atelectasis, chronic bronchitis, or emphysema.<br>***Special Considerations:*** *Including parents and children in plan of care ensures it is individualized for a particular child and enhances compliance. Both parents should be encouraged to participate and share this responsibility, if possible.* |
| 5. Assess ability of older child to do self-chest physiotherapy:<br>a. Level of maturity.<br>b. Ability to follow directions.<br>c. Ability and willingness to assume responsibility.<br>d. Level of understanding about the disease and rationale for therapy. | At about 12 years of age, children have the physical and emotional maturity to perform treatments on themselves. Responsibility for self-care prepares children for adulthood and fosters a sense of independence, positive self-worth, and control. |

## Planning and Goal Setting

| Steps | Rationale |
|---|---|
| 1. Check physician's order to determine number of treatments per day. | A physician determines initiation of CPT, specifies number of treatments per day, and may specify areas to be drained and percussed. |
| 2. Plan CPT around child's sleep, meal time, play schedule, family activities, and treatments each day. If possible, allow child to choose time of treatment. | Timing treatments is an important aspect in planning for a child's care. CPT should not conflict with other distracting activities. The child will cooperate better and resent the limitations treatment places on lifestyle less if consideration is given to individual needs and goals. |

| Steps | Rationale |
|---|---|
| | ***Special Considerations:*** *More than two treatments per day are difficult to plan around daily activities. However, physical needs of other family members and playtime must be considered when planning therapy to promote normal development of all family members, prevent resentments from developing, and enhance family functioning.* |
| a. Plan CPT in the morning on rising if receiving treatment once daily. | CPT in the morning mobilizes respiratory secretions that have accumulated in child's airway overnight and helps clear airways for daytime activities. |
| b. Plan CPT around bedtime, before meals, or 1½ hours after mealtime if recommended 2 or more times per day. | Treatments performed at bedtime clear airways for the period of inactivity. CPT should be done on an empty stomach to avoid vomiting or aspiration.<br>***Special Considerations:*** *The child with reflux may need a longer time of fasting before CPT (see Skill 63).* |
| c. For treatment given before meals, plan at least 30 minutes between the end of treatment and the meal for coughing and mobilization of secretions. | CPT may stimulate expectoration of copious amounts of thick, tenacious secretions, which may cause posttussive vomiting if a child eats immediately following therapy. Children may also experience nausea and vomiting following CPT from swallowing their secretions. |
| d. Allow 30 minutes for each treatment and 30 additional minutes if nebulization treatments are necessary. | ***Special Considerations:*** *Bronchodilators should be given 20 minutes before CPT when ordered to allow medication to take effect.* |
| e. Plan for periods of rest after CPT. Avoid major activities such as bath or exercise. | Children with severe lung disease may be exhausted after a treatment. |
| f. Stop tube feeding 30 to 45 minutes before CPT. If more than 100 ml of residual feeding remains in the stomach, hold the treatment for 30 minutes. | CPT should be done on an empty stomach to avoid vomiting and aspiration. |
| g. Provide for privacy. | Treatments and the resulting coughing and expectoration are often embarrassing to the older child. |
| 3. Assemble necessary equipment:<br>a. Tilt table, hospital bed, or chair.<br>b. One to four pillows. | Equipment and pillows provide for more accurate positioning and comfort for the child.<br>***Special Considerations:*** *Improvised equipment may be used to assist in positioning the child correctly for drainage by gravity (see the box at right). With infants, therapy is easiest when carried out on nurse's/parent's lap.* |
| c. Instruction sheet for CPT. | Written information, which enhances retention, is available for parents to review and refer to while learning how to perform CPT. |
| d. Glass of water or other fluids. | Fluids decrease tenacity of mucus so that it is easier to mobilize and cough out. Fluids also keep the mouth moist for comfort.<br>***Special Considerations:*** *High fluid intake should be encouraged unless medically contraindicated as in congestive heart failure or renal disease.* |
| e. Paper tissues, trash bags, or a clear plastic container with a cover for disposal of sputum. | Proper disposal of sputum promotes good sanitation and allows for quantity and consistency of sputum to be examined.<br>***Special Considerations:*** *It is not harmful for children to swallow their secretions. If thick tenacious mucus is swallowed, the child may experience some nausea.* |
| f. Mechanical percussor, vibrator, or rubber cups. | ***Special Considerations:*** *Mechanical devices can be used when parents are unable to perform manual method. Rubber cups are available for manual percussion. These are especially helpful if nurse's or parent's hands are too large to form a good cup on the child's chest.* |
| 4. Cover child's skin with thin cloth or shirt. Nurse or parents should remove rings from fingers. Teenage girls should remove bra and avoid tight-fitting clothes. | Percussing on the child's bare skin can cause local skin irritation. Rings interfere with a good cupping formation of the hand and can cause bruising if they come in contact with the child's skin during treatment. |
| 5. Determine areas to be drained according to assessment of lung fields, clinical findings, and chest x-ray data. | Treatment is individualized to improve congested areas in the lung. Children with localized disease require therapy to congested lung fields. The length of treatment will depend on extent of congestion. Children with diffuse progressive disease require therapy in all lung segments. |

### *IMPROVISED EQUIPMENT FOR CHEST PHYSIOTHERAPY*

1. The foot of the bed may be elevated. Some beds will be unsuitable for this method.

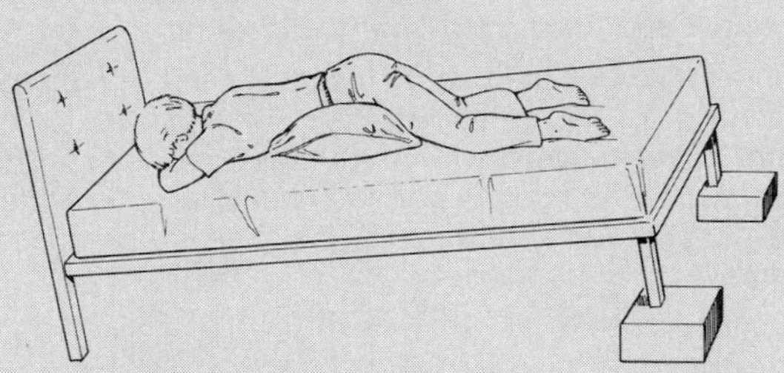

2. An upturned chair may be used.

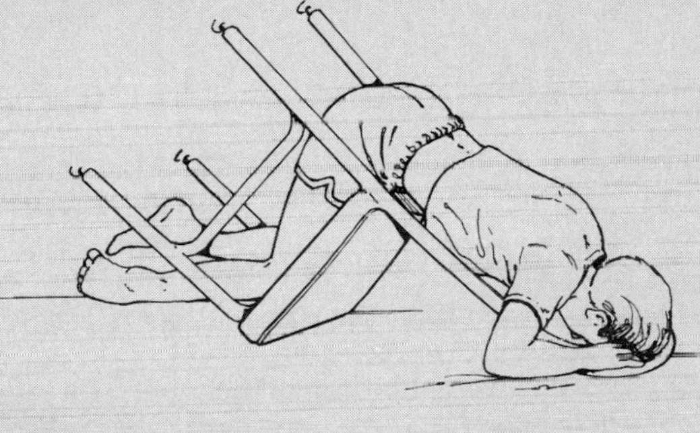

3. A pile of magazines or newspapers may be piled on a bed with one or two pillows on the top.

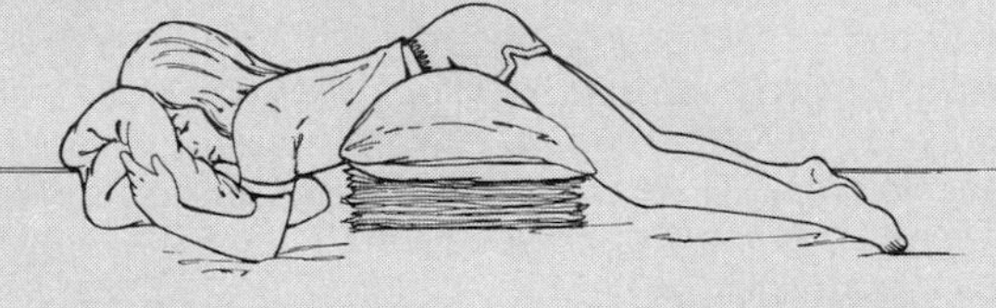

4. A child may lie over the side of the bed.

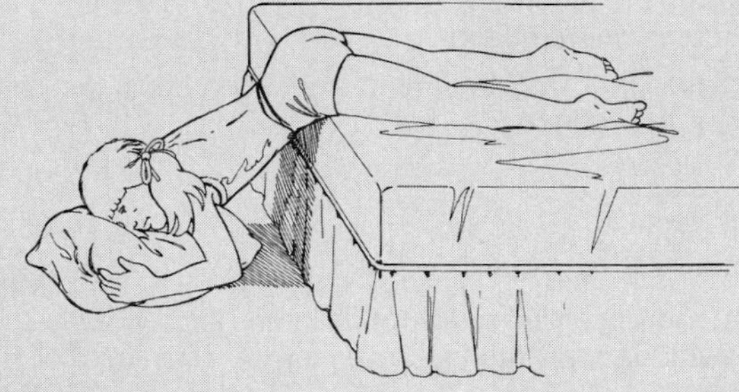

5. A board may be laid on a sofa with one end of the board on the sofa arm.

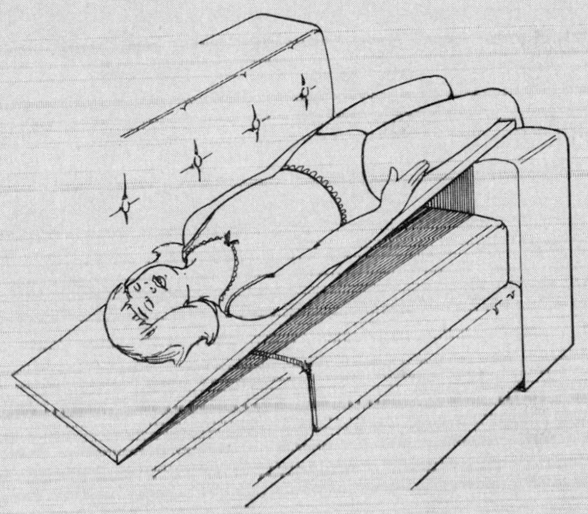

6. A six-way pillow may be used.

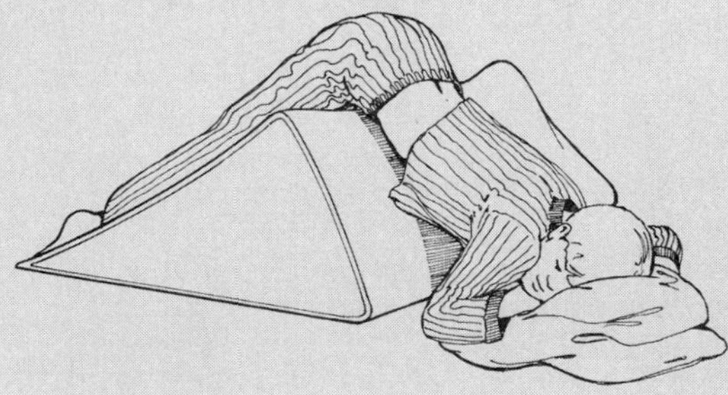

| Steps | Rationale |
|---|---|
| 6. Prepare child for treatment using developmentally appropriate methods. | A child who is well prepared can gather personal resources to help him or her deal with treatments. A child may cooperate better if relaxed and comfortable. |
| a. Explain procedure and reason for treatment in terms child can comprehend. | ***Special Considerations:*** *Use words such as "pounding" to "knock out" "mucus" or "germs" from the lungs.* |
| b. Explain length of treatment and discomfort the child might experience. | Discomforts of CPT are usually mild but can be frightening to a child. ***Special Considerations:*** *Discomforts include shortness of breath, increased cough during and following treatments, and nasal congestion and pressure in the head from placement in Trendelenburg position.* |
| 7. Develop individualized goals for child and family:<br>▪ Child will demonstrate improved airway clearance for secretions.<br>▪ Child will tolerate treatments with minimal discomfort.<br>▪ Parents or child will be able to perform CPT before discharge from hospital, if indicated.<br>▪ A reasonable home care plan for treatments will be developed that takes into consideration child's physical and psychosocial needs and other demands on the family. | |

## Implementation

| Steps | Rationale |
|---|---|
| 1. Have child cough or suction trachea before beginning treatment. | Secretions that have accumulated in the trachea should be removed before CPT. |
| 2. Therapist and parents should wash hands before treatment. | Good handwashing reduces the transmission of disease-producing organisms. |
| 3. Administer bronchodilators as ordered before CPT. | Bronchodilators help open bronchial tubes before treatment, facilitating drainage of secretions and mucus (Wong and Whaley, 1990). |
| 4. Select areas of lungs to be percussed. Treatments may be split up into sections and performed at various times throughout the day. | It may be difficult to keep child's attention and maintain cooperation for long periods. Children have variable attention spans. ***Special Considerations:*** *For children with diffuse, progressive disease the entire treatment may be required several times per day.* |
| 5. Place child in appropriate drainage position (see Fig. 89-1 for child and Fig. 89-2 for infant). Assist child in assuming proper positioning, placing pillows for comfort, support, and to maintain position. | The order of postures assumed varies according to selected areas to be drained. Usual order begins with upper lobes, then middle lobes, followed by lower lobes. Through entire treatment, mucus is directed toward main bronchus where it can be coughed or suctioned out. ***Special Considerations:*** *For middle and lower lobes, when child is placed in Trendelenburg position, make sure child's back is angled properly. Avoid propping child's buttocks without considering the angle of child's back.* |
| 6. Teach child and parent correct posture, positioning of pillows, and arm and leg positioning. | Teaching family members how to assume postures enables them to be self-sufficient and compliant with medical recommendations at home. ***Special Considerations:*** *If child is short of breath in Trendelenburg position, postures may need to be modified to meet individual needs. Lateral lobes may need to be done with child lying flat on side or in sidelying semi-Fowlers position (Perry and Potter, 1990).* |
| 7. Perform percussion using cupped hands (Fig. 89-3). Clap rhythmically over specific area to be drained. Mold hands side by side to form contour of chest. Alternate hands while clapping. Clapping should be vigorous, not painful. Speed and rhythm vary with experience and individual techniques. | Percussion with cupped hands on chest wall over segment to be drained sets up vibrations that are transmitted to the bronchi and help mobilize mucus and clear airways. Percussion is painless when performed properly. The cupped hand tends to trap a cushion of air, softening the impact of clapping. ***Special Considerations:*** *The entire circumference of the hand touches chest with each clapping motion. This should make a loud popping sound that resembles a galloping horse. It should not sound like slapping (Wong and Whaley, 1990).* |
| 8. Percuss 1 minute over lung segment to be drained. | ***Special Considerations:*** *Avoid percussing over breast tissue, backbone, stomach, or kidneys. Do not percuss below rib cage.* |

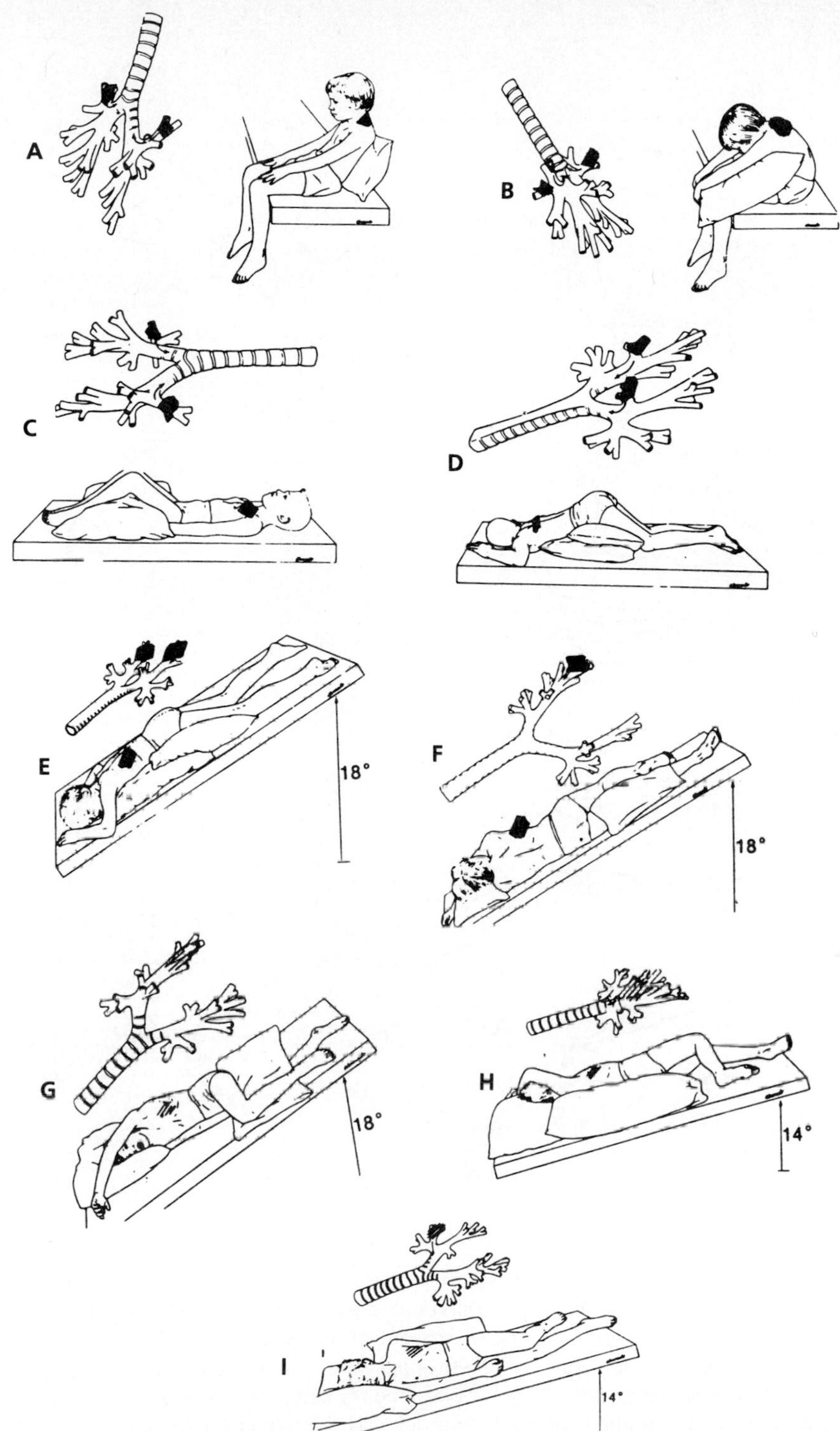


***FIG. 89-1*** Bronchial drainage positions for all major segments of child. For each position, model of tracheobronchial tree is projected beside child to show segmental bronchus being drained and pathway of secretions out of bronchus. Drainage platform is horizontal unless otherwise noted. Darkened area on child's chest indicates area to be cupped or vibrated by therapist. **A,** Apical segment of right upper lobe and apical subsegment of apical-posterior segment of left upper lobe. **B,** Posterior segment of right upper lobe and posterior subsegment of apical-posterior segment of left upper lobe. **C,** Anterior segments of both upper lobes; child should be rotated slightly away from side being drained. **D,** Superior segments of both lower lobes. **E,** Posterior basal segments of both lower lobes. **F,** Lateral basal segments of right lower lobe; left lateral basal segment would be drained by mirror image of this position (right side down). **G,** Anterior basal segment of left lower lobe; right anterior basal segment would be drained by mirror image of this position (left side down). **H,** Medial and lateral segments of right middle lobe. **I,** Lingular segments (superior and inferior) of left upper lobe (homologue of right middle lobe).

From Kendig EL Jr, editor: Disorders of the respiratory tract of children, ed 4, Philadelphia, 1983, WB Saunders.

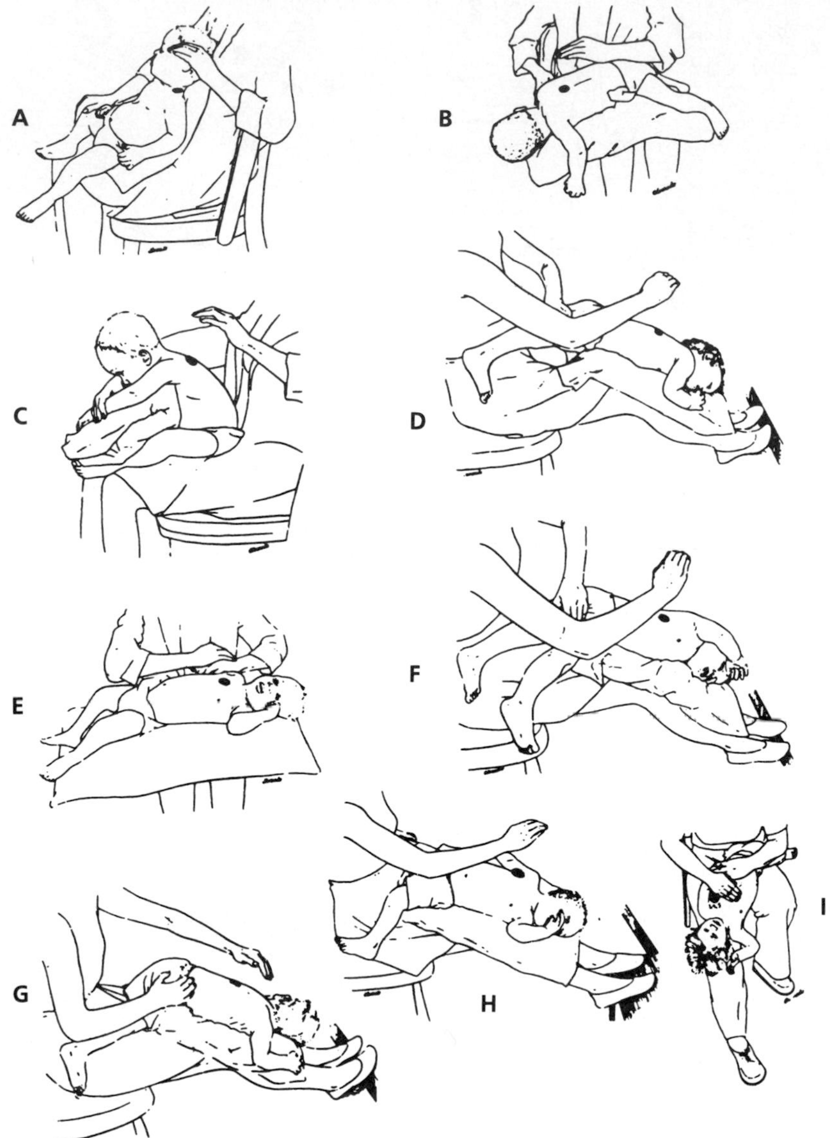


***FIG. 89-2*** Bronchial drainage positions for major sections of all lobes in infant. Procedure is most easily carried out in therapist's lap. Darkened area on child's chest indicates area to be cupped or vibrated by therapist. **A,** Apical segment of left upper lobe. **B,** Posterior segment of left upper lobe. **C,** Anterior segment of left upper lobe. **D,** Superior segment of right lower lobe. **E,** Posterior basal segment of right lower lobe. **F,** Lateral basal segment of right lower lobe. **G,** Anterior basal segment of right lower lobe. **H,** Medial and lateral segments of right middle lobe. **I,** Lingular segments (superior and inferior) of left upper lobe. Modified from Infant segmental bronchial drainage.

From Whaley L and Wong D: Nursing Care of Infants and Children, ed 4, St. Louis, 1991, The CV Mosby Co. Reprinted with permission of the Cystic Fibrosis Foundation, Rockville, MD.

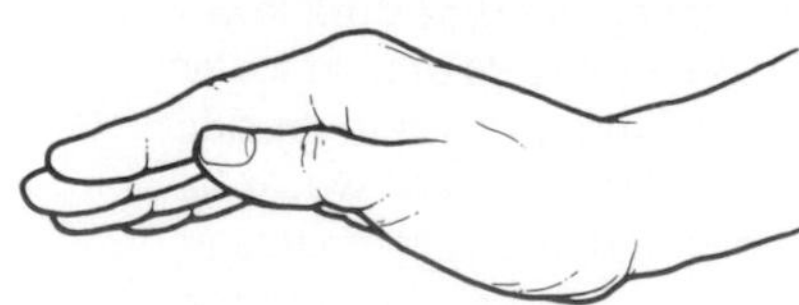

***FIG. 89-3*** The chest wall is percussed with a cupped hand.

From Wong DL and Whaley LF: Clinical manual of pediatric nursing, ed 3, 1990, St Louis, The CV Mosby Co.

| **Steps** | **Rationale** |
|---|---|

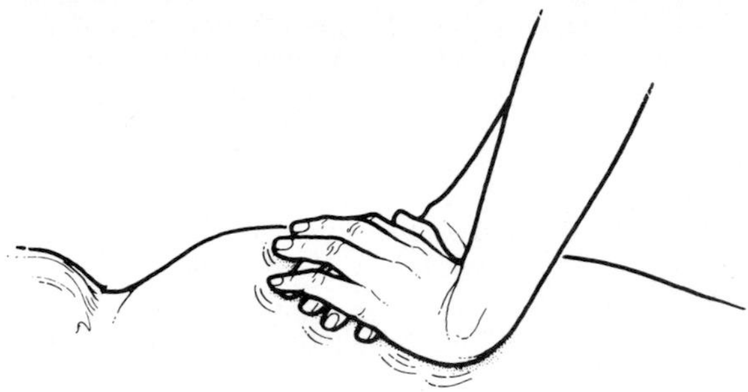

***FIG. 89-4*** Hand position for vibration.

From Wong DL and Whaley LF: Clinical manual of pediatric nursing, ed 3, 1990, St Louis, The CV Mosby Co.

| Steps | Rationale |
|---|---|
| 9. Vibrate 2 to 3 times.<br>a. Place hand over hand on area to be drained as child takes in a slow, deep breath.<br>b. Have child exhale through pursed lips, contract abdominal muscles, and relax chest wall muscles.<br>c. While child is exhaling, gently push down and perform isometric contractions of forearm with flat part of hand. Hold elbows slightly bent (Fig. 89-4).<br>d. Release pressure after child exhales.<br>e. Repeat vibrations 2 to 3 times.<br>f. Child should cough by taking deep breath and doing a series of small coughs. Vibrate chest as child coughs. | Vibration stimulates flow of secretions during prolonged, forced expiration. Pursed-lip breathing helps child slow down breathing so that more air moves into and out of lungs, keeping small airways from collapsing and trapping air in lungs. Coughing with vibration helps clear mucus from airways.<br>***Special Considerations:*** *Vibration is usually not performed manually on infants, although an electric vibrating tool may be used.* |
| 10. Percuss for another minute over same segment. Percussion should be done at a comfortable, effective, moderately fast rate. | |
| 11. Repeat vibration 2 to 3 times over the same segment during exhalation. | |
| 12. Allow child to sit up to cough between each segment being drained. | Any secretions mobilized should be removed by coughing or suctioning before beginning next position. Coughing is most effective when child is sitting up and leaning forward.<br>***Special Considerations:*** *If secretions are not expectorated after each posture, proceed to the next position. At times secretions are coughed up 1 to 2 hours after CPT when the mucus gradually becomes loosened from the sides of the smaller airways and moves to the larger airways where it can be coughed up.* |
| 13. Have child expectorate into a clear container or tissues. | Infants and small children usually swallow mucus that is brought up from the lungs. Swallowing the mucus is not harmful, but the mucus may upset the stomach and cause the child to vomit. At about 3 or 4 years of age, child may be taught to expectorate mucus coughed up from the lungs. |
| 14. Have the child rest between positions if necessary. | Individualize therapy to meet needs of each child. A child with more severe disease may require short rest periods between positions to prevent fatigue and enable child to better tolerate the treatment. Other children who do not tire easily may prefer to move through entire treatment without interruption. |
| 15. Change positions per Figs. 89-1 and 89-2 and repeat steps 7 to 14 until all congested areas have been drained. Treatment should take approximately 30 minutes if child is cooperative. | CPT is based on individual assessed needs. |
| 16. If long-term therapy is to be continued in the home, teach parents and child (if appropriate for child's age) positions for postural drainage, percussion, and vibration. | Long-term therapy at home may prevent the progression of chronic lung disease and maintain a clear airway. |
| 17. Carefully teach family members techniques of CPT, and observe them as they demonstrate. | |
| 18. If necessary, initiate referral to assess regimen through home health or outpatient follow-up care. | A home visit will validate proper performance of CPT and allow for further teaching, if needed. |

## Evaluation Outcomes

1. Child demonstrates improved airway clearance following CPT.

## Observational Guidelines

Observe gradual changes in chest assessment after CPT such as improved breath sounds with reduction of abnormal breath sounds; expectorated sputum becomes more normal, and sputum is coughed up more easily; decreased cough; less dyspnea and breathes more easily; improved pulmonary function studies, radiologic examinations and blood gases; and improved muscle stamina and flexibility.

2. Child tolerates the procedure with minimal discomfort.

Observe child's behaviors and verbal statements during procedure. Note level of fatigue following CPT. Ask child about level of discomfort.

3. Child (if age appropriate) and/or family demonstrates adequate knowledge base regarding CPT.

Interview child and family about indications for CPT, principles, and safety considerations.

4. Family members demonstrate CPT, percussion, and vibration correctly.

Observe family members perform procedure. Note proper positioning of child and use of techniques.

5. A plan is developed for implementation of CPT at home, including timing and rotation of responsibility.

View the written plan. Interview family members about their satisfaction with the plan.

## Documentation

Document pretreatment and posttreatment assessment of chest; frequency and duration of treatment and segments drained; effectiveness of cough; color, amount, and consistency of sputum; need for suctioning; child's cooperation and tolerance of treatment; any unexpected results of therapy such as hemoptysis, bronchospasm, or pneumothorax.

If parents, child, or significant others are taught CPT for home care, chart instructions given; understanding of rationale and skill; demonstration of proper positions, percussion and vibration; barriers to learning and compliance; referral for follow-up such as home care agency or pulmonary nurse specialist.

## Home Care Modifications

1. Parents may need to use improvised equipment for positioning in the home (see the box on p. 563).
2. Keep equipment and medications out of reach of children.
3. Parents may want to make a tilt-table for use in chest physiotherapy; tilt-tables may be purchased through most respiratory equipment companies.

# *SKILL* 90 Administering and Monitoring Oxygen

*Patricia A. Jamerson*

Oxygen is frequently administered to infants and children to correct hypoxia, minimize the work of breathing, and decrease myocardial work (Walters, Elmore, and Grandy, 1984). But like other drug therapies, it may be detrimental as well as beneficial. Low arterial oxygen tension may lead to cellular damage and death. Excessive oxygenation may result in pulmonary atelectasis and epithelial damage, brain and red blood cell destruction, and in infants, retinopathy of the premature (ROP), previously referred to as retrolental fibroplasia (RLF) (Rarey and Youlsey, 1981; Whaley and Wong, 1991).

Many delivery systems used for adults are also used with children—nasal cannulas, simple face masks, partial rebreather masks, nonrebreathing masks, Venturi masks, face tents, tracheostomy masks, and ventilators. Additional systems specifically designed for children are oxygen/croup tents and hoods.

## NURSING DIAGNOSES

Impaired gas exchange related to altered oxygen supply, alveolar hypoventilation; Anxiety related to unmet informational needs about purpose, procedure, and precautions of oxygen administration; Impaired skin integrity related to irritation of oxygen delivery system; Potential for injury related to adverse effects of hypoxia or hyperoxia; Potential altered body temperature related to exposure to cool or heated humidified oxygen; Fluid volume excess related to excessive fluid intake from humidification.

**Steps** | **Rationale**

## Assessment

1. Assess child for manifestations of hypoxia, including:
   a. Respiratory status, e.g., rate, effort, breath sounds, color.
   b. Neurologic status, e.g., level of consciousness, muscle tone, reflex response.
   c. Cardiovascular status, e.g., heart rate, blood pressure, perfusion, urine output.

Oxygen should not be used without specific indications (AAP/ACOG, 1988). Oxygen is an essential energy source needed to maintain cellular function; hypoxia may lead to cellular damage and eventually death. Baseline assessments are necessary to determine the need for and effectiveness of therapy.

   d. Laboratory data, e.g., arterial blood gases, hemoglobin and hematocrit.
   e. Noninvasive monitoring values, e.g., pulse oximetry, transcutaneous oxygen monitoring.

Blood gas values are the most accurate indicators of the need for therapy.
**Special Considerations:** *In severe respiratory distress, oxygen therapy may be instituted before obtaining baseline arterial blood gas values.*

2. Assess size and developmental status of child.

The type/size of delivery system needed is based on child's size and child's ability to cooperate (Lough, Doershuk and Stern, 1979).

3. Review medical history, and present respiratory status for factors that may influence oxygen therapy, e.g., chronic lung conditions (bronchopulmonary dysplasia, cystic fibrosis, asthma); acute conditions (respiratory syncytial virus, suspected epiglottitis); bypass of upper airway (tracheostomy); and nasal obstruction (nasogastric tube, copious drainage).

Preexisting disorders and respiratory status may influence the delivery system used, may determine if humidification is necessary, and may dictate the aggressiveness of oxygen therapy. For example, conservative administration of oxygen is necessary in children with cystic fibrosis to avoid elimination of the hypoxic respiratory drive (Whaley and Wong, 1991).
**Special Considerations:** *Mist tent therapy is not beneficial for lower airway disorders, as humidification seldom extends past the nasopharynx. It is also contraindicated when epiglottitis is suspected, since close observation of a child in a tent is not possible, and respiratory status can quickly deteriorate (Kleiber, 1989).*

4. Review physician's order for:
   a. Oxygen concentration and/or flow rate.
   b. Method of delivery.
   c. Therapy duration.
   d. Desired $SaO_2$.

Oxygen is a drug and, as with all medications, requires a physician's order and administration guidelines.
**Special Considerations:** *Although oxygen therapy is a medical decision, collaboration on the aspects of delivery based on nursing assessment is appropriate.*

5. Assess child/family's understanding of oxygen therapy.

Anxiety and lack of cooperation may result from misunderstanding or lack of information about administration techniques.

## Planning and Goal Setting

1. Assemble necessary equipment at child's bedside:

Gathering needed equipment allows oxygen delivery system to be set up quickly and efficiently.

   a. "Oxygen In Use" and "No Smoking" signs.

Oxygen supports combustion, therefore these signs alert family, staff, and visitors of necessary safety precautions.

   b. Oxygen source (one of the following):
      - 50 psi wall outlet.
      - Compressed oxygen (cylinder/tank).
      - Liquid oxygen concentrator.

**Special Considerations:** *In most institutions 100% oxygen is piped from a centralized store to the wall outlet under pressures of 50 pounds per square inch (psi). Other oxygen sources available may be used in the home. Compressed oxygen comes in four cylinder sizes (H, K, D, and E). Cylinders D and E are small and easily portable. Liquid oxygen is available in 40 to 90 lb reservoirs. Oxygen concentrators, which plug into standard electrical outlets, provide low flows (<5 L/min) of $O_2$ by extracting oxygen from room air. Delivery systems that require oxygen flow rates greater than 5 L/min rapidly deplete portable stores and are better used when wall outlet oxygen is available.*

   c. Flow meter.

A flow meter regulates the liter flow of oxygen, and therefore the fraction of inspired oxygen ($FiO_2$) in low flow devices.

   d. Humidification source (optional) and sterile water (one of following):
      - Pass-over humidifier.
      - Diffusion-head humidifier (bubbler).
      - Nebulizer.
      - Croupette.

Adding humidity counteracts the drying effect of supplemental oxygen and subsequent thickening of pulmonary secretions. Cool humidification provided by a croup tent may decrease laryngeal edema and tracheal irritation. Sterile water provides moisture while minimizing bacterial contamination and equipment damage.

| Steps | Rationale |
|---|---|
| | ***Special Considerations:*** *Humidity should be provided whenever the upper airway is bypassed such as in children with tracheostomies and in neonates, particularly premature infants, to minimize insensible water losses (Koff, Eitzman, and Neu, 1988). Otherwise, routine humidification is not indicated at flow rates less than 4 L/min when environmental humidity is adequate (Fulmer and Snider, 1984).* |
| e. Heating device (optional) (one of following): ▪ Wrap-around heater. ▪ Hot-plate device. ▪ Probe-type heating element. | Heat increases the relative humidity of supplemental oxygen. All newborns and children with tracheostomies need heated, humidified oxygen (Koff, Eitzman and Neu, 1988). Loss of body heat can be significant in small infants if cool aerosol is used (Hazinski, 1984). ***Special Considerations:*** *Temperature and water level in a humidifier should be monitored to avoid overheating.* |
| f. Device to regulate oxygen concentration (optional) (one of following): | These devices allow continuous delivery of specific oxygen concentrations. |
| ▪ Blender (mixer). | A blender mixes air and oxygen proportionately to yield a specific concentration. |
| ▪ Venturi system. | A Venturi system provides various $O_2$ concentrations by using different sized adaptors or entrainment ports, which mix room air with $O_2$ in a predetermined ratio to deliver a specific $FiO_2$. |
| g. Connective tubing: ▪ Large bore (22 mm) for nebulizers and heated humidifiers. ▪ Small bore for other delivery systems. | Large-bore tubing is necessary for devices that are susceptible to moisture buildup in the tubing because of condensation. This condensation in small-bore tubing would prevent $O_2$ flow. |
| h. Oxygen analyzer (optional). | Oxygen analyzers detect the concentration of environmental oxygen and allow monitoring to maintain consistent oxygen administration. |
| i. Delivery system (one of following): | |
| ▪ Appropriate-sized nasal cannula. | A nasal cannula is a vinyl tube with two small prongs that fit into the nares. Appropriate sized cannulas allow air to flow around the outside diameter of the prongs while in the nares (Koff, Eitzman, and Neu, 1988). ***Special Considerations:*** *If appropriate-sized cannula is unavailable or nasal prongs are not well tolerated, they may be trimmed or completely removed (Fig. 90-1) (Kloor and Carbajal, 1984; Koff, Eitzman, and Neu, 1988).* |

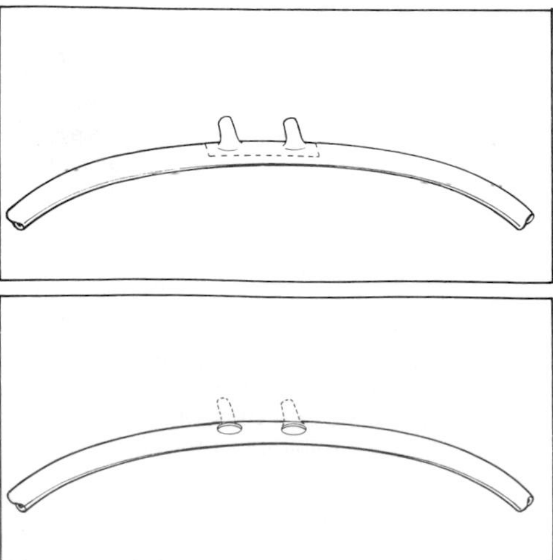

***FIG. 90-1*** Nasal cannula modifications.

| Steps | Rationale |
|---|---|
| ▪ Oxygen Mask: | Oxygen masks are soft, transparent vinyl reservoirs designed to fit snugly over the mouth and nose. ***Special Considerations:*** *There is a high risk of vomitus aspiration with a mask. For some children a mask may be a source of anxiety; using fantasy play (e.g., jet pilot) may elicit cooperation. Masks must be removed for eating and drinking, therefore an alternative delivery system may be necessary.* |
| (1) Simple face mask. | The simple face mask has open ports on each side, allowing exhalation of carbon dioxide and inspiration of room air if ventilatory needs exceed gas flow. This device provides a $FiO_2$ of 30 to 60% with oxygen flow rates of 6 to 10 L/min. |
| (2) Partial rebreather mask. | The partial rebreather mask is similar to a simple face mask with the addition of a reservoir bag. Gas flow may need to be adjusted to maintain bag volume one-third full during inspiration. $FiO_2$ values between 40% to 60% may be achieved with oxygen flow rates of 6 to 10 L/min. |
| (3) Nonrebreathing mask. | Similar to a partial rebreather mask; additional features include a one-way valve between the bag and mask, preventing inhalation of expired gas; and one-way valves or rubber flaps on the side ports allowing exhalation, but preventing inhalation of room air. Delivery of $FiO_2$ from 60% to 100% is possible with oxygen flow rates of 6 to 15 L/min. |
| (4) Venturi mask (Fig. 90-2). | The Venturi mask is similar to a simple face mask with the addition of wide-bore tubing connected to an adapter (cone) with a fixed orifice that allows a certain proportion of air to be entrained and mixed with oxygen to deliver a specific $FiO_2$. $FiO_2$ delivery is independent of liter flow. Different sized adapters allow $FiO_2$ from 24% to 50%. |

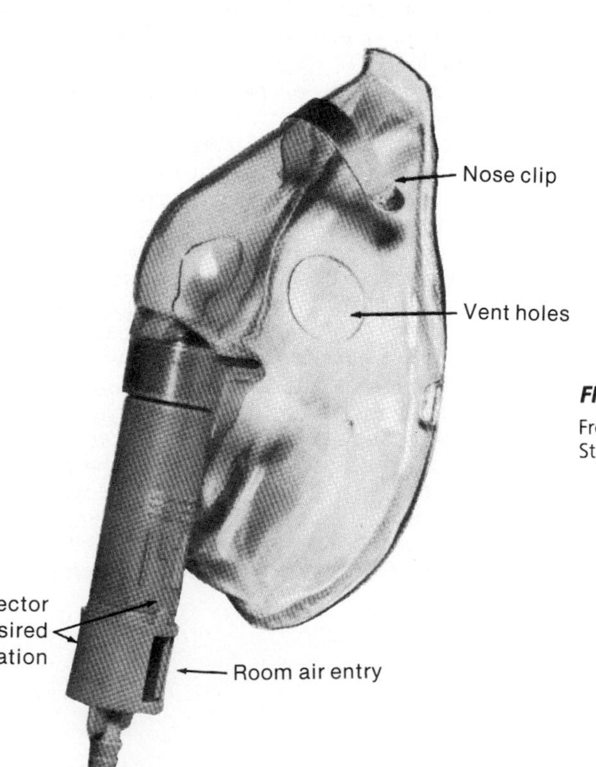


***FIG. 90-2*** Venturi Mask.

From Perry AG and Potter PA: Clinical nursing skills and techniques, St Louis, 1990, The CV Mosby Co.

| Steps | Rationale |
|---|---|
| 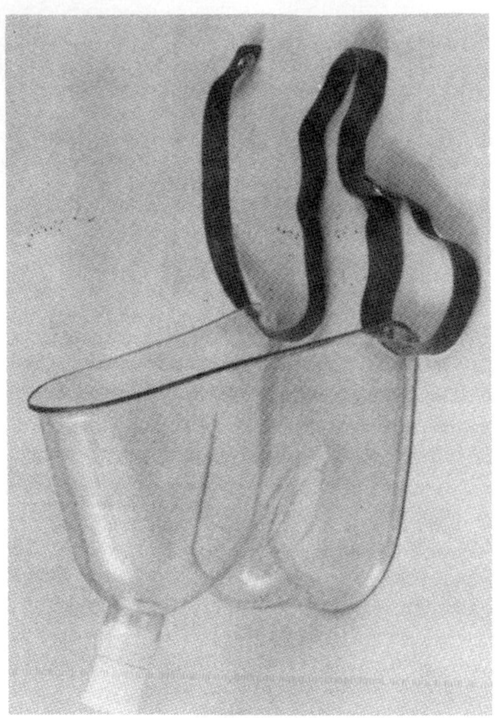 | ***FIG. 90-3*** Face Tent.<br>From Perry AG and Potter PA: Clinical nursing skills and techniques, ed 2, St Louis, 1990, The CV Mosby Co. |
| ▪ Aerosol masks with large-bore tubing: | Capable of providing high humidity and a wide range of oxygen concentrations (28% to 100% at flow rates of 8 to 12 L/min), aerosol masks are adaptations of the simple face mask. |
| (1) Face tent (Fig. 90-3). | More readily accepted than masks, a face tent made out of soft, transparent vinyl is contoured to fit loosely around the face and neck. |
| (2) Tracheostomy mask (collar). | A tracheostomy mask is a plastic cup with a large port contoured to fit a tracheostomy. |
| ▪ Oxygen/croup tent. | An oxygen tent is a large, clear plastic canopy designed to enclose the child in an oxygen-enriched environment. A built-in fan circulates air within the tent to help prevent overheating. The croup tent, a modification of the oxygen tent, is used to provide cool humidification in addition to oxygen. The croup tent may be an open or closed canopy that fits directly on the bed or is mounted at the head of the bed. Oxygen entering the tent is cooled by ice or a refrigeration unit. Oxygen concentrations up to 50% may be achieved using flow rates of 7 to 15 L/min. |
| ▪ Appropriate-sized oxygen hood with baffle and thermometer (Fig. 90-4). The hood should fit comfortably over the head and/or upper body of the infant or young child without rubbing against the neck, chin, or shoulders. | Oxygen hoods are Plexiglas cylinders/boxes or disposable porous vinyl huts designed to provide an oxygen-enriched environment. A baffle inside the hood provides circulation of airflow and diverts airflow away from the infant's head to minimize convection heat loss, and assists to maintain oxygen concentration to the child during inadvertent leaks. Temperature regulation is important to avoid overheating, as well as cooling, which can lead to increased oxygen consumption and apnea. |

| **Steps** | **Rationale** |
|---|---|

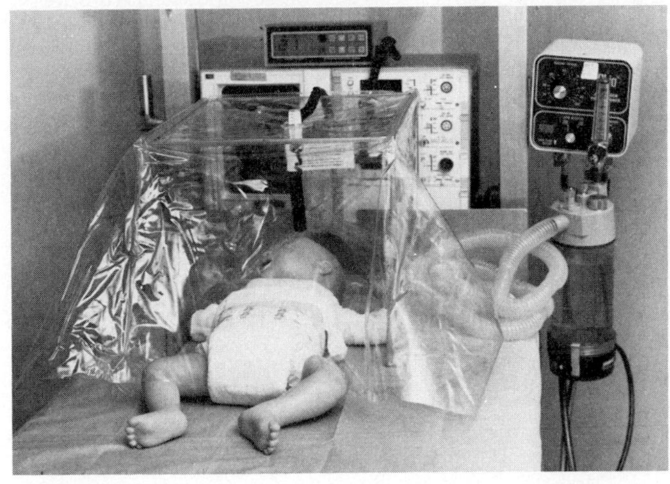

***FIG. 90-4*** Equipment used for oxygen administration: analyzer, hood, blender, flow meter, and nebulizer.

| Steps | Rationale |
|---|---|
| j. Additional linens such as sheets, gowns, blankets, diapers. | Frequent linen changes may be necessary to avoid evaporative heat losses attributable to moisture from aerosols or heated humidifiers. |
| k. Restraints (optional) (see Skill 51). | Restraints may be necessary if a child is uncooperative, and an alternative system cannot be used. |
| 2. Assemble equipment; select steps based on chosen system and variations: | Equipment assembly expedites initiation of treatment. |
| a. Secure oxygen/croup tent at head of or on bed/crib and attach to canopy, draping over bed/crib. Secure overbed frame with gauze strips and pad with rolled towel or bath blanket. | Securing tent to bed and using padding protects child from potential injury. Padding also helps absorb excess moisture. ***Special Considerations:*** *The child should not be in the bed/crib while the tent is being assembled and secured.* |
| b. Connect blender, if used, to oxygen and air sources. Select prescribed concentration. | |
| c. Attach flow meter to blender, or directly to oxygen source (Fig. 90-4). | |
| d. Attach humidifier/nebulizer, prefilled with sterile water to flow meter (Fig. 90-4). Add ice to croup tent reservoir, if applicable. Adjust nebulizer to prescribed concentration. | |
| e. For Venturi mask, select appropriate cone for prescribed concentration, and connect to mask. | |
| f. Attach connective tubing (large bore with or without water trap for oxygen hood) to humidifier/nebulizer if used, or flow meter and oxygen delivery system, e.g., cannula or mask. | ***Special Considerations:*** *If oxygen is used to power the aerosol generator of the oxygen tent, a second oxygen line should be attached to the gas unit to meet oxygenation needs. If the nebulizer cannot deliver a flow rate of 15 L/min, an additional* $O_2$ *or air source may be necessary to prevent* $CO_2$ *accumulation, even if supplemental* $O_2$ *is not required.* |
| g. Plug in fan/condenser for oxygen/croup tent. | |
| h. Place thermometer within oxygen/croup tent or hood. | Overheating is a potential hazard with enclosed systems, especially if the flow is inadequate or the cooling system is not functioning properly. |
| i. For tents/hoods, calibrate analyzer to room air (21%) and 100% (follow manufacturer's directions). | Calibration ensures accurate monitoring to maintain specific oxygen concentrations. |
| j. Analyze oxygen concentration within tent/hood after allowing probe to equilibrate. Adjust blender to achieve desired $FiO_2$. | ***Special Considerations:*** *If child cannot be oxygenated by an alternative method while equipment is calibrated, the blender should be adjusted to the prescribed setting and analyzed after the child is placed within the tent/hood.* |
| k. Set analyzer high and low alarm limits. | Alarm settings allow recognition of concentration changes. |
| l. Check integrity of system: ensure tubing is not kinked and all connections are tight; portholes/lid on oxygen hoods are closed; edges of oxygen/croup tent and hoods are sealed; and zippers on oxygen/croup tents are closed. | Kinked tubing will not allow free flow of oxygen and can lead to anoxia. Oxygen is heavier than air and will settle to the bottom of the tent or hood, where it may escape if leaks are present. Openings at the top of the hood/tent, and porous vinyl hood materials are designed to allow exhaled $CO_2$ to escape. |
| 3. Explain purpose and procedure to child and family for initiation of therapy (see Skill 1). | Explaining purpose and procedure reduces anxiety and promotes cooperation. |

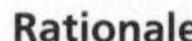

| Steps | Rationale |
|---|---|
| 4. Explain necessary safety precautions while oxygen is in use. Eliminate hazardous items from environment. | Oxygen supports combustion. Any objects that can create sparks and enhance combustion should be restricted (Swearingen, 1984). |
| a. No smoking in the room. | |
| b. No friction or battery-operated toys. | Sparks may be created and start a fire. |
| c. No nylon or wool materials. | Synthetic fabrics and wool tend to generate sparks of static electricity. Cotton fabrics are preferred. |
| d. No volatile, flammable materials, e.g., alcohol, oils, petroleum products, ether, or aerosols. | Flammable materials increase the risk of fire. |
| e. Only grounded electrical equipment that has been approved for use by appropriate department. | Grounded equipment is less likely to generate a spark in the event of a current leak or a wire fracture. |
| 5. Place "Oxygen in Use" and "No Smoking" signs at entrance to child's room and over head of bed. | These signs alert family, staff, and visitors to importance of oxygen safety. |
| 6. Develop individualized goals of nursing care:<br>▪ Improve oxygenation.<br>▪ Prevent complications of oxygen therapy. | |

## Implementation

| Steps | Rationale |
|---|---|
| 1. Initiate delivery of oxygen by adjusting flow rate to required amount. Flush masks, tents, and hoods before placing child in system. | Adequate flow rates of oxygen are necessary to avoid accumulation of carbon dioxide within the system. Flushing the system provides an oxygen-enriched environment. |
| a. Nasal cannula as prescribed.<br>b. Oxygen mask:<br>▪ Simple face mask: 6 to 10 L/min.<br>▪ Partial rebreather mask: 6 to 10 L/min.<br>▪ Nonrebreathing mask:<br>6 L/min = 55% to 60%<br>8 L/min = 60% to 80%<br>10 L/min = 80% to 90%<br>12-15 L/min = 90% to 100%. | ***Special Considerations:*** *Actual concentration of inspired oxygen when using a nasal cannula or simple face mask varies according to respiratory rate, tidal volume, minute ventilation, and gas flow rate. Increasing oxygen flow rates through nasal cannulas beyond 6 L/min does not increase the* $FiO_2$ *(Rarey and Youlsey, 1981).* |
| ▪ Venturi mask: 3 to 10 L/min. | ***Special Considerations:*** *The adapter (cone) used determines the* $FiO_2$ *delivered (from 24% to 50%), independent of liter flow.* |
| c. Oxygen tent: 7 to 15 L/min (see manufacturer's guidelines).<br>d. Oxygen hood: 7 to 15 L/min. | |
| 2. Institute oxygen therapy to the child, troubleshooting and correcting mechanical difficulties. | |
| a. Nasal cannula:<br>▪ Assess nares for patency; clear nasal passages of mucus. | A nasal cannula is ineffective if nasal obstruction exists.<br>***Special Considerations:*** *Mouth breathing is not a contraindication to cannula use as long as nasal obstruction is not present.* |
| ▪ Following the natural curve, insert prongs into nares after ensuring free flow of oxygen. | |
| ▪ Place cannula tubing over ears and under neck, or around back of head, and adjust to fit (Fig. 90-5). | ***Special Considerations:*** *Placing the cannula under the neck of infants/young children presents a strangulation hazard.* |

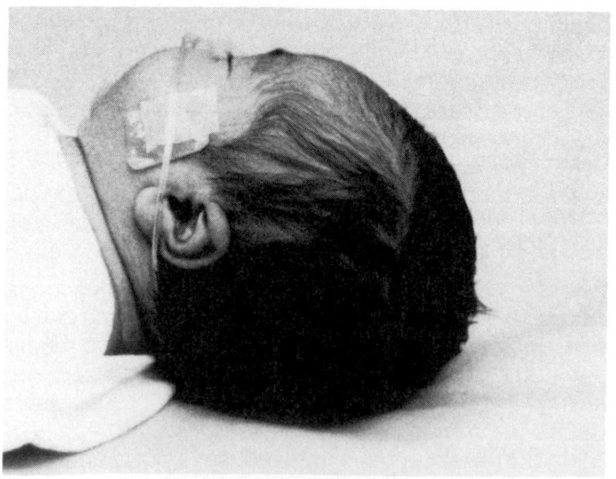

***FIG. 90-5*** Nasal cannula is secured with tape and placed around back of head.

| Steps | Rationale |
|---|---|
| ▪ If necessary, secure cannula to face with tape and a skin barrier such as Stomahesive. | A stable cannula decreases irritation and allows consistent oxygen delivery. Skin barriers may help protect the skin from tape irritation.<br>***Special Considerations:*** *Stomahesive adheres better if held to the skin for a few minutes to form a seal (Hagedorn and Gardner, 1989).* |
| ▪ Pad pressure areas if needed by placing gauze or cotton beneath tubing. | Padding prevents skin irritation and breakdown. |
| b. Oxygen mask:<br>▪ Slip mask over child's head, placing over chin, mouth, and nose. Adjust metal band to fit nasal bridge.<br>▪ Place elastic band around child's head. Adjust for a snug but comfortable fit.<br>▪ Pad pressure areas if needed with gauze or cotton under elastic band. | |
| c. Oxygen/croup tent:<br>▪ Place child in tent. Provide a favorite toy or blanket, or use fantasy such as pretend child is "camping." | A special toy or blanket can comfort the child and reduce anxiety concerning the tent. Fantasy play may also be helpful. |
| ▪ Tuck tent edges under mattress or fan fold with bedding. A bath blanket or draw sheet may also be used to secure front edge over child's legs. Ensure that zippers are closed. | Leaks in the system will diminish the concentration of oxygen. Greatest losses occur at tent bottom since oxygen is heavier than air. |
| ▪ If applicable, secure drainage tube of ice chamber. | Ice may melt onto floor, posing a safety hazard. |
| d. Oxygen hood:<br>▪ Place hood over infant's head/upper body.<br>▪ Close ports, lids. Pad base of hood, if needed. Do not pad neck opening. | ***Special Considerations:*** *Obstructing the neck opening with nonporous materials can lead to an accumulation of carbon dioxide within the hood (Walters, Elmore, and Grandy, 1984).* |
| 3. Assist child's emotional adaptation to delivery system. For example, use fantasy play (such as pretend camping or pilot), encourage a family member to remain close/hold hands or have photographs within sight, provide familiar comforting items such as a favorite toy or blanket. | Children are often fearful of oxygen equipment. Isolation from family and fears of suffocation can worsen respiratory distress. Following these suggestions may help relieve anxiety. |
| 4. Assess child's response to oxygen therapy in 15 to 30 minutes after initiation and on a regular basis throughout therapy. (See Assessment step 1.) | Frequent assessments help determine effectiveness of therapy, as well as the need for adjustment or discontinuation. Oxygen should not be used without specific indications (AAP/ACOG, 1988).<br>***Special Considerations:*** *Blood gas values should govern therapy, if possible; color, transcutaneous monitoring, and pulse oximetry are valuable but can be influenced by other variables. Mist in tents and hoods may hamper assessment; open them if needed to accurately assess child.* |
| 5. Monitor equipment function at least every 2 to 4 hours, and adjust as needed. | Equipment malfunction may lead to overheating, cold stress, dehydration, fluid overload, mucosal damage, hypoxia, oxygen toxicity, or hypercapnia. |
| a. Check flow liter rate. | Flow rates are easily and inadvertently altered by children, families, and other staff. Inappropriate flow rates may lead to hypoxia as well as hypercapnia. |
| b. Check water level in humidifier/nebulizer; ice in croup tent reservoir. | Inadequate fluid levels decrease available humidity, increasing the risk of overheating and thickened secretions. |
| c. If using portable oxygen source, check amount of oxygen remaining. | |
| d. Remove condensation from large-bore tubing by disconnecting and emptying onto a towel or other suitable receptacle. | As heated water vapor cools, "rain out" or condensation forms. Condensation decreases the amount of delivered oxygen and provides a bacterial growth medium (Lough, Doershuk, and Stern, 1979). Emptying water onto the floor poses a safety hazard for accidental falls. |
| e. Check connecting tubing for kinks or disconnection; check entrainment ports on mask for obstruction. | Inadequate gas flow may decrease oxygen concentration. Suffocation from anoxia can occur if gas flow is obstructed in closed systems (nonrebreathing masks, tents, hoods).<br>***Special Considerations:*** *Bed linens and gowns can obstruct entrainment ports.* |
| f. Check nasal prongs and nares for patency. | Nasal secretions may occlude prongs and nasal passages. |

| Steps | Rationale |
|---|---|
| g. Check integrity of tent/hood. Ensure snug fit of mask or cannula. | Oxygen concentration and humidity may be reduced if integrity is lost.<br>***Special Considerations:*** *Check more frequently if child is active or uncooperative.* |
| h. Check oxygen concentration of tent or hood with analyzer at child's face level at least every two hours (Walters, Elmore, and Grandy, 1984). Recalibrate analyzer every 8 hours (Rarey and Youlsey, 1981). | Sudden decreases in inspired oxygen concentration may result in serious clinical problem, e.g., hypertension, intracranial damage, or necrotizing enterocolitis (Walters, Elmore, and Grandy, 1984). Recalibration of analyzer is necessary to ensure precise concentration of oxygen is maintained.<br>***Special Considerations:*** *Humidity may affect accuracy of analyzer.* |
| i. Check child's temperature and temperature within tent/hood.<br>▪ *Tent:* 6° to 8°F lower than room temperature (Walters, Elmore, and Grandy, 1984).<br>▪ *Hood:* 34.4° to 35.6°/94° to 96°F (Kozier and Erb, 1986). | Overheating is a common problem with enclosed systems although cooling from convective and evaporative losses can occur. Hypothermia and hyperthermia may increase oxygen consumption threefold (Shreiner and Kisling, 1982). |
| 6. Tent/hood: change damp bedding and clothing as needed. | Wet bedding may lead to evaporative heat loss, chilling, and increased oxygen requirements. |
| 7. Dry the inside of mask as needed. | Moisture promotes skin irritation and breakdown. |
| 8. Organize nursing care to minimize disruption of oxygen therapy. | Opening tents/hoods can significantly decrease the $FiO_2$.<br>***Special Considerations:*** *Flush tent after loss of integrity to reestablish* $FiO_2$. |
| 9. Change oxygen equipment daily. | *Pseudomonas, Serratia,* and other microorganisms proliferate in the warm moist environment of respiratory therapy equipment (Lough, Doershuk, and Stern, 1979). |
| 10. Check pressure points, mouth, and nose at least every 8 hours. Cleanse and apply water soluble lubricant if needed. | Skin irritation and breakdown may occur from straps/tubing. Drying effect of oxygen may cause encrustations and cracked lips.<br>***Special Considerations:*** *Petroleum products could support combustion and should be avoided.* |
| 11. Suction airway as needed (see Skill 87 or 88). | Oxygenation is promoted by maintaining a patent airway.<br>***Special Considerations:*** *Humidification may increase secretions, necessitating frequent suctioning (Swearingen, 1984).* |
| 12. Monitor fluid status (see Skill 64). | Inappropriate humidification may lead to dehydration or overhydration. |
| 13. When removing child from oxygen source for feeding, bathing, comforting, or procedures:<br>a. Provide alternate oxygen source if child's condition warrants, e.g., cannula, face tent, flow-by.<br>b. Immediately return child to oxygen delivery system if change in respiratory status occurs, especially changes in color, increased respiratory effort, or restlessness (Whaley and Wong, 1991). | An alternate oxygen source is necessary to prevent hypoxia.<br>***Special Considerations:*** *Only remove from oxygen source if child's condition is stable and no blood gases are pending. Do not allow cold air to blow directly on an infant's face; it triggers a diving reflex, leading to bradycardia and shunting of blood from peripheral to central circulation (Whaley and Wong, 1991).* |
| 14. Obtain funduscopic eye exam for newborns before discharge or at 5 to 7 weeks of age if infant remains hospitalized (AAP/ACOG, 1988). | Funduscopic exams identify infants who may have acquired retinal damage from oxygen therapy.<br>***Special Considerations:*** *Examination should be repeated at 3 to 6 months of age (Walters, Elmore, and Grandy, 1984). A surgical procedure is available that may prevent blindness associated with retinopathy of the premature (ROP).* |

| Evaluation Outcomes | Observational Guidelines |
|---|---|
| 1. Child exhibits improved oxygenation. | Assess color. Monitor blood gases, pulse oximetry, and/or transcutaneous readings. |
| 2. Child demonstrates improved airway clearance. | Note thinning of secretions, productivity of cough, and decreasing congestion. Auscultate lung sounds. |
| 3. Respiratory distress is diminished. | Compare respiratory rate and effort, vital signs and color with baseline evaluation. |
| 4. Skin integrity remains intact. | Inspect areas under mask and prongs for signs of irritation. |
| 5. Fluid balance is maintained. | Monitor for signs of dehydration/overhydration. Note viscosity of airway secretions. |

### Evaluation Outcomes—cont'd

6. Temperature balance is maintained.

7. Complications of hypoxia and hyperoxia are prevented.

8. Child and family demonstrate understanding of oxygen therapy.
9. Child's anxiety regarding oxygen therapy is minimized.

### Observational Guidelines—cont'd

Monitor child's temperature. Observe for signs of chilling/overheating. Monitor temperature of delivered oxygen.
Monitor blood gases, pulse oximetry, transcutaneous monitor readings. Observe for signs of hypoxia/hypercapnia. Monitor chest x-ray (CXR), for signs of oxygen toxicity. Review results of funduscopic eye exam.
Ask child and family to explain reason for oxygen therapy and list precautions for safe administration of oxygen.
Observe child for signs of distress (crying, self-injury, tantrums, withdrawal). Note increased cooperation with therapy.

### Documentation

Record assessment findings, including laboratory and noninvasive monitoring values. Note time oxygen therapy was initiated and ended. Document type of oxygen delivery system; time and concentration or flow rate of oxygen; and time, humidification, and temperature of delivery system. Note changes in therapy and adverse reactions or side effects from oxygen therapy and corrective measures taken. Document child/family reactions and any teaching conducted.

### Home Care Modifications

1. Assist family to select oxygen source that will best meet their physical and financial needs and delivery method (Paulson, 1987).
2. Contact electric company, and explain child's needs; seek social service support if payment is a problem; arrange for emergency generator or other back-up system and priority service following power outage.
3. Make referral to home care agency and oxygen equipment vendor.
4. Provide child/family with written discharge instructions.
5. Arrange cardiopulmonary resuscitation training for family and/or caretakers (see Skill 126).

# *SKILL* 91 Measuring Oxygen Saturation by Oximetry

*Patricia A. Jamerson*

Pulse oximetry is a simple, continuous, noninvasive method of determining oxygen saturation to guide oxygen therapy. A sensor comprising a light emitting diode (LED) and a photodetector is placed in opposition around a foot, hand, finger, toe, or ear lobe. The diode emits red and infrared lights that pass through the skin to the photodetector. The photodetector compares the amount of blue light absorbed before and after leaving the arterial bed. Hemoglobin in the blood, which is saturated with oxygen, absorbs more blue light (Reidel, 1987). Therefore pulsatile blood flow is the primary physiologic factor that influences accuracy of the pulse oximeter; skin color, thickness, or edema do not affect the readings (Barker and Tremper, 1987; Fanconi et al, 1985; Reidel, 1987).

## NURSING DIAGNOSES

Impaired gas exchange related to altered oxygen supply, oxygen-carrying capacity of blood, or effects of anesthesia/medication; Potential impairment of skin integrity related to allergic response or shearing force with adhesive oximetry probe.

| Steps | Rationale |
|---|---|
| **Assessment** | |
| 1. Identify physiologic factors that may affect accuracy of reading.<br>a. Increased affinity of hemoglobin for oxygen (increased blood pH, decreased body temperature, decreased $PaCO_2$ levels, and decreased 2,3 diphosphoglycerate [DPG]).<br>b. Decreased hemoglobin or available binding sites (anemia, methemoglobinemia).<br>c. Decreased pulsatile blood flow (vasoconstrictors, thrombus proximal to probe).<br>d. Altered transmission of light in tissues (use of contrast dyes, increased bilirubin levels). | Oxygen saturation reflects the amount of oxygen that is combined with hemoglobin and carried in the blood. Factors that increase the affinity of hemoglobin for oxygen, result in a false elevation, since the oxygen saturation is increased at a lower $PaO_2$ value. Falsely increased levels are also obtained with factors that decrease the amount of hemoglobin or available binding sites. Factors that affect pulsatile blood flow may alter the ability of the photodetector to determine arterial vibrations. Contrast dyes in the blood stream and bilirubin levels greater than 20 mg/dl have been associated with false low readings (Barker and Tremper, 1987; Reidel, 1987). |

| Steps | Rationale |
|---|---|
| | ***Special Considerations:*** *Fetal hemoglobin, present in high levels in neonates, also has an increased affinity for oxygen. This characteristic produces a different oxyhemoglobin dissociation curve, which may result in falsely elevated oximeter readings (Pierce and Turner, 1989).* |
| 2. Determine child's age. | The child's age provides direction for probe selection, placement, and teaching. |
| 3. Review physician orders regarding pulse oximetry. | Physician orders may specify oxygen saturation limits and related interventions. |

## Planning and Goal Setting

| Steps | Rationale |
|---|---|
| 1. Assemble equipment:<br>a. Oximeter (see product references).<br>b. Sensor: ear clip, finger probe, or adhesive probe (Fig. 91-1). | ***Special Considerations:*** *The reusable ear clip and finger probes may be safely and reliably used in the older child, but are not as well tolerated as the disposable adhesive probe. Several sizes of probes are available.* |
| 2. Explain equipment and monitoring procedure to child and/or family. | Explaining purpose and actions eases anxiety. |
| 3. Develop an individualized goal of nursing care:<br>▪ To obtain accurate oxygen saturation readings. | |

## Implementation

| Steps | Rationale |
|---|---|
| 1. Turn on oximeter. | |
| 2. Select probe site, considering assessment factors and type of probe to be used. | Proper site selection will increase the accuracy of the measurements. |
| a. Wrap the adhesive probe around a finger or toe. In the neonate, use the hand or foot (Fig. 91-1). | ***Special Considerations:*** *Clubbing of the fingers does not affect accuracy (Schoni, Hurlimann, and Bruderer, 1987).* |
| b. For the clip probe, select digit large enough for the clip to remain firmly clamped in place. | |
| c. Avoid excoriated areas (especially with adhesive probe), the dominant hand, or a finger used for oral gratification. | |
| 3. Palpate for pulse proximal to selected sites. | Pulsatile blood flow is necessary for the photodetector to differentiate oxyhemoglobin in arterial blood.<br>***Special Considerations:*** *Placement of the probe distal to an inflated blood pressure cuff or indwelling arterial catheter may significantly restrict pulsatile blood flow and use of the pulse oximeter (Reidel, 1987). An advantage of the pulse oximeter over the transcutaneous oxygen monitoring method is its ability to work in low perfusion states as long as pulsatile flow is detected by the sensor (Fanconi et al, 1985).* |
| 4. Prepare site for probe placement. | |
| a. Wipe with alcohol if dirt or excess skin oil present. | Alcohol removes surface dirt and oil that may interfere with light transmission. |

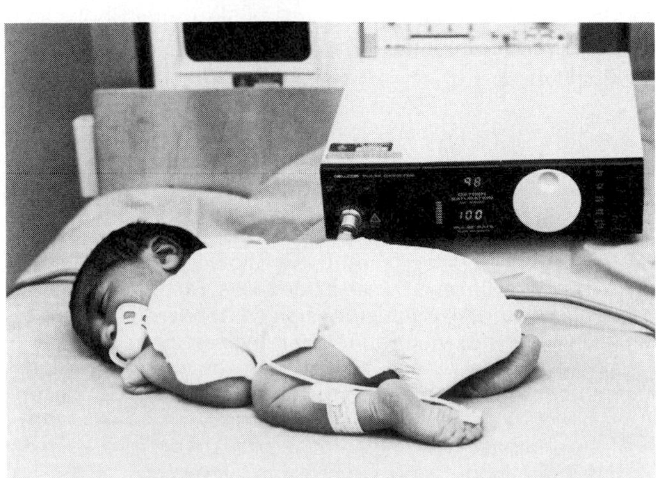

***FIG. 91-1*** Pulse oximeter with probe attached to child's foot.

| **Steps** | **Rationale** |
|---|---|
| b. Remove foot printing dye or nailpolish. | Foot printing dye and certain nailpolish colors (blue, black or green) also interfere with light transmission.<br>***Special Considerations:*** *Porcelain nail coverings and nail decorations such as jewels or gold also interfere with light transmission but are not easily removed. Select another site, if possible.* |
| 5. Align LED light source and photodetector opposite each other on the selected site. | Opposition of the LED light source and photodetector is necessary for proper sensing to occur. |
| 6. Securely attach probe on extremity. | Properly securing the probe prevents ambient light exposure and probe movement artifact, which may interfere wtih accuracy of readings.<br>***Special Considerations:*** *When using excessive sources of ambient light such as heat lamps or phototherapy lights, protect the probe with an opaque covering such as a towel, diaper, or aluminum foil (Reidel, 1987).* |
| 7. Plug probe into oximeter. | |
| 8. Set heart rate alarm limits within a range of 10 to 15 bpm below and above the child's normal range. | Realistic parameters limit false alarms while providing information about the child's heart rate. |
| 9. Set saturation alarm limits between 85% to 95%. | Maintaining an oxygen saturation between 85% to 90% is a safe range for the child. A saturation of 85% closely correlates with a $PaO_2$ of 50 mm Hg, whereas a saturation of 95% could range from 60 to 100 mm Hg. Above 95% saturation the $PaO_2$ value is unpredictable (Reidel, 1987; Fanconi et al, 1985, Hodgson et al, 1987). Hypoxia may lead to cellular damage and eventually death. Hyperoxia also is dangerous and may lead to retrolental fibroplasia (retinopathy of the premature), pulmonary and cerebral damage, and hemolysis (Whaley and Wong, 1991).<br>***Special Considerations:*** *The oxygen saturation percentage obtained is not a direct reflection of $PaO_2$, but can be correlated using the oxyhemoglobin dissociation curve (Fig. 91-2). Small decreases in oxygen saturation, especially in the upper part of the curve, can signal significant declines in $PaO_2$ (Fanconi et al, 1985).* |

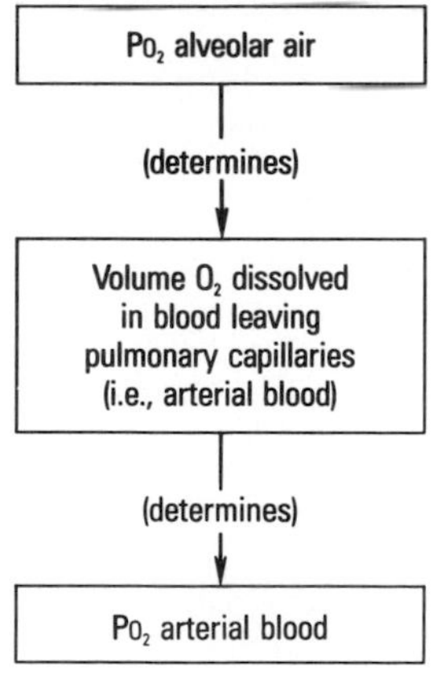


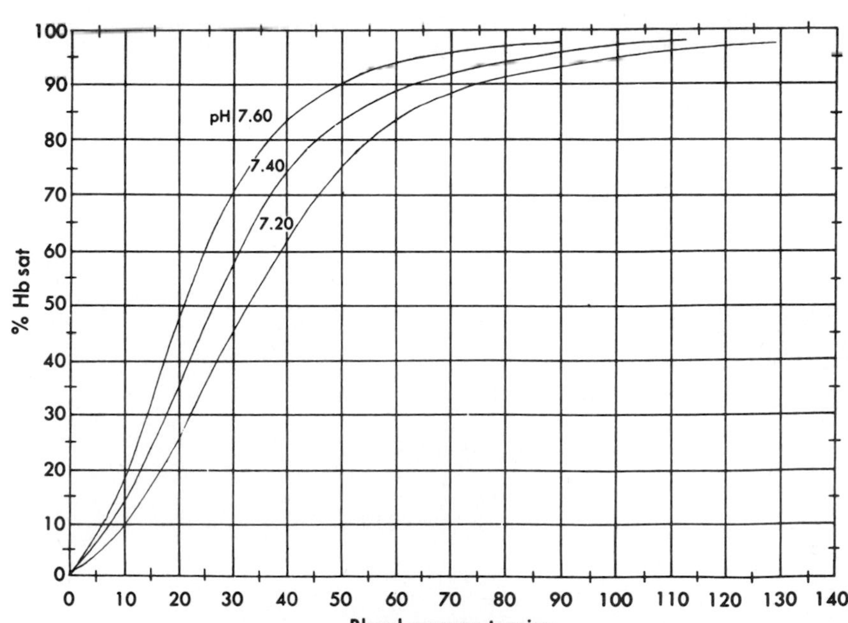


***FIG. 91-2*** Oxygen saturation curve of hemoglobin. For a given oxygen tension, the higher the blood pH, the more the hemoglobin holds onto its oxygen, maintaining a higher saturation.

From Anthony CP and Thibodeau GA: Textbook of anatomy and physiology, ed 12, St Louis, 1987, The CV Mosby Co.

| Steps | Rationale |
|---|---|
| 10. Limit movement of extremity; place on armboard; swaddle infant; or restrain extremity (see Skill 51). | Sensitivity of probe to spontaneous movements (motion artifact) affects accuracy of readings (Barker and Tremper, 1987; Reidel, 1987). |
| 11. Monitor saturation readings when obtaining vital signs, handling the child, suctioning, during activity, and when obtaining blood gas specimens; record time and events precipitating desaturations. | A written record provides a means of correlating oxygenation status during various activities. ***Special Considerations:*** *Verify an adequate thermal environment if saturation levels decrease for no apparent reason. A neonate is especially likely to become hypoxic as a result of cold stress (see Skill 83).* |
| 12. Assess probe placement site on a routine basis such as when obtaining vital signs. | Skin maceration, lacerations, and/or allergic reactions may occur, especially with the adhesive probe. |
| 13. Change site daily or more frequently if redness or other signs of skin trauma are noted. | ***Special Considerations:*** *Caution should be exercised while removing sensor from infants and children with fragile skin to avoid damage. As an alternative, the adhesive may be removed, and the probe secured by wrapping gauze around it. Tape in place using caution not to restrict blood flow (Reidel, 1987).* |

| Evaluation Outcomes | Observational Guidelines |
|---|---|
| 1. Accurate oxygen saturation measurements are obtained. | Compare blood gas $PaO_2$ values with oximeter readings. Note frequency of false alarms. Note factors that may influence reading (e.g., pH changes, bilirubin level, body temperature). |
| 2. Effect of activity and child's status on oxygen saturation is monitored. | Note saturation readings during various activities. Review record for events precipitating desaturations. |
| 3. Skin integrity remains intact. | Observe probe site for redness, blisters, macerated or lacerated areas. |

## Documentation

Record date and time pulse oximetry initiated and ended; time and events precipitating desaturations; response of child to oxygen therapy; blood gas results and corresponding oximetry reading.

# *SKILL* 92 Assisting a Child with Deep Breathing and Coughing

*Bobbie J. Mackay*

Deep breathing exercises use inspiratory muscles to produce a maximum sustained inhalation. Performed properly and sustained at least 3 seconds, deep breathing may improve ventilation and oxygenation. These exercises can be taught to children preoperatively to minimize postoperative pneumonia and/or atelectasis and to children immobilized with traumatic injuries. Incentive spirometry is an adjunct to breathing exercises that provides both visual, and at times, auditory feedback to the child, concerning the volume of air inspired during a deep breath.

Coughing is a highly coordinated natural defense mechanism. It cleanses and protects the airways and lungs from secretions and inhaled particles such as dust, bacteria, or toxic fumes. It may be induced reflexively by deposition of particles on tracheal mucosa or voluntarily through a controlled effort. A cough assists the mucociliary system and alveolar macrophages to maintain a patent airway. It also acts as an adjunct to chest physiotherapy. Effective coughing includes inspiratory, compressive, and expulsive phases.

Deep breathing exercises and controlled coughing are part of a regular pulmonary program for children with chronic lung conditions such as cystic fibrosis, asthma, chronic bronchitis, and with neuromuscular disease such as cerebral palsy or muscular dystrophy (Walsh, 1982).

## NURSING DIAGNOSES

Ineffective gas exchange related to respiratory muscle weakness; Ineffective gas exchange related to incisional pain; Ineffective gas exchange related to retained airway secretions; Knowledge deficit related to need for deep breathing and instruction in proper technique; Ineffective airway clearance related to fatigue, pain, tracheobronchial secretions/obstructions, neuromuscular impairment or lack of information about effective coughing techniques; Potential activity intolerance related to ineffective or uncontrolled coughing.

| Steps | Rationale |
|---|---|
| **Assessment** | |
| 1. Review child's medical history and present respiratory status for conditions associated with impaired/altered deep breathing or controlled coughing.<br>a. Chronic pulmonary conditions such as asthma, cystic fibrosis, bronchopulmonary dysplasia (BPD).<br>b. Conditions that affect chest wall movement such as kyphoscoliosis, pectus excavatum, body cast, broken ribs.<br>c. Neuromuscular diseases such as muscular dystrophy or cerebral palsy.<br>d. Anticipated surgery and type, postoperative status, including anesthetic induction.<br>e. Pain associated with surgical incision or trauma.<br>f. Debilitation from fatigue, malnutrition, or obesity.<br>g. Conditions that reduce the oxygen carrying capacity of the blood such as anemia. | Children with chronic lung conditions need to practice deep breathing to maintain chest wall compliance and proper function of the muscles involved in respiration. Children with spinal cord injuries or neuromuscular disorders have weak intercostal muscles. Deep breathing will increase the elastic qualities of the lung and strengthen intercostal muscles, thereby improving ventilation and oxygenation (Irwin and Tecklin, 1985). Postoperative trauma, inadequate lung expansion because of pain, restrictive dressings, narcotics, or bed rest may lead to hypoxemia, pneumonia, or atelectasis. Children with chest or upper abdominal incisions or injury are at risk for these complications. |
| 2. Assess respiratory signs and symptoms that indicate need to perform deep breathing exercises or controlled coughing.<br>a. Abnormal breath sounds:<br>▪ Crackles.<br>▪ Wheezing. | Inadequate lung expansion may lead to pneumonia, atelectasis, or other serious respiratory complications. If instituted early, deep breathing can prevent these developments. If complications are already present, deep breathing is an important adjunct to medical treatment. |

| Steps | Rationale |
|---|---|
| ■ Bronchial breathing.<br>■ Egophony (a nasal quality to speech when it is transmitted through consolidated lung tissue) (Lehrer, 1984).<br>b. Respiratory distress:<br>■ Dyspnea.<br>■ Tachypnea.<br>■ Nasal flaring.<br>■ Use of accessory muscles.<br>■ Stridor.<br>■ Shallow breathing.<br>■ Cyanosis.<br>■ Increased cough.<br>■ Intercostal and substernal retractions. | ***Special Considerations:*** *Consider whether coughing is necessary to clear secretions. The slow mucociliary transport or depressed cough reflex usually does not pose a problem postoperatively unless child has increased secretions from a chronic lung condition. A vigorous cough may collapse alveoli and small airways instead of opening them. A collapse of alveoli results in atelectasis, which interferes with proper oxygenation of the blood. Therefore if a child's lungs are not congested, routine coughing procedures are not recommended (Walsh, 1982). This recommendation is controversial as traditional practice has emphasized the need to cough following surgery (Perry and Potter, 1990). Check with the physician before initiating controlled coughing procedure if there is a question.* |
| c. Thick, tenacious, or foul smelling sputum. | Thick, tenacious, or foul smelling sputum indicates a need for coughing to mobilize these secretions. Deep breathing can assist this effort, although with less propulsive force. |
| 3. Assess child's ability to deep breathe. Have the child take a deep breath; observe shoulder and chest wall movement, and evaluate chest expansion. Use an incentive spirometer, if desired, to evaluate child's ability to sustain a maximal inspiration. | Assessment serves as a baseline to measure child's ability to sustain a maximal inspiration before instruction on deep breathing. A preoperative assessment establishes a baseline with which to compare postoperative results.<br>***Special Considerations:*** *Deep breathing is used cautiously in a child with hemodynamic or cardiac instability, because it may exaggerate a shift in the axis of the heart, which alters venous return. Also, a child with an air leak from a pneumothorax should not perform deep breathing because it may perpetuate the leak.* |
| 4. Assess character, features, and management of coughing associated with a chronic lung condition such as cystic fibrosis.<br>a. Type: dry, hacking, paroxysmal, moist, brassy, or barking. | Some coughs are characteristic of specific diseases. The character of the cough may help to establish a diagnosis or etiology and guide teaching and intervention. A brassy cough may indicate croup or foreign body aspiration. Children with generalized airway obstruction expel secretions through prolonged, exhausting bouts of coughing; the cough becomes weak and ineffective. Through this effort, mucosal swelling and irritation result in persistent, dry, hacking cough (Whaley and Wong, 1991). A paroxysmal, nonproductive cough stimulates the cough reflex and lowers cough threshold; a paroxysmal cough interferes with removal of particles and secretions by increasing intrathoracic pressure, causing airway collapse. |
| b. Productive cough: observe consistency, amount, color, and odor of sputum produced. | Types of secretions aid in determining the nature of disease. |
| ■ Loose productive cough. | A loose productive cough may indicate lung cancer, bronchitis, bronchiectasis, or emphysema (Whaley and Wong, 1991). |
| ■ Foul smelling sputum. | Foul smelling sputum indicates an infection. |
| ■ Copious amounts of frothy, pink-tinged sputum. | Copious, frothy, pink-tinged sputum indicates pulmonary edema. |
| ■ Brown mucus plugs. | Brown mucus plugs indicate presence of fungal infection such as *Aspergillus.* |
| ■ Post nasal drip. | Post nasal drip is indicative of sinus inflammation or infection. |
| ■ Presence of blood in sputum. Note if streaks of blood versus frank blood. | Severe coughing traumatizes walls of the larynx, trachea, and bronchi. Hemoptysis may also be a sign of infection or inflammation. |
| c. Progress: better, worse, unchanged, or persistent. | A persistent cough is a warning sign that indicates presence of cardiac or pulmonary disease. |
| d. Pattern of coughing: daytime, nighttime, different intensity with time or activity. | A child with chronic obstructive pulmonary disease often experiences episodes of severe coughing in the morning. Children with reflux, allergies, sinus disease, and ciliary dysfunction may experience nighttime coughing. |
| e. Factors that induce coughing. | Smoke, cold weather, and exercise are factors that can trigger coughing. Circumstances that induce coughing can be diagnostic. |
| f. Effects of coughing on respiratory rate, pulse, blood pressure, appetite, sleep, and physical stamina. | Chronic cough is exhausting, especially in debilitated children. It may cause loss of appetite, disturbed sleep, nausea and vomiting, tachycardia, elevated blood pressure, or dyspnea. Children may voluntarily limit food and fluid intake because of the fear that chewing or swallowing will trigger coughing spasm. |

**Steps** | **Rationale**

***Special Considerations:*** *If child experiences posttussive vomiting, he or she should be encouraged to eat again. An exhausting cough is often a decisive indication for using medication to suppress the cough at intervals.*

g. Symptoms associated with cough: sore throat, dyspnea, pain and its location.

Associated symptoms may help with diagnosis or treatment of the cough such as night coughing with dyspnea, indicating asthma.

h. Measures that child/family use to relieve coughing such as bronchodilators, cough suppressants, drinking water, or sucking on hard candy.

Measures that have been effective in relieving the cough may also help with diagnosis and treatment.

i. Concerns related to coughing and expectorating in the presence of others: "How do you manage when you need to cough up mucus?"

Children often find it embarrassing when they cough in front of others. They may also try to suppress a cough because they worry about posttussive vomiting, hemoptysis, or pneumothorax. Child may stifle a cough because of fear that it will precipitate an episode of breathlessness, or he or she is embarrassed to cough in public; having some dialogue about these feelings may help child deal with them more openly.

j. Method of disposing of secretions (e.g., swallowing sputum or hygiene measures used as sputum is expectorated).

Although it is not harmful for child to swallow sputum, it is beneficial to have them expectorate some sputum so that it can be examined. Child who is able to follow simple directions (usually by age 5) can be taught to expectorate their sputum.

k. Symptoms associated with cough such as presence of vertigo, syncope, paresis, and convulsions.

Changes in blood pressure associated with muscular effort and Valsalva maneuver may cause neurologic or circulatory symptoms. Pneumothorax, severe muscle spasms, pain, and ruptured aneurysm have been attributed to coughing (Irwin and Tecklin, 1985).

5. Determine child's age, developmental level, and ability to learn and cooperate with deep breathing and coughing instructions.

The child must be old enough to follow simple instructions, cognitively able to learn, and willing to cooperate, since the exercises require active participation.

***Special Considerations:*** *For a helpful behavior modification approach to teaching the child with developmental delay to cough, see Luedke (1986).*

6. Assess family members' willingness to learn deep breathing and coughing to encourage child.

The presence of family members encourages child to cooperate with treatments and is a motivating factor in recovery. Family members can coach child to perform deep breathing or coughing correctly.

7. Assess if child would benefit from incentive spirometry and has the ability to learn maneuvers. If not ordered, collaborate with practitioner/physician on an assessment of the child's condition and potential benefit from incentive spirometry.

Child's responsiveness to visual or auditory feedback indicates if incentive spirometry is a useful tool to use for training purposes or accomplishing maximal sustained inspiration.

***Special Considerations:*** *Preoperative training prepares child for proper use postoperatively when child may be in pain or anxious and less able to concentrate on learning a new technique.*

## Planning and Goal Setting

1. Assemble necessary equipment and materials:

a. A pillow and chair, depending on child's comfort needs.

A pillow and chair aid in securing child's position and promoting comfort. Pillows may be used to secure operative site. An upright position allows for better chest expansion.

b. Water pitcher and glass.

Oral mucosa may lose moisture from mouth breathing; a drink of water is a comfort measure and may help to mobilize secretions.

c. Tissues and paper bag at bedside; clear, screwtop container, and lined wastepaper basket for disposal of sputum.

Use tissues or jar to dispose of sputum. Hygiene measures used to dispose of sputum should be taught to child and family to reduce spread of bacteria and viruses.

d. Teaching materials or pamphlets.

e. Incentive spirometer if ordered.

f. Sterile specimen container (if sputum specimen needed).

***Special Considerations:*** *For the young child unable to cough, a sputum specimen must be obtained by suctioning (see Skill 87).*

2. Choose convenient time for teaching which does not interfere with other activities, e.g., rest, meals, therapies, play and when child is not in pain.

Cooperative planning with the child related to time for deep breathing exercises or controlled coughing, encourages compliance with treatment regimen and minimizes interference with other activities.

***Special Considerations:*** *Participation in planning should be according to child's developmental level.*

| Steps | Rationale |
|---|---|
| 3. Provide individualized, one-on-one attention in a quiet setting. | Individualized attention and an environment free of distractions helps child focus on learning the techniques. |
| 4. Provide privacy, especially for the child learning controlled coughing. | Coughing with production of sputum may be embarrassing for the child and he or she may become distracted or self-conscious in the presence of others. |
| 5. Develop individualized child and family goals:<br>▪ Child will be able to effectively perform deep breathing exercises or controlled coughing.<br>▪ Child will experience minimal pain during these maneuvers.<br>▪ Child and family will demonstrate understanding of the purposes of deep breathing or controlled coughing.<br>▪ Family will be able to assist child with deep breathing or controlled coughing. | |

## Implementation

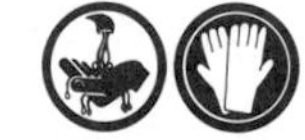

| Steps | Rationale |
|---|---|
| 1. Discuss with child and family members effective method of deep breathing or controlled coughing using developmentally appropriate methods. | Use of developmentally appropriate methods of preparation increases chances child will understand goals, cooperate with therapy, and desired goals will be achieved. |
| a. Explain that deep breathing prevents pneumonia and lung collapse. Deflate a balloon to demonstrate alveolar collapse. Explain the role of controlled coughing in airway clearance. | |
| b. Demonstrate techniques of deep breathing and controlled coughing. | Actual demonstration enables child to comprehend what is being taught and apply the information learned. It provides child with a role model and enables imitation of the behavior. |
| c. Hand out printed material and illustrations. | Age-appropriate teaching aids reinforce proper technique and help focus the child's attention on the task. |
| d. Assist child in setting a specified goal based on child's physical and personal needs. For example, child will cough effectively four times a day. | The desire to attain established goals serves as a motive for learning.<br>***Special Considerations:*** *Coughing and deep breathing are adjuncts to therapy; therefore child should not have choice about whether to participate but may choose times or location.* |
| e. Explain to child how technique is done and any discomfort child will experience. | Discomforts may include dyspnea, mild fatigue, or pain in a postoperative child. |
| 2. Discuss appropriate times: | |
| *Deep Breathing:* | |
| a. Every 1 to 2 hours in postoperative children with copious amounts of secretions. | A maximal deep inspiration will minimize the chances of atelectasis. It may loosen secretions and stimulate a spontaneous cough (Walsh, 1982). |
| b. Following administration of pain medication. | Medication lessens a child's pain and enhances cooperation with exercises.<br>***Special Considerations:*** *If pain medication is required, allow time for medication to take effect before starting exercises. Narcotics may reduce child's respiratory drive and number of spontaneous deep breaths.* |
| *Coughing:* | |
| a. In the morning on awakening. | Coughing in the morning clears airway of secretions that have accumulated in child's airway overnight. Morning coughing is especially important for children with chronic lung conditions. |
| b. Following chest physiotherapy (CPT) and after percussion and vibration of each lung segment. | Coughing after CPT with percussion and vibration removes secretions that have been mobilized into the bronchus. |
| c. Before bedtime. | Coughing before bedtime clears airways for the period of inactivity. |
| d. After administration of pain medication. | Pain medication will minimize child's discomfort and encourage more effective coughing. |
| e. After inhalation of bronchodilator, wetting solution, or mucolytic agent. | Bronchodilators help open airways. In children with chronic lung conditions such as cystic fibrosis or bronchopulmonary dysplasia, it allows secretions to be expectorated more easily. In children with asthma, bronchodilators reduce a child's cough. Wetting solutions and mucolytic agents help mobilize secretions. |
| f. Before meals or 1½ hours after mealtime. | Coughing should be done on an empty stomach to avoid aspiration or posttussive vomiting. |

| Steps | Rationale |
|---|---|
| g. Every 1 to 2 hours in postoperative children with copious amounts of secretions, crackles or wheezes, fremitus or fever. | A child with evidence of retained secretions needs to cough. **_Special Considerations:_** *A maximal sustained deep inspiration will minimize the chances of atelectasis in the postoperative patient (Walsh, 1982).* |
| 3. Administer aerosolized medications if ordered before coughing efforts (see Skill 103). | Inhalation of water particles or saline helps to thin secretions and makes them less adherent to airways. Inhalation of bronchodilators opens up airways and enables secretions to move more freely. Mucolytic agents break down and thin mucus. |
| 4. Position the child: | |
| a. Place child in a sitting position; head and shoulders relaxed and flexed, leaning slightly forward; feet on floor (Perry and Potter, 1990). | A sitting position relieves pressure on the diaphragm and provides for maximal lung expansion and expiratory efforts (the child may have difficulty coughing if in a dependent position). **_Special Considerations:_** *Chair should be appropriate size for child. A child confined to bed should lie on his or her back or side with the head of bed elevated. Position a pillow at the small of the back for comfort. Hold a small child or infant upright on a person's lap.* |
| b. Have child hug a stuffed toy or small pillow. As an alternative, encircle the child's chest with own hands, and compress the sides of the lower chest in synchrony with deep breathing or coughing efforts. | Hugging an object provides comfort and support during deep breathing exercises. This is less fatiguing and splints the chest for more effective deep breathing efforts (Whaley and Wong, 1991). |
| c. Sit facing child while teaching and practicing techniques. | It will be easier for the child to perform exercises while observing a role model. It also allows observation of the child during practice for proper technique and fatigue. **_Special Considerations:_** *If fatigue occurs, teaching session may need to be interrupted and rescheduled (Whaley and Wong, 1991).* |
| d. Have child and family member place palms of hands across from each other, along lower borders of child's anterior rib cage. Instruct and demonstrate technique. | Positioning hands as described allows them to feel movement of chest and abdomen as diaphragm descends and lungs expand. |
| 5. For deep breathing and controlled coughing: | |
| a. Starting from an upright position, have child drop head and bend forward while blowing air through pursed lips. | Lungs are cleared of as much air as possible in preparation for controlled, maximum inspiratory effort. Pursed lip breathing helps slow down child's breathing so that more air moves into and out of lungs. It keeps small airways from collapsing and trapping air in the lungs (Irwin and Tecklin, 1985). |
| b. Return child to upright position, then instruct to breathe in slowly and deeply through nose. | Slow deep inspiration dilates the bronchi and bronchioles to provide sufficient amounts of air behind mucus plugs to propel them from airways. Slow breaths also prevent hyperventilation, allow better gas distribution within lungs and are less likely to propel mobilized secretions deep into the tracheobronchial tree. Fast, gasping breaths do not aerate mucus-filled areas, but are directed to upper thorax. **_Special Considerations:_** *Children with spinal cord injuries often have weak intercostal muscles and a diminished cough reflex. Deep breathing will increase the elastic qualities of the lung, strengthen intercostal muscles, and therefore improve child's ability to achieve a productive cough (Whaley and Wong, 1991).* |
| ▪ Have child take in deep breath while pushing out abdomen. Place a small pillow in the child's lap to facilitate this action if desired. | This is the compression stage which begins with closure of the glottis. Both intrathoracic and intraabdominal pressure build with contraction of expiratory muscles (Irwin and Tecklin, 1985). |
| ▪ Explain to child that during inspiration, the diaphragm and abdominal organs descend and the chest wall expands. Chest and shoulders should not be used while deep breathing. Have child watch abdomen. | Explanation, demonstration, and practice focus on the correct method of deep breathing and reinforce teaching to help the child develop an understanding of how deep breathing feels. Understanding the sensations makes them easier to duplicate postoperatively (Whaley and Wong, 1991). Use of chest and shoulder muscles causes child to expend unnecessary energy. **_Special Considerations:_** *Children with chronic lung conditions may have difficulty minimizing chest and shoulder movements during inhalation (Perry and Potter, 1990).* |
| ▪ Have child hold slow, deep breath for slow count of 3 to 5, and then drop head and bend forward, slowly exhaling through pursed lips. | This technique allows for gradual expulsion of air. Pursed lip breathing increases alveolar ventilation and oxygenation, thus reducing the work of breathing (Irwin and Tecklin, 1985). |

| Steps | Rationale |
|---|---|
| ▪ Repeat slow, deep inspiration-pursed lip expiration cycle 3 to 4 times. Encourage child through each step. | Repetitions of inhalation and exhalation mobilize secretions toward the main bronchi (Irwin and Tecklin, 1985). Repeating several cycles allows child to become familiar with rhythm. |
| 6. For controlled coughing: a. Following repetition of inspiratory-expiratory cycle, instruct child to bend forward, use abdominal muscles and cough forcefully during expiration. Repeat until the airway is cleared at appropriate times (see Step 2). | Expiratory force should be sufficient to maintain maximum expiratory flow without causing airway collapse. The expulsive phase begins with opening of the glottis and expulsion of trapped air. Diaphragm relaxes to provide transmission of the increased intraabdominal pressure into the lungs (Irwin and Tecklin, 1985). |
| b. Instruct child and family about hygiene measures related to disposal of sputum. If a specimen is needed, collect expectorated sputum in a sterile container. | Correct hygiene measures reduce spread of bacteria and viruses. |
| 7. For deep breathing: Have child perform breathing exercises 5 to 10 times, as appropriate (see Step 2), until the child is no longer at risk. For children with chronic conditions, deep breathing should be a part of their regular therapy program. | Regular deep breathing will help prevent postoperative respiratory complications. ***Special Considerations:*** *Supervising the exercises or setting up a chart with a sticker reward system helps to reinforce the importance of the activity to the child and family.* |
| 8. Have child breathe normally for a few breaths in between deep breathing or coughing maneuvers. | This will prevent hyperventilation and fatigue. |
| 9. Provide positive reinforcement for successful attempts at deep breathing and/or coughing. | Positive reinforcement boosts child's self-esteem and encourages cooperation. It increases the probability that the behavior will be repeated. |
| 10. Have child practice the techniques several times. Provide verbal guidance as child practices. | Repetition of technique reinforces teaching. Practice is necessary to improve motor skills. ***Special Considerations:*** *Use gentle but firm guidance with child.* |
| 11. Use play therapy strategies: | Play therapy encourages cooperation and can make the exercises fun. |

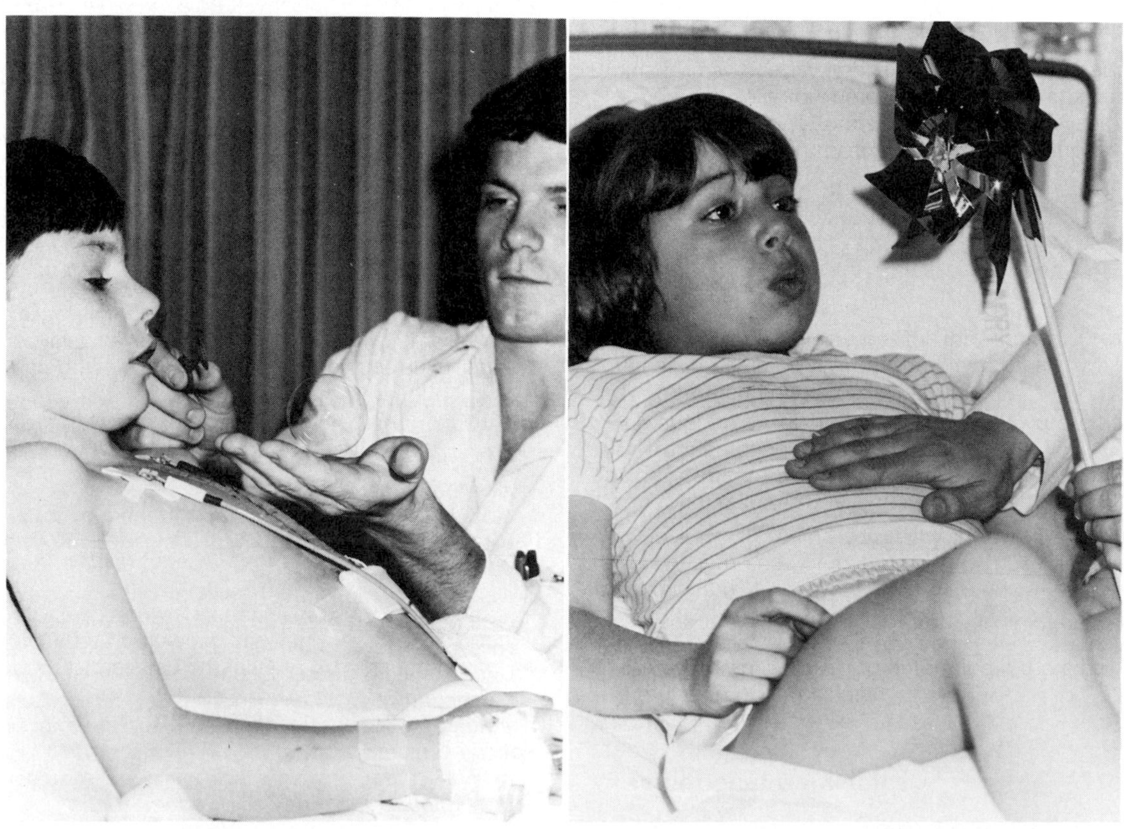

***FIG. 92-1*** Blowing bubbles or pinwheels can be fun for a child while also encouraging deep breathing.

From Irwin S and Tecklin JS: Cardiopulmonary physical therapy, ed 2, St Louis, 1990, The CV Mosby Co.

| Steps | Rationale |
|---|---|
| a. For deep breathing, examples of appropriate methods include: blowing soap bubbles; blowing through a straw into oral fluids; blowing up balloons or surgical gloves; blowing nail polished fingernails dry; blowing pinwheels, whistle toys, toy horn, and harmonicas; and using blow bottles designed to force liquid from one container to another (Fig. 92-1) (Whaley and Wong, 1991). | ***Special Considerations:*** *Incorporate these strategies with the breathing technique previously described. These strategies are appropriate as long as maximal inspiration is sustained for 3 to 5 seconds. An adult should always supervise when a child is playing with balloons because they pose an aspiration risk. Blow bottles can be constructed with bottles, stoppers, and tubing. Food coloring in the water makes the activity more interesting.* |
| b. For coughing, the child can practice the techniques with a doll or a friend. | Play therapy during coughing sessions may encourage cooperation and help child cope with feelings. |
| 12. If using incentive spirometry: | |
| a. Demonstrate to child how to place mouthpiece so that his or her lips cover it. Change to clean mouthpiece. | Demonstration is a reliable technique for teaching use of incentive spirometry. It enables child to ask questions and practice technique. |
| b. Have child exhale slowly through pursed lips, then inhale slowly while maintaining a constant flow through unit. | ***Special Considerations:*** *Flow-oriented spirometry produces elevation of one or more balls within a plastic cylinder. In volume-oriented spirometry, a light indicates when the correct volume has been reached (Perry and Potter, 1990).* |
| c. When the child reaches maximum inhalation, as evidenced by a signal light when the predetermined volume is reached, instruct child to hold his or her breath for 2 to 3 seconds, then have child exhale slowly through pursed lips. Have the child breathe normally for a few seconds before repeating the cycle. | |
| 13. Maintain increased fluid intake. | Adequate hydration keeps secretions thin and facilitates their removal from airways. |
| 14. Give medications as ordered by physician to control pain or paroxysmal coughing (see Skill 52). | Paroxysmal, ineffective coughing causes fatigue. To maximize cooperation, pain and discomfort must be minimized. |

| Evaluation Outcomes | Observational Guidelines |
|---|---|
| 1. The child effectively performs deep breathing or controlled coughing exercises. | Observe child's return demonstration. Note correct steps and inspiratory/expiratory/cough effort. Compare assessment findings with postprocedure findings. |
| 2. The child does not develop postoperative respiratory complications related to inadequate lung expansion. | Observe for abnormal lung sounds, shallow respirations, cyanosis, restlessness, irritability, elevated temperature, pain on inspiration, dyspnea, or thick, copious secretions. |
| 3. Ineffective, nonproductive, uncontrolled coughing is minimized. | Child rests better and demonstrates fewer episodes of posttussive vomiting or blood streaked sputum. |
| 4. Pain is minimized during deep breathing or coughing. | Note child's ability to inspire deeply, and observe behaviors of pain such as facial expressions, verbalizations, child's report of pain level, or restlessness. |
| 5. Child and family demonstrate adequate knowledge about deep breathing, coughing, or incentive spirometry. | Interview child and family members to discuss purpose of maneuvers, importance of treatment, timing, expected/unexpected outcomes, and actions to take. |
| 6. Family demonstrates an understanding of their role during deep breathing or coughing activity. | Observe family assisting child to deep breathe or cough in an effective manner. |

## Documentation

Document assessment related to child's respiratory status. Record any changes observed in child's status preoperatively and postoperatively, if applicable. Document any signs of atelectasis, pneumonia, or pneumothorax. Note presence of pain and child's response to analgesic agents and supportive care.

Document observations made related to character and frequency of cough; description of sputum including consistency, amount, color, and smell; circumstances that induce and relieve cough; anxiety, pain, dyspnea associated with cough; effect of coughing on appetite, sleep, and physical stamina; presence of hemoptysis or posttussive vomiting.

Document child's understanding of and ability to participate in deep breathing, coughing, or incentive spirometry exercises. Note family's ability to assist child with maneuvers.

Document place and time when teaching about deep breathing or coughing took place, who was present, instructional materials given, child's response and behavior during activity, and family's reaction.

# SKILL 93 Monitoring for Apnea

*Deborah S. Lammert*

Apnea in the infant or young child is defined as the cessation of spontaneous respirations exceeding a time period of 20 seconds, or a shorter pause associated with bradycardia, cyanosis, pallor, and/or marked hypotonia (Koff, Eitzman, and Neu, 1988). Without intervention, prolonged and/or frequent apneic events can seriously compromise the cardiopulmonary status of the infant. The initiation and maintenance of electronic apnea monitoring in the infant is therefore a primary nursing responsibility. Following an observed apparent life-threatening event (ALTE) in the home or community, the infant is often hospitalized for resuscitative intervention (if necessary), observation, evaluation, education, and family counseling.

Preterm infants discharged to the home from a special care or neonatal intensive care nursery may also require home apnea monitoring for associated apnea of infancy (AI). Apnea monitoring in both the acute-care facility and in the home has become a common intervention in the care of the infant with apnea of unknown etiology (Denson and Goldie, 1986). Correctly utilized, electronic apnea monitoring alerts the caregiver to a deterioration of the infant's condition and permits the prepared caregiver to intervene and possibly prevent death. Therefore it is essential that the nurse provide adequate monitoring of the infant, thorough teaching of the caregivers, and support to the family whose infant requires electronic apnea monitoring.

Because few infants demonstrate prolonged apnea after 12 months of age, home monitoring may be discontinued at that time by a physician or at an earlier age following a negative polysomnography test.

## NURSING DIAGNOSES

Ineffective breathing patterns related to recurrent apneic episodes; Anxiety related to unmet informational needs about apnea monitoring, and/or resuscitation techniques; Potential for altered family processes related to the experience of a crisis event, inadequate coping patterns, and/or inadequate support systems; Altered parenting related to caregiving responsibilities for technology-assisted child; Powerlessness related to infant's life-threatening event.

| Steps | Rationale |
|---|---|
| **Assessment** | |
| 1. Obtain baseline data from physical assessment, noting in particular: respiratory rate, depth, and rhythm; color of skin and mucous membranes; heart rate and rhythm; activity level; level of consciousness and response to stimuli; and any signs/symptoms of infection, respiratory difficulty, or seizure activity. | Determination of normal or current physical status provides basis for assessing normal versus abnormal findings, comparing data, and identifying actual or potential problems. Assessment focuses primarily on the respiratory and neurologic systems and identification of any infectious process, in order to assist in determining the etiology of the apneic event(s). |
| 2. Obtain health history from the family, including:<br>a. Prenatal/postnatal course.<br>b. Term status of infant at birth.<br>c. Any recent illness or injury of infant.<br>d. Sibling history of apnea or Sudden Infant Death Syndrome (SIDS).<br>e. Socioeconomic status.<br>f. Race/ethnic origin.<br>g. Type/quality of prenatal care.<br>h. History of gastroesophageal reflux (GER).<br>i. Age and sex of infant. | Associated characteristics that indicate high-risk factors for the infant with AI are: history of prematurity, low Apgar scores; respiratory infections, chronic or recurrent; two or more siblings with AI or SIDS; lower socioeconomic status; non-Caucasian race; poor or no prenatal care; GER-induced reflex laryngospasm; peak incidence age; 2 to 4 months; male gender; and higher incidence in winter months.<br>***Special Considerations:*** *Disorders associated with prolonged apnea in the infant include infection (sepsis, meningitis, pneumonia, bronchiolitis); CNS disorders (seizures); metabolic disorders (hypoglycemia, hyponatremia, hypokalemia, hypocalcemia, hypernatremia, toxic substance ingestion); cardiovascular disorders (shock, cardiac dysrhythmias); respiratory disorders (upper airway obstruction, aspiration, asphyxia); and gastrointestinal disorders (gastroesophageal reflux). Improvement in apnea caused by these conditions occurs only when the underlying etiology is treated or corrected (Koff, Eitzman, and Neu, 1988).* |
| 3. Obtain a detailed and comprehensive account of the apparent apneic event(s) from an adult that witnessed the episode. Ask questions and clarify answers regarding: | Data obtained through an account of the incident will assist in the determination of the etiology of the apneic episode. |

| Steps | Rationale |
|---|---|
| a. State of consciousness (awake, asleep, postictal).<br>b. Activity (feeding, burping, crying, sleeping).<br>c. Motor tone (stiff, limp, normal).<br>d. Color (pallor, cyanosis, facial rubor).<br>e. Duration of apnea.<br>f. Previous episodes.<br>g. Type of stimulation/resuscitation required.<br>h. Response of infant to intervention.<br>i. Relationship to feeding schedule; any emesis or reflux noted.<br>j. Any indication of seizure activity.<br>k. Other significant observations. | ***Special Considerations:*** *The family or caretaker may be experiencing emotional distress in relating the incident to the health care personnel. Specific questions and clarification of answers may provide guidance in the provision and gathering of important data, and will promote a complete and thorough account of the event.* |
| 4. Assess family coping skills, resources, and state of anxiety and/or crisis (see Skill 14). | Acute hospitalization of the infant following a suspected life-threatening event may predispose the family to crisis, with altered coping skills and an elevated level of anxiety. |
| 5. When appropriate, perform a thorough family assessment, including:<br>a. Family structure and support systems; primary caregiver.<br>b. Family financial status.<br>c. Characteristics of family dwelling, including electricity and telephones.<br>d. Lifestyle characteristics.<br>e. Health values and beliefs.<br>f. Level of education of family members/infant caregivers.<br>g. Ability to comprehend medical terminology, and understand purpose of therapies.<br>h. Ability to learn and adhere to medical therapies in the home.<br>i. Past experiences with home monitoring or other medical home care. | A family assessment provides data related to the family's knowledge and comprehension level and their ability to adhere to medical therapies for the infant. Home discharge plans are made in light of family abilities to carry out medically necessary monitoring and/or interventions.<br>***Special Considerations:*** *See also Skill 38.* |

## Planning and Goal Setting

| Steps | Rationale |
|---|---|
| 1. Plan to perform assessments in an organized manner. | Organization promotes efficiency in complete assessment and identification of actual and potential problems. |
| 2. Adapt family assessment to family ability to cope with situational crisis at hand. Use principles of crisis management when interacting with family. | Focusing on essential family assessment data during the initial interaction period permits the family to begin adapting and coping with the situational crisis. Following the acute crisis period, the family can be reassessed and additional data can be obtained. |
| 3. Gather necessary equipment and supplies: | Gathering equipment ensures efficiency in nursing care and prevents leaving the bedside while initiating apnea monitoring for the infant. |
| a. Apnea monitor with apnea and heart rate sensors that meet current Food and Drug Administration (FDA) performance standards. | Apnea monitors are most commonly the transthoracic impedance type, using either the chest strap (belt) with attached electrodes or adhesive electrode patches.<br>***Special Considerations:*** *The FDA issued mandatory regulatory standards for infant apnea monitors effective spring/summer 1990.* |
| b. Chest strap or pre-gelled electrodes and lead wires. | ***Special Considerations:*** *The chest-strap is generally easier for family members to use in the home. Adhesive electrodes are used as two or three electrode systems; each manufacturer includes specific instructions for electrode placement dependent on the particular monitor in use. These instructions should always be consulted before electrode placement.* |
| c. Cable connecting apnea monitor and lead wires.<br>d. Alcohol prep pads or dilute acetone solution; gauze pad or washcloth. | |
| e. Proper size oxygen mask and manual resuscitation bag at bedside. | ***Special Considerations:*** *Resuscitation bag should also accompany infant whenever absent from the nursing unit for tests, etc.* |
| 4. Prepare the equipment.<br>a. Inspect all wires, cables, and cords for intactness and the absence of broken and/or frayed areas with exposed wiring. | Electrical safety is promoted by using only equipment in good repair with proper electrical grounding.<br>***Special Considerations:*** *Keep the unit away from excessive moisture or any potentially wet areas.* |

| Steps | Rationale |
|---|---|
| b. Insert the three-pronged plug into an electric outlet marked for emergency back-up power in the event of a power outage. | |
| c. Place the monitor unit on a flat, stable, dry surface near the infant's crib. | |
| d. Set the alarm parameters:<br>▪ Upper limit heart rate—225 to 250 beats per minute (bpm).<br>▪ Lower limit heart rate—0 to 3 months, full term, 80 bpm; 0 to 4 months, preterm, 80 bpm; 3 to 6 months, 70 bpm; 6 months or older, 60 bpm.<br>▪ Apnea—15-20 seconds. | ***Special Considerations:*** *Measured apnea duration should activate alarm when duration is greater than a preset time not to exceed 20 seconds for infant apnea monitors (Center for Devices and Radiological Health, 1989).* |
| e. Inspect for the presence and operation of visual and audible alarm indicators. | ***Special Considerations:*** *Visual alarms will display continuous red (patient warning) and/or green (equipment advisory) lights. Audible patient alarms sound intermittently at one-second intervals, e.g., 10 beeps = 10 seconds.* |
| f. Place monitor so that visual indicators are not obscured from view. | |
| g. Place monitor 4 to 6 inches away from walls, curtains, or other articles that may muffle or absorb alarm sound. | |
| 5. Develop individualized child/family goals:<br>▪ Respiratory patterns will be accurately and safely monitored to permit early identification of and intervention during apneic episodes.<br>▪ The family will acquire knowledge of and ability to perform skills related to infant stimulation, resuscitation, and electronic apnea monitoring (if required) in the home.<br>▪ The family will develop coping skills to deal with increased stress in the home setting. | |

## Implementation

| Steps | Rationale |
|---|---|
| 1. Explain purpose of apnea monitor to family. Emphasize that the monitor is only a tool, not a "cure" for apnea; and does not prevent SIDS; it only alerts the caregiver to a situation that may require intervention. Explain the alarms and expected response to each alarm to the family. | Explanations help decrease anxiety related to fear of the unknown and increase family use of available coping mechanisms.<br>***Special Considerations:*** *Family teaching begun upon admission and continued throughout the hospitalization period enhances the learning abilities of the family and provides for ongoing reinforcement of learning.* |
| 2. Prepare the infant's skin. Cleanse and dry the mid-to-lower chest area, ensuring that the skin is free of oils, lotions, and talcum powder.<br>*Chest strap:*<br>Cleanse mid-to-lower half of the thorax around to the back with soap and water. Dry skin thoroughly. | Dead skin cells, oils, and other impurities must be removed since they interfere with passage of electrical signals to the electrodes.<br>***Special Considerations:*** *Avoid areas of obvious skin chafing or breakdown.* |
| *Adhesive electrodes:*<br>Cleanse sites where electrode patches will be placed (see step 3) with soap and water. Gently abrade the areas with a gauze pad or washcloth. | Proper cleansing and abrading of the skin for electrode placement ensures an optimal electrode/skin interface and promotes adherence of the electrodes to the skin. |
| 3. Properly place the electrode chest strap or adhesive electrodes:<br>*Chest strap:*<br>a. Place the reusable electrodes onto the chest strap so the Velcro surfaces of the belt and electrodes make contact. Aim inserts for lead wires toward the bottom of the belt. Position electrodes so that when the strap is fastened around the baby, each one will be located 1 to 2 fingerbreadths (fb) (depending on the size of the child) below the nipple at the mid-axillary line. | The electrode sensors must adequately contact the infant's skin, and be located where maximal respiratory movement can be detected and heart rate determined. Proper placement allows the monitor to sense changes in transthoracic impedance noted by the detection of small, high-frequency alternating current between two electrodes on the infant's chest or abdominal areas. Variations in electrical impedance correlate with changes in respiratory patterns.<br>***Special Considerations:*** *Some manufacturers recommend the application of an electrode gel or a drop of water to each electrode before securing the chest strap; this maximizes the conductivity of the current between skin and electrode surfaces.* |
| b. Attach lead wires into electrodes, correlating "RA" with the infant's right side, and "LA" with infant's left side (Fig. 93-1). | |

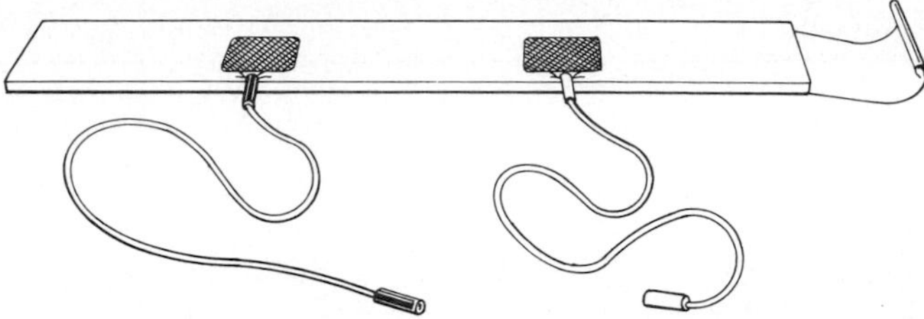

***FIG. 93-1*** Lead wires are attached to electrodes on chest strap.

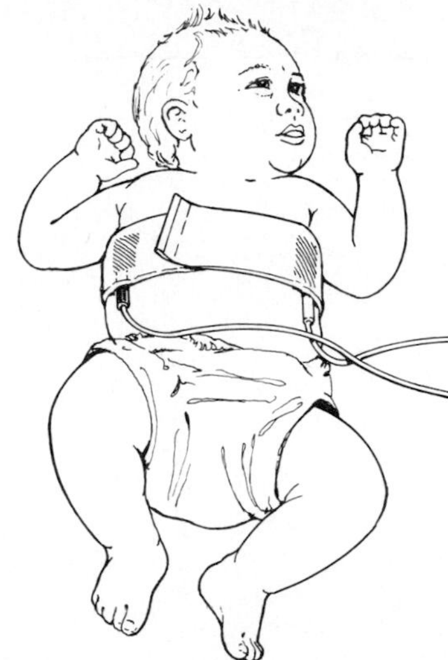

***FIG. 93-2*** Chest strap is secured around infant's trunk with electrodes positioned at the mid-axillary line.

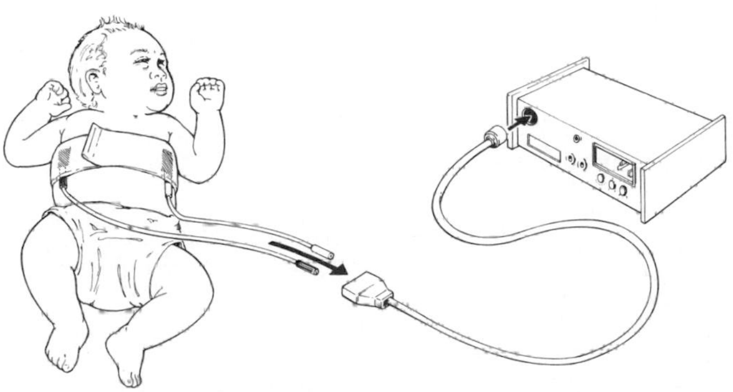

***FIG. 93-3*** Preattached lead wires are connected to monitor cable.

| Steps | Rationale |
|---|---|
| c. Wrap snugly and secure the strap around the infant's trunk with Velcro tab so that the electrodes are positioned correctly at the mid-axillary line 1 to 2 fb below the nipple line (Fig. 93-2). | ***Special Considerations:*** *The mid-thorax area is the usual site of maximal respiratory excursion. For convenience in securing and removing the electrode belt/strap, the belt is often secured anteriorly with the Velcro closure. As infants become older and are able to disengage the attachment and thus interfere with a secure, snug fit of the belt, the closure may be secured posteriorly, out of the infant's reach.* |
| d. Connect preattached lead wires to the cable of the monitor (Fig. 93-3). | |
| *Adhesive electrodes:* | |
| a. Connect button (snap-type) lead wires to the electrode patches *before* placing on the prepared skin surfaces of the infant. | Placing the electrode patches on the lead wire connectors before placing on the infant prevents undue force or pressure from being exerted on the infant's body surfaces. |
| b. Peel paper from the back of each electrode, and place the patch in the appropriate location. Place one electrode on each side of the chest 1 to 2 fb below the nipple line (Fig. 93-4). If three-electrode system used, place the remaining electrode on the lateral aspect of the abdomen, above the level of the umbilicus. Adhere to the designations "RA" and "LA" for placement on the right and left sides of the infant, respectively. | ***Special Considerations:*** *Three-electrode systems are infrequently used, especially in home settings.* |

| Steps | Rationale |
|---|---|

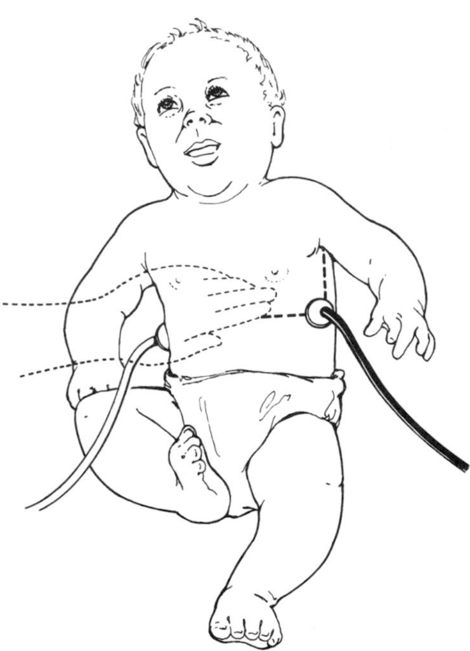

***FIG. 93-4*** Placing adhesive electrodes.

| Steps | Rationale |
|---|---|
| c. Firmly smooth the adhesive areas onto the skin; avoid heavy pressure directly on the center gelled area of the electrode patch. | Avoiding pressure on the center gelled surface of the electrode ensures that the conductive gel remains in the center, allowing maximal contact with the skin surface. |
| 4. Change the disposable electrode patches every 2 to 3 days, or when they become loose (Wong and Whaley, 1990). | Changing electrodes regularly prevents "drying" of the patches, which interferes with optimal conductivity, and decreases possibility of skin irritation. |
| a. Carefully peel electrodes off the infant's skin. | |
| b. Wash the skin with soap and water; dry thoroughly. | Washing the skin removes remaining traces of adhesive. |
| c. Note any signs of skin irritation at the electrode sites. | Careful attention to the skin is necessary since irritations and monilial infections under the site of electrode patches may occur (Andrews and Nielson, 1988). |
| d. Apply new electrodes using the previously described technique, placing them on an alternative skin site. | |
| 5. Ensure that the monitor is correctly functioning by testing alarms: | Testing of monitor alarms assists in verifying a correctly functioning monitor. |
| a. Determine if the "heart" or "pulse" indicator lights with each heartbeat palpated, and the "breath" or "respiratory" indicator lights with each observed breath of the infant. | ***Special Considerations:*** *Discrepancies in function can be corrected by slightly revising electrode placement and/or ensuring adequate skin/electrode interface. Follow manufacturer recommendations for other troubleshooting measures. If such interventions do not result in adequate monitor function, consult the monitor service/supply company for repair or replacement.* |
| b. Disconnect a monitor lead from the infant to simulate an accidental disconnect; ensure that the "loose electrode/disconnect" alarm sounds. | |
| 6. Determine that the audible alarm can be easily heard from a central location or establish that monitor is correctly connected to a remote alarm or a centralized monitoring system. | Audible alarms permit prompt response by nursing personnel. ***Special Considerations:*** *Some monitors and hospitals have the capability of hooking the monitor into the nurse call light system; in this case, activation of the monitor alarm sets off a priority nurse call light.* |

| Steps | Rationale |
|---|---|
| 7. Instruct the family members to notify the nursing staff immediately if audible and/or visual alarms occur and to note time, duration of apnea, and any symptoms such as change of color, unusual motor activity or facial expression. | Instruction of family members assists in identification of infant characteristics and/or symptoms surrounding the alarm event, and decreases anxiety and fear of monitor alarms. |
| 8. Promptly respond to alarms, using following procedure:<br>a. Check the time (Wong and Whaley, 1990).<br>b. For first 10 seconds (10 beeps), only observe the infant (Wong and Whaley, 1990):<br>▪ Color.<br>▪ Chest/abdomen movement.<br>c. If there is a change in color or infant does not resume breathing, stimulate infant by gently rubbing the back or chest, tapping sole of foot or calling name (Wong and Whaley, 1990). | Prompt response to alarms reduces the family's anxiety and allows accurate observation of the event and early intervention. Observation determines the correct course of action.<br>***Special Considerations:*** *Monitor alarms are not necessarily synonymous with apneic events. Either for technological reasons or because of incorrect usage, monitor alarms may sound when infant's respirations and heart rate are normal (Koff, Eitzman, and Neu, 1988).* |
| d. If apnea persists, vigorously stimulate infant with one hand or tap sole of foot (Wong and Whaley, 1990). Suction nose and oropharynx with bulb syringe (see Skill 87).<br>e. If infant is still not responding, administer artificial respirations using either mouth-to-mouth or manual resuscitation bag with oxygen until spontaneous ventilations are noted.<br>f. If pulse is compromised (bradycardic or absent) begin cardiopulmonary resuscitation (see Skill 126).<br>g. If no apnea or color change is observed upon initial observation, investigate possible causes of false alarm, e.g., faulty lead placement or connection, improper alarm setting, or mechanical failure. | Physical stimulation of the infant may initiate respiratory effort. Since neonates are obligatory nose breathers, suctioning the nose and oropharynx may also reinstitute respirations.<br>***Special Considerations:*** *Shaking is no longer an acceptable method of stimulation because of the risk for neck and/or brain injuries.* |
| 9. Following an apneic episode, explain to the family what has occurred and reassure them of continued surveillance of the infant. Clarify their perceptions and answer questions related to the apneic event and intervention required. | Family members will be anxious if present during the event and require reassurance and explanations about the apneic event, interventions required, and continued monitoring of the child. |
| 10. Prepare for discharge (see Skill 5):<br>a. If it is determined that the infant requires apnea monitoring in the home, review family assessment data and note areas of concern related to the ability of the family to carry out the medical plan of care. | The discharge of an infant from the hospital requiring home apnea monitoring creates a situational crisis for most families and requires a change in lifestyle to accommodate the needs of the infant. In addition, the stress of a potential life-threatening event with the infant in the home may be overwhelming to family members. Assessment of the family assists in identifying any areas that make the family ineligible for home apnea monitoring or that signify a need for special arrangements when discharging the infant to the home. |
| b. Notify appropriate services for assistance in acquiring needed equipment, supplies, and home nursing care. Provide referral to appropriate supportive and resource groups, e.g., social services, counseling center, or community health nurse. | Social services and/or discharge planning services may assist with the financial and practical aspects of acquiring the recommended monitor unit, supplies, and any additional home care services required by the family. Effective home monitoring calls for a coordinated, interdisciplinary effort. |
| c. Establish meeting times with the family members for instruction in home apnea monitoring. | Creating specific time periods for instruction allows the family to plan for attendance, and signifies to them the importance of the instruction. |
| d. Recommend that at least two persons from the immediate family attend the training sessions, as well as respite caregivers. Encourage participation from grandparents, other relatives, and significant others. Babysitters/child-care workers should also be required to attend. | Participation of several family members relieves the burden of constant, continual responsibility of the primary caregiver for the infant's care needs, decreasing feelings of isolation. Safety needs dictate that all persons who will care for the infant during monitoring are required to know pertinent information about infant resuscitation and monitoring. |
| e. Use a teaching checklist to instruct the family members/significant others and to document learning that has occurred (see Skill 43). | Use of a teaching checklist ensures that consistency and important aspects of care are covered during instructional periods and documents caregiver competency. |

| Steps | Rationale |
|---|---|
| f. Notify selected home apnea monitoring company of infant's anticipated discharge and need for appropriate monitor and supplies. Arrange for monitor delivery to the hospital at least 24 hours before discharge. Request that family members be present with infant upon delivery of monitor and during initial set-up. | Most home apnea monitoring companies will require advance notice to obtain adequate information and provide monitor and supplies. Use of the home apnea monitor for at least 24 hours prior to discharge will allow the family to adjust to the technical aspects of the home apnea monitor under supervision. |
| g. Ensure that the monitor company provides the family with printed instructions specific to the brand/make of monitor, and a phone number in case of need for repair or replacement. | Having the home monitor company representative instruct the family in specific technical use of the monitor and provide printed instructions along with a phone number for 24-hour repair/replacement provides reinforcement of learning and reassurance of needed assistance. |
| h. Provide the family with written information about home monitoring and related aspects of care, e.g., medications and feeding (see Skill 43). | Written information given to the family reinforces verbal instructions and provides a reference for home care. |
| 11. Explore with caregivers the infant's current developmental status and plans for continuation/initiation of developmental stimulation. Emphasize that the infant has psychosocial, emotional, and developmental needs not affected by apnea monitoring (see Skills 15 and 25). | Ongoing developmental needs of infants must be met to prevent delays or deficits. Attention to this area of infant care promotes caregiver response to the infant in a more "normal" fashion, encourages interaction and promotes caregiver/infant bonding and family functioning. |
| 12. Review other factors of infant's care that may precipitate or alleviate apnea, e.g.: | |
| a. Feeding (see Skill 63). | If an infant's apneic episode is related to gastroesophageal reflux, caregivers require teaching on reflux precautions. |
| b. Medication: dosage, schedule, side effects. | Many infants who demonstrate apnea receive theophylline at home (Norris-Berkemeyer and Hutchins, 1986). |
| c. Physiologic stressors: e.g., hypoglycemia, hypothermia, infection, fatigue. | ***Special Considerations:*** *Remind family members that drug dosages are based on weight; as infant grows, dose may need to be adjusted by the physician. Stressors such as hypoglycemia from inadequate intake, hypothermia from exposure of the young infant to cold stress, infection, and excessive fatigue may precipitate apneic episodes in the infant already predisposed to apnea.* |
| 13. Review safety measures needed for home monitoring, including: | Safety is a major concern since monitors can cause electrical burns and even electrocution (Whaley and Wong, 1991). |
| a. Remove electrode lead wires from infant when they are not attached to the patient cable or apnea monitor. | The FDA recommends this practice to avoid injury or death from inadvertently plugging the lead wires directly into the power cord. |
| b. Unplug power cord from electrical outlet when cord is not plugged into monitor. | ***Special Considerations:*** *Extension cords should not be used. Monitors should only be unplugged for transporting infant and during electrical storms. Leaving a monitor unplugged depletes the battery.* |
| c. Supervise siblings when near monitor or infant. | Sibling tampering with monitor and/or infant is a major cause of accidental disconnection and sibling injury (Andrews and Nielson, 1988). |
| d. *Always* disconnect infant from monitor for bathing or other immersion. | Immersion of the infant while connected to the monitor may cause electrocution. |

| Evaluation Outcomes | Observational Guidelines |
|---|---|
| 1. The infant remains free of cardiopulmonary compromise secondary to prolonged apnea. | Observe skin color, temperature, capillary refill, respiratory sufficiency, respiratory rate and pattern, and pulses. |
| 2. Effective and appropriate intervention is undertaken by nursing staff and/or family members during significant apneic events. | Observe nurse/family member response to apnea, using graded response to terminate apneic event. Observe infant for cessation of apnea/return of spontaneous, effective respirations. Note appropriate contact of emergency personnel/plans for notification. |
| 3. Electronic apnea monitoring is implemented correctly and utilized appropriately and safely. | Observe for correct use of apnea monitor on infant, including safety precautions, troubleshooting, and initiation of monitoring. |
| 4. Family members verbalize and demonstrate confidence in their abilities to provide a safe and therapeutic home environment for their infant requiring home apnea monitoring. | Observe family members' verbalizations and demonstrations when providing care to infant on the apnea monitor. Ask family members to verbalize an awareness of the infant's developmental needs, as well as physiologic and psychosocial needs. |
| 5. Family members are able to verbalize reasons for electronic apnea monitoring and ongoing medical care. | Ask family member(s) to state the reasons that the infant requires apnea monitoring and their plans for follow-up medical care. |

**Evaluation Outcomes—cont'd**

6. Family members are able to state internal and external resources/support systems available to them and plans for access of these support systems as needed to maintain an intact family unit.

**Observational Guidelines—cont'd**

Question family about available resources, coping mechanisms, plans for recreation and leisure, backup child-care plans, and utilization of support systems for assistance with care of the infant and family. Observe impact of infant on family system, and lifestyle modifications required to care for infant on apnea monitor.

## Documentation

Document timing, duration, and stimulation required to terminate apneic event(s). Record frequency of apneic episodes. Note infant color, respiratory rate and pattern, relation to feedings and other events. Document use of electronic apnea monitor and type and respiratory/cardiac parameters. Indicate verification of appropriate monitor functioning and alarms. Record instruction and verification of competencies of family/significant others in home apnea monitoring and related aspects of care and family's response to teaching. Document discharge instructions and provision of written information to the family. Identify any additional child-related events, actions taken, and resulting outcomes.

# *SKILL* 94 Maintaining an Endotracheal Airway and Mechanical Ventilation

*Pamela A. Brown*

Endotracheal intubation and mechanical ventilation are employed to relieve upper airway obstruction, maintain a patent airway, or to treat impending or actual respiratory failure from any cause. The special care needs of a child who is intubated and receiving mechanical ventilation include: (1) frequent assessment of respiratory status; (2) evaluation of the effects of mechanical ventilation; (3) maintaining patency of the endotracheal tube (ETT); (4) preventing dislodgment or displacement of the ETT; (5) prevention and/or early recognition of the complications of ETTs and mechanical ventilation; and (6) minimizing the adverse psychological effects for the child and family.

## NURSING DIAGNOSES

Fear/anxiety related to unmet informational needs about purpose for intubation and mechanical ventilation, inadequate ventilation, tube misplacement or obstruction; Impaired verbal communication related to the presence of an endotracheal tube; Ineffective airway clearance related to the presence of an endotracheal tube, limited ability to cough, and/or copious tracheobronchial secretions; Fluid volume excess related to excessive fluid intake from humidification and compromised regulatory mechanisms due to increased ADH and decreased insensible losses; Altered nutrition related to insufficient caloric intake for increased metabolic needs; Potential for impaired skin integrity related to irritation by endotracheal tube and pressure exerted to secure tube; Impaired physical mobility related to restraints needed to maintain endotracheal tube placement.

| Steps | Rationale |
|---|---|
| **Assessment** | |
| 1. Assess current respiratory status and history including:<br>a. Reason for intubation.<br>b. Reason for mechanical ventilation.<br>c. Response to intubation.<br>d. Response to mechanical ventilation. | Assessment of respiratory status provides data from which judgments about a child's condition are derived.<br>***Special Considerations:*** *With the increasing number of children with chronic respiratory illnesses, knowledge of a child's baseline facilitates realistic expectations for response to treatment and outcomes.* |
| 2. Assess adequacy of ventilation (see Skill 27). | Assessing the adequacy of ventilation is a priority responsibility in caring for the child receiving mechanical ventilation (Snow, 1984). |
| a. Auscultate breath sounds bilaterally. | Auscultation provides information about the child's respiratory status, fluid status, tube placement, and presence of atelectasis, pneumothorax, or consolidation.<br>***Special Considerations:*** *As the child's head is moved right to left, extended, or flexed, the position of the ETT may change. If the tube migrates into the right bronchus, breath sounds will be significantly diminished over the left lung.* |
| b. Evaluate respiratory effort (Brown et al, 1989):<br>▪ Respiratory rate.<br>▪ Respiratory pattern. | Use of a mechanical ventilator does not ensure that ventilation is adequate (Snow, 1984). Assessment of respiratory effort includes observation of both spontaneous (if any) and ventilated breaths. |
| ▪ Chest expansion: equal and bilateral. | Causes of unequal chest expansion include: tube displacement, significant atelectasis, or pneumothorax. |
| ▪ Effort exerted: nasal flaring or retractions (suprasternal, substernal, supraclavicular, intercostal or subcostal). | Normal breathing is effortless and silent. Chest retractions indicate the use of accessory muscles of respiration in an attempt to increase the amount of air brought into the lungs. |
| ▪ Resisting ventilator breaths. | Resistance or "fighting" a ventilator may be an indication of pneumothorax, tube misplacement or obstruction, or agitation. It also leads to inadequate ventilation.<br>***Special Considerations:*** *Muscle paralyzing drugs, e.g., pancuronium, may be used to eliminate ineffective resistance from agitation.* |
| c. Observe color and tissue perfusion. | Changes in color and perfusion may indicate hypoxemia caused by respiratory insufficiency.<br>***Special Considerations:*** *Cyanosis is a late sign and may not be a reliable indicator of hypoxemia.* |
| d. Assess heart rate. | Inadequate ventilation will initially cause tachycardia from the body's attempts to compensate, followed by bradycardia, in which the tissues and vital organs become increasingly hypoxic. |
| e. Assess activity and alertness, irritability, confusion, fatigue, lethargy, inappropriate behavior, somnolence, and coma. | Inadequate ventilation and hypoxemia may cause central nervous system disturbances. |
| 3. Assess patency of ETT:<br>a. Auscultate and observe chest for entry of air into the lungs synchronous with breaths delivered by the ventilator.<br>b. Assess ease of passing suction catheter through ETT. | Patency of the ETT is threatened by: limited ability to cough; presence of foreign body in the airway; and amount and characteristics of secretions.<br>***Special Considerations:*** *An endotracheal tube almost completely occludes the small airway of a child. Any further decrease in size can cause severe respiratory distress and inhibit efforts to effectively ventilate the child.* |
| 4. Determine if the ETT is properly secured, noting "landmark" at lip or nares. | Accidental extubation may cause serious or fatal consequences. Frequently assessing and ensuring security of the ETT helps minimize the risk of dislodgment. Accidental extubation may be caused by inadequate taping or tape loosened by copious secretions, excess movement in bed, emesis or cough, and/or accidental displacement of the tube by the child or by caretakers during the performance of a procedure (Kleiber and Hummel, 1989).<br>***Special Considerations:*** *Accidental or spontaneous extubations are more common in children because of their inability to understand why they are intubated and the consequences of extubation.* |

| Steps | Rationale |
|---|---|
| 5. Assess the presence and function of ventilation equipment:<br>a. Ventilator with appropriate settings and alarms.<br>b. Manual resuscitation bag.<br>c. Proper size mask.<br>d. Oxygen source.<br>e. Emergency intubation equipment. | Equipment failure may have a profound effect on a child's status, therefore assessing and troubleshooting the system is a priority responsibility.<br>***Special Considerations:*** *Always keep a manual resuscitation bag and mask system at the bedside for use in the event of an equipment or power failure, or accidental extubation. If the child's condition indicates fragile lung status, (e.g., neonates, children with adult respiratory distress syndrome), pressure manometers may be attached to the manual resuscitator. This allows monitoring of the pressure needed to inflate the lungs, preventing overinflation and possible pneumothorax.* |
| 6. Assess for complications of endotracheal intubation and mechanical ventilation (such as a decreased cardiac output, gastric distension, tracheal stenosis, or vocal cord paralysis). | Identification of potential risk leads to prompt interventions to prevent or minimize complications. |
| 7. Assess fluid balance (see Skill 64). | Ventilatory support decreases insensible water loss concurrent with an increase in water intake from humidified oxygen delivery, placing the child at considerable risk for overhydration. Mechanical ventilation also increases the risk for fluid imbalance, e.g., inappropriate ADH secretion. |
| 8. Assess skin integrity with special attention to dependent areas and tissue around the ETT (nares for nasal intubation or corners of mouth, lips for oral intubation). Also assess for presence of subcutaneous emphysema (crepitus) over the head and thorax. | Immobility imposed by mechanical ventilation and pressure exerted by ETT taping increase the risk for skin breakdown. Subcutaneous emphysema indicates alveolar rupture and escape of air into the tissues as a complication of mechanical ventilation. |
| 9. Assess nutritional status (see Skill 29). | Critically ill children have an increased need for calories, however, the presence of an ETT alters the feeding process. |
| 10. Assess child and family's understanding of need, purpose, and function of intubation and mechanical ventilation. | The greatest source of anxiety for the child and family is lack of understanding. |
| 11. Assess child's ability to communicate (see Skill 13). | The child who is intubated is unable to speak, therefore impairing verbal communication. Alternate means of communication will depend on child's developmental level, state of consciousness, and preexisting abilities. |

## Planning and Goal Setting

| Steps | Rationale |
|---|---|
| 1. Plan care with child and family, and discuss ways in which they can assist with care, including: bathing, comfort measures, diversional activities, changing diapers. | When a child is intubated and on a ventilator, the family and child feel especially vulnerable. Collaborative planning gives them some control, facilitates feelings of usefulness, and enhances understanding. |
| 2. Assemble equipment:<br>a. Retaping the ETT:<br>▪ Plastic or adhesive tape, three ½ to 1 inch wide pieces, sufficient length to reach cheek to cheek. | ***Special Considerations:*** *The tape must be able to maintain adhesive quality as it becomes wet with oral secretions.* |
| ▪ Benzoin or skin prep.<br>▪ Tape measure.<br>▪ 2 × 2 inch gauze pads.<br>b. Mouth care:<br>▪ 2 to 3 sponge-tipped applicators or toothbrush.<br>▪ Solution of one half mouthwash and one half hydrogen peroxide.<br>▪ Container of water.<br>▪ Oral suction equipment. | ***Special Considerations:*** *Benzoin may cause allergic dermatitis, especially in neonates (Rademaker and Kirby, 1987).* |
| 3. Develop individualized child and family goals:<br>▪ Patent airway and adequate ventilation will be maintained.<br>▪ Complications of endotracheal intubation and mechanical ventilation will be prevented.<br>▪ Child and family will be able to communicate needs. | |

| Steps | Rationale |
|---|---|
| **Implementation**  | |
| 1. Monitor adequacy of ventilatory support continuously and evaluate response to changes in ventilator settings using: | Constant monitoring, assessment, and evaluation of the effects of mechanical ventilation ensures that the child is receiving adequate and appropriate treatment. |
| a. Physical assessment (see Assessment step 2). | ***Special Considerations:*** *Many children will not respond immediately to a change in ventilator settings, therefore it is important to be alert to acute, as well as gradual, changes in respiratory status. If acute changes are noted, however, do not delay intervention while observing to see if response will gradually improve.* |
| b. Noninvasive monitoring devices—transcutaneous $O_2$ and $CO_2$, or pulse oximetry (see Skill 91). | Noninvasive monitoring devices continuously provide information about gas exchange.<br>***Special Considerations:*** *The accuracy of the various types of noninvasive monitoring devices can be affected by a number of factors. Therefore avoid interpretation of values as absolutes, and follow the trend of the values displayed over time.* |
| c. Arterial or capillary blood gas analysis. | Blood gases provide information about the effectiveness of gas exchange.<br>***Special Considerations:*** *Blood gases should be drawn no earlier than 20 minutes after a ventilator change has been made to allow time for an accurate picture of gas exchange with the new settings.* |
| 2. Maintain secure placement of ETT: | Security of the ETT must be carefully maintained to reduce tracheal irritation and edema, and lower the risk of accidental extubation.<br>***Special Considerations:*** *Frequency of retaping and use of other listed interventions is determined by individual need.* |
| a. Restrain the child, if necessary (see Skill 51). | To ensure the security of the endotracheal tube, it may be necessary to restrain child's hands. A child's immature cognitive ability and level of discomfort prevent understanding of the need for an ETT, and the child may attempt to remove it. |
| b. Sedate, if necessary. | The presence of an ETT can be irritating and cause the child to be agitated. The agitation and discomfort may stimulate the child to attempt to remove the ETT or may lead to damage of the trachea. Sedation may be necessary to reduce the effects of the agitation.<br>***Special Considerations:*** *Before sedating a child for agitation, rule out hypoxia as the cause. When administering sedation, closely monitor dosages and effects.* |
| c. Secure ventilator tubing. | The weight of the ventilator tubing combined with the child's movement may be a cause of accidental extubation.<br>***Special Considerations:*** *The ventilator tubing should be secured at the child's bedside in a manner that alleviates tension on the tube and allows enough slack to accommodate some movement. Swivel adapters are used for this purpose.* |
| d. Reposition and retape the ETT as needed. | The ETT must be retaped *every* time the security of the tube is in question.<br>***Special Considerations:*** *Do not reinforce loose tape.* |
| ▪ Recruit an assistant. | Retaping an ETT requires two people; one person removes and replaces the tape while the second person holds the ETT and child's head in position. |
| ▪ Split two pieces of tape two thirds of the length. | |
| ▪ Have the assistant hold the ETT in place and stabilize the child's head. | It is imperative that the child remain still during the retaping procedure or accidental extubation may occur.<br>***Special Considerations:*** *It may be necessary to sedate the child before the procedure.* |
| ▪ Measure the length of the tube from the child's lip or naris to the end of the tube (Fig. 94-1). | This measurement will be used to ensure that the tube is retaped in the same position.<br>***Special Considerations:*** *ETT markings may also be used to verify positioning.* |

| **Steps** | **Rationale** |
|---|---|

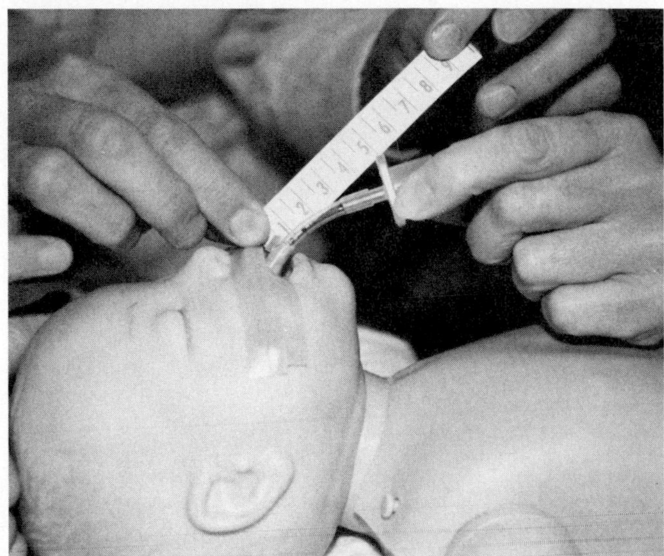

***FIG. 94-1*** Measuring the tube ensures that placement is maintained.

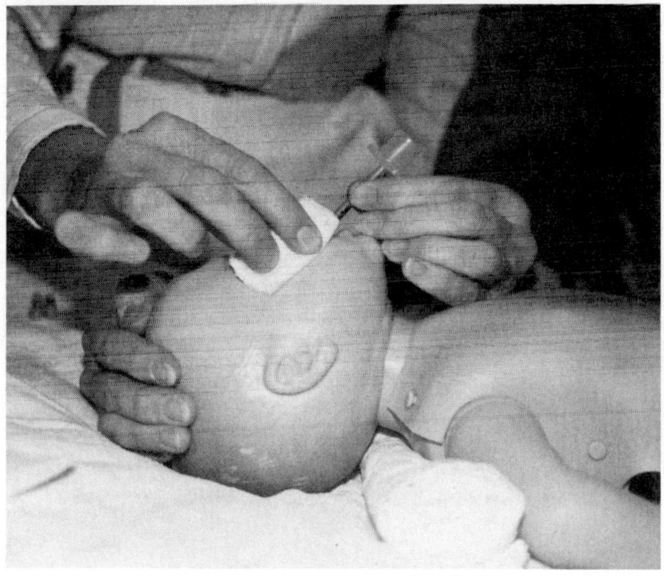

***FIG. 94-2*** Gauze pads are used to cleanse and dry the child's face.

| Steps | Rationale |
|---|---|
| ▪ Remove the old tape. Clean and dry the face with 2 × 2 gauze pads (Fig. 94-2). | |
| ▪ Apply benzoin or skin preparation to cheeks and allow to dry. | These products serve to protect the skin and promote adherence of tape. |
| ▪ Check the position of the tube with the tape measure. | Measuring ensures that the tube is in the same position as before the old tape was removed. |
| ▪ Apply the upper portion of the first piece of split tape on the upper lip (Fig. 94-3).<br>▪ Wrap the bottom portion of tape around the ETT (Fig. 94-4).<br>▪ Apply the second split piece of tape, repeating the two previous steps, beginning from the opposite side.<br>▪ Place the third solid piece of tape over the upper lip, covering the other two pieces (Fig. 94-5). | ***Special Considerations:*** *To minimize skin irritation, place the tape on a slightly different area of skin each time the tube is retaped. Avoid excess layering of tape around the tube, so that loosening may be easily detected.* |
| ▪ Double check tube placement by measuring as described previously and auscultate breath sounds. Note landmarks on ETT at lips or naris. | Measuring provides a final check that the tube was retaped in the correct position. Breath sounds should be equal bilaterally. ETTs are sometimes trimmed to eliminate deadspace, altering the measurement of the tube. Noting tube markings provides an additional method of ensuring placement. |

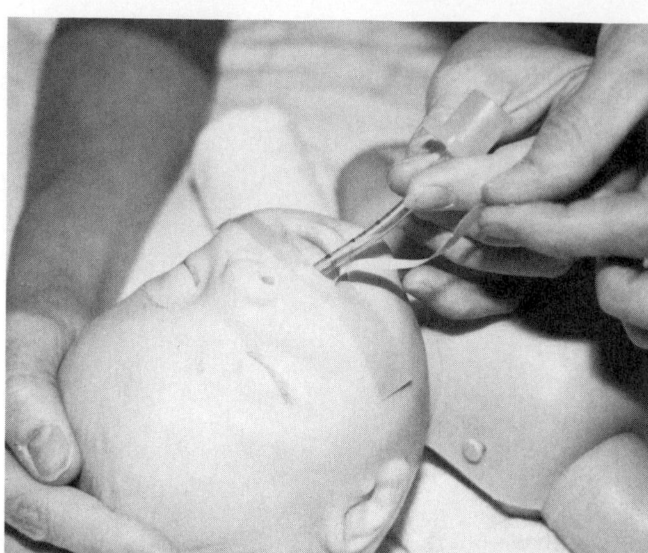

***FIG. 94-3*** The first piece of split tape is applied to the upper lip.

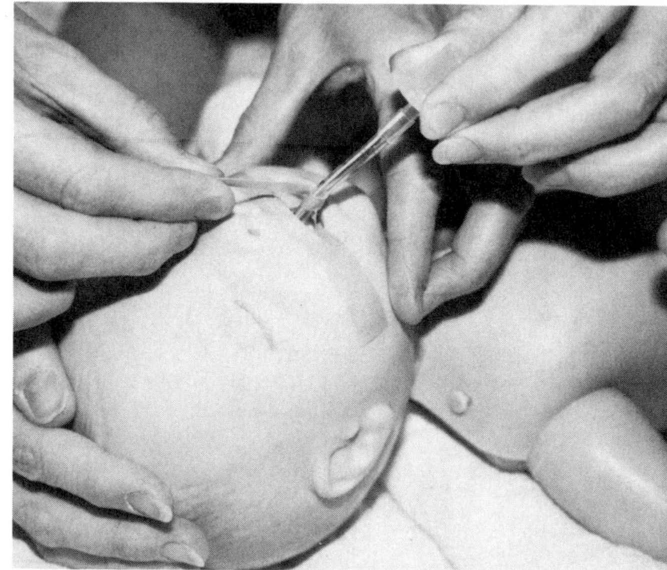

***FIG. 94-4*** The bottom portion of tape is wrapped around the endotracheal tube.

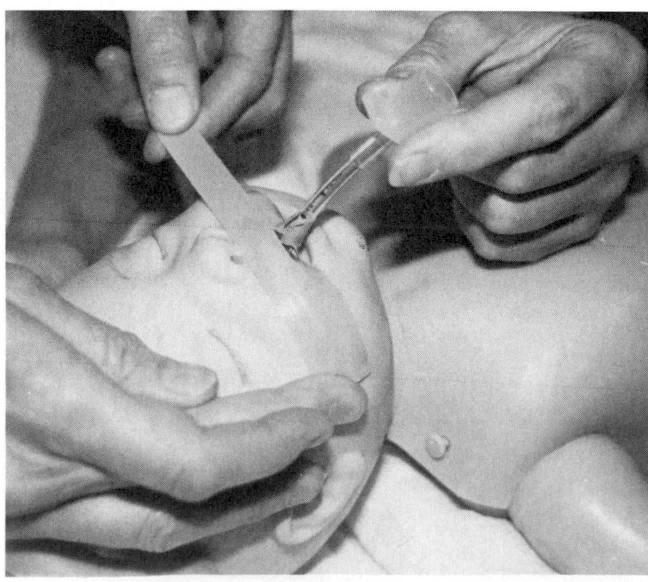

***FIG. 94-5*** A solid third piece of tape is placed over the upper lip.

***TABLE 94-1*** Ventilator Settings

| Term | Definition | Purpose/Parameters | Nursing Responsibilities |
|---|---|---|---|
| Continuous Positive Airway Pressure (CPAP) | Continuous pressure delivered to a spontaneously breathing, intubated child | Increase tissue oxygenation, provide residual volume air in intubated child<br>3-4 cm $H_2O$ | Monitor level of CPAP<br>Assess child's response to therapy |
| Fraction of inspired oxygen ($FiO_2$) | Amount of oxygen delivered | Increase tissue oxygenation titrated to child's response<br>Range: .21-1.0 | Monitor $FiO_2$<br>Assess response<br>Monitor for signs and symptoms of hypoxemia and oxygen toxicity |
| Peak Inspiratory Pressure (PIP) | Maximum pressure delivered to child during a ventilator breath | Provide pressure to expand the lungs or to deliver a preset tidal volume<br>15-30 cm $H_2O$ (Dependent on age and clinical condition) | Monitor amount of PIP<br>Assess response, including chest expansion<br>Volume ventilated children: increasing PIP—decreasing lung compliance |
| Positive End Expiratory Pressure (PEEP) | Application of positive pressure at end expiration in intubated and ventilated child | Maintain functional residual volume and increase tissue oxygenation<br>3-4 cm $H_2O$ | Monitor amount of PEEP<br>Assess response |
| Positive Pressure Ventilation (PPV) | Delivers a volume of air into the lungs until a predetermined pressure limit is reached | Create an airway pressure greater than intraalveolar pressure. Mode of choice in children with small tidal volumes and noncompliant lungs | Assess response |
| Intermittent Mandatory Ventilation (IMV) | Preset number of breaths regardless of spontaneous respirations | Provide adequate respiratory rate to oxygenate and remove $CO_2$<br>Rate: appropriate for age | Monitor respiratory rate, spontaneous and ventilator breaths<br>Assess response |
| Synchronized Intermittent Mandatory Ventilation (SIMV) | Preset rate of breaths delivered in synchrony with spontaneous breaths | Provide adequate respiratory rate to oxygenate and remove $CO_2$<br>Rate: appropriate for age | Monitor respiratory rate, spontaneous and ventilator breaths<br>Assess response |
| Tidal Volume | Volume of gas delivered to the child during inspiration | Provide volume of air sufficient to expand lungs<br>10-15 ml/kg | Observe for chest expansion<br>Assess response |
| Volume Cycled Ventilation | Delivers a predetermined tidal volume regardless of the pressure required | Terminate inspiration after predetermined volume delivered. Mode of choice in children with large tidal volumes and noncompliant lungs | Assess response |

| Steps | Rationale |
|---|---|
| 3. Maintain mechanical ventilation and monitor ventilatory parameters at least every 2 hours (see Table 94-1). | |
| 4. Maintain patency of endotracheal tube. | Maintenance of a patent airway is essential to adequate ventilation.<br>***Special Considerations:*** *If obstruction of the ETT is suspected, the child should immediately be removed from the ventilator and ventilated using a manual resuscitation bag.* |
| a. Suction ETT as needed (see Skill 88). | Suctioning removes secretions and ensures patency of the ETT.<br>***Special Considerations:*** *If unable to easily pass an appropriate size suction catheter through the ETT, remove the tube and begin to ventilate the child using a manual resuscitator and a mask. Notify the physician immediately so that the child can be reintubated as soon as possible.* |

| Steps | Rationale |
|---|---|
| b. Ensure adequate humidity in ventilator circuit. | The upper airway passages are bypassed when a child is intubated, therefore it is important that gases delivered from a ventilator be adequately humidified.<br>***Special Considerations:*** *Inadequate humidification may contribute to the formation of thick, tenacious secretions and increase the risk of airway obstruction. Overhumidification may lead to condensation of fluid in the ventilator circuit and increase the risk of aspiration.* |
| c. Ensure that intubation equipment is readily accessible. | All equipment required to intubate a child must be available for rapid, efficient, and adequate response should the need arise. |
| 5. Perform oral care at least every 4 hours. | Frequent oral care prevents pooling of secretions in the mouth, promotes oral hygiene, and reduces risk of infection.<br>***Special Considerations:*** *Children with copious secretions or active infection may need oral care more frequently.* |
| a. Suction oral cavity (see Skill 87). | Suctioning removes secretions in the mouth before giving care. |
| b. Cleanse mouth, gums, and teeth with mouthwash solution using sponge-tipped applicators or toothbrush. | ***Special Considerations:*** *Securely hold ETT to prevent dislodgement while cleansing the mouth.* |
| c. Suction oral cavity. | |
| d. Rinse mouth with water, using a sponge-tipped applicator or syringe. | Rinsing ensures that all the mouthwash solution has been removed. |
| e. Suction oral cavity. | ***Special Considerations:*** *If a child has thrush, notify physician for appropriate antifungal agent to add to the oral care regime.* |
| 6. Implement measures to maintain skin integrity: | |
| a. Reposition oral ETT from one side of the mouth to the other, each time the tube is retaped. | Repositioning an oral ETT helps to reduce pressure exerted by the ETT on any one side of the mouth.<br>***Special Considerations:*** *When repositioning ETTs, be careful to not change the depth of the tube (refer to the instructions on retaping). Nasal ETTs may also be repositioned to vary pressure points slightly. However, if breakdown is seen around the naris, notify physician. The child may need to be reintubated to prevent permanent damage.* |
| b. Reposition child frequently, moving side to supine to side. Be careful to avoid accidental extubation during repositioning. Use eggcrate, airflow, or sheepskin mattresses. | Position changes relieve pressure on any one area of the body.<br>***Special Considerations:*** *The child may sit in a chair or be held.* |
| 7. Monitor fluid status: intake and output, signs of overload/deficits, daily weights, and urine specific gravity (see Skill 64). | The child who is being mechanically ventilated is at risk for developing fluid imbalances because of: decreased insensible water loss; increased water intake from humidification of air in ventilator circuit; and increased ADH secretion from effects of positive pressure ventilation. |
| 8. Monitor nutritional status:<br>a. Ensure adequate caloric intake.<br>b. Provide gastric, enteral, or parenteral alimentation (see Skills 66 and 67). | When a child is critically ill, nutritional needs are increased. The child must receive adequate nutrition to promote healing. |
| 9. Provide comfort measures: | Having an ETT in place is anxiety producing for a child, and may increase the pain and discomfort the child feels. |
| a. Encourage presence of family members when possible. Allow family members to hold the child, if permitted. | The presence of family members or a trusted adult is immensely comforting for a child. |
| b. Provide age appropriate stimulation/distraction (see Skill 15). | Much discomfort comes from immobility and boredom associated with intubation and hospitalization.<br>***Special Considerations:*** *Ask the child and family about specific activities that are fun and comforting for the child; include these in nursing plan of care.* |
| c. Provide pain relief and sedation as needed. | Anxiety and discomfort are often expressed in agitation. In addition, the child may have other injuries that contribute to pain and discomfort. Analgesics and sedatives are often used in conjunction with muscle relaxants to ensure that the child is free of pain and rests comfortably. |
| 10. Provide information to child and family regarding intubation and ventilation.<br>a. Discuss purpose of mechanical ventilation and interventions directed at maintaining ETT and ventilation, e.g., suctioning, retaping the ETT, frequent blood gas sampling. | Frequent explanation, given in a manner in which both the child and family can understand, can serve to decrease anxiety, assist coping, and improve compliance with treatment. |

| Steps | Rationale |
|---|---|
| b. Encourage child and family to ask questions and verbalize fears and concerns. | Assisting the child and family in verbalizing their concerns is helpful in clarifying misconceptions and incorrect information, therefore reducing stress on the child and family. |
| 11. Allow family to assist with care when possible. | Involving parents in the care of the child is helpful in reestablishing their parental role, therefore reducing anxiety. The child's anxiety also diminishes when care is provided by the person the child most trusts. |
| 12. Provide the child with age appropriate alternative means of communication: pointing to objects on a poster or writing on a piece of paper or a magic slate (see Skill 13). | Not being able to communicate needs adequately can be immensely frustrating for all. Interventions aimed at reducing communication impairment will serve to decrease the child's frustration and facilitate provision of care. |

| Evaluation Outcomes | Observational Guidelines |
|---|---|
| 1. Adequate ventilation is maintained. | Auscultate lung fields bilateral and anterior/posterior. Observe peripheral perfusion, skin and mucous membrane color, quality of chest movements, and amount of effort required to breathe. Observe level of consciousness and compare with baseline. Perform and interpret arterial blood gases and follow oxygen saturation readings and vital signs. |
| 2. ETT remains secure, patent, and in proper position. | Observe tape around tube for adherence and stability. Auscultate breath sounds when ventilator breath is given for equal sounds bilaterally. Observe for symmetrical chest excursion with ventilator breaths. Evaluate ease with which catheter passes through tube during suctioning. |
| 3. Skin integrity remains intact. | Inspect skin for redness, blisters, or abrasions. Note especially skin around the ETT insertion site. |
| 4. Fluids remain in balance. | Observe body for edema or signs of dehydration, especially face and dependent areas. Review output and intake records, daily weights, electrolyte levels, and urine specific gravities. |
| 5. Adequate nutritional status is maintained. | Calculate caloric intake. Observe for gradual weight gain or loss. Note skin turgor, hemoglobin levels, and wound healing. |
| 6. Discomfort is minimized. | Observe for agitation and other signs of stress or anxiety. Observe responses to interventions aimed at increasing comfort such as calm appearance, ability to rest and sleep. |
| 7. Child/family's anxiety is minimized. | Interview family to determine understanding. Note decrease in anxiety. Family asks appropriate questions and responds correctly to questions. |

## Documentation

Record size, type, location, and length of ETT. Note frequency and specific measures taken during performance of ETT care. Also note frequency with which ETT suctioning is performed, including description of secretions and tolerance of procedure. Document the type of ventilation and ventilator settings. Record laboratory results and results of respiratory assessment, including evaluation of therapy. Note interventions performed to ensure tube remains in place, e.g., sedation, restraints. Record efforts to increase comfort and child's response to those efforts. Document teaching/interventions performed to decrease fear/anxiety related to therapy.

## Home Care Modifications

1. Teach family, and observe for demonstration of proficiency in all steps of observation and care in skill related to mechanical ventilation, except for endotracheal tube care. Teach family care for tracheostomy (see Skill 95) and how to modify other care needs in relation to maintaining mechanical ventilation.
2. Problem solve with family on issues related to home care such as initial adjustment; home health care nursing; social and psychological support of the child, primary caregivers, siblings and extended family; and financial burden (Aday, Aitken, and Wegener, 1988).

# SKILL 95 Maintaining a Tracheostomy Site and Airway

Carolyn Testi

Tracheostomy site maintenance provides a stable, secure airway, while preventing obstruction and decannulation of the tracheostomy tube. Tracheostomy site maintenance allows a child to have a continuous alternate airway for an indefinite time. With frequent cleaning of site and changing of the tracheostomy tube, infections can be prevented or minimized. Tracheostomies can often provide a stable airway, allowing discharge from the hospital for children with extenuating unstable airway difficulties, and be maintained by the family at home.

This skill addresses uncuffed tracheostomy tubes because cuffed tubes are usually not used in children under 8 years of age. The anatomic differences between children and adults make it possible to secure an airway in a child without the use of a cuffed tracheostomy tube (Koff, Eitzman, and Neu, 1988).

## NURSING DIAGNOSES

Ineffective airway clearance related to excessive or thick secretions or intubated trachea; Potential for infection (respiratory) related to direct pathway to lower respiratory tract due to tracheostomy; Anxiety related to procedure for suctioning, cleaning, and changing tracheostomy tube; Potential for infection (skin) related to warm, moist environment around stoma.

| Steps | Rationale |
|---|---|
| **Assessment** | |
| 1. Assess tracheostomy site for:<br>a. Skin breakdown—redness, rash, or breakdown of stoma; or soiled tracheostomy ties.<br>b. Infection—increased amount, thick consistency, foul odor, or purulent coloring of secretions.<br>c. Insecure attachment—loose or twisted tracheostomy ties. | Presence of one or more of these complications may indicate a need for more frequent cleaning, suctioning, or tube changing. |
| 2. Assess for signs of lower respiratory infection: low grade to moderate temperature elevation, cough, tachypnea, respiratory distress, cyanosis. | Children with tracheostomies are at higher risk for contracting respiratory infections, including pneumonia and bronchitis, because of a direct pathway to the lower respiratory tract. |
| 3. Assess child's history:<br>a. Age and developmental level of child.<br>b. Type of tracheostomy tube.<br>c. Length of time tracheostomy tube has been indwelling.<br>d. Reason for tracheostomy.<br>e. Need for supplemental oxygen, humidity, or mechanical ventilation. | Knowledge of a child's history will help determine type and steps in maintenance and the child's ability to cooperate with care.<br>***Special Considerations:*** *Infant tracheostomy tubes do not have inner cannulas. Uncuffed tubes are used with children up to 8 years of age. Refer to an adult procedure manual for care of a cuffed tube.* |
| **Planning and Goal Setting** | |
| 1. Determine steps of procedure to implement:<br>a. Clean tracheostomy site and inner cannula.<br>b. Change tracheostomy ties.<br>c. Change tracheostomy tube. | Performing tracheostomy care on a regular basis decreases the risk of infection, skin breakdown, and plugged tube (Lawrence, 1984).<br>***Special Considerations:*** *Tracheostomy ties need to be changed daily and when soiled. The tracheostomy site and inner cannula (if applicable) need to be cleaned twice a day. If gauze dressing is required, it should be changed twice a day or when moist with secretions. Lichenstein (1986) recommends that tracheostomy tubes need to be changed every other day. Others recommend changing all types of tracheostomy tubes at least once a week. If secretions become thickened and an infection occurs, changes may need to be more frequent.* |

| Steps | Rationale |
|---|---|
| 2. Gather supplies: | Having all supplies collected and within reach improves efficiency and safety. |
| a. Cleaning tracheostomy site and inner cannula: | |
| ▪ Cotton-tip applicators. | |
| ▪ Sterile water or saline. | |
| ▪ Hydrogen peroxide. | Hydrogen peroxide is helpful in removing encrustations. |
| ▪ Tracheostomy cleaning kit, which includes: | |
| (1) Disposable sterile containers. | The disposable container is used for soaking and cleaning inner cannula. |
| (2) Sterile pipe cleaners or small tube brush. | |
| (3) Sterile, precut trach dressing or sterile gauze pads. | If a gauze dressing is necessary, noncotton filled gauze pads are used to avoid cotton fibers in the stoma where they can promote bacterial growth. |
| (4) Sterile latex gloves. | |
| (5) Moisture proof bag. | A moisture proof bag is used to discard soiled dressing and prevent the spread of nosocomial infections. |
| ▪ Additional supplies for ventilator dependent child. | |
| (1) Spare inner cannula in a sterile container. | A spare cannula is needed because ventilation cannot be discontinued long enough to clean the inner cannula. |
| (2) Clean towel. | A clean towel is draped across the child's chest to place the disconnected ventilator tubing on it. |
| (3) Manual resuscitator. | A manual resuscitator is used to hyperventilate the child before and after suctioning. |
| b. Changing tracheostomy ties:<br>▪ Twill tape ties or tracheostomy tube holder.<br>▪ Scissors and hemostat or forceps (optional).<br>▪ Sterile gloves. | ***Special Considerations:*** *A commercially available tracheostomy tube holder, which is a cotton-lined adjustable neck band with Velcro fasteners, can serve as an alternative to traditional twill ties in children who are cooperative or unable to pull on the fasteners (see Product References). Another technique to prevent skin breakdown from twill ties is to thread ¼ inch rubber surgical tubing onto the ties to encircle the back of the neck.* |
| c. Changing tracheostomy tube:<br>▪ Tracheostomy tubes (size currently in use and one size smaller), either metal with inner cannula and obturator or plastic tube with obturator.<br>▪ Clean container with screwtop lid.<br>▪ Water-soluble lubricant.<br>▪ Suction equipment.<br>▪ Sterile gloves. | One size smaller tube should be available in case of difficulty with insertion of new tube.<br>***Special Considerations:*** *Use type of tube to which the child is accustomed. Also, an additional sterile tube should be taped to head of bed for emergency use.* |
| 3. Recruit an additional person for assistance, if needed. | An additional person can assist with restraining the infant or child and securing tracheostomy tube.<br>***Special Considerations:*** *If no one is available to assist, mummy-wrap infant or child securely (see Skill 51).* |
| 4. Plan an appropriate time for completing procedure. Change tubes before meals or about 1 to 2 hours after meals. | Proper timing can enhance cooperation and safety. Avoid performing procedure at meal times to reduce the risk of vomiting and aspiration, which may result if tube changes produce gagging sensations. |
| 5. Prepare supplies: | Preparation of supplies increases efficiency and safety. |
| a. Mix hydrogen peroxide with sterile water in equal parts in a sterile container. An adequate amount for most cases is 15 cc hydrogen peroxide and 15 cc water. | Half-strength hydrogen peroxide decreases skin irritation. |
| b. If cleaning an inner cannula, fill the other sterile container with hydrogen peroxide. | |
| c. Open tie package and place supplies within reach.<br>d. If changing tracheostomy tube, attach ties to new tube.<br>e. Assemble and check proper functioning of suction equipment. | ***Special Considerations:*** *It is recommended to use one long piece that loops through the tube end and ties on the side of the neck. If cutting ties from a continuous roll, cut the tie a sufficient length to wrap around neck twice.* |
| 6. Prepare child/family for procedure (see Skill 1):<br>a. Discuss reasons for keeping site and tracheostomy tube clean.<br>b. Describe procedure and possible sensations: a feeling of choking when inner cannula is removed, tracheostomy tube is moved, or suctioned.<br>c. If mechanically ventilated, reassure child/family that disconnection time will be minimal (Persons, 1987). | When the child and family know what to expect, their fears decrease and their cooperation increases.<br>***Special Considerations:*** *Infants also need to be prepared. A gentle, kind voice is soothing to them.* |

| Steps | Rationale |
|---|---|
| 7. Develop individualized child and family goals: ▪ Child's airway will remain intact and patent. ▪ The skin integrity of the tracheostomy site will be maintained. ▪ Infection and trauma of the tracheostomy site and lower respiratory tract will be prevented. ▪ Child and family will experience minimal discomfort and anxiety as a result of the procedure. | |

## Implementation 

1. Position child with towel or blanket roll under shoulders (see Fig. 95-1).

A shoulder roll allows the head to hyperextend, promoting maximum exposure of the tracheostomy site.
***Special Considerations:*** *Many infants, depending on how agitated they become and how much assistance is available, will need to be mummy-wrapped in addition to the shoulder roll (see Skill 51).*

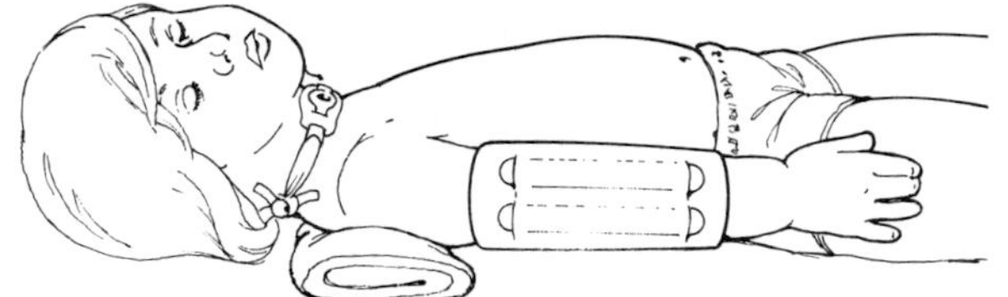

***FIG. 95-1*** A shoulder roll provides maximum exposure of tracheostomy site.

2. Remove tracheostomy collar. Continue mechanical ventilation if applicable.

Removing collar allows for maximum exposure of the tracheostomy site.
***Special Considerations:*** *If tracheostomy collar is used to provide supplemental oxygen to the child, an assistant is needed to hold collar in place. If dressing is present, remove and dispose of it in moisture proof bag. Some agencies recommend wearing a clean (not sterile) glove to remove the soiled dressing.*

3. Put on gloves. Keep dominant hand sterile and nondominant hand clean.

Although a sterile field cannot be maintained around a tracheostomy site because of bronchial secretions and exudate, sterile gloves are worn during tracheostomy care to minimize cross contamination of the lower respiratory tract. Wearing gloves also reduces the risk of herpetic whitlow and HIV infection (Soule, 1983).

4. Suction the length of the inner cannula (see Skill 88).

Suctioning removes secretions that may obstruct the airway.
***Special Considerations:*** *Increase fluid intake whenever secretions are tenacious.*

5. Remove and cleanse the inner cannula (if applicable).
   *Non-ventilator-dependent child:*
   a. Using the nondominant hand, unlock the inner cannula and remove it.
   b. Soak the inner cannula for several minutes in sterile disposable container.

   Soaking the cannula moistens and removes dried secretions.

   c. Remove the cannula from the soaking solution, thoroughly cleanse the lumen and entire inner cannula with a moistened brush or pipe cleaners.

   Cleansing with a brush or pipe cleaner provides the friction needed to remove accumulated encrustations, which can obstruct or narrow the cannula's lumen.

   d. Thoroughly rinse the cannula by pouring sterile water or saline over it, then gently tap on edge of sterile container to remove excess solution.

   Hydrogen peroxide should be thoroughly rinsed from the cannula since it can cause tracheal and stomal irritation. Rinsing also provides a thin layer of moisture for insertion lubrication. Excess solution is removed to prevent possible aspiration.

   e. Holding the cannula to the light at eye level, inspect for cleanliness. Repeat the cleaning steps if encrustations remain.
   f. Suction the outer cannula remaining in the tracheostomy site.

   Suctioning removes secretions that may cause adherence of the two tubes when the inner cannula is inserted.

   g. Grasp the outer flange of the inner cannula, and insert into the outer cannula in the direction of its curvature.
   h. Lock the inner cannula in place, and gently pull to ensure it is positioned and securely locked.

| **Steps** | **Rationale** |
|---|---|
| *Ventilator-dependent child:* | |
| a. Using nondominant hand, remove the lid of the container holding the spare cannula. | Use of the nondominant hand to open the container maintains the sterility of the dominant hand. |
| b. Using nondominant hand, unlock the inner cannula, and remove it by gently pulling it out in line with its curvature. | |
| c. Using the dominant hand, insert the spare cannula and lock it in place, ensuring that it is secure. | Use of the sterile gloved hand maintains sterility of the inner cannula. |
| d. Use the nondominant hand to reattach the child to the ventilator. | The ventilator dependent child will require continuous ventilation during the cleaning procedure. |
| e. Clean the soiled cannula following steps 5b-5e in non-ventilator-dependent section. Store in clean container. | |
| 6. Clean area around stoma and flanges of outer cannula with cotton-tipped applicators moistened with half-strength hydrogen peroxide. Rinse the cleansed area with applicators moistened in sterile water. Gently pat area dry with sterile gauze. | Cleansing around the stoma removes secretions and encrustations and helps prevent infection. ***Special Considerations:*** *If the child has excessive tracheal secretions, clean around the stoma more often than twice a day.* |
| 7. If secretions are excessive, apply a dressing around the stoma and cannula. | The dressing may help to absorb the secretions and reduce irritation and risk of infection. |
| a. Use a precut tracheostomy dressing or a refolded gauze square (see Figs. 95-2 and 95-3). | |

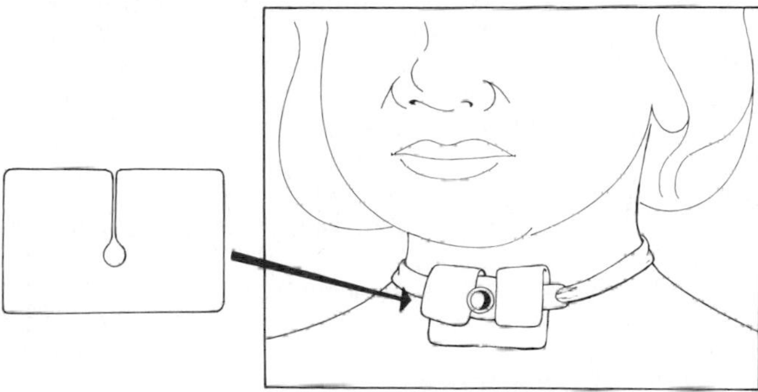

***FIG. 95-2*** Use of the precut tracheostomy dressing.

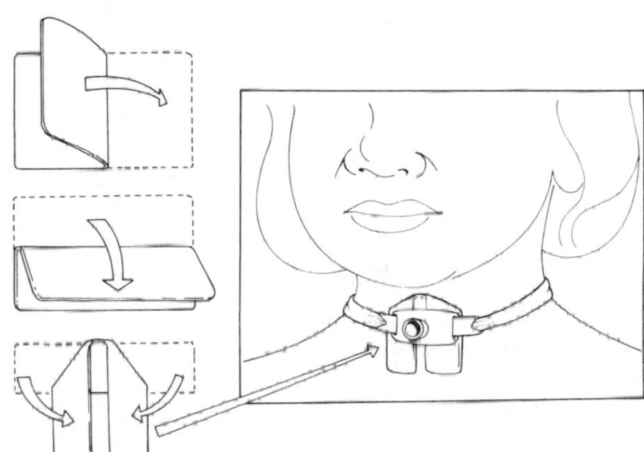

***FIG. 95-3*** A refolded gauze square can help to absorb excessive secretions.

| **Steps** | **Rationale** |
|---|---|
| b. Do not cut the gauze or use cotton-filled gauze dressings. | Aspiration of cotton lint or frayed fibers can result in tracheal abscess. |
| c. Provide secure support for the tracheostomy tube while applying dressing. | Excessive movement of the tracheostomy tube could cause tracheal irritation or accidental extubation. |
| 8. Change tracheostomy ties: | |
| a. Have an assistant wear a sterile glove, and hold the tracheostomy tube in place with gentle, but firm pressure on the flanges of the tube. | Once the ties are removed, the tracheostomy cannula can be easily coughed out. To prevent accidental decannulation, an assistant will need to hold the tracheostomy tube securely in place. ***Special Considerations:*** *If unable to recruit an assistant, the new ties will need to be placed on the tracheostomy cannula before removing the old ties.* |
| b. Cut using bandage scissors or untie the old tracheostomy ties and remove them from the flanges. | Removal of the old ties is helpful to make room to pull the new tracheostomy ties through the flanges. ***Special Considerations:*** *A hemostat or forceps may be needed to pull the ties through the flanges, especially if the new ties need to be threaded before removing the old ties.* |
| c. Clean the back of the neck with soap and water at this time and inspect the skin for pressure sores from the ties. | Changing tracheostomy ties provides a good opportunity to clean and inspect the skin. ***Special Considerations:*** *If changing the tracheostomy ties without assistance, clean the neck before placing the new ties on.* |

| Steps | Rationale |
|---|---|

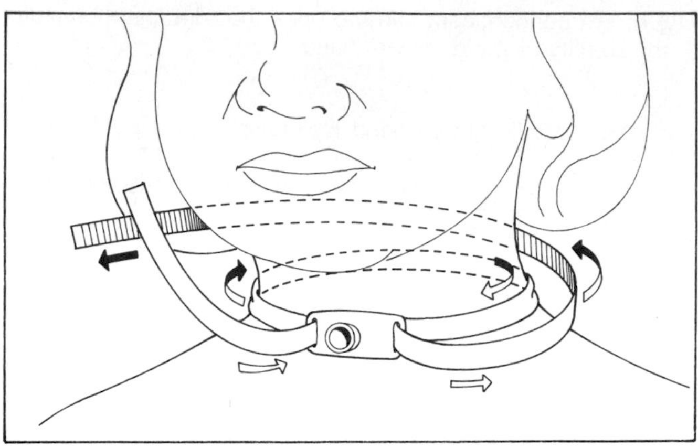

***FIG. 95-4*** A doubled tie increases the security of the tracheostomy cannula.

| Steps | Rationale |
|---|---|
| d. Insert new tracheostomy tie into one flange, around the back of the neck, and through the opposite flange (Russell, 1984) (see Fig. 95-4). | Using one long tie prevents raveling of a cut tracheostomy tie end and increases the security of the tracheostomy cannula by providing two layers of ties behind the neck. |
| e. With the assistant holding the tracheostomy cannula in place, help the child to sit up. | With the child in a sitting position, the entire neck area can be observed for gaps in the ties and placement around the neck. ***Special Considerations:*** *If placing tracheostomy ties without assistance, or on a child who is comatose or on mechanical ventilation, turn child from side to side.* |
| f. Bring the tracheostomy tie back around to the original side where the tie was inserted, and tie the two ends together in a single square knot to check fit. | This provides two layers behind the neck, without having the knot directly behind the head. The knot should be on the side of the neck for comfort and to decrease the risk of pressure sores. |
| g. Check the tightness of the ties by inserting index finger between the ties and the neck when the head is slightly flexed. It should fit snugly. | Flexion of the neck simulates an increase in neck circumference, which also occurs with coughing. The cannula needs to be held securely in place, but an excessively tight fit will restrict circulation or cause choking. |
| h. Finish securing the ties into a triple square knot. Alternate the side of the knot with each tracheostomy tie change. | A triple knot holds the ties securely and provides an extra knot in case one accidentally comes untied. Alternating the site of the knot prevents formation of pressure sores. |
| i. Leave an inch surplus tie past the tied knot. | An inch of surplus tie provides room for readjustment of the ties, if needed. |
| j. Frequently check ties. | Checking the ties ensures that the tracheostomy tube is secure, but circulation is not impaired. |
| 9. Change tracheostomy cannula (plastic or metal):<br>a. Put on sterile gloves.<br>b. Attach ties to the new tracheostomy cannula, and insert the obturator (with a metal tracheostomy tube, the inner cannula must be removed to insert the obturator). | Frequent cannula changes decrease the amount of granulation tissue that may form within the trachea and around the stoma, obstructing the airway and delaying cannulation (Lichenstein, 1986). |
| c. Apply small amount of water-soluble lubricant to end of tracheostomy tube. | Lubrication of the end of the tube enhances ease of insertion. ***Special Considerations:*** *If a water-soluble lubricant is not available, a small amount of water may be used for lubrication.* |
| d. Clean the tracheostomy site as described previously. Suction airway, if needed. With the assistant gently holding the tracheostomy tube in place, cut the ties. | ***Special Considerations:*** *Children with excessive secretions should have the tracheostomy suctioned just before cutting the tracheostomy ties. If possible, it is best to avoid suctioning because of the agitation it may cause, making the tube change more difficult. Children on mechanical ventilation should be hyperventilated just before changing the tracheostomy tube.* |
| e. With the new assembled tracheostomy cannula in the dominant hand, remove the old tracheostomy tube with the other hand, and immediately insert the new tracheostomy cannula at a right angle. Rotate it in a semicircular manner until completely in place (see Fig. 95-5). | Use of the dominant hand to insert the new tracheostomy cannula allows maximum dexterity. A right angle approach with semicircular rotation enhances ease of insertion. ***Special Considerations:*** *Some procedures advise having the assistant remove the old tracheostomy tube. The advantage in having the same person removing the old and inserting the new cannula is better orientation for placement, rhythmic motion, and minimizing the time span between removal and insertion of tracheostomy tube.* |

| **Steps** | **Rationale** |
|---|---|

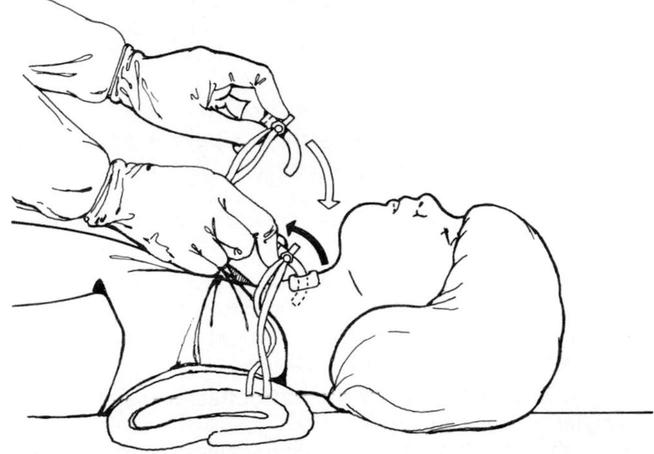

***FIG. 95-5*** The old tracheostomy tube is removed and the new cannula is quickly inserted at a right angle.

| **Steps** | **Rationale** |
|---|---|
| f. Immediately remove the obturator from the newly inserted tracheostomy cannula. If a metal tracheostomy tube, insert the inner cannula and twist into place. | The removal of the obturator allows air to pass through the cannula. |
| g. Reattach ventilator dependent child to mechanical ventilation. | |
| h. Assess child's respirations. | Correct placement of the new tracheostomy tube can be determined by observing respiratory effort and auscultating breath sounds.<br>***Special Considerations:*** *If the child is having difficulty breathing after the tube is inserted, remove it and reinsert. If continued difficulty, a new tracheostomy cannula may be needed. A tracheostomy tube that has not been in place long enough to establish a tract may accidentally be inserted into the soft tissues of the neck rather than into the trachea (Persons, 1987).* |
| i. Suction tracheostomy airway (see Skill 88). | Most children are stimulated to cough during the tracheostomy tube change. Suctioning removes secretions coughed into the tube during the change. |
| j. Tie the tracheostomy ties as described in step 8. | |
| k. Keep the obturator accessible, at the bedside or in the room at all times. | Having the obturator available is a safety precaution in event of accidental decannulation. |
| 10. Reapply tracheostomy collar and humidification. | Humidification prevents thickening of secretions. Oxygen should be delivered by tracheostomy collar with humidification.<br>***Special Considerations:*** *If a compressor is not available to deliver humidity by tracheostomy collar, several room humidifiers can be used. At least 50% humidity should be achieved (Lichenstein, 1986).* |
| 11. Clean tracheostomy tubes:<br>*Plastic Shiley tubes:* | Cleaning and reusing the tracheostomy tubes helps reduce the cost involved with frequent tube changes. |
| a. Clean tube thoroughly with mild detergent, water, and pipe cleaners or small tube brush. | |
| b. Rinse thoroughly with water. | Rinsing removes soap and pipe cleaner fibers from the tube. |
| c. Soak in hydrogen peroxide for 8 hours or overnight. | Hydrogen peroxide is effective for disinfecting the tube.<br>***Special Considerations:*** *Boiling in water will melt a plastic tracheostomy tube.* |
| d. Rinse completely with water or saline. | Hydrogen peroxide should be rinsed completely from the tracheostomy tube because it can irritate the tracheal lining and stoma.<br>***Special Considerations:*** *If stoma irritation is noted after thorough rinsing, half-strength hydrogen peroxide may be needed for future cleaning.* |
| e. Dry with a clean paper towel, and gently shake tube to remove water from tube shaft. Allow to air dry completely. | If the tube is stored while still damp, mildew growth can occur. |

| Steps | Rationale |
|---|---|
| f. Store in a clean container after attaching twill tape. | Tracheostomy tubes should be stored in a clean container to reduce exposure to infection-causing organisms. **Special Considerations:** *Tracheostomy tubes should never be stored in a plastic bag because of possible mildew growth.* |
| *Metal tubes:* | |
| a. Clean and rinse as with plastic tubes (steps 11a-11b). | |
| b. Remove any tarnish with silver polish. Thoroughly rinse polish. | Tarnish is a prime medium for bacterial growth and is extremely irritating to the trachea and stoma, therefore it must be completely removed. **Special Considerations:** *Silver polish is the only effective cleanser to remove tarnish.* |
| c. Clean tube again with soap, water, and pipe cleaners. | **Special Considerations:** *If child breaks out in a rash around the stoma as a result of using a metal tracheostomy tube that has been cleaned with silver polish, wash and rinse a second time. Also notify the child's physician.* |
| d. Boil the pieces of the tube in water for 15 minutes. | Boiling in water is the easiest and most effective way to sterilize a metal tracheostomy tube. |
| e. Cool the tracheostomy tube on sterile gauze, attach twill ties, then store in clean container. | Cooling the metal tracheostomy tube prevents accidental burns and avoids condensation in the storage container. |
| 12. Emergency care for the child with a tracheostomy: | |
| a. If respirations cease, remove the inner cannula (if present), and immediately suction the tracheostomy. | An obstruction of thickened secretions can cause cessation of breathing. **Special Considerations:** *After the child has fully recovered, it is advisable to change the tracheostomy tube because thickened secretions may have collected at the base of the cannula.* |
| b. If breathing is not reinstituted, change the tracheostomy tube—remove old one, suction stoma, and place a second tube. | Continued cessation of respirations may be due to plugged secretions. A clean tube provides a patent airway and breathing should be fully restored. **Special Considerations:** *The cause of the plug should be identified. The child may need more humidification or more frequent changes of the tracheostomy tube.* |
| c. If the child does not breathe when the new tracheostomy tube is inserted, begin artificial respiration (see Skill 126). | Ventilation must be reestablished to avoid damage from hypoxia. **Special Considerations:** *The physician should check the child's tracheostomy site after breathing has been restored.* |
| d. If unable to reinsert the tracheostomy tube when routinely changing the tube or accidental decannulation: | |
| ▪ Calmly reposition the head, relubricate the tube, and again attempt insertion. | A slight adjustment of the position of the trachea may permit insertion of the tube. Also a bronchial spasm may have occurred, preventing tube insertion during previous attempt. |
| ▪ If the tube will still not insert, reinsert the old tracheostomy tube, after inserting the obturator. | The new tracheostomy tube may have a defect preventing its insertion. Using the old tube, which previously fit in the tracheal stoma, allows time to identify the problem. **Special Considerations:** *A size smaller tube may be needed to pass into the tracheal opening.* |
| ▪ As an alternative technique when insertion is difficult, place a suction catheter through the tube to be inserted, place the suction catheter into the stoma, and thread the trach tube along the suction catheter until in place (Donaghy, 1986). | |
| ▪ If insertion continues to be unsuccessful, cut a suction catheter to approximately 6 inches in length, insert into stoma, and hold in place until assistance is available. | A tube with a lumen will establish an airway until assistance is available. **Special Considerations:** *A suction catheter is usually the most accessible tube with a lumen in this situation, but any lumened object will maintain an airway. A mature stoma (one that has completely healed) will usually stay open by gently extending the head and neck.* |
| ▪ If respirations are absent, and repeated attempts to reinsert tracheostomy tube are unsuccessful, seal stoma with sterile dressings, and ventilate child with mask and manual resuscitation bag. Perform mouth-to-trach ventilation, if necessary. | It is imperative to establish respirations to avoid a hypoxic insult. |

## Evaluation Outcomes

1. The tracheostomy tube remains securely in place.
2. The tracheostomy tube provides a patent airway, free of mucus plugs and excess secretions.
3. The stoma site remains clear, free of secretions, skin breakdown, odor, and purulent drainage.
4. The child remains free of signs and symptoms of lower respiratory tract infection.
5. The child and family experience minimal discomfort and anxiety as a result of the procedure.

## Observational Guidelines

Note securely knotted ties with no visible gaps. Accidental decannulation does not occur.

Observe amount of secretions. Respirations are regular and nonlabored.

Observe stoma for pink, healthy skin with no secretions. No purulent drainage or foul odor is noted. Temperatures afebrile.

Note character of suctioned secretions. Observe for signs and symptoms of respiratory distress or auscultate breath sounds. Measure temperature.

Observe the child's responses during the procedure. Ask child and family to identify their feelings concerning the procedure.

## Documentation

Record observations of skin integrity, secretions, and presence and quality of breath sounds. Record changing of tracheostomy ties and tube changes. Record child's response to procedures, any emergencies that arise, and actions taken.

## Home Care Modifications

1. Clean technique for suctioning a tracheostomy is used in the home as compared with the sterile suctioning done in a hospital setting.
2. Families may use a suction catheter more than one time. The suction catheters can be soaked in full strength hydrogen peroxide overnight and thoroughly rinsed with tap water.
3. Normal saline can be made at home by adding 1½ teaspoons of noniodized salt to one quart of water brought to a boil for 5 minutes. Store in a clean container and keep in refrigerator.
4. Half-inch hemming tape or seam binding can be used for tracheostomy ties and is available at most fabric stores.
5. Plain paper cups for suctioning can be used rather than a sterile container. Use the bottom cup each time, and seal the box again to keep the cups clean and dry (Kozier and Erb, 1987).
6. The child should take tub baths and not showers.
7. If a tracheostomy collar is not available to supply humidity to the tracheostomy, several humidifiers in a room may be used at home. Provide humidity for infants, especially during naps and night sleeping.
8. If needing humidity immediately, run a hot shower to steam an enclosed area.
9. Place gauze over site on windy days when outdoors. When playing outdoors on dry, cold days, increase humidity by dampening gauze.
10. Use bibs without plastic liner when feeding infant (McCrory, 1986).
11. Metal tubes do not need to be sterilized for a mature stoma (McCrory, 1986).
12. Infants and children who are 2 years of age or younger should be connected to cardiac/apnea monitors any time they are not in the caregiver's presence.
13. Any person responsible for the care of an infant or child with a tracheostomy must know how to suction the tracheostomy and perform pediatric cardiopulmonary resuscitation (McCrory, 1986).
14. For home care instructions that may be photocopied and given to families, see Wong and Whaley: Clinical manual of pediatric nursing, ed 3, Caring for a child with a tracheostomy, St Louis, 1990, The CV Mosby Co.

# SKILL 96 Assisting with Insertion, Maintenance, and Removal of a Chest Tube

*Joan Young Kemper*

When the integrity of the pleural space is disrupted, and intrapleural vacuum is lost or decreased, ventilation is impaired and respiratory distress occurs. This disruption can occur as a result of an accumulation of air (pneumothorax), blood (hemothorax), and/or serous fluid (pleural effusion) in the pleural space. This accumulation may occur spontaneously, especially in neonates, or develop as a result of trauma, surgery, or ventilatory assistance (barotrauma).

Insertion of a chest tube connected to an evacuation device is often necessary if the pneumothorax is greater than 10% (Hazinski, 1984), if a significant amount of fluid is accumulated, or if significant respiratory distress is present. A chest tube is often required after thoracic surgery to prevent the accumulation of serosanguineous fluid and air. The chest tube evacuation system removes accumulated air and fluid by creating negative pressure, greater than that of the pleural space.

Chest tubes are inserted and removed by the physician with nursing assistance. Maintenance of the chest tube evacuation system is a nursing responsibility. The first priority in nursing care is the maintenance of adequate cardiopulmonary function of the infant or child.

## NURSING DIAGNOSES

Ineffective breathing pattern related to decreased lung expansion; Impaired gas exchange related to altered oxygen supply; Anxiety related to change in breathing pattern, procedures for insertion, maintenance, and removal of chest tube system and/or protective restraint; Pain related to difficulty breathing and/or chest tube insertion/removal; Potential for respiratory infection related to direct pathway of chest tube to pleural cavity.

| Steps | Rationale |
|---|---|
| **Assessment** | |
| 1. Assess respiratory status for signs and symptoms of pneumothorax, hemothorax, or pleural effusion, including: | Baseline assessments are necessary to determine the need for and effectiveness of treatment. ***Special Considerations:*** *Diagnosis of a pneumothorax, hemothorax, hemopneumothorax, or pleural effusion is confirmed by chest radiograph. Transillumination of the chest with a fiberoptic probe and/or thermography may be used in neonates to confirm a pneumothorax.* |
| a. Breath sounds: hyperresonance; dull, decreased or absent; differences in quality or pitch. | The affected lung field may be hyperresonant with decreased breath sounds if a pneumothorax is the cause of impaired ventilation. A hemothorax may produce dull, decreased or absent breath sounds on the affected side. ***Special Considerations:*** *The thin chest wall of the neonate and infant allows breath sounds to be referred from other areas of the lung, therefore decreased breath sounds may not be noted, but a difference in the quality or pitch of breath sounds may be heard over the affected area (Hazinski, 1984).* |
| b. Increased respiratory rate and effort. | Assessment of these symptoms may indicate an extraneous air syndrome (air leak). ***Special Considerations:*** *Early manifestations of extraneous air syndrome in neonates include restlessness and irritability, tachypnea, lethargy, grunting, flaring nares, and retractions (Whaley and Wong, 1989).* |

| Steps | Rationale |
|---|---|
| c. Chest movements: unequal thoracic wall movement with decreased movement on affected side; paradoxical movement (chest wall retracts during inspiration and moves outward with expiration). | Pneumothorax may produce unequal thoracic wall movement with decreased movement on the affected side (Moore, Mills, and Mast, 1984). Fractures of the ribs producing flail chest cause paradoxical respirations. |
| d. Tracheal shift. | An accumulation of trapped air or fluid may cause the mediastinal contents to shift, compromising the contralateral lung. |
| e. Percussion and palpation of thorax: hyperresonance; dullness; crepitus. | Pneumothorax may produce a hyperresonance to percussion on the affected side (Moore, Mills, and Mast, 1984). Hemothorax may result in a dullness to percussion of the involved area (Hazinski, 1984). Subcutaneous emphysema caused by air leaking into the subcutaneous tissues results in crepitus being palpated over affected area. **_Special Considerations:_** *Percussion of the chest as an assessment method is less useful in infants because of their relatively small chest size (Koff, Eitzmann, and Neu, 1988).* |
| f. Dusky or cyanotic skin color, mucous membranes, nailbeds. | Abrupt and profound duskiness or cyanosis is a late sign of respiratory distress and may indicate a tension pneumothorax. **_Special Considerations:_** *In the neonate, a sudden change in color may be indicative of pneumothorax, especially if on mechanical ventilation.* |
| 2. Assess cardiovascular status. | Cardiovascular assessment helps detect tension pneumothorax, which causes a mediastinal shift that may produce a significant reduction in cardiac output. **_Special Consideration:_** *Tension pneumothorax is a life-threatening situation that requires emergency decompression for lung re-expansion.* |
| a. Decreased blood pressure, pulse pressure, heart rate, and peripheral perfusion. | A significant reduction in cardiac output is caused by the shift of mediastinal contents. |
| b. Cardiac sounds: point of maximum impulse (PMI) shifts toward unaffected side; diminished and/or muffled. | Changes in cardiac sounds are also indicative of tension pneumothorax. |
| 3. Determine the child's age, developmental level, and possible need for restraint. | Age and development influence the ability to cooperate with the procedure, as well as the selection of chest tube size. Unexpected movement of the child significantly increases the risk of injury to the lung during the procedure (Moore, Mills, and Mast, 1984). |
| 4. Review the physician's orders for consent wording, type of chest tube and drainage system, suction requirements, premedication, preprocedure and postprocedure chest radiography, supplemental oxygen, and/or mechanical ventilation needs. | Reviewing the physician's orders facilitates efficient completion of procedure. **_Special Considerations:_** *The majority of infants with compromising pneumothorax require ventilatory support (Fletcher and Eichelberger, 1983).* |
| 5. Assess for allergies, particularly to antiseptic, anesthetic, or analgesic agents. | Povidone-iodine, lidocaine, and various analgesics are commonly used in this procedure. Determining allergies permits avoidance of allergic substance and subsequent adverse effects. |

## Planning and Goal Setting

| Steps | Rationale |
|---|---|
| 1. Gather and assemble necessary supplies and equipment: | Preparing equipment allows procedure to be performed quickly and efficiently. |
| *Sterile supplies:* | |
| a. Sterile thoracostomy tray containing: ▪ 4 × 4 inch gauzes. ▪ Surgical drapes. | Many physicians request a thoracostomy tray so that surgical instruments are available during chest tube insertion (Hazinski, 1984). **_Special Considerations:_** *If tray is unavailable, gather listed items.* |
| ▪ Local anesthetic ampule, e.g., lidocaine—1% without epinephrine. | Lidocaine is used to anesthetize the insertion site intradermally, subcutaneously, and into the muscles of the chest wall. |
| ▪ Scalpel handle with no. 11 and no. 15 scalpel blades. | The no. 11 blade is used to make the skin incision. The no. 15 blade may be used to make an incision in the chest wall. |
| ▪ Two curved mosquito hemostats. | One curved hemostat is used to spread the subcutaneous tissue, and the other is used to thread the chest tube into the thorax. |
| ▪ Needle holder and suture materials. | Suture type is based on child's size and physician's preference. |
| ▪ Scissors. | Scissors are used to cut suture. |

| Steps | Rationale |
|---|---|
| b. Additional supplies: | |
| ▪ Mask, sterile gown, and gloves for physician. | |
| ▪ Antiseptic solution, e.g., povidone-iodine. | |
| ▪ Syringes: 5 ml, 10 ml, and 50 ml. | The 5 ml syringe is used for the lidocaine injection; the 10 ml for evacuation of fluid and/or air; the 50 ml for adding saline to the evacuation system. |
| ▪ Needles: 25 gauge and 22 gauge. | The 25 gauge needle is used to administer local anesthetic subcutaneously. The 22 gauge is used to add saline to the evacuation system. |
| ▪ Sterile saline. | Saline is used to lubricate the trocar of the thoracostomy tube and to fill the water seal unit of the drainage system. It is unlikely that saline will cause cell hemolysis if it comes in contact with lung tissue (Persons, 1987). |
| ▪ Occlusive dressing, e.g., petrolatum gauze, adhesive bandage. | |
| ▪ Cotton-tip applicators. | Applicators are used to apply antibiotic ointment or benzoin. |
| ▪ Y-connector (optional). | Y-connector is needed if two chest tubes are inserted. |
| ▪ 5-in-1 connector. | The 5-in-1 connector is used to join connective tubing to chest tube in all systems. |
| ▪ Appropriate size thoracostomy tube.<br>(1) Newborns: 8 to 12 French.<br>(2) Infants: 8 to 14 French.<br>(3) Child: 14 to 28 French.<br>(4) Adolescent: 28 to 38 French. | |
| ▪ Evacuation system: | The type of system selected is determined by the child's condition, physician preference, and institutional availability. |
| (1) Bottle drainage. | ***Special Considerations:*** *Bottle systems have largely been replaced by plastic disposable units in most institutions (Perry and Potter, 1990).* |
| (2) Commercially-available disposable drainage system: water-seal system (e.g., Pleur-Evac) or non-water seal system (e.g., Thora-Klex). | ***Special Considerations:*** *Advantages of a disposable unit are its compactness, reduced maintenance, suitability for both gravity and suction drainage, reduced risk of spillage and enhanced portability and safety. The disadvantages are cost and units with collection chambers calibrated in only 10 ml increments, since neonates' and infants' drainage is often less than 10 ml per hour. Disposable units are similar to the three-bottle drainage system.* |
| *Non-sterile supplies:* | |
| a. Suction source: Emerson or wall suction. | ***Special Considerations:*** *Either Emerson or wall suction may be used. Emerson chest-suction system is a three-bottle system that removes large amounts of fluid and air while maintaining low controlled negative pressure from 9 cm $H_2O$ to 60 cm $H_2O$.* |
| b. Tincture of benzoin. | Benzoin promotes dressing adherence.<br>***Special Considerations:*** *Benzoin may cause allergic skin dermatitis, especially in neonates.* |
| c. Antibiotic ointment. | |
| d. ½ inch or 1 inch nonpaper occlusive tape and/or banding ties. | Tape or bands are used to secure the chest tube and connections. Tape will also be needed to secure the dressing. |
| e. Large safety pin or hemostat. | |
| f. Specimen tubes. | Laboratory analysis of fluid drainage may be required. |
| g. Rubber-tipped clamps (optional). | The clamps are used to seal off the chest tube in the event of accidental disconnection. Rubber tips prevent damage to the plastic tube.<br>***Special Considerations:*** *Clamping the chest tube is controversial because it may increase the risk of a tension pneumothorax, a more serious condition than a simple pneumothorax caused by an unclamped tube. Check institution's policy regarding clamping.* |
| h. Moisture-proof bag. | A moisture-proof bag is used to dispose of contaminated dressings. |

| Steps | Rationale |
|---|---|
| 2. Using aseptic technique, prepare evacuation drainage system. Open packaging and prepare according to manufacturer's directions. | Aseptic technique prevents microorganisms from entering the child's pleural cavity via the drainage system. |
| 3. Place disposable units on frame of child's bed/crib. | Placing unit below the level of the child's chest prevents liquid from entering the pleural cavity. |
| 4. Prepare child and family for procedure (see Skill 1). Include the following information:<br>a. A local anesthetic will be given, but a feeling of pressure may be experienced when the tube is inserted.<br>b. If breathing has been difficult, considerable relief may occur shortly after insertion. | Preparing the child and family for procedure enhances knowledge and thus decreases anxiety and increases cooperation. |
| c. Instruct the child not to cough or move when the tube is being inserted. | Coughing or movement may result in lung or other visceral organs being punctured. |
| 5. Obtain informed signed consent if required by institution (see Skill 8). | Invasive procedures often require signed consents. |
| 6. Recruit assistant(s) as needed. | Assistance is usually needed to ensure proper positioning and prevent movement during procedure, which could lead to injury. |
| 7. Select a location for performing procedure with adequate lighting and emergency equipment. | Proper lighting facilitates the physician's performance of the procedure. Life support equipment must be available since a tension pneumothorax may result in cardiovascular and respiratory collapse. |
| 8. If child's condition permits, administer premedication before procedure as ordered, allowing time for peak effect during procedure. | Controlling pain enhances the child's ability to remain still during the procedure. |
| 9. Develop individualized child and family goals:<br>▪ Child will have minimal discomfort or distress associated with chest tube placement, maintenance or removal.<br>▪ Positioning-related injury during the procedure will be prevented or minimized.<br>▪ Complications of chest tube placement, maintenance or removal will be prevented or minimized.<br>▪ Lung expansion and respiratory status will improve. | |

## Implementation

| Steps | Rationale |
|---|---|
| 1. Position infant/child as directed by physician. Maintain this position throughout insertion. Restrain as necessary (see Skill 51). Common positions: | ***Special Considerations:*** *Move any electrodes present for cardiopulmonary monitoring from operative site. Incision is usually made in the mid-axillary line just above the nipple in the 4th or 5th intercostal space.* |
| a. For fluid evacuation: Position infant/child supine, without elevating affected side. Secure the arm over the head.<br>b. For air evacuation: Position the infant/child so that point of entry is the most elevated area of chest (Fletcher and Eichelberger, 1983). Elevate the upper arm so that axilla is exposed (Fig. 96-1). | Positioning child with point of entry elevated allows air to rise and provides protective space between lung and chest wall when tube is inserted. |
| 2. Open sterile supplies, arranging them so they are accessible to physician. Assist physician with gown and gloves as necessary. Adjust lighting as needed. Maintain sterile technique throughout procedure. | Empyema may result if sterile technique is not used (Moore, Mills, and Mast, 1984). |
| 3. Assist with anesthetic preparation and other supplies as needed. | If using a multidose vial, nursing assistance will be required to maintain asepsis. |

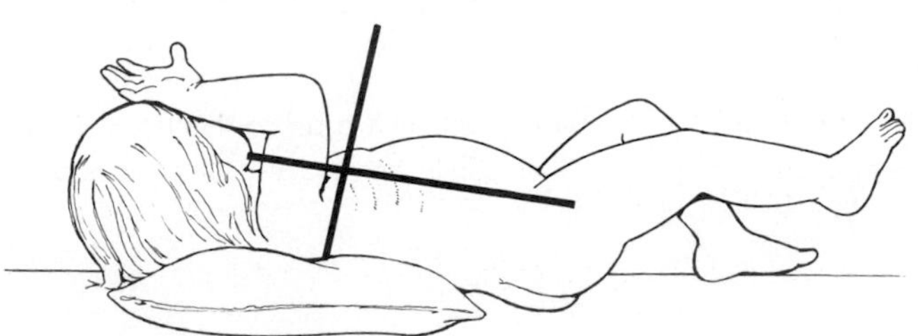

***FIG. 96-1*** Positioning of child for chest tube placement.

| Steps | Rationale |
|---|---|
| 4. Monitor the child's cardiopulmonary status during the procedure, including heart and respiratory rate, blood pressure, respiratory effort, and color of skin, mucous membranes, and nailbeds. | Monitoring the child during the procedure facilitates early detection of increasing respiratory distress. The child's respiratory status may also be compromised by the positioning and discomfort of the procedure. |
| 5. Provide verbal comfort to child. Use a soothing voice with infant, and keep the older child informed on procedure's progress. | Verbal comforting enhances the child's ability to remain relaxed during the procedure. |
| 6. After tube insertion is complete, connect to evacuation drainage system using sterile 5-in-1 connector and connecting tube. | ***Special Considerations:*** *Air bubbles in the water seal unit indicate air escaping from pleural space and confirm tube patency.* |
| 7. If applicable, connect drainage system to suction, and apply ordered amount of suction.<br>a. Infants with lung disease on ventilators: 10 to 20 cm $H_2O$ (Fletcher and Eichelberger, 1983).<br>b. Older infants and children: 20 to 40 cm $H_2O$ (Moore, Mills, and Mast, 1984). | Suction applies additional negative pressure on the pleural space and thus facilitates removal of air and fluid. |
| 8. Observe for gentle bubbling in the suction-control bottle or chamber. Observe the suction level float ball in the Thora-Klex unit. | Gentle bubbling indicates that the system is working correctly. Vigorous bubbling may interfere with chest auscultation and increase evaporation of fluid in the drainage system.<br>***Special Considerations:*** *Incorrect connection of the suction system may cause air to remain in chest under tension (Moore, Mills, and Mast, 1984).* |
| 9. If two chest tubes are inserted, connect both to same drainage unit using sterile Y-connector. | Use of one drainage system is recommended with two tubes to avoid fluid from one system being suctioned through chest into a second system (Persons, 1987). |
| 10. After physician has sutured tube to child's skin, put on sterile gloves, and apply occlusive dressing, or assist physician. | Applying dressing in a sterile manner prevents introduction of microorganisms at the insertion site. |
| a. Apply sterile petrolatum gauze or antibiotic ointment depending on physician preference.<br>b. Cover with small, sterile gauze dressing.<br>c. Remove gloves, and secure dressing in place, completely covering with tape. | Petrolatum gauze provides an airtight seal at insertion site. A large, bulky dressing restricts chest-wall movement, obscures tube position, and prevents adequate auscultation and observation of chest wall movement (Fletcher and Eichelberger, 1983; Moore, Mills, and Mast, 1984). |
| 11. Assist with obtaining chest radiograph immediately on completion of procedure. | Chest radiography verifies the position of the tube and evacuation of intrapleural air and fluid. |
| 12. Observe additional safety precautions as follows: | |
| a. Do not elevate drainage system above child's chest level. | Raising the unit above the child's chest allows liquid in the system to enter pleural cavity. |
| b. Secure all tubing connections by taping or banding, without completely covering connections with tape (see Fig. 96-2). | Secure connections prevent accidental separation, which would disrupt negative pressure system and allow air to enter chest cavity. Completely taping the connections may obscure a possible air leak or a loose connection (Persons, 1987). |
| c. Keep rubber-tipped clamps at bedside or at head of bed for emergency use in accidental disconnection of tubing or for changing drainage system. | Clamping the chest tube is rarely done and only as an emergency measure to prevent air from entering pleural space, because clamping may result in tension pneumothorax.<br>***Special Considerations:*** *Do not clamp chest tube for disconnection if child is on positive pressure ventilator. Most institutions allow clamping for specific circumstances for a brief period only.* |
| d. Maintain fluid in various chambers at proper levels. | Improper fluid levels may be detrimental to functioning of the system. |

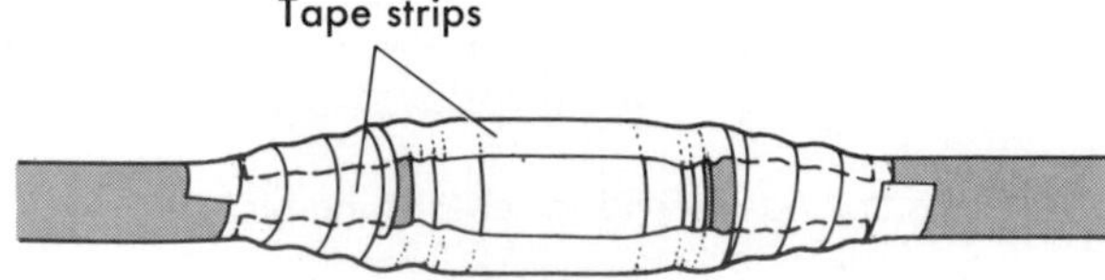


***FIG. 96-2*** Method for wrapping chest tube connections.

From Beare P and Myers J: Principles and practice of adult health nursing, St Louis, 1990, The CV Mosby Co.

| Steps | Rationale |
|---|---|
| 13. Secure excess tubing by coiling flat on bed: | Coiling excess tubing prevents kinks, which would impair drainage system. |
| a. Make a tape tab on tubing by folding a 2 inch piece of 1 inch-wide adhesive tape over tubing. | |
| b. Coil excess tubing on top of bed with no dependent loops hanging over side. | A dependent loop of tubing with fluid in it can obstruct drainage and increase intrathoracic pressure. |
| c. Secure tubing by using a safety pin or hemostat to attach tape tab to bed linen. | |
| d. Ensure that adequate slack is present in tubing to allow child to turn and move in bed. | Accidental dislodgement could occur if movement created tension on the tubing. |
| 14. Monitor respiratory status and vital signs every 15 minutes for first hour following insertion and then as ordered or per routine, noting same factors as in initial assessment. | Monitoring respiratory status and vital signs allows for evaluation of the therapeutic effect of the procedure and enables early detection and intervention for possible complications. ***Special Considerations:*** *Possible complications of chest tube insertion include lung laceration, perforation of major blood vessels or visceral organs, injury to intervertebral or phrenic nerves, hypotension, infection and subcutaneous emphysema.* |
| 15. Assess child's comfort level and administer analgesics as needed (see Skill 52). | ***Special Considerations:*** *Chest tube may be uncomfortable but should not be extremely painful. Continuous acute pain may be an indication of other problems.* |
| 16. Note the amount and color of drainage in collection bottle or chamber: | |
| a. Check drainage every 30 minutes for the first 2 hours after insertion, then every hour. | Closely monitoring drainage aids in early detection of bleeding complications. |
| b. Mark time, date, and drainage level on adhesive tape strip on bottle or directly on disposable unit every 8 hours. | Marking ensures more accurate measurement of drainage amount for output records and determining fluid replacement. |
| c. Note and report to physician any sudden change in amount of drainage. | Sudden increases in amount of drainage may indicate hemorrhage. Decreases may indicate an occluded tube. ***Special Considerations:*** *If blood loss exceeds 30 cc/kg in first 8 hours following injury, surgical intervention may be required (Hazinski, 1984).* |
| 17. If the chest tube is inserted for purpose of fluid evacuation, "milk" the chest tube every hour only if indicated. | Alternating compression-release cycles help maintain patency by breaking up clots and facilitate drainage by forcing air and fluid through the tube. |
| a. With nondominant hand, occlude the chest tube near insertion site and hold securely. | Pinching the chest tube near insertion site prevents excess changes in negative pressure from occurring intrathoracically during "milking" and secures the tube to prevent dislodging. |
| b. With dominant hand, compress tubing gently, quickly, and repeatedly along the length of tubing between index finger and thumb. | ***Special Considerations:*** *"Stripping" chest tubes (a more vigorous compression of tubing) remains controversial and should be performed only with a physician's order and if institutional policy allows (Krauss, 1985; Johanson et al, 1988). Stripping increases intrathoracic negative pressure significantly and may pull lung tissue or pleura into the chest tube (Duncan and Erikson, 1982; Duncan, Erikson, and Wiegel, 1987).* |
| c. Mark the collection unit with marking pen and record amount of drainage when milking is completed. | |
| 18. Check for proper functioning of the drainage system. | |
| a. Monitor respiratory status. | Equipment malfunction may result in development of pneumothorax. |
| b. Gravity (water-seal) drainage method: | |
| ▪ Air evacuation—observe the water-seal chamber for fluctuations in fluid level corresponding with child's respirations; observe water-seal chamber for silent versus noisy, intermittent versus continuous, and placid versus turbulent bubbling. | Fluctuations represent the normal pressure changes in the pleural space during respirations. Fluid level rises during inhalation and falls during exhalation. ***Special Considerations:*** *This pattern is reversed if child is on positive-pressure ventilator.* |
| ▪ Fluid evacuation—Observe for fluid fluctuations corresponding with respirations in the chest tube itself between insertion site and collection chamber. | Absence of fluctuation may indicate tubing obstruction (kink, dependent loop, blood clot, pressure on tube or tubing), or it may indicate that the lung has fully reexpanded. |
| c. Suction drainage method: | |
| ▪ Temporarily remove from suction source, and observe for bubbling in water-seal chamber. Check manufacturer's instructions for each specific device's indicators of normal functioning (e.g., Thora-Klex contains a pleural air leak indicator). | Bubbling in the water-seal chamber when suction is removed usually indicates presence of an air leak caused by either a leak in the drainage system or by evacuation of air from pleural space. ***Special Considerations:*** *Bubbling usually subsides a short time after the tube is inserted and the air is evacuated. In neonates, it may subside within a few hours of insertion.* |

| Steps | Rationale |
|---|---|
| ▪ Observe suction control chamber for activity indicative of normal functioning specific to the type of unit such as audible bubbling, proper fluid level, or negative reading on system pressure indicator. | Improper functioning of the suction control unit may result in accumulation of air or fluid in the chest, causing increased cardiopulmonary compromise. ***Special Considerations:*** *A detailed troubleshooting guide for chest tube systems is available in Hazinski (1984).* |
| 19. If immobilized, reposition the infant/child frequently (at least every 2 hours). | Positioning facilitates lung drainage and adequate lung expansion. |
| 20. Change the chest tube dressing every 24 to 48 hours or more often, if necessary. | |
| a. Wearing nonsterile gloves, remove old dressing, taking care not to dislodge tubing. | |
| b. Note the presence and nature of drainage on dressing, then discard in moisture-proof bag. | Purulent drainage indicates wound infection. Excessive serosanguineous drainage may indicate improper tube placement. Properly discarding dressing prevents transmission of pathogens from contaminated dressing. |
| c. Assess the insertion site for evidence of erythema, excessive or abnormal drainage, or subcutaneous emphysema. Wearing sterile gloves, palpate area around insertion site for crepitus. | Erythema or foul-smelling drainage may indicate the presence of an infection. Subcutaneous emphysema can result from a poor seal at the insertion site. |
| d. Using sterile technique, reapply occlusive dressing. | |
| 21. Change the collection bottle or disposable unit when it is full or if the system is disrupted. | ***Special Considerations:*** *When collection chamber is full in a Pleur-Evac unit, the excess drainage may be withdrawn with a 50 cc syringe through rubber stopper in unit.* |
| a. Prepare a new unit. | Preparing the system before clamping the tube ensures rapid transfer and reestablishment of drainage system. |
| b. Clamp the chest tube using rubber-tipped clamps or have child perform Valsalva maneuver to switch to the new unit. | Clamping is done to prevent air from entering the pleural space. The Valsalva maneuver increases intrathoracic pressure and prevents air from reentering the pleural space (Persons, 1987). |
| 22. Assist practitioner in removal of chest tube when it is no longer functioning or needed. | ***Special Considerations:*** *A Heimlich valve attached to chest tube may be used if drainage has decreased sufficiently and suction is no longer required. A Heimlich valve allows drainage of fluid and air out of pleural space but does not permit air to enter space.* |
| a. Time administration of ordered analgesic to allow for peak effect during tube removal. | |
| b. Place a linen protector under the child and beneath the chest tube. | Drainage may occur when tube is removed; it also provides a temporary place for the chest tube after removal. |
| c. Wearing sterile gloves, prepare an occlusive dressing, e.g., petrolatum gauze placed on 4 × 4 inch gauze pads. | An occlusive dressing forms an airtight seal over the chest tube wound, preventing recurrence of pneumothorax. |
| d. Remove soiled dressings and discard in moisture-proof bag. | |
| e. Cleanse skin around chest tube insertion site with antiseptic solution. | |
| f. Position infant/child in a semi-Fowler's position or in a lateral position on unaffected side. Restrain as necessary. | |
| g. If possible, have child perform Valsalva maneuver by bearing down as tube is removed by the physician. | A Valsalva maneuver increases the intrathoracic pressure, forcing remaining fluid or air from the pleural space while preventing air from reentering (Persons, 1987). |
| h. Quickly apply occlusive dressing over insertion site. Completely cover dressing with air-occlusive tape. | Quick application of occlusive dressing is necessary to prevent air from entering chest. ***Special Considerations:*** *Dressing should remain intact for 48 to 72 hours until sufficient wound closure occurs.* |
| i. If ordered, use a sterile swab to obtain drainage from inside the chest tube. | A swab for culture and sensitivity is sometimes needed to determine presence of pathogens in tube, which may require antimicrobial therapy. |
| j. Monitor respiratory status and vital signs following same protocol used following insertion. | |
| k. Assist with chest radiograph 1 or 2 hours after removal. | Chest radiograph is taken to determine if there has been a reaccumulation of air or fluid. |
| l. Properly dispose of chest tube and drainage system. | |

| Evaluation Outcomes | Observational Guidelines |
|---|---|
| 1. Discomfort is minimized throughout procedure and while chest tube is in place. | Note both verbal and behavioral indications of discomfort or pain, e.g., irritability, restlessness, crying. Note frequency of analgesics administered and child's response to medication. |

## Evaluation Outcomes—cont'd

2. Child remains free of complications from procedure and therapy.

3. Child exhibits improved expansion of affected lung.

## Observational Guidelines—cont'd

Monitor vital signs and cardiopulmonary status. Observe insertion site for signs of infection. Palpate insertion site for crepitus. Note type of sputum produced by child. Note amount and type of drainage from chest tube. Review chest radiographs for complications.

Auscultate breath sounds in bilateral lung fields. Assess respiratory status. Note results of chest radiographs.

## Documentation

Document date and time of chest tube insertion/removal; location and appearance of insertion site; drainage system used and amount of suction applied. Note presence, and describe bubbling and fluctuations in water-seal and suction control unit. Record vital signs and cardiopulmonary function assessments; amount, color, and consistency of drainage; medications administered and child's response. Document child's tolerance of procedure; obtained consents; laboratory tests performed (e.g., culture and sensitivity); date dressings applied and changed; and drainage on dressings.

## UNIT XIV

### PRODUCT REFERENCES AND TEACHING RESOURCES

#### Books

Wong DL and Whaley LF: Clinical manual of pediatric nursing, 1990, ed 3, St Louis, The CV Mosby Co.
Offers information on home care instructions for apnea monitoring and CPR, and performing postural drainage.

#### Products

Dale Medical Products, Inc
7 Cross Street
PO Box 1556
Plainville, MA 02762-0556
Offers Dale Tracheostomy Tube Holder.

Nellcor Inc
25495 Whitesell Street
Hayward, CA 94545
1-800-NELLCOR
Manufactures pulse oximeters.

### REFERENCES

Aday LA, Aitken M, and Wegener D: Pediatric home care: results of a national evaluation of programs for ventilator-assisted children, Chicago, 1988, Pluribus.

American Academy of Pediatrics and American College of Obstetrics and Gynecology: Guidelines for perinatal care, ed 2, Evanston, Ill, 1988, American Academy of Pediatrics and American College of Obstetrics and Gynecology.

American Heart Association: Pediatric basic life support: basic principles of BLS in infants and children. In Healthcare provider's manual for basic life support, Dallas, 1988, AHA.

American Heart Association and American Academy of Pediatrics: Instructors manual for pediatric advanced life support, Dallas, 1988, AHA.

Andrews M and Nielson D: Technology dependent children in the home, Pediatr Nurs 14(2):111-114; 151, 1988.

Bailey C et al: Shallow versus deep endotracheal suctioning in young rabbits: pathologic effects on the tracheobronchial wall. Pediatrics 82(5)746-751, 1988.

Barker S and Tremper K: Pulse oximetry: applications and limitations, Int Anesthesiol Clin 25:155-175, 1987.

Baun MM and Flones MJ: Cumulative effects of three sequential endotracheal suctioning episodes in the dog model, Heart Lung 13:148-154, 1984.

Birdsall C: What suction pressure should I use? Am J Nurs 85:866, 1985.

Bostick J and Wendelgass ST: Normal saline instillation as part of the suctioning procedure: effects on $PaO_2$ and amount of secretions, Heart Lung 16(5):532-537, 1987.

Breslin EH: Prevention and treatment of pulmonary complications in patients after surgery of the upper abdomen, Heart Lung 10:511, 1981.

Brooks JG: Sudden infant death syndrome and apnea of infancy. In Levin DL, editor: A practical guide to pediatric intensive care, ed 2, St Louis, 1984, The CV Mosby Co.

Brown PA et al: Quick reference to pediatric intensive care nursing, Rockville, Md, 1989, Aspen.

Burgess WR and Chernick V: Respiratory therapy in newborn infants and children, ed 2, New York, 1986, Thieme Medical Publishers Inc.

Burton GG, Gee GN, and Hodgkin JE: Respiratory care, ed 2, Philadelphia, 1984, JB Lippincott Co.

Center for Devices and Radiologic Health: Second draft proposed standard for the infant apnea monitor, Washington, DC, 1989, Food and Drug Administration.

Chameides L: Textbook of pediatric advanced life support, American Heart Association and American Academy of Pediatrics, Dallas, 1988, AHA.

Dean PG: Monitoring the apneic infant: impact on the infant's mother, 15(2):65-76, 1986.

Demers RR and Saklad M: Minimizing the harmful effects of mechanical aspiration, Heart Lung 2:544, 1973.

Denson SE and Goldie WD: SIDS: possible causes and strategies for intervention for some infants at risk, Perinatology/Neonatology 10(4):21-26, 1986.

Donaghy B: Letter to the editor: pediatric home tracheostomy care alternatives, Pediatr Nurs 12(3):223-224, 1986.

Duncan C and Erickson R: Pressures associated with chest tube stripping, Heart Lung 11(2):166, 1982.

Duncan C, Erickson R, and Weigel RM: Effect of chest tube management on drainage after cardiac surgery, Heart Lung 16(1):1, 1987.

Fanconi S et al: Pulse oximetry in pediatric intensive care: comparison with measured saturations and transcutaneous oxygen tension, J Pediatr 107:362-366, 1985.

Fletcher M and Eichelberger M: Thoracostomy tubes. In Fletcher M, MacDonald M, and Avery G: Atlas of procedures in neonatology, Philadelphia, 1983, JB Lippincott Co.

Fuchs P: Streamlining your suction techniques, Nursing 14(5):55-61, 1984.

Fulmer J and Snider G: ACCP-NHLBJ National Conference on oxygen therapy, Chest 86:234-247, 1984.

Hagedorn M and Gardner S: Physiologic sequelae of prematurity: the nurse practitioner's role, J Pediatr Health Care, 3(6):288-297, 1989.

Hanson J: Parent guide to bronchopulmonary dysplasia, Albuquerque, NM, 1987, The American Lung Association of New Mexico.

Hazinski MF: Nursing care of the critically ill child, St Louis, 1984, The CV Mosby Co.

Hodgson A et al: The accuracy of the pulse oximeter in neonates, Adv Experim Med and Biol 22:177-179, 1987.

Hoffman L and Maszkiewicz R: Airway management: the basics of suctioning, Am J Nurs 87:39-53, 1987.

Irwin S and Tecklin JS: Cardiopulmonary physical therapy, St Louis, 1985, The CV Mosby Co.

Jensen M and Bobak I: Maternity and gynecologic care, St Louis, 1985, The CV Mosby Co.

Johanson B et al: Standards for critical care, ed 3, St Louis, 1988, The CV Mosby Co.

Kendig EL Jr, editor: Disorders of respiratory tract of children, ed 4, Philadelphia, 1983, WB Saunders Co.

Kigin CM: Chest physical therapy for the postoperative or traumatic injury patient, Physical Therapy 61:724, 1981.

Kleiber C: How beneficial is mist tent therapy? Pediatr Nurs 15(3):314-315, 1989.

Kleiber C and Hummel PA: Factors related to spontaneous endotracheal extubation in the neonate, Pediatric Nursing 15(4):347-351, 1989.

Kleiber C, Krutzfield N, and Rose EF: Acute histologic changes in the tracheobronchial tree associated with different suction catheter insertion techniques, Heart Lung 17(1):10-14, 1988.

Kloor T and Carbajal D: Infant oxygen administration by modified nasal cannula, Clin Pediatr 23:477-479, 1984.

Knipper J: Evaluation of adventitious sounds as an indicator of the need for tracheal suctioning, Heart Lung 13(3):292-293, 1984.

Koff P, Eitzman D, and Nev J: Neonatal and pediatric respiratory care, St Louis, 1988, The CV Mosby Co.

Kozier B and Erb G: Techniques in clinical nursing, Menlo Park, Calif, 1987, Addison-Wesley Publishing Co, Inc.

Krauss T: Chest tube stripping: is it necessary? Focus on Critical Care 12(6):41, 1985.

Kuzenski B: Effect of negative pressure on tracheobronchial trauma, Nurs Res 27:260-263, 1978.

Lawrence PA: Home care for ventilator dependent children: providing a chance to live a normal life, Dimens Crit Care Nurs 3(1):42-50, 1984.

Lehrer S: Understanding lung sounds, Philadelphia, 1984, WB Saunders Co.

Lichenstein M: Pediatric home tracheostomy care: a parent's guide, Pediatric Nurs 12(1):41-48; 69, 1986.

Lichenstein M: Author's response: pediatric home tracheostomy care alternatives, Pediatric Nurs 12(3):223, 1986.

Lough M, Doershuk C, and Stern R: Pediatric respiratory therapy, ed 2, Chicago, 1979, Year Book Medical Publishers.

Luedke J: Simple cough: how complex (letter), Am J Nurs 86(2):129, 1986.

Mark KB and Zahr LC: Parental anxiety related to the care of a child with apnea, Issues Compr Pediatr Nurs 9(4):223-228, 1986

McCrory L: Letter to the editor: pediatric home tracheostomy care alternatives, Pediatr Nurs 12(3):113, 1986.

Moore G, Mills M, and Mast C: Thoracentesis and chest tube insertion. In Levin D, Morriss F, and Moore G: A practical guide to pediatric intensive care, ed 2, St Louis, 1984, The CV Mosby Co.

Norris-Berkemeyer S and Hutchins KH: Home apnea monitoring, Pediatr Nurs 12(4):259-262, 1986.

Part V: Pediatric advanced life support, JAMA 255:2961-2968, 1986.

Patel D et al: Bacterial colonization of plastic bulb syringes, J Pediatr 112:466-468, 1988.

Paulson P: Nursing considerations for discharging children home on low-flow oxygen, Issues Compr Pediatr Nurs 10:209-214, 1987.

Perry AG and Potter PA: Clinical nursing skills and techniques, ed 2, St Louis, 1990, The CV Mosby Co.

Persons C: Critical care procedures and protocols: a nursing process approach, Philadelphia, 1987, JB Lippincott Co.

Pfaff S and Terri B: Discharge planning: infection prevention and control in the home, Nurs Clin North Am 15:893-908, 1980.

Pierce JB and Piazza DE: Differences in postsuctioning arterial blood oxygen concentration values using two postoxygenation methods, Heart and Lung 16(1):34-38, 1987.

Pierce JR and Turner BS: Physiologic monitoring. In Merenstein GB and Gardner SL, editors: Handbook of neonatal intensive care, ed 2, St Louis, 1989, The CV Mosby Co.

Rademaker M and Kirby J: Contact dermatitis to a skin adhesive, Contact Dermatitis 6(5):297-298, 1987.

Rarey K and Youlsey J: Respiratory patient care, Englewood Cliffs, NJ, 1981, Prentice-Hall Press.

Reidel K: Pulse oximetry: a new technology to assess patient oxygen needs in the neonatal intensive care unit, J Perinat Neonat Nurs, 1(1):49-57, 1987.

Rhoades C, Adcock M, and Jovanovich J: Prevention of nosocomial infections in critical care units, Nurs Clin North Am 15:803-815, 1980.

Riegel B and Forshee T: A review and critique of the literature on pre-oxygenation for endotracheal suctioning, Heart and Lung 14:507-518, 1985.

Russell E: Unknotting a tying problem, Nursing 14(1):16, 1984.

Schoni M, Hurlimann R, and Bruderer K: Pulse oximetry, digital clubbing, and cystic fibrosis, Lancet 1(8546):1371, 1987.

Sexton DL: Chronic obstructive pulmonary disease: care of the child and adult, St Louis, 1981, The CV Mosby Co.

Shapiro BA, Harrison RA, and Trout CA: Clinical application of respiratory care, Chicago, 1982, Year Book Medical Publishers.

Shekleton M and Nield M: Ineffective airway clearance related to artificial airway, Nurs Clin North Am 22:167-178, 1983.

Shreiner R and Kisling J: Practical neonatal respiratory care, New York, 1982, Raven Press.

Simmons BP and Wong ES: CDC guidelines for the prevention and control of nosocomial infections, Am J Infect Control 11:230-238, 1983.

Snow J: Pulmonary disorders. In Hazinski MF, editor: Nursing care of the critically ill child, St Louis, 1984, The CV Mosby Co.

Soule B, editor: The APIC curriculum for infection control practice, vol 2, Dubuque, Iowa, 1983, Kendall/Hunt Publishing Co.

Sporing E, Walton M, and Cady C: The Children's Hospital of Philadelphia manual of pediatric nursing policies, procedures, and personnel, Oradell, NJ, 1984, Medical Economics Books.

Swearingen P: The Addison-Wesley photo-atlas of nursing procedures, Menlo Park, Calif, 1984, Addison-Wesley Publishing Co, Inc.

Tafuro P and Ristuccia P: Recognition and control of outbreaks of nosocomial infections in the intensive care setting, Heart and Lung 13:486-495, 1984.

Walsh M: To cough or not to cough? Nursing 12(6):124-126, 1982.

Walters P, Elmore G and Grandy M: Oxygen administration. In Levin D, Morris F, and Moore G, editors: A practical guide to pediatric intensive care, St Louis, 1984, The CV Mosby Co.

Whaley LF and Wong DL: Nursing care of infants and children, ed 4, St Louis, 1991, The CV Mosby Co.

Whaley LF and Wong DL: Essentials of pediatric nursing, ed 3, St Louis, 1989, The CV Mosby Co.

Whaley LF and Wong DL: Clinical manual of pediatric nursing, ed 3, St Louis, 1990, The CV Mosby Co.

Wong DL and Whaley LF: Manual of pediatric nursing, ed 4, St Louis, 1991, The CV Mosby Co.

# UNIT XV Circulation

## SKILL 97 Inserting Intravenous (IV) Catheters

*Anna L. Summerfield*

Nurses have increasingly become responsible for initiating and making judgments about IV therapy. An intravenous catheter provides ready access to safely deliver nutrients, fluids, electrolytes and/or medications as required by the child's current health state.

**NURSING DIAGNOSES**

Anxiety related to unmet informational needs about purpose and procedure for IV therapy; Pain related to insertion of IV catheter; Impaired physical mobility related to restraint of IV site.

| Steps | Rationale |
|---|---|
| **Assessment** | |
| 1. Determine the reason the IV has been ordered.<br>a. Volume deficit or maintenance.<br>b. Medication administration.<br>c. Nutrition deficit. | Knowing the reason for the IV enhances explanation to child/family and facilitates planning phase for selection of catheter size and type, site for IV, and tubing type.<br>***Special Considerations:*** *Consistent information from health care professionals promotes rapport with family.* |
| 2. Review the child's history. | If admission history is not specific to IVs, then a further session should be scheduled with the family. |
| a. Culture and religion. | There may be specific customs that are in conflict with medical intervention, such as IV therapy. Complete discussion—nurse/physician/family—is conducted when conflicts arise to reach a reasonable solution to benefit the child. |
| b. Past experiences with IVs. | Knowledge of previous experiences is important in the approach needed to establish trust and understanding. Although many children have never had an IV, those who have usually retain memories of the experience and the pain associated with it (Whaley and Wong, 1991). Procedures involving needles are painful for children (Wong and Baker, 1988).<br>***Special Considerations:*** *Play sessions with children in a history-taking phase assist in identifying the child's perception of IVs. Clarify misperceptions before starting IV.* |
| 3. Assess child's developmental level, including:<br>a. Age. | Age is one determinant for site choice.<br>***Special Considerations:*** *Preferred sites (Figs. 97-1 A and B).*<br>*Infants: hands, arms, feet, and scalp.*<br>*Toddlers, older child and adolescents: hands and arms.* |
| b. Cognitive ability. | The child's ability to understand guides explanations and needed emotional support. |
| c. Degree of mobility/immobility. | The site should restrict activity as little as possible. In the older child, this lack of restriction allows the child to continue self-care. |

| Steps | Rationale |
|---|---|

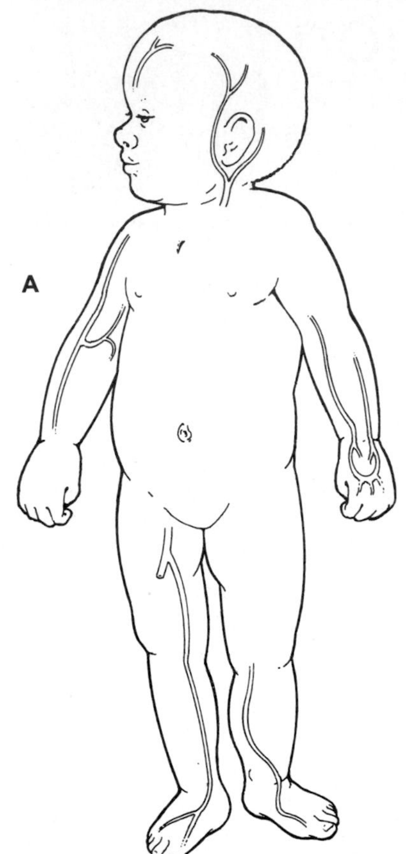


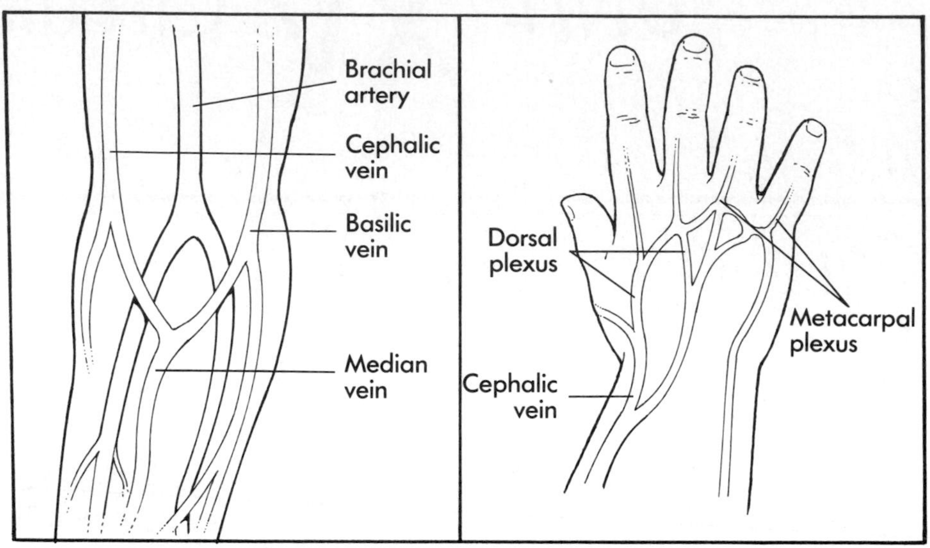


***FIG. 97-1*** **A,** Preferred sites for venous access in infants. **B,** Preferred sites for venous access in toddlers, older children, and adolescents.

4. Review physical assessment, especially:
   a. Fluid and electrolyte status (see Skill 64).

Assessing fluid and electrolyte status establishes baseline data before initiating therapy; also, a child who is dehydrated or has an elevated temperature may be more difficult to cannulate.
***Special Considerations:*** *Data that are helpful in this assessment are the medical diagnosis, treatment the child is receiving (especially medications and fluid therapies), lab reports, history, and records of intake and output.*

   b. Clinical diagnosis.

Existing conditions may rule out use of a site.
***Special Considerations:*** *Hydrocephalus, ventriculoperitoneal (VP) or ventriculoatrial (VA) shunt, anencephaly, or skull fracture exclude scalp vein usage. Arteriovenous (AV) shunts in extremities exclude use of that extremity. Edema of extremity excludes usage of that limb. Burns require IV access in a nonburned site. Moles, hematomas, scar tissue, or inflammation of tissue surrounding a potential site exclude using the site.*

   c. Previous IV sites.

Cannula change is recommended every 48 to 72 hours routinely to prevent phlebitis unless contraindicated by limited vein access.

5. Review physician's order for:
   a. Type of solution.
   b. Amount of solution.
   c. Rate.
   d. Time specifications.
   e. IV additives.

The Five Rights of Medication Administration apply to IV therapy.

## Planning and Goal Setting

1. Communicate with the child/family that the physician has ordered IV therapy.

Connotations of "serious illness" go with the sight of an IV. Understanding may result in decreased anxiety and increased cooperation.

| Steps | Rationale |
|---|---|
| 2. Prepare the child/family for the procedure (see Skill 1). Teaching should include:<br>a. Reason for IV use.<br>b. Description and functioning of equipment.<br>c. Approximate length of procedure and how long the child will need an IV.<br>d. Planned time of the procedure.<br>e. Possible sites where the IV will be placed.<br>f. Sensations or feelings the child may experience.<br>g. Potential need for restraints on arms and legs to prevent the child from pulling on the tubing and catheter site. | Information assists the child to maintain as much control as possible.<br>***Special Considerations:*** *The older child should be allowed to assist in the site selection. If a scalp vein site selection is possible, explain to the family the proximity of the veins in the scalp to the skin surface and that the needle does not penetrate the skull bone. Assure them that other sites will be considered first, but a scalp site will allow hand and foot freedom. Also, reinforce that a minimum of hair will be shaved and that it grows back quickly. Offer to save the shaved hair if they desire. If a parent still objects strongly, respect their wishes.* |
| 3. Plan emotional support based on child's age and cognitive ability (see Skill 1). | Relaxing the child as much as possible promotes vasodilation.<br>***Special Considerations:*** *Many parents find the procedure too stressful and become upset because they are unable to comfort and protect the child from pain during the procedure (Whaley and Wong, 1991). Parents are encouraged to be present but given the option to remain outside. The best approach is skillful, quick venipuncture, then have parents hold and comfort child. Egocentricity may lead the 4 to 6 year old to believe he or she has done something bad to deserve the pain of the IV start. Adolescents may be critical of the professional's venipuncture technique.* |
| 4. Consider additional strategies to minimize pain and anxiety during venipuncture: | |
| a. Use intradermal lidocaine. | The use of intradermal lidocaine at the venipuncture site can significantly reduce insertion pain (Dickey, 1988).<br>***Special Considerations:*** *A more promising intervention is the topical application of lidocaine and prilocaine. The cream, EMLA (eutectic mixture of local anesthetics), is applied to the insertion site with an occlusive dressing for 60 minutes before vein cannulation (Manner et al, 1987; Maunuksela and Korpela, 1986). The cream is currently under investigation for use in the United States by Astra Pharmaceuticals.* |
| b. Establish a "2-stick policy" limiting the number of unsuccessful venous insertions to 2, after which the professional "takes a break" and asks for assistance from the most proficient person available (Jimenez, Turley, and Quiggins, 1988). | This policy helps to minimize the child's pain and anxiety by limiting the number of attempts by one person. Numerous factors may affect proficiency in any particular instance. |
| 5. Assemble equipment:<br>a. Obtain ordered solution.<br>b. Select tubing according to agency policy; an inline filter and a calibrated volume control chamber (Buretrol, Soluset) are recommended for pediatric patients (Whaley and Wong, 1991); minidropper or microdropper that delivers 60 drops of solution per ml.<br>c. Assemble and flush tubing (Fig. 97-2) using aseptic technique. Follow manufacturer's guidelines, being careful to eliminate air from line. | Preparing tubing out of direct sight of child minimizes anxiety. Inline volume control sets prevent large amounts of fluid from infusing in the event of pump failure.<br>***Special Considerations:*** *Double check solution with physician orders (e.g., prescribed solution, rate of flow, additives [if any], time, and amount). Check expiration date and clarity of solution. Discard expired or cloudy solution. Also discard solution if cracks or pinholes are noted in the bottle/bag. Filters most commonly used are 0.22 μm (micron) in pore size (Weinstein, 1987). Prevent fluid overload by placing no more than one third the daily requirement of fluid in the chamber at one time (Streckfuss, 1985).* |
| d. Label bag and tubing before leaving medication room. Agency policy varies regarding labeling. | ***Special Considerations:*** *Label on bag should indicate patient name, expiration date, date and time assembled for administration, and additives. Label on tubing indicates date and time assembled for administration. Solutions are generally left hanging for 24 hours while tubing is changed every 48 to 72 hours (Bryan, 1987; Messner, 1987; Maki, 1987).* |
| 6. Select location for venipuncture procedure considering adequate lighting, accessibility of child, ease of restraint and presence of roommates. | ***Special Considerations:*** *Performing a painful procedure away from the child's room provides a more comforting atmosphere when child returns.* |

| Steps | Rationale |
|---|---|

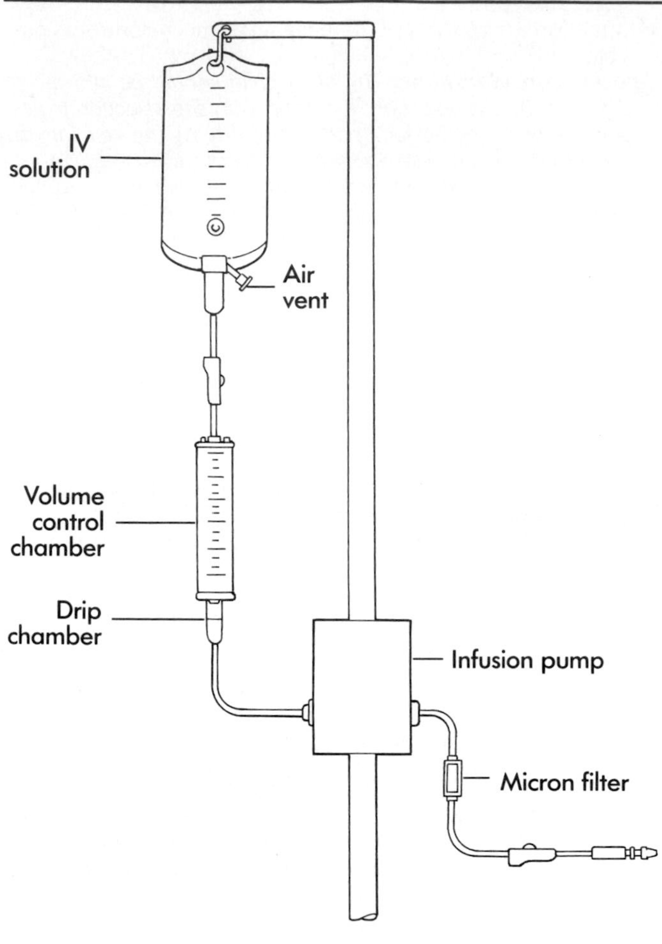


***FIG. 97-2*** IV tubing set-up for infants and children.

7. Review appropriate IV sites for child considering:
   a. Clinical diagnosis.
   b. Age.
   c. Duration of therapy.
   d. Assessed mobility/immobility.
   e. Solution and rate of flow.
   f. Condition of veins.
   g. Comfort of child.

An IV appropriately placed will have increased duration, although the average IV may only last 24 hours for an infant (Arthur, 1984).

***Special Considerations:*** *Maximize utilization of veins by beginning insertion as far to the periphery of the vein as possible. Subsequent venipunctures may be performed proximally on the same veins (Scranton, 1977; Millam, 1987); this is especially important in long-term therapy. Hypertonic solutions, acidic solutions, and viscous fluids require larger veins to quickly dilute these elements as they enter the bloodstream. The higher the rate of flow, the larger the vein needed. Determine refill capacity of the vessel by placing the tourniquet above the proposed site and gently strip the vessel proximal to distal. If there is no refill, choose another site. If the child is febrile, administer an antipyretic, if possible, as veins tend to be more fragile when temperature is elevated. Try not to place IV in dominant hand. Avoid flexion areas of extremities whenever possible. Also consider child's self-comforting habits such as thumbsucking. Scalp veins offer the best sites for an IV in children under 9 months (Arthur, 1984). Select a long, straight vein that is not near a joint (Feldstein, 1986).*

8. Distinguish veins from arteries by palpating vessel without a tourniquet for a pulse.

Arteries are contraindicated because of the risk of decreasing or obliterating blood flow to the body part supplied by the particular vessel.

***Special Considerations:*** *Veins are more superficial in most peripheral sites, however veins and arteries are equally superficial in the scalp.*

| Steps | Rationale |
|---|---|
| 9. Select the smallest cannula (needle/catheter) capable of delivering the solution and/or medications ordered at the required rate. Recommended gauge:<br>a. Infant and toddler (0 to 4 years): 23 to 25 gauge steel needle; 22 to 24 gauge catheter.<br>b. Young child (4 to 6 years): 22 to 24 gauge catheter.<br>c. Older child (6 to 12 years) and adolescent: 18 to 24 gauge catheter. | Correct cannula selection helps prevent phlebitis and infiltration (Feldstein, 1986). Small cannulas make insertion easier (Millam, 1987). This smallest cannula-largest vein combination allows maximum blood flow around the cannula and minimizes cannula contact with vein wall (Feldstein, 1986).<br>***Special Considerations:*** *The use of Teflon cannulas instead of steel needles, and placement of small bore (e.g., 22 to 24) cannulas prolongs the time that peripheral venous lines are functional by as much as 24 to 48 hours (Phelps, 1987).* |
| 10. Gather and organize supplies for venipuncture:<br>a. Appropriate infusion pump (set at ordered rate) and volume counter reset at zero.<br>b. Tape: ½, 1 and 2 inches (adhesive or micropore).<br>c. Isopropyl alcohol and povidone-iodine swabs.<br>d. Adhesive bandage appropriate to child's size (small dot for infants; regular size for all others); or nonocclusive dressing (OpSite, Tegaderm).<br>e. Cotton balls, 2 × 2 or 4 × 4 inch gauze dressings.<br>f. Medicine cup (optional; cut in half, cover edges with tape).<br>g. Gloves. | Infusion pumps are used in pediatric patients (especially children under 12 years of age) as a safety measure to significantly decrease the risk of fluid overload. Infants are especially vulnerable to fluid overload (see Skill 64).<br>***Special Considerations:*** *Even when a pump is used, it is recommended that the volume control set be time taped to double check correctness of pump function. Syringe pumps are used when small volumes are infused. Cassette pumps are more accurate than peristaltic or roller type pumps, but are also more expensive (Runciman, 1987). Pumps are preferred delivery systems for children as opposed to gravity-driven controllers since a constant infusion rate can be maintained (Streckfuss, 1985). Protective covering (medicine cup) may be needed for an infant scalp IV, although some feel the protective covering can be used by the child during normal activity to "rake out" the IV (Streckfuss, 1985).* |
| h. Extension tubing; and extension set with a T-port (T-connector) if using a catheter. | T-connectors on catheters allow manipulations such as tubing change to occur without actual movement of the cannula. Motion of cannula against vein wall is a cause of mechanical phlebitis (Feldstein, 1986). They also provide a convenient access for administration of emergency medications. |
| i. Age-appropriate padded leg/armboard (if using extremity).<br>j. Tourniquet:<br>▪ ½-inch penrose drain.<br>▪ Rubberband for infants.<br>▪ Blood pressure cuff. | An armboard may be used to stabilize an insertion site close to a joint. Padding an armboard with an absorbent substance such as Webril or Stockinette assists in keeping the skin drier and prevents skin breakdown. |
| k. Syringe (3 to 5 ml) filled with normal saline (without preservative for infants).<br>l. Scissors.<br>m. Razor (for shaving hair). | Preservatives (e.g., methyl and propylparabens/benzyl alcohol) can cause seizures in infants and neonates when administered intravenously. |
| 11. Prepare all other items.<br>a. Tear the tape: 1 piece of ½ inch tape, 2 inches long; 2 pieces of ½ inch-tape, 3 inches long; 3 pieces of 1-inch tape, 2½ inches long; 1 piece of 1-inch tape, 2½ inches long<br>b. Open adhesive bandage or non-occlusive dressing package.<br>c. Open alcohol and povidone-iodine swabs.<br>d. Flush steel needle device/T-connector/extension set with appropriate saline preparation from 3 to 5 ml syringe.<br>e. Open catheter case and visually inspect catheter tip for burrs or splits. | Varying lengths are necessary depending on site.<br>***Special Considerations:*** *Avoid use of adhesive tape in child with known allergy. Tincture of benzoin, although often used to increase adherence of tape to skin, is not recommended because it is drying and can promote skin breakdown (Bryant, 1988). Applying a skin sealant, (protective film) immediately before taping helps to prevent skin breakdown. The sealant must be allowed to dry before attempting to place tape (Bryant, 1988). If skin is denuded, do not use skin sealant.* |
| 12. Develop individualized goals for nursing care:<br>▪ Establish child/family understanding of the need for IV therapy and the procedure.<br>▪ Insert IV successfully with a minimal number of attempts.<br>▪ Promote child/family comfort and safety.<br>▪ Stabilize IV to maintain the site. | |

**Steps** | **Rationale**

## Implementation 

1. Take the child to the treatment area that has been prepared for the procedure.

Child's room or bed should not be used for painful procedures. Utilizing treatment rooms preserves the bed/room as a "safe" place (Piercy, 1981).
***Special Considerations:*** *Respect the older child's wishes to have the procedure performed in his or her room.*

2. Stabilize the site.
   a. If desired, apply an armboard or footboard at this point (see Skill 51).

Securing the site ahead of time increases the likelihood of successful vein puncture.
***Special Considerations:*** *With the infant, toddler, and preschool child, a second nurse or health care worker is needed to help the child hold still. Parents, when they choose to be present, are to provide support and should not be asked to restrain the child. Children usually cooperate better and feel more in command if they are allowed to sit up during this process, although this may not be possible even with some older, normally cooperative children (Whaley and Wong, 1991).*

3. Explain what is being done during each step and tell older children how they can participate, allowing them some control.

Explanations help to obtain cooperation and reduce stress.
***Special Considerations:*** *Examples of directions include "I need you to hold your arm very still" or "You can cry or shout 'Ouch!' as many times as you need to."*

4. Distend the vein by method of choice.
   a. Tourniquet:
      - Extremity: Apply 2 to 6 inches above the site.
      - Scalp: Apply tourniquet like a headband. If using a rubber band, fold a piece of tape over one side.

The piece of tape provides a pull tab for removing the band.
***Special Considerations:*** *Compression on the vein by means of a finger may be preferred instead of a tourniquet especially when using a scalp vein.*

   b. Blood pressure cuff:
      - Determine child's blood pressure.
      - Pump cuff to above systolic for 30 seconds and then drop pressure until it is between systolic and diastolic.
      - Have child clench and relax hand.
      - Release cuff pressure immediately on entering the vein.
   c. Hand as a tourniquet: Have another nurse apply pressure above the site.

***Special Considerations:*** *Tourniquet should constrict venous return but not arterial flow. Check pulse distal to site. If child has fragile veins that "blow" when punctured and form a hematoma, it is best to use no tourniquet at all or only light pressure (Arthur, 1984). If using scalp vein, the area should be shaved for purposes of visualization, asepsis, and properly securing tape. Save the hair for the family.*

   d. Other tips if unable to visualize or palpate vein:
      - Hold extremity in a dependent position.
      - Lightly tap site.
      - Massage area in direction of flow.
      - Wrap extremity in warm moist packs for 10 to 15 minutes.

These techniques promote vasodilation.
***Special Considerations:*** *Warm moist packs work especially well in the dehydrated child. Avoid rapid cooling of packs because this may produce vasoconstriction. The Landry Vein Light is a useful new device that can transilluminate otherwise nonvisible veins through the use of dual fiberoptic lights (see Product References on p. 645).*

5. Prepare the site according to agency policy.
   a. Cleanse the site with povidone-iodine. Allow to dry 30 seconds, then swab with alcohol.

Cleansing the site with an antiseptic and antiinfective decreases skin surface microorganisms. Following povidone-iodine with alcohol allows better vein visualization. Povidone-iodine must dry on the skin for at least 30 seconds before removal with alcohol to be effective (Axnick, 1984).
***Special Considerations:*** *Avoid iodine preparations, because of its harshness, in those children with an allergy and in premature babies. Instead, scrub with alcohol only.*

6. Put on gloves.

Wearing gloves prevents potential contamination and transmission of infectious diseases found in blood (see Skill 50).

7. Perform venipuncture:
   a. Hold skin taut and anchor vein with thumb.
   b. Puncture skin at 20 to 30 degree angle with bevel of needle facing up (Fig. 97-3).
   c. Adjust the degree of angle and ease the needle into vein.

The soft tissue assists in supporting the needle/catheter.
***Special Considerations:*** *Enter the skin about ¼ to ½ inch distal to entry to the vein for both steel needle and catheter insertion.*

   d. Watch for blood return—flashback indicating successful venipuncture.
   e. When blood return is seen—STOP—push catheter off the needle and into the vein. Push up to insertion site if no resistance is met.

Blood return occurs when the stylet enters the vein.
***Special Considerations:*** *Blood return in the infant is not as fast as blood return in an adult. It may merely consist of the appearance of blood at the tip of the opening of the needle (Arthur, 1984). Advance catheter only as far as possible without meeting resistance.*

| Steps | Rationale |
|---|---|
| 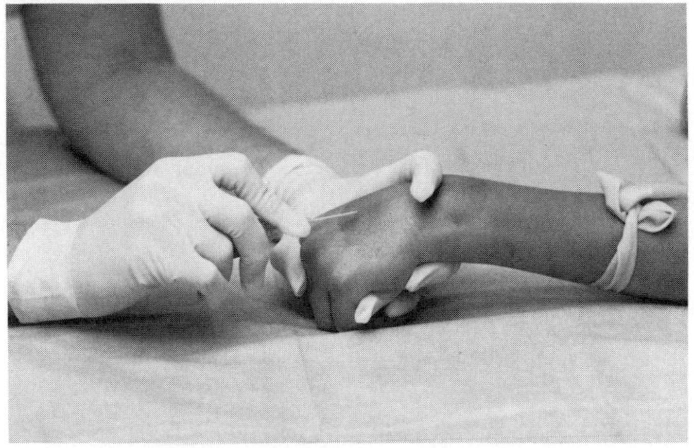 | ***FIG. 97-3*** Puncture skin with needle at 20° to 30° angle. |
| f. Do not advance steel needles (butterflies). | Advancing a steel needle risks puncturing vein in a second area. |
| g. Remove needle (stylet) from catheter. | ***Special Considerations:*** *Never reinsert stylet into catheters. The catheter tip could accidentally be severed.* |
| 8. Connect (one of the following):<br>a. Normal saline-flushed T-connector (extension set) with normal saline-filled syringe to catheter hub.<br>b. Normal saline-filled syringe to steel needle hub (tubing of needle is flushed with normal saline before insertion). | ***Special Considerations:*** *It may be helpful to place a fingertip over the vein proximal to the end of the catheter or needle to prevent a backflow of blood when attaching T-connector.* |
| 9. Release tourniquet with one hand while stabilizing catheter/needle with other hand. | |
| 10. Slowly and gently flush catheter/needle with 1 to 3 ml of normal saline. Observe site for puffing or redness and immediately discontinue if any is noted.<br>11. Periodically flush the catheter/needle during taping. | Flushing ensures proper placement of device in vein and prevents clotting before infusion is started.<br>***Special Considerations:*** *If solution will not infuse easily, pull back on catheter/needle slightly in case it is lodged against vein wall. Discontinue IV if flushing continues to be difficult. The flushing syringe should be left in place to check proper location after taping is complete.* |
| 12. Remove gloves if no more contact with blood/body secretions is anticipated. | It is difficult to tape with gloves on. |
| 13. Secure IV in place.<br>a. Tape wings or hub of catheter/needle first by placing 3 inches of ½ inch tape adhesive side up under the wings or hub.<br>b. Diagonally fold tape over the wing(s) or over on itself to leave margin of adhesive on each side of hub (see Fig. 97-4*A*).<br>c. Place 1 inch of ½-inch tape over the wing(s) or hub adjacent to insertion site and first piece of tape (see Fig. 97-4*B*).<br>d. Place third piece of tape (3 inches of ½-inch tape) adhesive side up under T-connector just above second piece of tape. Fold over hub in chevron style (Fig. 97-4*C*).<br>e. Press tape firmly in place during each step. | A securely taped IV prevents dislodgement and mechanical phlebitis.<br>***Special Considerations:*** *Do not place tape over actual insertion site. Proper placement of tape rather than the amount of tape used assures stability. Adequate taping and support should permit a child to leave the bed and maintain as active a daily routine as possible (Streckfuss, 1985). A portion of a cotton ball may be needed to support an angled insertion site. Different IV needle/catheter brands may require adaptation of the basic steps. Never encircle the extremity with tape as this could restrict circulation, especially if infiltration or swelling occurs.* |
| f. Apply topical antimicrobial ointment and adhesive bandage over the insertion site as indicated by agency policy (Fig. 97-4*D*).<br>g. If using transparent dressing (Tegaderm, OpSite), place this over the insertion site first, then tape as described above. | Insertion sites are potential sites for infection and should be protected with a sterile adhesive bandage or transparent dressing.<br>***Special Considerations:*** *The small dot adhesive bandages work best for infants' IVs. The prepared medicine cup can be used to protect scalp sites in infants. Tape the cup in place over the site, being certain not to impede vein patency.* |
| h. Use remaining tape strips to secure T-connector tubing or steel needle tubing at a point distal to the site to prevent tension on actual site. | Securing tubing prevents tension on actual site. |
| 14. Check patency following taping with flush syringe. | The taping procedure and/or small change in catheter position may hamper patency. |
| 15. Remove flush syringe, connect IV tubing, release the clamp and begin infusion. Double check rate on pump for correctness. | ***Special Considerations:*** *Begin the infusion only after determining that the IV site continues to be patent.* |

| Steps | Rationale |
|---|---|

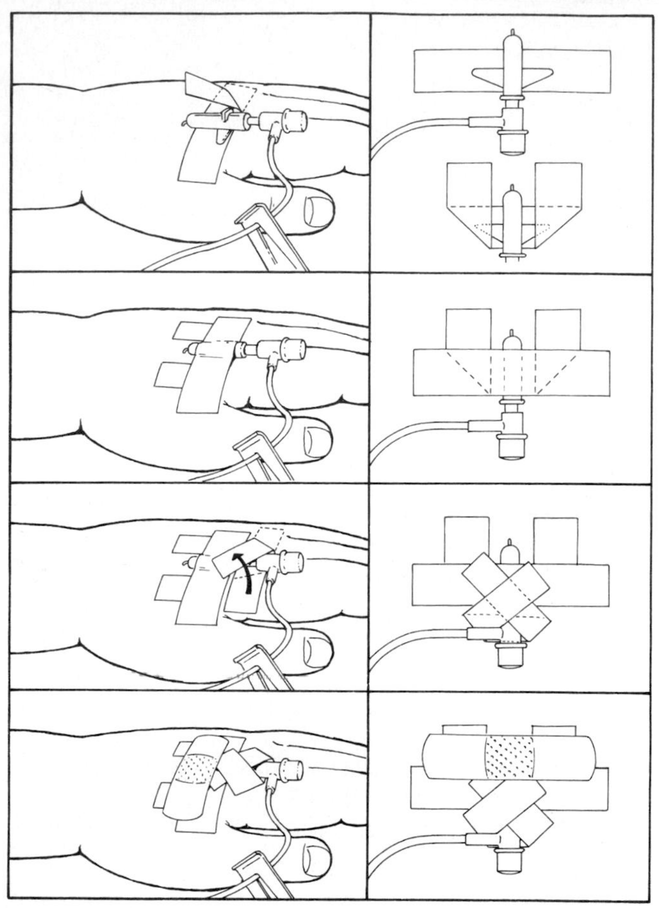


***FIG. 97-4*** **A,** Diagonally fold tape over the wing(s) and over on itself. **B,** Place next strip of tape over the wing(s) or hub and over first piece of tape. **C,** Apply third piece of tape, folding chevron style and **D,** Apply adhesive bandage over insertion site.

16. Apply armboard/footboard if needed and not already in place (Fig. 97-5).

***Special Considerations:*** *Apply tape snugly but not tight enough to constrict circulation. Coban may be used to secure the armboard/footboard.*

17. Write on tape: date and time started, gauge of needle/catheter, and initials of individual inserting device.

Labeling provides instant reference to the date for site change (Messner, 1987) or site care.

***Special Considerations:*** *To brighten the tape, paste colorful stickers on it, draw pictures on the tape, or write the child's name (Piercy, 1981).*

18. Return child to family and own room if venipuncture was performed in another location.
19. Restrain child appropriate to supervision for protection of IV (see Skill 51).

Restraining may be necessary for the protection of the IV site and the safety of the child.

20. Teach family and/or child:
    a. Signs of infiltration (swelling, pain, leakage, or coolness at the site).
    b. Signs of phlebitis (pain, redness, swelling, or heat at the site).
    c. How to protect tubing while picking child up (Fig. 97-6) or when assisting child to play.
    d. To notify nurse for:
        - Signs of infiltration or phlebitis.
        - Large air bubbles in the tubing.
        - Disconnected tubing.
        - Near empty bag or volume control set.
        - Pump alarms sounding.

Explanations increase knowledge, feelings of control, and decrease anxiety. Family may feel uneasy about holding an infant with an IV in place.

***Special Considerations:*** *Show family how to unfasten restraints, if they are used, perform range of motion exercises, pick child up or move child, and refasten restraints properly.*

***Special Considerations:*** *The family needs to be reassured that they are not entirely responsible for the IV but are helping their child and the health team.*

21. Praise the child for his or her help, praise family for support during procedure, and provide cuddle time for the infant/toddler.

Praise allows child to feel he or she actively participated in helping with procedure.

***Special Considerations:*** *Reward the child with stickers or an IV therapy coloring book. Honestly answer family's questions about number of attempts to establish IV to maintain trust.*

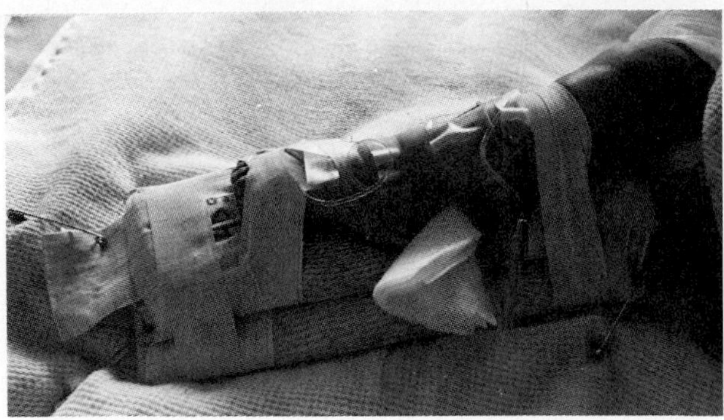

***FIG. 97-5*** Extremity immobilized with board and firmly secured to bedding with pins.

From Whaley LF and Wong DL: Nursing care of infants and children, ed 4, St Louis, 1991, The CV Mosby Co.

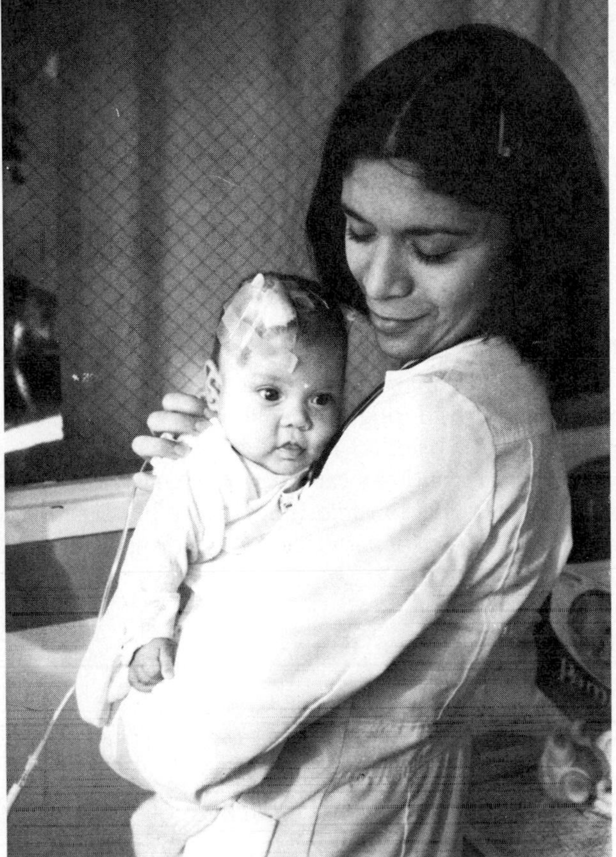

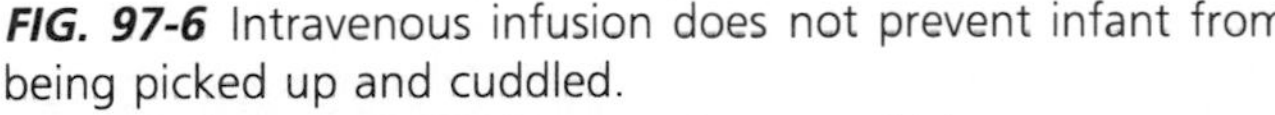

***FIG. 97-6*** Intravenous infusion does not prevent infant from being picked up and cuddled.

From Whaley LF and Wong DL: Nursing care of infants and children, ed 4, St Louis, 1991, The CV Mosby Co.

| Evaluation Outcomes | Observational Guidelines |
| --- | --- |
| 1. Preparation of the child and family for the IV therapy procedure is completed. | Ask the child/family to identify why the IV is necessary, what having an IV means, what to expect during the procedure, and what their role is during and after the procedure. |
| 2. The IV is successfully started with minimum number of attempts. | Observe number of attempts. Observe patency of IV. Verify that IV drips well off the pump with no diffuse or localized swelling at site. |
| 3. Comfort and safety measures relating to IV therapy are implemented. | Check armboard/footboard for presence of absorbent covering; check tape, making sure it is not too tight; check circulation distal to restraints for presence of capillary refill; observe pump for proper functioning; observe behavior and listen to child's comments of discomfort regarding IV therapy. |
| 4. IV remains in place until it is discontinued per order or scheduled site change. | Check to see that tape at IV site is intact; check to see that armboard/footboard or other protective devices are intact; check restraints for proper placement. Check connecting joints of tubing for security. |
| 5. Activities of daily living (ADL) are maintained as much as possible during IV therapy. | Check child during play for inadvertent dislocation of IV; note continuance of ADLs with adaptation as needed. Ask the child/family to identify when to call the nurse. |

### Documentation

Record assessment data and preparation given to child/family; date and time IV started; gauge and type of needle/catheter inserted; site of IV; number of attempts in general terms (e.g., IV placed on third attempt); type of solution, any medications, and rate of flow; type of restraints, if any used; pump or other equipment utilized; reaction of the child/family to the procedure.

# SKILL 98 Maintaining and Discontinuing IVs

*Anna L. Summerfield*

Intravenous maintenance facilitates continued access to the circulatory system by ensuring a patent line at all times without causing injury to the child. One of the major concerns when considering the maintenance of IVs is infection, either local or systemic. Key issues such as fluid change, tubing change, and site care all are effective measures to protect the child from infection. The IV line and site are closely monitored for early detection of complications such as occlusion, infiltration, and phlebitis, so that early intervention can occur.

## NURSING DIAGNOSES

Impaired skin integrity related to insertion of IV catheter; Potential for infection related to invasive IV catheter; Potential for fluid volume excess related to excessive IV fluid intake.

| Steps | Rationale |
|---|---|
| **Assessment** | |
| 1. Review at beginning of each shift:<br>a. Physician order for solution and rate change or discontinue order.<br>b. Present solution infusing and rate.<br>c. Date IV inserted.<br>d. Date of tubing and solution expiration.<br>e. Date dressing placed. | A review of factors concerning the IV guides planning and implementation of IV maintenance.<br>***Special Considerations:*** *Replacing tubing sets and changing site on peripheral IV every 48 to 72 hours is safe and cost effective (Maki, 1987). Change IV fluid bottle or bag every 24 hours (Messner, 1987; Bryan, 1987). Check agency policy for infection control guidelines.* |
| 2. Assess every 1 to 2 hours:<br>a. Flow rate.<br>b. Tubing free of air and kinks.<br>c. Pump operation.<br>d. Tubing connections.<br>e. Restraints, if in use (see Skill 51). | Assessing these factors provides safeguards against potential hazards.<br>***Special Considerations:*** *Certain types of IV pumps continue to infuse fluid even after infiltration has occurred. Large air bubbles could cause an embolus. "Time Taping" volume control sets provides a quick visual check that the IV pump is functioning properly. Most pumps on the market do have air detection devices as part of the pump or as a feature that can be connected to the tubing. Know limitations of equipment and always double-check its functioning.* |
| 3. Assess child/family behavior and verbalized complaints about the site. | Behavioral changes and verbalized complaints can indicate the development of complications.<br>***Special Considerations:*** *In infants, observe for fussy or irritable behavior not consolable by standard measures. Ask the older child how the IV feels and observe for signs of discomfort.* |
| 4. Assess IV site hourly for:<br>a. Infiltration—edema, slight burning or pain, blanching, coolness, leakage from insertion site.<br>b. Phlebitis—swelling, tenderness or pain, erythema, warmth, slight induration or palpable venous cord (Feldstein, 1986).<br>c. Occlusion—pump alarming, signs of infiltration, tubing/catheter kinked. | Early detection of a problem with early intervention prevents complications.<br>***Special Considerations:*** *Develop a routine for each check, e.g., start at the solution container and work down the line to the IV site (Feldstein, 1986). It may be necessary to remove elastic coverings such as Coban to adequately inspect the site. Teach the older child and/or family to recognize signs of infiltration, phlebitis, or occlusion. Elicit their help by asking them to call if they notice any of the signs. Instruct the child and family not to adjust fluid drip rate or manipulate pump controls, but to call for assistance.* |
| 5. Assess circulation hourly when the IV site is located in an extremity. | Infiltration of fluid can cause enough pressure on vascular system to decrease/constrict blood flow to the extremity.<br>***Special Considerations:*** *Tape or dressings should never cover fingers or toes completely. Inform the child and family that hourly IV checks need to continue during the night.* |

| Steps | Rationale |
|---|---|
| 6. Assess hydration status (see Skill 64). | Detecting changes in fluid and electrolyte balance decreases incidence of fluid overload or volume deficit. ***Special Considerations:*** *Children receiving IV therapy should automatically be on intake and output with daily weights. Review hydration status every 4 to 8 hours.* |

## Planning and Goal Setting

1. Gather and organize supplies:
   a. Appropriate IV tubing/fluid (review orders).
   b. IV expiration labels for solution and tubing.
   c. Adhesive bandage or transparent dressing.
   d. Antibacterial ointment (according to facility policy).
   e. Povidone-iodine/alcohol prep.
   f. 2 × 2 inch sterile gauze (2).
2. Develop individualized goals for nursing care:
   - To maintain a patent IV access.
   - To prevent complications such as infiltration, infection or occlusion.
   - To maintain fluid and electrolyte balance.
   - To discontinue IV catheter/needle promptly when indicated and prevent hematoma formation at insertion site.

## Implementation

| Steps | Rationale |
|---|---|
| 1. Tubing/solution change and daily care: a. Prepare and prime new IV tubing/fluid setup using aseptic technique and bring to the child's bedside at appropriate time. b. Loosen and remove any tape on the old tubing connections. | Changing tubing and IV solution on a recommended schedule prevents nosocomial infection. ***Special Considerations:*** *New tubing/solution should be ready at least 1 hour before needed to prevent last minute delays. All solutions with additives are to be labeled as to content.* |
| c. Turn off infusion pump and clamp off infusing fluid. Remove tubing from pump. | When the old tubing is removed from the pump, the fluid would continue to flow. |
| d. Disconnect the old IV tubing from T-connector extension tubing and connect the sterile end of new tubing. | ***Special Considerations:*** *Avoid contamination of sterile end of tubing.* |
| e. Rethread tubing according to pump directions, unclamp, and resume infusion at prescribed rate. Label tubing and new solution container with expiration labels. | ***Special Considerations:*** *Some facilities use color-coded stickers for each day of the week to provide an easy method of knowing when tubing and solutions are to be changed.* |
| f. Change solution bag every 24 hours using aseptic technique. | ***Special Considerations:*** *If there is any question as to sterility of fluid, change both tubing and fluid.* |
| 2. Daily care and/or site care: a. Replace secondary tape that is soiled, as needed. b. Replace armboard/footboard if soiled. c. Observe for skin irritation around tape and site. | Daily care provides opportunity to closely inspect site. ***Special Considerations:*** *Because peripheral IV sites in the pediatric population are usually maintained until electively discontinued or until infiltration occurs (Phelps, 1987), actual site care and the frequency of such are controversial. Check agency policy as to site care regimen. It is difficult to provide site care to an infant and not dislodge the IV.* |
| d. If performing site care, remove adhesive bandage/dressing directly over IV insertion site. Do not remove transparent dressing. | Transparent dressings act as a one-way barrier against infection. Therefore, they are not routinely changed. |
| e. Inspect site for drainage or redness. f. Gently clean site with povidone-iodine prep pad, allow to dry, and cleanse gently with alcohol. g. Replace tape as needed. h. Apply antibacterial ointment at catheter insertion site, if it is facility policy. | Redness and drainage are complications that indicate the need for a site change. ***Special Considerations:*** *Ask a second nurse to help stabilize the IV during site care or have the child/family assist. This helps prevent inadvertently dislodging the IV. If possible, IVs should not be left in place longer than 72 hours, because the incidence of site infection increases significantly at this point (Messner, 1987).* |
| i. Reapply adhesive bandage/dressing. | IV dressings provide protection from gross contamination from the environment and allow easy inspection of the site (Axnick, 1984). |

| Steps | Rationale |
|---|---|
| ***Complications*** | |
| 1. Suspected IV infiltration: | |
| a. Check if the IV will drip off the pump by removing the tubing from pump and slightly elevating volume control set. | An IV that does not drip spontaneously or freely may be infiltrated. |
| b. Observe for edema at the site. If the IV is in an extremity, compare the site to the other extremity.<br>c. Determine presence of pain at the site.<br>d. If infiltration is defined, stop infusion and discontinue the IV. | ***Special Considerations:*** *IV catheters and small gauge needles do not always give a blood return even when they are in the vein. Some pumps indicate an infiltration, which may actually be a pump malfunction. If a blistering substance (e.g., calcium, potassium, vancomycin) infiltrates, notify the physician immediately.* |
| e. Wrap the extremity in a warm, moist compress.<br>f. Elevate the extremity and encourage motion. | Warm compresses increase fluid absorption through vasodilation (Guhlow, 1979).<br>***Special Considerations:*** *Some controversy exists about the use of warm soaks depending on the substance/fluid infiltrated. Check with physician. Neonates and infants may be especially prone to tissue necrosis related to infiltration because of their inability to communicate pain and because of limited extravascular tissue space on the scalp and dorsum of the hand and foot (Phelps, 1987).* |
| 2. Suspected IV phlebitis: | |
| a. Gently palpate the IV site and observe child's reaction; compare temperature of affected IV site to unaffected site. | Palpation provides information necessary to confirm a phlebitic or inflamed vessel.<br>***Special Considerations:*** *Warmth can indicate phlebitis even before skin is red or tender (Feldstein, 1986).* |
| b. If phlebitis is defined, stop infusion and discontinue the IV. | Phlebitis is defined when pain and tenderness are present upon palpation of the site, site is warmer than nonaffected site and redness is present along vein. |
| c. Place cold compress over site; follow in 1 to 2 hours with a warm one (Guhlow, 1979). | Cold compresses will decrease pain and inflammation at the site.<br>***Special Considerations:*** *Use extra caution in applying cold or warm compresses on young children unable to verbalize discomfort.* |
| 3. Suspected occlusion:<br>a. Straighten the tubing.<br>b. Reposition the child.<br>c. Attempt to drip IV off the pump.<br>d. Release tape above the site and retape. | |
| e. If patency is not established by simple intervention, discontinue the IV. | ***Special Considerations:*** *The risk of pulmonary embolism precludes irrigation of an occluded IV catheter/needle (Barrus, 1987).* |
| 4. Air in the line (Boykoff, 1988):<br>a. Hold IV tubing taut and tap tubing to remove bubbles near top of IV line.<br>b. Curl tubing around a pen/syringe when bubbles are present near top of IV line. Fill drip chamber before releasing pen and tubing. | ***Special Considerations:*** *Careful priming of tubing and not allowing the volume control set to completely empty prevents air in line. The use of an air eliminating filter prevents air in line from reaching child. Another measure to prevent air in the line is to maintain the drip chamber upright at all times. The chamber may be taped upright to the tubing itself or to the IV pole.* |
| c. Withdraw air with needle and syringe at Y site when air is just above Y site. | ***Special Considerations:*** *Explain procedure to child and family to decrease anxiety.* |
| d. Inject IV solution into Y site when air is above Y site (especially effective if drip chamber is collapsed).<br>▪ Aseptically withdraw 5 to 10 ml IV solution from solution container using a 10 ml syringe and a small gauge needle.<br>▪ Clamp tubing with hemostat below Y site and below air.<br>▪ Clean Y site latex port with alcohol and insert above prepared syringe/needle.<br>▪ Slowly inject solution into tubing; air is pushed up to drip chamber.<br>▪ Remove syringe.<br>▪ Release hemostat/clamp. | ***Special Considerations:*** *Be sure drip chamber is filled before releasing the hemostat/clamp.* |

| Steps | Rationale |
|---|---|
| e. Flush IV line when air is located between Y site and child. | |
| ▪ Clamp T-connector with hemostat/clamp proximal to child and below air. | Clamping prevents backflow of blood into cannula. |
| ▪ Aseptically disconnect the tubing from the T-connector. | ***Special Considerations:*** *Do not contaminate the open end of the T-connector. Placing a sterile syringe into the T-connector prevents contamination.* |
| ▪ Allow enough fluid to flush through tubing into a receptacle to remove air. | ***Special Considerations:*** *The tubing end must not be contaminated.* |
| ▪ Reconnect tubing to T-connector and release hemostat/clamp. | |
| ***Discontinue IV*** | |
| 1. Remove tape down to site. 2. Place 2 × 2 inch gauze over IV entry site and gently ease the catheter or needle from the skin. | ***Special Considerations:*** *Gently pull tape away from skin to prevent tissue damage, skin breakdown, and child's discomfort. Gloves should be worn for the actual removal of the catheter/needle. Allow child to help remove tape.* |
| 3. Fold a second 2 × 2 inch piece of gauze and place over site, applying firm pressure for 1 to 3 minutes. | Some bleeding may occur. Applying pressure at site reduces likelihood of hematoma formation. |
| 4. Apply adhesive bandage or tape over 2 × 2 inch gauze. | A dressing is applied for prevention of nosocomial infection. ***Special Considerations:*** *Physician's orders are not usually necessary before discontinuing or resiting phlebitic/infiltrated IVs, although checking with the physician may prevent an unnecessary restart.* |

| Evaluation Outcomes | Observational Guidelines |
|---|---|
| 1. IV access is safely maintained. | Observe patency and security of access. Note documentation of tubing/solution changes and daily care/site care. |
| 2. Complications such as infiltration, infection, or occlusion are promptly identified. | Check site for coolness, warmth, erythema, edema, pain, blanching, palpable cord, or leakage. Observe for potential occlusion situations, e.g., kinked tubing, child lying on tubing, or pump malfunction. |
| 3. Rehydration is provided with IV therapy. | Check intake and output, electrolyte reports, and weight curve for significant changes. |
| 4. IV is safely removed if infiltrated or phlebitic. | Note removal of IV immediately if signs of infiltration/phlebitis are noted. Observe site for resolution of infiltration/phlebitis. |
| 5. IV site is free of hematoma after removal. | Review site for signs of hematoma, i.e., firm blue hue at or above insertion site. |

## Documentation

Document in the nurses' notes at the beginning of each shift the type of IV solution hanging and additives; rate of solution; site of IV and condition of site; and changes in any of these factors. Note amount infused on intake and output record every 1 to 2 hours or in accordance with agency policy and procedure. (The child's condition may require more frequent documentation and a continous running total [e.g., for ICU patients]). Record site condition every 1 to 2 hours. Indicate fluid and tubing changes, noting date and time. Document site care and any necessary interventions. Record discontinuation of the IV, noting condition of the site and the nursing care given after IV is discontinued (e.g., wrap with warm soaks or extremity elevated). If an IV is resited, document the ease or difficulty with which it is accomplished.

# SKILL 99 Administering Blood and Blood Products

*Christina Algiere Kasprisin*

Blood components are administered when the child has a deficiency of that product. This deficiency can result from increased loss, increased destruction, or decreased production of blood components. The physician must weigh the benefits of the transfusion against the risk of transfusion reaction and disease transmission. The role of the nurse is to minimize the risks through careful assessment, monitoring, and evaluation of the child's response to the component therapy.

## NURSING DIAGNOSES

Anxiety related to unmet informational needs about risks and benefits of blood transfusion therapy; Potential for injury related to transfusion of incompatible blood components.

| Steps | Rationale |
|---|---|
| **Assessment** | |
| 1. Assess child's pretransfusion status:<br>a. Clinical condition.<br>b. Weight.<br>c. Developmental status.<br>d. Laboratory values.<br>e. Indication for component therapy.<br>f. Previous transfusions. | This baseline information aids in evaluating the effectiveness of the component therapy.<br>***Special Considerations:*** *Although component therapy is ordered by the physician, any discrepancies should be questioned.* |
| 2. Verify physician order for type and quantity of blood component and any special administration concerns, e.g., warmed blood and infusion rate. Check if autologous or directed donor blood requested. | Legally, a physician's order is required to administer blood components.<br>***Special Considerations:*** *A double check of the physician's order ensures that right child receives the correct components in the correct quantity.* |
| 3. Assess child/family's understanding of the transfusion process, including any concerns they may have. | |
| a. Teach signs and symptoms of transfusion reaction to report. | The informed child and family assist in the early detection of transfusion reactions. |
| b. Ensure signed consent is obtained if required by institution. | As with all medical therapy, the physician is responsible for obtaining informed consent for the administration of blood components. Some institutions may require a signed consent form for the medical record.<br>***Special Considerations:*** *Explain the reasons for component therapy to the child. If the need for the transfusion is not critical, allow the child* some *flexibility in scheduling. Some religions, e.g., Jehovah's Witnesses, prohibit blood transfusions. If the parent refuses to give consent and the child cannot be medically managed without the transfusion, then a court order may be obtained.* |
| 4. Determine preparation necessary for this transfusion: | Appropriate preparatory measures help ensure efficient, timely, and safe administration of the transfusion. |
| a. Laboratory testing, including blood typing, testing for antibodies to blood groups, and cross matching with the donor's blood. | |
| b. Intravenous access established and patent, preferably with a large diameter needle. | If an IV site is not present or patent, access must be established before the blood component is obtained from the laboratory. A large diameter needle or catheter minimizes hemolysis of red blood cells. |
| c. Required blood component available in laboratory. | If a blood component is ordered that requires special preparation, additional time is required by the laboratory.<br>***Special Considerations:*** *A child who has received multiple transfusions may require washed or leukocyte-poor red blood cells to minimize risk of transfusion reaction. Blood that has been irradiated is often given to children who are immunosuppressed.* |

| Steps | Rationale |
|---|---|

## Planning and Goal Setting

1. Gather supplies:
   a. Blood administration set with calibrated chamber.
   b. Y-type blood administration set for older children.
   c. Syringe and tubing for neonates.
   d. Normal saline for intravenous use.
   e. Micropore filter per institution policy.

All supplies should be ready when the blood component is obtained from the laboratory. The risk of bacterial colonization increases as the red blood cells remain at room temperature. Storage on the nursing unit is not acceptable because the required controlled temperature is not available.

***Special Considerations:*** *An administration set with filter (usually 170 microns) must be used for all blood products. Some institutions may require that a microaggregate filter be used. They have a pore size of approximately 40 microns and are indicated for massive transfusion (usually defined as a transfusion greater than the child's total blood volume within 24 hours). Some laboratories supply washed, prefiltered blood in syringes for neonates. If the red cells have been filtered by the laboratory, additional filtration is not necessary.*

   f. Infusion pump if required by institutional policy or child's status.

A pump helps provide a steady infusion rate.

***Special Considerations:*** *Check with manufacturer to determine if red cells can be infused through that system. Hemolysis has been reported with some pumps.*

   g. Blood warmer if indicated.

Blood warmers are indicated for children who are hypothermic, at risk for hypothermia, or are receiving comparatively large volumes of blood in a short period of time. This will decrease the likelihood of a hypothermic transfusion reaction.

***Special Considerations:*** *If an electronic blood warmer is used, check to ensure that the alarms are set and the unit has been routinely inspected by biomechanical engineering.*

2. Develop individualized goals of nursing care:
   - Blood components will be infused using correct technique.
   - Any adverse reaction to the blood component administration will be rapidly identified.

## Implementation

1. Obtain the blood component just before starting the transfusion. Hang blood within 30 minutes after it is obtained from the laboratory. (See Table 99-1 for Guidelines on Administration of Non-Red Cell Components.)

Blood that has warmed to 10° C cannot be returned to the blood bank for reuse (Widman, 1985).

***Special Considerations:*** *Each institution should have a procedure on transfusion therapy. This may include restrictions on who can obtain the components from the laboratory, how the component and child should be identified, etc.*

***TABLE 99-1*** Administration Guidelines for Non-red Cell Components

| Components | Equipment | Considerations |
|---|---|---|
| Fresh Frozen Plasma (FFP)—should be ABO compatible. | Standard blood administration set (70 to 120 micron filter); can be straight, calibrated or syringe. | Circulatory overload can occur if volume is too large/fast for child's condition.<br>Possible transmission of blood borne diseases.<br>Infuse per child's clinical status.<br>Possible allergic and febrile reactions. |
| Platelets | Standard blood administration set (70 to 120 micron filter); can be straight, calibrated or syringe. | Circulatory overload can occur if volume is too large/fast for child's condition.<br>Transmission of blood borne diseases is possible.<br>Infuse per child's clinical status.<br>Possible allergic and febrile reactions.<br>If large red cell contamination, initially infuse slowly. |
| Cryoprecipitate | Standard blood administration set (70 to 120 micron filter); can be straight, calibrated or syringe. | Circulatory overload can occur if volume is too large/fast for child's condition.<br>Possible transmission of blood borne diseases.<br>Infuse per child's clinical status.<br>Possible allergic and febrile reactions. |
| Plasma Protein Fraction/Albumin | Tubing usually supplied by manufacturer. | Virtually no risk of disease transmission.<br>Infuse per child's status to avoid circulatory overload. |

| Steps | Rationale |
|---|---|
| 2. Verify that blood component received is what was ordered, is compatible with the child, and is not expired. | *Do not* administer blood component if any discrepancies exist. **Special Considerations:** *Blood products expire at the date/time stamped. If no time is given, the component expires at midnight of the date stamped. The Food and Drug Administration establishes the length of time a blood component can be stored.* |
| 3. Identify child, check ID bracelet/blood ID bracelet for hospital number. These must be identical to the numbers on the transfusion form and compatibility tag. Many institutions require this be done by two individuals. Asking the child or family "What is your name?" is an extra safeguard. | Because of the harm that can result from an error, patient identification is essential. **Special Considerations:** *Human error contributes to severe transfusion reactions and death. Of the deaths associated with blood transfusions reported to the FDA, 61% were caused by human error (Myhre, 1980). In another study, 12 deaths resulted from lack of positive patient identification (Schmidt, 1981).* |
| 4. Compare child's ABO/Rh group with that of blood component label and compatibility tag to determine appropriateness. | |
| 5. Measure the child's vital signs, including temperature, immediately before beginning infusion. | These provide a baseline to determine if a transfusion reaction is occurring. |
| 6. Assemble blood bag/syringe and tubing: | |
| *Y set* | |
| a. Close the clamps. | |
| b. Remove the protective covering from one arm of the Y set and aseptically insert the spike into the normal saline. | Normal saline flushes the air from the filter and tubing. Normal saline is the solution of choice. |
| c. Open the clamp on both arms of the Y tubing. | **Special Considerations:** *Blood should not be in prolonged contact with solution such as Lactated Ringer's (LR). The calcium in the LR may interfere with the anticoagulant and the high concentration of dextrose may cause changes in the red cells.* |
| d. Close the clamp on the free arm of the set (the blood side of the filter) and open the clamp below the filter, thus flushing the tubing. | **Special Considerations:** *Y sets can be used with older children where fluid volume is not a critical concern.* |
| e. After the tubing has been flushed, connect it to child's IV site. | |
| f. Gently agitate the unit of red blood cells. | Agitation resuspends the red cells in the anticoagulant. |
| g. Remove the protector cap from the free arm of the Y set. | |
| h. Aseptically insert the spike into an outlet in the red cell unit. Use steady, firm pressure in a straight line with the outlet port and bag to complete the insertion. Do not force the connector or insert it at an angle. | The spike from the IV tubing must be carefully inserted to guard against accidentally puncturing the unit of red blood cells. If the integrity of the unit is compromised, it cannot be used for transfusion. |
| i. Invert the unit of red cells and suspend from IV pole. Place tubing in infusion pump. Open clamp to blood and close clamp to normal saline. | |
| *Straight set with or without graduated chamber* | |
| a. Gently agitate the blood component. | Agitation resuspends the red cells in the anticoagulant. |
| b. Close the clamps. | |
| c. Remove the protective covering from the tubing and aseptically insert the spike into an outlet in the red cell unit. Use steady firm pressure in a straight line with the outlet port and bag to complete the insertion. | |
| d. Invert the unit of red cells, open the clamps, fill the calibrated chamber, filter and tubing. | The red blood cells are used to flush the tubing of air. **Special Considerations:** *Calibrated infusion chambers are used when exact fluid volume administration is a concern.* |
| e. Shut the lower clamp. Connect tubing to a patent IV site, then open clamp slightly. | |
| *Syringe set* | |
| a. Connect the smallest amount of tubing necessary to administer transfusion. Using the blood product, flush the tubing of air. | The tubing is "dead space." Therefore the shortest amount of tubing to safely administer the blood component should be used. **Special Considerations:** *Note the volume of component in the syringe before and after clearing the tubing of air. Syringes are used when small volumes are transfused. Determine by consultation with the laboratory if the blood requires filtration before beginning the infusion.* |

| Steps | Rationale |
|---|---|
| b. Place the syringe in the appropriate infusion control device. | |
| 7. Regulate initial rate for administration. The initial rate should be slow, with approximately one fifth of the volume to be transfused in the first 15 minutes. | This slow rate will minimize the child's exposure should a severe transfusion reaction occur. **Special Considerations:** *If the child is in borderline congestive heart failure (due to anemia) no more than 2 ml/kg/hr should be infused, with a concomitant diuretic if indicated.* |
| 8. Monitor vital signs per hospital policy. Every 15 minutes for first hour and every hour thereafter until infusion is completed is recommended. | |
| 9. If no transfusion reaction occurs in the first 15 minutes (see step 10), increase rate to complete infusion in 1½ to 2 hours. | The rate can be increased as dictated by the child's clinical condition. Most institutions require that blood be infused within 4 hours to minimize the possibility of bacterial growth. **Special Considerations:** *If the child cannot tolerate an infusion in 4 hours or less, notify the blood bank in advance. The blood component may be divided and a portion can remain in the blood bank in controlled temperature.* |
| 10. Observe the child carefully during the transfusion. Signs of a transfusion reaction are:<br>a. Urticaria.<br>b. Fever (1° C rise above baseline).<br>c. Chills.<br>d. Extreme pain at infusion site.<br>e. Dyspnea, wheezing.<br>f. Low back pain.<br>g. Hemoglobinuria. | Careful observation ensures rapid detection of any reaction. **Special Considerations:** *If the only manifestation of reaction is urticaria, some physicians will medicate the child with an antihistamine and continue the transfusion.* |
| 11. If a change in the child's condition occurs, stop the transfusion and keep the IV patent with normal saline or maintenance fluids (switch to new tubing if necessary). | When a transfusion reaction is suspected, the infusion is stopped immediately to limit the child's exposure to the blood component. **Special Considerations:** *Most hospitals require a sample of blood and urine from the patient for identification of the cause of the reaction.* |
| 12. If no reaction occurs, discontinue the transfusion when the required volume has been infused. | **Special Considerations:** *When multiple units of blood components are to be infused, the filter must be checked and found free of debris. Change the tubing and filter as required.* |
| 13. Obtain posttransfusion vital signs. | |
| 14. Dispose of blood container and tubing per hospital policy. | **Special Considerations:** *Handle carefully because of the risk of contamination by blood borne diseases.* |
| 15. Praise child for cooperating during the transfusion. | |

| Evaluation Outcomes | Observational Guidelines |
|---|---|
| 1. The child and family are taught the risks/benefits of transfusion therapy. | Interview the family to confirm their understanding of the need for the therapy and the risks involved. |
| 2. The child and family are taught the signs and symptoms of a transfusion reaction, both immediate and delayed. | The child and family state they will notify the nurse immediately if rash, fever, chills, pain at infusion site, dyspnea, wheezing, low back pain, or blood in the urine is noted. Family states they will also be alert for fever or jaundice 3 to 7 days after the transfusion. |
| 3. Blood component is infused safely. | The component is verified to be what was ordered, is compatible with the child, and is not expired. Child is properly identified by hospital bracelet, blood ID bracelet, or hospital number; these numbers should be identical to the numbers on transfusion form and compatibility tag. Nurse takes protective precautions according to hospital policy. |
| 4. Blood component is infused properly to maximize component benefit. | Component is not expired, is properly stored, and is hung within 30 minutes of arrival on unit. The component is filtered and given through a patent, large catheter IV access. If a pump is used, it does not cause hemolysis. A warmer, if used, maintains proper temperature. Component is infused preferably in 1½ to 2 hours but no more than 4 hours. |

### Evaluation Outcomes—cont'd

5. Adverse reactions to component therapy are prevented or minimized.

### Observational Guidelines—cont'd

Component is properly prepared (e.g., washed, irradiated) and correctly matched to the child. Vital signs are taken before initiating infusion, every 15 minutes for 1 hour, then every 1 hour through completion. Infusion rate is slow for first 15 minutes. Child is observed frequently for signs and symptoms of reaction, and if noted, transfusion is stopped immediately and physician is notified.

### Documentation

Record initiation date, time, venipuncture sites, blood component infused, identification number, and patient baseline assessment data including vital signs. All child and family teaching should be noted. During the transfusion, document any pertinent observations. When the transfusion is completed, the date and time, the child's vital signs, and response to the therapy should be noted.

# *SKILL* 100 Providing Continuous Electrocardiographic Monitoring

*Patricia A. Jamerson*

Electrocardiographic (ECG) monitoring assists the health care provider to identify infants and children with alterations in cardiac electrical activity as a result of hypoxia, metabolic or acid-base imbalance, improper neurologic or cardiac functioning, and/or medications. Specifically, ECG monitoring provides information about rate, rhythm, and intracardiac conduction (Hazinksi, 1984). Respiratory monitoring is frequently used in conjunction with cardiac monitoring to alert the caregiver to apnea and respiratory embarrassment which may compromise cardiac function. The most common dysrhythmias seen in infants and children are bradycardias and supraventricular tachycardias (Chameides, 1988).

## NURSING DIAGNOSES

Decreased cardiac output related to prematurity, fluid/electrolyte imbalances or congenital/acquired defects; Altered cardiopulmonary tissue perfusion related to hypovolemia/hypervolemia, medications or Rh incompatibility; Anxiety related to unmet informational needs about equipment and purpose for electrocardiographic monitoring; Potential for impaired skin integrity related to electrode placement site, frequent electrode removal/replacement, or allergy to electrode adhesive or products used for skin preparation.

| Steps | Rationale |
|---|---|
| **Assessment** | |
| 1. Determine child/family's previous experience with ECG monitoring and level of fear and anxiety related to procedure. | Previous experiences with monitoring influence perceptions and attitudes toward the procedure and thus may affect cooperation. |
| 2. Review history and present condition for factors influencing ECG monitoring: | |
| a. Age and size of child. | Preparatory steps and lead placement may need to be altered for infants and small children. |

| Steps | Rationale |
|---|---|
| b. History of or high risk for apnea, bradycardia, reflux, or choking. | Infants identified as at risk include those who are premature, have had a documented episode of apnea or bradycardia, have had episodes of reflux/choking, have breathing difficulty or color change at home, have abnormal pneumograms or are siblings of Sudden Infant Death Syndrome (SIDS) victims (Dunne and Matthews, 1987; Southall, 1983). ***Special Considerations:*** *Respiratory monitoring should also be provided for infants/children at risk.* |
| c. Presence of acid-base or electrolyte imbalances, especially calcium and potassium. | Cellular metabolism and pH levels affect cardiac conduction. |
| d. Medications. | Digoxin, Inderal, and quinidine decrease the heart rate; caffeine, theophylline, atropine, and epinephrine increase heart rate (Naulty, 1983). |
| e. Presence of a pacemaker:<br>▪ Fixed rate.<br>▪ Demand. | Alarm limits should be determined by pacemaker settings. Firing and capturing should be assessed. |
| f. Dextrocardia (heart located on the right side of the body) or dextroposition (heart rotated such that the apex is on the right instead of the left). | Lead placement needs to be altered to reflect the direction of cardiac conduction. |
| g. Congenital heart defect or acquired heart disease. | Dysrhythmias may develop postoperatively or secondary to cardiac disease or congenital defect. Emergency measures may be necessary if cardiac output is compromised, or if the potential for further deterioration of the electrical rhythm exists (Chameides, 1988). |
| 3. Assess for additional measures that may be needed in order to achieve optimal monitoring. | All variables that interfere with monitoring children are not possible to control, however, inadequate ECG monitoring should not be tolerated for long periods, especially if the child is at risk for developing cardiac dysrhythmias. |
| a. Restraints (see Skill 51).<br>b. Sedation.<br>c. Therapeutic play.<br>d. Diaphoresis electrodes (commercially available). | ***Special Considerations:*** *Infants' and children's movements are not always possible to control. A combination of interventions may be necessary to minimize waveform interruption.* |
| 4. Assess heart rate and respiratory rate (see Skills 31 and 32). | Assessing baseline heart and respiratory rates facilitates setting alarm parameters on the monitor. |

## Planning and Goal Setting

| Steps | Rationale |
|---|---|
| 1. Obtain necessary equipment:<br>a. ECG monitor, hard-wire bedside console, and oscilloscope.<br>b. ECG cables.<br>c. Lead wires.<br>d. Pre-gelled disposable electrodes (infant, child, adult) OR | The ECG device consists of a sensor system, an amplifier, a filter, and a recorder. Because infants and children are so active, the monitoring system should minimize movement artifact. ***Special Considerations:*** *Of the three types of electrodes available, the floating disc electrode is the type most commonly used with infants and children. An electrode plate rests upon a cushion saturated with electrolyte gel which is surrounded by an adhesive ring.* |
| e. Electrode vest and electrolyte gel. | An electrode vest is available for infants, to decrease skin breakdown from frequent electrode changes. Electrolyte gel is used to promote conduction. |
| f. Alcohol or washcloth with soap and water.<br>g. 4 × 4 gauze (optional).<br>h. Benzoin (optional).<br>i. Razor (optional).<br>j. Monitor paper (optional). | These items are used to prepare the skin for the electrodes to improve adherence and conductivity. ***Special Considerations:*** *Benzoin may cause an allergic contact dermatitis (James, White, and Yanklowitz, 1984).* |
| k. Respiratory monitor (optional). | Respiratory monitoring is frequently used in conjuction with cardiac monitoring. ***Special Considerations:*** *Respiratory monitoring equipment must be capable of accurately measuring respiratory rates even when chest movement is minimal (Hazinski, 1984).* |
| 2. Determine electrical safety of system. | Electrical safety precautions reduce the risk of fire hazard and/or electrocution (Hazinski, 1984). |
| a. Identify potential electrical hazards: | |
| ▪ Broken cords or lead wires.<br>▪ Loss of insulation on wires or cables. | Loss of integrity may lead to equipment malfunction and increases the risk of electrocution and fire. |
| ▪ Leads, wires, cables in contact with stray current or wet surfaces. | Stray currents may be conducted through liquids. |

| Steps | Rationale |
|---|---|
| b. Check to see if equipment is properly grounded. | Grounding prevents electrical shock and enhances the quality of the ECG tracings. |
| 3. Prepare child and family for monitoring:<br>a. Familiarize with equipment and purpose of monitoring.<br>b. Allow child to place electrodes on favorite doll/stuffed animal (see Skill 1). | Preparation decreases anxiety, allays fears, and promotes co-operation.<br>***Special Considerations:*** *Child may need reassurance that monitoring causes no pain or discomfort. Family may need reassurance that there is no danger of electrocution, that cardiac rhythm is continuously monitored, and that help is immediately available if rhythm problems occur.* |
| 4. Develop individualized goals of nursing care:<br>▪ Continuously monitor cardiac rhythm and rate safely and accurately.<br>▪ Document cardiac dysrhythmias.<br>▪ Provide a quality ECG tracing with minimal extraneous artifact. | |
| 5. Develop individualized child and family goals:<br>▪ Child's skin integrity will remain intact.<br>▪ Child and family will experience minimal anxiety. | |

## Implementation

| Steps | Rationale |
|---|---|
| 1. Turn on bedside ECG monitor and calibrate according to manufacturer's instructions. | Turning on monitor before attaching electrodes to the child allows static energy to dissipate. |
| 2. Attach cable to monitor and insert lead wires into cable. In most systems: RA (right arm) lead is white; LA (left arm) lead is black; and LL (left leg) lead is green or red. | ***Special Considerations:*** *The proximal end of the cable is usually color-coded to facilitate connection with color-coded lead wires.* |
| 3. Attach electrodes to lead wires if snap-on type. | Connecting the electrodes on the lead wires before attaching them to the chest eliminates exerting pressure on the chest in an attempt to connect electrodes and wires. |
| 4. Select lead placement that provides the best recording of electrical activity and reflects information desired (see box at right). Avoid muscle masses, nipples, recent surgical incisions and areas of the chest that may be frequently x-rayed. | Placement over muscle masses may lead to movement artifact. Skin irritation and trauma may be caused by electrode placement over nipples and surgical incisions, or frequent electrode removal to obtain x-rays.<br>***Special Considerations:*** *In dextroposition/dextrocardia, the leads need to be positioned to reflect the path of conduction (left to right).* |
| 5. Set the lead selector on the monitor. | ***Special Considerations:*** *Lead II is generally the lead that most closely follows the conduction pathway, yielding wave forms that are positively deflected (upright).* |
| 6. Prepare the skin:<br>a. Shave, if necessary. | Adhesion of electrodes and conduction of electrical signals are enhanced by proper skin preparation. |
| b. Swab skin with alcohol and allow to air dry, or wash with soap and water; dry skin thoroughly. | Swabbing with alcohol minimizes skin oils and removes tissue debris, thus enhancing stable contact of electrodes and minimizing impedance (Decker, 1987).<br>***Special Considerations:*** *Avoid the use of alcohol in the premature infant because it can burn the skin (Naulty, 1983).* |
| c. Abrade skin with 4 × 4 gauze or abrasive pad of electrode until slightly reddened (optional). | Abrasion further decreases resistance of skin to electrical conduction.<br>***Special Considerations:*** *Abrasive techniques should not be used in infants and children with thin, fragile skin. Benzoin may be used to help electrodes adhere to a diaphoretic child.* |
| 7. Remove protective paper backing from electrode and check gelled pad for moistness. | Dried gel is a poor conducter of electrical potential. |
| 8. Place electrodes adhesive side down on preselected sites (see box at right). Press firmly into place, ensuring good skin contact. Attach clip-type lead wires, if not previously attached. | |
| 9. Evaluate clarity of image on the oscilloscope and make necessary adjustments to improve quality according to manufacturer's directions. General guidelines include: | A quality tracing eliminates false alarms and facilitates visual monitoring of electrical activity. |
| a. Set trace sweep speed at standard 25 mm per second. | Trace speed is the rate that the electrocardiographic pattern moves across the screen. |
| b. If the monitor has adjustable gain capability, set gain so that each QRS complex is recognized by tachometer. | *Gain* indicates the degree of amplification of the signal from the voltage of the QRS complex. The tachometer computes the heart rate. |

| Steps | Rationale |
|---|---|

### THE MECHANICS OF MONITORING

Electrical activity in the heart is monitored by using a combination of leads. The various leads reflect depolarization as it is conducted through the heart. A lead that parallels the conduction pathway will be reflected as a positive deflection in the electrocardiographic tracing. A lead opposite to conduction yields a negative deflection (e.g., the patterns noted if routine placement were used for a child with dextrocardia). Lead placement perpendicular to conduction yields no deflection. Exact lead placement is not necessary when using Limb or Augmented leads since only potential differences of the extremities are being measured. The most commonly used placement is Lead II because it most closely follows conduction through the heart, yielding a positive deflection. Lead II measures the differences between the right arm and left foot.

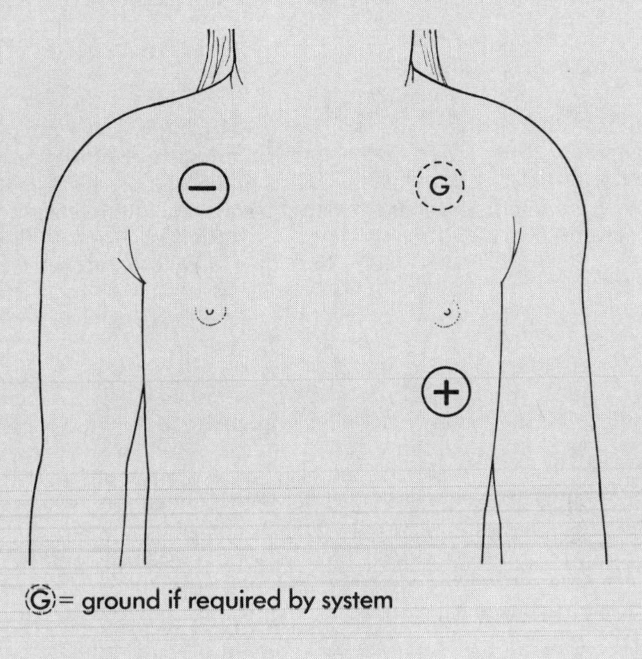


(G)= ground if required by system

c. Adjust the intensity or brightness of the display for optimal visualization in working space.

Many monitors have brightness adjustment dials. Brightness is usually determined by the type of phosphorescent chemical used to coat the screen.

10. Troubleshoot and correct artifacts (see Table 100-1). Initially check the following factors:
    a. Electrode patches:
       - Dried.
       - Poor or absent skin contact.
    b. Lead wires:
       - Disconnected.
       - Broken.
    c. Movement of child:
       - Seizures.
       - Respirations.

Removal of artifacts that can mimic dysrhythmias improves reliability of monitoring, minimizes false alarms that may result in incorrect treatment, and facilitates accurate assessment of cardiac electrical activity.

***Special Considerations:*** *Always treat the child, not the monitor.*

11. Set high and low heart rate alarms 10 to 15 bpm above and below child's heart rate range (Decker, 1987). Verify limits during each work shift.

Individualized heart rate alarm limits allow recognition of changes and help to limit false alarms.

12. Enter patient data into computer system (optional).

Computerized sytems have the capabilities of generating printouts pre-labeled with the child's name and other statistics.

13. Turn on monitor at central station (optional).

Central station monitoring extends capability to detect changes in the ECG.

14. Obtain baseline rhythm strip, noting:
    a. Rate.
    b. PR interval.
    c. Ectopy.

Obtaining an initial rhythm strip provides documentation of ECG pattern at onset of monitoring and also may be useful for standardizing the recording and optimizing the tracing quality.

15. Continuously monitor child for changes in rate or rhythm.
    a. Obtain strip every 4 hours and upon observation of changes, if recorder available; otherwise, document ECG pattern.

***Special Considerations:*** *Information obtained from the bedside monitor should not be considered diagnostic except for dysrhythmias. A 12-or 14-lead rhythm strip should be obtained if there is concern about other changes in the ECG pattern.*

**TABLE 100-1** Troubleshooting Cardiac Monitors

| Problem | Possible Causes | Nursing Actions |
|---|---|---|
| Wandering baseline (Fig. 100-1*A*) | Lead placement. | Move electrodes away from muscle masses. |
| | Sensing respirations. | Move electrode away from diaphragm; increase or decrease sensitivity of respiratory module. |
| | Dangling wires or cable. | Secure lead wires and cable. |
| | Damaged or broken lead wires or cable. | Replace lead wires or cable. |
| | Dried or loose electrode. | Replace electrode. |
| Sixty-cycle interference (alternating current) (Fig. 100-1*B*) | Electrical interference from other equipment due to leakage of electrical power or faulty grounding. | Ensure all equipment attached to common ground.<br>Change other equipment to a different outlet.<br>Remove equipment one by one to identify faulty grounding.<br>Replace lead wires.<br>Check plugs for broken prongs.<br>Check and rearrange overriding cords or wires, including IV tubing.<br>Change lead selector to another lead. Remove and send faulty equipment for repair. |
| | Poor electrode contact. | Remove and replace dried electrodes.<br>Reprep skin. |
| Jittery tracing (see Fig. 100-1*C*) | Muscle movement, e.g., shivering. | Move electrodes away from muscle masses. |
| | Poor electrode contact. | Remove and replace dried electrodes. |
| | Dangling cables. | Secure cables and lead wires. |
| | Electrical short circuit. | Replace broken or damaged lead wires. |
| | Interference from static electricity. | Regulate room humidity. |
| High rate alarm | Tachycardia. | Check the child's pulse. |
| | Movement including seizures, respirations. | Decrease sensitivity.<br>Secure child's cable.<br>Change lead setting or placement. |
| | Gain too high. | Readjust sensitivity.<br>Select another lead. |
| | Loose electrodes. | Check and reapply electrodes. |
| | Improper cable connection. | Check integrity of child's cable.<br>Check for physiologic conditions contributing to problems (liquid accentuates baseline signals, therefore pulmonary atelectasis, consolidation, or effusion may be present) (Naulty, 1983). |
| | Tall T-waves, as seen in hyperkalemia or spikes from muscle activity. | Monitors determine the heart rate by counting R-wave amplitude. Muscle activity may falsely increase detection of high amplitude signals. |
| Low rate alarm | Bradycardia. | Check the child's pulse. |
| | Loose or dry electrodes. | Check and reapply electrodes. |
| | Improper cable connection. | Check integrity of child's cable. |
| | Gain too low. | Readjust gain setting.<br>Select another lead.<br>Check for physiologic conditions contributing to problem (air impedes the passage of electrical currents, therefore pneumothorax or other air leak may be present) (Naulty, 1983). |
| Straight line | Asystole. | Check the child's pulse. |
| | Disconnection of equipment. | Check connections between electrodes, lead wires, child's cable, and monitor. |
| | Faulty equipment. | Check and replace dried electrodes; broken wires. |

Adapted from Decker S: Continuous EKG monitoring systems, Nurs Clin North Am 22:1-13, 1987.

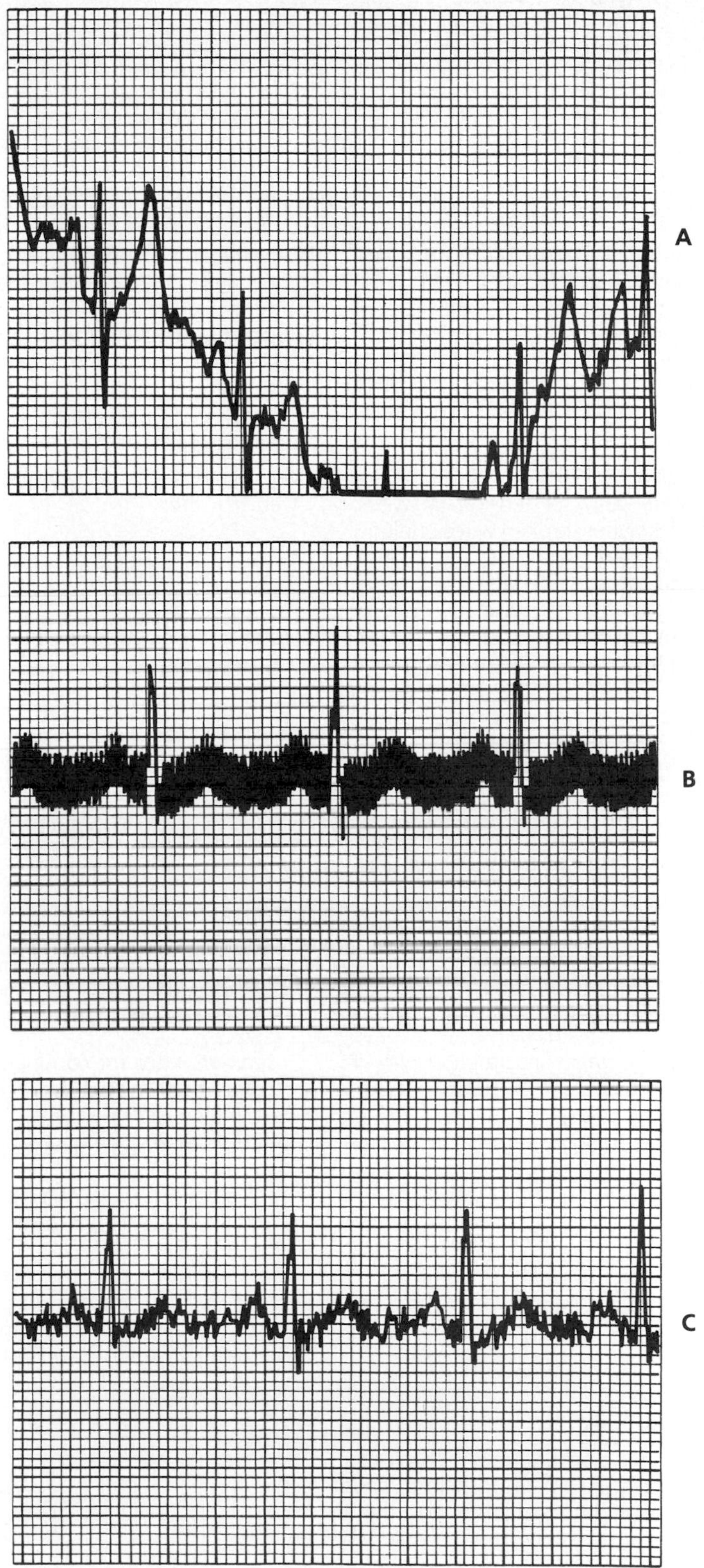


***FIG. 100-1*** Irregular ECG tracings require troubleshooting for artifacts. **A,** Wandering baseline. **B,** Alternating current. **C,** Jittery tracing.

| Steps | Rationale |
|---|---|
| b. Auscultate apical heart rate at regular intervals.<br>c. Palpate peripheral pulses at regular intervals. | Presence of ECG monitor readout does not eliminate the need for direct auscultation of heart rate and palpation of pulses.<br>***Special Considerations:*** *Discrepancies between auscultated rate and readout rate is due to the 2- to 5-second lag through the amplifier between the signal and the readout device. Record the auscultated rate as the more accurate and current of the two (Hazinski, 1984).* |
| 16. Change electrodes and rotate sites every 24 to 48 hours. Check skin integrity after removing electrodes. | Cellulitis and chemical burns may develop with prolonged application. Dried electrode gel may result in poor conduction of signals.<br>***Special Considerations:*** *In neonates and children with fragile skin, daily removal of electrodes may lead to skin maceration. An individualized schedule should be incorporated to avoid irritation or maceration. An electrode vest is an alternative for neonates.* |
| 17. Monitor electrical safety (Hazinski, 1984):<br>a. Inspect monitoring system daily for tension on wires, loss of insulation on cables/wires, broken wires or plugs, or loose outlet-plug connection.<br>b. Avoid catching cables and cords in siderails or bed mechanisms. | Maintaining electrical safety standards prevents physiologic harm and/or fire. |
| c. Remove lead wires from child while bathing. Prevent equipment from coming into contact with wet surfaces.<br>d. Closely monitor children in high humidity environments (e.g., mist tent) or those with invasive catheters interrupting skin resistance.<br>e. Keep invasive catheter lines away from direct contact with ECG leads. | Water is an electrolyte solution and rapidly conducts electrical current. |
| f. Never touch the child and an electrical device simultaneously. | A path may be provided for stray current to travel from device to child. |
| g. Never touch two electrical devices simultaneously. | If there is a current leak, touching two devices provides a path to the ground from the broken instrument. |
| 18. Decrease audible alarm in child's room if central monitoring is available. | Reducing alarm volume facilitates rest and decreases anxiety caused by unexpected, loud noise of alarm. |

| Evaluation Outcomes | Observational Guidelines |
|---|---|
| 1. Monitoring of cardiac rhythm and rate is accurately displayed with minimal interruption or artifact. | Observe monitor for continuous quality tracing of ECG pattern. Obtain rhythm strip every 4 hours if possible. Note if artifacts are minimized or absent. |
| 2. Early detection of dysrhythmias and/or electrical instability is provided. | Note documentation and reporting of dysrhythmias. |
| 3. Electrocardiographic monitoring is conducted safely. | Check electrode wires and cables daily for breaks, loss of grounding and breaks in insulation. Observe for tension on electrodes that may lead to breaks. |
| 4. Skin integrity remains intact. | Assess electrode sites for redness, rashes, or skin breakdown. |
| 5. Minimal anxiety is experienced by child and family. | Note if signs of anxiety are present in the child and/or family, e.g., frequently watching monitor, panic if alarm sounds, asking many questions, or restlessness. |

## Documentation

Record time monitoring initiated and discontinued; lead placement; rhythm strip, and/or description of rate, rhythm, and ECG patterns every 4 hours. Document dysrhythmias as they occur; alarm limits; electrode changes and new lead placements; child and family response to monitoring; changes in skin integrity.

## UNIT XV

## PRODUCT REFERENCES AND TEACHING RESOURCES

Applied Biotech Products, Inc
PO Box 52703
Lafayette, LA
(318) 234-8993
1-800-284-7655
Offers Landry Vein Light.

## REFERENCES


Arkansas Children's Hospital: Nursing procedure manual, Little Rock, Ark, 1987, Arkansas Children's Hospital.

Arthur G: When your littlest patients need IVs, RN 9:30-35, 1984.

Axnick KJ: Infection control, St Louis, 1984, The CV Mosby Co.

Barrus D: Should you irrigate an occluded IV line? Nursing 17:63-64, 1987.

Boykoff S: Six ways to clear the air from an IV line, Nursing 18:46-48. 1988.

Brunner LS: The Lippincott manual of nursing practice, Philadelphia, 1986, JB Lippincott Co.

Bryan CS: CDC says. . . : the case of IV tubing replacement, Infection Control, 8(6):255-256, 1987.

Bryant R: Saving the skin from tape injuries, AJN 88(2):189-191, 1988.

Caplan M and Ranieri C: What's his ECG telling you?: a guide for nurses, RN 52:42-51, 1989.

Chameides L: Textbook of pediatric advanced life support, Dallas, 1988, American Heart Association.

Decker S: Continuous EKG monitoring systems, Nurs Clin North Am, 22:1-13, 1987.

Dickey J: Effectiveness of intradermally injected lidocaine hydrochloride as a local anesthetic for intravenous catheter insertion, J Emerg Nurs 14(3):160-163, 1988.

Dunne K and Matthews T: Near-miss Sudden Infant Death Syndrome: clinical findings and management, Pediatrics, 79:889-893, 1987.

Feldstein A: Detect phlebitis and infiltration before they harm your patient, Nursing, 16(1):44-47, 1986.

Guhlow LJ: Pediatric IVs, RN 42(3):40-51, 1979.

Hazinski MF: Nursing care of the critically ill child, St Louis, 1984, The CV Mosby Co.

James WD, White SW, and Yanklowitz B: Allergic contact dermatitis to compound tincture of benzoin, J Am Acad Dermatol, 11(5):847-850, 1984.

Jimenez J, Turley C, and Quiggins C: A quality circle improves pediatric phlebotomy, Medical Laboratory Observer 20(7):85-87, 1988.

Kasprisin CA: Care of the patient receiving transfusion therapy and transfusion therapy for the pediatric patient. In Rutman RC and Miller WV, editors: Transfusion therapy principles and procedures, ed 2, Rockville, Md, 1985, Aspen Publications.

Maki G: Prospective study of replacing administration sets for intravenous therapy at 48 vs 72 hour intervals, JAMA 258(13):1777-1781, 1987.

Manner T et al: Reduction of pain at venous cannulation in children with a eutectic mixture of lidocaine and prilocaine (EMLA cream): comparison with placebo cream and no local premedication, Acta Anaesthesiol Scand 31:735-739, 1987.

Maunuksela EL and Korpela R: Double-blind evaluation of a lidocaine-prilocaine cream (EMLA) in children: effect of the pain associated with venous cannulation, Br J Anaesth, 58:1242-1245, 1986.

Messner RL: Nursing management of peripheral IV sites, Focus on Critical Care 4(2):25-33, 1987.

Millam DA: Tips for improving your venipuncture techniques, Nursing, 17(6):46-49, 1987.

Myhre BA: Fatalities from blood transfusions, JAMA 244:1333-1335, 1980.

Naulty C: Cardiac monitoring. In Fletcher MA, MacDonald M, and Avery G, editors: Atlas of procedures in neonatology, Philadelphia, 1984, JB Lippincott Co.

Nelson R and Miller H: Keeping air out of IV lines, Nursing 16(3):57-59, 1986.

Phelps SJ: Risk factors affecting infiltration of peripheral venous lines in infants, J Pediatr 111(3):384-389, 1987.

Piercy S: Children on long-term IV therapy, Nursing 11(9):66-69, 1981.

Runciman WB: An evaluation of intravenous infusion pumps and controllers, Anaesth Intens Care, 15(2):217-228, 1987.

Schmidt PJ: Transfusion mortality, AORNJ 34:1114-1122, 1981.

Scranton PE: Practical techniques in venipuncture, Baltimore. 1977, Williams & Wilkins Co.

Southall D: Home monitoring and its role in the Sudden Infant Death Syndrome, Pediatrics 72:133-138, 1983.

Streckfuss BL: Communicating with pediatric patients, NITA 7:94-95, 1984.

Streckfuss BL: Pediatric IV care, NITA 8:75-82, 1985.

Weinstein S: Intravenous filters, Infection Control 8(6):220-221, 1987.

Whaley LF and Wong DL: Nursing care of infants and children, ed 4, St Louis, 1991, The CV Mosby Co.

Widman FK, editor: Technical manual of the American Association of Blood Banks, ed 9, Arlington, VA, 1985, American Association of Blood Banks.

Wildblood RA: The how-to's of home IV therapy, Pediatr Nurs 13(1):42-46,68, 1987.

Wong DL and Baker C: Pain in children: comparison of assessment scales, Pediatr Nurs 14(1):9-17, 1988.

# UNIT XVI Medications

# SKILL 101 Administering Oral Medications

*Kristie S. Nix*

Oral medications are frequently prescribed for children because of their relative ease of administration by comparison with other routes. Despite this convenience, a nurse must exercise attention to detail to prepare and administer oral medications safely. As families commonly give medications in the home, nurses have a responsibility to teach safe practices about storage, preparation, and administration of oral medications.

## NURSING DIAGNOSES

Altered health maintenance related to lack of knowledge about medication administration; Potential for injury related to adverse effects of medication; Noncompliance with oral medication therapy regimen related to denial of illness, insufficient finances, or cultural/spiritual health beliefs.

| Steps | Rationale |
|---|---|
| **Assessment** | |
| 1. Determine child's age, height, weight, and developmental status. | These parameters determine the dose and form of medication needed for the child. Age and developmental status assist in determining if the child is capable of chewing and/or swallowing oral medication. |
| 2. Using health history, note factors that affect drug therapy. | |
| a. Allergies. | Administration of a drug to which the child is allergic may result in an anaphylactic reaction. |
| b. Current and past medications, prescribed and OTC. | Medications and diet are assessed to determine possible drug and/or food interactions. |
| c. Diet history (see Skill 29). | Some foods may interact with medications and, therefore, are contraindicated. Medications may contain food ingredients, e.g., lactose fillers, to which the child is allergic. |
| d. Cultural beliefs about medication (see Skill 41). | Cultural beliefs influence willingness to follow prescribed regimen and indicate significant family members to whom teaching should be directed. |
| 3. Assess for contraindications to oral medications, e.g., NPO (nothing by mouth) status, recent surgery, swallowing difficulty, or nausea/vomiting. | The child who is NPO to undergo procedures should not take oral medications because of aspiration risk. After surgery, other routes are used until the child can tolerate oral intake. Oral medications are not effective if the child is vomiting. |
| 4. Assess family knowledge about medication. Determine any problems experienced in past with oral medications in general or for specific drug ordered. Ask family about child's preferences for medication administration (e.g., spoon, cup, or syringe). | Determination of family's knowledge gives a baseline for identification of teaching needs. Information gathered about past problems and current requests may modify approach or technique. |
| 5. Determine child's preferences for liquids or foods. | Giving liquids after medications aids in swallowing. Some medications are more palatable and more easily taken if mixed in a small amount of food or liquid.<br>***Special Considerations:*** *Ask older child to choose from foods and liquids such as applesauce, pudding, or juice for mixing with medications.* |

| Steps | Rationale |
|---|---|

## Planning and Goal Setting

1. Gather equipment.
   a. Medication cards or Kardex with correct drug order transcribed from physician's order.

***Special Considerations:*** *Follow agency policy about use of medication cards, Kardex or other recording forms. Always verify these with physician's order.*

   b. Medication tray.

A tray provides an organized method for transporting medications.

   c. A mortar and pestle (if needed).

A mortar and pestle are used for crushing tablets.

   d. Container(s): measuring spoon, dropper, syringe, calibrated spoon, or medicine cups (Fig. 101-1).

***Special Considerations:*** *Choice of container depends on age and ability of child to drink medication from cup. If developmentally unable to drink from a cup, a syringe or calibrated dropper is preferred.*

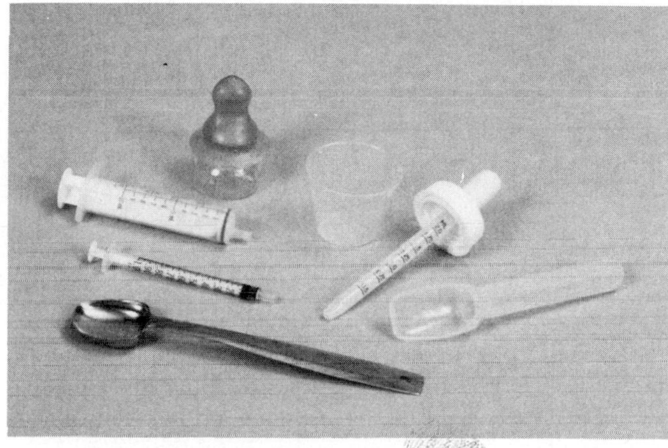

***FIG. 101-1*** Acceptable devices for measurement and administration of medications to children. Unacceptable devices for measurement are paper cups, household spoons, and uncalibrated droppers.

   e. Liquid to drink after administration.

***Special Considerations:*** *Check with child about preferences, diet restrictions, or allergies.*

   f. Drinking straw or nipple (optional).

An infant may take medicine easily by sucking medication from a bottle nipple. A preschooler often prefers drinking through a straw.

   g. Food with which to mix medication (optional).
2. Review information for each medication to be administered.
   a. Usual dose.
   b. Intended effects.
   c. Administration method.
   d. Possible side effects (acceptable and unacceptable).
   e. Time of onset and peak effect.
   f. Nursing considerations.

In addition to preventing errors, a sound knowledge base enables one to anticipate intended effects of the drug, observe child for untoward effects, and monitor child to help determine needed changes in therapy.

3. Compare physician's order/Kardex/medication cards for the following information.
   a. Child's name.
   b. Medication name.
   c. Dose.
   d. Route of administration.
   e. Time of administration.

There must be a written physician's order for every medication given.

***Special Considerations:*** *These five elements are called the Five Rights of Medication Administration and should be checked at least three times during medication preparation.*

4. Confirm the name of each drug carefully.

Names of different drugs have similar spellings.

***Special Considerations:*** *Question any medication name or dose that is not exactly as ordered (e.g., digoxin and digitoxin seem similar in name but have significant differences). A name is easily confirmed by checking a drug reference manual or consulting with a pharmacist. Never give a medication that has not been verified.*

5. Calculate safe doses before preparing a drug (see Appendix C).

This information serves as a guide for comparing the physician's order with recommended safe doses. When remarkably different, orders should be clarified to avoid possible errors.

***Special Considerations:*** *All pediatric nurses have responsibility to determine that prescribed doses fall within recommended ranges. Follow facility policy to question a drug order after checking standard drug references. Verify orders and discuss questions with prescribing physician. After discussion, follow original or revised orders and document conversation in child's record (Regan, 1980).*

| Steps | Rationale |
|---|---|
| 6. Develop individualized child and family goals:<br>▪ Child ingests oral medications following guidelines for safe preparation and administration.<br>▪ Child is monitored for response to medication.<br>▪ Family demonstrates an adequate knowledge base about oral medications. | |

## Implementation

### *Preparation*

| Steps | Rationale |
|---|---|
| 1. Read the medication label to ensure correctness of medication on hand. Review Five Rights of Medication Administration at this time.<br>a. Right child.<br>b. Right medication.<br>c. Right dose.<br>d. Right route.<br>e. Right time. | ***Special Considerations:*** *Never use medication from a container with an illegible label.* |
| 2. Prepare appropriate amount of oral medication. | |
| *Liquid medications:* | Liquid medications are frequently prescribed for a child as they are more easily swallowed than other oral medications. |
| a. Select measuring spoon, dropper, calibrated spoon, syringe, or medicine cup to measure dose (Fig. 101-1). | Small amounts, frequently prescribed for children, require the use of calibrated devices with incremental markings.<br>***Special Considerations:*** *To ensure accurate doses, use a container that is relative to dose needed, e.g., for 0.5 ml, use a 1.0 ml syringe; for 5.0 ml, use 5 or 6 ml syringe.* |
| b. Uncap medication bottle and place cap topside down. | Cap remains clean and free from countertop contamination. |
| c. Hold measuring container at eye level to locate correct measurement marking. Place container on level countertop. | ***Special Considerations:*** *Some measuring devices—e.g., measuring spoons or droppers—do not require placement on level countertop.* |
| d. After label recheck, turn label to palm of hand to prevent spillage on the label. | Label remains legible. |
| e. Fill container with medication to the correct amount.<br>*OR*<br>If using a syringe, first pour approximate dose of medication into a plastic medication cup. Then, draw up correct amount into syringe. | |
| f. At eye level, read the amount at the bottom of the meniscus.<br>*OR*<br>If using a syringe, hold it upright (tip up) at eye level and read the measurement from the top edge of the rubber stopper. | Liquid in a container forms a meniscus; correct dose should be read at the bottom of the meniscus. |
| g. Discard any excess medication, never returning it to the bottle. | This precaution prevents possible contamination or insertion of incorrect medication into container. |
| h. Clean bottle lip and container with a damp paper towel, if necessary. | Liquid medications often have a sugar base, which can leave the bottle sticky, messy, and difficult to open. |
| *Tablets/capsules:* | |
| a. Pour medication from bottle into the bottle's lid. Transfer the medication from the lid to medication cup. Never return unwanted tablets or capsules to the stock bottle from the medication cup. | This method ensures that a medication is not accidently placed in the wrong container, thus preventing errors. |
| b. If necessary for correct dose, break tablet using manufacturer's score. Do not try to divide a medication that is not scored. A scored tablet is easily broken with a safety-edge razor blade, scalpel, or sterile needle. Clean blades between use and return to protective covering. Dispose of needle in receptacle. | Unscored medications may break into unequal portions, resulting in inaccurate dose.<br>***Special Considerations:*** *Consult with the pharmacist first for providing the correct dose when a partial dose is needed from an unscored tablet. Unresolved problems may then be referred to the prescribing physician.* |
| c. If necessary, crush the tablet using a mortar and pestle. Check that medication can be crushed and mixed with food or beverages. Never crush a sustained-release or enteric-coated tablet or capsule contents. Capsules may be opened and mixed gently in a small amount of food. | Crushing capsule contents or a sustained release tablet may result in immediate release of the medication, modifying its intended effect. An enteric-coated tablet will be released in the stomach instead of the duodenum if crushed, resulting in altered therapeutic effects or untoward effects, such as gastric upset or inactivation of medication. |

| Steps | Rationale |
|---|---|
| | ***Special Considerations:*** *Check with a standard drug reference or pharmacist if unsure whether medication can be crushed or mixed with food.* |
| d. If needed, mix medication with a small amount (less than 1 tablespoon) of child's preferred food, e.g., applesauce, pudding, jelly, ice cream, crushed popsicle, peanut butter, pureed baby foods. A commercially available syrup base may also be well accepted. | Medication is often more acceptable to child when mixed with preferred food. Use only a small amount so that child is more likely to consume entire dose. ***Special Considerations:*** *Avoid essential foods, such as milk, for mixing with medications, as the child may refuse the food as a result of the taste of the combination. An alternative dose form is the troche, an artificially sweetened lozenge compounded with the drug. It is excellent for children who can chew or suck but resist other dose forms (Wong and Redding, 1987).* |
| 3. Place all tablets or capsules for the same child in the same medication cup, except those that may require preadministration assessments (e.g., obtaining apical pulse). Keep liquid medications in separate containers for administration. | Separated medications serve as a reminder that preassessments must be completed before medication is administered. |
| 4. Recheck Five Rights of Medication Administration: compare medication label with medication form and prepared medication. | |
| 5. Return medication containers and unit dose medications to storage site; recheck label for Five Rights of Medication Administration. | |
| ***Administration*** | |
| 1. Confirm identity of child using identification bracelet, comparing information from medication card/Kardex. | Bracelets provide reliable identification. ***Special Considerations:*** *Do not ask a younger child, "Is your name ________ ?" as child may say yes or no unreliably or even deny identity to avoid medication (Whaley and Wong, 1991). Although family member may be asked to give child's name, using bracelet is best means of identification.* |
| 2. Inform the child that it is time to take medicine; use this time for any teaching needs or questions that family may have about medication. | Information lets the child know what is happening and provides the opportunity for education (see Home Care Modifications). ***Special Considerations:*** *Never tell a child that a medication is candy or candylike. If the medication is mixed with a food or liquid, tell the child so that he or she does not think the food always tastes like the medicine-food combination (Wong and Whaley, 1990).* |
| 3. Perform any preadministration nursing assessments that relate to drug, e.g., take pulse or blood pressure. | Medication may be withheld, depending on assessment. |
| 4. As possible, offer the child choices about administration of medication, e.g., "You may take the red or the purple medicine first. Which will it be?" | Offering choices gives child an opportunity to exercise control. |
| 5. Ask family's advice about approach to administer medication, e.g., "How does your child take this medication best?" | Family provides valuable information related to the child's preferences. Medication may be accepted more easily when preferences are considered. ***Special Considerations:*** *Family members may not always know of alternative methods for administration. Use opportunities for teaching, e.g., "Have you ever tried giving the baby the medication through a nipple?" Sometimes it is less traumatic for the child if the parent administers the medication while the nurse observes, as long as the practice is consistent with agency policy.* |
| 6. Administer medication considering the child's developmental level and ability to cooperate. Use restraint technique if necessary: With child in lap, place his right arm behind you then hug left arm and hand with your left hand; immobilize child's head between your arm and body; if necessary, grasp child's legs between yours (Fig. 101-2). | Developmental level guides approach to administering medication. Properly restraining the child allows for safe administration. |

| Steps | Rationale |
|---|---|

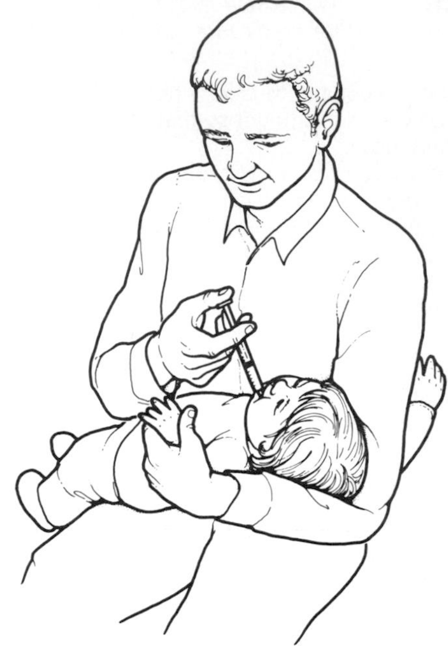

***FIG. 101-2*** Proper restraint for administration of oral medication.
From Wong DL and Whaley LF: Clinical manual of pediatric nursing, ed 3, 1990, St Louis, The CV Mosby Co.

*Liquid medications:*

a. Place dropper or syringe in mouth along the buccal area.

Aiming medication toward cheek instead of back of throat prevents gagging and/or possible aspiration.

b. Slowly squeeze a small amount of medication (about 0.5 ml) into the mouth or allow the child to suck medication from the syringe or dropper.

***Special Considerations:*** *A gentle puff of air in the infant's face may elicit a reflexive swallow (Orenstein et al, 1988).*

c. Another method with infants is to use a bottle nipple filled with the medication (Fig. 101-3). Allow child to suck medication from nipple.

In early infancy, sucking occurs reflexively and medication will be easily taken.

***Special Considerations:*** *Certain thick medications may require enlarging the nipple hole for proper administering. To enlarge a hole, insert a round, wooden food toothpick to the desired diameter and boil in water for 2 minutes. Holes may also be enlarged with a hot needle.*

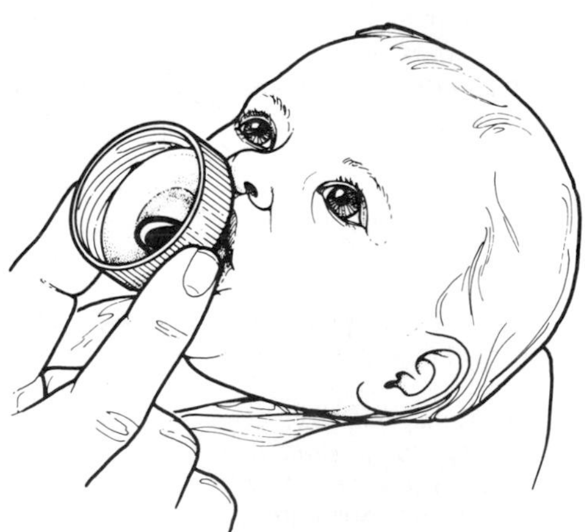

***FIG. 101-3*** A bottle nipple may be used to administer oral medication to infants.
From Wong DL and Whaley LF: Clinical manual of pediatric nursing, ed 3, 1990, St Louis, The CV Mosby Co.

d. Have child sip medication from cup or use a straw cut in half.

Some medications (e.g., iron preparations) stain the teeth and should be given through a straw. Other medications are more readily accepted because opportunity to drink with a straw is enjoyable and may help unpleasant tasting medication to be swallowed more easily, bypassing taste buds. Cutting a straw in half lessens suction required.

*Tablets/capsules:*

a. Place medication in mouth or feed child medication/food mixture. Give older child the medication to put in mouth.

***Special Considerations:*** *When tongue thrust is prominent, medication may have to be retrieved from infant's chin and refed.*

b. If necessary, assist child to swallow medication.
   - Offer drink.

| Steps | Rationale |
|---|---|
| ▪ Have child hold nose while medicine is placed in mouth. | This action may help mask an unpleasant-tasting medication. |
| ▪ With child's head slightly tilted back, massage anterior neck downward. | This action sometimes stimulates swallowing mechanism. |
| 7. Offer child liquid of preference after medication is taken. | Fluids will aid in removal of medication tastes from mouth and assist passage of medication to stomach. ***Special Considerations:*** *Liquid of preference must be acceptable for drug it accompanies.* |
| 8. Confirm that medications have been swallowed before leaving child. | Older children and adolescents may delight in "tricking" those in authority by concealing medication in mouth then spitting it out later. |
| 9. Praise child for cooperation. | |
| 10. Reinforce expected therapeutic benefit and need to notify nurse immediately should any unexpected reactions occur. Provide necessary teaching about medications (see Home Care Modifications). | The child and family should be active participants in monitoring reaction to medication. Untoward reactions are often noticed earlier by family members who know the child best. |
| 11. Rinse or wipe the teeth and gums with plain water after sweetened liquid or chewable medications (Hill, Flaitz, and Frost, 1988). | Cariogenic substances in medications are cleansed from teeth. |
| 12. Return to check child to evaluate response to medications. | Monitoring child provides information about medication's therapeutic effect or onset of side effects or allergic reactions. |
| a. If child vomits after medication administration, note time emesis occurred and call physician. | If emesis occurs soon after administration and before the medication is absorbed, it may be readministered or omitted at the discretion of the physician. If readministered, another route should be considered until the child is able to tolerate oral intake. ***Special Considerations:*** *The palatability of some medications is improved by the use of sweeteners. Sorbitol, a sugar alcohol, may cause side effects (stomachaches, cramps, gas, and diarrhea), which may be confused with a reaction to the medication itself. Sorbitol content of medications should be investigated for children sensitive to this sweetener (Hill, Flaitz, and Frost, 1988; Hyams et al, 1988).* |

| Evaluation Outcomes | Observational Guidelines |
|---|---|
| 1. Child or family demonstrates adequate knowledge about oral medications. | Interview or ask child or family to discuss purpose of medication and place in overall medical plan; timing of medications; possible expected side effects; actions to take in case of unexpected side effects. |
| 2. Child is monitored for response to medication. | Observe for improvement in child's condition (e.g., relief of pain or decreased temperature). Observe for side effects. |
| 3. Family demonstrates appropriate methods of oral administration. | Observe family administer medication in a safe and effective manner to child using appropriate equipment for child's capability; restraining child gently, if needed; and holding child in upright position. |

## Documentation

Follow agency policy about documentation; Most require that medications are charted *after* administration. On medication administration record, note all medications given: routine, PRN, STAT or one-time doses. Include date, time, medication, dose, route. Sign initials next to time of administration and sign full name in appropriate section. Nonroutine medications (e.g., PRN, STAT, or one-time orders) should also be documented in the nurse's notes; a follow-up evaluation of medication's effectiveness should be documented within 1 hour (e.g., "Tylenol elixir 60 mg PO given at 1430 for axillary temperature of 102.4°F. Axillary temperature at 1530: 99°F"). The following should also be documented in the nurse's notes: refusal to take medication; evidence of side effects or complications experienced, e.g., vomiting or evidence of therapeutic effects.

**Steps** | **Rationale**

## Home Care Modifications

1. Help family identify a safe area to lock medications out of the reach of curious children. Remind them that medications in purses are easily accessible and potentially dangerous.
2. Family members should reinforce that medication is not candy and should never entice a child to take medication by saying that it is like candy. Overdoses can easily occur when a child thinks that medicine is candy.
3. Inform family of high content of sweetening agents added to children's liquid or chewable oral medications (Hill, Flaitz, and Frost, 1988). Recommend rinsing mouth with water or toothbrushing after medication administration.
4. Assist family to identify acceptable containers for measuring liquid medication, such as measuring spoons (not dinnerware), syringes, or calibrated medication spoons. These and other medication administration devices, such as medicine nursers, are commonly available in pharmacies or infant products section of grocery stores (see Fig. 101-4 and Product Information). Basic information about measurements should be discussed, e.g., that 5 ml = 1 teaspoon, as labeling practices vary.
5. Show the family how to crush a tablet between two teaspoons.
6. Give the family specific written instructions for each medication. Discuss timing of medications to be given around the clock in intervals.
7. Help family to determine a record-keeping system, e.g., a calendar posted on the refrigerator, to keep track of times medications were administered.
8. Discuss use of Ipecac for treating accidental poisoning by ingestion. Teach family to keep Ipecac as part of a first-aid kit and how to use it properly.
9. Discuss proper steps to take when a child must take a medication at babysitter, day-care center, camp, or school. Family should understand that since uniform policies are often lacking, they should investigate medication policies. The following guidelines (Yankovich, 1987; National Association of School Nurses, 1981) may be of help:
   a. Prescription medication must be ordered by a physician/dentist and taken to the babysitter, day-care center or school by the parent/guardian (child in secondary school may deliver the medication to the appropriate school personnel).
   b. Permission for administration of prescription and nonprescription medication must be given in writing by parent/guardian on appropriate authorization forms (Fig. 101-5).
   c. If facility has OTC medication, the parent should notify school personnel in writing that no medication (e.g., aspirin or acetaminophen) is to be given without parental permission.
   d. Medication must be in its original container with the label intact.
   e. Medications at the facility should be stored in a locked cabinet.
   f. Medications administered at school should be documented appropriately.

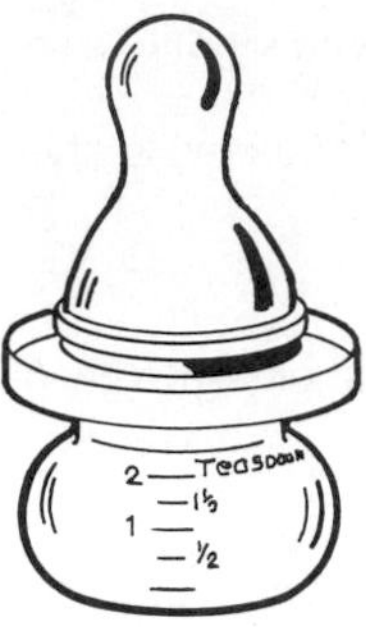

***FIG. 101-4*** The medicine nurser is another acceptable container for measuring and administering liquid medication.

**WILLIAMSBURG-JAMES CITY COUNTY PUBLIC SCHOOLS**
**Williamsburg, Virginia 23185**

**PARENT MEDICATION CONSENT FORM**

NOTE: If possible, parents are advised to give medication at home and on a schedule other than during school hours. If it is necessary that a medication be given during school hours, the following regulations must be followed:

- Medication must be ordered/advised by physician/dentist and permission granted to R.N. at school to contact physician/dentist if necessary.
- Medication must be brought to school by parent/guardian in original container with appropriate label intact. (Secondary students may bring necessary medication to school; must give to R.N. at beginning of school day, and medication must be kept in the locked medicine area of the clinic.) **If medication is not properly labeled, it will NOT be given.**
- Parent/guardian **must** sign this form, granting R.N. permission to administer medication, according to regulations set herein.

The R.N. at ____________ School has my permission to administer the following medication to my child, ____________________ as recommended by Dr. ____________________ for the purpose of treating ____________________ (condition) and I give my permission for the R.N. to contact the physician/dentist, if necessary.

Name of medication: ____________________

Dose to be given: ____________________

Time to be given: ____________________

____________________
Signature of parent/guardian

____________________
Date

H.S. #9 (Revised 1-83)

***FIG. 101-5*** Sample authorization form for medication administration.

From Yankovich AR: Medication usage in public schools: policy recommendations and procedural guidelines, School Nurse 3(3):32-37, 1987.

# *SKILL* 102 Administering Metered-Dose Inhalers

*Kristie S. Nix*

Metered-dose inhalers (MDI) are most commonly used in children with chronic respiratory dysfunctions such as asthma. While inhaled medications, such as bronchodilators and steroids, are relatively easy and inexpensive to use and have the benefit of local versus systemic effects, they may be difficult to administer to children because of the need to coordinate medication delivery with breathing cycle. As families usually give these medications at home, nurses have a responsibility to teach safe and effective administration of metered-dose medications.

## NURSING DIAGNOSES

Altered health maintenance related to lack of knowledge about metered-dose-inhalant administration; Potential for injury related to adverse effects of inhalant medications; Noncompliance with inhalant therapy regimen related to denial of illness, insufficient finances, or cultural/spiritual health beliefs.

| Steps | Rationale |
|---|---|
| **Assessment** | |
| 1. Determine child's age, height, weight, and developmental status. | Age, height, and weight parameters guide dose of medication appropriate for the child. Developmental status provides insight into child's ability to understand medication and its use, and participate in its administration. Until a child is able to coordinate breathing and timing necessary for administration by MDI, use of a spacer device, or holding chamber, allows effective delivery of inhalant medications. |
| 2. Using health history, note factors that affect drug therapy. | |
| a. Allergies. | Administration of a drug to which the child is allergic may result in an anaphylactic reaction. |
| b. Current and past medications, prescribed and OTC. | Many children with respiratory dysfunction do not equate OTC inhalers with medicine and fail to report it in their drug history (Abundis, 1985).<br>***Special Considerations:*** *When reviewing history with family, specifically ask about the use of OTC inhalers or other medications.* |
| c. Diet history (see Skill 29). | Medications and diet are assessed to determine possible drug and/or food interactions. |
| d. Cultural beliefs about medication (see Skill 41). | Cultural beliefs influence willingness to follow prescribed regimen and indicate significant family members to whom teaching should be directed. |
| 3. Assess for contraindications to medications. | As many medications have some systemic as well as local effects, contraindications should be carefully checked (e.g., sympathomimetics affect the cardiac system and should not be given to persons with cardiac dysfunction). Freon, often used as the propellant in MDIs, should be avoided in conditions such as hypoxia, lung disease, or others affecting potential for heart dysrhythmias (Lourenco and Cotromanes, 1982).<br>***Special Considerations:*** *There is some controversy about the effect of MDI fluorocarbon propellants on the cardiorespiratory system, as freon has been reported to produce cardiac muscle damage (Burgess and Chernick, 1986). However, the dose of propellant inhaled with therapeutic nebulizers is usually too small to produce any adverse effect (Lourenco and Cotromanes, 1982).* |
| 4. Assess child's respiratory status (see Skill 27). | Respiratory assessment gives baseline information valuable for later comparisons and indicates need for MDI. |

| Steps | Rationale |
|---|---|

### USING THE PEAK FLOW METER

To use a peak flow meter to assess symptoms of respiratory distress:

1. Place either the disposable or plastic mouthpiece on the flowmeter.
2. Check that the indicator is at the bottom of the numbered scale before taking a measurement.
3. Hold the meter so that the mouthpiece and cylinder are parallel to the floor and the numbered scale extends vertically from the cylinder. Be careful not to cover the opening at the end of the tube with your finger.
4. Have the child inhale as deeply as possible.
5. Then, with lips closed tightly around the outside of the mouthpiece, have the child blow out as hard and fast as possible into the mouthpiece. This will cause the indicator to move up the scale.
6. The final position of the indicator is the peak flow or PEFR (peak expiratory flow rate).
7. Gently push the marker to the lower end of the scale and repeat the test two more times.
8. Record the highest PEFR achieved, along with the date and time on a trend chart. (Do *not* record the average of the three measurements!)

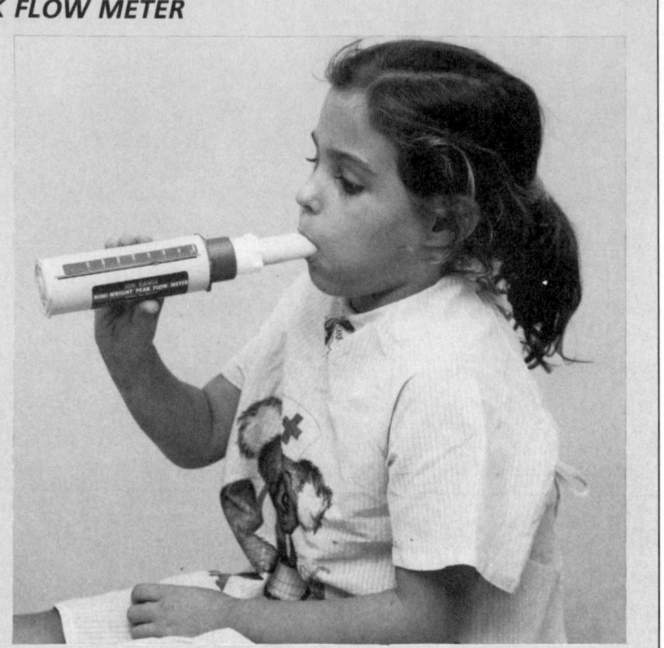

Specific instructions pertaining to the individual models of peak flow meters are also provided by the manufacturers.
From Garcia MK: Asthma: old problems and new strategies, School Nurse 5(3):25-38, 1989.

***Special Considerations:*** *A peak flow meter, an inexpensive hand-held device, is a valuable tool used to determine the need for and response to asthma medications. The easy-to-use device measures the child's ability to breathe out quickly, called the peak expiratory flow rate (PEFR) (see box above). A drop in PEFR can be detected much earlier than wheezing or other signs of narrowed airways (Plaut, 1988).*

5. Assess family knowledge about MDI. Determine any problems experienced in past with metered-dose medications or specific drug ordered. Ask family about child's preferences for MDI administration.

Determining family's knowledge gives a baseline for identification of teaching needs. Information gathered about past problems and current requests may modify approach or technique.
***Special Considerations:*** *Evidence suggests an association between excessive use of sympathomimetic inhalers and a rise in asthma mortality rates (Abundis, 1985). Parents should be cautioned about overdosing with OTC and/or prescribed MDI medications.*

## Planning and Goal Setting

1. Gather equipment.
   a. Medication card(s) or Kardex with correct drug order transcribed from physician's order.

***Special Considerations:*** *Follow agency policy about use of medication cards, Kardex, or other recording forms. Always verify these with physician's order.*

   b. Medication tray.

A tray provides an organized and safe method for transporting medications.

   c. Medication canister, inhaler mouthpiece unit, and spacer device (optional).

A spacer device, also called a holding chamber (Fig. 102-1), is a reservoir into which the spray is released before inhalation. Besides simplifying the timing and coordination required for MDI use, spacers allow medication droplets to become smaller as alcohol solvents evaporate, facilitating deposition in the lungs. Thus, the amount of medication deposited in the oropharyngeal and laryngeal areas is lessened, helping to reduce side effects associated with systemic absorption (Cahill, 1988).

**Steps** | **Rationale**

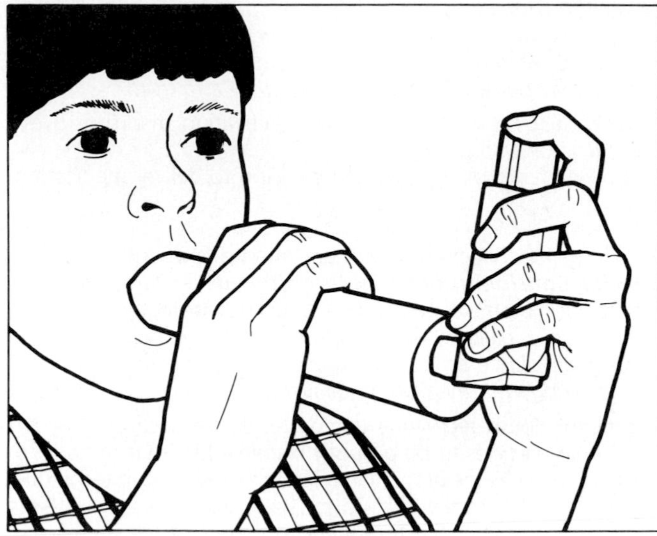

***FIG. 102-1*** Child using spacer device.

From Plaut TF: Children with asthma: a manual for parents, ed 2, Amherst, Mass, 1988, Pedipress.

***Special Considerations:*** *Children as young as 3 years have successfully used spacer devices. The spacer eliminates gagging and spasm that often accompany the forceful impact of the spray on the back of the throat. Spacers are available commercially or may be homemade.*

d. Emesis basin and water or other solution appropriate for rinsing mouth.

To reduce incidence of oral thrush, rinsing mouth after steroid MDI medication is recommended.

2. See Skill 101, Planning steps 2 through 5.
3. Confirm that amount prescribed is the same that inhaler delivers.

An MDI delivers a measured dose of medication with each compression of the canister; physician's order must specify exact dose or number of puffs to be delivered by inhaler.

4. If two MDI medications are to be given, determine if order of administration is significant.

In some cases, order of administration improves therapeutic effect of medications; e.g., inhaled steroids, such as beclomethasone, should be preceded by inhaled bronchodilator.

5. Develop individualized child and family goals:
   - Child receives metered dose medications following guidelines for safe preparation and administration.
   - Child is monitored for desired and undesired effects.
   - Family demonstrates an adequate knowledge base about medications and MDI administration.

## Implementation

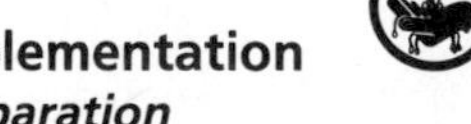

### *Preparation*

1. Read the medication label to ensure correctness of medication on hand. Review Five Rights of Medication Administration at this time.

***Special Considerations:*** *Never use medication from a container with an illegible label.*

2. Assemble inhaler equipment.
   a. Remove dustcap and mouthpiece from medication container.
   b. Insert metal container tip into the short end of the plastic mouthpiece if not already assembled.

Nozzle engages in small hole, connecting the two-piece unit.

***Special Considerations:*** *Some MDIs simply require removal of dustcover, whereas others must be assembled. For commercially available spacer devices, follow manufacturer's instructions.*

### *Administration*

1. See Skill 101, Administration steps 1 through 4.
2. If parent has given MDI before, determine approach used previously to administer medication, e.g., "How does your child prefer to have the metered-dose inhalant given?"

Parents provide valuable information related to the child's preferences. Medication may be accepted more easily when preferences are considered.

***Special Considerations:*** *Sometimes it is less traumatic for the child if the parent or child administers the inhalant while the nurse observes as long as the practice is consistent with agency policy.*

| Steps | Rationale |
|---|---|
| 3. If child has not previously used MDI, provide demonstration of what child is expected to do. | The child is an active participant in MDI administration and should practice exhalation and inhalation before administration. ***Special Considerations:*** *To facilitate correct technique, the child may benefit from watching self in a mirror.* |
| 4. Shake inhaler for 2 to 5 seconds. | Inhaler must be shaken with every activation in order to mix medication and propellant. |
| 5. Position inhaler with canister above mouthpiece (upside down). Hold canister with index finger on top and thumb on bottom. Remove mouthpiece cover. | This position allows for easy compression to deliver medication. |
| 6. Have child sit and exhale normally to the end of a breath. | Exhaling allows inspiration of medication deeper into airways. ***Special Considerations:*** *To help younger children with this step, ask them to pretend to blow out birthday candles or blow up a balloon. The child should not exhale entirely to residual volume as this may cause collapse of smaller airways, interfering with medication delivery.* |
| 7. Hold canister mouthpiece about 1 to 1½ inches in front of the open mouth. Do not place the mouthpiece in child's mouth. *Or* If a spacer device is used, have the child place the mouthpiece on the tongue, making a seal with the lips (see Fig. 102-1). | The open mouth technique is most effective because it allows solution particles to be properly dispersed so that more medication reaches the bronchial tubes. A closed-mouth technique, often recommended in drug package inserts, causes a large portion of medication to adhere to tissues of the mouth and throat (Lourenco and Cotromanes, 1982). |
| 8. Instruct child to breathe in through the mouth for a count of "One, two." Firmly press the canister down into the mouthpiece (see Fig. 102-2) to administer the puff at the count of "three, four, five" when the child inhales deeply. *Or* With a spacer, administer puff; then have child breathe in slowly. | This action releases exact dose of medication for inhalation and increases likelihood of medication deposition in the lungs instead of the mouth. ***Special Considerations:*** *The opposing inhalation/exhalation actions can be confusing and difficult to coordinate for a young child or any child who has never used MDI. Assist learning with use of props such as balloons, and demonstration/return demonstration techniques. Some children may benefit from use of a nose clip or from pinching nose shut.* |
| 9. Ask child to hold breath for a few seconds (up to 10) after the medication has been released. | Slow inhalation followed by a breath hold maximizes deposition of medication in lung (Traver and Martinez, 1988). ***Special Considerations:*** *If a fine mist can be seen escaping from child's mouth or nose, inhaler technique is incorrect. A young child using a spacer may need to hold breath for 5 seconds and repeat inhale/exhale sequence three more times to benefit from all of medication.* |

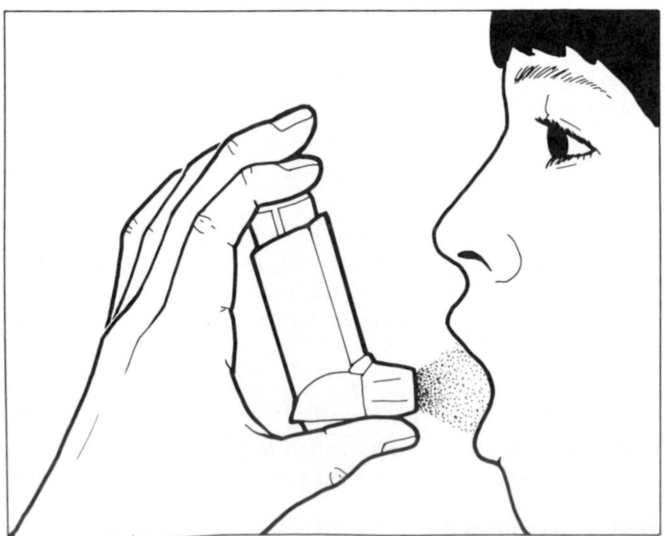

***FIG. 102-2*** Canister is depressed for release of medication.

From Plaut TF: Children with asthma: a manual for parents, ed 2, Amherst, Mass, 1988, Pedipress.

| Steps | Rationale |
|---|---|
| 10. Remove mouthpiece and have child breathe out slowly through pursed lips. | Exhaling against pursed lips keeps distal bronchioles open, allowing increased absorption and diffusion of medication. ***Special Considerations:*** *Show child how to puff out cheeks for pursed-lip breathing.* |
| 11. If second puff (dose) of a bronchodilator MDI is prescribed, wait 2 to 10 minutes (follow drug manufacturer's recommendations or physician's instructions) before administering it. | Time delay allows medication to dilate airways, allowing second puff to penetrate more deeply into bronchial tree (Dunlap and Marchionno, 1983). |
| 12. Have child rinse mouth, gargle, and spit out fluid, particularly after beclomethasone MDI. | Continuous use of beclomethasone is known to cause appearance of *Candida* sp., representing colonization of the respiratory tract (Burgess and Chernick, 1986). Rinsing helps to prevent fungal infections (Dunlap and Marchionno, 1983). |
| 13. Praise child for cooperation. | |
| 14. Reinforce expected therapeutic benefit and need to notify nurse immediately if any unexpected reactions occur. Provide necessary teaching about inhalers and medications (see Home Care Modifications). | The child and family should be active participants in monitoring reaction to medication. Untoward reactions are often noticed earlier by family members who know the child best. |
| 15. Replace dustcap. | The dustcap prevents valve from getting dirty. |
| 16. Return to check child to evaluate response to medications. The timing of return will vary, depending on the medication. | Monitoring child provides information about medication's therapeutic effect or onset of side effects or allergic reactions. A common side effect of MDI medications is airway irritation and cough. |
| 17. Clean MDI daily by taking apart and rinsing mouthpiece under warm water for 1 minute. Allow parts to air dry. | Daily cleaning prevents bacterial growth and obstruction of inhaler mouthpiece. |

| Evaluation Outcomes | Observational Guidelines |
|---|---|
| 1. Child or family demonstrates adequate knowledge about inhaled medications. | Interview or ask child or family to discuss purpose of medication and place in overall medical plan; timing of medications; possible expected side effects; actions to take in case of unexpected side effects. |
| 2. Child receives medications by MDI correctly. | Observe that no puff escapes; child performs exhalation and inhalation and pursed-lip breathing properly. |
| 3. Child achieves desired response to medication. | Observe for improvement in child's condition (e.g., improved respiration). Observe for side effects. |
| 4. Family members demonstrate appropriate use of MDI. | Observe that family members administer medication in a safe and effective manner to child. |

## Documentation

Document after administration unless contrary to agency policy. Include date, time, medication, dose, and route. Sign initials next to time of administration and sign full name in appropriate section. In the nurse's notes, document teaching sessions and child/family's ability to use MDI correctly, refusal to take medication; evidence of side effects or complications, e.g., vomiting or evidence of therapeutic effects.

## Home Care Modifications

1. Suggest that child with respiratory dysfunction who needs frequent medications may benefit from a medication-alert bracelet or necklace.
2. Inform family that contents of MDI canister are under pressure and should never be punctured or incinerated.
3. As with all medications, keep MDI out of reach of small children.
4. Spacers may be homemade with zippered plastic bags, a rolled 8½ × 11 sheet of paper, or a cardboard toilet paper tube (Traver and Martinez, 1988; Plaut, 1988).
5. Inform family that one canister contains 200 to 300 puffs. Assist family in determining amount of inhalant left in canister (see Fig. 102-3).

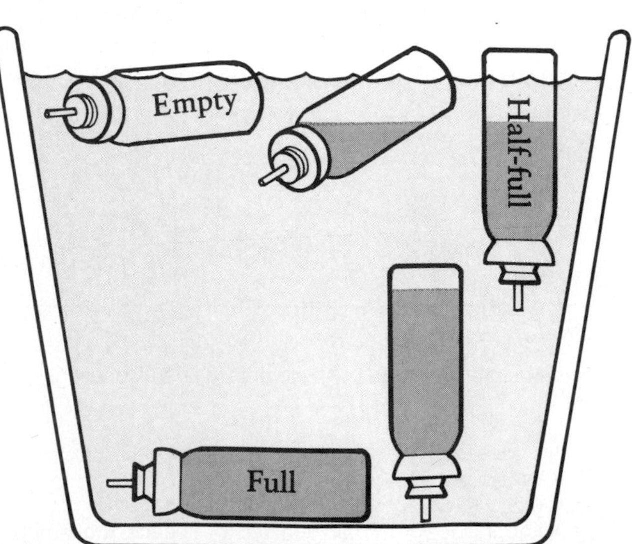


***FIG. 102-3*** Measuring the amount of inhalant in canister.

From Plaut TF: Children with asthma: a manual for parents, ed 2, Amherst, Mass, 1988, Pedipress.

### Home Care Modifications—cont'd

6. Instruct child and family in the use of peak flow meter (see box on p. 654). Peak flow monitoring is easily used at school or at home. Detecting reductions in peak flow, often before the child is aware of narrowed airways, permits early treatment with MDIs for improved asthma control. It also allows monitoring of exercise-induced asthma, demonstrates the effectiveness of medication, and provides objective information the family can use when communicating with the health care professional about the child's status (Garcia, 1989). Several models and sizes are available to accommodate the family's needs.

# *SKILL* 103 Administering Medications by Nebulization

*Bobbie J. Mackay*

Nebulizers produce aerosol particles that deposit water or medications along the tracheobronchial tree. Aerosol treatments can decrease the viscosity of sputum and improve its mobilization by mixing it with fluid or coating it with water. The size of the particles, ability of the particles to remain in suspension for a significant period of time, and the velocity of the air stream affect the distribution of aerosols. Aerosol medications are most often used in children with chronic lung conditions such as asthma, cystic fibrosis, or bronchopulmonary dysplasia. Aerosol therapy effectively delivers bronchodilators, mucolytic agents, wetting solutions, and antibiotics topically to the tracheobronchial tree, although the use of some of these medications is controversial.

Although bronchodilators are frequently given by metered-dose inhalers, nebulization administration is often used for acute episodes, children too young to use inhalers, and medications not available in inhalers. Families often give nebulized treatments at home. Therefore, nurses need to teach families proper administration of aerosol medications, side effects of medications, and maintenance of equipment.

## NURSING DIAGNOSES

Altered health maintenance related to lack of knowledge about medications administered by nebulization; Potential for injury related to adverse effects of inhalant medications; Noncompliance with inhalant nebulization medication regimen related to denial of illness, insufficient finances, or cultural/spiritual health beliefs.

| Steps | Rationale |
|---|---|
| **Assessment** | |
| 1. Assess respiratory status of child before and after each treatment. | Presence of symptoms indicates necessity for treatments. Symptoms determine number of treatments needed and appropriate medication. |
| a. Auscultate breath sounds:<br>▪ Wheezing.<br>▪ Crackles.<br>▪ Egophony (a nasal quality to speech transmitted through consolidated lung tissue).<br>▪ Bronchial breathing.<br>▪ Snoring.<br>▪ Grunting.<br>▪ Diminished breath sounds. | Presence of wheezing indicates need for bronchodilator or steroid preparation, to be determined by physician. Egophony indicates consolidation of secretions in the lung. Adventitious (accidental) sounds, e.g., crackles, wheezes, and pleural rubs; and abnormally transmitted sounds, e.g., egophony breath sounds, bronchial breathing and bronchophony, indicate pathology and assist physician in prescribing medication (Lehrer, 1984).<br>***Special Considerations:*** *For the child with asthma, an objective method to assess respiratory status is with a peak flow meter (see box in Skill 102, p. 654).* |

| Steps | Rationale |
|---|---|
| b. Observe for signs of respiratory distress:<br>▪ Tachypnea.<br>▪ Dyspnea.<br>▪ Nasal flaring.<br>▪ Use of accessory muscles.<br>▪ Stridor.<br>▪ Shallow breathing.<br>▪ Cheyne-Stokes respiration.<br>▪ Cyanosis.<br>▪ Intercostal and substernal retractions.<br>▪ Increased cough. | These signs indicate evidence and degree of respiratory distress. These signs may indicate a need for bronchodilators or other aerosol medications. |
| c. Observe sputum:<br>▪ Consistency.<br>▪ Amount.<br>▪ Odor.<br>▪ Color. | Thick, tenacious or foul-smelling sputum indicates need for wetting solutions, mucolytic agents, or antibiotics. |
| 2. Determine child's age, height and weight, developmental level, and ability to cooperate. | Age, height, and weight parameters guide medication dose appropriate for the child. Child's age and developmental level provide insight into child's ability to understand nebulization treatments, comprehend the rationale for medications and their side effects, and participate in procedure. Knowledge of these factors assists in planning, teaching, selecting equipment, and performing the procedure. Nebulized medications are easier to administer to younger children than metered-dose inhalers as less coordination is required (Brims, 1988). |
| 3. Review health history; note factors that may affect drug therapy. | |
| a. Medication allergies, as noted on the child's chart and arm band. | Administration of drug to which child is allergic will cause a mild to severe allergic reaction. |
| b. Side effects previously experienced. | Some children may experience hypersensitivity reactions to preservatives in aerosol medications. Any previous side effects such as nausea, vomiting, fine motor tremors, nervousness, and headache should be noted. |
| c. Current and past medications, prescribed or OTC. | Current medications may alter or potentiate effects of aerosolized medications. A history of previous therapy provides insight into medications to which child has had beneficial responses. Nebulized medications often interact with OTC inhaled medications. Many medications have local and systemic effects. Contraindications for use should be carefully checked.<br>***Special Considerations:*** *Specifically ask parents about any OTC medications child is using and the response to this medication.* |
| 4. Determine family's understanding of and ability to administer aerosolized medications at home. Assess:<br>a. Health beliefs and behaviors that might interfere with family's willingness to comply with therapy.<br>b. Perceived need for nebulization treatments.<br>c. Barriers to learning.<br>d. Willingness to learn. | Assessment allows for appropriate discharge planning. Accurate assessment of family's ability to learn allows development of an individualized education program that encompasses three components essential to learning: motivation, experiential background, and ability to learn (Burns, 1983). |
| 5. Assess older child's ability to administer self-aerosol therapy.<br>a. Level of maturity.<br>b. Ability to draw up and measure medications and to follow directions.<br>c. Ability and willingness to assume responsibility.<br>d. Level of understanding about the disease and rationale for therapy. | Children age 8 years and older can begin to learn about their medications, what they do, how to measure and administer medications, and how to clean their equipment. Responsibility for self-care prepares children for adulthood by fostering a sense of independence, positive self-worth and control. |
| 6. If child received aerosols at home, determine successful approaches family has used. | Child will cooperate better if established routine and individual preferences are considered when planning therapy. |

| Steps | Rationale |
|---|---|

## Planning and Goal Setting

1. Review physician's order to determine medications prescribed, doses, and number of treatments/day. Sometimes a combination of medications is administered simultaneously.

A physician order must be written for every medication given.

2. Assemble necessary equipment (Fig. 103-1):
   a. Clean nebulizer.
   b. Air compressor.
   c. Clean mask, mouthpiece, T-piece, or spacer.
   d. Tubing.

Infants and young children need to have a face mask held over their nose and mouth because they are nose breathers, and therefore are unable to coordinate deep breathing through the mouth. A mask minimizes the amount of medication lost to the environment. Children age 5 years and older can be taught how to deep breathe through a mouthpiece for better distribution of medication. Equipment need not be sterile but must be cleaned after each use (see Home Care Modifications).

***Special Considerations:*** *At times, aerosols are administered by holding the T-piece in front of the infant's face and nose. However this method allows medication to be lost to the air and provides less control of amount that reaches the child than does delivery by mask. Various devices are available for aerosol therapy, including ultrasonic nebulizers, electric pump nebulizers, and nebulizers with a client-demand system. A client-demand nebulizer is a new method that distributes medication as the child inhales, reducing loss of medication to the air.*

3. Assemble medication as prescribed (follow Five Rights of Medication Administration (see Skill 101, Planning step 3).
4. Assemble additional supplies.
   a. Emesis basin and water or other solutions appropriate for rinsing mouth.

Rinsing the mouth is a comfort measure and can reduce the potential for developing oral yeast infections from inhaled steroids (Weinstein, 1987).

***Special Considerations:*** *A child may have emesis after treatment. Reassure him or her that it is not caused by the treatment.*

   b. Age-appropriate toys or diversional objects, e.g., books, TV, or toys for younger children.

Providing diversional activity while administering aerosols distracts the child so that treatment is more tolerable.

***Special Considerations:*** *The older child who is better able to cooperate may receive more benefit from treatment by concentrating on effective breathing.*

   c. Instruction sheet for nebulization.

An instruction sheet provides a good review for skills and a reinforcement tool for patient-family education.

5. Review treatment and medication information about nebulization therapy.

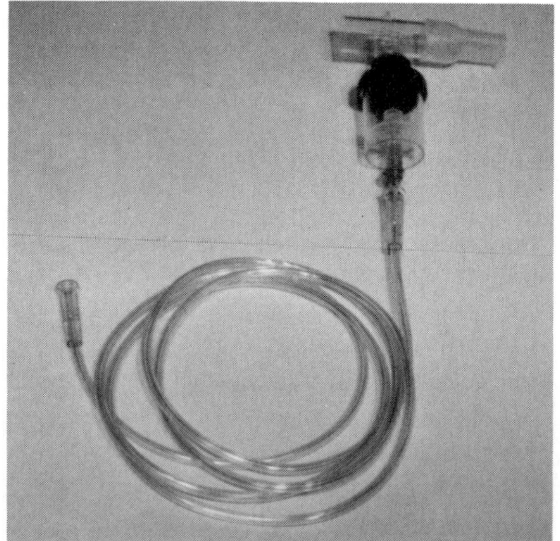

***FIG. 103-1*** Equipment used to administer medication by nebulization: nebulizer chamber, mouthpiece, T-piece, and tubing.

| Steps | Rationale |
|---|---|
| a. Review child's symptoms and compare them to the medications used to ensure appropriateness. | Children with chronic lung conditions may be receiving the same medications for years, even though recommendations for therapy have been updated. Verifying that treatment corresponds with child's symptoms ensures that the child gets the most up-to-date treatment.<br>***Special Considerations:*** *Aerosol medications are used to treat a number of problems in children, e.g., asthma, inflammation, and infection. Medications used most often in nebulizers include: (1) bronchodilators to prevent bronchospasm and dilate bronchial tubes; (2) steroids to reduce inflammation of bronchioles; (3) decongestants to shrink swollen membranes; (4) antibiotics to topically treat bacteria colonized in tracheal airway (Plaut, 1988); (5) cromolyn administered prophylactically to block the release of chemical mediators, which precipitate asthma; (6) wetting solutions to dilute and mobilize secretions; and (7) mucolytic agents to liquefy mucus.* |
| b. Coordinate use of aerosols in conjunction with other forms of therapy (e.g., chest physiotherapy, exercise, or coughing maneuvers) as indicated. Determine if aerosol is to be given before or after each therapy or both. The physician should specify how medications are to be combined and administered. | Aerosol treatments must be administered correctly in conjunction with other forms of therapy for maximum benefit. Bronchodilators, wetting solutions, or mucolytic agents are usually nebulized before other forms of therapy to open bronchial tubes and loosen secretions. At times, antibiotics are administered after other treatments to deposit the medication after airways have been cleared. |
| c. Review information for each medication to be administered.<br>▪ Usual dose.<br>▪ Expected outcome.<br>▪ Side effects.<br>▪ Method of administration.<br>▪ Rationale for use.<br>▪ Nursing considerations. | Reviewing information about medications helps prevent errors, and enables one to anticipate effects of the medications. The child should be observed for response to therapy and side effects experienced from medication. |
| d. Note length of aerosol treatment. | Nebulization treatments usually take between 10 and 15 minutes. If it takes longer to administer the medication, the filter may need to be changed, the nebulizer may be occluded, or the compressor may need to be serviced. |
| 6. Choose a convenient time for aerosol therapy. If possible, allow child choices about timing of treatment. | Aerosol therapy is usually performed in conjunction with other forms of physical therapy. Cooperative planning with the child/family related to therapy times encourages compliance with therapy and minimizes interference of child/family experiences with other activities. Choices give the child an opportunity to exercise control and foster cooperation. |
| 7. Provide for privacy during aerosol therapy. | Children often become embarrassed or self-conscious in the presence of others. Privacy also minimizes distractions for the child. |
| 8. Develop individualized goals for child and family:<br>▪ Child and family will be prepared for aerosol therapy including techniques and possible discomforts.<br>▪ Child receives aerosol medications properly.<br>▪ Child achieves desired response to medications such as relief of bronchospasm, airway clearance, or reduction of bronchial infection.<br>▪ Child and family will demonstrate knowledge and ability to administer treatment and care for equipment. | |

## Implementation

| Steps | Rationale |
|---|---|
| 1. See Skill 101, Administration steps 1 through 5. | |
| 2. Inform child and family that it is time to take nebulization therapy. This time can be used to answer questions and for teaching about aerosol medications or treatments. | This prepares child for what is happening and provides opportunity for patient-family education. |
| a. Provide teaching tools or pamphlets for family performance of this procedure at home (see Home Care Modifications). | |
| b. Discuss proper setup of equipment and supplies. | |

| Steps | Rationale |
|---|---|
| c. Discuss and demonstrate proper method of inhaling medication.<br>d. Discuss side effects of medications and criteria for notifying health care professional of side effects.<br>e. Describe any discomforts child may experience, such as a bad taste in the mouth or emesis. | Teaching aids reinforce other types of approaches such as verbal instruction and demonstration. They provide written information for child and family to refer to later.<br>***Special Considerations:*** *Teaching may need to be reinforced on several occasions.* |
| f. If child and family are unfamiliar with procedure, demonstrate what child is expected to do, then have child practice.<br>g. Explain and demonstrate proper cleaning and maintenance of equipment. | Demonstration and practice are valuable teaching interventions. The child observes proper technique then has the opportunity under supervision to repeat what he or she has observed. Child should practice deep-breathing techniques before administration. |
| 3. Initiate treatment. | |
| a. Verify that power switch is in *off* position on the compressor. | Having the switch in the *off* position prevents nebulization of solution before mouthpiece is positioned and child is ready.<br>***Special Considerations:*** *Some hospitals use compressed air from a wall unit. In this case, connect the tubing to the compressed air nozzle in the wall and regulate by a meter flow unit.* |
| b. Plug portable compressor into appropriate power source (a grounded wall outlet). | A grounded wall outlet is recommended to avoid an electrical hazard.<br>***Special Considerations:*** *For travel or in case of power failure, compressors are available that use alternate power sources such as battery pack or auto cigarette lighter.* |
| c. Place medication or wetting solution in nebulizing chamber. | ***Special Considerations:*** *Most nebulizers take 2 to 5 ml of solution; do not exceed amount of solution recommended by manufacturer. Medications can be measured, poured into nebulizer, and sealed securely with cork so that the nebulizer can be carried safely for activities away from home.* |
| d. Connect one end of air tubing to compressor at hose connector; turn hose connector clockwise to tighten. | ***Special Considerations:*** *If using ultrasonic nebulizer, secure connector plug to receptacle; engage locking lever on top of connector.* |
| e. Connect other end of tubing to small end (nozzle) at bottom or side of nebulizer. | |
| f. Insert bottom part of mask into top of nebulizer. Place mask over mouth and nose. If using mouthpiece, insert T-piece into top of nebulizer, and slide mouthpiece on either end of T-piece. The tongue should be below the opening of the mouthpiece. | |
| g. With child in sitting position, instruct to inhale deeply and slowly and to hold his or her breath for 10 seconds; then exhale slowly through mouthpiece or mask. Child can breathe through the nose or mouth if using a mask. If a mouthpiece is used, child should inhale through the mouth. | Deep breathing will ensure maximum intake and distribution of medication; breath holding for 10 seconds allows for more even distribution of solution along airway. A sitting position relieves pressure on the diaphragm and provides for maximal lung expansion and expiratory efforts.<br>***Special Considerations:*** *Should child need to pause to cough, tilt the medication cup to the side so that the solution will not be nebulized and wasted. If using client-demand ultrasonic nebulizer, have child exhale through nose or remove mouthpiece from mouth while exhaling. If the child is severely dyspneic and cannot hold breath for 10 seconds, begin with 6 seconds, gradually increasing to 10 as possible.* |
| h. Turn on nebulizer and observe for proper mist formation. | A fine, steady mist is necessary to effectively deliver the solution to the airway. |
| i. Gently tap side of nebulizer chamber periodically during treatment. Treatment is finished when all medication is used and no mist is seen. | It is normal during course of operation for some of the nebulized solution to accumulate on sides of the chamber. Tapping side of the chamber allows solution to drain back into bottom of nebulizer to be recycled. |
| j. Provide diversion as planned. | |
| 4. Turn power off and unplug compressor from power source. | Leaving compressor plugged into an electrical outlet is a fire hazard. |
| 5. In a hospital setting, disposable supplies, such as nebulizers, mask, and tubing, are discarded after each use. | ***Special Considerations:*** *Some disposable supplies such as nebulizer tubing, masks, or mouthpieces can be saved and sent home with the child and family. They can be cleaned and safely reused in a home setting.* |

| Steps | Rationale |
|---|---|
| 6. Praise child for cooperation. | Praising child fosters cooperation and improves child's positive feelings. |
| 7. Reinforce expected therapeutic benefit and need to notify nurse or physician of side effects experienced. | If family members are knowledgeable about side effects, they can monitor child's response. Unexpected reactions are often noted earlier by family members. |

| Evaluation Outcomes | Observational Guidelines |
|---|---|
| 1. Child's status improves after aerosol use. | Observe respiratory rate, frequency of cough; auscultate breath sounds. Note cyanosis, nasal flaring or retractions. Compare to prenebulization symptoms. Observe for signs of known side effects of medications. |
| 2. Child and family verbalize and demonstrate understanding and adequate knowledge about aerosol medications.<br>a. Uses.<br>b. Rationale and treatments.<br>c. Side effects.<br>d. How to administer aerosol correctly. | Interview child (if age appropriate) and family to discuss purpose of medication, timing of medication, possible side effects, rationale, and proper administration. Note that family members ask appropriate questions and give appropriate answers. Observe child and family members as they demonstrate technique. |
| 3. Family members and child (if age appropriate) verbalize understanding of how to clean and maintain equipment. | Family members are able to provide return demonstration of procedure and verbalize steps. |

## Documentation

Record assessment data, particularly observations of respiratory distress; family and/or child's ability to administer aerosolized medications, child's response to medication, family and child's understanding of symptoms of respiratory distress, and verbalizations of family and child's feelings related to treatments and the disease process. Note date and time of medication administration and record appropriately. Document clinical response to nebulized medication.

## Home Care Modifications

1. After each use, wash nebulizer chamber and mask, mouthpiece, T-tubes, and spacer under warm tap water for 30 seconds. This removes excess medication left after treatment.
2. Shake off excess moisture and allow rinsed parts to air dry on clean towel or drain.
3. Put compressor, nebulizer, and all medications in safe place, out of reach of children.
4. Perform cleaning, daily disinfection, and maintenance of equipment and parts.
   a. Wash mouthpiece, T-tube, mask, spacer, and nebulizer in warm soapy water at least once a day. It is unnecessary to wash tubing as only filtered, compressed air flows through.
   b. Rinse thoroughly in warm water.
   c. Mix solution of 1 part vinegar and 2 parts water. Immerse washable parts daily in this solution to soak for 30 minutes to disinfect them and remove soap deposits. To prevent mold growth in humid areas of the country, add bleach to the solution. *Note:* If using medical disinfectants, follow manufacturer's instructions.
   d. Rinse washable parts with tap water after soaking in vinegar solution. Although washable parts can be cleaned and disinfected in the dishwasher, they should still be soaked in vinegar and water to remove soap deposits.
5. Change filter on air intake valve monthly or when filter turns gray in color. Do not use cotton or other material as a filter or attempt to wash or clean felt filters. It may damage compressor.

# SKILL 104 Administering Eye, Ear, and Nasal Medications

*Kristie S. Nix*

Medications administered in the eye, ear, or nose are a special nursing challenge, as these routes are often unfamiliar to children and their families. Because eye, ear, and nasal medications are frequently administered at home, it is important that families are instructed in proper administration techniques. This skill provides general guidelines; each medication to be administered should be investigated for any special administration techniques required.

## NURSING DIAGNOSES

Altered health maintenance related to lack of knowledge about eye, ear, or nasal medication administration; Potential for injury related to adverse effects of eye, ear, or nasal medications; Noncompliance with eye, ear, or nasal medication regimen related to denial of illness, insufficient finances, or cultural/spiritual health beliefs; Alteration in sensory perception related to side effects of eye, ear, or nasal medications.

| Steps | Rationale |
|---|---|
| **Assessment** | |
| 1. Review health history; note factors that affect drug therapy. | A review of these factors can prevent untoward physiologic or psychologic reaction to drug administration. |
| a. Age, developmental level, and general health status. | These factors provide information about ability of child to cooperate and appropriateness of dose. |
| b. Allergies. | Administration of a drug to which the child is allergic may result in a local or systemic reaction. |
| c. Cultural beliefs about medication (see Skill 41). | Cultural beliefs influence willingness to follow prescribed regimen and determine significant family members to whom teaching should be directed. |
| d. Home remedies or OTC medications used previously. | Home care treatments may have undesirable side effects or combination effects with other medications. For example, nasal decongestants may have a rebound effect or aggravate mucous membranes. Eye drops may have a similar effect with chronic use. |
| 2. Inspect condition of the eye, ear, or nose and related structures (e.g., sinuses) and assess if child has experienced any sensory alterations (sight, hearing, or smell). Determine if there are contraindications to medication administration, e.g., ruptured eardrum or pressure equalization tubes in the tympanic membrane. | Assessment permits baseline information to evaluate therapy and identify contraindications. ***Special Considerations:*** *Crusted secretions on the eyelashes, ear, or nose, or previous applications of medication may require removal by washing or soaking to permit inspection. A physician's order should be obtained for cleansing of the ear canal by irrigation. Even with an order, irrigation should be approached cautiously and is contraindicated if rupture of the tympanic membrane has occurred or if a pressure equalization (PE) tube is in place.* |
| 3. Assess family knowledge about medication. Determine any problems experienced in past with eye, ear, or nose medications in general or for the specific drug ordered. Ask family about child's preferences for medication administration. | Determining family's knowledge permits identification of teaching needs. Information gathered about past problems and current requests may guide or modify approach/technique. |
| **Planning and Goal Setting** | |
| 1. Gather equipment. | |
| a. Medication card or Kardex with correct drug order transcribed from physician's order. | ***Special Considerations:*** *Follow agency policy for use of medication cards, Kardex, or other recording forms. Always verify these with written order.* |
| b. Medication tray. | A tray provides an organized and safe method for transporting medications. |

| Steps | Rationale |
|---|---|
| c. Gloves (optional). | Gloves should be used whenever body fluid contact is possible, according to facility policy (see Skill 50). If not recommended by barrier precaution system, gloves should be used when drainage may be due to an infectious process that could be transmitted, e.g., conjunctivitis. |
| d. Cotton ball or facial tissue. | Medication drips can be absorbed with these items. |
| e. Basin, washcloth, towel, and soap. | Cleansing may be necessary before application of medication. **Special Considerations:** *Be cautious not to transfer organisms from one eye/ear/naris to the other; use a clean washcloth for each side. Removal of cerumen or drainage should be approached cautiously; if done improperly, e.g., with cotton-tipped applicators or hairpins, the canal may be occluded or tympanic membrane injured. A warm, wet washcloth is the safest way to remove cerumen or drainage from the outermost portion of the ear canal.* |
| f. Dressing supplies (optional) such as cotton balls for the ear or eye patch and tape. | Dressings may be used to occlude or protect the site. |
| 2. See Skill 101, Planning steps 2 through 5. | **Special Considerations:** *For the eyes, the following abbreviations are common:*<br>▪ *OU, both eyes.*<br>▪ *OS, left eye.*<br>▪ *OD, right eye.* |
| 3. Determine amount and type of medication prescribed for application. | **Special Considerations:** *Verify medication concentration carefully because higher concentrations provide more available drug for absorption per unit area. For example, a 1% concentration is 10 times that of the same medication with a 0.1% concentration.* |
| 4. Develop individualized child and family goals:<br>▪ Medications are administered following guidelines for safe preparation and administration.<br>▪ Child is monitored for desired response and side effects of medication.<br>▪ Family demonstrates an adequate knowledge base about administration of eye, ear, or nasal medications. | |

## Implementation

### *Medication preparation*

| Steps | Rationale |
|---|---|
| 1. Read the medication label. Review Five Rights of Medication Administration. | Check ensures that correct medication is given. As with oral medications (see Skill 101), Five Rights of Medication Administration should be checked three times before administration. **Special Considerations:** *Never use medication from a container with an illegible label.* |
| 2. Prepare medication, following any special instructions, e.g., shaking container or warming medication. | **Special Considerations:** *Eye, ear, and nose medications are often brought to the child's room and dispensed from the original container.* |

### *Administration*

| Steps | Rationale |
|---|---|
| 1. See Skill 101, Administration steps 1 through 5. | |
| 2. Explain administration to child, including positioning and sensations to expect, e.g., eye medications may blur vision briefly. | **Special Considerations:** *Refer to Skill 1 for tips on preparing the child/family.* |
| 3. As possible, offer the child choices about application of medication. | Offering choices gives child an opportunity to exercise control and may improve compliance. **Special Considerations:** *The child may prefer to have the parent administer the medication while the nurse observes as long as practice is consistent with agency policy.* |
| 4. Soak or wash affected area, removing previous medication, crusts, exudate, or debris. Pat or air dry. For nasal medications, assist the child to blow his or her nose, or remove secretions with a bulb syringe. | Removal of secretions enhances penetration of medication through mucous membranes. |
| 5. Assist child to a comfortable position that provides access to area to be treated. If necessary, secure additional persons to assist or use restraint technique (see Skill 51). | Immobilization of child permits safe application. |

| Steps | Rationale |
|---|---|
| a. Eye: Have child lie supine with head tilted slightly backward. | |
| b. Ear: Position child on side with ear to be treated facing up. | |
| c. Nose: With child supine, tilt head backward. Place a pillow or rolled towel under the child's shoulders or let child's head slightly hyperextend over the edge of bed. | |
| 6. Instill medication. | |
| *Eye medications* | |
| a. Place finger on bony orbital rim under the lower eyelid; pull the lid down. | This action exposes the conjunctival cul-de-sac. |
| b. Instruct the child to look up and turn head to same side as eye to be treated. | Having child look up prevents blepharospasm (spasm of the orbicular muscle of the eyelid), which may occur when child tries to see what is being done as the eyedrop approaches the eye (Boyd-Monk and Steinmetz, 1987; Kovalesky, 1985). Having the child's head turned minimizes systemic absorption through the lacrimal duct. |
| c. For drops, squeeze correct number into the cul-de-sac, being careful not to contaminate dropper by touching the eye. Repeat with other eye if ordered (Fig. 104-1). | ***Special Considerations:*** *If both drops and ointments are ordered, begin with drops first (Wong and Whaley, 1990). If both eyes are to be treated, always begin with the right eye; if the procedure is interrupted, there will be no confusion as to which eye was already treated. An alternative approach for an uncooperative child is to place the drops at the inner corner of the closed eye. When the child eventually opens the lid, the drops will flush the eye surface.* |
| d. For ointments, place a half-inch strip of ointment in the cul-de-sac, beginning at the inner canthus and moving outward (Fig. 104-2). Give the tube a half-turn to "cut" the ribbon of medicine (Wong and Whaley, 1990). Have child close eye gently. Repeat steps for other eye if ordered. | Ointments increase contact time of medication to the external ocular surface. ***Special Considerations:*** *Ointments blur vision considerably and, therefore, are preferably used at bedtime (Boyd-Monk and Steinmetz, 1987). Prevent curling of ointment as it leaves the tube by warming it before administration.* |
| e. Instruct child to keep eyes closed for a few seconds. If capable, ask the child to roll the closed eyes and/or blink. | Lid and eye movement helps to distribute the medication. |
| *Ear drops* | |
| a. Check temperature of container: ear drops should be at body temperature. | Cold eardrops may cause vertigo, nausea, and pain while ear drops that are too warm may burn the ear canal. |
| b. For children under three years, pull the auricle down and back (Fig. 104-3); for older children, pull the auricle up and back (Fig. 104-4). | The ear canal is curved; this maneuver straightens the ear canal for optimal medication delivery. ***Special Considerations:*** *If both ears are to be treated, always begin with the right ear; if the procedure is interrupted, there will be no confusion as to which ear was already treated.* |
| c. Instill number of drops ordered, holding dropper 1 cm above canal (Fig. 104-5). | Dropper is less likely to become contaminated if a safe distance above canal is maintained. |
| d. Gently massage tragus with finger (Fig. 104-6). Assist child to remain on side for 5 minutes. | Massage promotes distribution of medication. Ear drops remain in canal rather than draining out when the child remains on the side. |
| e. If ordered, place a cotton ball or portion of cotton ball at canal opening. Do not insert cotton ball into the canal. | Packing the ear canal may result in pressure on the eardrum. ***Special Considerations:*** *Remove cotton ball after specified time period.* |
| f. If ordered, repeat steps with other ear. | |
| *Nasal medications* | |
| a. Drops. | |
| ▪ If necessary, withdraw correct amount of medication in dropper. | Some medications are packaged in dropper bottles while others are two-piece units. The dropper frequently has incremental markings. |
| ▪ Holding child's head secure, push up the tip of the child's nose slightly and place the correct number of drops in the nostril. For drops to reach the eustachian tube opening, tilt the head to the affected side. Repeat for other nostril. | In order to prevent injury to the mucous membranes, the child's head must be immobilized. ***Special Considerations:*** *Prevent contamination of the dropper; do not touch the dropper to the nares.* |
| ▪ Keep the child's head tilted back for 1 minute. | Keeping the head tilted back promotes local absorption and prevents gagging and tasting the medication. |

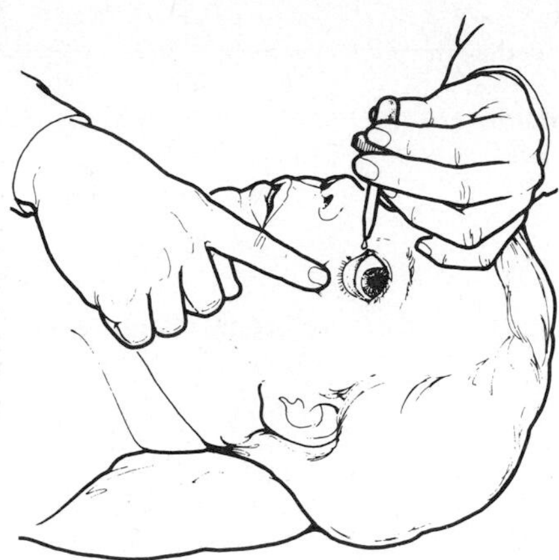

***FIG. 104-1*** Squeeze correct number of drops into the cul-de-sac.

From Wong DL and Whaley LF: Clinical manual of pediatric nursing, ed 3, 1990, St Louis, The CV Mosby Co.

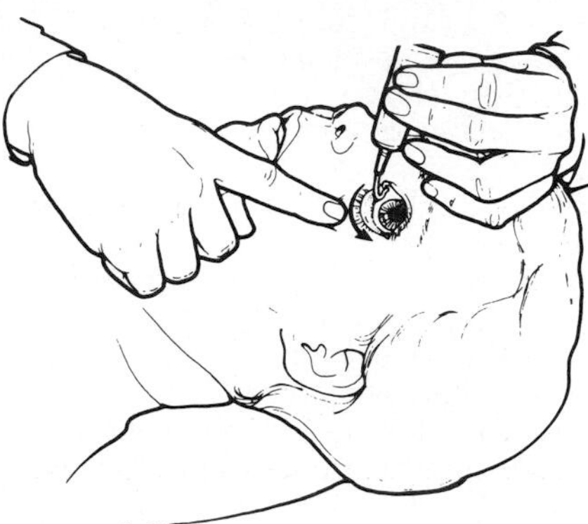

***FIG. 104-2*** To instill eye ointments, begin at the inner canthus and move outward.

From Wong DL and Whaley LF: Clinical manual of pediatric nursing, ed 3, 1990, St Louis, The CV Mosby Co.

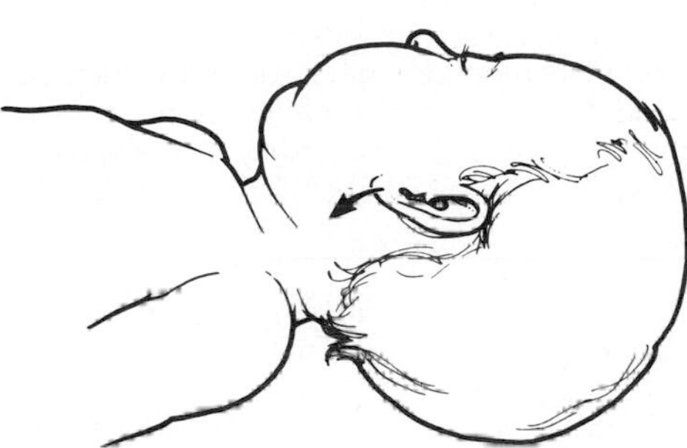

***FIG. 104-3*** Straighten the ear canal in children under 3 years of age by pulling the outer ear down and back.

From Wong DL and Whaley LF: Clinical manual of pediatric nursing, ed 3, 1990, St Louis, The CV Mosby Co.

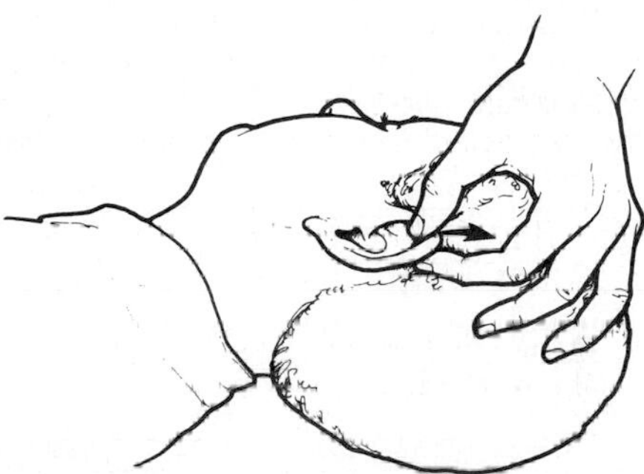

***FIG. 104-4*** For older children the auricle is pulled up and back.

From Wong DL and Whaley LF: Clinical manual of pediatric nursing, ed 3, 1990, St Louis, The CV Mosby Co.

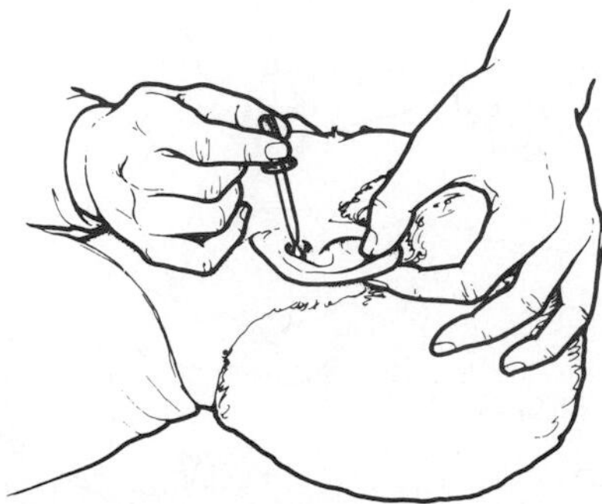

***FIG. 104-5*** Medication dropper is held 1 cm above ear canal.

From Wong DL and Whaley LF: Clinical manual of pediatric nursing, ed 3, 1990, St Louis, The CV Mosby Co.

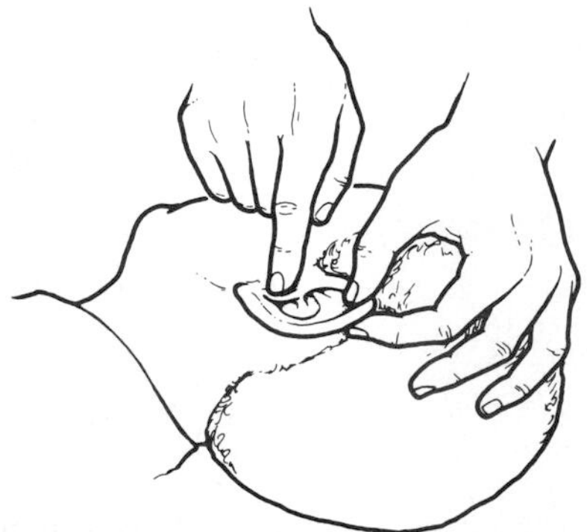

***FIG. 104-6*** Massage of tragus promotes distribution of medication.

From Wong DL and Whaley LF: Clinical manual of pediatric nursing, ed 3, 1990, St Louis, The CV Mosby Co.

| Steps | Rationale |
|---|---|
| b. Spray.<br>■ Occlude one nostril and instruct child to inhale.<br>■ Administer spray. | ***Special Considerations:*** *Practicing techniques with the child facilitates understanding of procedure.* |
| (1) Atomizer: Insert atomizer tip into unoccluded nostril. Following manufacturer's instructions, squeeze the atomizer quickly and firmly during inhalation. | |
| (2) Aerosol: If necessary, assemble cartridge according to manufacturer's instructions. Shake well before use and remove cap from adapter tip. Holding unit between thumb and index finger, press adapter and cartridge together firmly to release one measured dose of medication during inhalation. | Medication and propellant are evenly distributed with shaking. |
| ■ Repeat steps with other nostril if ordered. | |
| ■ Instruct child to keep head tilted back for 1 minute and to breathe through the nose if possible. Do not allow the child to blow the nose during this time. | Maximal contact with nasal membranes permits absorption.<br>***Special Considerations:*** *Provide diversionary activities during 1-minute wait. An older child may participate by "counting down" the minute.* |
| 7. Using clean tissue or cotton ball, wipe away any excess medication. | |
| 8. Apply dressings if indicated. | Dressings protect the site, absorb excess medication, or are used as part of therapy, e.g., an eye patch. |
| 9. Praise child for cooperation. | |
| 10. Reinforce expected therapeutic benefit and need to notify nurse immediately should any unexpected reactions (local or systemic) occur. | The child and family should be active participants in monitoring reaction to medication. Untoward reactions are often noticed earlier by family members who know the child best. |
| 11. Return to check child to evaluate response to medications. | Monitoring child provides information about medication's therapeutic effect or onset of side effects or allergic reactions. |

| Evaluation Outcomes | Observational Guidelines |
|---|---|
| 1. Child or family demonstrates adequate knowledge about eye, ear, or nose medications. | Child or family can discuss purpose of medication and place in overall medical plan; timing of medications; possible expected side effects; actions to take in case of unexpected side effects. |
| 2. Child achieves desired response to medication. | Observe for improvement in child's condition (e.g., decreased redness or pain at site). Observe for local or systemic side effects. |
| 3. Family demonstrates appropriate methods of medication administration. | Observe while family members apply eye, ear, or nose medication in a safe and effective manner. |

## Documentation

Record assessment and care of site (such as cleansing), noting any changes in site from previous assessment. Follow agency policy for documentation of medications. On medication record, include date, time, medication, strength, and site of application. Record teaching related to drug administration. Document evidence of side effects, complications, or therapeutic effects.

## Home Care Modifications

1. Teach parents about proper cleansing of ears and to avoid inserting cotton-tipped applicators, hairpins, or other sharp objects into canal. Advise that only the visible outer portion of the canal should be cleaned with a washcloth. Discuss role modeling, suggesting that child will attempt what the parent does.
2. Discuss methods of restraint, such as a mummy wrap, or straddle restraint (see Fig. 104-7), which may be successfully used by one person when administering medications to the eye, ear, or nose.
3. See also Skill 101.

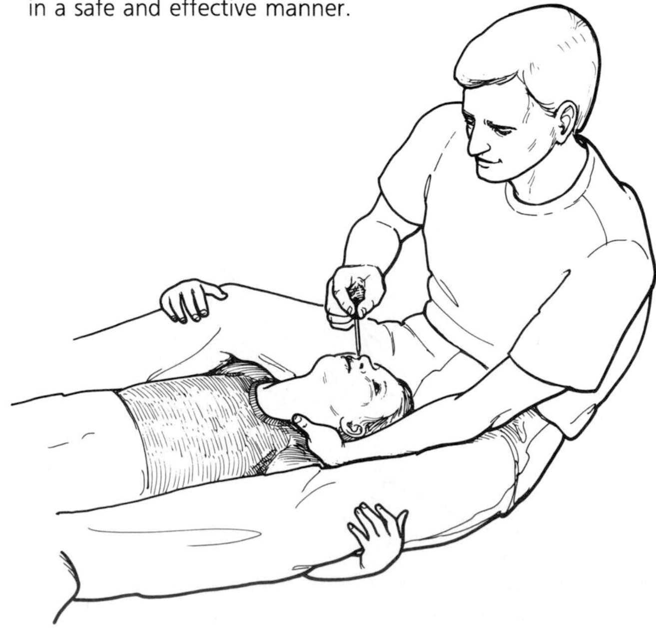

***FIG. 104-7*** The straddle restraint may be used when one person is administering eye, ear, or nasal medications.

From Wong DL and Whaley LF: Clinical manual of pediatric nursing, ed 3, 1990, St Louis, The CV Mosby Co.

# SKILL 105 Administering Intradermal, Subcutaneous, and Intramuscular Injections

*Midge Elliott*

Parenteral medication administration is the process of administering drugs by injection into body tissues. Types of parenteral injection include:

- *Intradermal (ID):* injection into the dermis just under the epidermal layer of the skin.
- *Subcutaneous (SC):* injection into connective tissues just below the dermal layer of the skin.
- *Intramuscular (IM):* injection into the body of a muscle.
- *Intravenous (IV):* injection into a vein (see Skill 108 for intravenous route).

Each injection type requires a specific set of nursing skills to ensure that the medication reaches the appropriate anatomic site for optimal absorption, intended action, and safety. Medications injected parenterally are more invasive, produce more discomfort, act more quickly, and carry greater risk than do medications administered orally. Many nursing responsibilities are associated with administering parenteral drugs safely and effectively.

## NURSING DIAGNOSES

Anxiety/fear related to unmet informational needs about parenteral medications and/or anticipatory discomfort of medication via injection; Pain related to needle injection of parenteral medication; Potential for injury related to adverse effects of parenteral medications; Noncompliance related to denial of illness, insufficient finances, or cultural/spiritual health beliefs.

| Steps | Rationale |
|---|---|
| **Assessment** | |
| 1. Assess child's overall condition of health. | Assessment identifies contraindications for injections and promotes safe and effective administration of parenteral medication. Data gathered may indicate medication should be withheld, injection equipment or technique should be altered, or administration routes or sites must be modified. |
| a. Nursing and medical history. | A review helps to determine child's ability to understand and cooperate with procedure, level of consciousness, and degree of mobility, which influence the plan for assistance with turning, positioning and restraining child during injection. A review can also identify any special injection techniques or nursing approaches needed. Problems with previous injections, such as hematoma formation, pain, abscess formation, or other untoward reactions may also be revealed. |
| b. Written and verbal history of allergies and drug reactions. | A past drug allergy or reaction to the ordered drug contraindicates administration. ***Special Considerations:*** *Do not rely solely on information in a child's record. Question child and parent and if report of a drug reaction contradicts the medical record, always investigate before administering drug. Drug allergies can be noted in red ink or on special stickers so they are highly visible.* |
| c. Amount of muscle mass. | Adequate muscle mass is necessary for deposition of medication with IM injections. It may be necessary to use a shorter needle, divide the dose, or use an alternate route, e.g., IV. ***Special Considerations:*** *See the box on p. 670 for possible sites.* |
| d. Tissue perfusion. | Venous congestion and reduced cardiac output may impair absorption and require modifications in route or site. |
| e. Condition of skin. | Skin areas with lesions, inflammation, edema, excessive hair, or birthmarks are unsuitable for injection sites due to unpredictable absorption rates. |

**Steps** | **Rationale**

### *COMPARISON OF INTRADERMAL, SUBCUTANEOUS, AND INTRAMUSCULAR INJECTIONS*

**INTRADERMAL INJECTIONS**

*Indications:* The intradermal route is used for administering small doses (0.01 to 0.1 ml) of agents for allergy testing, tuberculin testing, and immunotherapy for cancer.
*Syringe used:* 1 ml tuberculin (TB) syringe.
*Needle used:* ⅜ to ½ inch length, 25 to 27 gauge; short bevel.
*Injection sites:* Ventral forearm; secondary choices include scapular area, upper chest, or medial aspect of thigh.

**SUBCUTANEOUS INJECTIONS**

*Indications:* The subcutaneous route is used when the child cannot take medications orally, when medication would be destroyed or inactivated by gastrointestinal juices or when a more rapid drug action is desirable than that possible using the oral route. *Medications frequently given subcutaneously include:* allergens, epinephrine, heparin, insulin, narcotics, tetanus toxoid, some vaccines and vitamin $B_{12}$.
*Syringe used:* 1 ml insulin or TB syringe.
*Needle used:* ⅜ to ⅝ inch length, 23 to 26 gauge; medium bevel.
*Injection sites:* Subcutaneous injections may be given in essentially any part of the child's body where relatively few sensory nerve endings are present and large blood vessels and bones are relatively deep. The most common injection sites include the upper arm, lower abdomen, anterior thigh; secondary choices include scapular area and upper buttocks (above the iliac crest) (see Skill 106).

**INTRAMUSCULAR INJECTIONS**

*Indications:* The intramuscular route is used when a more rapid action is desired, when the volume is less than or equal to 1.0 to 2.0 ml for each injection site, or when the medication is in an oil preparation. *Medications frequently given intramuscularly include:* analgesics, antibiotics, steroids, sedatives, muscle relaxants, and some vaccines.
*Syringe used:* 1 to 3 ml syringe.
*Needle used:* ⅝ to 1½ inch length; 20 to 25 gauge; medium bevel.
*Injection sites:* Infants (0 to 2 years): Primary choice is vastus lateralis, secondary choice is ventrogluteal; children (2 to 12 years): primary choices for most injections are vastus lateralis and ventrogluteal, secondary choices are deltoid for small-volume injections and dorsal gluteal. The ventrogluteal site should be evaluated as a primary site for injection in children (Beecroft and Redick, 1990).

f. Child's age and weight.

Weight is important in calculating safety of drug dose orders and both age and weight are used to select appropriate IM injection sites.

2. Note previous injection sites in child's medical record, especially insulin rotation administration sites.

A specific rotation plan is best especially when multiple injections are needed, e.g., insulin administration (see Skill 106).

3. Note factors interfering with site selection and availability such as casting, traction, infection, injury.

Presence of these factors would contraindicate injection at that site.

## Planning and Goal Setting

1. See Skill 101, Planning steps 2 through 5.
2. Assess child's/family's knowledge about the medication, its action, side effects, reason child is receiving it, and any past problems with injections or ordered drug.

Gaps noted in knowledge base hold important implications for health education. Information gathered about past problems or current requests may modify approach or technique.

***Special Considerations:*** *For the child who has experienced excessive stress with injections, therapeutic play can facilitate expression of feelings and improve the ability to cope with future injections (see Skill 16).*

3. Develop individualized child and family goals.
   - Child is prepared for injection and experiences minimal anticipatory anxiety or distress before injection.
   - Child and/or family are knowledgeable about medication.
   - Child is safely administered medication into correct tissue.
   - Child experiences minimal pain or discomfort with injection.

## Implementation

### *Preparation*

1. Wash hands and prepare necessary equipment and supplies in the medication room.

Preparing parenteral medications before entering child's room minimizes anticipatory anxiety from child observing injection preparation.

   a. Drug card/medication Kardex with correct drug order.
      - Use the Five Rights of Medication Administration for drug preparation/administration.

The Five Rights of Medication Administration are used to prevent errors in administering any drug (see Skill 101).

| Steps | Rationale |
|---|---|
| b. Medication as ordered, in vial, ampule, or prefilled cartridge. | Parenteral medications come in several different forms: powders that must be reconstituted, premixed in vials or ampules, or in prefilled cartridges. |
| c. Bottle of diluent, if necessary. | Powdered medications in vials require reconstitution with a diluent specified on medication label. |
| d. Equipment for transporting medication to child's room such as tray or cart. | A tray or cart provides safe and efficient means for transporting injection equipment and supplies. |
| e. Alcohol wipe and 2 × 2 inch sterile gauze pad. | Alcohol is the most commonly used topical antiseptic for cleansing vials and preparing skin for injection. The gauze pad is used to stabilize skin when removing needle after injection. It can also be used to gently massage site after injection, unless contraindicated, and to stop any bleeding. Dry gauze facilitates blood clotting and avoids alcohol sting. |
| f. Adhesive bandage strip. | Adhesive bandages are used to cover the injection site as younger children often believe blood or body tissues will "leak out" of the puncture site. Also, drawing a happy face or other picture on the strip is a distractor and stress reliever. |
| g. Award sticker (optional). | The award sticker can be used for a younger child to reinforce a positive outcome. |
| h. Syringe to accommodate type and volume of medication: (see box at left)<br>▪ *Intradermal:* 1 ml tuberculin (TB) syringe.<br>▪ *Subcutaneous:* 1 ml insulin syringe or 1 ml TB syringe.<br>▪ *Intramuscular:* 1 to 3 ml syringe. | Although the choice of syringe may vary, these represent the most commonly used syringes for each type of injection.<br>***Special Considerations:*** *The barrel of syringe should be marked in increments of measurement appropriate to the medication ordered, i.e., units or ml. For volume less than 1.0 ml, use a tuberculin syringe, calibrated in 0.01 increments. Very minute doses may require the use of a 0.5 ml low-dose syringe. These syringes are specially constructed to reduce dead space (Whaley and Wong, 1991).* |
| i. Needle appropriate for intended route, site, viscosity of medication and child's size (see also box at left):<br>▪ Intradermal: Range: ⅜ to ½ inch; 25 to 27 gauge; short bevel.<br>▪ Subcutaneous: Range: ⅜ to ⅝ inch; 23 to 26 gauge; medium bevel.<br>▪ Intramuscular: Range: ⅝ to 1½ inch; 20 to 25 gauge; medium bevel. | Age and weight, fatty tissue and muscle mass, condition and turgor of skin, viscosity of medication and injection site should be used to determine needle size and gauge.<br>***Special Considerations:*** *Dehydrated or emaciated children may not have adequate tissue to absorb fluid by injection. An alternate route may be necessary.*<br>***Special Considerations:*** *A 1-inch needle is needed for adequate muscle penetration in infants 4 months old and possibly in infants as young as 2 months (Hicks et al, 1989). Use of a needle longer than 1 inch in infants and small children is discouraged (Beecroft and Redick, 1989).* |
| (1) Choose needle long enough to reach intended tissue, allowing ¼ to ½ inch of needle exposed above skin. (For example, with a subcutaneous injection, choose needle long enough to deposit medication into fatty tissue but not so long that it reaches into muscle mass. For an IM injection, choose needle that will deposit medication deep into muscle body, not into bones or nerves.) | Although a rare complication, the needle may break off from the hub and is more easily retrieved if a portion of the needle is left above the skin.<br>***Special Considerations:*** *The pinch test may be used to ascertain appropriate needle length for IM injections: Grasp muscle (of deltoid or vastus lateralis) between thumb and index finger. One half that distance will approximate the length of needle necessary to penetrate the muscle. Add sufficient needle length to pass through excessive subcutaneous tissue in the obese child receiving an IM injection (Lenz, 1983).* |
| (2) Choose the smallest diameter needle appropriate for the medication to be given. | Small-gauge (larger diameter, e.g., 20- or 22-gauge) needles are used with viscous medications; large-gauge (smaller diameter, e.g., 25- or 26-gauge) needles are used with watery solutions. Smaller diameter needles are less painful but may bend or break during injection. |
| (3) Also obtain filtered needle if drawing up medication from an ampule. | A filtered needle prevents glass fragments from being drawn up into the medication.<br>***Special Considerations:*** *The needle is used for withdrawal of medication only; it is not used for injection.* |
| j. Latex gloves (optional). | The possibility of encountering blood exists with injection administration.<br>***Special Considerations:*** *Use individual judgment and refer to institutional policy and current CDC guidelines to decide when to wear gloves.* |

| Steps | Rationale |
|---|---|
| 2. Check the medication label three times for Five Rights of Medication Administration.<br>a. When medication is removed from cabinet or drawer.<br>b. When measuring the medication or when comparing the prepackaged cartridge with the medication card or Kardex.<br>c. Immediately before returning the medication container to the cabinet or drawer or before discarding the container. | Triple checking the medication with the order helps reduce the possibility of error. |
| 3. Check medication card/Kardex for ordered dose. Perform any necessary calculations. | Calculations ensure that ordered dose does not exceed safe recommended dose for child's weight. |
| 4. Remove syringe and needle from packaging, and attach or change needle aseptically as needed. Secure needle hub and syringe tightly in place. | Handling syringe carefully avoids contamination of the plunger, inside of barrel, and syringe tips, which are to remain sterile. |
| 5. Check expiration date on medication container and inspect medication. If medication is expired or discolored or if it contains precipitate, discard and obtain another vial or ampule. | After the expiration date, the medication may lose its potency or become contaminated. Changes in color, consistency, or odor may also mean the medication is no longer stable and may not produce desired results.<br>***Special Considerations:*** *Do not use medications from illegibly labeled or unlabeled containers.* |
| 6. Draw the correct dose into the syringe from the ampule or vial, or use prefilled cartridge containing the ordered drug. | Measuring the correct volume is necessary to deliver the prescribed dose. |
| 7. *Optional:* For IM injections, draw up 0.2 ml of air into syringe, if appropriate, after correct dose of medication is obtained. | The use of an air bubble may be beneficial with certain drugs such as iron dextran, diphtheria or tetanus toxoid to avoid irritation caused by tracking the drug through the tissues.<br>***Special Considerations:*** *Syringes are calibrated to deliver a prescribed drug dose and the amount of medication left in the hub and needle is not part of the syringe barrel calibrations. Thus a hazard of the air bubble technique is potential overdose (Chaplin, Shull, and Welk, 1985; Wong, 1982).* |
| 8. If more than one injection is to be administered at a time, label each syringe accurately to ensure correct identification. | Labeling syringes and sites facilitates administration. |
| 9. Verify Five Rights of Medication Administration, correct syringe, and needle. | Verification prevents medication errors. |
| ***Administration*** | |
| 1. At designated time for medication administration, proceed to child's room with assistance for restraint as needed (see Skill 51). | Routine medications may be administered within 30 minutes of the designated time. Certain medications such as antibiotics must be administered at the designated time to maintain therapeutic blood level. Stat and preoperative medications must be given at the exact time designated by the physician's order. |
| 2. Check child's name on identification bracelet. | Verifying the name ensures correct identification for safe administration of correct medication.<br>***Special Considerations:*** *Asking the child his or her name is unreliable. A young, drowsy, or confused child may respond to someone else's name. An older child may give someone else's name to avoid an injection.* |
| 3. Prepare the child and family for the procedure (see Skill 1).<br>a. Explain procedure to child in a calm, confident, reassuring manner using developmentally appropriate language. Tell the child it is time for an injection and explain the purpose of the medication; e.g., "this will help relieve your hurt" or "this will help fight what is making you sick." Additional instructions may be necessary, e.g., if the injection is a preoperative medication. If the medication is to have a relaxing or sedating effect, have the child void before giving the injection. If the medication is an antibiotic or narcotic, always ask again about past history of allergic or other untoward reaction. | A calm approach helps to minimize the anticipatory anxiety associated with injections. Injections are generally painful and frightening procedures for children. Preparation should be sensitive and well timed, based on child's developmental level, previous experience, and current level of stress.<br>***Special Considerations:*** *The younger child often fears body mutilation and may perceive the injection as punishment for real or imagined bad behavior.* |
| b. Practice coping techniques (see Skills 1 and 52) and, if possible, give the child a choice of injection sites. | Strategies and choices enhance the child's sense of control.<br>***Special Considerations:*** *If the child or family refuses medication, report to immediate supervisor and/or physician (depending on institutional policy), discard the medication according to facility policy and chart reason for refusal.* |
| 4. Close child's door and/or curtains. | This ensures privacy and minimizes distractions. |

## *INTRAMUSCULAR INJECTION SITES IN CHILDREN*

| SITE | DISCUSSION |
|---|---|
| **Vastus lateralis** | **Location**<br>Palpate to find greater trochanter and knee joints; divide vertical distance between these two landmarks into quadrants; inject into middle of upper quadrant<br>**Needle insertion and size**<br>Insert needle at 45 degree angle toward knee in infants and in young children or needle perpendicular to thigh or slightly angled toward anterior thigh<br>22 to 25 gauge, ⅝ to 1 inch*<br>**Advantages**<br>Large, well developed muscle that can tolerate larger quantities of fluid (0.5 ml [infant] to 2.0 ml [child])<br>No important nerves or blood vessels in this location<br>Easily accessible if child is supine, side-lying, or sitting<br>A tourniquet can be applied above injection site to delay drug hypersensitivity reaction if necessary<br>**Disadvantages**<br>Thrombosis of femoral artery from injection in midthigh area<br>Sciatic nerve damage from long needle injected posteriorly and medially into small extremity |
| **Ventrogluteal** | **Location**<br>Palpate to locate greater trochanter, anterior superior iliac tubercle (found by flexing thigh at hip and measuring up to 1 to 2 cm above crease formed in groin), and posterior iliac crest; place palm of hand over greater trochanter, index finger over anterior superior iliac tubercle, and middle finger along crest of ilium posteriorly as far as possible; inject into center of V formed by fingers<br>**Needle insertion and size**<br>Insert needle perpendicular to site but angled slightly toward iliac crest<br>22 to 25 gauge, ½ to 1 inch<br>**Advantages**<br>Free of important nerves and vascular structures<br>Easily identified by prominent bony landmarks<br>Thinner layer of subcutaneous tissue than in dorsogluteal site, thus less chance of depositing drug subcutaneously rather than intramuscularly<br>Can accommodate larger quantities of fluid (0.5 ml [infant] to 2.0 ml [child])<br>Easily accessible if child is supine, prone, or side-lying<br>Less painful than vastus lateralis<br>**Disadvantages**<br>Health professionals' unfamiliarity with site<br>Not suitable for use of a tourniquet |

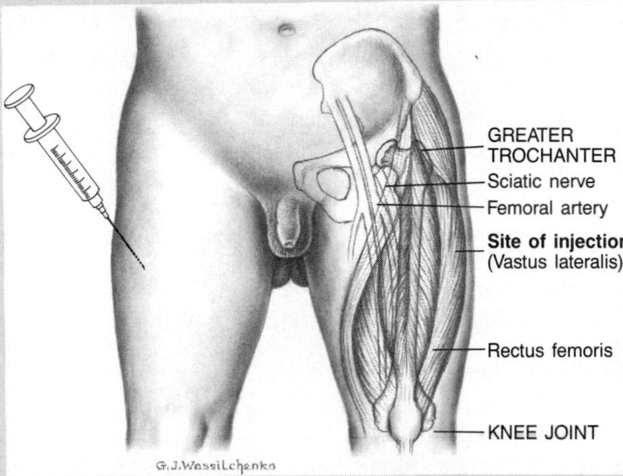


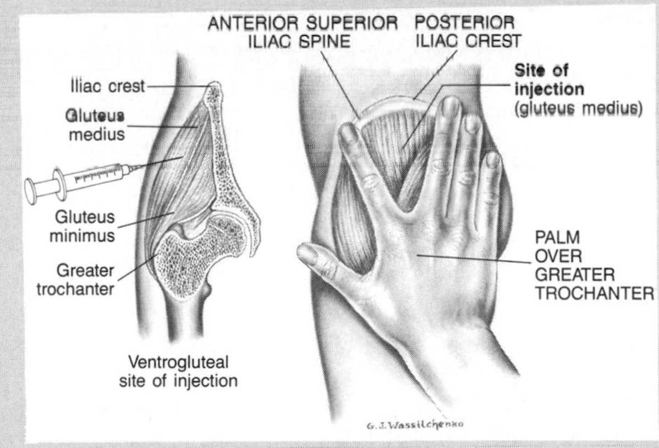


*Research has shown that a 1-inch needle is needed for adequate muscle penetration in infants 4 months old and possibly in infants as young as 2 months (Hicks J et al, 1989). Other recommendations for needle size and volume of fluid are based on traditional practice and have not been verified by research.

*Continued.*

## *INTRAMUSCULAR INJECTION SITES IN CHILDREN—cont'd*

### Dorsogluteal

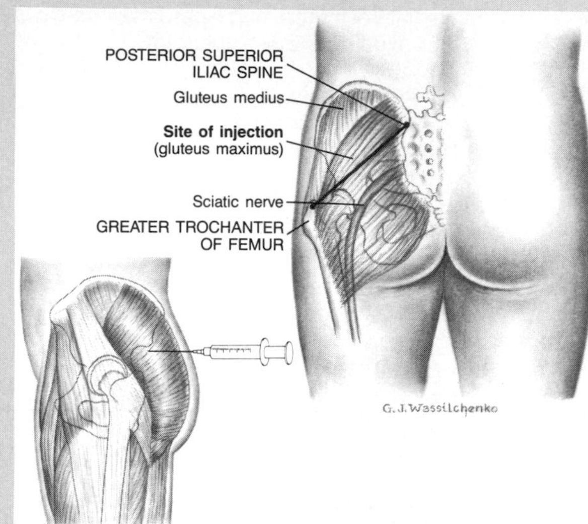


**Location**

Locate greater trochanter and posterior superior iliac spine; draw imaginary line between these two points and inject lateral and superior to line into gluteus muscle

**Needle insertion and size**

Insert needle perpendicular to surface on which child is lying when prone

20 to 25 gauge, ½ to 1½ inches

**Advantages**

In older child large muscle mass; well-developed muscle can tolerate greater volume of fluid (1.0 ml [young child] to 2.0 ml [child])

Child does not see needle and syringe

Easily accessible if child is prone or side-lying

**Disadvantages**

Contraindicated in children who have not been walking for at least 1 year

Danger of injury to sciatic nerve

Thick, subcutaneous fat, predisposing to deposition of drug subcutaneously rather than intramuscularly

Not suitable for use of a tourniquet

Inaccessible if child is supine

Exposure of site may cause embarrassment in older child

### Deltoid

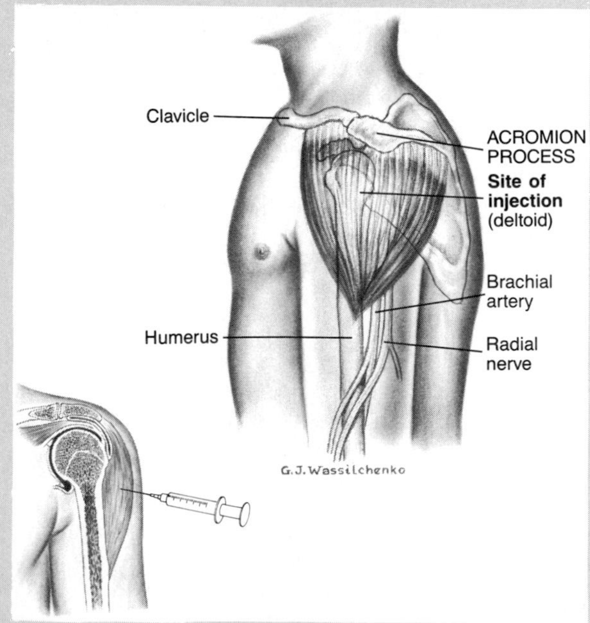


**Location**

Locate acromion process; inject only into upper third of muscle that begins about 2 finger-breadths below acromion

**Needle insertion and size**

Insert needle perpendicular to site but angled slightly toward shoulder

22 to 25 gauge, ½ to 1 inch

**Advantages**

Faster absorption rates than gluteal sites

Tourniquet can be applied above injection site

Easily accessible with minimal removal of clothing

**Disadvantages**

Small muscle mass; only limited amounts of drug can be injected (0.5 to 1.0 ml)

Small margins of safety with possible damage to radial nerve

Pain with repeated injections

Modified from Wong DL and Whaley LF: Clinical manual of pediatric nursing, ed 3, St Louis, 1990, The CV Mosby Co.

| Steps | Rationale |
|---|---|
| 5. Select site based on assessment of anatomic landmarks. Make sure lighting is adequate and entire injection site is exposed (see boxes on pp. 670 and 673). | Inspection provides information about any bruises, hematomas, rashes, or other visible contraindications to a specific site. Palpation validates bony landmarks and allows differentiation between subcutaneous and muscle tissue and assessment of tender or knotty areas to avoid. |
| 6. When ready to administer injection, ask child to avert eyes, if he or she prefers, and use distraction to minimize anxiety. Encourage child to squeeze your hand, hum a song, or count; engage the child in conversation on a topic of interest to him or her. | The child who is afraid of needles and/or potential pain may benefit from distraction. Distraction tends to temporarily lower the child's awareness of pain and often increases tolerance (Potter and Perry, 1987). |
| ***Intradermal injections*** | |
| 1. With the child either sitting or lying, expose the ventral forearm with elbow flexed, on a flat surface (e.g., over bed, table). | The ideal injection site for an intradermal injection is the middle third of ventral or volar aspect of the forearm. ***Special Considerations:*** *If both forearms are unacceptable for injection, other acceptable injection sites include the scapular area of the back, the upper chest, and the medial aspect of the thigh.* |
| 2. Locate the ventral forearm injection site by measuring to identify the middle third of the forearm. Avoid obvious superficial veins in site selection. | ***Special Considerations:*** *In a toddler, 2 to 3 finger widths away from the antecubital fossa and the wrist may be used to identify the site. In an older child or adolescent, a handsbreadth away from the antecubital fossa and wrist may be necessary for site determination.* |
| 3. Cleanse site with alcohol swab working from center outward in a circular manner. Allow to dry thoroughly. Do not use Betadine or any colored antiseptic. | Cleansing with alcohol produces an antibacterial action, maintaining aseptic technique. Colored antiseptics may mask subtle reactions, making interpretation of skin reaction results more difficult. |
| 4. Hold child's forearm in nondominant hand, stretching skin over site with thumb. Hold syringe between thumb and forefinger in dominant hand, resting plunger against the heel of palm, so that syringe is nearly parallel to skin. | Stretching the skin tautly over the injection site enables easy entry of needle through epidermis. ***Special Considerations:*** *Use distraction/coping techniques at this time to relax arm.* |
| 5. Press the tip of the needle against the skin with the bevel up. Insert the needle, then advance the needle through the epidermis, so that the needle point is visible under the skin. Some resistance should be felt during insertion. | If the needle moves too easily or is not visible under the skin it has been inserted too deeply. |
| 6. Inject the medication slowly and gently, using firm, steady pressure. A pale wheal—5 to 10 mm in diameter—should form over the tip of the needle as soon as the medication is injected (Fig. 105-1). | Slow injection minimizes discomfort. If no wheal forms, the medication has been administered too deeply into subcutaneous tissues. Injection will need to be repeated. |
| 7. After the wheal forms, withdraw needle. Wipe site gently with sterile gauze pad. *Do not rub.* | Rubbing can interfere with interpretation of test results. |
| 8. If administering more than one intradermal injection at a time at the same site, space them at least 2 inches apart or use two different injection sites. | Spacing injections in this manner prevents overlap of skin reactions, minimizing the possibility of confusion about results. ***Special Considerations:*** *If multiple antigens are administered, as in allergy testing, it may be necessary to number the skin sites with the corresponding antigen.* |

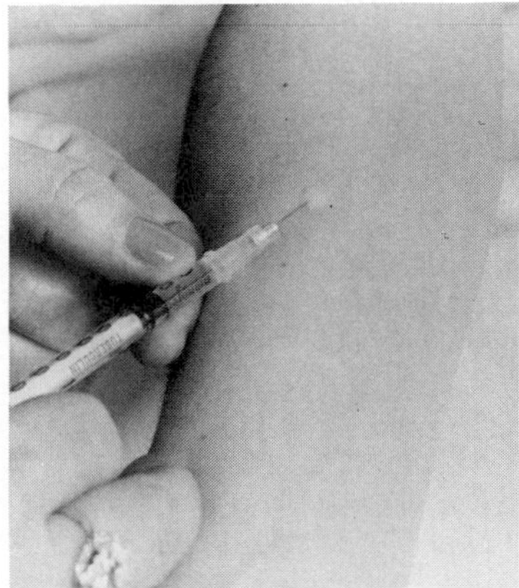

***FIG. 105-1*** If injected correctly, medication forms wheal when deposited in dermis.

From Perry AG and Potter PA: Clinical nursing skills and techniques, ed 2, St Louis, 1990, The CV Mosby Co.

| Steps | Rationale |
|---|---|
| 9. Assist child to comfortable position. Praise cooperation with statements such as "holding still helped us finish faster." | Positive reinforcement rewards child's cooperation. |
| 10. Monitor child for expected therapeutic effect and/or untoward reactions. Provide necessary teaching about medications. | The child and family should be active participants in monitoring reactions to medication. Untoward reactions are often noted earlier by family members who know the child best. |
| ***Subcutaneous injections*** | |
| 1. Determine rotation site for subcutaneous injection:<br>a. Insulin (see Skill 106).<br>b. Heparin: lower abdominal area below belt line to either side of umbilicus is preferred, but subcutaneous sites above the belt line may be used if needed.<br>c. Allergens. | Frequent injections of insulin, heparin, and allergens are usually administered on a special rotation basis.<br>***Special Considerations:*** *If giving two allergens, do not rotate arms. Mark allergen vials as "Left" or "Right" to give consistently on appropriate side.* |
| 2. Locate subcutaneous injection site carefully. Identify anatomic landmarks:<br>a. Upper arm: center third of the lateral aspect of the upper arm in a line from the point of the shoulder to the bony protuberance of the elbow.<br>b. Abdomen: rectangular area formed by the horizontal line between the right and left anterior superior iliac spines and between the tenth ribs, excluding the belt line and the area immediately surrounding the umbilicus.<br>c. Anterior thigh: center third of anterior thigh. | Careful site selection and rotation of injections promotes optimal drug absorption and distribution and reduces the possibility of lipodystrophy (atrophy of adipose tissue) and hypertrophy (thickening of subcutaneous tissue).<br>***Special Considerations:*** *If the infant's or child's skin is soiled, clean with soap and water and dry thoroughly before cleansing skin site with alcohol.* |
| 3. Position child in a comfortable seated, semirecumbent, or supine position with muscles relaxed. | Child should not stand for injections: landmarks are more difficult to assess; restraint is more difficult; and, child may faint or fall. |
| 4. Engage child in conversation and encourage distraction by humming a song, counting, etc., throughout procedure. | Distraction reduces discomfort and anxiety associated with the procedure, tends to temporarily lower the child's awareness of the pain and often increases pain tolerance (Potter and Perry, 1987). |
| 5. Cleanse injection site with alcohol wipe, using circular method, working from center outward. Allow alcohol to dry. Open dry gauze pad and place on child's skin near injection site. | Cleansing with alcohol produces an antibacterial action, maintaining aseptic technique. Allowing alcohol to dry prevents irritation by introducing alcohol into subcutaneous tissue. The dry gauze pad will be available to stabilize skin before needle removal on completion of injection. |
| 6. Stabilize injection site.<br>a. Grasp skin and subcutaneous tissues between thumb and finger of nondominant hand<br>*OR*<br>b. Spread skin tautly over subcutaneous tissues between thumb and finger of nondominant hand. | ***Special Considerations:*** *Stabilization of the subcutaneous injection site in small- to average-sized children is usually best accomplished with the grasping method. In obese children, it is advisable to stabilize the injection site by stretching the skin tautly over the layer of fat and subcutaneous tissue. For heparin injections, use the grasp method but do NOT pinch tightly, as this increases bruising.* |
| 7. Hold syringe in dominant hand between thumb and fingers and insert needle quickly in a dartlike fashion at a 45-degree angle in the small- to average-sized child or at a 90-degree angle in the obese child (Fig. 105-2). | A dartlike motion avoids excessive pulling or dragging of tissues and reduces discomfort. |
| 8. Leave a small portion (at least ⅛ inch) of the needle shaft exposed above the skin. | If the needle accidentally breaks off at the hub, it can be readily retrieved if a small portion is exposed above the skin. |
| 9. After insertion of the needle, release grasp on skin with nondominant hand. Aspirate to check for blood return. If blood flows into the needle or syringe, withdraw and place dry gauze over the injection site, applying gentle pressure. Inform child/family that there might be bruising at site. Discard syringe and medication. Prepare new injection. | Injection into compressed tissues irritates nerve fibers, increasing discomfort for the child. Checking for blood return avoids inadvertent intravascular injection.<br>***Special Considerations:*** *Do not aspirate when administering heparin as this is thought to increase bruising. Some diabetic educators have discontinued teaching the aspiration technique for insulin injection (see Skill 106). Check institutional policy.* |
| 10. Slowly and steadily inject medication. | Rapid injection does not allow the tissues to distend gradually to accept the medication and increases the pain of injection. |
| 11. When completed:<br>a. Place the dry gauze pad next to the needle.<br>b. Gently withdraw the needle at the same angle as it was inserted.<br>c. Apply gentle pressure to the site with the dry gauze pad. | Stabilizing the skin prevents excess tissue pulling as the needle is withdrawn. Pressure helps seal the puncture site and prevents medication leakage. |

| **Steps** | **Rationale** |
|---|---|

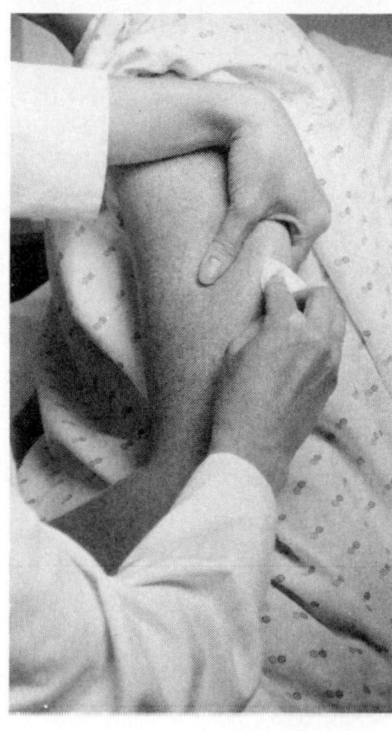
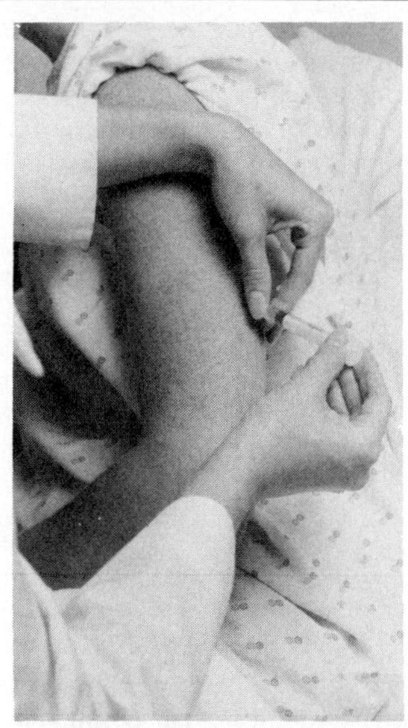
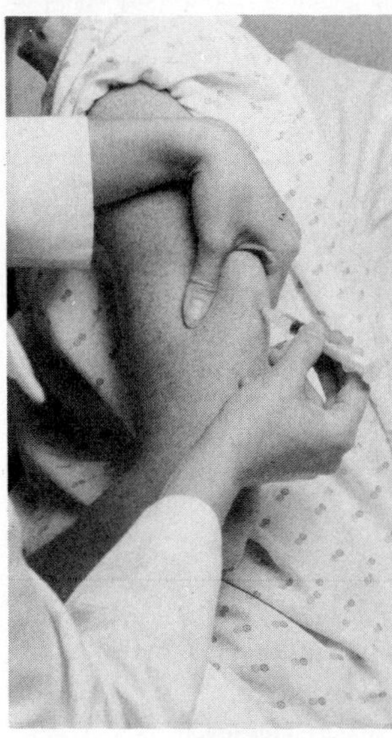
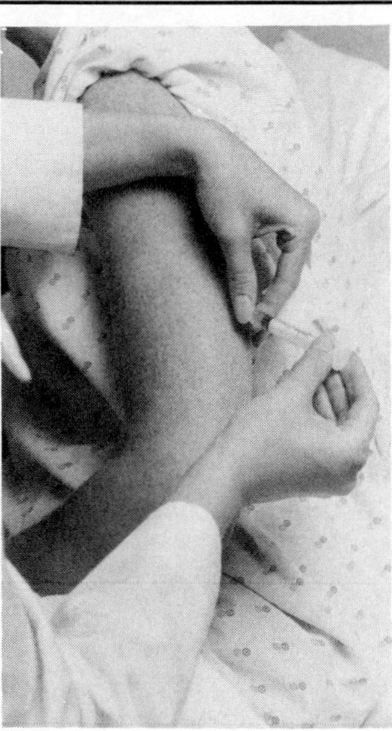

***FIG. 105-2*** Correct technique for administering subcutaneous injection.
From Perry AG and Potter PA: Clinical nursing skills and techniques, ed 2, St Louis, 1990, The CV Mosby Co.

12. Use dry gauze pad to gently massage the site. Observe for superficial bleeding at puncture site. Apply adhesive bandage if indicated or desired.

Massage helps distribute medication within the tissue and promotes absorption by increasing blood flow.
***Special Considerations:*** *Massage is contraindicated in heparin injections due to bruising. Excessive massage is contraindicated in insulin injections due to inappropriate increase in insulin absorption rate.*

13. Refer to Steps 9 and 10 under Intradermal Injections, to complete administration.

### *Intramuscular and Z-track injections*

1. Locate intramuscular injection site carefully (see the box on p. 673).
   a. Identify anatomic landmarks.
   b. Inspect intended site for skin irritation, rashes, pimples, and bruising; palpate area for masses, tenderness, edema, and hardened areas. Provide privacy during site exposure.

Careful site selection promotes optimal drug absorption and distribution.
***Special Considerations:*** *The ventrogluteal site should be evaluated as a primary site for IM injection (Beecroft and Redick, 1990).*

2. Assist child to correct position (see the box on p. 673). Ensure child's comfort and relaxation of body part. Engage child in conversation to facilitate distraction.

Comfortable positioning and relaxation reduce additional discomforts during the injection. Child should not stand for injections.
***Special Considerations:*** *Internal rotation of the femur during injection into the dorsogluteal site, in either the prone or side-lying position, results in dorsogluteal muscle relaxation and reduced discomfort from the injection (Rettig and Southby, 1982).*

3. Gently tap the site (optional).

Tapping the site reduces pain perception. Cutaneous stimulation activates the large-diameter sensory nerve fibers in the skin and alleviates pain by reducing painful stimuli (carried in small-diameter sensory nerve fibers), reaching higher centers of the brain (Potter and Perry, 1987).

4. Cleanse injection site.
   a. Apply alcohol wipe, using a circular method, working from center outward.

Cleansing with alcohol produces mechanical and chemical antibacterial action.

   b. Allow alcohol to dry.

If skin is wet when the medication is injected, alcohol may be introduced into the subcutaneous tissue and/or the muscle.

   c. Hold dry gauze pad between fingers of nondominant hand or place on child's skin near the injection site.

This ensures dry gauze pad is available to stabilize the skin before needle withdrawal.

| Steps | Rationale |
|---|---|
| 5. With nondominant hand *grasp* the muscle around the injection site (for vastus lateralis and deltoid injections) *OR* *stretch* skin tautly over injection site (for dorsogluteal and ventrogluteal injections). | Stabilization of the skin and tissues facilitates needle penetration. ***Special Considerations:*** *Sometimes, the muscle must be grasped to increase penetrable muscle mass. Obese clients may require stretching of skin and displacement of subcutaneous tissue in combination with grasping of the muscle for injection.* |
| a. *For Z-track injection* pull skin laterally away from the injection site and maintain this position throughout the injection procedure (Fig. 105-3). | Lateral traction displaces the skin and subcutaneous tissues during the injection, allowing closure of needle track to maintain medication in the muscle when tissue resumes normal position after injection. ***Special Considerations:*** *Inferon and many antibiotics are commonly given Z-track. Research indicates that the incidence and severity of IM injection site lesions and subsequent discomfort can be reduced by using the Z-track method (Keen, 1986). The use of the Z-track method can be particularly helpful for children receiving multiple IM injections.* |

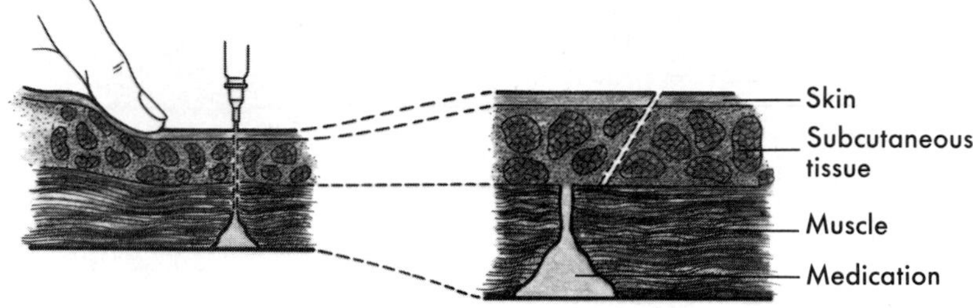


***FIG. 105-3*** Lateral displacement of skin and tissues during Z-track injection maintains medication in the muscle.

From Perry AG and Potter PA: Clinical nursing skills and techniques, ed 2, St Louis, 1990, The CV Mosby Co.

| Steps | Rationale |
|---|---|
| 6. Hold the syringe between the thumb and forefinger of the dominant hand, using the injection angle designated for the specific injection site (see the box on p. 673). Explain to child that he or she may feel something but it is important to remain still. | This hold ensures appropriate injection technique. Preparation readies the child for discomfort, although child may involuntarily move. ***Special Considerations:*** *Always use restraint measures to ensure a safe injection (see Skill 51).* |
| 7. Quickly pierce skin and subcutaneous tissue, inserting needle deep into the center of the muscle, using a dartlike motion. Expect to feel some resistance. | Using a dartlike motion inserts the needle quickly through the skin and subcutaneous tissues, reduces tissue pulling/dragging, and reduces discomfort. |
| 8. Grasp lower end of syringe barrel with nondominant hand and gently pull back on plunger of syringe with dominant hand, for 2 to 3 seconds, observing for any discoloration in the medication or in the needle hub. Hold syringe steady while needle remains in tissues. *For Z-track injection,* maintain lateral traction on skin with nondominant hand and grasp lower portion of syringe with same hand while gently pulling back on plunger of syringe with dominant hand for 2 to 3 seconds observing for any discoloration in the medicine or in the needle hub. Hold syringe steady while needle remains in tissues. If blood return occurs, withdraw needle, apply gentle pressure to site with dry gauze, dispose of injection equipment, and start again. | Checking blood return avoids inadvertent intravascular injection. A steady hold on the syringe prevents unnecessary discomfort from movement of the needle within the tissues. If blood is aspirated, direct pressure is needed to stop the bleeding. The equipment is contaminated and is not reused. ***Special Considerations:*** *Explain situation to child/parent so they understand reason for repeated injection.* |
| 9. Slowly inject the medication and remove needle (see steps 11 and 12 in Subcutaneous Injection section). | A slow, steady rate of injection allows the muscle to distend gradually and enhances absorption of the medication. Too rapid an injection increases pain. |
| 10. For *Z-track injection:* | |
| a. Wait 10 seconds after injecting the medication before withdrawing the needle. | Delaying withdrawal allows complete absorption of medication into muscle and prevents medication seepage from site. |
| b. While gently withdrawing the needle, gradually relax the lateral traction of the skin over the injection site in one smooth motion. *OR* Withdraw the needle at the same angle as it was inserted and then allow the skin to return to its normal position. | Either method achieves displacing the needle tract made into deeper muscle from the subcutaneous tissue and skin. ***Special Considerations:*** *A small-diameter needle may bend if using the first method.* |

| Steps | Rationale |
|---|---|
| c. Use a sterile gauze pad to apply gentle pressure to the site. *Do not massage area.* | Massage could force medication to move from intramuscular tissue, causing undue irritation. Encouraging physical activity, if appropriate, will facilitate absorption and distribution of medication. |
| 11. Refer to steps 9 and 10 under Intradermal Injections to complete IM injection. | |

| Evaluation Outcomes | Observational Guidelines |
|---|---|
| 1. Child demonstrates minimal anticipatory anxiety and expected level of distress during procedure. | Child demonstrates coping techniques during injection and is easily comforted after procedure or easily returns to previous activities. |
| 2. Child and family verbalize accurate understanding of purpose and need for medication and consent to injection. | Ask child and family to describe need and purpose for medication. Note verbal or behavioral consent for injection. |
| 3. Child is safely administered medication into correct tissue. | Review medication administration record for documentation. |
| 4. Child experiences little or no pain during and after injection. | Question child about discomfort after injection. Assess level of discomfort with a pain assessment tool (see Skill 52). |
| 5. Child is monitored for desired effects, undesired reactions, and complications after injection. | Observe child after administration for therapeutic effects or adverse side effects. *Intradermal:* Observe 15 minutes after injection for pain, extensive erythema and induration (greater than 8 mm diameter), blisters, and necrosis. Note aching or swelling around elbow or axilla. Evaluate after 48 hours for erythema and induration (Hermann, 1983). *Subcutaneous and Intermuscular:* Note presence of superficial bleeding, minor irritation, or mild burning as common sequelae. Observe for unusual redness, swelling, burning, itching, or excessive pain indicating allergic response or local nerve injury. Systemic complications: observe for tachycardia, general malaise, low-grade fever, anaphylactic reaction. Note child's therapeutic response to medication. |

## Documentation

### *Intradermal injections*

Immediately after the procedure note on the child's medical record the date, time, and location of the injection site(s) and the medications/allergens administered. Draw a picture in notes to clarify positioning of labeled sites or number the antigens if multiple injections are administered simultaneously. Document reassessment 15 minutes later, noting signs or symptoms of an anaphylactic reaction and any treatment administered. One hour later (for allergy injections) or 48 hours later (for skin tests) document the diameter of induration horizontally and vertically. Note the degree of erythema and induration (see grading scales below).

| *Erythema* | *Induration* |
|---|---|
| Trace (tr) = faint discoloration | Trace (tr) = barely palpable |
| + = pink | + = palpable, but not visible |
| + + = red | + + = easily palpable, visible to the naked eye, buckles when squeezed gently |
| + + + = purplish red | + + + = easily palpable, easily visible, does not buckle when squeezed gently |
| + + + + = vesiculation/necrosis | + + + + = vesiculation/necrosis |

### *Subcutaneous and intramuscular injections*

Immediately after the procedure note the medication, dose, route, site, date, and time of administration. Note any evidence of complications and report untoward effects to appropriate person, as well as any actions taken. Recheck site 30 minutes to 1 hour later for any signs of untoward effects and document and report presence of any noted complications. Note child's therapeutic response to the medication (e.g., pain relief with intramuscular injection of analgesic).

# SKILL 106 Administering Insulin

*Kristie S. Nix*

Administering insulin requires unique skills. The nurse is frequently responsible for administering and teaching families about insulin, whether in situations in which the child has been newly diagnosed or in which a child has management problems. This skill outlines conventional insulin preparation and administration and references some newer administration technologies (see box at bottom right).

## NURSING DIAGNOSES

Altered health maintenance related to lack of knowledge about insulin administration; Potential for injury related to hypoglycemic/hyperglycemic insulin reactions; Impaired tissue integrity (subcutaneous) related to frequent insulin injections; Noncompliance with insulin therapy regimen related to denial of illness, insufficient finances, or cultural/spiritual health beliefs.

| Steps | Rationale |
|---|---|
| **Assessment** | |
| 1. Review information pertinent to insulin(s) ordered: composition, purpose, time of onset, peak effect, duration, and usual dose recommendations (Table 106-1). | Understanding characteristics of insulin is essential for safe administration. |
| 2. Determine child's/family's knowledge about preparation and administration of insulin, including previous dose and methods of administration. | A child may have tried one or more methods of administration, including twice daily injections, multiple daily injections, or continuous subcutaneous insulin injection (CSII), which is also called insulin pump therapy. Information obtained from the family may be helpful in determining compliance with therapy or motivation for involvement (see the box at right). |
| 3. Inspect subcutaneous injection sites. | Problems with insulin therapy include lipohypertrophy or lipoatrophy, an increase or loss of subcutaneous fat that occurs as a local response to insulin. The areas may be unsightly and children often prefer these sites for injection because of decrease in pain perception. However, erratic insulin absorption from these sites results in difficulty with diabetic regulation.<br>***Special Considerations:*** *The best prevention of lipodystrophy is proper site rotation.* |
| 4. Determine blood glucose as appropriate (see Skill 120). | Diabetic management depends on this finding, which is usually performed before insulin administration. |
| 5. Request and analyze any family records about insulin administration. | Records may help determine patterns that relate to insulin dose, site selection, and general diabetic management knowledge base of the caretaker (e.g., food intake and activity level).<br>***Special Considerations:*** *Commend the family for record-keeping efforts. Reward the child appropriately with stickers, recognition, or awards.* |
| **Planning and Goal Setting** | |
| 1. Prepare necessary equipment and supplies.<br>a. Insulin (check expiration date).<br>b. Insulin syringes (0.5 to 1.0 ml; calibrated in units).<br>c. Alcohol swabs.<br>d. Band-Aid (optional). | Organization saves time and effort.<br>***Special Considerations:*** *Insulin strength must match syringe units: e.g., U-100 insulin must be used with a U-100 syringe. Disposable insulin syringes come with a preattached needle designed for accurate insulin dose preparation. A 0.5 ml syringe is marked in 1-unit increments, and a 1.0 ml syringe is marked in 2-unit increments. Syringes produced by different manufacturers may vary in the amount of space between the bottom line and needle. For this reason, use the same model and brand of syringe for consistent insulin dose.* |
| 2. Select an optimal time and place for educational interventions. | Learning to give injections is anxiety provoking to a family: controlling environmental factors improves teaching climate. |

**TABLE 106-1** Characteristics of Insulin Preparations

| Class/Name | Appearance | Source* | (Approximate Time in Hours) Onset | Peak | Duration |
|---|---|---|---|---|---|
| **RAPID-ACTING** | | | | | |
| Regular | Clear | B, P, B-P, H | 0.5 | 2-4 | 4-6 |
| Velosulin | Clear | P, H | 0.5 | 1-3 | 4-8 |
| Semilente | Cloudy | B, B-P | 0.5-1.5 | 5-10 | 12-16 |
| **INTERMEDIATE-ACTING** | | | | | |
| NPH | Cloudy | B, P, B-P, H | 1.5-2 | 4-12 | 16-24 |
| Lente | Cloudy | B, P, B-P, H | 1.5-2.5 | 6-15 | 16-24 |
| Insultard | Cloudy | P, H | 1.5-2 | 4-12 | 16-24 |
| **BIPHASIC** | | | | | |
| Mixtard | Cloudy | P, H | 0.5-1.0 | 3-4/4-8 | 16-24 |
| Novolin 70/30 | Cloudy | H | 0.5-1.0 | 2-12 | 16-24 |
| **LONG-ACTING** | | | | | |
| PZI | Cloudy | B, P, B-P | 4-8 | 14-24 | 36+ |
| Ultralente | Cloudy | B, B-P, H | 4-8 | 18-24 | 36+ |

*B, Beef; P, Pork; B-P, Beef and pork; H, Human.
Adapted from Travis B, Brouhard BH, and Schreiner BJ: Diabetes mellitus in children and adolescents, Philadelphia, 1987, WB Saunders Co.

## *ALTERNATIVE INSULIN DELIVERY METHODS*

### CONTINUOUS SUBCUTANEOUS INSULIN INFUSION (CSII)

Also known as insulin pump therapy (IPT), CSII allows insulin delivery through a pumping device attached to tubing and a needle placed in abdominal subcutaneous tissue and changed daily or up to every 3 days. The pump, with a cartridge of regular insulin, is programmed to provide a continuous infusion (basal rate) supplemented with a self-programmed bolus of insulin before meals and snacks. Although CSII most closely simulates nondiabetic insulin physiology, only a highly motivated child is a candidate for pump therapy due to the requirements for frequent blood glucose monitoring, knowledge of insulin dose adjustment and pump programming, care of an indwelling needle site, and troubleshooting problems with the pump. For detailed information about pump therapy, see Travis, Brouhard, and Schreiner (1987), and Tomky and Weinrauch (1987).

### MANUALLY OPERATED INFUSERS

Manually operated infusers are similar to CSII in that a needle remains in the abdomen; however, the protocol is similar to multiple daily injections because only bolus doses are administered manually. This method offers an alternative to expensive pumps and is an option for children who resist multiple injections. However, it may also be necessary to continue daily conventional injections of modified insulins, as the infuser administers only regular insulin (Orzeck, 1987).

### INJECTION PENS

Injection pens hold a cartridge containing insulin and are manually set with the dose to be delivered. Conveniently, pens eliminate the need for filling syringes and carrying bottles of insulin while continuing conventional insulin regimen. Adolescents especially may appreciate ease of use when in inconvenient environments, thus increasing compliance.

### PRESSUREJET INJECTION DEVICES

Although expensive, this method offers needleless pressurejet injection of insulin, useful for children terrified of needles. Some users report less pain with this type of injection, whereas others find them comparable to standard injections (Orzeck, 1987).

| Steps | Rationale |
|---|---|
| 3. Develop individualized child and family goals:<br>▪ Insulin will be correctly prepared and administered.<br>▪ Child and family will demonstrate adequate knowledge base and skill about insulin administration. | |

## Implementation

| Steps | Rationale |
|---|---|
| 1. Prepare insulin for administration. | |
| a. Double-check for correct insulin type, source, strength, and expiration date. | Double checking prevents errors. Insulins vary by their onset and peak action: short, intermediate and long; source: human, beef, pork, or beef/pork; and strength: U-100, with 100 units/ml as standard, although other strengths are available.<br>***Special Considerations:*** *Never substitute type, species, or strength for another without a physician's order.* |
| b. Inspect insulin for proper appearance (see Table 106-1). | Regular insulin is clear while modified insulins are usually milky or cloudy in appearance. Regular insulin that appears cloudy may indicate contamination with another insulin or a defective product. |
| c. Store and administer insulin at room temperature. | Injecting cold insulin can lead to subcutaneous atrophy, reduced rate of absorption, and local reaction. In the past, when insulin was less stable, it was stored in the refrigerator. |
| d. Turn vial upside down and roll gently between palms to mix. Do not shake. | Insulin is a protein substance, which bubbles when shaken. Rolling the vial allows crystals, which settle on the bottom, to mix.<br>***Special Considerations:*** *A modified insulin should not be used if it remains clear after it has been mixed.* |

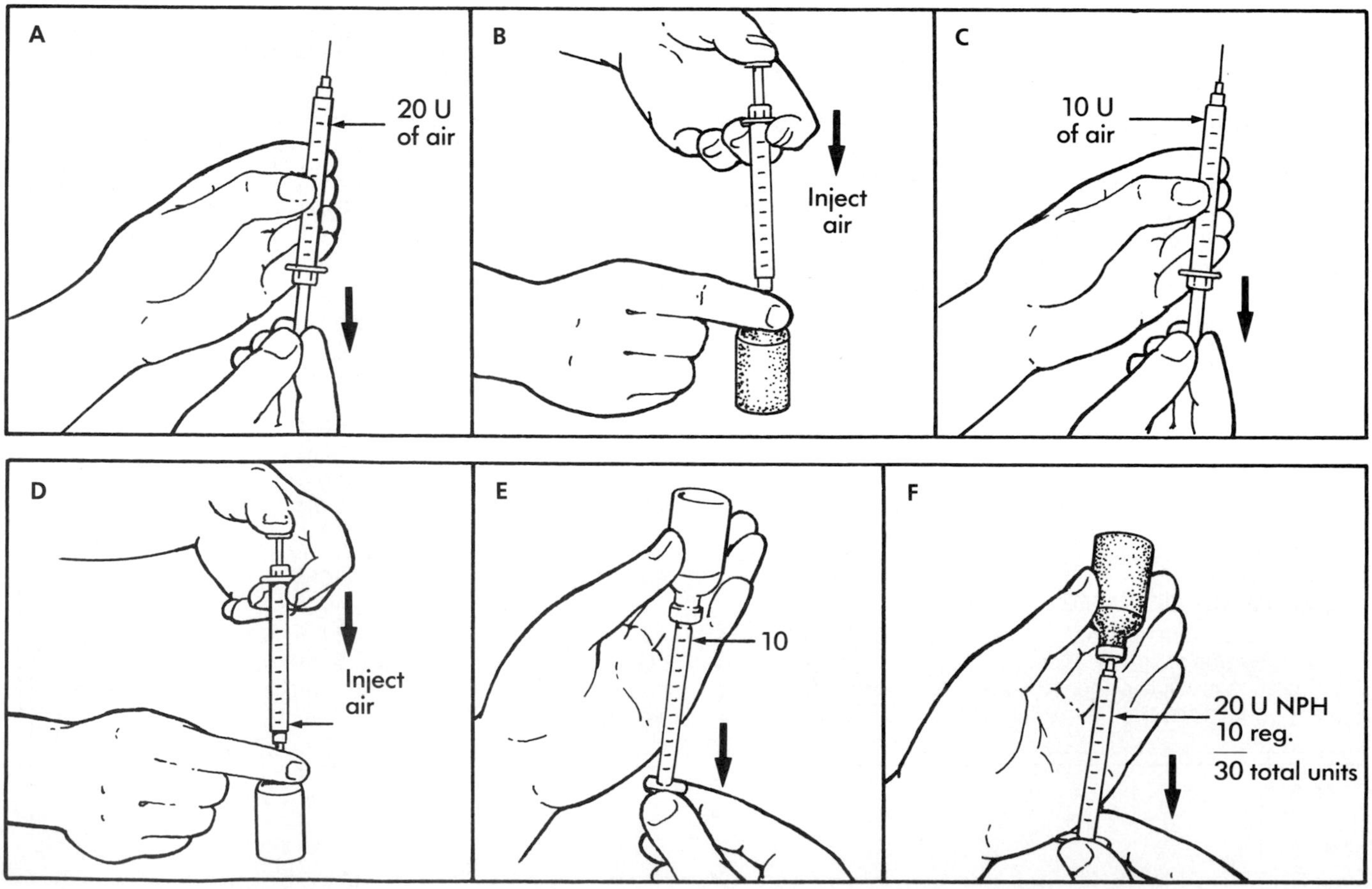

***FIG. 106-1*** **A,** Draw air into syringe equal to dose of cloudy insulin. **B,** Insert needle into cloudy insulin and inject air into vial. **C,** Fill syringe with air equal to dose of clear insulin. **D,** Insert needle into clear insulin and inject air. **E,** With needle still in clear insulin, turn vial upside down and withdraw correct dose. **F,** Insert needle in cloudy insulin and withdraw correct dose.

| **Steps** | **Rationale** |
|---|---|
| e. Withdraw ordered dose from vial into insulin syringe. To mix two types of insulin (e.g., regular and NPH) in one syringe for a single injection (Fig. 106-1): | Mixed insulins are given to provide glycemic control for a longer period. The most commonly prescribed mixture used with children is a combination of intermediate (usually NPH) and short-acting (usually regular) insulins. Preparing two insulins by this one syringe method ensures that the short-acting insulin, which is often needed in emergencies, does not accidently contain any intermediate product. |
| ▪ Clean the rubber stopper of each vial with an alcohol swab.<br>▪ Into vial of intermediate insulin, inject air equivalent to units to be withdrawn, then remove syringe. (Do not withdraw any of the insulin.)<br>▪ Into short-acting insulin vial, inject air equivalent to units to be withdrawn, then withdraw the units ordered. Remove any air bubbles.<br>▪ Insert needle into intermediate vial. Do not push any of the short-acting insulin back into the intermediate vial.<br>▪ Slowly withdraw ordered units of intermediate insulin. Remove air bubbles. | ***Special Considerations:*** *Families should be advised not to mix insulin more than 5 minutes ahead of time because of the binding characteristic of regular with modified insulin, leading to unpredictable onset and peak action times. A newer insulin product, which eliminates dual mixing, is 70/30, a mixture of 70% NPH and 30% regular insulin, which has predictable onset and peak action times.* |
| f. Always have a second nurse (or family member during teaching sessions) check insulin preparations. | This is a safe practice to prevent life-threatening dose errors. An adult should check a child's preparations. |
| 2. See Skill 101, Administration steps 1 through 5. | |
| 3. Select rotation sites for injection, palpating for masses, edema or tenderness (Fig. 106-2). | Although regular insulin may be given intravenously, most replacement therapy will be given subcutaneously. Because absorption rate varies with site (shortest in arm, longest in thigh) (Whaley and Wong, 1991), it is recommended that all sites in an area (e.g., right arm) be used before moving to another area, thus reducing erratic absorption patterns (Thatcher, 1985). |

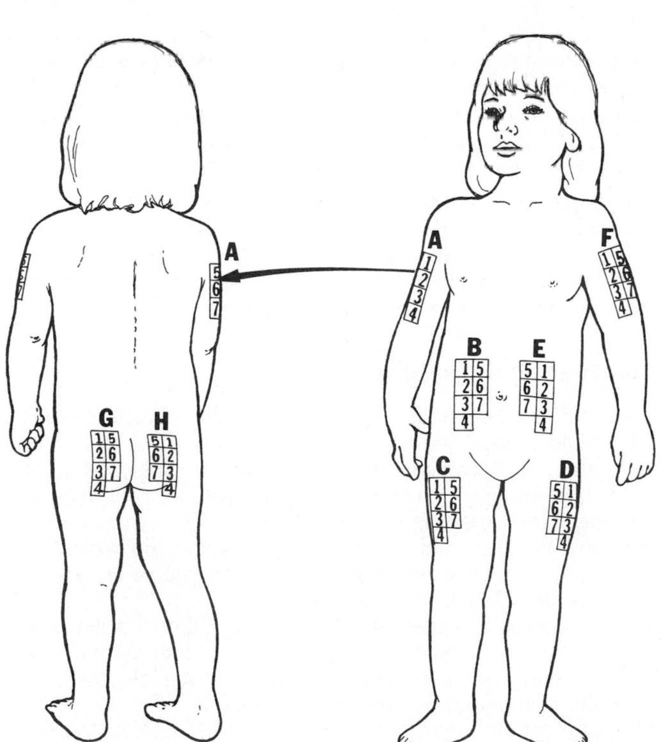


***FIG. 106-2*** Rotation sites for insulin injections.

**Steps** | **Rationale**

| Injection record | | | | | | | | |
|---|---|---|---|---|---|---|---|---|
| SITE | | 1 | 2 | 3 | 4 | 5 | 6 | 7 |
| right arm | A | | | | | | | |
| right abdomen | B | | | | | | | |
| right thigh | C | | | | | | | |
| left thigh | D | | | | | | | |
| left abdomen | E | | | | | | | |
| left arm | F | | | | | | | |
| left buttock | G | | | | | | | |
| right buttock | H | | | | | | | |

***FIG. 106-3*** Anatomical injection record.

From Perry AG and Potter PA: Clinical nursing skills and techniques, ed 2, St Louis, 1990, The CV Mosby Co.

***Special Considerations:*** *Check records for last administration site. An anatomic chart may be kept in medication Kardex or care plan for easy reference (Fig. 106-3).*

4. Inject insulin, following guidelines for subcutaneous administration (see Skill 105).

***Special Considerations:*** *Because of the rare possibility of entering a blood vessel, aspirating for blood after needle has been inserted is optional (Lewis and Smalldon, 1984).*

5. Dispose of needle and syringe properly. Do not recap needle unless it is to be reused.

***Special Considerations:*** *Although controversy exists about reusing disposable equipment at home, many diabetics do so to reduce costs. After each injection, the needle is wiped off with a new alcohol swab before recapping, then stored in the refrigerator (Fawbush, 1984). Some diabetics reuse a disposable for only one day, but it is accepted practice to reuse for 7 days (Whaley and Wong, 1991) as long as needle condition is acceptable. Poteet, Reinert, and Ptak (1987) found a low incidence of normal flora contamination on cultures of disposable needles and syringes reused by diabetics, suggesting that such low-risk calls for reconsideration of Centers for Disease Control (CDC) guidelines and most agency policies dictating that disposable syringes are strictly for one-use only.*

6. Teach child and family preceding steps.

Parents are often anxious about their lack of diabetic regimen knowledge, particularly that related to insulin and its administration (Hodges and Parker, 1987). Although a young child may not be capable of administering injections, he or she can usually participate in some aspect of care.

## Evaluation Outcomes

1. Correct type, dose, and mix of insulin are properly prepared and administered to the appropriate rotation site.
2. The child and family demonstrate knowledge of insulin.
3. The child or family correctly prepares and administers insulin.
4. The child or family demonstrates proper care of insulin and equipment.
5. The child or family keeps an accurate record of insulin administration.

## Observational Guidelines

A second person checks insulin preparation. Proper rotation schedule is documented.

Ask questions to validate knowledge about types, dose, and action of insulin. The child may enjoy a question/answer game format rather than direct questions.

Observe while the child or family demonstrates the procedure.

Assess use of aseptic technique, proper storage of insulin, and syringe unit disposal or storage.

Analyze records for essential elements: date, time, insulin type(s) and dose, site, reactions, and comments. Other diabetic management records kept simultaneously include glucose determination, food intake, and activity level.

## Documentation

Include date, time, blood glucose, insulin type and dose given, site, food intake, activity level, reactions, and comments. Note any teaching completed, including receptiveness to teaching, comments by the family, and degree of goal achievement.

### Home Care Modifications

1. Determine that child and family have the visual acuity and physical dexterity required to accurately prepare the correct insulin dose.
2. Family must understand what supplies/equipment are needed, where and how to obtain them, and financial resources to procure them.
3. Family must identify a clean, safe area in the home for preparing and storing insulin and injection equipment.
4. Teach family to prepare and administer insulin correctly.
5. Discuss importance of using the same brand of needle and syringe consistently.
6. Teach family essential insulin characteristics (e.g, appearance, onset and peak action times, expiration date) and interrelationships with diet, exercise, stress, growth and development, and emergency treatment guidelines.
7. Emphasize importance of a rotation site plan.
8. Assist the family to establish and maintain a record-keeping system.
9. Assist family to obtain diabetic identification for the child to wear should complications occur away from home.

# *SKILL* 107 Converting and Maintaining a Heparin Lock

*Anna L. Summerfield and Krena Hunter White*

A heparin lock provides a viable alternative to infusing fluids at a slow, keep-open rate when venous access is required or desired, but additional fluids are not. A heparin lock is especially advantageous in the care of children; these advantages include greater mobility and avoidance of unnecessary infusion of fluids. Heparin locks are most often used with children for short-term medication administration. Children requiring long-term therapy (e.g., with chemotherapeutics) often have central venous access devices placed (see Skill 110). Sometimes heparin locks are maintained for rapid venous access in an emergency, e.g., a child who may seizure, or to prevent an additional venipuncture for a child who may need to have a fluid infusion restarted at a later time.

An established IV site can easily be converted to a heparin lock, or IV access can be initiated and maintained exclusively as a heparin lock. Maintaining the lock consists of intermittent flushes of a dilute heparin solution or normal saline, per facility protocol, to maintain patency of the device.

### NURSING DIAGNOSES

Anxiety related to unmet informational need about purpose and procedure for heparin lock; Potential for infection related to invasive heparin lock catheter; Potential for injury related to adverse effects of intravenous medications.

| Steps | Rationale |
|---|---|
| **Assessment** | |
| 1. Review chart for the following information.<br>a. Order for heparin lock or conversion to heparin lock.<br>b. Time of last flush if already converted.<br>c. Documentation about site appearance.<br>d. Date and time of last site change.<br>e. Existing device, e.g., intravenous catheter with or without extension set, or butterfly (scalp vein) needle. | A physician's order is necessary to establish a heparin lock or to convert an existing infusion to a heparin lock. Additional information guides indicated interventions, e.g., site change, administering flush, and provides a baseline for further observations, e.g., site appearance.<br>***Special Considerations:*** *Follow facility policy about frequency of flushes and site changes. Heparin locks are usually flushed every 6 to 8 hours or after medication infusion.* |
| 2. Assess insertion site.<br>a. Intravenous catheter or butterfly (scalp vein) needle is intact and patent; tape is secure but not constrictive.<br>b. Signs/symptoms of infiltration, phlebitis, leakage, discomfort.<br>c. Child/family observations of the site. For example, ask, "Does the skin look any different to you from the last site check?" | Presence of one or more of these complications usually requires removal of the intravenous catheter and reinsertion at a different site. Validating assessment with the child/family promotes collaboration and instills confidence.<br>***Special Considerations:*** *Signs/symptoms of complications: redness (localized or along vein); pain; changes in skin color and/or temperature; swelling, burning, or stinging sensation; moisture on dressing at insertion site.* |

| Steps | Rationale |
|---|---|

## Planning and Goal Setting

1. Gather and organize supplies:
   a. Conversion.
      - Alcohol or Betadine swabs.
      - Injection cap (latex port adapter).
      - Extension tubing with injection site (T-connector) (optional).
      - Normal saline in a syringe to prime extension tubing.
      - 1 to 2 ml of normal saline in a syringe with a 25-gauge, ⅝ to 1 inch needle.
      - ½ to 1 inch tape.

Having all supplies collected improves efficiency of nursing care.
***Special Considerations:*** *An extension set minimizes manipulation of the catheter hub, preventing vein trauma during medication administration or flushes. An extension set may have been attached to the hub when the catheter was placed, requiring only an injection cap for conversion. Extension tubing is preattached to a butterfly needle; therefore, additional tubing is not needed.*

   b. Maintenance.
      - One syringe (3 ml or prefilled cartridge with flush solution) with 25-gauge needle (⅝ to 1 inch).
      - Flush solution: dilute heparin (10 to 100 units heparin/1 ml normal saline) *or* normal saline.
      - Alcohol or Betadine swabs.

A small-diameter needle helps maintain the integrity of the latex injection cap.
Instillation of a flush solution into the lock device and catheter/needle prevents a backflow of blood, thereby maintaining patency (Shearer, 1987).
***Special Considerations:*** *Follow facility policy as to recommended flush solution. See the box below for a comparison of heparin solution and normal saline flush techniques. Normal saline is recommended as the flush solution for a child with hemophilia (Gardner, 1986).*

2. Prepare equipment in medication room.

Preparing equipment out of direct sight of the child helps to minimize anxiety.

   a. Conversion: open injection cap and extension tubing package(s) and remove protective caps, using aseptic technique. Prime the extension set (if using) with normal saline syringe, attaching directly to extension set hub.

Expelling air from the extension set prevents an air embolus from entering the vein.

   b. Maintenance: assemble prefilled flush solution cartridge into reusable syringe case. Expel air from the cartridge.
      *OR*
      Draw 1 ml of flush solution into 3 ml syringe/needle.

1 ml is recommended to assure clearance of the needle or catheter (Hanson, 1976).
***Special Considerations:*** *Use Five Rights of Medication Administration (see Skill 101).*

3. Develop individualized goals of nursing care:
   - Prevent or minimize discomfort and/or anxiety associated with heparin lock conversion/maintenance.
   - Maintain venous access.
   - Prevent or minimize complications of a heparin lock, e.g., phlebitis/infection, infiltration.

### *HEPARIN OR SALINE FLUSH: STUDY COMPARISONS*

The original flush solution determined to be most suitable for heparin locks in the 1970s was a dilute heparin solution of 10 to 100 units of heparin/1 ml of normal saline (Taylor et al, 1989). Recent studies comparing traditional heparin flush with a flush of normal saline solution without heparin arose out of concern for potential systemic effects of heparin on clotting factors, needle stick injuries, cost, and nursing time considerations. The latter three concerns were related to the common practice of also flushing with normal saline before and after medication administration to avoid drug incompatibilities with the heparin flush.

Cyganski, Donahue, and Heaton (1987) compared the two methods and found that significantly more restarts were necessary in the saline-only flush group, and a higher incidence of phlebitis occurred. However, other studies have found the normal saline-only flush method to be at least as effective as heparin solution flushes, in terms of length of time the sites lasted and development of complications such as clotting, phlebitis, infiltration, and leakage at the site (Dunn and Lenihan, 1987; Shearer, 1987; Taylor et al, 1989). Significant cost and nursing time savings were reported as a substantial advantage for use of the saline flush (Dunn and Lenihan, 1987; Taylor et al, 1989).

One study (Shearer, 1987) reported use of the positive pressure technique as a possible factor for the success of the saline flush, as this technique was not a part of the heparin flush procedure. Taylor et al (1989), however, did not use positive pressure techniques with either method, and still found the saline flush to be adequate. More study of the effectiveness of this technique is indicated.

| **Steps** | **Rationale** |
|---|---|

## Implementation

1. Prepare the child/family for the procedure: explain the lock, how it works, and the conversion/flush procedure. Demonstrate on a model (see Skill 1).

Preparation increases knowledge, decreases anxiety, and assists the child/family to maintain as much control as possible.

***Special Considerations:*** *Include ways the child can help (if age-appropriate), such as cleaning the injection cap with a swab.*

### *Conversion*

1. Stop the fluid infusion on the pump and/or clamp the delivery set tubing.

When the delivery set tubing is detached, fluid will continue to flow if not obstructed by a roller clamp or the infusion pump.

2. Swab the connection site between delivery set tubing and extension tubing (or catheter hub) with alcohol or Betadine.

Swabbing the connection mechanically and chemically removes microorganisms, minimizing the risk of infection.

3. Maintaining asepsis, disconnect the delivery set tubing from the catheter hub/extension tubing.

***Special Considerations:*** *If tubing and fluids have not expired and will be used for intermittent medication administration, place a capped needle on the end of the delivery set tubing. The needle will need to be primed before use.*

4. Insert the primed extension set adapter into the catheter hub (if adding to the site). Securely connect by carefully pushing or locking adapter and catheter hub together (Fig. 107-1).
5. Attach the injection cap to the distal hub of the extension set or the catheter hub. Tighten by turning injection cap clockwise while stabilizing hub of catheter/extension set (Fig. 107-2).

The Luer-Lok feature of the injection cap allows a secure connection.

6. Firmly swab the injection cap with alcohol or Betadine.

Cleaning the cap with an antiseptic decreases the risk of introducing microorganisms into the vein. A firm swabbing motion assists in mechanical removal of microorganisms.

7. Insert needle/syringe of normal saline into the center of injection cap, stabilizing the catheter or extension set hub with the nondominant hand (Fig. 107-3).

The direct center of the injection cap permits easier needle entry. Stabilization of the hub prevents perforation of the catheter or extension tubing, and, if extension tubing is not present, decreases movement of the catheter in the vein lumen, minimizing trauma.

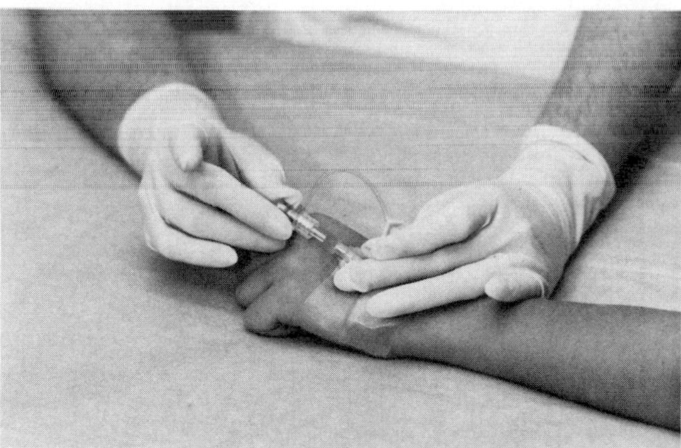

***FIG. 107-1*** Extension set adapter is attached to catheter hub.

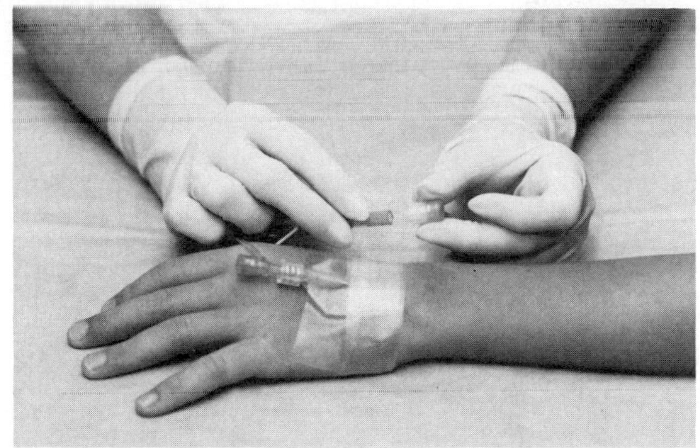

***FIG. 107-2*** Injection cap is connected to distal hub of extension set.

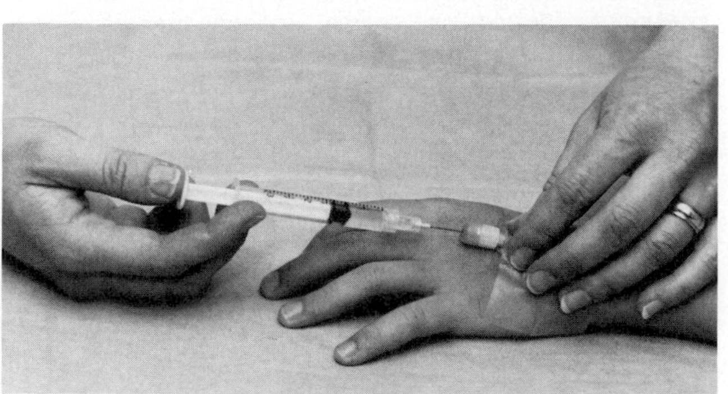

***FIG. 107-3*** Syringe is inserted into center of injection cap, while catheter hub is stabilized.

| Steps | Rationale |
| --- | --- |
| 8. Slowly inject 1 to 2 ml of normal saline. Observe site closely for tissue distension or "puffing." Note ease of flushing. | Excessive force or rapid injection may cause pain and/or infiltration. A normal saline flush following conversion allows verification that the catheter/needle is patent and positioned in the vein; absence of edema and ease of flushing are appropriate indicators.<br>***Special Considerations:*** *Do not verify patency by aspirating for a blood return, since blood may coagulate in the lock.* |
| 9. Withdraw needle, stabilizing catheter hub or injection cap. Follow with maintenance flush. | Stabilization avoids trauma to vein and/or tension on the extension tubing, and facilitates needle removal.<br>***Special Considerations:*** *If facility protocol is for normal saline flushes only, no additional flush is necessary.* |
| 10. Secure injection cap with tape (optional). Fold a small part of the tape end over to make a tab. Apply dry, sterile covering such as gauze or clear adhesive dressing to lock insertion site. If desired, apply stretchable, elasticized self-adherent covering (Coban) or additional gauze wrappings over site/extension tubing. | Covering the insertion site with a dressing protects from possible dislodgment or other trauma, and infection. Opaque coverings may help discourage the child from manipulating the site.<br>***Special Considerations:*** *Position coverings to allow easy access to the site for frequent assessment. An armboard may be needed to stabilize joint near the insertion site.* |
| 11. Reward the child's cooperation with statements such as, "Holding still helped us get finished faster." | Positive reinforcement increases self-esteem and interest in participating in personal health care.<br>***Special Considerations:*** *Visible reinforcers, such as stars or stickers, are usually effective with children.* |
| ***Maintenance*** | |
| 1. Inject flush solution, every 6 to 8 hours or after medication infusion, per facility protocol (see Conversion steps 6 to 9). | ***Special Considerations:*** *Heparin flush solution may cause burning or stinging if injected rapidly, or as a sign of irritation or infiltration. If the lock does not flush easily, do not use force, as a clot could be dislodged. Facility policy may specify a normal saline flush before and after medication administration to prevent possible drug incompatibilities, if dilute heparin is the flush solution.* |
| 2. Withdraw the flush syringe from the injection cap while injecting the last 0.5 ml of flush solution (optional). | Withdrawal of the needle while still injecting is a positive pressure technique, which helps prevent backflow of blood into the device (Shearer, 1987). |
| 3. Inspect site for complications at least every 1 to 2 hours, or according to facility procedure, removing coverings and dressings as needed (see Assessment step 2). | Although infiltration may only be noted during fluid infusion, other complications may develop, e.g., trauma/dislodgment, especially in an active child.<br>***Special Considerations:*** *Taylor et al (1989) reported significantly more leakage at the insertion site with heparin than with saline-only flush solutions.* |
| 4. Change heparin lock site according to facility policy or if complications develop. | Scheduled change of the lock and site decreases the potential for complications such as infiltration, phlebitis, and infection. |
| 5. Praise child for cooperation with each aspect of care. | |

| Evaluation Outcomes | Observational Guidelines |
| --- | --- |
| 1. Discomfort and/or anxiety associated with heparin lock conversion/maintenance is prevented or minimized. | Note child's level of cooperation with procedure. Listen to verbal statements, and observe nonverbal responses during procedure, such as crying when heparin solution is injected. Question about anxiety/discomfort after procedure. |
| 2. Patency of venous access is maintained. | Heparin lock flushes easily, with no signs of infiltration. |
| 3. Complications of heparin lock placement are prevented or minimized. | Observe site for redness, edema, leakage, burning or pain, blanching, coolness or warmth, or slight induration to palpable venous cord. |

## Documentation

Document conversion of continuous fluid infusion to a heparin lock. Follow facility policy for documenting flushes, indicating solution used. Describe assessment of the site; time of flush administration; amount, type, dilution (if any) of solution; type of dressing used, if any; any unusual response from child. Document family teaching and results of return demonstration, if the family will be performing the procedure.

## Home Care Modifications

See Wong and Whaley (1990) for instructions "Caring for a Heparin Lock" that may be photocopied and given to families.

# SKILL 108 Administering IV Medications

*Barbara Martin*

The intravenous route allows instantaneous and total drug absorption into the venous circulation, with almost immediate distribution to tissues and prompt physiologic action. With consecutive doses, predictable drug levels can be achieved to maintain therapeutic effects. In addition, after initial insertion, IV administration is more comfortable for the child than are other routes of parenteral injection.

The IV route, however, is also most hazardous. Untoward responses are more likely to occur, as high concentrations of the drug in serum and tissues are attained so rapidly. The drug, once injected, cannot be recalled, and patient responses may be grave. Therefore, extreme caution must be exercised when administering drugs IV, with attention paid to the Five Rights of Safe Medication Administration. Careful monitoring and immediate recognition of any adverse consequences are essential so that remedial actions can be instituted.

This skill outlines a variety of mechanical and manual techniques for administering drugs into an existing intermittent or continuous IV system; these include admixture; piggyback; delivery by volume control device; and injection: IV push by syringe pump, manual antegrade, and manual retrograde.

## NURSING DIAGNOSES

Anxiety related to lack of knowledge about purpose and procedures for intravenous medication administration; Potential for injury related to adverse effects of intravenous medications; Potential for fluid excess related to excessive intravenous fluid/medication intake; Potential for infection related to invasive intravenous catheter.

| Steps | Rationale |
|---|---|
| **Assessment** | |
| 1. Gather and analyze relevant data. | |
| a. History and nature of allergic reactions in the child and mother, if giving the drug to an infant under 3 months of age. | Allergic responses may be immediate with IV drug administration. Allergy to one drug may indicate allergy to another in the same class or one that is chemically similar. Antibodies to a drug to which the mother is allergic may be present in the infant under 3 months (Sager, 1980). |
| b. Child's responses relevant to the current drug regimen, including serum drug levels and levels of their active metabolites, if indicated. | The regimen can be evaluated by noting if clinical goals are being met, e.g., diuresis. Responses indicating toxicity or undesired side effects may be noted and should be reported before giving the drug. If appropriate responses are not being achieved, changes in the regimen may be indicated.<br>***Special Considerations:*** *The upper limit of the therapeutic range for a particular drug is fixed by toxicity, rather than efficacy. The level desired is usually in the center of the range (Goodman and Gilman, 1985).* |
| c. Child's status prerequisite to giving the drug: weight, vital signs, laboratory values, relevant medical orders or medical condition that would influence tolerance to or excretion of the drug such as low serum albumin and impaired hepatic, cardiac, or renal function. | Dose is frequently based on the child's weight. Condition of child may contraindicate giving the particular medication.<br>***Special Considerations:*** *If the drug seems inappropriate, further inquiry is essential.* |
| d. Assess the existing IV site for<br>▪ Redness.<br>▪ Swelling.<br>▪ Pain/tenderness. | Repeated IV drug administration depends on the ability to maintain vein patency. Any sign of phlebitis or infiltration indicates the need to establish a new IV site. Extravasation of some medications (e.g., chemotherapy, adrenergics) can result in tissue necrosis. |
| 2. Gather specific information pertinent to the IV use of the medication ordered. Refer to current, accurate, and complete guidelines for IV administration of the drug. | Safe administration of IV medications requires knowledge of pharmacologic guidelines.<br>***Special Considerations:*** *Clarify information about medication with pharmacist or physician before administering.* |

| Steps | Rationale |
|---|---|
| a. Action, indications and use, peak onset, length of action, and features of metabolism and excretion. | An understanding of the goals of treatment allows evaluation of the medication's efficacy in meeting them. Specifics about the drug are useful in appraising outcomes.<br>***Special Considerations:*** *Actual onset of drug action will vary depending on site of drug injection, dose volume, IV flow rate, and tubing size (Leff and Roberts, 1985).* |
| b. Precautions and contraindications: Consult the pharmacist or physician about precautions or contraindications that apply to child. | Any special precautions and/or contraindications referred to on the manufacturer's insert provide direction for assessment information needed before administration.<br>***Special Considerations:*** *Some drugs are not indicated for IV use or are not recommended for use with children. Insoluble substances, drugs with an oily base, and those that precipitate or hemolyze blood constituents (e.g., sterile water) should not be given IV (Goodman and Gilman, 1985). IM preparations often contain components that are contraindicated for IV administration (Plumer, 1987).* |
| c. Usual pediatric dose range: Validate any dose based on child's body weight or body surface area (BSA). Doses should be specifically stated if they vary from mg/kg or BSA determinations. (See pediatric dosage calculations, Appendix C.) | IV doses are frequently less than with other routes since all barriers to absorption are bypassed (Burman and Berkowitz, 1986). Pediatric doses have not been determined for all medications, so extrapolations from adult dose recommendations must be made cautiously.<br>***Special Considerations:*** *Doses calculated on edematous weight may be inappropriate (Gahart, 1985). If possible, determine pre-illness weight for greatest accuracy.* |
| d. Suitable dilution for IV use: Consult the package insert for specific directions for dilution. All diluents, and solutions must be suitable for IV use. | A drug that is soluble in one solution may precipitate another. Some drugs are incompatible with diluents containing preservatives or bacteriostatic agents. The incidence of phlebitis may be related to drug concentration and acidity. Drugs with low pH or those that are hypertonic should be diluted.<br>***Special Considerations:*** *The dose volume following dilution may exceed the child's hourly fluid restriction needs and overload may result (see Skill 64). The final dose volume will influence injection site selection. Small volumes may be completely trapped in Y-sites, T-sites, or stopcocks, and remain there or be bolused to the child when the site is flushed (Glass and Giacoia, 1987) (Fig. 108-1).* |

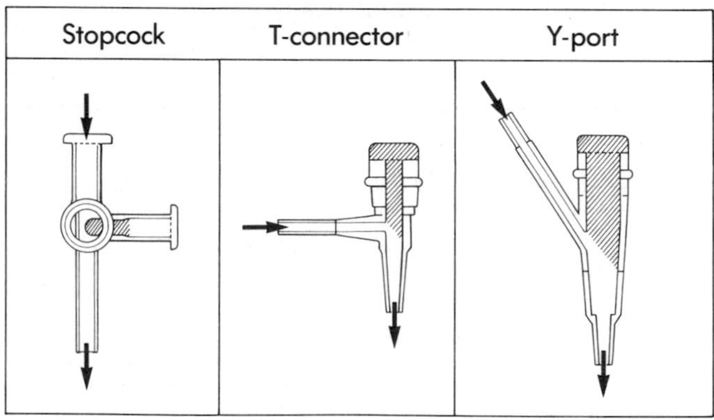


▨ Sites of dead space drug trapping

***FIG. 108-1*** Small drug volumes may become trapped in stopcocks, T-connectors, and Y-ports.

| Steps | Rationale |
|---|---|
| e. Compatibility and stability of all components of infusion system, including brand of IV solution, additives, flush solutions, type of container, filters, and tubing. | All components as well as rate of mixing, pH, and temperature affect solubility and compatibility of IV medications (Gahart, 1985). Once reconstituted, drug potency and compatibility may be limited. Inline filters are recommended for drugs that form particulate matter (e.g., mannitol), whereas others (e.g., digoxin, nitroglycerine, insulin) adhere to filters, glass, and plastic, thus reducing the amount available to child (Plumer, 1987).<br>***Special Considerations:*** *When a heparin lock is used, verify medication compatibility with heparin. If incompatible, use normal saline to flush the lock before and after the IV injection. Medication compatibility with hyperalimentation solutions must be verified before administration. Never mix additives with blood or blood products. Some drugs are light-sensitive and must be protected with an opaque covering, as, for example, in the case of medicating a neonate with phototherapy lights (Glass and Giacoia, 1987). If specific information is unavailable, clarify any questions about compatibility of components according to facility policy.* |

| Steps | Rationale |
|---|---|
| f. Rate: Check the manufacturer's recommendations or authoritative drug reference for rate of infusion. Most intermittent infusions should be given within 30 minutes to 1 hour. | The rate of drug delivery is an important determinant of drug disposition and action and should not vary from dose to dose. ***Special Considerations:*** *Distal injection sites and slow IV rates greatly prolong drug delivery time because dose volumes do not travel as a unit, but disperse within tubing, and may layer out (Leff and Roberts, 1985). Individualized problem-solving and consultation with the physician are indicated if dose volume and recommended rate of delivery exceed the child's fluid needs.* |
| g. Side effects. | Information about side effects enables recognition of reactions that may be associated with a drug. Undesirable side effects are more likely to occur with the IV route, particularly with rapid delivery rates, and must be reported immediately so that appropriate remedial actions can be taken (Gahart, 1985). |
| 3. Assess the existing infusion system. a. Type of infusion control device. | Familiarity with the system is essential to prevent errors in drug delivery. ***Special Considerations:*** *Infusion pumps with peristaltic action should not be used to deliver drugs with very short half-lives, such as dobutamine, as extremes in vital signs may result (Schulze et al, 1983).* |
| b. Existing lines and type of solution. | Fluid in an established line must be compatible with the drug. Medications often require separate secondary lines because of incompatibility with other drugs being given. ***Special Considerations:*** *The use of large-bore tubing with small-dose volumes greatly prolongs delivery rate and promotes drug layering. Small-bore tubing may be indicated (Glass and Giacoia, 1987). Polyethylene tubing is preferred over polyvinyl-chloride tubing, which binds with many drugs.* |
| c. Rate of primary infusion. | When the rate is slow and drug volume is small, a port close to the child should be selected for drug administration. However, if the maintenance rate is over 50 ml/hr, a distal volume control device or minibag piggyback setup is appropriate (Axton and Fugate, 1987). |
| d. Expiration date of system component(s) (see Skill 98). | Each component (e.g., IV solution, tubing) represents a potential vehicle for infection. ***Special Considerations:*** *Tubing change time should be standardized. Significant amounts of drug doses may be discarded with random changes of IV tubing (Lunn and Wilson, 1986). Any discontinued medication that remains in secondary lines must be discarded to prevent inadvertent overdoses.* |
| e. Drug injection port. | Flashballs, Y-sites, and injection caps become damaged with repeated use and may need to be replaced. |

## Planning and Goal Setting

| Steps | Rationale |
|---|---|
| 1. See Skill 101, Planning steps 2 to 5. | ***Special Considerations:*** *Validate that IV drug administration falls within the scope of nursing practice. Note any agency restrictions or exemptions about IV drug administration to children and administer only those medications approved in writing by the agency (Plumer, 1987).* |
| 2. Know availability and location of antidotes/emergency supplies (e.g., Benadryl, epinephrine, drug-specific antidotes). | Familiarity with recommended antidotes and the location of emergency supplies is essential to treat adverse responses. |
| 3. Determine the drug delivery method most appropriate for the child, based on assessment data (Table 108-1). | Decisions about method used should be based on the individual child's needs and type of medication ordered. ***Special Considerations:*** *Delivery rate, dose volume, and drug delivery site should be consistent to ensure that therapeutic results are predictably maintained. Calculating approximate drug delivery time to coordinate serum drug concentrations determinations is often the responsibility of several nurses who administer doses around the clock. If administration rates vary, serum drug levels may be inaccurate and adjusted drug doses may be inappropriate.* |

***TABLE 108-1*** **Planning Guide for IV Medication Administration**

| Method | Description | Indications for Use | Supplies |
|---|---|---|---|
| Admixture | Solution to which a drug has been added. | Continuous infusion to maintain a steady serum level of the drug that has been added, e.g., aminophylline nitroprusside, KCl, vitamins. CDC recommends that admixtures be performed by a pharmacist if possible (Sager, 1980). | IV medication and appropriate diluent, sterile syringes and needles, compatible IV fluid (250 to 1000 ml), IV tubing, alcohol swabs, label, 20-gauge 1½- or 2-inch needle. |
| Piggyback | IV medication dose is diluted in a separate container with a small amount of compatible solution (25 to 50 ml NS or $D_5W$). Container is attached to primary existing IV line and infused while primary solution is discontinued momentarily, then restarted when drug delivery is completed. | Intermittent infusion over a short period of time (20 to 60 min) so that peak drug levels are achieved. The drug may be given once or may be repeated at regular intervals to maintain desired therapeutic effect. Antibiotics are often administered by this method. | Drug in labeled minibag, secondary infusion tubing, date label for tubing, 20-gauge 1-inch needle, alcohol swabs, extension hook for primary bag (optional), compatible flush solution (if indicated) with administration setup. |
| Volume control set | Calibrated container that holds a small volume of compatible fluid to which IV medication can be added. | Less expensive than disposable minibags, but carry a greater risk of contamination with repeated entries (Sager, 1980). Useful in preventing inadvertent administration of a large amount of fluid, so with children used not only for drug administration, but also for primary infusion. | Syringe with prepared IV medication, label with child's name, room number, drug, dose, date and time, and rate of delivery; volume control container, date labels, ordered IV solution or flush solution (if indicated), alcohol swabs. |
| Manual IV push | Direct injection of prepared medication into an injection site over a calculated time period. In contrast to IV push, an IV bolus is rapidly injected when immediate drug serum levels are desired, usually in emergency situations. | When dose volumes are small or when IV medications cannot be diluted in large volumes (e.g., digoxin). Also if the IV rate is <50 ml/hr and cannot be increased for drug administration, since slow infusion rates (<25 ml/hr) are associated with significant drug trapping and drug dispersion and retention along the tubing resulting in unpredictable and prolonged drug delivery time. | Labeled syringe with prepared IV medication, 20-gauge, 1-inch needle, additional syringes with NS for flushing if necessary, alcohol swabs, watch with second hand. |
| Manual antegrade injection | An IV medication dose is injected toward the child into special microbore tubing that is attached to the end of the primary infusion tubing. An equivalent volume of primary fluid is displaced toward the child. The medication mixes with and is infused along with the primary solution at the existing fluid infusion rate. | For reliable drug delivery with slow primary infusion rates. It is advantageous when the following situation exists: IV flow rate is less than 20 ml/hr, the dose volume is 2.5 ml or less, and injection toward the child is safe (Fig. 108-2). Medication and primary solution must be compatible. | Syringe with prepared IV medication and label, extension of small-volume (microbore) tubing with three-way stopcock at distal end. (The low volume extension tubing must hold a fluid volume that is greater than twice the dose volume to prevent inadvertent delivery of medication by rapid bolus.) Sterile plug or injection cap for stopcock sideport, alcohol swabs. |

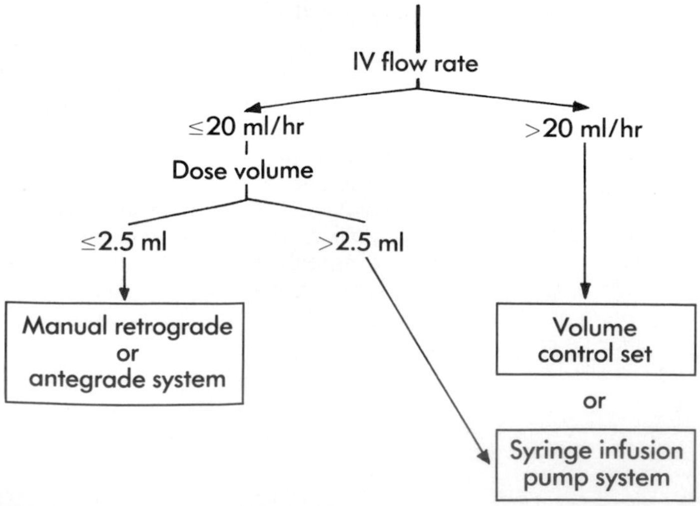

***FIG. 108-2*** Algorithm for selection of appropriate intravenous administration.

***TABLE 108-1*** Planning Guide for IV Medication Administration—cont'd

| Method | Description | Indications for Use | Supplies |
|---|---|---|---|
| Manual retrograde injection | IV medication dose is injected away from the child into special microbore tubing connected to the end of the primary infusion tubing with a stopcock. Medication mixes with and is infused along with the primary solution at the existing primary infusion rate. Use of multiple connections with this method increases risk of contamination. | Similar to the antegrade method, is useful when the IV flow rate is <20 ml/hr and the dosage volume is 2.5 ml or less (Fig. 108-2). The dose volume should not exceed half the hourly flow rate of the primary infusion. Prevents trapping of small dose volumes in Y- or T-sites, or in filter reservoirs. Medication and primary solution must be compatible. Retrograde is preferred over antegrade when primary fluid displaced by the dose volume cannot be injected toward the child. | Syringe with prepared IV medication and label, extension of small-volume (microbore) tubing with three-way stopcock at each end. (The low volume extension tubing must hold a fluid volume that is greater than twice the dose volume). Two sterile plugs or injection caps for stopcock sideports, empty sterile syringe to receive displaced primary solution, alcohol swabs, T-connector extension set. |
| Mechanical syringe infusion pump | Mechanical method allows dependable drug delivery at a precisely controlled rate independent of the primary infusion rate. The syringe pump, operated by battery or line power, administers the medication into an established IV line. | Expensive initially, but has many advantages: no adjustment of IV rates, no additional fluids administered with priming or flushing, visible drug delivery, and less time involvement. Recommended when the medication cannot be given by IV push, when the dose volume is small, but >2.5 ml (to prevent trapping), when the primary IV flow rate exceeds 20 ml/hr, and when the drug's specific gravity is higher or lower than that of primary solution (Leff and Roberts, 1985) (Fig. 108-2). Pump infusion may be preferable to retrograde and antegrade methods when absolute control over rate of drug delivery is a concern (Geyer, 1989). | Labeled Luer-Lok syringe with prepared IV medication (see model-specific instruction guide), syringe pump device connected to microbore or extension tubing with a three-way stopcock or four-way stopcock if used simultaneously with a primary infusion. See manufacturer's guide for storage instructions, battery charging calibration, alarm checks, and precautions. |

| Steps | Rationale |
|---|---|
| 4. Assemble necessary equipment for the selected technique of drug administration (see Table 108-1). | Equipment will vary with the method selected. |
| a. Medication (verify that drug is intended for IV use). | Not all medications are intended for IV use and are labeled accordingly. |
| b. Tubing: in-line 0.22 mm filter. | A 0.22 mm filter safely controls particulate and bacterial contamination (Glass and Giacoia, 1987). |
| c. Syringes (a separate one for each drug; size appropriate with volume prepared). | |
| d. Needles (large-bore needle to prepare drug in vial, e.g., 18-gauge and a smaller bore or filtered needle for drug withdrawal). | Entering the vial with a small needle may produce rubber fragments that are impossible to detect (Sager, 1980). Withdrawal of medication with a smaller-bore needle will prevent aspiration of particulate, possibly created by large-bore needle. |
| e. Sterile diluent as specified for drug preparation. | |
| f. Sterile IV solution as ordered or indicated for administration (e.g., normal saline). If IV medication is to be administered into compatible primary infusion, validate that ordered solution is infusing. | |
| g. Labels for containers and tubing. | |
| h. Tape for securing system components. | |
| 5. If necessary, establish infusion (see Skill 97). | |
| 6. Develop individualized goals of nursing care:<br>▪ IV drug administration is accurate, safe and timely.<br>▪ Child is monitored for desired response and undesirable side effects.<br>▪ Optimal therapeutic response is achieved.<br>▪ Fluid balance is maintained. | |

| Steps | Rationale |
|---|---|

## Implementation

### *Preparation*

1. Prepare label directly from original order: child's name, room number, drug, dose, solution, rate of infusion.
   As errors may occur in transcription, refer to original order.
2. Note expiration date on drug.
   Stability is not guaranteed if drug has expired.
3. Inspect medication for discoloration or turbidity.
   A cloudy or discolored solution may indicate intrinsic contamination, and the drug should be returned to the pharmacy.
4. In clean, isolated area, prepare medication according to manufacturer's instruction.
   Traffic generates airborne contamination (Plumer, 1987).
   ***Special Considerations:*** *A laminar flow hood is recommended to prevent airborne contamination during preparation (Plumer, 1987). Specific diluents and recommended volumes for reconstitution vary among preparations. The medication must be completely dissolved before adding to the IV solution.*
   a. Use noncoring technique for vial (Fig. 108-3).
   Noncoring technique prevents creation of dangerous particulate.
   b. Withdraw drug from glass ampule with filter aspiration needle and inspect prepared medication for particulate matter.
   This special needle filters glass particulate entering the syringe (Plumer, 1987). Visual inspection confirms solution integrity.

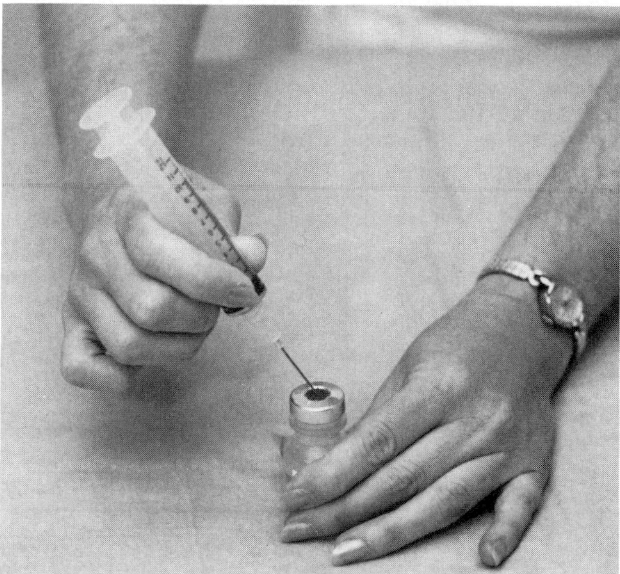

***FIG. 108-3*** Noncoring technique.

5. Recheck prepared label with empty medication vial or ampule.
   Rechecking verifies accuracy of preparation.
   ***Special Considerations:*** *It is helpful to have another nurse verify preparation. Agency policy may require a second check on certain IV drugs such as digoxin.*
6. Dispose of single-dose medicine container. If a multiple-dose container has been used, any remaining medication must be labeled with the following: child's name, date and time reconstituted, mg/ml in vial. Check drug label or insert for product-specific storage instructions.
   ***Special Considerations:*** *There is currently no CDC recommendation about discarding drug remaining in a multidose vial. The vial should be discarded when empty or on manufacturer's expiration date. Storage in a dark place or refrigeration may be necessary. Bacterial growth in some containers may be promoted by refrigeration (Garner et al, 1984).*

### *Administration*

1. Take prepared medication to child's room as soon as possible.
   Once reconstituted, medications deteriorate over time (Sager, 1980).
2. Assure child that needlestick is not necessary. Provide any necessary teaching about medication and its administration to child/family (see Skill 1).
   This assurance will prevent unnecessary anxiety and fantasizing. Perceptions should be explored, as many associate IV therapy with a grave condition.
3. Substantiate child's identity by checking ID band.
   Proper identification prevents error in administration.
4. Proceed with method of IV administration (see specific method section below).
   ***Special Considerations:*** *Wear protective gloves if exposure to blood is likely.*
5. Cover fluid container and tubing with opaque covering if indicated.
   Medications, such as amphotericin B and nitroprusside, deteriorate when exposed to light.

| **Steps** | **Rationale** |
|---|---|

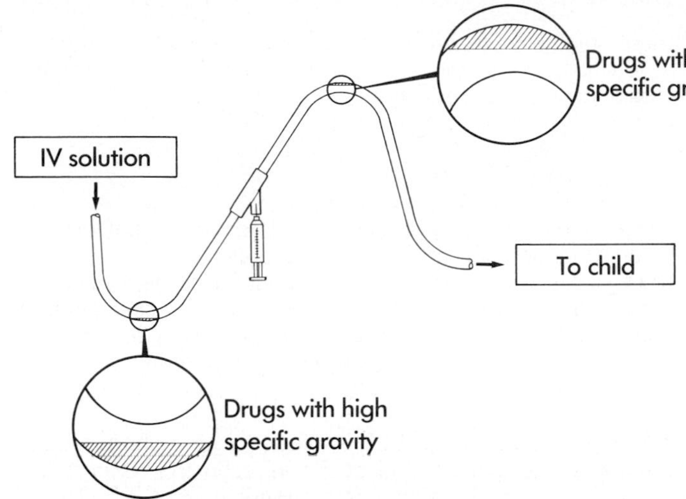


***FIG. 108-4*** Layering effect in IV tubing due to specific gravity. Drugs with low specific gravity accumulate at high points; drugs with high specific gravity accumulate at low points.

| Steps | Rationale |
|---|---|
| 6. If a mechanical infusion method is used, regulate infusion rate, and place infusion device out of child's reach. | Regulation prevents overdose and fluid overload. Access to the device may result in tampering. |
| 7. Position the child's arm/foot and hand so that they are level and ensure that no tubing hangs below the level of the child's arm/foot. If the tubing is very long, arrange it in a coil level with the child (Lunn and Wilson, 1986). | Drugs with high-specific gravity (e.g., KCl) will separate and layer in dependent loops, remaining trapped rather than moving toward the infusion site (Fig. 108-4) (Motz-Harding and Good, 1985). Drugs with low specific gravity will remain trapped in upward loops of tubing. |
| 8. Observe the child frequently during drug infusion. If this is the first time the drug is administered, remain with the child for several minutes. If the drug is being infused mechanically, check the child and inspect infusion site every 5 to 15 minutes. | Adverse reactions are more apt to occur the first time the drug is given, early in the infusion. Control pumps continue to infuse fluid for a period of time after fluid has infiltrated. Frequent checking for signs of overload or undesired response ensures child's safety. |

### *Adding medication to an IV solution (admixture)*

| Steps | Rationale |
|---|---|
| 1. Follow Preparation steps 1 to 6. | |
| 2. Prepare IV fluid container. | |
| a. For bag, remove injection port cover. | |
| b. For bottle, remove cap and latex overseal, setting cap down, inside facing upward. | Setting cap upward preserves sterility. |
| 3. Cleanse bag injection port or bottle rubber stopper with alcohol swab. | Cleansing assures antisepsis: sterility of rubber stoppers is not assured (Sager, 1980). |
| 4. Inject prepared IV drug into IV fluid container through:<br>a. Injection port of bag.<br>b. Rubber stopper of bottle at the designated injection site. | ***Special Considerations:*** *Injection with a long (1½ or 2 inch) needle prevents drug trapping at the injection site (Motz-Harding and Good, 1985).* |
| 5. Cover rubber stopper of bottle with swab and recap with cover or manufacturer's sterile additive cap. | The bottle should be covered to prevent touch contamination or loss of fluid during mixing. |
| 6. Agitate bag or bottle gently but thoroughly to mix drug with fluid. For bag, squeeze injection port. | The additive and fluid must be completely mixed to form a new solution. Squeezing port assures that the full dose is added.<br>***Special Considerations:*** *If there is to be more than one additive, each medication is injected and mixed thoroughly before another is added. The greater the number of additives, the greater the chance of instability.* |
| 7. Inspect admixture against both light and dark backgrounds for particulate matter. | If particulate is present, the solution must not be used |
| 8. Attach prepared label to container, adding date and time of admixing, date of expiration, and signature. | The label identifies the new solution and the person responsible for admixture.<br>***Special Considerations:*** *Never attach the label before adding the drug, as this would falsely identify the solution and might result in an administration error (Cohen, 1988).* |
| 9. For subsequent steps see Administration steps 2 through 8. | |

| Steps | Rationale |
|---|---|
| ***Adding medication to an infusing IV solution*** | |
| 1. Determine how much volume remains in infusing bag to calculate amount of medication to prepare. Example: if KCl 10 mEq is ordered to be added to 500 ml of solution and 300 ml remain, then proper dilution would require 6 mEq of KCl. | These steps prevent errors in preparation and administration. Adequate volume for dilution is necessary to prevent phlebitis, pain, or untoward effects. |
| 2. See Preparation steps 1 through 6 and Administration steps 1 to 3. | |
| 3. Validate that infusing solution is compatible with admixture by checking it against the prepared label. | Checking for appropriate solution will assure compatibility of admixture and prevent errors in preparation. |
| 4. Close flow clamp on tubing of infusing solution or stop infusion device. | The medication must be admixed thoroughly. If the medication is injected while the fluid is running, a bolus of concentrated drug could be delivered with grave consequences (e.g., a bolus of KCl could cause cardiac arrest) (Plumer, 1987). |
| 5. Remove infusion container from hook. | |
| 6. Swab bag injection port or bottle's rubber stopper. | |
| 7. Inject the prepared medication from the syringe to which 1½- to 2-inch needle has been attached. | If a dense solution (e.g., KCl) is injected with a short needle, some will remain trapped at the injection site, even if the solution is properly agitated (Motz-Harding and Good, 1985). |
| 8. Squeeze the injection port to expel all medication and gently, but thoroughly, agitate the fluid container. | Squeezing the port ensures that full dose is admixed and the intended solution is created. |
| 9. Affix prepared label to container, adding time of admixture, expiration date, and signature. | All fluid infusions must be changed every 24 hours (Plumer, 1987). ***Special Considerations:*** *Some institutions use a red label to readily identify presence of additives.* |
| 10. Rehang container. | |
| 11. Open clamp or start infusion device and proceed with IV administration. | |
| 12. Continue with Administration steps 5 through 8. | |
| ***Intermittent infusion of IV medication by minibag (piggyback)*** | |
| 1. Follow Preparation steps 1 through 6 and Administration steps 1 through 3. | |
| 2. If the intermittent IV medication is incompatible with the primary infusion, initiate and piggyback a compatible "flush" solution into the primary line at injection port near the child. | The "flush" is used to temporarily replace the primary infusion to assure compatibility during drug delivery. The volume required to "flush" the primary tubing will be dictated by the tubing volume between the site of piggyback and the child. Standard tubing holds approximately 1 ml/10 inches. |
| 3. Attach a 20-gauge, 1-inch sterile needle to end of secondary tubing. | A 20-gauge, 1-inch needle is preferred, as longer needles can puncture the primary tubing and smaller diameters may break and travel through the tubing (Plumer, 1987). |
| 4. Close roller clamp on secondary tubing. | If the roller clamp is not closed, medication and air flow uncontrollably on spiking. |
| 5. Attach expiration date label to tubing. | A date label provides information as to when next tubing change is needed. ***Special Considerations:*** *Tubing must be changed every 48 hours.* |
| 6. Using aseptic technique, spike minibag with secondary tubing. | |
| 7. Swab distal injection port of primary (or flush) tubing with alcohol. | Swabbing provides antisepsis for introducing needle into the system. ***Special Considerations:*** *If a heparin lock is used for administering IV medication, the needle on the administration set must be replaced each time. Use hemostat to remove and dispose needle, then replace with a capped sterile needle. This assures antisepsis with needle entry, but prevents needle stick injury.* |
| 8. Remove cap from needle on secondary line and insert needle fully into primary (or flush) tubing port near primary container (above the infusion pump). | This port location allows infusion pump control of drug delivery rate. |
| 9. Tape needle securely in place. | In and out movement of the needle can result in contamination and/or a safety hazard. |
| 10. Lower secondary bag and tubing and carefully open clamp to secondary tubing so that primary (or flush) solution back primes secondary tubing. Fill drip chamber less than half full, then close secondary tubing clamp. | Priming secondary tubing with the primary solution prevents loss of medication dose and inadvertent contamination of personnel and environment (e.g., antibiotics or chemotherapeutic agents) (Plumer, 1987). |

| Steps | Rationale |
|---|---|
| | ***Special Considerations:*** *With subsequent dose of the same medication, the same secondary tubing can be used and cleared of air, if necessary, in this same manner.* |
| 11. Suspend minibag:<br>a. At same level as primary solution,<br>*OR*<br>b. Lower primary container with extension hook so that it is 6 to 8 inches below minibag. | Lowering the primary container allows the medication to infuse and the primary line to automatically restart after drug in the secondary line falls below the solution level in the drip chamber of the primary container.<br>***Special Considerations:*** *A backcheck valve on the primary tubing is necessary with this technique. The one-way valve prevents the medication from flowing back into the primary container and eliminates the risk of air entering the line when the secondary bottle empties.* |
| 12. Clamp off main infusion above injection port if not using a lowered primary setup. | If the main infusion hangs at the same elevation as the minibag and is left open while the medication tubing is opened, primary solution will flow up into the medication minibag. |
| 13. Open clamp of minibag secondary tubing, noting time the medication starts infusing. | This allows the medication to start infusing into the primary line and permits prediction of completion time. |
| 14. Adjust the rate of infusion on the infusion control device or primary tubing below the injection port where the medication is infusing. | The rate of medication delivery should be consistent with each dose so that predictable outcomes are achieved. |
| 15. See Administration steps 5 to 8. | |
| 16. When the medication has completed infusing, clamp the minibag secondary line and open the primary (or flush) line, unless using a lowered primary setup. | Leaving the secondary line in place allows its use for subsequent doses of the same medication and reduces risk of contamination.<br>***Special Considerations:*** *A different drug would require its own secondary line, or complete flushing of any remaining drug from the secondary tubing if drug incompatibility exists.* |
| 17. Readjust the primary infusion rate as indicated. If heparin lock was used, allow flush infusion to clear the line of medication, then discontinue and flush according to agency policy (see Skill 107). | This rate may differ from the rate at which the drug was infused.<br>***Special Considerations:*** *If the primary rate is very slow, or if a flush solution substitutes for the primary infusion, maintain drug infusion rate to clear tubing of medication before resuming ordered rate. This assures that the complete drug dose is administered in a timely manner.* |
| ***Intermittent infusion with volume control set*** | |
| 1. Follow Preparation steps 1 through 6 and Administration steps 1 through 3. | |
| 2. If necessary, add volume control chamber to primary infusion.<br>*OR* | A volume control chamber may or may not be part of the existing tubing. |
| Assemble secondary line volume control chamber, tubing, and flush solution. Fill chamber with amount of solution sufficient to clear tubing of air, then attach 20-gauge, 1-inch needle to end of tubing and purge. Label tubing with expiration date. | A separate flush solution is necessary when medication is incompatible with the primary solution. |
| 3. Fill volume control chamber to one-half the volume rate/hour minus medication volume, then close clamp. For example, if volume rate = 30 ml/hr and medication volume = 5 ml, fill chamber with 10 ml of solution. When medication is added, total amount will equal 15 ml, one-half the hourly amount. | This method permits drug delivery in 30 minutes, an appropriate dilution unless specified differently on drug information or physician order (Axton and Fugate, 1987).<br>***Special Considerations:*** *Specify amount of dilution in nursing care plan to standardize administration.* |
| 4. Cleanse injection port of container with alcohol and inject prepared IV medication. Gently but thoroughly mix medication by rotating container between hands. | Injection site permits addition of medication in chamber. Vigorous agitation may cause air vent filter to become wet, resulting in container malfunction.<br>***Special Considerations:*** *If the medication is of high specific gravity, container should be rotated frequently during administration to ensure proper mixing of medication and dilution fluid.* |
| 5. Indicate time admixture prepared on label and attach to volume control chamber. | The label provides information about infusion and expected time of completion. |
| 6. If using secondary flush solution, piggyback into primary tubing line near child and attach needle securely with tape. | Less flush solution is required when piggybacked into port near child. |

| Steps | Rationale |
|---|---|
| 7. Install tubing on infusion pump (if not already done) and set rate and volume according to manufacturer's instructions. Start infusion pump. | |
| 8. Follow Administration steps 5 to 8. | |
| 9. When drug delivery is complete: | |
| a. For primary solution, fill volume control chamber with amount equal to hourly infusion rate. Resume ordered hourly rate. b. For flush solution, fill volume control chamber with desired amount solution for flush of tubing. Allow this amount to infuse, then resume primary infusion at ordered rate. | Amount of flush solution required to clear medication will depend on type and length of IV tubing used. ***Special Considerations:*** *If primary hourly rate is slower than medication administration rate, maintain drug infusion rate to clear tubing of medication before resuming primary rate. This assures that complete drug dose is administered in a timely manner.* |
| ***Administration of IV medication by direct injection (IV push)*** | |
| 1. See Preparation steps 1 through 6 and Administration steps 1 through 3. | |
| 2. Use alcohol to cleanse heparin lock site or injection port nearest the child on the primary infusion line. | ***Special Considerations:*** *The catheter hub on a heparin lock should be stabilized to prevent discomfort and vein irritation during swabbing.* |
| 3. For heparin lock, verify patency by injecting 1 to 2 ml of normal saline, observing the site during flush. | Patency assures that extravasation, tissue injury, and pain will not occur. The drug should not be given if patency is uncertain. ***Special Considerations:*** *Pressure may be applied on the vein an inch or so above the cannula insertion site while observing for a decrease in infusion rate or resistance to injection, indicating that the cannula is within the vein. Resistance or infusion slowing will not occur if the fluid extravasates. Observe the site for extravasation (Millam, 1988).* |
| 4. Insert needle of syringe with IV medication into the center of the site/port. | ***Special Considerations:*** *Although small-bore needles are less traumatic to the port, they are more apt to break off (Plumer, 1987). There has been no confirmed relationship between needle size and incidence of contamination of IV systems (Eggleston, 1984). Injection into a flashball is preferred over Y-sites or T-ports for small dose-volumes to prevent drug trapping (Leff and Roberts 1985).* |
| 5. Using the second hand of a watch, inject the IV medication slowly at evenly spaced intervals over the indicated time period. Assure that tubing is positioned level with IV insertion site. | IV push medications are usually given over a period of minutes (1 to 10 minutes or more). ***Special Considerations:*** *IV push should not be confused with a bolus injection, which is a discrete mass of medication injected rapidly when immediate drug action is desired in emergency situations (Zenk, 1986). When the injection rate equals the drug's clearance rate, serum levels are never achieved. Emergency drugs with very short half-lives, therefore, must be given by bolus injection (Roberts, 1981).* |
| 6. Observe the child closely during the IV drug push. | IV injection of concentrated drug presents a higher risk of adverse complications. As the medication is being injected manually, adverse reactions can be noted immediately. |
| 7. Upon completion of injection, withdraw syringe and needle (do not recap) and discard into proper container. | Proper disposal prevents inadvertent injury. |
| 8. For heparin lock, flush according to agency policy. | ***Special Considerations:*** *If the drug dose volume is very small (less than 0.5 ml), flush injection port to reduce trapping (Leff and Roberts, 1985).* |
| ***Administration of IV medication by manual retrograde injection*** | |
| 1. Follow Preparation steps 1 through 6. | |
| 2. Connect a three-way stopcock to the end of primary infusion tubing and attach microbore extension (Fig. 108-5). | The closer to the child the drug is given, the nearer actual delivery time is to calculated delivery time (Hargrove, 1987). ***Special Considerations:*** *Specialty sets such as the Benzing Retrograde Set (Medfusion Systems, Inc., Marietta, Ga.), or the Pediatric Retrograde Set (Quest Medical, Inc., Carrollton, Tex.) provide shear forces and velocity necessary to prevent small-dose dispersion, layering, and trapping that occur with slow primary infusion rates and standard size tubing.* |

**Steps** | **Rationale**

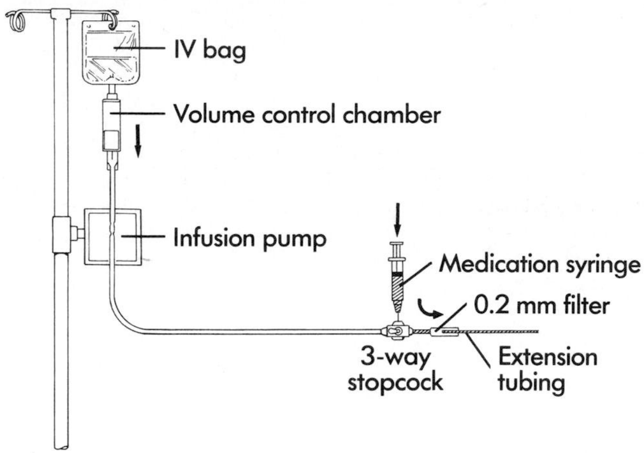


***FIG. 108-5*** Antegrade infusion.

3. Attach male adapter plug or injection cap to additive sideport of stopcock while not in use.

This maintains sterility of the sideport and prevents air from being sucked into the line during infusion.

4. Prime tubings and connect to catheter hub or heparin lock.

This prevents the inadvertent delivery of air during the infusion.

5. Follow Administration Steps 1 through 3.

***Special Considerations:*** *A variety of extension sets and injection ports are available. Dead space volumes of injection ports can equal a substantial portion of the drug dose when small volumes are administered.*

6. For medication administration, carefully remove protective male adapter or cap from sideport and insert and tighten medication syringe hub;

   *OR*

   swab injection site with alcohol at distal end of extension tubing (if there is no stopcock) and insert needle of medication syringe.
7. Turn stopcock to shut off IV flow to the child, or clamp tubing distal to the attached extension tubing.

This prepares the line for antegrade injection toward the child and into the microbore extension tubing.

8. Inject prepared IV medication.

This allows the drug to mix with the primary fluid in the tubing as it moves toward the child.

***Special Considerations:*** *An equivalent volume of primary solution will be displaced toward the child. If this volume is prohibited due to fluid restriction, use the retrograde method of injection.*

9. Remove syringe and reinsert protective sterile adapter into stopcock terminal if removed, then open stopcock to allow primary infusion to flow.

The sideport plug maintains sterility and prevents air embolism.

***Special Considerations:*** *Flushing is recommended at the side port to minimize drug trapping, although it adds steps to the process and increases fluid administration.*

10. Attach prepared medication label at injection site near child for duration of drug infusion.

This alerts others to the nature of the infusion.

***Special Considerations:*** *Drug infusion rate depends on dose volume and established primary flow rate; therefore, the tubing length/volume must be able to accommodate this.*

11. See Implementation section, Administration steps 5 through 8 on p. 694.

### *Administration of IV medication by manual retrograde injection*

1. Follow Preparation steps 1 through 6.
2. If necessary, assemble microbore extension tubing and stopcocks (Fig. 108-6). Attach distal stopcock to proximal end of primary infusion line. Attach proximal stopcock to extension set with T-port if it is not already attached to IV catheter.

Microbore tubing is preferred for delivery of small-dose volumes.

***Special Considerations:*** *Stopcocks are packaged with protective caps on injection ports. Extension set permits proximal stopcock placement close to but not directly at IV catheter hub.*

3. Prime tubing and connect to IV catheter hub or heparin lock.

Priming prevents inadvertent delivery of air during infusion.

4. Follow Administration steps 1 to 3.
5. Regulate IV flow rate with roller clamp, then release tubing from infusion pump.

Some infusion pumps will not allow the pressure created by retrograde injection. Manual regulation of IV flow rate is necessary to prevent fluid surge to child.

| Steps | Rationale |
|---|---|
| 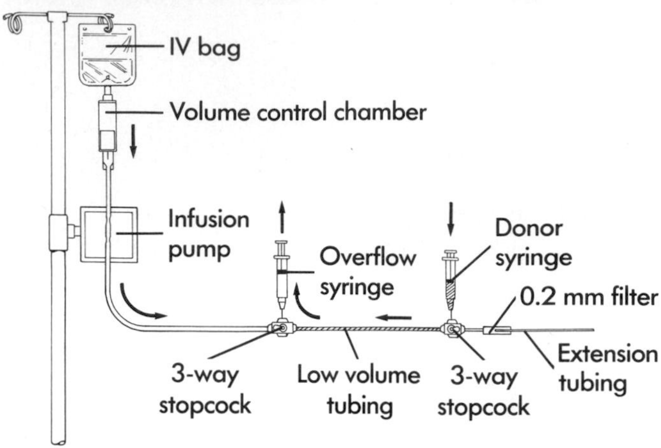 | ***FIG. 108-6*** Retrograde infusion. |
| 6. Attach medication syringe to proximal stopcock, and empty syringe to distal stopcock. Remove side-port adapter from stopcock and insert syringe hub into stopcock. Tighten syringe, using Luer-Lok if available. | Setup includes donor and receiving syringes. ***Special Considerations:*** *Different specialty sets will have various types of injection sites, such as injection caps, which will require modification in technique. Luer-Lok syringes are less apt to accidentally disconnect.* |
| 7. Adjust stopcocks.<br>a. Discontinue IV flow to the child via proximal stopcock, opening toward medication syringe.<br>b. Discontinue primary solution flow and open distal stopcock to empty syringe. | Adjustment prepares the line for retrograde injection and prevents forward flow of drug toward child. |
| 8. Inject IV medication using retrograde method into the low volume tubing, away from the child. At the same time, the empty syringe will passively accept backflow. Discard this solution. | Displaced primary solution volume is accepted into empty syringe. |
| 9. Remove syringes and replace sterile protective plug into each stopcock side port. | Plug maintains sterility of the side port. |
| 10. Reopen tubing by turning stopcock or releasing tubing at the proximal end of the extension tubing and at the distal end to reestablish primary flow.<br>11. Reinsert primary tubing into infusion pump and resume original IV flow rate for primary infusion. | This procedure reestablishes fluid flow toward the child. ***Special Considerations:*** *The fluid mixes with the drug and delivers it toward the child. No flushing is needed. The volume of the tubing and the primary infusion rate will determine the rate at which the drug is delivered to the child (Leff and Roberts, 1985).* |
| 12. Attach prepared medication label at injection site close to child while drug infuses.<br>13. See Administration steps 6 through 8. | The label alerts others to the nature of the infusion. |
| ***Administration of IV medication by mechanical syringe infusion pump*** | |
| 1. Follow Preparation steps 1 through 6.<br>2. Prepare IV medication using Luer-Lok syringe for the desired volume. The appropriate size syringe for the anticipated volume provides the most accuracy in delivery.<br>3. See Administration steps 1 to 3. | Luer-Lok syringes help keep dead space fluid volume to a minimum and are less apt to disconnect accidentally. |
| 4. Program the pump indicating:<br>a. Amount of fluid (total volume) to be infused.<br>b. Desired infusion period (total time). | These parameters establish the time it will take to dispense the loaded syringe. ***Special Considerations:*** *Different methods for calculating and programming are necessary for different pumps (see model-specific instruction guide).* |
| 5. Connect syringe to low-volume microbore tubing and prime tubing. | Syringe and tubing must be purged of air bubbles. |
| 6. Use 1-inch needle for inserting tubing into prepped injection cap or port, or connect tubing to T-connector with Luer-Lok. | ***Special Considerations:*** *For intermittent medication administration with a continuous IV, low-volume tubing may be connected to the primary infusion (if solution is compatible with drug to be given) or the syringe pump can be added at the stopcock terminal (Fig. 108-7).* |

| Steps | Rationale |
|---|---|

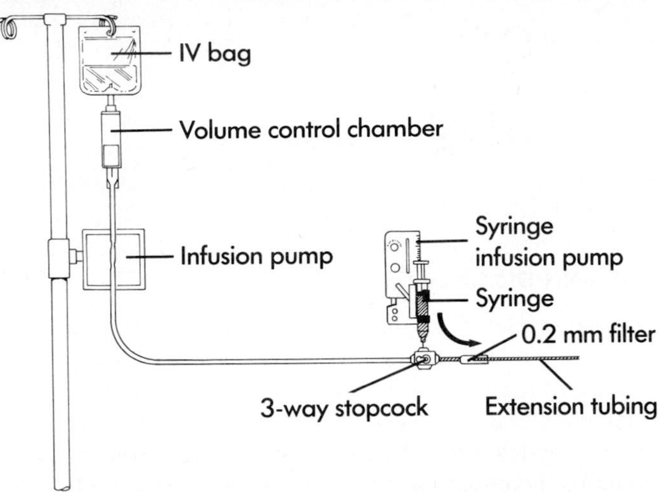


***FIG. 108-7*** Syringe pump infusion.

| Steps | Rationale |
|---|---|
| 7. Insert syringe into pump according to manufacturer's directions. | Following manufacturer's instructions assures correct placement of syringe into the pump. |
| 8. Affix prepared label to the assembly. | The label alerts others of the nature of the infusion. |
| 9. Turn on pump and begin infusion. | Infusion period timer begins as soon as the power is switched to ON position. |
| 10. Turn alarm switch to the ON position. | Alarm will sound when the syringe is empty, or if occlusion occurs (see manufacturer's instructions).<br>***Special Considerations:*** *If overdelivery is suspected, do not use; request servicing.* |
| 11. Follow Administration steps 6 through 8. | |
| 12. When infusion alarm sounds:<br>a. Remove empty syringe and replace with syringe of flush solution. Infuse according to previous steps. Upon completion, disconnect infusion. Follow agency policy for heparinizing.<br>*OR*<br>b. Continue primary infusion. | Alarm provides notification of infusion status. Flush assures complete dose delivery.<br>***Special Considerations:*** *Some pumps give a near-empty alarm, which signals that infusion will soon be complete.* |

| Evaluation Outcomes | Observational Guidelines |
|---|---|
| 1. The IV drug is administered safely and accurately. | Essential qualifying data are obtained before drug delivery: vital signs, serum levels, laboratory data, etc. Prepared dose is checked by another nurse. No signs of inadequacy or toxicity of dose are noted. No signs of injury related to drug delivery are noted: extravasation, phlebitis, infection. |
| 2. IV drug administration is consistent and reliable. | The drug is administered in a timely manner. Serum drug levels remain within therapeutic range. Therapeutic patient responses are consistently observed. |
| 3. Anticipated therapeutic effects (corrective or preventive) are observed. | Expected drug effects are noted: laboratory data, vital signs, other subjective or objective therapeutic outcomes specific to the drug administered. |
| 4. Child is monitored for untoward effects. | No signs of hemodynamic or respiratory compromise are noted. |
| 5. Fluid balance is maintained. | No signs of fluid overload are observed: tachycardia, tachypnea, adventitious lung sounds, edema, altered neurologic function, weight gain. |

## Documentation

In documentation, include date, time, any pertinent qualifying preadministration data assessed (e.g., vital signs) as well as IV medication, dose, type of diluent, prepared dose volume, site of administration, rate of administration, type of flush solutions and their amount (add all solution volumes to the intake and output record), and observable outcomes. Note frequent verification of vein patency, especially with vasoactive or vesicant medications.

# SKILL 109 Administering Chemotherapy

*Cecilia E. Shaw*

Administering chemotherapy is a skill increasingly needed by general pediatric nurses, as well as those working in specialized oncology settings. This skill focuses on safety features of administering chemotherapy via a free-flowing solution at a peripheral IV site. For administration of chemotherapy via a central line, steps of this skill specific to chemotherapy may be applied to Skill 111. This skill is intended to provide general guidelines; the nurse is encouraged to seek out specialized information needed to administer specific drugs and follow facility policies.

## NURSING DIAGNOSES

Anxiety related to invasive procedure, anticipation of pain and/or lack of knowledge about chemotherapeutic medications; Potential for injury related to side effects, adverse effects, and/or vesicant extravasation; Potential fluid volume deficit related to excessive losses from nausea/vomiting; Potential for infection related to invasive IV catheter.

| Steps | Rationale |
|---|---|
| **Assessment** | |
| 1. Assess: | |
| a. Child's age, height, weight, and developmental level. | Developmental factors must be considered when administering IV medications. The child's height and weight are essential for body surface area (BSA) dose calculations. |
| b. Willingness and ability to cooperate. | ***Special Considerations:*** *Information about procedures must be presented at a level which the child can understand.* |
| c. Previous experience with chemotherapy.<br>▪ Drugs given.<br>▪ Antiemetic regimen.<br>▪ Physical and emotional reactions. | Chemotherapy history provides information about tolerance and toxicity experiences. Prior techniques that worked well and with which the child is comfortable may be revealed. |
| d. Allergy/anaphylaxis or previous toxicity history. | Previous drug hypersensitivity reactions place children at high risk for anaphylactic reactions. |
| 2. Assess physiologic readiness for chemotherapy. | |
| a. Laboratory data such as red blood cell, white blood cell, hemoglobin, hematocrit, platelets, and absolute neutrophil count (ANC) (Walters, 1990): $\text{ANC} = \dfrac{\text{WBC} \times \%\ (\text{segs} + \text{bands})}{100}$ | Protocols specify parameters of these tests for chemotherapy administration. Guidelines for chemotherapy modifications or deletions are included in the protocol. |
| b. Hydration status (see Skill 64). | Adequate hydration is essential for circulation, metabolism, and excretion of chemotherapy. |
| c. Kidney and liver function. | Pretreatment tests evaluate the organ systems involved in drug metabolism and excretion, as well as those vulnerable to toxic drug effects.<br>***Special Considerations:*** *Tests ordered are often drug/protocol specific, e.g., blood urea nitrogen, creatinine, SGPT, SGOT, 24-hour creatinine clearance, alkaline phosphatase.* |
| d. Cardiac function (if anthracyclines are to be given). | Baseline as well as ongoing studies for cardiac function are required with anthracycline administration. |
| e. Vital signs. | Vital signs provide baseline data for future comparison. |
| 3. Assess peripheral IV site carefully for location, duration, and signs of integrity and patency. If an IV line needs to be established, see Skill 97. | A site with maximal soft tissue coverage and distance from joints minimizes impairment and loss of function if extravasation occurs. Sites older than 48 hours have increased incidence of infection and phlebitis, although the age of site does not automatically exclude its use. A good blood return is preferable, but does not guarantee vein integrity. |

**Steps** | **Rationale**

***Special Considerations:*** *Routine site changes are unrealistic when veins are scarce and extensive chemotherapy is anticipated. However, careful monitoring of vein status is essential. Placement of a central venous access device is generally recommended when veins are scarce or if intensive chemotherapy with vesicants is planned (see Skill 111). Scalp vein use in infants is strongly contraindicated with vesicants.*

## Planning and Goal Setting

1. Review orders or protocol and drug information for chemotherapy ordered:
   a. Accuracy of dose based on child's BSA (see Appendix C).
   b. Timing of medications.
   c. Dilution requirements.
   d. Rate of infusion.
   e. Usual side effects.

Research protocols are designed to compare varying durations of infusion, time sequence and dilution methods, and drug combinations in relation to effects and efficacy. Adherence to protocol specifications helps to ensure accurate research results.

   f. Vesicant potential (drugs that may cause tissue necrosis if infiltrated).

Vesicant drugs are those that, if infiltrated, may cause tissue necrosis, e.g., doxorubicin, dactinomycin, vincristin.

   g. Drug stability and light sensitivity.

After reconstitution, drugs have variable stability. A light-sensitive drug must be protected with a brown or opaque paper or plastic covering.

2. Gather supplies.
   a. Antiemetic and chemotherapy medications (for preparation of IV medications, see Skill 108). Label syringes with child's name, date, drug name, and dose.

***Special Considerations:*** *If chemotherapy reconstitution/mixing is necessary, it should be done under a laminar flow hood. Avoid using positive pressure within vials in order to prevent the escape of drugs into the environment. Dispensing pins, which filter outgoing air, should be used during drug preparation (APON, 1987). Two qualified persons should double check all medications as a safety precaution. Pregnant staff should not prepare, administer, or dispose of cytotoxic agents.*

   b. Extravasation tray (for vesicants). Have appropriate emergency drugs (e.g., Adrenalin, Solu-Cortef, and Benadryl) and resuscitation equipment available according to facility's protocol.

Prompt intervention will help minimize tissue damage as a result of infiltration of chemotherapeutic agents.

***Special Considerations:*** *A high incidence of anaphylaxis has been reported with asparaginase, bleomycin, and cisplatin.*

   c. Povidone-iodine, iodophor and/or alcohol prep pads.

***Special Considerations:*** *If using iodophor instead of iodine, do not follow with alcohol wipe due to the neutralizing effect of alcohol (Knobf, 1982).*

   d. Tape and self-adherent bandage.
   e. Compatible IV flush solution and tubing (primed and connected).

***Special Considerations:*** *If tubing is primed directly with chemotherapy, avoid contamination of self, others, and environment.*

   f. Surgical latex or designated chemotherapy administration gloves (nonpowdered).

Surgical latex gloves are less permeable to chemotherapy drugs than polyvinyl chloride (PVC) and provide the best protection available from exposure to possible carcinogens (OSHA, 1986). The danger to hospital personnel from handling a cytotoxic drug is a combination of its inherent toxicity and the extent to which workers are directly exposed to the drug in the course of carrying out their duties (Powers, 1985).

   g. Gown (optional).

***Special Considerations:*** *If a gown is used, the guidelines published by the Occupational Safety and Health Act (OSHA, 1986) recommend one that is disposable, made of lint-free, low permeability fabric with a closed front, long sleeves, and elastic or knit cuffs.*

   h. Luer-Lok syringes.

The Luer-Lok feature ensures tight connections and lessens chance of accidental leakage/spills.

   i. Adhesive bandage.
   j. Plastic-backed absorbent pad.

In case of accidental leakage or spill, the pad will contain the spread of drug and minimize exposure.

   k. Toxic waste container.

A toxic waste container prevents contamination of the outside environment with cytotoxic waste materials produced in the course of using cytotoxic drugs (Powers, 1985).

| Steps | Rationale |
|---|---|
| | ***Special Considerations:*** *Legislation about toxic waste disposal varies greatly with state, county, and city laws. Consult as needed with local hospital occupational hygienist, agency attorney, or Environmental Protection Agency (EPA) representative.* |
| 3. Time administration of antiemetic for when maximum effect is desired. | Administering antiemetic within sufficient time preceding chemotherapy provides maximum beneficial effect. |
| 4. Provide teaching about drugs, including purpose and expected and/or potential toxicities. Instruct child and family to immediately report discomfort at site, burning, or unusual sensations, e.g. itching or tightness in throat. | The family should be equipped with information about the child's regimen. Enlisting assistance in detecting treatment side effects or classic signs and symptoms of vesicant extravasation or anaphylaxis allows early intervention to prevent complications and facilitate dose/drug modification. |
| 5. Develop individualized nursing goals of care:<br>▪ Chemotherapy drugs are administered without incidence of extravasation, anaphylaxis or unacceptable side effects.<br>▪ Chemotherapy is prepared and administered safely, preventing exposure of staff and others to cytotoxic substances. | |

## Implementation

| Steps | Rationale |
|---|---|
| 1. See General Implementation steps for IV medication administration in Skill 108. | |
| 2. Put on gloves and place absorbent pad beneath injection site. | Gloves and pad provide protection from exposure to cytotoxic drugs. |
| 3. Connect primed IV tubing with flush solution to peripheral IV catheter hub. Allow flush solution to infuse rapidly for 2 to 3 minutes. | A rapid bolus of solution will quickly reveal infiltration. |
| 4. Secure IV tubing with liberal use of tape or self-adherent bandage, maintaining visibility of insertion site. | Well-secured tubing prevents inadvertent dislodgment or disconnection. Insertion site should be easily visible to detect infiltration. |
| 5. Position child comfortably, allowing for movement to recumbent position. | In case of anaphylaxis, the child's position can be easily changed. |
| 6. Swab most distal Y-port of IV tubing with povidone-iodine prep followed by alcohol. | Cleansing promotes aseptic entry. |
| 7. Insert needle of chemotherapy syringe into port. | |
| 8. Aspirate for blood return. | Patency should be verified before administering vesicant drugs due to potential for tissue damage.<br>***Special Considerations:*** *Although desired, blood return is not always obtained even though vein may be patent. If large amounts of flush solution infuse without infiltration, consider giving nonvesicant chemotherapy. If vesicant drugs are to be administered and blood return is not obtained, restart IV.* |
| 9. Slowly administer chemotherapy over recommended time via free-flowing IV solution. | The rate of injection varies with each drug, based on dose dilution, volume, and potential for adverse reaction.<br>***Special Considerations:*** *This information is often provided on the medication label, in chemotherapy texts, or by a pharmacist.* |
| a. If administering several drugs, give the vesicants first. | More caustic drugs should be given before the vein has been subjected to any other irritants, although this practice is controversial (Oncology Nursing Society, 1988). |
| b. Verify blood return after every 1 to 2 ml of vesicant drug, observing for infiltration, listening for reports of pain/burning, and assessing for signs/symptoms of anaphylactic reaction. | If infiltration occurs, chemotherapy must be immediately discontinued.<br>***Special Considerations:*** *If infiltration occurs, leave the needle in place to maintain access for protocol treatment. Proceed with facility extravasation or anaphylactic protocol as indicated.* |
| c. If the child reports burning, check for blood return. If good blood return is obtained, slow the flow rate. | Certain drugs use an alcohol diluent and are irritating, e.g., carmustine. A slower rate may decrease burning sensation. |
| d. Do not inject chemotherapy so forcefully that flow of solution in the drip chamber stops. | This indicates excess pressure, which may cause the vein to rupture, resulting in extravasation of drug (Goodman, 1981). |
| 10. When infusion is complete, withdraw needle from injection port. | |
| a. Use alcohol pad to absorb any fluid that escapes from the port/needle. | This precaution minimizes the spread of chemotherapy drugs and protects others from unnecessary exposure (Powers, 1985). |

| Steps | Rationale |
|---|---|
| 11. Repeat steps 5 to 10 for each drug prescribed, allowing flush solution to clear tubing between drugs and after last drug. | A flush prevents inadvertent drug interaction. ***Special Considerations:*** *Amount of flush solution should be individualized to child's needs, e.g., older child may be able to tolerate a 25 ml flush, an amount which would be excessive for an infant (see Skill 64).* |
| 12. Dispose of equipment and/or any contaminated laundry according to facility policy. | Proper handling protects the facility, staff, and outside environment from contamination with cytotoxic waste materials produced in the course of using cytotoxic drugs (Powers, 1985). |
| 13. Praise child for cooperation. | |
| 14. Reinforce expected effects and need to notify nurse immediately should any unexpected reactions occur. | The child and family should be active participants in monitoring reactions to medication. Untoward reactions are often noticed earlier by family members who know the child best. |
| 15. Check child periodically to evaluate response to medications. | Monitoring child provides information about medication's therapeutic effect or onset of side effects or allergic reactions. ***Special Considerations:*** *Treatment side effects may appear 7 to 10 days after administration and following discharge; provide adequate teaching for families about side effects and appropriate interventions. Telephone contact following discharge provides valuable support for families.* |

| Evaluation Outcomes | Observational Guidelines |
|---|---|
| 1. Prescribed chemotherapy is administered safely and without complications related to administration technique. | Review medication administration record and compare to orders/protocol. Note intact IV site without evidence of extravasation (redness, infiltration) or reports by the child of burning or pain at the site. The child does not exhibit any immediate skin reactions or change in respiratory rhythm, rate, or depth attributable to drug administration. |
| 2. Exposure of staff and others to cytotoxic substances is prevented. | Monitor chemotherapy preparation and administration for technique, use of gown, gloves, spill pad, and proper handling of contaminated laundry or disposable equipment. |

## Documentation

Record drug(s) and dose of each medication administered; flush solution and amount infused; blood return, including frequency of verification; duration of infusion; prescribing physician, RN administering; child and family response; any expected side effects or unexpected events during administration and interventions taken.

# SKILL 110 Maintaining Central Venous Access Devices

Janet Ludgar

Central venous access devices (VADs) are catheters or infusion ports designed to provide prolonged and frequent access to venous circulation for treatment requiring long-term administration of medications, nutrients, or blood transfusions, as well as frequent blood sampling. There are two types of VADs, each type having unique advantages and disadvantages. Partially implanted devices (PIDs), such as Hickman, Broviac, or Groshong catheters, are more visible and more accessible but require more maintenance care. Totally implanted devices (TIDs), such as Port-A-Cath, Infus-A-Port, or Mediport, require skin puncture for access but are less visible, requiring less care.

PIDs, also known as right atrial catheters, are threaded internally to a major blood vessel, leaving the distal end protruding from the skin. Devices are available for both long- and short-term use, with or without valves, and with single or multiple lumens in assorted sizes (Marcoux, Fisher and Wong, 1990). The long-term PID is inserted more commonly under general anesthesia in children and threaded subcutaneously from the desired exit site to the vein insertion site where a small incision is made. The proximal end of the catheter is usually inserted into the subclavian vein to the junction of the superior vena cava and right atrium of the heart. One or two Dacron cuffs located on the catheter section placed in the subcutaneous tunnel help secure the catheter once tissue adheres to the cuff, usually within 2 to 4 weeks. The cuff also provides a barrier for bacteria, thus decreasing the incidence of infection. Short-term PIDs are not tunneled subcutaneously nor do they have Dacron cuffs. They have been used as long as 6 months, as opposed to PIDs, which can be used 2 or more years.

The TID's catheter placement is similar to the long-term PID; however, the catheter does not exit the skin. Instead, the catheter attaches to a port, which is placed in a subcutaneous pocket. The port septum is thick silicone and is self-sealing when punctured with a noncoring needle. Ports are available in a variety of materials and designs as well as single or double reservoirs. The skin parallel port has a side septum rather than a top entry. Side entry access ports have various advantages such as decreased resistance to flow rate, easier aspiration of blood, and improved ability to secure needle placement. TIDs are thought to have decreased risk of infection over PIDs because they are not continually exposed to the external environment. This issue remains debatable and requires further research (Marcoux, Fisher and Wong, 1990).

This skill describes one systematic, principle-based approach to VAD care that may vary considerably with different facilities and agencies. Proven standards of care for these devices have yet to be developed. If available, consult policy on VAD care for agency variations.

## NURSING DIAGNOSES

Anxiety related to unmet informational needs about the purpose, care and prevention of complications for venous access devices; Potential for impaired skin integrity related to tape allergy or body rejection of venous access device; Potential for infection related to continual exposure of partially implanted devices to external environment; Body image disturbance related to venous access catheter placement.

| Steps | Rationale |
|---|---|
| **Assessment** | |
| 1. Assess the child's medical diagnosis, history, primary purpose for using venous access device, type of device used, and any allergies, e.g., iodine. | Assessing data about child's medical history and purpose for venous access device allows evaluation of child's responses, provides a helpful teaching plan for the family, and promotes appropriate care planning related to specific device. |
| 2. Assess child for elevated temperature or other generalized symptoms of infection such as lethargy or anorexia. | Elevated temperature, lethargy or anorexia, could indicate infection at insertion or exit site as well as systemically. |
| 3. Review child's record for information on:<br>a. Previous observations of site and catheter.<br>b. Date and time of last dressing change. | Previous observations provide a baseline for comparing sites and catheter placement.<br>***Special Considerations:*** *PID gauze dressings should be changed at least three times a week and when wet or soiled; once a week is suggested for transparent dressings. Postoperatively, TIDs have a dressing, which is usually removed 1 to 2 days after surgery. Some agencies require that immunosuppressed children have insertion and exit site care with dressing change daily. Refer to specific agency policy.* |
| c. Date and time of last irrigation. | If not receiving continuous infusion of fluids, venous access device must be flushed to prevent blood from clotting and obstructing the catheter (Wong and Whaley, 1990).<br>***Special Considerations:*** *PIDs should be flushed daily, Groshong catheters weekly, and TIDs every 3 to 4 weeks (Marcoux, Fisher, and Wong, 1990). Some agencies require more frequent flushing; refer to agency procedure manual. Central venous access devices should also be flushed after blood is withdrawn, after medication is administered, and/or anytime blood is noted in the catheter.* |
| d. Date and time of last injection cap change on PIDs. | Injection caps should be changed weekly to prevent leaking from frequent punctures.<br>***Special Considerations:*** *A convenient time for changing the injection cap is during routine flushing of catheter or during dressing change.* |
| 4. Assess the child's and family's knowledge and attitude toward the device. | Adolescents may experience a negative alteration in body image as a result of catheter placement that may require nursing intervention.<br>***Special Considerations:*** *The child's ability to cope with the device depends on developmental level, ability to understand need for device, visibility of the device, and parental response to it (Vogel and McSkimming, 1983).* |
| 5. Assess for signs of venous access device complications.<br>a. Infection.<br>b. Occlusion.<br>c. Accidental removal or displacement.<br>d. Cardiac tamponade (Marcoux, Fisher, and Wong, 1990). | Early detection of complications allows prompt intervention. |
| **Planning and Goal Setting** | |
| 1. Set appropriate time with child for site care and dressing procedure. | Asking for the child's input about time of procedure gives child a sense of control and helps gain cooperation during procedure. |
| 2. When possible, have family member at bedside to observe procedure. | Observation of procedure facilitates family member's learning. |
| 3. If necessary, obtain an assistant to help restrain and comfort the child. | If the child is not cooperative, restraining is necessary to prevent injury to the child or damage to the device and to ensure asepsis. |
| 4. Assemble equipment: | |
| ***Insertion and exit site care*** | |
| a. Adhesive remover pads. | |
| b. Six povidone-iodine or antiseptic swabs. | ***Special Considerations:*** *If child is allergic to iodine, use hexachlorophene swabs.* |
| c. Four sterile cotton-tipped applicators. | |
| d. Hydrogen peroxide or alcohol. | ***Special Considerations:*** *Some agencies recommend use of alcohol/acetone swabs instead of hydrogen peroxide.* |

| Steps | Rationale |
|---|---|
| e. Plastic bag for disposal of used supplies and dressing. | |
| f. Two culturettes. | Culturettes should be available in the event drainage is present. |
| g. Sterile gloves, mask, and gown (optional). | ***Special Considerations:*** *The use of mask and gloves with site care of TIDs and PIDs is controversial. Refer to agency procedure manual for protocol.* |
| h. For PID also need: | ***Special Considerations:*** *Short-term PIDs require sterile technique, as they have no Dacron cuffs, thus increasing the risk of infection.* |
| ▪ Antibacterial ointment.<br>▪ Skin preparation pads (optional).<br>▪ One sterile 2 × 2 inch preslit gauze pad.<br>▪ Alcohol swabs. | ***Special Considerations:*** *Do not use ointment if transparent dressing is used; apply antibacterial solution instead.* |
| ▪ Sterile 4 × 4 inch gauze dressing or nonocclusive transparent plastic dressing. | ***Special Considerations:*** *Transparent dressings are normally changed once a week, although more frequent changes may be indicated for children at higher risk for infection, such as in intensive care areas (Young et al, 1988).* |
| ▪ 1-inch tape.<br>▪ Smooth cannula clamp (except for Groshong). | ***Special Considerations:*** *Do not use scissors, pins, or other sharp objects near central venous catheters. Use of sharp objects can damage catheter with subsequent risk of infection, air emboli, or hemorrhage.* |
| ***Irrigation/flushing*** | |
| *Totally implanted device:* | |
| a. Three alcohol swabs. | |
| b. Three povidone-iodine swabs. | |
| c. 10 ml Luer-Lok syringe containing 3 to 5 ml heparinized saline (100 units/ml). | A syringe smaller than 10 ml puts excessive pressure on port's reservoir and may cause the catheter to dislodge from port internally (Wezel-Bolen, 1986). Totally implanted devices are flushed with a higher concentration of heparinized saline than partially implanted devices because TIDs are flushed less frequently than PIDs (Marcoux, Fisher, and Wong, 1990).<br>***Special Considerations:*** *For children weighing less than 25 kg, the dose of heparinized saline will need to be decreased. Consult physician for exact dose.* |
| d. One sterile 22-gauge *straight* Huber needle. | A Huber needle prevents coring of portal septum. Conventional needles will damage the septum's self-sealing capability (Marcoux, Fisher, and Wong, 1990).<br>***Special Considerations:*** *A straight Huber needle is safe for side access ports, and for irrigation or flushing only of top access ports. For long-term infusion of top access ports, a 90-degree bent Huber needle is needed.* |
| e. Sterile gloves. | |
| *Partially implanted device:* | |
| a. Alcohol swabs. | |
| b. One 23-gauge 1-inch needle. | |
| c. 1-inch waterproof tape. | |
| d. Hickman/Broviac also need:<br>▪ One syringe containing 3 to 10 ml heparinized saline (10 units/ml). | ***Special Considerations:*** *Refer to agency policy to determine specific amount of heparinized saline. In infants with pediatric Broviac catheters, the catheter should be flushed with only 3 ml heparinized saline (10 units/ml). Multiple lumen catheters should be flushed with 3 ml of solution into each port.* |
| ▪ Smooth cannula clamp. | Hickman and Broviac catheters must be clamped to prevent backflow of blood. Smooth clamps are used to avoid damage to the catheter. |
| e. Groshong also needs:<br>▪ One syringe containing 5 to 10 ml normal saline. | Normal saline instead of heparinized saline is used with the Groshong because a valve prevents backflow of blood into the catheter. |

| Steps | Rationale |
|---|---|
| ***PID injection cap change*** | |
| a. Sterile Luer-Lok injection cap. | |
| b. 1-inch waterproof tape. | |
| c. One alcohol swab. | |
| d. Smooth cannula clamp. | ***Special Considerations:*** *As Groshong catheters have a two-way valve on the distal end, a cannula clamp is not needed and can damage the catheter.* |
| 5. Develop individualized child and family goals: ▪ Venous access device complications will be prevented or minimized. ▪ The venous access device will remain patent and functional for its designated use. ▪ Child and/or family will be knowledgeable in the care of specific device. ▪ Child and family will experience minimal anxiety as it relates to the care of device. | |

## Implementation

| Steps | Rationale |
|---|---|
| 1. Prepare child and family for procedure (see Skill 1). | ***Special Considerations:*** *Children often dislike the smells of the preparations used, especially for insertion/exit site care. Some suggestions to help the child tolerate the procedure include turn the head away from the dressing site and lightly place a towel over head, use a small fan to blow the smells away from face, involve the child in the procedure to provide distraction, or familiarize the child with the smells in play therapy before the procedure.* |
| 2. Instruct family of each implemented step while they observe. | Venous access devices are often used for long-term venous access. It is often necessary for family members to care for child with a venous access device at home. |
| ***Clamping partially implanted device (Broviac/Hickman)*** | |
| 1. Cut approximately 1½- to 2-inch strip of 1-inch waterproof tape. Fold each end approx ⅛ inch over on itself. | Folding tape ends facilitates later removal of tape. |
| 2. Fold tape over approximately half way down the catheter, forming a tape tab. | Taping the catheter prevents damage to the catheter from clamping. |
| 3. Apply smooth catheter clamp over the tape tab. | Clamping over the tape tab is an added precaution against damaging the catheter. ***Special Considerations:*** *Groshong catheters are not clamped.* |
| 4. Change tape tab location with injection cap change (see p. 714). | Periodically changing tape tab site prevents catheter damage. |
| ***Insertion and exit site care*** | |
| 1. Clamp the catheter on PID (except Groshong). | Catheters must be clamped to prevent hemorrhage, air emboli, or the introduction of microorganisms into the bloodstream. |
| 2. Gently remove old dressing using adhesive remover pads. Note any discharge. Place in plastic bag, seal, and discard. | Disposal of old dressing in plastic bag minimizes transmission of microorganisms from the dressing. ***Special Considerations:*** *Allowing child to assist in removing dressings will help gain cooperation during procedure.* |
| 3. Observe insertion site (Fig. 110-1) and exit site if present for: a. Redness. b. Swelling. c. Drainage/odor. d. Skin irritation. e. Discomfort/tenderness. f. Exposure of Dacron cuff on PIDs or of port with TIDs. | Redness, swelling, or drainage at insertion or exit site may indicate catheter-related infection and necessitate the use of systemic antibiotics, antibiotic-lock technique, or removal of venous access device. Body rejection of the TID may result in skin breakdown and exposure of the port. ***Special Considerations:*** *If excessive redness, swelling, or drainage is noted, notify the physician. The antibiotic-lock technique involves instilling a high concentration of antibiotic inside an infected catheter at periodic intervals (Messing et al, 1988). If catheter is removed, the tip of catheter should be cultured. If skin irritation occurs, determine source of irritation. It may be necessary to change type of tape.* |

| Steps | Rationale |
|---|---|

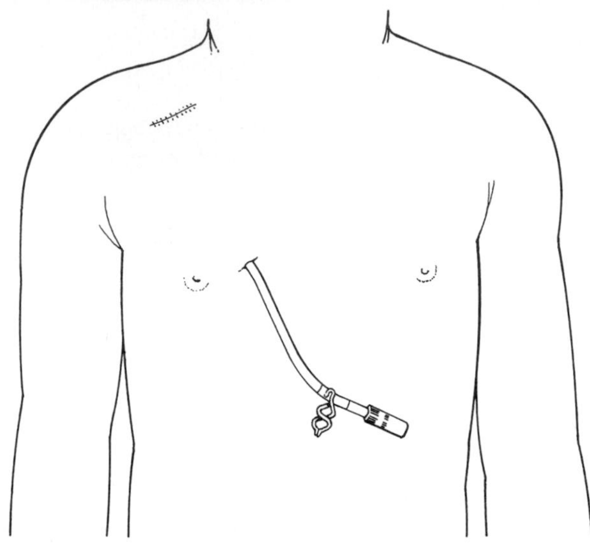

*FIG. 110-1* Insertion and exit sites for partially implanted central venous access device.

4. Inspect catheter and hub to determine intactness. Measure the length of the exposed catheter and compare to base measurement.

Catheter can become damaged with cracks or splits. It can also be partially dislodged.

5. Wash hands for 1 minute using antibacterial soap or don sterile gloves.

Washing hands removes bacteria that may have been introduced during removal of dressing.

6. Cleanse insertion/exit site(s):

*Totally implanted device:*

a. Using three povidone-iodine swabs, clean upper insertion site. With first swab, clean across incision; with second swab, clean above incision; with third swab, clean below incision. Use each swab only once.

Transient organisms on the skin can only be removed by chemical and mechanical methods. Using each swab only once prevents contamination of the incision.

***Special Considerations:*** *Steri-strips may be in place and should not be removed until 7 to 10 days post-insertion when site is healed. Cleansing swabs will not loosen the Steri-strips.*

b. With a povidone-iodine swab, clean lower insertion site in a spiral motion working outward for a diameter of 2 to 3 inches. Using new povidone-iodine swabs, repeat this step twice. Use each swab only once (Fig. 110-2).

Cleaning in this manner avoids cross-contamination of incision by microorganisms from other areas of the skin.

***Special Considerations:*** *The lower insertion site is the location of the implant. Some surgeons place TIDs using a procedure that results in only one insertion site.*

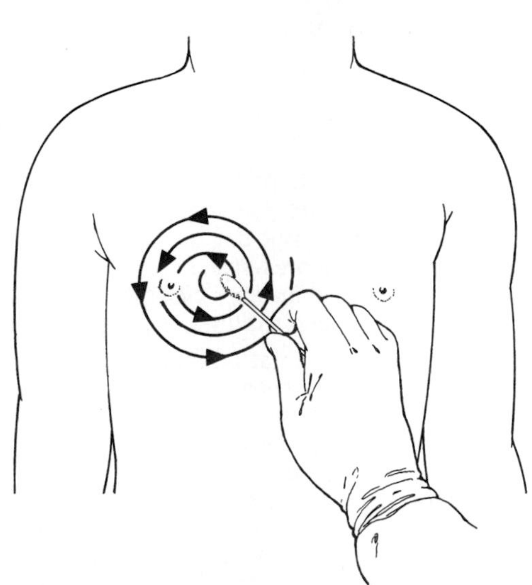

*FIG. 110-2* Insertion site of totally implanted device is cleaned with a spiral, outward motion.

c. With sterile cotton swab tips soaked in hydrogen peroxide, remove povidone-iodine from skin around lower insertion site (site of implant) in a spiral motion, working from inside to outside. Allow area to air dry.

Allowing povidone-iodine to remain on skin may cause irritation (Doran, 1983). Hydrogen peroxide also has an antiseptic action and helps remove encrustations.

***Special Considerations:*** *If port is not being accessed, a dressing over either insertion site will not be necessary once the initial dressing is removed (usually 1 to 2 days).*

| **Steps** | **Rationale** |
|---|---|
| *Partially implanted devices:* | |
| a. Using three povidone-iodine swabs, clean insertion site in manner identical to method for TID cleaning. | Cleaning in this manner prevents cross-contamination of incision. ***Special Considerations:*** *Sutures at the insertion site may be removed 7 to 10 days after placement. Once insertion site is healed, care of insertion site may be discontinued. It is not necessary to redress insertion site after initial dressing is removed.* |
| b. Clean exit site of PIDs in same manner insertion site of TID is cleansed (Fig. 110-3). | ***Special Considerations:*** *After approximately 4 weeks, tissue will adhere to the Dacron cuff in the subcutaneous tunnel. Dressings may not be required once this occurs, but the exit site should continue to be cleansed daily (Marcoux, Fisher, and Wong, 1990). Some agencies recommend the use of alcohol/acetone swabs to clean and "defat" the skin.* |

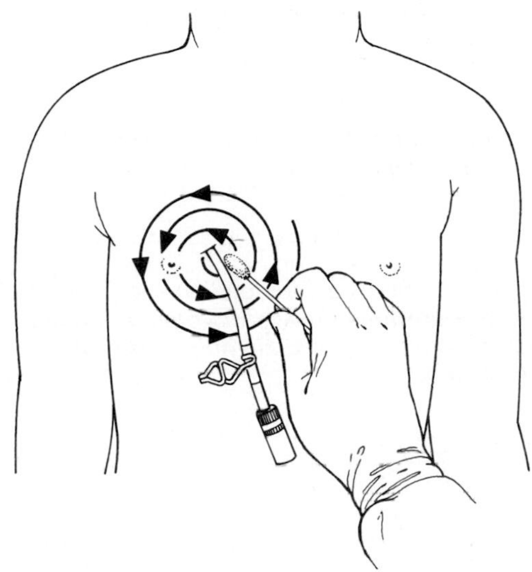

***FIG. 110-3*** Cleaning site of partially implanted device.

| **Steps** | **Rationale** |
|---|---|
| c. With alcohol swab, firmly wipe catheter from exit site distally to connection end. Clean butterfly tab/sutures on Groshong using clean povidone-iodine and hydrogen peroxide swabs as in insertion/exit site care. | Cleaning catheter from exit site distally helps remove microorganisms from exit site (Vogel and McSkimming, 1983). ***Special Considerations:*** *Groshong catheters have a butterfly tab located on the catheter a few inches from the exit site. The tab is sutured to the skin to secure the catheter while the Dacron cuff adheres. The sutures are removed 4 weeks after the catheter is placed.* |
| d. Apply antibacterial ointment to exit site with a sterile cotton-tipped applicator. | An antibacterial ointment provides a barrier to the entrance of microorganisms. Use of a sterile applicator maintains asepsis and prevents excess application. |
| e. Apply skin preparation product (if desired) to areas of the skin where tape will be applied (a "window frame" pattern) (Fig. 110-4). | Skin preparation products may protect the skin where tape is applied and promote tape adherence. ***Special Considerations:*** *Change position of tape on the skin with each dressing change or discontinue use if skin irritation develops.* |

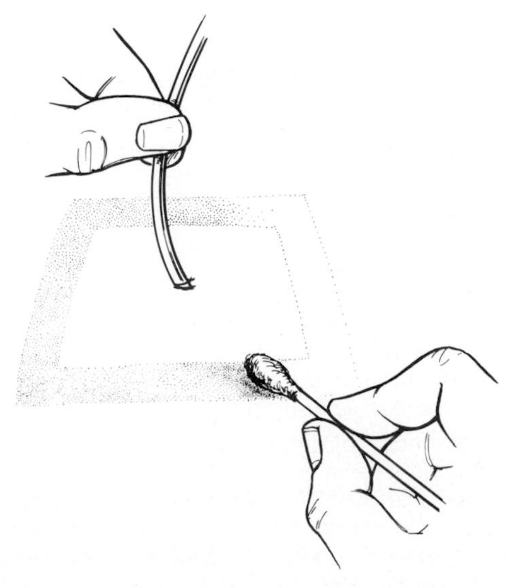

***FIG. 110-4*** Skin preparation improves dressing adherence and provides protection.

From Wong DL and Whaley LF: Clinical manual of pediatric nursing, ed 3, St Louis, 1990, The CV Mosby Co.

| Steps | Rationale |
|---|---|
| f. Position catheter downward so it lies on child's abdomen. | Positioning catheter downward reduces tension on catheter during taping. |
| g. Touching only corner of gauze, cover exit site with preslit sterile 2 × 2 gauze, bringing catheter through slit. | The preslit gauze protects the skin from catheter irritation. |
| 7. Touching only corner of sterile dressing, apply 4 × 4 gauze or transparent dressing over insertion site of TID and insertion/exit sites of PID. Tape gauze edges securely. | The gauze or dressing provides an additional barrier to microorganisms. **Special Considerations:** *Make dressing waterproof with plastic, self-adhering drape if contamination may be a problem, e.g., tracheostomies, draining wounds, nasogastric tubes, high humidity oxygen apparatus or showering (Persons, 1987). Follow manufacturer's directions for application of transparent dressing.* |
| 8. Label the dressing with date, time, and initials. For PID, if no other procedures planned (e.g., flushing/irrigation or injection cap change), loop catheter and tape (see General Measures step 1). | Dressing is labeled to facilitate maintenance of dressing change schedule. **Special Considerations:** *Institutional policy dictates the frequency of dressing changes.* |

### *Irrigation/flushing*

*Totally implanted device:*

| Steps | Rationale |
|---|---|
| 1. Palpate port with two fingers, placing one on each side of port (Fig. 110-5). | Palpating device is necessary to determine location of port. **Special Considerations:** *The most common location of ports is the upper right or left quadrant of the anterior chest between the clavicle and breast.* |

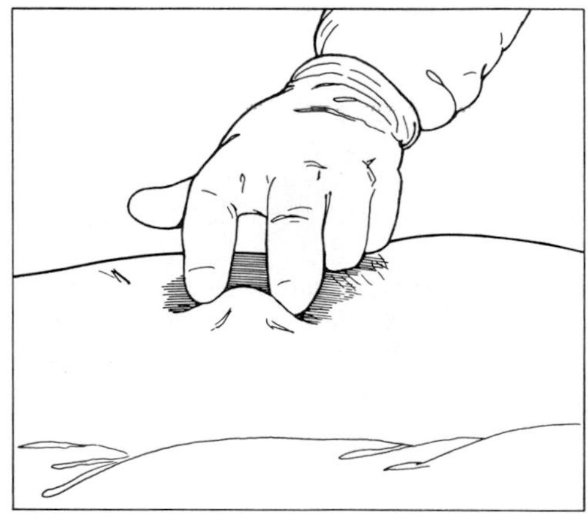

***FIG. 110-5*** Palpation of port under the skin.

| Steps | Rationale |
|---|---|
| 2. Clean skin over port septum using alcohol swabs in a spiral motion, working from inside outward for a diameter of 3 inches (see Fig. 110-2). | Alcohol has antiseptic properties in addition to those of povidone-iodine (Perry and Potter, 1990). |
| 3. Using one povidone-iodine swab, clean area over port in a spiral motion, working from inside outward for a diameter of 3 inches. Repeat this step twice using a new swab each time. | Transient organisms on the skin can only be removed by chemical and mechanical methods. Using each swab only once prevents contamination of the incision. |
| 4. Open Huber needle package, keeping needle sterile and inside package. | Contamination of needle or end of syringe will introduce microorganisms into infusion port and child's bloodstream. |
| 5. Hold Huber needle by package and attach Luer-Lok syringe of heparinized saline into hub. | |
| 6. Once syringe is locked onto needle securely, remove needle from package, maintaining its sterility. | |
| 7. Prime needle by expelling a small amount of heparinized saline from syringe. | Priming needle prevents air from being injected into port, reducing risk of air embolus. |
| 8. With nondominant hand, palpate port again, being careful not to contaminate area over center of port. | The port septum, located in the center of the port, must be identified for correct needle placement. **Special Considerations:** *Topical or subcutaneous local anesthetic may be used at this time to minimize the child's discomfort during needle insertion.* |
| 9. While stabilizing the port with nondominant hand, use dominant hand to push Huber needle firmly through skin into the center of the silicone septum at a 90-degree angle to the port, until the needle rests firmly against the needle stop. A "click" sensation will be felt. Do not tilt or angle needle once it is in place. | The "click" sensation indicates proper placement. Tilting the needle may dislodge it. **Special Considerations:** *The needle is always inserted at a 90-degree angle to the port. It is also at a 90-degree angle to the skin for the top entry port, but parallel to the chest surface for the side access port.* |

| **Steps** | **Rationale** |
|---|---|

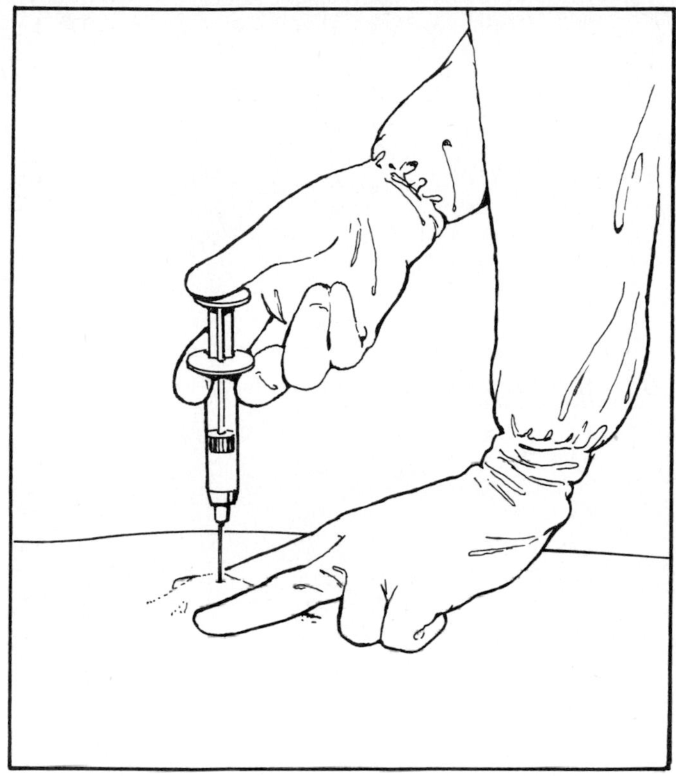

***FIG. 110-6*** Port is stabilized while needle is slowly withdrawn.

| **Steps** | **Rationale** |
|---|---|
| 10. Keeping nondominant hand in place, flush port rapidly but not forcefully with heparinized saline. As last 1 ml of solution is being injected, slowly withdraw needle from port (Fig. 110-6). Stabilize port while removing needle. | Flushing ensures patency of infusion port and catheter. Pushing last ml of heparinized saline while removing needle maintains positive pressure within infusion port, preventing backflow of blood into port with subsequent clotting. Forceful flushing may dislodge clot into the child's vascular system.<br>***Special Considerations:*** *If port does not flush easily, reposition child on either side or with arms above head, then try to flush again. If resistance is felt, withdraw needle and notify physician.* |
| *Partially Implanted Device:* | |
| 1. Remove tape that is holding loop in catheter. | Untaping the catheter improves handling of the injection port. |
| 2. If injecting through the injection cap, scrub with alcohol swab for 1 minute. | Scrubbing injection cap reduces risk of introducing microorganisms into the system as needle passes through port. |
| 3. Insert needle with attached syringe of solution into center of cap (see Fig. 110-7)<br>*OR*<br>Remove cap and attach hub of syringe (with needle removed) directly to catheter, twisting the syringe to lock it (Fig. 110-8). | Irrigating through cap helps maintain a closed system to reduce risk of infection. Attaching the hub of the syringe directly eliminates needle resistance to the flush.<br>***Special Considerations:*** *Follow facility policy as to method to use.* |
| 4. Unclamp catheter. | ***Special Considerations:*** *Groshong catheters should not be clamped. When irrigating Groshong catheters, eliminate steps 4 and 7.* |
| 5. Inject solution rapidly but not forcefully. | Injecting irrigation solution rapidly clears blood from inside catheter. Forceful irrigation could dislodge a clot. Resistance being met while flushing catheter may indicate that a clot has formed inside the catheter.<br>***Special Considerations:*** *If resistance is met, reposition child on either side or with arms above head and reattempt flushing. If resistance continues, clamp catheter, withdraw needle, and notify physician.* |
| 6. If catheter is multilumen, inject each port with a syringe of heparinized saline using same procedure. | Multilumen catheters are usually flushed with 3 ml into each port.<br>***Special Considerations:*** *Refer to agency procedure manual to determine specific amount.* |

| Steps | Rationale |
|---|---|

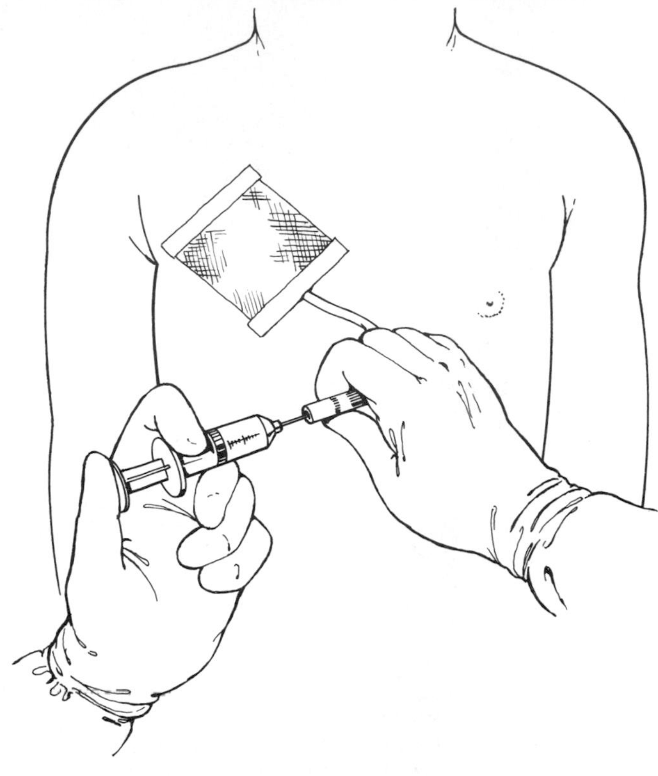

*FIG. 110-7* Needle is inserted into center of cap.

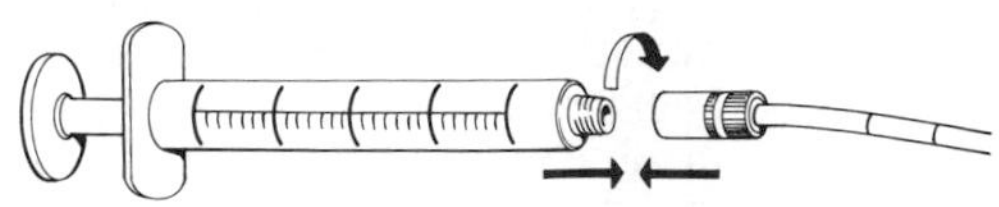

*FIG. 110-8* Syringe hub is attached directly to catheter.

7. Clamp catheter over tape tab as last ½ to 1 ml of solution is injected.

Clamping catheter while solution is being injected maintains positive pressure within catheter, preventing backflow of blood into catheter tip and subsequent clot formation.
***Special Considerations:*** *With Groshong catheters, withdraw needle as last ½ to 1 ml of solution is being injected.*

***PID injection cap change***

1. Remove tape holding looped catheter.
2. Apply a new tape tab for clamping to catheter at different location from current tape tab.

Moving tape tab site to different locations prevents one area from being damaged.

3. Clamp catheter over new tape tab.

Catheter must be clamped before removal of injection cap to prevent air embolus and hemorrhage.
***Special Considerations:*** *Groshong catheters have a valve that prevents backflow, and should not be clamped; therefore, eliminate steps 2 through 4.*

4. Remove old tape tab.
5. Clean outside of old injection cap and catheter tip with alcohol swab.
6. Open injection cap package maintaining sterility.
7. Remove old injection cap and discard (Fig. 110-9).
8. Apply new injection cap (Fig. 110-10).
9. Using 1-inch waterproof tape, apply tape around injection cap and catheter, folding each end of tape over on itself ⅛ inch.

Placing tape around injection cap and catheter is a safety measure to prevent injection cap from becoming dislodged (Wezel-Bolen, 1986). Overlapping the end provides a tab for easier removal.

**Steps** | **Rationale**

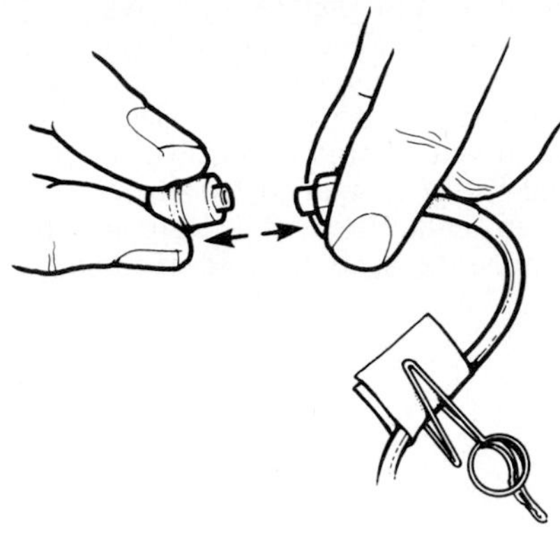

***FIG. 110-9*** Remove old injection cap and discard.

From Wong DL and Whaley LF: Clinical manual of pediatric nursing, ed 3, St Louis, 1990, The CV Mosby Co.

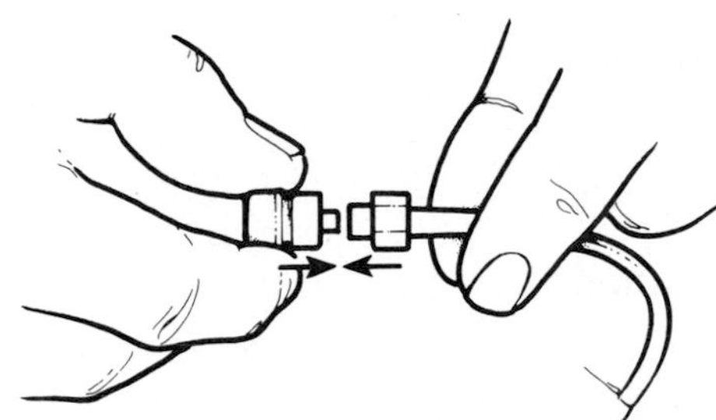

***FIG. 110-10*** Apply new injection cap.

From Wong DL and Whaley LF: Clinical manual of pediatric nursing, ed 3, St Louis, 1990, The CV Mosby Co.

### *General measures*

1. After each aspect of care, secure the device with small dressing, tape, or clothing.
   a. Partially implanted device: Loop catheter once over top of dressing and tape catheter securely, leaving injection cap exposed (see Fig. 110-11). If desired, protect the catheter from tape adhesive by placing a ¼-inch piece of tape, sticky side in to the tape where it passes over the catheter.

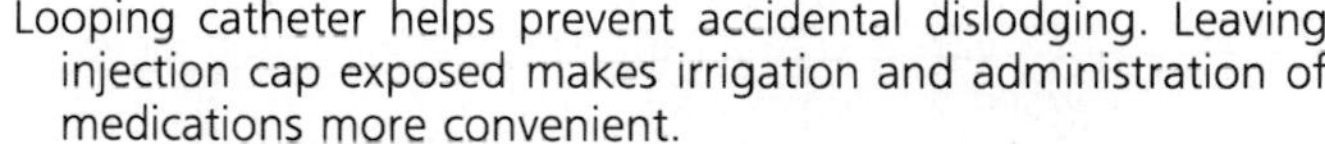

Looping catheter helps prevent accidental dislodging. Leaving injection cap exposed makes irrigation and administration of medications more convenient.

***Special Considerations:*** *In infants and small children, an extra 4 × 4 gauze should be placed over the looped catheter, clamp, and injection cap to prevent access. Young children should wear pullover shirts or one-piece outfits to discourage them from playing with or biting the catheter (Doran, 1983).*

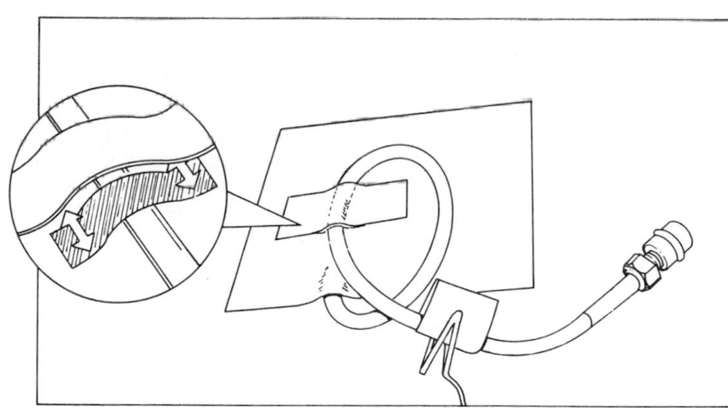

***FIG. 110-11*** Catheter is looped over top of gauze dressing, secured, and protected from tape adhesive.

   b. Totally implanted device: Discourage touching the port site.

The child may play with the bulge under the skin, an activity referred to as "twiddler's syndrome," resulting in port-catheter separation (Gebarski and Gebarski, 1984).

2. Give positive reinforcement to child for cooperation during procedure.

Positive reinforcement gives child a sense of accomplishment and may help gain cooperation with other procedures related to care of the device.

## Evaluation Outcomes

1. Skin integrity is maintained at insertion and/or exit site.
2. The child remains free of complications related to central VAD.

## Observational Guidelines

Assess skin integrity at insertion and exit site with each dressing change for redness, swelling, drainage, or irritation.

Monitor for fever, chills; shortness of breath, chest pains; pain, numbness, or tingling in neck, shoulder, arm, or hand on the same side of the body as catheter or at suture line; increase in length of exposed catheter; leaking of fluid.

## Evaluation Outcomes—cont'd

3. Central VAD remains patent and functional.
4. Child and/or family member performs VAD care correctly and demonstrates understanding of complication prevention and intervention.
5. The child and family experience minimal anxiety related to VAD care.

## Observational Guidelines—cont'd

Note amount of pressure required to flush VAD. Note the ease of infusions, as well as blood withdrawals.

Observe child and/or family member performing VAD care before child's discharge. Ask family to verbalize preventive procedures and action to take related to possible complications.

Ask child and family to express feelings about performing the task. Note any behaviors that indicate anxiety related to VAD or its maintenance, such as avoidance behaviors, crying, and agitation.

## Documentation

Record name of procedure; date and time of procedure; family members observing procedure; child's reaction (response) to procedure; family's reaction to procedure; return demonstration by family; indications of complications and corrective actions taken. Note type of dressing used and appearance of insertion and exit sites. Document amount, type, and concentration of irrigation solution; note ease with which venous access device was flushed.

## Home Care Modifications

1. To protect family from accidental needle sticks, used syringes and needles should be stored in a metal or opaque glass container (e.g., a coffee can). The top should be taped securely when the can is full.
2. Antibacterial soap, e.g., Dial or Safeguard, may be used for handwashing at home before procedures involving care of the VAD.
3. The child should carry some type of identification such as a medical alert card or jewelry about the VAD.
4. Adults who supervise child, e.g., teachers, school nurse, coach, and baby sitters, should be provided with instructions and information about the VAD (Meeske and Davidson, 1988).
5. To prevent the dressing from becoming wet while the child is showering, a piece of plastic (e.g., plastic wrap) should be taped occlusively over the dressing and a fresh dressing applied immediately after getting out of shower. Consult with physician before permitting showers (Whaley and Wong, 1991).
6. The child with a PID may be restricted in some activities. Swimming is usually prohibited but may be allowed with certain modifications. If the exit site is healed and the cuff is adhered to the tissue, a transparent plastic dressing may be placed over the site and catheter to allow swimming for an hour or less in a chlorinated pool. Swimming is allowed with a TID but only after 2 to 4 weeks when the suture line is well healed (Marcoux, Fisher, and Wong, 1990).
7. Most contact sports are prohibited with a PID because of the possibility of the catheter being hit or dislodged. Children with TID are less restricted but should still refrain from soccer, football, or hockey.
8. It is often useful to introduce children and family to other children and families who are using devices successfully. Families are able to share concerns and helpful management tips (Whaley and Wong, 1991).
9. Parents should be cautioned to keep scissors and other sharp objects away from the child to prevent accidental cutting of catheter.
10. Long-term PIDs can be repaired if torn. The family should be given a repair kit if unable to return to the institution for repair (Marcoux, Fisher, and Wong, 1990). If leak develops in catheter, instruct parents to tape it above the leak and then clamp catheter at taped site. This is not considered an emergency, but the child should be taken to physician as soon as possible after a leak to prevent infection or clotting of catheter (Vogel and McSkimming, 1983).
11. Children with VADs who require dental work may need to receive antibiotics prophylactically. Bacteria released into the blood during the dental work may attach to the VAD. Antibiotics decrease the risk of infection occurring (UCLA TPN Newsletter, 1986).
12. See "Home Care Instructions: Caring for a central venous catheter" (Wong and Whaley, 1990) for information that can be photocopied and distributed to families.

# SKILL 111 Administering Medications Through Central Venous Access Devices

*Janet Ludgar*

Children with cancer or other chronic illnesses often require frequent and prolonged administration of numerous intravenous medications or fluids. Central venous access devices (VADs) provide an easier means of access, allowing more freedom of movement during infusions and increasing availability of home treatment. VADs also eliminate or minimize the need for multiple venipunctures and thus may decrease the child's anxiety. Solutions of high concentration, such as hyperalimentation, may be given through the VAD because the accessed vessels have larger volume and turbulence than peripheral veins, providing rapid dilution. The disadvantages include the need for surgical insertion, risk of complications and additional care, and expense depending on the type of VAD. Refer to Skill 110, Maintaining Central Venous Access Devices for further information.

## NURSING DIAGNOSES

Anxiety related to unmet informational needs about purpose and administration of medications; Potential for injury related to adverse effects of intravenous medications.

| Steps | Rationale |
|---|---|
| **Assessment** | |
| 1. Review chart to determine date and time medication was last administered. Note if any adverse reactions were observed. | A brief review of the child's record will prevent errors in administering medications. |
| 2. If a new medication order has been written, review medication dose, route, dilution, child's allergies, and medication's compatibility with heparin. | Reviewing medication includes amount of dilution, type of infusion, administration time and duration of infusion. |
| 3. Determine the type of VAD being used. | The type of VAD will influence both planning and implementation of the procedure. |
| 4. Check for the Five Rights of Medication Administration:<br>a. Right drug.<br>b. Right patient.<br>c. Right route.<br>d. Right dose.<br>e. Right time. | Verification of the Five Rights of Medication Administration helps prevent medication errors. |
| **Planning and Goal Setting** | |
| 1. See Skill 108 for other steps related to IV medication administration. | |
| 2. When possible, have family members at bedside to observe procedure. | Family's repeated observation of the procedure facilitates teaching of the skill for home care, as they may be responsible for administering medications when child is discharged. |
| 3. Prepare child for the procedure (see Skill 1). | Preparing the child reduces any fears or anxiety associated with the procedure. |
| 4. Assemble equipment. | |
| ***Partially implanted device*** | |
| *IV push and continuous infusion:* | |
| a. Two or three alcohol swabs. | |
| b. Smooth cannula clamp. | Only smooth cannula clamps should be used to prevent damaging catheter.<br>***Special Considerations:*** *Because Groshong catheters have a valve on the distal end to prevent blood reflux, a clamp is not needed for these catheters.* |

| Steps | Rationale |
|---|---|
| c. 1-inch waterproof tape. | |
| d. 1-inch hypoallergenic tape. | |
| e. One syringe with 3 to 10 ml heparinized saline (10 units/ml). | ***Special Considerations:*** *Refer to agency procedure manual to determine specific amount and concentration of heparinized saline.* |
| f. Two syringes with 3 to 5 ml sterile normal saline. | ***Special Considerations:*** *Air bubbles must be removed from all prepared syringes to prevent introduction of air emboli.* |
| g. 23-gauge, 1-inch needle. | A sterile needle is used to attach to primed IV tubing.<br>***Special Considerations:*** *When infusions are given at rapid rates or when blood products are administered, a larger bore needle is needed.* |
| h. Prepared medication in syringe for push or with tubing for continuous infusion. | ***Special Considerations:*** *Tape all tubing connections to prevent accidental disconnection, which can result in hemorrhage, emboli, or infection.* |
| ***Totally implanted device*** | |
| *IV push medications:* | |
| a. Three alcohol swabs. | |
| b. Three povidone-iodine swabs. | ***Special Considerations:*** *Check for sensitivity to iodine products.* |
| c. 10 ml Luer-Lok syringe with 3 to 5 ml heparinized saline (100 units/ml). | Use of a smaller than 10 ml syringe puts excessive pressure on port's reservoir and may cause the catheter to dislodge from port internally (Wezel-Bolen, 1986). TIDs are irrigated with a stronger heparinized saline solution than PIDs because of less frequent maintenance flushes (Marcoux, Fisher, and Wong, 1990).<br>***Special Considerations:*** *Refer to agency procedure manual to determine specific amount and concentration of heparinized saline. For children weighing less than 25 kg, the dose of heparinized saline will need to be decreased. Consult with physician for exact dose.* |
| d. 10 ml Luer-Lok syringe with 5 ml normal saline. | Normal saline is used to flush before and after medication to remove heparin that may be incompatible with medication. |
| e. 20- or 22-gauge straight or 90-degree, prebent Huber needle. | Huber needles are necessary to prevent coring of portal septum. Conventional needles will damage the septum's self-sealing capability. A 90-degree bent Huber needle is safer when accessing for longer infusions and at a perpendicular angle (Marcoux, Fisher, and Wong, 1990). Straight needles are useful when accessing side entry access ports, which are parallel to the skin.<br>***Special Considerations:*** *Huber needles are available in a variety of styles, including with or without extension tubing, with or without a clamp, with injection port, or with wings to improve maneuverability. There is also a catheter-over-needle design in which the needle is removed and the catheter remains in the port.* |
| f. Extension tubing with Luer-Lok, if not already attached to needle. | |
| g. Clamp, if not part of needle attachment. | |
| h. Sterile gloves. | |
| i. Prepared medication in syringe. | |
| *Continuous infusion medications:* | |
| a. Three or four preslit sterile 2 × 2 inch gauze pads. | |
| b. Antibacterial ointment. | |
| c. Sterile cotton-tipped applicator. | |
| d. Sterile 4 × 4 inch gauze dressing or transparent dressing. | |
| e. 20-gauge Huber needle, straight or 90-degree bent. | |
| f. 1-inch hypoallergenic tape. | |
| g. 1-inch waterproof tape. | |
| h. IV tubing primed with prepared medication. | ***Special Considerations:*** *Tape all tubing connections to prevent accidental disconnection.* |
| i. IV infusion device with output pressure of less than 15 pounds/square inch (Ecoff, Barone, and Simons, 1983). | A higher output pressure can cause the tubing to dislodge from the port internally. |

| Steps | Rationale |
|---|---|
| 5. Develop individualized goals of nursing care.<br>▪ Safely and accurately administer medication(s).<br>▪ Teach procedure to child/family.<br>▪ Maintain patency of central VAD. | |

## Implementation 

| Steps | Rationale |
|---|---|
| 1. Instruct family about administration of medications while having family observe procedure. | Family may be responsible for administration of medications when child is discharged. |
| 2. Wash hands for 1 minute using antibacterial soap. | |

***Partially implanted device***

| Steps | Rationale |
|---|---|
| 1. Remove tape that may be holding loop catheter. | Untaping the catheter improves handling of injection cap. |
| 2. If injecting through the cap, scrub with alcohol swab for 1 minute. | Scrubbing injection cap reduces risk of introducing microorganisms into system as needle passes through port.<br>***Special Considerations:*** *If device is multilumen, the larger lumen is usually used for blood sampling and administration of blood products (Perry and Potter, 1990).* |
| 3. Insert needle of the syringe with saline into center of injection cap (see Fig. 110-7)<br>*OR*<br>remove cap and attach hub of syringe (with needle removed) directly to catheter, twisting the syringe to lock it. | |
| 4. Unclamp catheter (except Groshong) and gently aspirate to verify blood return. | Aspiration is used to verify blood return. Blood return affirms placement in vessel.<br>***Special Considerations:*** *Blood should enter syringe with aspiration. If unable to obtain blood return or if catheter does not irrigate easily, the catheter may be against the wall of the right atrium. Reposition child on either side with arms above head and try again. A fibrin sheath may develop at the tip of the catheter causing the catheter to fail to give a blood return when aspirated, but it can be irrigated. In this case, the catheter can be used for administration of medications (Goodman and Wickham, 1984). Do not administer medications that are vesicants or irritants through a central VAD that does not have a blood return.* |
| 5. Inject normal saline rapidly but not forcefully. | Forceful irrigation may dislodge a clot. Irrigating confirms patency and removes any heparin in the catheter, which may be incompatible with some medications. |
| 6. Clamp catheter (except Groshong) over waterproof tape tab. | Clamping of the catheter prevents reflux of blood into catheter. Groshong catheters have a valve that prevents reflux. Clamping over waterproof tape tab prevents damage to catheter. |
| 7. Remove normal saline needle and/or syringe from injection cap or catheter tip. Dispose of properly. | |
| 8. Administering IV push:<br>a. Insert needle of medication syringe into cap port<br>*OR*<br>attach medication syringe hub to catheter, twisting to lock it.<br>b. Unclamp catheter and inject medication over period of time prescribed. | |
| 9. Administering continuous infusion:<br>a. Attach sterile needle to primed IV tubing. Prime the needle then insert into injection cap<br>*OR*<br>attach IV tubing directly to catheter, twisting to lock it. | IV tubing and needle should be primed to prevent danger of air embolus. |
| b. Turn on IV infusion pump, set at desired rate, then unclamp catheter. | Turning on infusion pump before unclamping catheter helps maintain positive pressure within catheter to prevent reflux of blood. |
| c. Secure needle to port or IV tubing to catheter with waterproof tape. | Securing the needle/IV tubing prevents accidental dislodging. |
| d. Loop and securely tape catheter with hypoallergenic tape. | Taping securely prevents accidental dislodging of catheter. |

| Steps | Rationale |
|---|---|
| 10. On completion of medication administration, clamp catheter (except Groshong) and remove needle and/or syringe or tubing from port. Turn off infusion pump. | Catheter is always either clamped or attached to infusion per push or pump to reduce risk of air embolus. |
| 11. If injecting flush through injection cap, scrub with alcohol for 1 minute. | Scrubbing injection cap port reduces risk of introducing microorganisms into system as needle passes through cap. |
| 12. Insert needle with syringe of 3 to 5 ml normal saline and inject slowly (see Fig. 110-7) *OR* attach hub of syringe (with needle removed) directly to catheter, twisting to lock it. | All blood or medications that may clog catheter lumen should be flushed. ***Special Considerations:*** *Many medications are not compatible with heparin. Blood precipitates with most fluids other than normal saline (Perry and Potter, 1990).* |
| 13. Clamp catheter (except Groshong) over waterproof tape tab while last ½ to 2 ml of saline is being injected. | Clamping catheter as last ml is being administered helps maintain positive pressure within catheter, preventing reflux of blood into catheter tip and subsequent clot formation. |
| 14. If no other IV fluids are to be administered, follow irrigation procedure as described in Skill 110. | |
| ***Totally implanted device*** | |
| 1. Connect extension tubing to Huber needle (unless preattached), being careful not to contaminate Huber needle or end of extension tubing. | Contamination of needle or end of extension tubing will introduce microorganisms into infusion port and child's bloodstream. |
| 2. Attach the 10 ml saline syringe to extension tubing and needle and prime. | Priming tubing and needle prevents air embolus. |
| 3. Clamp extension tubing. | |
| 4. Palpate port with two fingers, placing one on each side of port (see Fig. 110-5). | Palpation identifies parameters of port and area to be cleaned. |
| 5. Clean skin over port using alcohol swabs in a spiral motion working from inside outward for a diameter of 3 inches. Repeat this step twice using a new alcohol wipe each time (see Fig. 110-2). | Rigorous skin preparation is necessary to prevent introducing microorganisms into the system. Cleaning in a spiral outward direction prevents contaminating areas that have been cleaned. |
| 6. Using one povidone-iodine swab, clean area over port in a spiral motion working from inside outward for a diameter of 3 inches. Repeat this step twice using a new povidone-iodine swab each time (see Fig. 110-2). | Povodine-iodine possesses some additional antiseptic qualities to enhance disinfecting the skin. ***Special Considerations:*** *Hexachlorophene swabs may be substituted if child is allergic to Betadine (povidone-iodine).* |
| 7. Put on sterile gloves. | Gloves are worn since the sterile needle will require handling. |
| 8. With nondominant hand, palpate port again as in step 4, being careful not to touch area over center of port. | Palpating port helps to determine edges so that port center (the injection site) can be easily identified. |
| 9. While stabilizing device with nondominant hand, use dominant hand to insert Huber needle firmly through skin into the center of the silicone septum at a 90-degree angle to the port until needle rests firmly against needle stop inside the port. A "click" sensation will be felt. Do not tilt or angle needle once it is in place. | When needle is inserted completely into port, a "click" sensation will be felt, which ensures proper fit. ***Special Considerations:*** *The needle is always inserted at a 90-degree angle to the port. It is also at a 90-degree angle to the skin for the top entry port, but parallel to the chest surface for the side parallel access port.* |
| 10. Release clamp on extension tubing. | |
| 11. Check placement by aspirating for blood return. | Port-catheter separation is suspected when air or small amounts of serous fluid are aspirated. Occlusion is suspected if complete resistance is encountered when attempting aspiration (Marcoux, Fisher, and Wong, 1990). ***Special Considerations:*** *The port-catheter connection can be palpated in children with minimal subcutaneous tissue.* |
| 12. Irrigate port with normal saline. | Irrigating port with saline flushes heparin through port, preventing incompatibility with medication, while verifying proper needle insertion and port functioning. ***Special Considerations:*** *If normal saline cannot be flushed through port, reposition child and try again. If difficulty continues, withdraw needle from port and notify physician. Do not administer medications through port that does not irrigate easily.* |
| 13. Clamp extension tubing. | Clamping extension tubing when changing syringes helps prevent air embolus. |
| 14. Remove syringe from extension tubing. | |

| Steps | Rationale |
|---|---|
| 15. For administering IV push medications: | |
| a. Attach prepared medication syringe to extension tubing. | |
| b. Unclamp extension tubing and inject medication at prescribed rate. Clamp tubing and remove medication syringe when completed. | |
| 16. For administering continuous infusions: | |
| a. Attach primed IV set to clamped extension tubing. | Priming and clamping are both measures to reduce air emboli risk. |
| b. Using sterile cotton-tipped applicator, apply antibacterial ointment to site of needle insertion. | Applying antibacterial ointment further reduces risk of infection at site. |
| c. Apply sterile preslit 2 × 2 gauze around needle insertion site, bringing gauze under angle of needle. Apply ample sterile 2 × 2 pads under needle and secure needle in place. | Applying 2 × 2 gauze pads under needle provides stability to needle. |
| d. Apply sterile 4 × 4 gauze or transparent dressing over needle. Tape gauze securely (Fig. 111-1). | Application of sterile dressing over needle is necessary to prevent contamination of needle. ***Special Considerations:*** *During continuous infusions, a gauze dressing should be changed three times a week and a transparent dressing and Huber needle weekly.* |

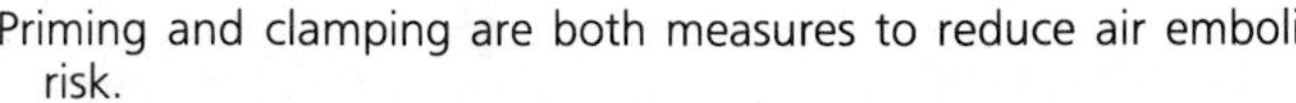

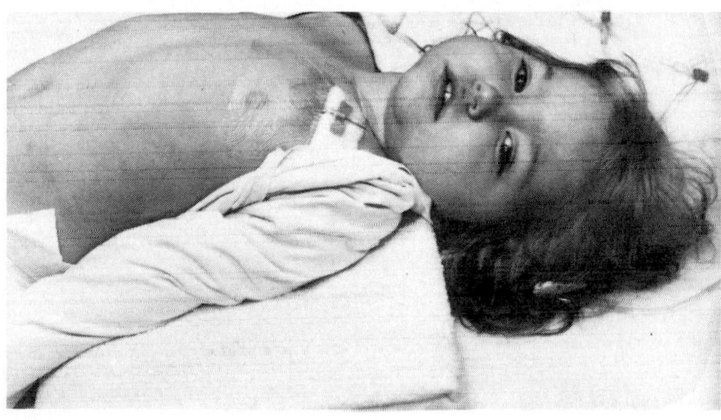

***FIG. 111-1*** Child receiving medication by way of an implantable port. Note the bent Huber needle inserted into the port and secured with a transparent dressing.

From Whaley L and Wong D: Essentials of pediatric nursing, ed 3, 1989, St Louis, The CV Mosby Co.

| Steps | Rationale |
|---|---|
| e. Coil extension tubing and tape securely. | Coiling tubing reduces tension on the needle and prevents accidental dislodging. |
| f. Turn on IV infusion pump. Set at desired rate. | Turning IV infusion pump on before opening clamp on extension tubing helps maintain positive pressure within port preventing reflux of blood into port. |
| g. Open clamp of extension tubing. Administer medication. | |
| 17. Upon completion of medication administration, close clamp on extension tubing. | Clamping extension tubing before turning off pump helps maintain positive pressure within port, preventing reflux of blood. |
| 18. Remove medication syringe or turn off IV infusion pump, then remove IV tubing set. | |
| 19. Following medication administration (IV push or continuous infusion): | |
| a. Attach syringe of normal saline to extension tubing, unclamp tubing, then irrigate. Flush after every medication given. | A normal saline flush administers the remaining medication in the tubing, and prevents mixing with the heparin. ***Special Considerations:*** *After administering blood products, irrigate port with 20 ml sterile normal saline before heparinization to remove fibrin from port (Goodman and Wickham, 1984).* |
| b. Clamp tubing and remove saline syringe. | |
| c. Connect 10 ml heparinized saline syringe to extension tubing and release clamp. | |
| d. If no other IV fluids are to be administered, stabilize port between two fingers of nondominant hand and irrigate with heparinized saline, slowly withdrawing needle from port as last ½ to 1 ml of solution is being injected. | Port must be stabilized while removing needle to prevent dislodging of port. Withdrawing needle as last ½ to 1 ml of fluid is being injected maintains positive pressure within port and prevents reflux of blood into port. |

## Evaluation Outcomes

1. Medication is administered safely.
2. At least one family member is able to safely administer medication with supervision after observing procedure twice.
3. Patency of central VAD is maintained.

## Documentation

Record date and time of medication or fluid administration; name, dose, and route of medication or fluid administration; medication side effects experienced by child; patency of catheter and any difficulty with irrigation, aspiration, or infusion; amount and concentration of heparinized saline flush used; measures taken to educate child or family in care and their responses; any adverse conditions observed, such as local signs of infection at site or damage to catheter.

## Home Care Modifications

See Skill 110.

## Observational Guidelines

Observe for side effects of medication, note correct dose, route, time, dilution.

Observe family member return demonstration. Observe for maintenance of aseptic technique. Observe for proper administration of medication.

Assess ease with which central VAD irrigates, note blood return with aspiration applicable to device.

UNIT XVI

## PRODUCT REFERENCES AND TEACHING RESOURCES

### Books

Wong DL and Whaley LF: Clinical manual of pediatric nursing, ed 3, St Louis, 1990, The CV Mosby Co.
Home care instructions: Giving eye medications; Giving ear medications; Giving nose drops; Giving subcutaneous (Sub Q) injections; Caring for heparin lock; Caring for a central venous catheter; Giving oral medications; and Giving intramuscular (IM) medications.

### Products

Apex Medical Corporation
PO Box 1235
Sioux Falls, SD 57101-1235
1-800-328-2935
Manufactures medication administration devices: spoons, cups.

Gerber Products Corporation
445 State Street
Fremont, MI 49412
1-800-4-GERBER
Manufactures Nuk Medi-Nurser and other medication administration devices.

Groshong, Hickman and Broviac Catheters
Davol Specialty Access Products
3385 West 1820 South
Salt Lake City, UT 84104
(801) 975-1700
1-800-443-3385—Technical information on catheters.
1-800-556-6275—Patient education literature.

Port-a-Cath
Pharmacia Nutech, Inc.
800 Centennial Avenue
Piscataway, NJ 08854
1-800-526-3619
Pharmacia Laboratory has a patient information manual available and a videotape available titled "Living with your Port-a-Cath."

### Organizations

American Diabetes Association (ADA)
National Service Center
1660 Duke Street
PO Box 25757
Alexandria, VA 22314
1-800-232-3472, (703) 549-1500
Offers patient education and audiovisual materials, community information, reference list of summer camps nationwide; publishes *Diabetic Forecast,* a magazine for diabetics and their families.

Asthma and Allergy Foundation of America
1717 Massachusetts Avenue NW #305
Washington, DC 20036
1-800-7-ASTHMA
Offers a variety of educational materials for children and support groups for parents of children with asthma and allergy.

### REFERENCES


Abundis J: Hazards of metered-dose bronchodilator inhalers, J Emerg Nurs 11(5):262-264, 1985.

APON: APON cancer chemotherapy handbook, McLean Va, 1987, Association of Pediatric Oncology Nurses.

Axton SE and Fugate T: A protocol for pediatric IV meds, AJN 87(7):943-945, 1987.

Beecroft PC and Redick SA: Possible complications of intramuscular injections on the pediatric unit, Pediatr Nurs 15(4):333-336, 1989.

Beecroft PC and Redick SA: Clarification of ventrogluteal site (letter), Pediatr Nurs 16(4):396, 1990.

Boyd-Monk H and Steinmetz CG: Nursing care of the eye, Norwalk, Conn, 1987, Appleton & Lange.

Brims S: Aerosol therapy: a nurse's guide, Home Healthcare Nurse 6(6):37-40, 1988.

Burgess WR and Chernick V: Respiratory therapy in newborn infants and children, ed 2, New York, 1986, Thieme, Inc.

Burman R and Berkowitz H: IV bolus: effective but potentially hazardous, Crit Care Nurse 6(1):22-27, 1986.

Burns MD: Pulmonary care: a guide for patient education, Norwalk, Conn, 1983, Appleton-Century-Crofts.

Cahill M, editor: Treatments: the nurses' reference library, Springhouse, Penn, 1988, Nursing 88 Books.

Centers for Disease Control: Recommendations for prevention of HIV transmission in health-care setting, MMWR:36(25):3-18, 1987.

Chaplin G, Shull H, and Welk PC III: How safe is the air-bubble technique for IM injections? Nursing 15(9):59, 1985.

Chow MP et al: Handbook of pediatric primary care, New York, 1984, John Wiley & Sons.

Cohen MR: Medication errors, Nursing 18(3):10, 1988.

Cyganski JM, Donahue JM, and Heaton JS: The case for the heparin flush, AJN, 87(6):796-797, 1987.

Doran EM: Care of the Hickman catheter in children, Nurs Clin North Am, 18(3):579-583, 1983.

Dunn DL and Lenihan SF: The case for the saline flush, AJN 87(6):798-799, 1987.

Dunlap CI and Marchionno P: Help your COPD patient take a better breath with inhalers, Nursing, 13(5):42-43, 1983.

Ecoff L, Barone RM, and Simons RM: Implantable infusion port (Port-a-Cath), NITA 6(6):406-408, 1983.

Engle V: Turning a patient into a manager. In Managing diabetics properly, Springhouse, Penn, 1983, Intermed Communications, Inc.

Eggleston M: Focus on vial sterility, Infect Control 5(4):163-164, 1984.

Fawbush MW: Reuse of disposable syringe-needle sets in the diabetic patient: fact or fiction? Florida Nurse 32(10):15, 1984.

Fischer D and Knobf T: The cancer chemotherapy handbook, Chicago, 1989, Year Book Medical Publishers.

Ford DC, Leist ER, and Phelps SJ: Guidelines for administration of intravenous medications to pediatric patients, ed 3, Bethesda, Md, 1988, American Society of Hospital Pharmacists.

Gahart BL: Intravenous medications: a handbook for nurses and other allied health personnel, ed 4, St Louis, 1985, The CV Mosby Co.

Garcia MK: Asthma: old problems and new strategies, School Nurse 5(3):25-38, 1989.

Gardner C: Spartanburg General Hospital policy book on IV therapy administration (part II), NITA 9:352-384, 1986.

Garner JS et al: CDC recommendation clarified, Infect Control 5(9):419, 1984.

Gebarski S and Gebarski K: Chemotherapy port "Twiddler's Syndrome": a need for preinjection radiography, Cancer 54(1):38-39, 1984.

Geyer J: Response to letter on IV infusions of gentamycin and ampicillin, Pediatr Nurs 15(5):514-515, 1989.

Glass SM and Giacoia GP: Intravenous drug therapy in premature infants: practical aspects, JOGNN 16(5):310-318, 1987.

Goodman L and Gilman A, editors: The pharmacological basis of therapeutics, ed 7, New York, 1985, Macmillan.

Goodman M: Cancer: chemotherapy and care, part II, Evansville, Ind, 1981, Bristol Laboratories Division.

Goodman MS and Wickham R: Venous access devices: an overview, Oncol Nurs Forum 11(5):16-23, 1984.

Hanson RL: Heparin lock or keep open IV, AJN 76(7):1102-1103, 1976.

Hargrove C: Administration of IV medications in the NICU: the development of a procedure, Neonatal Network 5(10):41-49, 1987.

Hermann CS: Performing intradermal skin tests the right way, Nursing 13(10):50-53, 1983.

Hicks J et al: Optimum needle length for diphtheria-tetanus-pertussis inoculation of infants, Pediatrics 84(1):136-137, 1989.

Hill EM, Flaitz CM, and Frost GR: Sweetener content of common oral liquid medications, Am J Hosp Pharm 45(1):135-142, 1988.

Hockenberry M: Pediatric oncology: perspective on care, St Louis, 1986, The CV Mosby Co.

Hodges LC and Parker J: Concerns of parents with diabetic children, Pediat Nurs 13(1):22-24; 68, 1987.

Home care of Hickman and Broviac catheters, Memphis, 1984, St Jude Children's Research Hospital.

Hughes C: Giving cancer drugs IV: some guidelines, AJN 86(1):34-38, 1986.

Hyams JS et al: Carbohydrate malabsorption following fruit juice ingestion in young children, Pediatrics 82(1):64-68, 1988.

Intramuscular injections: a guide to sites and technique. Philadelphia, 1986, Wyeth Laboratories.

Keen MF: Comparison of intramuscular injection techniques to reduce site discomfort and lesions, Nurs Res 35(4):207-210, 1986.

Knobf T: IV therapy guidelines for oncology practice, Oncol Nurs Forum 9(2):30-34, 1982.

Kovalesky A: Nurses' guide to children's eyes, Orlando, Fla, 1985, Grune & Stratton.

Leff RD and Roberts RJ: Practical aspects of intravenous drug therapy techniques, Bethesda, Md, 1985, American Society of Hospital Pharmacists.

Lehrer S: Understanding lung sounds, Philadelphia, 1984, WB Saunders Co.

Lenz CL: Make your needle selection right to the point, Nursing 13(2):50-51, 1983.

Lewis KH and Smalldon M: Simplify insulin injection: omit pull-back, AJN 84(4):426, 1984.

Lourenco RV and Cotromanes E: Clinical aerosols: characterization of aerosols and their diagnostic uses, Arch Intern Med 142(11):2163-2172, 1982.

Lunn JK and Wilson A: Retrograde medication administration: a predictable and simple system for pediatric drug delivery, Focus Crit Care 13(6):59-63, 1986.

Managing IV therapy, Nursing Photobook, Springhouse, Penn, 1985, Springhouse Corp.

Marcoux C, Fisher S, and Wong D: Venous access devices in children, Pediatr Nurs 16(2):123-133, 1990.

Maul-Mellott S and Adams J: Childhood cancer: a nursing overview, Boston, 1987, Jones & Bartlett.

McConnell EA: The subtle art of really good injections, RN 45(2):25-34, 1983.

McGovern K: Some pointers on needle safety, Nursing 16(10):58-59, 1986.

McGowen E and Whipple TJ: Medicate aerosol delivery, Drug Letter 28(1):1-4, 1989.

Medication administration and IV therapy manual, Springhouse, Penn, 1988, Springhouse Corp.

Meeske K and Davidson L: Teacher's reference on right atrial catheters, J Pediatr Nurs 3(5):351-353, 1988.

Messing B et al: Antibiotic-lock technique: a new approach to optimal therapy for catheter-related sepsis in home parenteral nutrition patients, J Parenter Enteral Nutr 12(2):185-189, 1988.

Millam D: Managing complications of IV therapy, Nursing 18(3):34-42, 1988.

Motz-Harding E and Good F: The right solution: mixing IV drugs thoroughly, Nursing 15(2):62-64, 1985.

National Association of School Nurses: Guidelines for a model school nurse program, Scarborough, Me, 1981, National Association of School Nurses.

Newton DW and Newton M: Route, site and technique: three key decisions in giving parenteral medication, Nursing 9(7):18-24, 1979.

Oncology Nursing Society: Cancer chemotherapy guidelines, modules II, III, V, Pittsburgh, Penn, 1988, Oncology Nursing Society.

Orenstein S et al: The Santmyer swallow: a new and useful infant reflex, Lancet 1(8581):345-346, 1988.

Orzeck EA: Injection aids, Diabetes Forecast 40(10):40-42, 1984.

OSHA Publication 81.1: Guidelines for cytotoxic drugs, Washington DC, 1986, Office of Occupational Medicine.

Perry AG and Potter PA: Clinical nursing skills and techniques, ed 2, St Louis, 1990, The CV Mosby Co.

Persons CB: Critical care procedures and protocols: a nursing process approach, Philadelphia, 1987, JB Lippincott Co.

Plaut TF: Children with asthma: a manual for parents, ed 2, Amherst, Mass, 1988, Pedipress.

Plumer AL: Principles and practice of intravenous therapy, ed 4, Boston, 1987, Little, Brown & Co.

Poteet GW, Reinert B, and Ptak HE: Outcome of multiple usage of disposable syringes in the insulin-requiring diabetic, Nurs Res 36(6):350-352, 1987.

Potter PA and Perry AG: Basic nursing: theory and practice, St Louis, 1987, The CV Mosby Co.

Powers L: American Society of Hospital Pharmacy technical assistance bulletin on handling cytotoxic drugs in hospitals, Am J Hosp Pharm 42(1):131-137, 1985.

Price S: Port-a-Cath: implantable drug delivery system, Memphis, 1986, St Jude Children's Research Hospital.

Regan WA: Doctor's orders and nursing judgement, The Regan Report on Nursing Law 21(4):1, 1980.

Rettig FM and Southby JR: Using different body positions to reduce discomfort from dorsogluteal injections, Nurs Res 31(4):219-221, 1982.

Roberts RJ: Intravenous administration of medication in pediatric patients: problems and solutions, Pediatr Clin North Am 28(1):23-34, 1981.

Sager DP: Intravenous medications: a guide to preparation, administration and nursing management, Philadelphia, 1982, JB Lippincott Co.

Schulze KF et al: Physiologic oscillations produced by an infusion pump, J Pediatr 103:796-798, 1983.

Shapiro BA, Harrison RA, and Trout CA: Clinical application of respiratory care, Chicago, 1982, Year Book Medical Publishers.

Shearer J: Normal saline flush versus dilute heparin flush: a study of peripheral intermittent IV devices, NITA 10(6):425-427, 1987.

Smith S and Duell D: Clinical nursing skills, ed 2, Los Altos, Calif, 1988, National Nursing Review.

Taylor N et al: Comparison of normal versus heparinized saline for flushing infusion devices, J Nurs Qual Assur 3(4):49-55, 1989.

Thatcher G: Insulin injections: the case against random rotation, AJN 85(6):690-692, 1985.

Tomkey D and Weinrauch S: Insulin pumps, Diabetic Forecast 40(10):43-45, 1987.

Traver GA and Martinez M: Asthma update part II: treatment, J Pediatr Health Care 2(5):227-233, 1988.

Travis LB, Brouhard BH, and Schreiner BJ: Diabetes mellitus in children and adolescents, Philadelphia, 1987, WB Saunders Co.

UCLA TPN Newsletter, January, 1986.

Vanbree NS, Hollerback AD, and Brooks GP: Clinical evaluation of three techniques for administering low-dose heparin, Nurs Res 33(1):15-19, 1984.

Vogel TC and McSkimming SA: Teaching parents to give indwelling CV catheter care, Nursing 13(1):55-56, 1983.

Walters P: Chemotherapy: a nurse's guide to action, administration, and side effects. RN 53(2):52-57, 1990.

Wezel-Bolen GV: Technological advances in the care of children with chronic illnesses, Pediatrics: nursing update 1(11), Princeton, NJ, 1986, Continuing Professional Education Center, Inc.

Weinstein AM: Asthma: the complete guide to self-management for asthma and allergies for patients and their families, New York, 1987, McGraw-Hill Inc.

Whaley LF and Wong DL: Nursing care of infants and children, ed 4, St Louis, 1991, The CV Mosby Co.

Wong DL: Significance of dead space in syringes, AJN 82(8):1237, 1982.

Wong DL and Redding B: Lozenges can be lifesavers, AJN 86(9):1129-1130, 1986.

Wong DL and Whaley LF: Clinical manual of pediatric nursing, ed 3, St Louis, 1990, The CV Mosby Co.

Yankovich AR: Medication usage in public schools: policy recommendations and procedural guidelines, School Nurse 3(3):32-37, 1987.

Young G et al: Catheter sepsis during parenteral nutrition: the safety of long-term OpSite dressings, J Parenter Enteral Nutr 12(4):365-370, 1988.

Zenk KE: Administering IV antibiotics to children, Nursing 16(12):50-52, 1986.

# UNIT XVII Surgery

# SKILL 112 Preparing the Child Psychologically for Surgery

*Deborah Kay Brantly and Judy Holt Rollins*

Without information and psychologic preparation, children facing surgery often develop misconceptions not only of the surgical event itself, but of any in the series of events leading up to or after surgery. Fantasies may lead to fears, which can lead to negative reactions and often long-term consequences (e.g., behavioral problems, fears, inability to trust others). Riffee (1981) reported that although a decrease in self-esteem occurred in all children who were hospitalized, there was a greater decrease in children hospitalized for surgery.

Although preparing children for surgery is similar to preparation for any procedure or hospitalization, the numerous preoperative and postoperative routines require a series of preparatory sessions to prevent overstressing the child with too much information (Whaley and Wong, 1991). Anticipatory anxiety is common, because children find the anticipated loss of or entry into a part of the body very threatening (Junenker, 1977). Thus, psychologic preparation for surgery includes both education and expressive components.

## NURSING DIAGNOSES

Anxiety related to unmet informational needs about surgical procedures and/or perioperative experience; Fear related to separation from family/peers during hospitalization; Ineffective coping related to unrealistic expectations or inadequate coping methods.

| Steps | Rationale |
|---|---|
| **Assessment** | |
| 1. Review information about the type of surgery, scheduled time, and child's admission status. | This information provides a beginning framework for timing preparation activities. Some surgical procedures require simple and brief psychologic preparation; others require an extensive series of sessions. More time is available to prepare a child when surgery is elective or scheduled. For emergency surgery, simple explanations and assurance of emotional support can be given concurrently with each step. |
| 2. Determine the child's age, developmental level, cognitive functioning, and physical condition. | These factors provide guidelines for timing preparation activities and planning age-appropriate preparation techniques. Developmental level also offers predictive clues to the fears and anticipated reaction the child may have to surgery (see Table 112-1). Because the stress of surgery compounds cognitive difficulties of the mentally retarded child, more concrete preparation and frequent repetition of instructions will be required (Benchot, 1986). The child in poor physical condition may lack the energy to concentrate on preparation activities. |
| 3. Ask about recent significant life experiences the child/family has encountered, the child's previous experiences with health care and/or surgical procedures, and what the child has been told by family members, friends, neighbors, and the physician. | The child who has recently experienced a significant life change (e.g., birth of a sibling or parental divorce) may need time to master the event before facing the trauma of surgery. The child may have acquired conditioned fears about the hospital setting through previous personal experiences or those of others (Demarest, Hooke, and Erickson, 1984). |

**TABLE 112-1** Age-Related Fears Associated with Surgery

| Age | Primary Concerns | Intervention |
|---|---|---|
| Under 5 years | What will happen when they wake up<br>Where they will be<br>Who will be with them | Show recovery room, if possible<br>Tell when their parents will visit them after surgery<br>Encourage parents to be with them as soon as possible |
| School-age | | |
| Younger | Anesthesia<br>That they might wake up during surgery<br>How doctor knows when or if doctor knows how to awaken them | Show mask<br>Explain "gas" or "medicine" and how it works<br>Stress concept of "special sleep"<br>Explain that it is a special person's job to control the sleep |
| Older | Same as above plus<br>Operation itself<br>Mutilation<br>Possible death | Same as above<br>Provide knowledge about procedure |
| Adolescents | Same as above plus<br>Special anxiety for change in body image<br>Loss of control while under anesthesia (in terms of behavior and for body integrity)<br>Peer reaction to scars<br>Impact on sexuality<br>Impact on adolescent mode of dress | Same as above<br>Reassure that only what is supposed to be done will be performed<br>Introduce to peer with similar surgery |

Adapted from Gustafson, 1982; Whaley and Wong, 1991.

| Steps | Rationale |
|---|---|
| 4. Identify the child's general psychologic state and usual coping methods when anxious. | Generally, the more psychologically healthy the child, the better equipped he or she is to handle the stress of surgery. When surgery is expected to improve the child's quality of life, for instance, to relieve pain, to correct a deformity, to lessen fatigue or shortness of breath, the child may be eager for the procedure. The child will use more familiar methods of coping during times of high stress. |
| 5. Assess availability of the child's family and other support systems. | The child will need situational support during surgery and hospitalization, whether by family members or other appropriate persons. |
| 6. Determine parental preference for involvement with the preparation and during surgery, e.g., reading preparation material to the child, assisting in tours, practicing deep breathing, rooming-in, presence during anesthesia induction (see box at right and Fig. 112-1), or presence in postanesthesia care unit (PACU). | Parents are a great source of support, particularly for the younger child. Learning may be enhanced by participation of a familiar person. Continuation in a normal parenting role often relieves some of the sense of hopelessness or helplessness parents may feel. Allowing the parents to determine their involvement maintains their sense of power in the health care setting while giving them an opportunity to decline or limit participation in activities in which they are uncomfortable. |
| 7. With the surgeon and anesthesiologist, review details of surgery and its preoperative and postoperative implications for the child. | Consulting with the surgeon and anesthesiologist provides an opportunity to ask questions. The discussion will frequently reveal additional information not present in orders. These details allow for a more complete and individualized preparation. |
| 8. Determine the role of other members of the health care team in preparing the child for surgery. | Physicians, anesthesiologists, child life specialists, physical therapists, and other professionals often perform preparation activities. Coordinated efforts among professionals enhances the likelihood that the child will be successfully prepared for the surgery and surrounding events. |
| 9. Review common stress points surrounding surgery and additional ones specific to the child's surgery (Visintainer and Wolfer, 1975).<br>a. Admission.<br>b. Blood tests.<br>c. The afternoon of the day before surgery. | Using the stress points to guide interventions increases the likelihood that the child will be adequately prepared.<br>***Special Considerations:*** *The afternoon of the day before surgery is stressful for the child who is admitted for preparatory events such as x-rays, bowel preparation, physical examinations by physicians in training, and special baths or shampoos.* |

## *PARENTAL PRESENCE AT INDUCTION*

Hospitals have traditionally separated parents and their child before the child enters the surgical unit. It is sometimes argued that parents will bring infectious agents to the area or will become upset when they see their lifeless child after induction, or that children will "behave" better without their parents. Others list disadvantages such as disruption of operating room routine and increased time and cost (Gauderer, Lorig, and Eastwood, 1989). With proper preparation and precautions, there is minimal theoretical basis for any of these arguments. However, the effects of separation on children at this stressful time and the benefits of parental presence are well documented (Thompson, 1985). In a recent study, parental presence in the operating room during anesthesia induction resulted in decreased psychologic trauma for the child, smoother induction, and decreased parental anxiety (Gauderer, Lorig, and Eastwood, 1989).

Wearing gown, hat, mask, and shoe covers, parents can hold small children, or stand close to the older child in the operating room. Induction is usually performed via a mask. Once the child is asleep, the parent(s) is escorted to a waiting area.

Some hospitals use induction rooms, a small room close to the operating room where the child is given anesthesia, usually by mask or rectum. Parents are present, again, often holding their child in their arms. Deeper induction (e.g., IV anesthesia), if necessary, occurs after the child is transported to the operating room.

Gauderer, Lorig, and Eastwood (1989) demonstrated the feasibility, safety, and acceptance of parental presence for anesthesia induction:

> With appropriate selection and preoperative preparation, parental presence in the operating room during the induction of anesthesia is a positive factor in the delivery of surgical care to children. We feel that in this age of multiple choices in health care delivery, there is a place for parents during the induction of anesthesia in an appropriate setting.

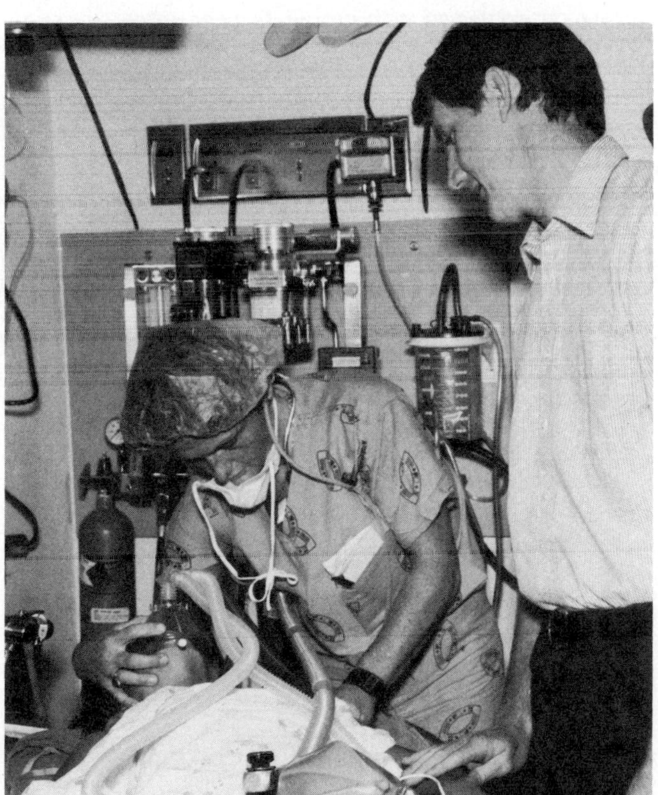

***FIG. 112-1*** Parent present during anesthesia induction.

| Steps | Rationale |
|---|---|
| d. Injection of preoperative medication.<br>e. Before and during transport to the operating room.<br>f. Return from the PACU. | |
| 10. Review the sensations the child may encounter at common stress points (see the box at right). | Children who receive information about what they may see, hear, smell, and feel are more prepared to cope with surgery. Some health care facilities use induction rooms; therefore, it is more important to be familiar with the common sensations of the induction room rather than those of the operating room the child may never actually see. The key to good preparation is taking the time to think through each stress point from the child's perspective.<br>***Special Considerations:*** *As an advocate for children, encourage minimizing or eliminating as many frightening sensations as possible, e.g., keeping strange equipment out of sight until the child is asleep.* |

## Planning and Goal Setting

| Steps | Rationale |
|---|---|
| 1. Plan timing of interventions based on age-appropriateness.<br>a. With the mature toddler and preschooler, plan shorter, more frequent preparation sessions (Evans and Hansen, 1985).<br>b. Plan time to include practice of postoperative recovery techniques.<br>c. Plan time for play after preparation sessions. | Preparation of the younger child is optimally begun a couple of days in advance of the surgery, whereas for the older child, 1 to 3 weeks is preferred (Blacher, 1987). |
| 2. Whenever possible, schedule work hours to coincide with the critical stress points surrounding the child's surgery. | Preparation, combined with encouragement, reassurance, and reinforcement from a single caregiver who attends the child and family throughout hospitalization, and especially at critical points, enables the child to cope more effectively with and adjust to the various stresses encountered (Wolfer and Visintainer, 1975). |
| 3. Decide the most appropriate teaching setting: individual or group setting. | Group teaching is frequently used to save time and resources. Groups can also supply peer support. However, some children may best be prepared individually.<br>***Special Considerations:*** *With a stress point approach, the child would still be prepared and supported individually at certain critical times.* |
| 4. Gather needed materials for preparation for each of the common stress points and events specific to child's surgery that may be stress producing. | Gathering materials in advance facilitates an efficient, accurate, and orderly preoperative preparation.<br>***Special Considerations:*** *Materials may include medical equipment, dolls, play materials, and photographs (see Product References and Teaching Resources), informative booklets, films, videos, or tape recordings.* |
| 5. Develop individualized child and family goals.<br>▪ Child/family will demonstrate understanding of the surgical procedure and the expected preoperative, intraoperative, and postoperative course.<br>▪ Child/family will exhibit minimal anxiety about anticipated surgery.<br>▪ Child will demonstrate mastery of preoperative and postoperative coping skills and rehabilitative measures. | |

## Implementation

| Steps | Rationale |
|---|---|
| 1. Provide parents with literature about the surgery and hospitalization. Include:<br>a. Basic information about the hospital or outpatient facility (see Skill 2).<br>b. Information about preparation activities such as puppet shows and tours before or after admission.<br>c. General guidelines about what to expect preoperatively, intraoperatively, and postoperatively, and the parents' role at each stage. Include information about parents rooming-in, presence in induction or PACU areas, and general expectations of the child's condition and behavior after discharge. | Providing parents with information in advance may reduce their level of stress, allowing them to take a more active role in helping their child to experience less stress and a more positive response to surgery (Smallwood, 1988). Advance information also permits parents the opportunity to make arrangements, e.g., child care for siblings or time off from work.<br>***Special Considerations:*** *If time permits, information may be provided at the surgeon's office or mailed to the family. It is helpful to list a telephone number and contact person for parents to contact with questions.* |

## *SENSATIONS THE CHILD MAY ENCOUNTER AT SELECTED COMMON STRESS POINTS*

### BEFORE AND DURING TRANSPORT TO OPERATING ROOM

**Emotions or feelings such as:**

Fear ("of waking up, or will wake up when they cut and it will hurt;" "of where you will be when its over;" fear that its going to hurt; fear that they'll do the wrong thing or more than they should; fear of death; fear of falling off stretcher; fear of talking in sleep)
Anxiety ("anxious to get it over with")
Guilt (being punished)
Powerlessness
Curiosity
Hunger
Thirst
Embarrassment from exposure
Perhaps dizzy or nauseated from preoperative medication and movement

**Smells such as:**

Strange place, "hospital smells," antiseptic cleaning solutions

**Sights such as:**

Strangers, in scrubs
Unfamiliar surroundings
Gurney, straps
The ceiling of halls and unfamiliar rooms
People in masks, gowns, gloves, "funny shoes"
Some familiar people, some unfamiliar
Strange equipment, tanks, monitors
Bright lights

**Sounds such as:**

Strange voices of transporters and others along the way
Clang of siderails
Wheels of gurney
Elevator sounds
Automatic door sounds
Parents' reassuring voices
Beeps
Hums
Clicks
Muffled voices under masks, some familiar, some not
People talking to each other

**Taste such as:**

Maybe dry mouth

**Touch such as:**

Straps to "help you hold still"
People "helping you move"
Perhaps cold
Hard operating room table

### RETURN FROM THE RECOVERY ROOM

**Emotions or feelings such as:**

Dizzy
Uncomfortable
Nauseated
In pain
Cold
Relief that operation is over
Joy at seeing parents
Anxiety ("Will I ever feel right again")
Fear
Guilt (being punished)
Powerlessness
Inability to move
Hunger
Thirst
Sore throat from intubation

**Smells such as:**

Gases, medications, or cleaning solutions

**Sights such as:**

Parents
IV tubing, bags or bottles, pump
Catheter
Dressings
Drainage tubes and bottles
Changes in body image (missing limbs, disfigurement, swelling, discoloration)
BP cuff
Monitors
Clips and leads to monitors
Blood
Siderails

**Sounds such as:**

Voices of transporters and others along the way
Wheels of gurney
Elevator sounds
Automatic door sounds
Parents' reassuring voices
Beeps
Hums
Clicks
Clang of siderails
People talking to each other
Voice of familiar nurse or other health care professional

**Taste such as:**

Dry mouth
Perhaps ice chips

**Touch such as:**

Pressure of BP cuff on arm
Pressure from hands and equipment for examination and monitoring
IV, catheter, or drainage tubing resting against skin
Pressure from dressings and tape
People "helping you move"

See Sensations Chart in Skill 1, pp. 2-3, and Skill 2 for sensations of other procedures that may be associated with preoperative care.

| Steps | Rationale |
|---|---|
| d. A list of helpful books or pamphlets for parents to begin preparing their child for surgery (see Product References and Teaching Resources). | |
| e. Literature for the child, e.g., an invitation to a puppet show, booklet about coming to the hospital for surgery. | Addressing the child makes him or her feel expected and welcome. |
| 2. On admission, orient the child and family to the hospital or outpatient facility, if not already done (see Skill 3). | This may be the first hospital stay for the child and he or she will need information about both the hospitalization and the surgery, whether it is to be performed on an inpatient or outpatient basis.<br>***Special Considerations:*** *If the child will go to a different unit or area after surgery, at the appropriate time in preparation activities be certain to show the child and family the new unit, introducing the unfamiliar nurses who will be providing care.* |
| 3. Explore the child's understanding of the surgery and the reason for it. Clarify misconceptions by using child's own terms whenever possible or by asking parents to express what was said in more familiar words. | The child's past experiences, information from other children or family members, the media, or school may precipitate preconceived ideas of the surgery. Assessing the accuracy of such information provides a foundation for clarifying misconceptions, reducing fears, and promoting a sense of mastery.<br>***Special Considerations:*** *Children under 4 years have difficulty understanding relationships or may have no interest in the reason for surgery. They may think that the surgery is a punishment and need to be reassured that this is not true.* |
| 4. Prepare the child and family for each stressful event: (1) admission, (2) blood tests, (3) preoperative medication, (4) transport to the operating room, and (5) return from the PACU room, as well as additional stressful events specific to the child's surgery, e.g., bowel preparation and bath or shower with special medicated soap. | Systematic preparation, rehearsal of the forthcoming events, and supportive care at each of the stress points is more effective than the traditional single session preparation or consistent supportive care without systematic preparation and rehearsal (Whaley and Wong, 1991). When children and parents receive systematic psychologic preparation and continued supportive care, children show less upset behavior and more cooperation in the hospital, and few posthospital adjustment problems (Wolfer and Visintainer, 1975).<br>***Special Considerations:*** *Although infants are too young for elaborate preparation, they can be prepared by practicing "peek-a-boo" with surgical caps, masks, and gowns as well as an anesthesia mask, if it will be used. (Parents are ideal facilitators of this play.) Provide opportunities for infants to handle IV tubing, oxygen cannulas, nasogastric tubes, syringes, and stethoscopes. This helps satisfy their curiosity and reduces subsequent disturbance of equipment (Goldberger, 1988).* |
| a. Provide information about what to expect, describing the sequence of events and arranging material so that frightening information is presented last (refer to Guidelines for selecting nonthreatening words or phrases on p. 7). Include:<br>▪ When the procedure or event will take place.<br>▪ What will happen, e.g., preoperative injection, bath, or shower.<br>▪ What parts of the body are involved; emphasize that no other parts of the body will be touched.<br>▪ Why it is necessary.<br>▪ Where it will occur.<br>▪ If transported somewhere, how and by whom and what will they be wearing.<br>▪ What the child will be wearing and if he or she can wear underwear.<br>▪ What can be taken with child (stuffed animal, doll).<br>▪ What child will see, hear, smell, feel (refer to the box on p. 729). Describe in detail; use pictures, video, or tour areas such as induction or operating room, PACU. Demonstrate sensations when possible, e.g., wet alcohol sponge to skin.<br>▪ What people will be there, who the child may know, and what the people will be wearing. | Information about what to expect removes or minimizes the series of real, imagined, or potential threats for the child. Vague, undefined threats are more upsetting than threats that are known and understood. Unexpected stress is more upsetting than expected stress. The child is under stress to the extent that these threats are not removed, minimized, or coped with more or less effectively (Visintainer and Wolfer, 1975). If frightening information is presented first, children may be upset and unable to focus on subsequent information.<br>***Special Considerations:*** *A story form using a doll and hospital equipment works well for the young child. The same materials may be used for an older child, giving more details with special attention to the mechanics of the procedure.* |

| **Steps** | **Rationale** |
|---|---|
| ▪ What are the people's roles (e.g., anesthesiologist's job is "to make sure you don't feel or hear anything and to know when to wake you up").<br>▪ Who will be performing ("in charge of") the surgery.<br>▪ If parents will be present; if not, where they will be (show where in tour or photograph) and when child will see them again. | |
| b. Provide information about what to expect after the event. Include:<br>▪ Anything about the child that will look different or feel different after surgery such as catheters, an IV, monitoring electrodes, a sore throat from intubation.<br>▪ Expected dressing(s) (even Band-Aids) and that the surgeon or other health care professional will want to look frequently at it.<br>▪ Anticipated dressing changes.<br>▪ What will be temporary and what will not.<br>▪ When child can eat or drink again.<br>▪ Anticipated pain and its management.<br>▪ The reason to begin walking as soon as possible (if appropriate).<br>▪ When the child can walk, go to playroom. | Changes, either temporary or permanent, that the child may experience after the event may confuse or frighten him or her, e.g., waking up after surgery with an IV. |
| c. Provide information about the child's role, helping child identify role and expected behaviors. Include:<br>▪ Choices available to child, e.g., choice of which arm to use to draw blood, choice of anesthesia flavor or soda flavor when able to take liquids postoperatively, choice of toy after procedure or surgery.<br>▪ Role in positioning, and deep breathing, stressing the reason and importance of it even if uncomfortable (see Skill 92).<br>▪ Expected behaviors, e.g., crying is permissible as well as other alternatives, such as counting or giving verbal commands such as "hurry up." Muscle relaxation can work well for older children.<br>▪ Role in expressing needs. Child should know when it is permissible to talk or move, what person is available to meet needs, and what to do if necessary to void; should know that questions are encouraged. | Information about role and behaviors increases feelings of control and involvement in the event. Clarifying limits and expected "acceptable" behaviors provides a sense of control, autonomy, and competence. It also allows the child to direct efforts to realistic goals, e.g., recognizing that a blood test is unavoidable but that being cooperative may shorten the length of time it will take. |
| d. Provide an opportunity for the child to express feelings and concerns. Attempt to identify fears and clarify misconceptions, e.g., ask, "Most people tell me they have a special worry—can you tell me or draw me a picture about yours?" (see Skill 16). | Children of all ages find surgical events fearful (Slaw, Stephens, and Holmes, 1986). Visintainer and Wolfer (1975) categorized the types of fears or threats experienced by pediatric patients hospitalized for surgery as (1) physiologic harm or bodily injury in the form of discomfort, pain, mutilation, or death; (2) separation from parents or trusted friends, familiar surroundings, or security objects; (3) the strange, unknown, and the possibility of surprise; (4) uncertainty about limits and expected "acceptable" behavior; and (5) relative loss of control, autonomy, and competence.<br>***Special Considerations:*** *Older children may not exhibit overt manifestation of fear as readily as younger children (Katz, Kellerman, and Siegel, 1980), thus questioning is essential to elicit true feelings.* |
| e. Discuss fears of bodily harm. Answer questions about disfigurement or death honestly and realistically. | Children need to know the outcomes of the surgery. Honest discussion of the questions posed will facilitate the therapeutic relationship and establish trust.<br>***Special Considerations:*** *A psychiatric clinical nurse specialist or other mental health professional should be contacted immediately to participate in preparation activities with the child and family when the anticipated consequences of surgery will result in significant changes in body image such as disfigurement or amputation; or if death may occur.* |

| Steps | Rationale |
|---|---|
| f. Encourage child to rehearse the event.<br>▪ Exchange roles with the nurse and conduct the procedure on a doll, while repeating the story (see Skill 16).<br>▪ Practice procedures such as deep breathing and turning (see Skill 92). | Rehearsal provides the opportunity to assess the child's understanding of the event and makes it more familiar. Handling the anesthesia mask and other medical equipment increases familiarity and reduces anxiety (Siaw, Stephens, and Holmes, 1986). Performing a procedure on a doll allows the child to assume an active role and helps him or her gain a sense of control and mastery of the situation.<br>***Special Considerations:*** *Some facilities give each child going to surgery a doll, puppet, or stuffed animal to take to surgery. The child awakens after surgery to the doll that has received the same procedure (e.g., an IV, dressings, cast) as the child. The doll is updated to match the child's postoperative course.* |
| 5. Encourage parents to be available for the child as much as possible, particularly during the identified stress points. | Surgery is a stressful event in the life of the child; parents can offer support and help the child cope with the stress. Separation from parents adds more stress, especially for the young child.<br>***Special Considerations:*** *If parents will not be available during significantly stressful times, encourage them to designate an appropriate family member or other person to assume the role.* |
| 6. Encourage parents to participate with the child as they are comfortable and offer support for parents in learning hospital comfort measures or skills associated with their child's needs. | Generally, maximal parental involvement and interaction is viewed as beneficial to the child. Supporting the parents' learning eases their fears of becoming involved with unfamiliar activities. |
| 7. Offer child and parents support and reassurance during and/or after the stressful events (see Guidelines during and after the procedure on p. 7). | Supportive care reduces emotional distress (Wolfer and Visintainer, 1975).<br>***Special Considerations:*** *After surgery, reassure the child that the operation is over (see Skill 16 for postoperative or postprocedure activities).* |
| a. Keep parents updated on the progress of their child's surgery on a regular basis. | In the absence of information that everything is all right, parents may be subject to needless anxiety. |
| b. Help parents maintain their basic needs.<br>▪ Provide comfortable waiting areas.<br>▪ Use communication systems, such as a message book in the surgery waiting area, where parents can note their whereabouts, e.g., "We've gone to the cafeteria to eat." | Parents will frequently go without eating or taking care of other basic needs, afraid they will miss news about the child, or afraid to leave the child immediately after surgery or a stressful procedure. |
| 8. Reunite child and parents as soon as possible. | The period when the child awakens from anesthesia can be very stressful for the child, e.g., may feel confused, in pain. Parents are a significant source of support for the child. Hospitals that recognize this concept are permitting parents in the PACU whenever possible.<br>***Special Considerations:*** *Parents are typically anxious about their child's surgery and seeing the child as soon as possible also provides relief for them.* |
| 9. After surgery discuss with parents and child their roles, what they can expect for the remainder of the recovery period, and from whom to seek help. | Information allows child and parents to assume their expected roles, facilitating the best possible outcome for the child. Knowing what to anticipate provides markers for recovery, permits the child and parents to experience progress, eliminates the unexpected, and alerts the family to unusual occurrences. When parents know whom to call for help, aid can be summoned quickly. |
| 10. As soon as the child is physically able, provide opportunities for therapeutic play (see Skill 16). | It is common for the child to have aggressive feelings after surgery, which can be frightening for the child and parents. Therapeutic play allows the child to safely release aggression or anger often experienced after being in a passive role, particularly when painful or frightening events have occurred. The child has the opportunity to master the series of events through play (Pass and Pass, 1987). |

### Evaluation Outcomes

1. The child and family demonstrate understanding of the surgical procedure and the expected preoperative, intraoperative, and postoperative course.
2. The child and family exhibit minimal anxiety about the anticipated surgery.
3. Child demonstrates mastery of preoperative and postoperative coping skills and rehabilitative measures.

### Observational Guidelines

Child correctly demonstrates the surgical procedure on a doll. Older child verbally relates sequence of events. Parents discuss their role in supporting the child throughout the course.

Child and parents discuss the surgery openly and with relative ease. Child's behavior is free of angry outbursts or withdrawal.

Child correctly demonstrates deep breathing and positioning. Child chooses and demonstrates a coping technique.

### Documentation

Describe the knowledge level of the child before and after the preparation, using direct quotations when possible. List fears the child has expressed and if, on evaluation, these fears seem alleviated. Document type of preparation (group, individual, or both) and materials used. Document the parents' role during preparation and anticipated role during and after surgery.

# *SKILL* 113 Physically Preparing the Child for Surgery

*Donna Phillips Smith*

The significance of the physical preparation of a child for surgery is often overlooked with the emphasis on preoperative teaching and psychologic preparation. However, adequate physical preparation and documentation of preoperative routines can prevent intraoperative and postoperative complications.

### NURSING DIAGNOSES

Anxiety related to unmet informational needs about preoperative procedures; Potential for injury related to altered mobility and cerebral function due to preoperative sedatives.

| Steps | Rationale |
|---|---|
| **Assessment** | |
| 1. Review orders and/or consult with physician on the type of surgery to be performed, timing, and admission status, e.g., elective, emergency, outpatient, morning of surgery admission. | The type, timing, and admission status of surgery has implications for the physical preparations needed, their urgency, and the general condition of the child. ***Special Considerations:*** *Children with conditions requiring elective surgical procedures are usually in good health except for the surgical problem. Other types of surgery may require interventions to improve the child's overall physical condition and nutritional status before surgery (Leape, 1987).* |
| 2. Determine if the physician has obtained informed consent from family for the surgery, and that written authorizations have been signed and witnessed (see Skill 8). | Obtaining informed consent for a surgical procedure is the physician's responsibility, although the nurse may witness the written authorization. ***Special Considerations:*** *For elective surgical procedures, the authorization papers may have been signed at the preoperative visit to the surgeon's office.* |
| 3. Determine special preparation orders and/or facility protocol for surgical pediatric patients, e.g., lab tests, skin preparation, bowel cleansing, prophylactic antibiotics, IV initiation, timing of NPO (nothing by mouth) status and x-rays. | Physical preparation will be guided by facility protocol and/or special physician orders. ***Special Considerations:*** *Diagnostic studies may be limited in children, consisting only of a complete blood count (CBC) and urinalysis (UA). Routine chest x-rays, electrocardiograms (ECG), and bleeding studies, often performed on adult patients, are usually not necessary in children unless clinically indicated.* |

| Steps | Rationale |
|---|---|
| 4. Determine if preoperative anesthesia assessment has been completed and if preoperative medication(s) are ordered. | A preoperative assessment is performed by an anesthesiologist or nurse anesthetist to determine risk factors and plan course of anesthesia. Preoperative medication may be ordered to decrease anxiety, sedate, minimize secretions, and protect the cardiovascular system by blocking vagal nerve response (King, Wieck, and Dyer, 1983).<br>***Special Considerations:*** *A preoperative injection is generally the most upsetting event for the child before surgery. Unfortunately, the injection may do little to relieve anxiety, and may not have the desired sedation effect (Whaley and Wong, 1989). A recent trend is toward either not using preoperative medications, or using oral mixtures and other nonparenteral medications to produce sedation (Brzustowicz et al, 1984; Nelson et al, 1989).* |
| 5. Obtain nursing history (if not previously done). Assessment information significant to obtain for the preoperative child includes: | The nursing history may reveal significant information that will influence preparation for surgery, and intraoperative and postoperative care by the entire health care team. |
| a. Allergies. | Knowing allergies to medications and skin preparation products allows an alternate selection to prevent a reaction. |
| b. Medication history and current regimen. | Certain medications may cause complications during surgery and/or anesthesia by producing undesirable drug interactions or exacerbation of an underlying disease process. |
| c. Previous surgeries, including serious reactions or complications. | Knowledge about tolerance of previous surgical procedures can identify potential risks and prevent future complications. |
| d. Serious reaction or unexplained death of any family member to anesthesia. | The potential for malignant hyperthermia, one of the most life-threatening complications of certain anesthetics, is genetically inherited (Marshall and Wollman, 1985).<br>***Special Considerations:*** *Notify the surgeon or anesthesiologist immediately if there is a suspected or known positive family history for malignant hyperthermia.* |
| e. Time of last food ingestion if surgery impending. | Recent food ingestion increases the risk for vomiting and aspiration during surgery and recovery. Delay of the surgery and/or gastric decompression may be necessary. |
| f. Presence of braces, loose teeth, or permanent or removable prosthetic devices. | Braces, loose teeth, and permanent oral prosthetic devices require careful handling during intubation to avoid injury and/or breakage, leading to possible aspiration. Removable devices must be taken out before surgery.<br>***Special Considerations:*** *Inform the anesthesiologist if any of these oral conditions exist.* |
| 6. Determine body weight (see Skill 28). | Safe and effective preoperative and anesthetic drug doses are based on an accurate body weight. |
| 7. Perform a physical assessment (see Skill 27). | A preoperative physical assessment provides a baseline for postoperative evaluation and can identify potential risk factors for intraoperative and postoperative complications.<br>***Special Considerations:*** *Astute assessment and monitoring of all body systems is essential in the neonate undergoing surgery (Rushton, 1988). Children with mental or physical impairments comprise another population with special assessment needs. They are often prone to more respiratory problems and may have contractures or other mobility problems requiring special handling in the perioperative and postoperative period.* |
| 8. Review existing data and/or assess for risk factors related to surgical procedures: | Presence of these conditions denotes a higher risk of complications from surgery and anesthesia. If possible, surgery is postponed until the condition can be improved. |
| a. Age: premature or full-term newborn after first 2 days of life, especially if multiple congenital anomalies are present. | Immaturity of the organ systems of premature infants makes them a higher surgical risk (Rushton, 1988). After the first 2 days of life, the full-term newborn begins the transition from neonatal hematologic status through physiologic jaundice to a lowered hemoglobin level, increasing the surgical risk (Fochtman and Raffensperger, 1976). |
| b. Poor nutritional status from inadequate intake or poor absorption related to disease process. | Diminished nutritional reserves prevent optimal coping with surgical stressors and interfere with wound healing. |

| Steps | Rationale |
|---|---|
| c. Dehydration, fluid, and electrolyte imbalance from diuretics, steroids, laxatives, enemas, barium studies, mechanical bowel obstruction, or inflammatory bowel disease, etc. | Uncorrected dehydration increases the risk for hypotension, hypovolemia, and inadequate perfusion during surgery. ***Special Considerations:*** *Total fluid replacement should be gradual (more than 24 hours) to allow compensatory mechanisms to adjust (McConnell, 1987).* |
| d. Compromised respiratory status, such as chronic lung diseases, recent pneumonia, and immobility. | Diminished respiratory capacity can reduce oxygenation and perfusion during anesthesia and lead to postoperative complications. |
| e. Preexisting infection such as acute otitis, sepsis, appendicitis, wound abscess. | Physiologic stress from an existing infection limits the body's ability to cope effectively with surgical stress. ***Special Considerations:*** *Although surgery can sometimes be delayed to treat a bacterial infection, there are times when it is the treatment, e.g., appendicitis.* |
| f. History of treatment with anthracycline drugs (doxorubicin and daunorubicin). | There is an increased risk of cardiomyopathy and anesthesia complications if the cumulative dose of these drugs approaches 450 mg/m$^2$ (Hall, 1984). |

## Planning and Goal Setting

| Steps | Rationale |
|---|---|
| 1. Coordinate physical preparation with psychologic preparation and preoperative teaching. | Preoperative teaching and both physical and psychologic preparation will help the child and family cope with the planned procedure. |
| 2. Time special procedures and tests to coordinate with planned time for surgery when possible, e.g., obtain laboratory results for review, feed an infant before NPO status, administer prophylactic antibiotic for highest blood levels during operative phase. | Careful timing makes the preoperative phase progress smoothly, avoiding delays and providing optimum conditions during surgery. For example, antibiotics are most effective if administered within 2 hours before surgery to provide optimum drug levels intraoperatively, where maximal bacterial contamination occurs (American Academy of Pediatrics, 1984). |
| 3. Review child's current medication regimen with physician to determine if any changes will be needed because of the surgery and NPO status. | To prevent adverse drug interactions or other complications during anesthesia and surgery, certain medications may need to be discontinued, tapered, or increased, or the route of administration may need to be changed due to NPO status. ***Special Considerations:*** *Medications that are particularly significant to consider are insulin, corticosteroids, thyroid drugs, digoxin, diuretics, theophylline, aspirin, and anticonvulsant agents (Emergency Medicine, 1987). For example, the dose of anticonvulsant agents may need to be increased to control for possible seizures associated with the trauma and increased stress of the surgical procedure.* |
| 4. Review facility protocol for surgical patients. | Facility protocol may require tests and procedures not ordered by the physician. |
| 5. Gather supplies needed for specific preparations to be done, such as skin preps, IV supplies, preoperative medications. In the immediate preoperative period, obtain hospital gown, paper cap (if required), blankets, current medical chart, previous medical records if available, and identification labeling card or plate. | Gathering supplies in advance facilitates an efficient, accurate, and orderly preoperative preparation. It also ensures that all the required items are readily available to transport with the child to surgery. |
| 6. Develop individualized goals of nursing care:<br>▪ Provide physical preparation of the child for the planned surgery.<br>▪ Assist in preventing or minimizing operative complications.<br>▪ Document pertinent information for safe transfer of child's care to surgery personnel. | |

## Implementation

### *Preliminary preparation (may be done several days to 1 hour before surgery)*

| Steps | Rationale |
|---|---|
| 1. Obtain and witness written authorization (if not already obtained). | Written authorization to perform the surgery is required by most facilities for legal protection of involved parties. |

| Steps | Rationale |
|---|---|
| 2. Review results of laboratory tests and other diagnostic examinations and report abnormal results to physician. | Abnormal test results indicate conditions that may increase the risks of surgery or anesthesia. Surgery may be cancelled or postponed based on this information. For example, low hemoglobin, indicating reduced capacity to carry oxygenated blood to the tissues, and low hematocrit, possibly indicating hypovolemia, may be corrected before surgery by the administration of fluids/blood. |
| 3. Provide operative site cleansing as ordered: antibacterial agent, frequency, and length of time. | Preoperative site cleansing removes both transient and resident flora and/or confers residual bacteriocidal activity to decrease the incidence of postoperative wound infection (Craig, 1986).<br>***Special Considerations:*** *Site cleansing before the surgical prep is often done for orthopedic surgery, in which a postoperative infection is difficult to eradicate. Shaving the operative site, although usually not done in children, is done if necessary in the operating room to decrease the incidence of postoperative wound infection. Clipping hair or the use of depilatories is preferable to shaving (Craig, 1986).* |
| 4. Bathe or assist child to bathe or shower with an antibacterial agent (if ordered) the night before or morning of elective surgery, or as possible or indicated before emergency surgery. | Preoperative bathing with hexachlorophene or chlorhexidine has been shown to significantly reduce the incidence of postoperative wound infections, although it is unknown if similar results would be achieved with plain soap and water (Craig, 1986). |
| 5. Shampoo hair if indicated, such as for cranial surgery, or when the hair might not be shampooed for several days postoperatively. | Shampooing is indicated to decrease transient bacteria and facilitate comfort postoperatively. |
| 6. Explain the impending NPO status to the child and family. Ask the family to refrain from eating or drinking in front of the child during this time. | Understanding how NPO status contributes to a safe surgical outcome will encourage participation and compliance. |
| 7. Initiate NPO status at the designated time. Remove all cups, pitchers, and food from the bedside. Also remove these items from drawers and trash containers. Prominently display a sign at the bedside stating "Nothing by mouth" or "I can't eat or drink."<br>a. No milk or solids after midnight for a scheduled surgery.<br>b. Clear liquids may be given up to the following hours preoperatively:<br>▪ 0 to 3 years: 4 hours<br>▪ 3 to 6 years: 6 hours<br>▪ 7 and older: 8 hours<br>(Committee on Drugs, 1985).<br>c. Provide a snack and liquids at bedtime if child will be asleep at the initiation of NPO status.<br>d. Place a nasogastric tube if ordered to assist stomach emptying. | The stomach must be empty of food and fluids to prevent vomiting and aspiration due to a depressed gag reflex and gastroesophageal reflux during anesthesia and in the early postoperative period. In addition, fluid can silently reflux and be aspirated during anesthesia causing postoperative pneumonia (Fochtman and Raffensperger, 1976). The infant, however, is especially prone to glycogen depletion if not receiving IV glucose. A last oral feeding of a clear liquid will help prevent this.<br>***Special Considerations:*** *Gastric emptying normally occurs in 4 hours for infants under 1 year of age, in 8 hours for older children. However, fear, trauma, gastrointestinal disease, or prematurity may delay emptying (Fochtman and Raffensperger, 1976). If surgery is unexpectedly delayed, an infant without an IV infusion is especially prone to hypoglycemia. Notify the physician.* |
| 8. Initiate a peripheral or central (if existing access) intravenous infusion if ordered. | Intravenous infusion may be necessary to prevent dehydration and hypoglycemia during NPO status.<br>***Special Considerations:*** *Warm infusion fluids if child is at risk for hypothermia due to age, size, trauma, environmental exposure, or brain damage (Rushton, 1988; Temple and Katz, 1987; Benchot, 1986).* |
| 9. Initiate other therapeutic measures as ordered such as nasogastric tubes, Foley catheters, bowel preparation and/or irrigation, hyperalimentation, blood and platelet transfusions, or vitamin K administration at indicated times. | Nasogastric tubes empty the stomach and decompress the intestines, making them easier to handle and less subject to trauma during intestinal surgery. Saline enemas are indicated before a repair for Hirschsprung's disease to clear fecal impactions and reduce surgical field contamination. Hyperalimentation may be ordered to improve nutritional status. Transfusions may be ordered to correct anemia and/or thrombocytopenia preoperatively. In neonates, vitamin $K_1$ administration immediately after birth and/or before surgery is necessary because of low coagulation levels from hepatic immaturity (Rushton, 1988). |

| Steps | Rationale |
|---|---|
| | ***Special Considerations:*** *A polyethylene glycol electrolyte solution (GoLytely) is often used for bowel preparation when indicated preoperatively. As the taste is not well accepted by children and the addition of sweeteners is contraindicated, it is usually given by nasogastric tube (Konings, 1989; Tuggle et al, 1987). The usual dose is 25 to 60 ml/kg/hr or 1 L/hr for older children. Monitor the child closely. Metoclopramide (Reglan), an antinauseant that speeds gastric emptying, may be ordered prophylactically or if nausea/vomiting occur (Konings, 1989).* |
| 10. Administer prophylactic antibiotics as ordered. | Antimicrobial prophylaxis decreases the incidence of postoperative infection in procedures with a significant risk (e.g., bowel surgery or compound fracture), or those in which the occurrence of infection can be catastrophic (e.g., open heart or neonatal surgery). However, the benefits for prevention of wound infection need to be weighed against the risks of drug reaction and emergence of resistant bacteria (American Academy of Pediatrics, 1984).<br>***Special Considerations:*** *Administration of antimicrobial prophylaxis more than 48 hours before surgery has not been shown to be beneficial; often a single dose is sufficient (American Academy of Pediatrics, 1984).* |
| 11. Remove makeup and nail polish if present. | Nail polish and makeup can interfere with the assessment of oxygenation during anesthesia by obscuring cyanosis. |
| 12. Review records for documentation required by facility such as signed surgical consent form, known allergies, body weight, physician's history and physical, nursing care plan, typed and cross-matched blood available, laboratory and other diagnostic reports. | Most facilities have documentation requirements for operative patients that must be easily accessible to the surgical team.<br>***Special Considerations:*** *A checklist for surgical patients is typically used to ensure all required documentation is available.* |
| ***Immediate preparation (approximately 1 hour before surgery)*** | |
| 1. Attire child according to facility policy: hospital gown, diaper for infant, pajama bottoms, or underwear for older child, if permitted. | Hospital gowns are used for surgical patients because they are less confining and can be easily removed as required for the procedure or emergency care.<br>***Special Considerations:*** *Not wearing underwear is often very distressing for children, especially if the planned surgery is for an area on the upper body. Underwear is not easily removed from the anesthetized patient; however, some policies allow children to wear underwear to surgery.* |
| 2. Verify that child has a legible and accurate identification bracelet, allergy alert, and blood bracelets if applicable. | Proper identification and allergy notification is essential for safe care. |
| 3. Remove all jewelry, hair ornaments, and any removable prosthetics, including dental retainers and contact lenses. Give to the family or provide for safekeeping according to facility policy. | Removal and safekeeping of all personal items prevents damage or loss. In addition, metal items can pose a burn hazard with some surgical equipment. |
| 4. Measure and record vital signs. Report any deviations to physician. | Measurement of vital signs provides a baseline for assessment during surgery. It also provides a last minute comparison with admission measurements so that a change in status that might cause complications can be detected, such as a fever indicating an unrelated infection.<br>***Special Considerations:*** *Every degree centigrade of temperature elevation increases body metabolism by 10% which requires more anesthetic drugs (Fochtman and Raffensperger, 1976).* |
| 5. Verify that the child has been NPO since the designated time. For example, ask "Has your baby had anything to eat or drink since 4 AM?" Ask the preschooler or older child, "Have you eaten or drunk anything this morning?" Report any ingestion, known or suspected to the physician. | A last minute verification that the NPO status has been maintained will help to avoid the serious complication of vomiting and aspiration. A parent may have unwittingly allowed a small drink, or a small child may have obtained food unobserved. Surgery is usually postponed if suspected or known ingestion occurs. |
| 6. Ask the toilet-trained and older child to void if possible. If unable, record the time of the last voiding if known. | An empty bladder reduces the risk for accidental trauma and avoids incontinence during surgery. |

| Steps | Rationale |
|---|---|
| 7. Administer the preoperative medication at the scheduled or notified time. See skills 101 or 105. Inform the family and child of any expected side effects, and advise them to report any unexpected effects that could indicate a reaction, such as severe agitation or difficulty breathing. | Preoperative medication is timed to provide the optimum effects at the time of anesthesia induction. Informing the family of expected and unexpected side effects allays concerns and promotes prompt notification if a significant reaction occurs. ***Special Considerations:*** *One common harmless side effect of atropine is a flushed face with circumoral blanching. An undesirable side effect of some sedatives or narcotics in children is a paradoxical reaction of agitation.* |
| 8. Provide for the child's safety by raising bed or stretcher rails, and have family or a staff member remain with the child until transfer of care to operating room personnel. Inform the attending person to call for assistance if the child needs to void. | A sedated child may become frightened if alone, or may attempt to get up despite instructions to call for assistance. ***Special Considerations:*** *Depending on the facility and nature of the surgery (emergency or elective), the child may be transported directly to operating room or may be received in a holding area.* |
| 9. Provide a warm environment appropriate to the child's needs by increasing room temperature, or using a prewarmed incubator, radiant warmer, or warmed blankets. | Maintaining an optimal thermal environment prevents cold stress, which can lead to hypoxia and severe acidosis, and is potentially fatal when added to surgical stress (Rushton, 1988). Also, platelets do not function normally in very low body temperatures (below 94° F) leading to coagulation problems (Temple and Katz, 1987). ***Special Considerations:*** *Neonates, trauma victims, and children with brain damage are especially vulnerable to cold stress.* |
| 10. Document all actions taken, including administration of medications on the medical record. | Careful documentation of immediate preoperative preparation communicates essential information to the operating room team. |
| 11. Gather all items to accompany child to operating room such as medical records, identification labeling cards, x-ray films, or previous medical records. | Gathering all items to accompany the child to surgery prevents unnecessary delays when the surgical team is ready to receive the child. ***Special Considerations:*** *If the child is wearing underwear or taking a personal item to surgery, clearly label the item with the child's name on a piece of adhesive tape.* |
| 12. Accompany child and family to operating room or transfer child to operating room personnel according to facility policy and child's condition.<br>a. Use safety restraints on transport carriers.<br>b. Verify child's identification with operating room staff. | Safe transfer of care to the surgical team ensures that a qualified person is attending to the child's condition at all times. ***Special Considerations:*** *Encourage the parents to accompany the child as far as possible, preferably through the induction of anesthesia to provide support and minimize anxiety (Whaley and Wong, 1991). In a 4-year experience of allowing parental presence during induction with over 3000 patients in an ambulatory surgical center, Gauderer, Lorig, and Eastwood (1989) reported advantages of not needing to use premedication, decreased psychologic trauma to the child, smoother induction, and decreased parental anxiety. Possible disadvantages proposed were seldom experienced.* |
| 13. Direct the family to where they may wait for the surgeon to contact them with a report on the child's condition after surgery. | Even though the family may have received this information previously, anxiety and emotions may prevent them from remembering at this time. |

| Evaluation Outcomes | Observational Guidelines |
|---|---|
| 1. All ordered and routine physical preparation is completed in a timely manner. | Review physician orders for completion, review preoperative checklist documentation. |
| 2. Physical preparation assists in preventing or minimizing operative complications such as untoward drug reactions, hypothermia, postoperative wound infection, or delayed wound healing. | Review surgery record for complications in the perioperative period. Monitor temperature postoperatively. Monitor wound healing. |
| 3. Safety precautions are maintained in the immediate preoperative phase and during transfer to operating room personnel. | The child does not experience a fall in his or her patient room or from transport equipment and is properly identified for transfer to operating room personnel. |
| 4. The operating room team receives all necessary information to provide appropriate care for the child. | Review accompanying documents for completeness according to agency policy and physician orders such as signed consent, baseline vital signs, preoperative medication given (if any), history and physical, old medical records, or radiographic films. Existing allergies are clearly noted. |

### Documentation

Document nursing history and physical assessment for a baseline comparison. Follow facility policy for documentation of all preoperative measures such as bowel preparation, skin cleansing routines, initiation of IV therapy, prophylactic antibiotics, vital signs, preoperative medication administered (if any) and safety precautions observed. Note personal items accompanying the child. Note time of transfer to operating room personnel.

# *SKILL* 114 Providing Postoperative Care for the First 24 Hours

*Donna Phillips Smith*

Postoperative care requires careful planning, preparation, and organization to successfully manage the initial phase of intense need through early convalescence. This skill addresses postoperative care of the child following transfer from the postanesthesia care unit (PACU) through the first 24 hours. The first 24 hours postoperatively are particularly crucial with infants and children because they lack the physiologic reserves to readily compensate for alterations in ventilation, fluid and electrolyte balance, temperature, and energy requirements related to the surgical event.

Although general principles apply to surgery and recovery from anesthesia for any child, nursing care becomes very individualized depending on the nature of the surgery and preoperative status. Some potential postoperative complications that apply in almost every situation include airway obstruction, nausea/vomiting/aspiration, shock, fluid and electrolyte imbalances, abdominal distension, and respiratory and wound infection. These risks require frequent, comprehensive assessment accompanied by appropriate preventive measures and interventions.

The nurse, child, and family must cope with a variety of circumstances surrounding surgery including: if surgery was planned or an emergency, if the child was hospitalized overnight or admitted the morning of surgery, or if the surgery was done on an outpatient basis. In addition, the type of support provided for children and families such as allowing parental presence during induction and in the PACU varies considerably with different facilities. All of these factors influence the complications of surgery, both physiologic and psychologic.

### NURSING DIAGNOSES

Potential for aspiration related to depressed gag reflexes due to general anesthesia; Ineffective airway clearance related to tracheo-bronchial obstruction/secretion; Fluid volume deficit related to hypovolemia, blood losses, or electrolyte imbalances; Altered tissue perfusion related to hyperkalemia or hypokalemia, blood losses, or circulatory obstruction; Impaired skin integrity related to surgical incision and/or invasive catheters/tubes/drains; Pain related to nerve endings injury at incision site, constrictive dressing, restrictive positioning, or complications with invasive catheters/tubes/drains; Hypothermia related to compromised thermoregulatory mechanisms and/or anesthetic vasodilation; Altered patterns of urinary elimination related to sensory motor impairment from general anesthesia or catheter placement; Ineffective individual family coping related to lack of information about postoperative course and/or inadequate coping methods.

| Steps | Rationale |
|---|---|
| **Assessment** | |
| 1. Determine age and developmental level (if information is available). | Chronologic and developmental age guide assessment, interventions, monitoring concerns, and teaching efforts during postoperative care. |
| 2. Determine preparation conditions related to this surgery, e.g.: emergency or planned; if preoperative teaching was performed, content, and by whom; admitted to unit before surgery or direct surgical admission; and primary nurse assigned and extent of this relationship (new or established). | Preparation conditions and the establishment of a professional relationship before surgery influence planning and effectiveness of postoperative care. Emergency surgery is often performed with minimal or no psychologic preparation and a less than optimum physiologic status. Lack of preparation may increase risk of postoperative complications. Knowledge of preoperative teaching content helps maintain consistency with the child's preparation. If a new admission, additional assessment data and procedures may be necessary, along with initial postoperative assessment and care. For the child and family, the unfamiliar environment and caregivers add additional anxiety at a stressful time. |
| 3. Obtain a telephone report from PACU nurse before the child arrives, if possible. | A pretransfer report provides an overview of the perioperative course, and any special preparation measures or monitoring concerns needed to appropriately plan for the child's arrival to the unit and subsequent care. |
| a. Surgical procedure performed, postoperative diagnosis, status during surgery and immediate postanesthesia phase of recovery, including estimated blood loss and presence of drains, tubes. | Postoperative care varies to some extent based on the type of procedure performed, perioperative physiologic status, and anesthetics/reversal agents/other medications administered. Knowledge of these factors allows appropriate planning for special support measures and identifies potential complications. |
| b. Vital signs/trends in PACU. | This information allows appropriate interpretation of vital signs obtained postrecovery, and guides observation for complications. |
| c. Postoperative care orders, including special equipment, systems, or supportive measures required, e.g., nasogastric (NG) suctioning, electrocardiographic (ECG) monitoring, ventilator settings. Also measures initiated in PACU such as prophylactic antibiotics and drainage bags. | Advance notice of postoperative orders allows appropriate preparations, e.g., obtaining special equipment or preparing medications, to be made before the child arrives. |
| d. Method of transport, e.g., carrier, incubator, crib, or bed. | This information allows appropriate preparation of the room or provides notification to deliver the child's bed to PACU, e.g., a warmed incubator. |
| e. Preexisting problems, handicaps, disabilities. | If the child was not previously admitted, communicating special needs allows appropriate preparation. |
| **Planning and Goal Setting** | |
| 1. Gather or arrange for necessary equipment such as: | Gathering equipment in advance facilitates a smooth transfer to the unit. **_Special Considerations:_** _Necessary equipment may vary with type of surgery, age, and planned postoperative measures._ |
| a. Stethoscope, temperature measuring device, BP device. | This equipment is needed to monitor postoperative vital signs. |
| b. Emesis basin, washcloths, towels, extra linens. | These items are helpful should vomiting occur postoperatively. |
| c. Positioning aids: pillows, blanket and towel rolls, bed cradle, etc. | Positioning aids help maintain comfortable and appropriate positioning postoperatively. |
| d. Oxygen administration or humidification device, airway suction, catheters, bulb syringes (see related skills). | Maintaining a patent airway and preventing hypoxia are priority interventions postoperatively. |
| e. Infusion pumps, continuous suction devices for NG or chest tube, analgesia control devices, arterial monitoring lines (see related skills). | Immediate availability of these devices (if needed) facilitates safe and efficient transfer of care. |
| f. Cardiorespiratory monitoring devices if needed (see related skills). | **_Special Considerations:_** _Young infants may require monitoring even for minor procedures because of a greater risk of apnea from airway obstruction, neurologic dysfunction, or incomplete reversal of anesthesia (Rushton, 1988)._ |
| g. Restraints if necessary (see Skill 51). | **_Special Considerations:_** _Situations for which the need for restraints should be evaluated include cleft lip repair, hypospadius repair with a suprapubic catheter, and NG tube placement._ |
| h. Postoperative assessment and care forms, vital sign and intake and output flowsheets, etc. | Having forms available is efficient and facilitates accurate recording. |

| Steps | Rationale |
|---|---|
| 2. Prepare room/area for child's arrival: place full size bed in high position; remove or turn down outer covers; assemble/prepare equipment, arrange within easy reach, and test functioning as appropriate. | An organized and prepared room with properly functioning equipment helps ensure an efficient and safe transfer. |
| 3. Recruit additional staff to assist with initial arrival. | Initial arrival requires simultaneous observation and completion of urgent tasks. Assistance helps maintain safety and control and may be reassuring to child/family. |
| 4. Develop individualized child and family goals:<br>▪ Postoperative complications will be prevented or minimized.<br>▪ Child's pain/discomfort will be minimized.<br>▪ Child/family will experience minimal anxiety regarding postoperative phase.<br>▪ Child/family will participate in postoperative recovery. | |

## Implementation

### *Initial postoperative assessment*

| Steps | Rationale |
|---|---|
| 1. If family is available, inform them of child's expected arrival. Update them on the child's condition while in PACU. Explain preparation and procedure for child's arrival, including priority interventions of safe transfer to bed/crib, vital signs, and initial assessment. | Informing the family of anticipated events and the child's condition may allay anxiety and prepare them for the initial postoperative phase when assessment and intervention to stabilize/maintain stability of the child is the priority concern (Ogilvie, 1990).<br>***Special Considerations:*** *Return of child from PACU is one of six identified stress points when children have surgery (see Skill 112).* |
| 2. Greet child (and family if accompanying child) on arrival to unit. | A brief acknowledgment in a busy situation conveys concern and respect for the individual child. If relationship has been established previously, a familiar voice can be reassuring, even if the child is not fully conscious. |
| 3. Transfer to bed/crib (if needed). Move child slowly and smoothly. Raise the side rails (see Skill 73). | A smooth and safe transfer minimizes discomfort to the child. |
| 4. Position sleepy or semiconscious child on side with head turned downward. If supine position must be maintained, e.g., traction, turn head to the side. Do not use a pillow. Elevate head 30 degrees if not contraindicated. Explain to family importance of turning the child's head to the side should vomiting occur. | Children are especially prone to postoperative vomiting and aspiration because of depressed reflexes, difficulty coordinating swallowing and breathing, closer proximity of the trachea and esophagus, small size of the stomach, tendency to reflux, compression of abdominal organs, and diaphragmatic breathing (Addleman, 1988). Prone or side position and elevation promote drainage from the mouth, decreasing the risk of aspiration. |
| 5. Assess airway patency. Reposition if necessary to provide patent airway, taking care to not hyperextend the neck. Suction to clear airway if needed. If an oral airway is in place, leave it until the gag reflex returns. | Airway obstruction can rapidly lead to serious or fatal complications. Hyperextension can obstruct the airway especially in the young child because of a flexible trachea that easily collapses. Other anatomic differences that predispose children to airway obstruction include a large head, short neck, a large tongue in relation to size of mouth, enlarged tonsils and adenoids, and narrow air passages (Addleman, 1988).<br>***Special Considerations:*** *Because young infants are obligate nose breathers, obstruction of the nares can result in significant airway obstruction.* |
| 6. Connect/hang/position all fluids, suction, oxygen equipment, monitoring leads, drainage bags, etc. Raise side rails. Apply restraints if ordered or need assessed. | Therapeutic and safety measures should be continued with minimal disruption or promptly initiated upon transfer.<br>***Special Considerations:*** *If the IV solution ordered postoperatively differs from the fluids the child was receiving in PACU, change to the ordered solution even if existing fluids remain.* |
| 7. Obtain vital signs. Compare to those obtained in PACU and preoperative baseline vital signs. Recheck according to facility policy, or as indicated by child's status. A common routine is every 15 minutes times 4, every 30 minutes times 2, then every hour times 4 (see Skills 30-33). | Vital sign measurement assists in detecting common early postoperative complications, e.g., inadequate intravascular volume, hypoxia and hypothermia or hyperthermia (see Table 114-1).<br>***Special Considerations:*** *Leaving the BP cuff in place avoids disturbing the child during frequent measurements.* |

**TABLE 114-1** Potential Causes of Postoperative Vital Sign Alterations

| Alteration | Potential Cause | Comments | Alteration | Potential Cause | Comments |
|---|---|---|---|---|---|
| **HEART RATE** | | | **BLOOD PRESSURE** | | |
| Increase | Decreased perfusion (shock)<br>Elevated temperature<br>Pain<br>Respiratory distress (early)<br>Medications (atropine, morphine, epinephrine) | Heart rate may increase to maintain cardiac output | Increase | Excess intravascular volume<br>Increased intracranial pressure<br>Carbon dioxide retention<br>Pain<br>Medications (ketamine, epinephrine) | Serious condition in premature infants because it increases risk of intraventricular hemorrhage |
| Decrease | Hypoxia<br>Vagal stimulation<br>Increased intracranial pressure<br>Respiratory distress (late)<br>Medications (prostigmine) | Bradycardia is of more concern in the young child than tachycardia | Decrease | Vasodilating anesthetic agents (halothane, isoflurane, and enflurane)<br>Opioids (morphine)<br>Shock (late sign) | Decreased BP is a late sign of shock due to elasticity and constriction of vessels to maintain cardiac output |
| **RESPIRATORY RATE** | | | **TEMPERATURE** | | |
| Increase | Respiratory distress<br>Fluid volume excess<br>Hypothermia<br>Elevated temperature<br>Pain | Body responds to respiratory distress primarily by increasing rate | Increase | Infection<br>Environmental causes (warm room, excess coverings) | Fever associated with infection usually occurs later than fever of noninfectious origin<br>Absence of fever does not rule out infection, especially in infants<br>Malignant hyperthermia requires immediate treatment |
| Decrease | Anesthetics, opioids | Neonate prone to apnea due to CNS immaturity<br>Decreased respiratory rate from opioids may be compensated for by increased depth of respiration | Decrease | Vasodilating anesthetic agents (see above) and muscle relaxants<br>Environmental causes (cool room)<br>Infusion of cool fluids/blood | Neonates especially susceptible to hypothermia with serious or fatal consequences |

| Steps | Rationale |
|---|---|
| 8. Conduct an initial postoperative assessment: (for detail on physical assessment, see Skill 27). | An initial postoperative assessment identifies existing/potential complications and provides a baseline for ongoing observations. Early complications of greatest concern are hemorrhage and a nonpatent airway.<br>***Special Considerations:*** *Vary type and depth of assessment according to risk for complications based on age, surgical procedure and preoperative status.* |

| **Steps** | **Rationale** |
|---|---|
| a. Respiratory status: Note airway patency, rate, depth, breath sounds, secretions, and color of mucous membranes and nailbeds. Signs of distress include nasal flaring, tachypnea, use of accessory muscles, paradoxical movement, stridor, croupy cough, hoarseness, and restlessness. | Adequate respiratory function is a priority concern. All anesthetics are depressants that may interfere with respiratory function. Because of narrow airways and anatomic differences of the epiglottis and larynx, children are prone to laryngeal spasm, and laryngeal edema (postextubation croup). Due to CNS immaturity, neonates are prone to periodic apnea, hypoventilation or delayed onset of respirations following anesthesia (Rushton, 1988). |
| b. Cardiovascular status: Note heart rate and rhythm; perfusion (capillary refill, urinary output, peripheral pulses, warmth of extremities, and skin color); and blood pressure. Compare perfusion between extremities, especially distal to cast, splint, or any incision for vascular or musculoskeletal surgery. | Poor perfusion may signal impending shock more reliably than vital sign changes, which may be caused by other factors. Inadequate intravascular volume may result from blood loss, external fluid loss, or third-spacing (loss of intravascular fluid into interstitial compartment). Cardiac dysrhythmias may indicate hypoxia. Unequal perfusion indicates circulatory obstruction requiring immediate attention to prevent tissue necrosis.<br>***Special Considerations:*** *Significant blood loss may occur during cardiac surgery. Third-spacing is likely to occur following abdominal procedures (Hedenkamp and Howell, 1988).* |
| c. Skin integrity: Inspect all dressings, visible surgical incisions, drains, tubes, IV or access sites, and donor sites for appearance, amount of drainage, and intactness. Check under child for wound hemorrhage, which may collect undetected. For oral/throat surgery, inspect oral cavity with a light source (not a tongue blade). Inspect skin distal to casts/splints for swelling, pressure, and neurovascular impairment. | Bright red blood, evidence of wound hemorrhage, will usually occur within the first few hours postoperatively. Swelling and discoloration under the incision in the early postoperative phase may indicate internal hemorrhage. Restriction of circulation can lead to irreversible tissue damage. All disruptions in skin integrity, e.g., an IV or chest tube, are potential sites for infection.<br>***Special Considerations:*** *Traditional practice is to outline drainage on dressings and casts to monitor any increases. However, if drainage is expected this practice may cause undue anxiety for the child/family.* |
| d. Neurologic status: Determine level of awareness, pupillary size and response, behavior, spontaneous neuromuscular movement, reflexes, response to environment, suck reflex, and characteristics of cry. Also assess for presence of pain (see Skill 52). | Assessing neurologic status helps to determine appropriate emergence from anesthesia and presence of pain. Children usually have a more rapid emergence from anesthesia than adults because of a higher cardiac output and greater alveolar ventilation (Addleman, 1988). Impaired neurologic function may be caused by hypoxemia, inadequate cerebral perfusion, hypoglycemia, residual anesthesia/drugs, fluid and electrolyte imbalances, cold stress, sepsis, or pain (Rushton, 1988). Residual anesthetics may inhibit pain response. Untreated pain, especially in the neonate, may result in physiologic instability (Rushton, 1988). |
| e. Fluid balance: Note IV infusion, type of fluids, and rate. Observe for signs of fluid volume deficit/overload (see Skill 64). If indwelling catheter placed in bladder, note amount and appearance of urinary output. | Early postoperative complications include inadequate intravascular volume from excess fluid losses (third spacing, hemorrhage, or insensible losses), and fluid volume overload from inappropriate replacement (excess amount, hypotonic solution).<br>***Special Considerations:*** *The infant has a greater blood volume (85 ml/kg) than an adult (65 ml/kg), therefore blood losses represent a greater portion of total blood volume (Addleman, 1988).* |
| f. Gastrointestinal status: Note presence of nausea/vomiting, and amount and appearance of emesis. Auscultate for presence of bowel sounds; note abdominal distension. If an NG tube is placed, note type, size, patency, and consistency and amount of drainage. | Common complications of vomiting and abdominal distension are related to diminished or absent gastric motility and intestinal peristalsis in response to anesthetics, narcotics, and manipulation of the bowel during abdominal surgery. A patent NG helps maintain gastric decompression to prevent vomiting secondary to ileus. Abdominal distension may inhibit respiratory effort since children are abdominal breathers. Dark, old blood in emesis or NG drainage is expected following oral/nasal/throat surgery; bright red blood may indicate hemorrhage. |

| Steps | Rationale |
|---|---|
| g. Thermal regulation: Note body temperature and warmth and color of extremities. Signs of cold stress in the neonate are apnea, respiratory distress, and tachycardia (see Skill 83). | An increased risk for hypothermia exists postoperatively related to decreased responsiveness of thermoregulatory centers and vasodilation from some anesthetic agents. Oxygen consumption is greatly increased in the hypothermic neonate, leading to hypoxia, metabolic acidosis, depletion of glycogen stores, and peripheral/pulmonary vasoconstriction (Rushton, 1988). The young child (1 to 4 years of age) with a high metabolic rate may easily become pyrexic from environmental causes or a postoperative response (Addleman, 1988). |
| 9. Explain and discuss with family the child's general status; anticipated frequency of postoperative vital signs and ongoing assessments; equipment being used for monitoring purposes and therapeutic drains, lines, support systems, etc.; and the family's desired role in postoperative care (see also Skill 112). | Helping the family to understand the child's physiologic status, postoperative procedures, and equipment prevents undue anxiety related to standard care. For example, the family might believe the child's condition is worsening because vital signs are being obtained frequently. |
| 10. Answer family/child's questions. Gather additional patient data if a new admission. | Answering questions conveys a respect for their concerns, and helps to clarify misconceptions (Ogilvie, 1990). Gathering additional data helps develop an individualized care plan. |
| 11. Review postoperative orders and additional information pertaining to surgery and preoperative status on child's medical record. Collaborate with surgeon regarding anticipated care needs. | Reviewing orders helps verify their implementation. Additional information from the surgeon and the child's medical record assists in developing care plan. ***Special Considerations:*** *In some facilities, all preoperative orders are automatically voided.* |
| 12. Develop an individualized plan of postoperative care in collaboration with the child/family. | Collaborative planning promotes participation and cooperation in postoperative care, to minimize complications. |
| ***Early postoperative care*** | |
| 1. Monitor vital signs and perform ongoing assessments per facility routine and as indicated by child's condition. Compare with baseline assessments. | Vital sign changes/trends and ongoing assessments assist in identification of potential complications in the early convalescent phase (see Table 114-1). |
| 2. Monitor respiratory status and perform measures to prevent complications: | |
| a. Assess for respiratory distress (increased or irregular rate, shallow depth, increased effort, crackles/wheezes, cough, increased secretions, cyanosis) and temperature elevation. | Increasing respiratory distress and temperature elevation may indicate respiratory infection. Suddenly increased distress may signal atelectasis or pulmonary embolus. ***Special Considerations:*** *Cyanosis is a late sign of hypoxia.* |
| b. Encourage deep breathing, incentive spirometry or stimulate infant to cry every 1 to 2 hours; perform chest physiotherapy every 3 to 4 hours; reposition every 2 hours; suction or assist with expectoration as needed (see Skills 89 and 92). | Anesthetics, dependent positioning, splinting of respirations, narrow air passages, and preexisting respiratory conditions contribute to inadequate lung expansion and collection of secretions. These measures counteract such effects to help prevent postoperative respiratory infection and airway obstruction. |
| c. Encourage early mobility/ambulation (see step 9c). | Early ambulation assists in preventing respiratory complications. |
| d. Provide humidification, supplemental oxygen, ventilatory support as needed/ordered (see Skills 90 and 94). | ***Special Considerations:*** *Neonates especially may require oxygen or mechanical ventilation postoperatively to prevent episodic hypoxemia (Rushton, 1988).* |
| 3. Monitor cardiovascular status and maintain fluid balance (see Skill 64): a. Assess for poor perfusion, dehydration, or fluid volume overload. b. Monitor intake and output and fluid balance. Include fluids administered in PACU. c. Provide appropriate fluid replacement. Administer volume expanders as ordered. | Decreased intravascular fluid volume from hemorrhage and fluid losses (external or interstitial) may lead to decreased perfusion in the early convalescent phase. Inadequate intravascular volume requires immediate intervention to prevent progression to shock. Surgical trauma triggers a stress response, which may lead to water and sodium retention. |
| 4. Monitor incisions, dressings, drains and tubes. Change/reinforce dressings as ordered/needed using sterile technique. Fold diapers low to prevent contamination of abdominal dressings. | Monitoring disruptions in skin integrity allows prevention and detection of possible complications such as hemorrhage, wound infection, and wound dehiscence. A wound infection may not be evident in the first 24 hours. A greater risk for wound dehiscence exists if the child is emaciated, obese, has poor circulation, or with excess tension on the suture line (Kozier and Erb, 1987). ***Special Considerations:*** *Dressings are usually not changed for at least 24 hours postoperatively unless gross contamination occurs, e.g., with a stool.* |

| Steps | Rationale |
|---|---|
| 5. Monitor neurovascular status for impairment distal to cast/splint, or abdominal, orthopedic, or vascular surgical site (see Skill 77). | Circulatory impairment, thrombus or embolus formation are complications associated with these types of procedures that can result in severe tissue damage or death.<br>***Special Considerations:*** *If a thrombus/embolus lodges in the pulmonary, coronary, or cerebral arteries, acute changes in cardiac, respiratory, or neurologic status may be noted.* |
| 6. Monitor gastrointestinal function and provide measures to prevent complications. | Delayed return of peristalsis, obstruction from paralytic ileus, and abdominal distension are postoperative complications. |
| a. Auscultate for presence of bowel sounds, note passage of flatus/stool, observe for abdominal distension, and measure abdominal girth. | Abdominal distension may contribute to respiratory distress because lung capacity is decreased from upward pressure of the diaphragm.<br>***Special Considerations:*** *Elevate the head of the bed to ease respiratory effort if abdominal distension is present (Hedenkamp and Howell, 1988).* |
| b. Perform oral care if NPO. Provide sips of liquids if ordered when fully awake and bowel sounds/flatus present. Avoid red or brown liquids, or juices with oral/throat surgeries. | Preoperative NPO status, medications and fluid losses contribute to dry mucous membranes and thirst. Small amounts of ice chips/fluids may be better tolerated with decreased gastric motility. Brown or red liquids may obscure/be mistaken for blood in vomitus. Juices may irritate an oral surgical wound.<br>***Special Considerations:*** *Criteria for resuming oral intake vary considerably with type of surgery and surgeon preference.* |
| c. Monitor NG for patency, placement and appropriate suction (usually low intermittent). Irrigate with saline as needed/ordered (see Skill 65). | A patent NG may prevent abdominal distension and vomiting.<br>***Special Considerations:*** *Gravity drainage may be used in place of low intermittent suction in neonates and infants (Hedenkamp and Howell, 1988).* |
| d. Resume nutritional intake as tolerated per orders. | Resuming feedings promotes normal fluid and electrolyte balance, restores nutritional intake, and normal GI function.<br>***Special Considerations:*** *In preterm infants and neonates, since digestive and absorptive functions may not be optimal postoperatively, dilute feedings; hyperalimentation or enteral supplementation are often used initially (Rushton, 1988).* |
| 7. Monitor temperature. Administer antipyretics and provide appropriate environmental measures, e.g., adding or removing coverings, warmed blankets, stockinette cap for neonate, and warmed blood/fluids (see Skills 83 and 84). | Maintaining an appropriate thermal environment for the child will minimize oxygen consumption and metabolic rate alterations for hypothermia or hyperthermia to avoid serious or fatal consequences.<br>***Special Considerations:*** *A preexisting infection is more likely to be responsible for fever in the first 24 hours than a wound infection or a postoperative pneumonia.* |
| 8. Assess for presence of pain. Manage pain appropriately with nonpharmacologic and pharmacologic measures (see Skill 52). | Untreated pain is physiologically and psychologically distressing. Appropriate pain management makes it easier for the child to cooperate with measures to prevent postoperative complications.<br>***Special Considerations:*** *Do not assume pain/discomfort is because of the surgical incision. Investigate other possible causes such as an infiltrated IV, constrictive dressing, or an embolus.* |
| 9. Provide for positioning and mobility needs: | Positioning and mobility can promote comfort and prevent postoperative complications such as atelectasis and pressure sores.<br>***Special Considerations:*** *Time pain medication for optimum effect during positioning/mobility to enhance cooperation and comfort.* |
| a. Elevate an extremity, elevate head of the bed, straighten alignment, provide support for body position with pillows, rolls, etc., as ordered/needed (see Skill 74). | Appropriate positioning minimizes the risk of aspiration, promotes venous drainage, and reduces stress on the incision. A comfortable position helps relaxation (Perry and Potter, 1990).<br>***Special Considerations:*** *Extremity support for neonates and infants is often overlooked, yet may increase comfort.* |
| b. Change position every 1 to 2 hours if the child is unable to do so. | Repositioning helps maintain skin integrity and promotes respiratory function.<br>***Special Considerations:*** *If a lengthy period of immobility is anticipated or the child has a large amount of edema (from third-spacing), obtain a pressure reduction mattress.* |
| c. Encourage activity and ambulation as soon as possible, e.g., afternoon or evening of surgery, if not contraindicated. | Early ambulation prevents respiratory, circulatory, urinary, and gastrointestinal complications (Kozier and Erb, 1987). |

| Steps | Rationale |
|---|---|

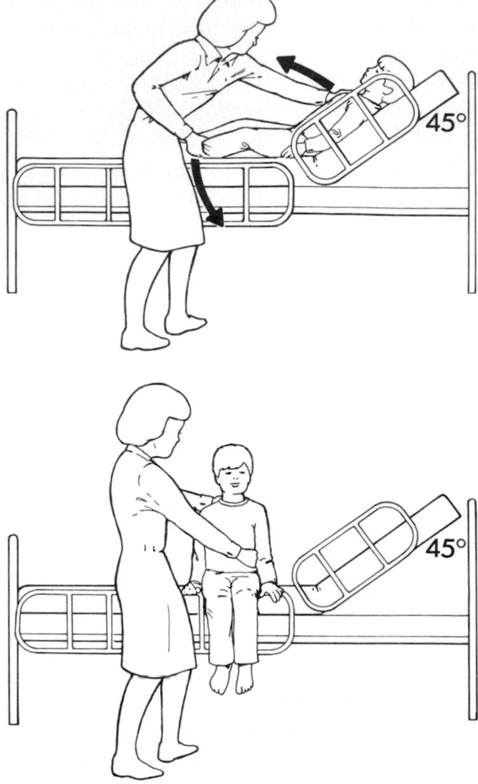


***FIG. 114-1*** Child is assisted to sitting position.

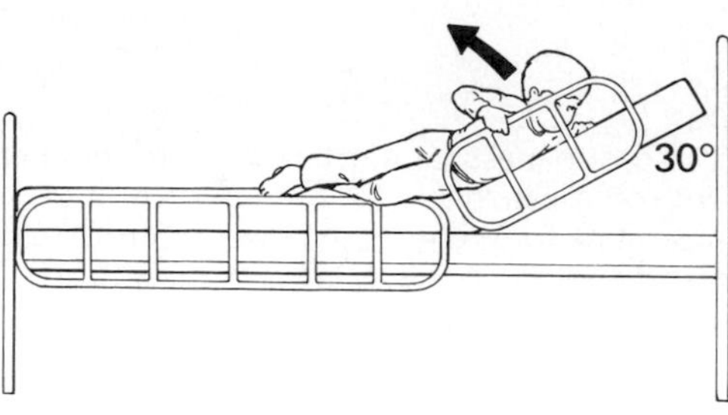


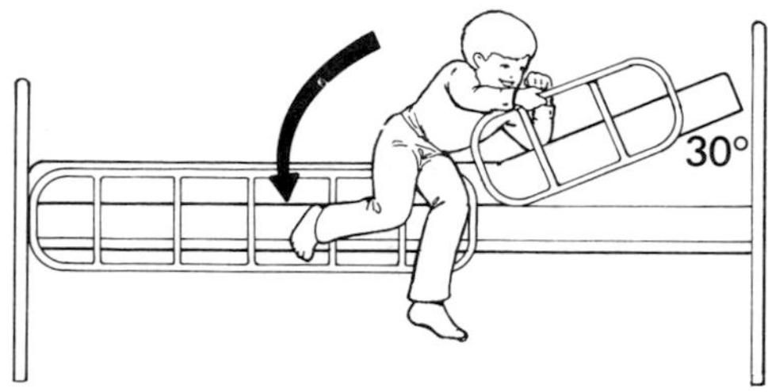


***FIG. 114-2*** Child pushes from side-lying position to sitting position.

- With bed at lowest position, assist child to sitting position.
  (1) With child supine, elevate head of bed and then assist child to pivot to a sitting position with legs over side of bed (Fig. 114-1).

  *OR*

  (2) Assist child to sidelying position and then assist to sitting position (Fig. 114-2).

***Special Considerations:*** *This method is recommended for a child with abdominal surgery because it minimizes abdominal strain.*

- Allow child to sit on side of bed and dangle legs before standing. Question child about dizziness, faintness, unsteadiness, and allow these sensations to resolve before continuing. Perform vital signs if necessary to assess stability.

Sitting and dangling legs allows body to reach equilibrium and reduces risk of falling.

***Special Considerations:*** *Postural hypotension is common. If symptoms, e.g., dizziness, tachycardia, nausea, and faintness, do not resolve, return to bed and try again later.*

- Assist child to put on nonrestrictive, safe clothing and nonskid footwear.

Allowing child to dress self as much as possible fosters independence and allows self-participation in care. Ask family to bring child's usual walking shoes or nonskid houseshoes. Avoid long, full robes, and gowns which could trip the child.

- Secure safety belt around child's waist.

Use of safety belt is essential to provide a secure hold on the child and prevent falls.

***Special Considerations:*** *A safety belt is not necessary for a toddler/preschooler.*

10. Monitor for urinary retention if not catheterized. For the toilet trained child, suggest attempting to void, and promote normal positioning as possible to help voiding, e.g., boys may stand at the bedside with a urinal, girls may sit up on a bedpan if unable to be out of the bed. If the child has not voided 4 to 6 hours postoperatively, palpate for a distended bladder. Notify physician or catheterize per protocol if unable to void and bladder is distended (see Skill 68).

Narcotics and anesthetics may depress bladder tone and sensation of the urge to void. Also, genitourinary or abdominal surgery may traumatize urinary organs. Normal voiding position may facilitate relaxation of the urinary sphincter. If the bladder is distended and the child unable to void, catheterization may be necessary.

| Steps | Rationale |
|---|---|
| 11. Obtain postoperative blood specimens for testing as ordered, e.g., hemoglobin, hematocrit, electrolytes, and blood gases. | Blood analysis is often ordered postoperatively to determine extent of blood loss, fluid and electrolyte balance, and respiratory status. |
| 12. Assist child/family in beginning to resolve feelings related to surgical experience (see Skills 16 and 112).<br>a. Facilitate a review of the event for the older child.<br>b. Provide therapeutic play, drawing, or storytelling for the younger child. | Providing support for the child/family or helping to correct misconceptions can assist in developmental mastery concerning body image changes and a stressful experience (Whaley and Wong, 1989).<br>***Special Considerations:*** *Resolution of feelings is a gradual process. A referral may be indicated.* |
| 13. Implement discharge planning as appropriate (see Skill 5). | The family often needs to administer medications, perform procedures, care for therapeutic devices, and monitor for complications after discharge. Discharge planning ideally begins upon admission. |

## Evaluation Outcomes / Observational Guidelines

| Evaluation Outcomes | Observational Guidelines |
|---|---|
| 1. Postoperative complications are prevented or minimized. | Review record or assess for signs/symptoms of postoperative complications, e.g., airway obstruction, vomiting/aspiration, respiratory infection, abdominal distension, inadequate intravascular volume, or fluid excess. If complications developed, note early identification and prompt intervention. |
| 2. Child's pain is appropriately managed. | Review pain assessment and intervention record; note behaviors and child's verbal comments regarding effectiveness of interventions; note compliance with measures such as activity and respiratory therapy. |
| 3. Child/family are prepared for postoperative course. | Note participation of child/family in recovery and preventive measures and use of effective coping mechanisms. Note verbal statements and behaviors regarding expectations and actual postoperative course. |
| 4. Child/family begin to resolve feelings associated with surgery. | Note participation in therapeutic discussion or play. Observe verbal statements or behaviors regarding surgical incision and body image. |

## Documentation

Document time child received from PACU and postoperative vital signs per protocol. Record initial assessment and intervention measures. Use appropriate forms as required by facility. Record all ongoing assessment for postoperative complications and notification of surgeon if appropriate. Document interventions to prevent or minimize complications. Record any discharge planning and teaching.

## UNIT XVII

### PRODUCT REFERENCES

See p. 37 in Unit I for Teaching Resources.

#### Books

Note: Create a valuable resource by assembling a book of photographs of the sights and sounds surrounding surgery at the individual health care facility. Separate books can be made for each major age group. An additional book for parents is also helpful.

### REFERENCES

Addleman CD: What do you look for in the pediatric postanesthesia patient? J Post Anesth Nurs 3(1):3-10, 1988.

American Academy of Pediatrics: Antimicrobial prophylaxis in pediatric surgical patients, Pediatrics 74(3):437-439, 1984.

American Academy of Pediatrics, Committee on Drugs: Section on Anesthesiology: Guidelines for the elective use of conscious sedation, deep sedation, and general anesthesia in pediatric patients, Pediatrics 76(2):317-321, 1985.

Benchot R: Mentally retarded patients: special needs before and after surgery, AORN J 44(5):768-780, 1986.

Blacher R: The psychological experiences of surgery, New York, 1987. John Wiley & Sons.

Brzustowicz RM et al: Efficacy of oral premedication for pediatric outpatient surgery, Anesthesiology 60:475-477, 1984.

Craig C: Preparation of the skin for surgery, Infect Control 7(5):257-258, 1986.

Crawford C, Finke L, and Henning M: Nursing management of the postoperative pediatric patient, Issues Comp Pediatr Nurs 6(3):157-165, 1984.

Demarest D, Hooke J, and Erickson M: Preoperative intervention for the reduction of anxiety in pediatric patients, Child Health Care 12(4):179-183, 1984.

Evans M and Hansen B: A clinical guide to pediatric nursing, ed 2, Norwalk, Conn, 1985. Appleton-Century-Crofts.

Ferguson B: Preparing young children for hospitalization: a comparison of two methods, Pediatrics 64(5):656-664, 1979.

Fochtman D, and Raffensperger J: Principles of nursing care for the pediatric surgery patient, ed 2, Boston, 1976. Little, Brown & Co.

Gauderer ML, Lorig JL, and Eastwood D: Is there a place for parents in the operating room? J Pediatr Surg 24(7):705-707, 1989.

Goldberger J: Issue-specific play with infants and toddlers in hospitals: rationale and intervention, Child Health Care 16(3):134-141, 1988.

Gustafson M: Ideas for activities with hospitalized children, Washington, DC, 1982, Association for the Care of Children's Health.

Hall SC: The pediatric cancer patient and general anesthesia, J Assoc Pediatr Oncol Nurse 1(2):8-14, 1984.

Hedenkamp E and Howell L: Assessment of the acutely ill child. In Weeks L, editor: Advanced cardiovascular nursing, Boston, 1988, Blackwell Scientific Publications.

Juneker D: Play as a tool of the nurse. In Steele S, editor: Nursing care of the child with a long-term illness, ed 2, New York, 1977, Appleton-Century-Crofts.

Katz E, Kellerman J, and Siegel S: Behavioral distress in children with cancer undergoing medical procedures: developmental considerations, J Consult Clin Psychol 48:356-365, 1980.

King E, Wieck L, and Dyer M: Quick reference to pediatric nursing procedures, Philadelphia, 1983, JB Lippincott Co.

Konings K: Preop use of GoLytely in pediatrics, Pediatr Nurs 15(5):473-474, 1989.

Kozier B and Erb G: Techniques in clinical nursing, ed 2, Menlo Park, Calif, 1987, Addison Wesley Publishing Co.

Leape L: Patient care in pediatric surgery, Boston, 1987, Little, Brown & Co.

Marshall BE and Wollman H: General anesthetics. In Gilman AG et al, editors: The pharmacological basis of therapeutics, ed 7, New York, 1985, Macmillan Publishing Co.

McConnell E: Fluid and electrolyte concerns in intestinal surgical procedures, Nurs Clin North Am 22(4):853-860, 1987.

Nelson PS et al: Comparison of oral transmucosal fentanyl citrate and an oral solution of meperdine, diazepam, and atropine for premedication in children, Anesthesiology 70(4):616-621, 1989.

Ogilvie L: Hospitalization of children for surgery: the parent's view, Child Health Care 19(1):49-56, 1990.

Pass M and Pass C: Anticipatory guidance for parents of hospitalized children, J Pediatr Nurs 2:250-258, 1987.

Perry AG and Potter PA: Clinical nursing skills and techniques, ed 2, St Louis, 1990, The CV Mosby Co.

Riffee D: Self-esteem changes in hospitalized school-age children, Nurs Res 30(2):94-97, 1981.

Rushton CH: The surgical neonate: principles of nursing management. Pediatr Nurs 14(2):141-150, 1988.

Siaw S, Stephens L, and Holmes S: Knowledge about medical instruments and reported anxiety in pediatric surgery patients, Child Health Care 14(3):134-141, 1986.

Smallwood S: Preparing children for surgery: Learning through play, AORN J 47(1):177-185, 1988.

Temple A and Katz J: Management of acute head injury: implications for perioperative nurses, AORN J 46(6):1066-1076, 1987.

Thompson R: Psychosocial research on pediatric hospitalization and health care: a review of the literature, Springfield, Ill, 1985, Charles C Thomas, Publisher.

Tuggle DW et al: The safety and cost-effectiveness of polyethylene glycol electrolyte solution on bowel preparation in infants and children, J Pediatr Surg 22(6):513-515, 1987.

Visintainer M and Wolfer J: Psychologic preparation for surgical pediatric patients: the effects on children and parents' stress responses and adjustment, Pediatrics 56:187-202, 1975.

Whaley L and Wong D: Essentials of pediatric nursing, ed 3, St Louis, 1989, The CV Mosby Co.

Whaley L and Wong D: Nursing care of infants and children, ed 4, St Louis, 1991, The CV Mosby Co.

Will surgery complicate your patient's drug therapy? Emerg Med 19(18):57-93, 1987.

Wolfer J and Visintainer M: Pediatric surgical patients' and parents' stress responses and adjustment as a function of psychologic preparation and stresspoint nursing care, Nurs Res 24(2):244-255, 1975.

# UNIT XVIII Specimens

## SKILL 115 Applying a Urine Bag for Specimen Collection

*Patti J. Tombridge*

Urine collection bags are used for infants and small children who are unable to follow directions or control urination. This method enables clean urine specimens to be collected without invasive procedures. The bags are clear plastic and disposable, with adhesive material around the opening at the point of attachment.

### NURSING DIAGNOSES

Potential for impaired skin integrity related to adhesive irritation and/or removal of urine bag; Total incontinence related to developmental age of patient.

| Steps | Rationale |
|---|---|
| **Assessment** | |
| 1. Review physician's order for urine specimen (e.g., timed specimen, or urine culture). | A review facilitates prompt, accurate collection of specimen and prevents repetition of procedure. |
| 2. Review facility's policy as to amount of urine required to complete test. | Amount of urine necessary for accurate test results varies with the type of test and laboratory capabilities. |
| 3. Determine if child has skin allergies or is sensitive to tape. | Knowledge of allergic responses helps guide procedure methods. |
| 4. Determine age and size of child. | Age and size help determine bag selection. Use age as a general guide to frequency of voiding and amount.<br>***Special Considerations:*** *Urine collection bags are available in two sizes: newborn and pediatric.* |
| 5. Inspect perineal area. | A break in the skin (e.g., diaper rash) may contraindicate the use of a collection bag. Application of bag to broken skin would contribute to breakdown and could lead to inaccurate results.<br>***Special Considerations:*** *Notify the physician if this condition exists.* |
| 6. Determine the last time the child voided. | The application of the urine collection bag may be delayed if the child has recently voided, except for newborns who void small, frequent amounts. |
| **Planning and Goal Setting** | |
| 1. Offer fluids, if not contraindicated. | Increased fluid intake will help increase the frequency and amount of voiding. |
| 2. Gather supplies:<br>a. Urine collection bag.<br>b. Mild soap, warm water and a washcloth.<br>c. Towel.<br>d. Diaper.<br>e. Skin preparation product (e.g., Skin Prep, tincture of benzoin). | ***Special Considerations:*** *Tincture of benzoin has been reported to cause allergic contact dermatitis in varying degrees of severity (James, White, and Yanklowitz, 1984; Rademaker and Kirby, 1987). Its use should be avoided if possible, especially on premature infants, and inflamed skin.* |

| Steps | Rationale |
|---|---|
| f. Label—complete with child's identification. | |
| g. Lab requisition—complete with child's identification and test desired. | |
| h. If collecting urine for a culture, the following additional supplies will be needed:<br>▪ Sterile pads (e.g., 2 × 2 inch gauze) or cotton balls.<br>▪ Antiseptic solution (e.g., povidone-iodine).<br>▪ Sterile water. | ***Special Considerations:*** *Though the urine obtained this way cannot be considered sterile, it is often tried first in hopes of obtaining interpretable results to avoid catheterization or suprapubic urine aspiration (see the box below).* |
| 3. Recruit an assistant. | ***Special Considerations:*** *Family member may be willing to help but should have option of not helping.* |
| 4. Develop individualized goals of nursing care:<br>▪ To obtain a clean urine specimen in sufficient amount for testing.<br>▪ To prevent perineal skin irritation as a result of the procedure. | |

## Implementation

| Steps | Rationale |
|---|---|
| 1. Explain procedure to family and child, if appropriate (see Skill 1). | Explanation of procedure facilitates coping skills of family and child. |
| 2. Place the infant on back and remove diaper. | |
| 3. Wash the genital area, rinse thoroughly, and pat dry. | Cleansing with particular attention to skin folds removes powder, oils, and lotions that could contaminate the specimen (Kozier and Erb, 1987). |
| *For collecting a urine culture:*<br>a. Soak the sterile cotton ball or pad with antiseptic solution. | Cleansing the perineum may remove microorganisms that could contaminate specimen for culture. |
| b. Cleanse the perineum with the soaked sterile pad:<br>*Girls:*<br>▪ Using at least 2 pads, wipe from front to back only once with each pad.<br>*Boys:*<br>▪ Using at least 2 pads, cleanse the penis from the tip to the scrotum, retracting the foreskin gently in uncircumcised males. | ***Special Considerations:*** *Despite traditional recommendations that the perineum be thoroughly cleansed with an antiseptic to yield a reliable urine culture, several studies on infants and children have questioned this practice (see the box below).* |
| c. Wipe the perineum with sterile water and allow to dry. | Rinsing with sterile water will prevent any remaining antiseptic solution from contaminating the urine (Kozier and Erb, 1987).<br>***Special Considerations:*** *In a study of adults, Moore and Bauer (1976) found that minute amounts of cleansing antiseptic in the urine specimen did not alter results.* |

### *THE EFFECT OF COLLECTION METHODS ON RATES OF CONTAMINATION*

McDonald et al (1985) found no significant difference in contamination rates of bagged urine specimens from infants whose perineum was cleansed with an antiseptic and those who were not cleansed before the urine bag application (N = 62). The contamination rates were 69% and 73%, respectively. The antiseptic used was chlorhexidine gluconate-cetrimide. The results suggest that for urine cultures from bagged specimens, only about one-third provide interpretable results, whether or not the child is well-cleansed before bag application. Further study is indicated on the effect of other antiseptics on contamination rates.

Two similar studies on toilet-trained children have also found that perineal cleansing did not have a significant effect on the rate of suspicious or positive urine cultures. Lohr, Donowitz, and Dudley (1989), in a study of toilet-trained girls ages 2 to 10 (N = 102), reported that perimeatal cleansing (with soap and sterile water) had no statistical significance over not cleansing (1% vs. 2%) on rates of contamination of urine cultures. In addition, there was a lack of statistical significance between midstream (voiding a few milliliters in one container, then collecting the rest of the void in another sterile container), and non-midstream urine contamination rates. An important feature was that each girl was asked to sit in the reverse position on the toilet for specimen collection, which provides separation of the labia from the urethral meatus without manual assistance. The other study (Saez-Llorens et al, 1989) also investigated the effect of perimeatal cleansing (with 2% castile soap and water) on uncircumcised boys (N = 99). The results of the effect of perimeatal cleansing on contamination rates between the cleansed and the uncleansed boys (5% vs. 9%) was also not statistically significant. Only midstream specimens were collected in this study. The marked improvement of the ability of a urine specimen to provide interpretable results once the child is toilet trained is clearly evident in comparing the contamination rates of these two studies to the study of bagged urine specimens.

| **Steps** | **Rationale** |
|---|---|
| 4. Have the assistant hold the infant's legs apart in the frog position. | Holding the legs in frog position will eliminate skin folds, allowing better adherence of the bag. |
| 5. Apply skin preparation (if used) and allow to dry. | Skin preparations may protect the skin and improve adherence of the bag. |
| 6. Remove the bottom half of the adhesive backing of the collection bag and apply the bag as follows:<br>a. Stretch the perineum taut.<br>b. Attach the bag at the perineum (Fig. 115-1).<br>c. Press the adhesive firmly to the skin working outward. | |
| d. Remove the protective paper from the top half of the adhesive backing and press it firmly in place over the symphysis working outward. | This outward application ensures a leakproof fit (Whaley and Wong, 1991).<br>***Special Considerations:*** *For males, place penis and scrotum inside the bag (Fig. 115-2).* |
| 7. Cut a small slit in the center of the diaper and pull the bag through. | The slit allows room for the urine to collect and facilitates checking for urine. |
| 8. Check the urine collection bag every 15 to 30 minutes. | After voiding, the weight of the urine and wetness may cause the bag to pull away from the skin, leaking the specimen.<br>***Special Considerations:*** *Alert family to frequently check the bag for urine. If specimen leaks out or the child has not voided within 45 minutes, remove the bag and repeat the cleansing process (Whaley and Wong, 1991).* |
| 9. After the child has voided gently remove the bag from the skin. Start at the front edge of the bag. | Removal of the bag starting at the front facilitates the ease of bag removal and eliminates any urine loss from the bag. |
| 10. Inspect the urine for stool contamination. | |

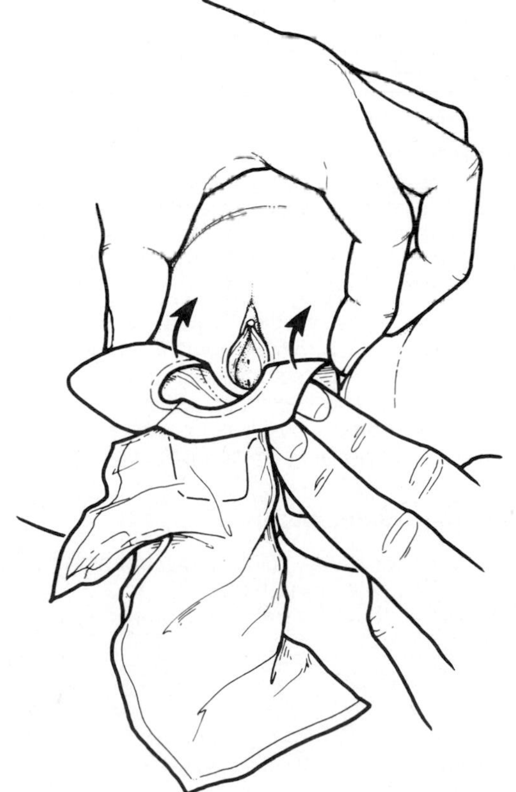

***FIG. 115-1*** Urine bag is attached to the female perineum.

From Wong DL and Whaley LF: Clinical manual of pediatric nursing, ed 3, St Louis, 1990, The CV Mosby Co.

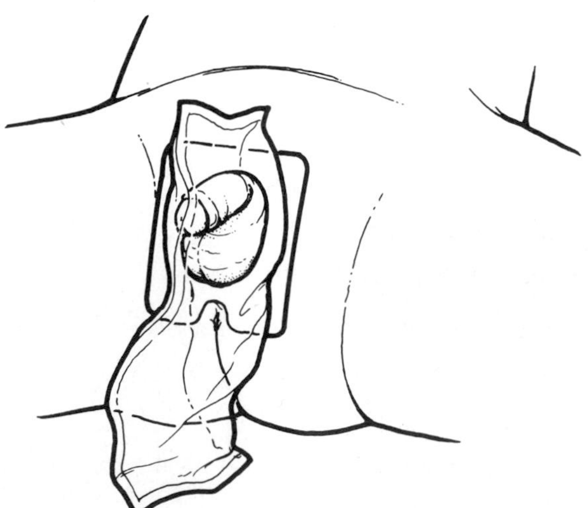

***FIG. 115-2*** Urine bag in place on a male child.

From Wong DL and Whaley LF: Clinical manual of pediatric nursing, ed 3, St Louis, 1990, The CV Mosby Co.

| Steps | Rationale |
|---|---|

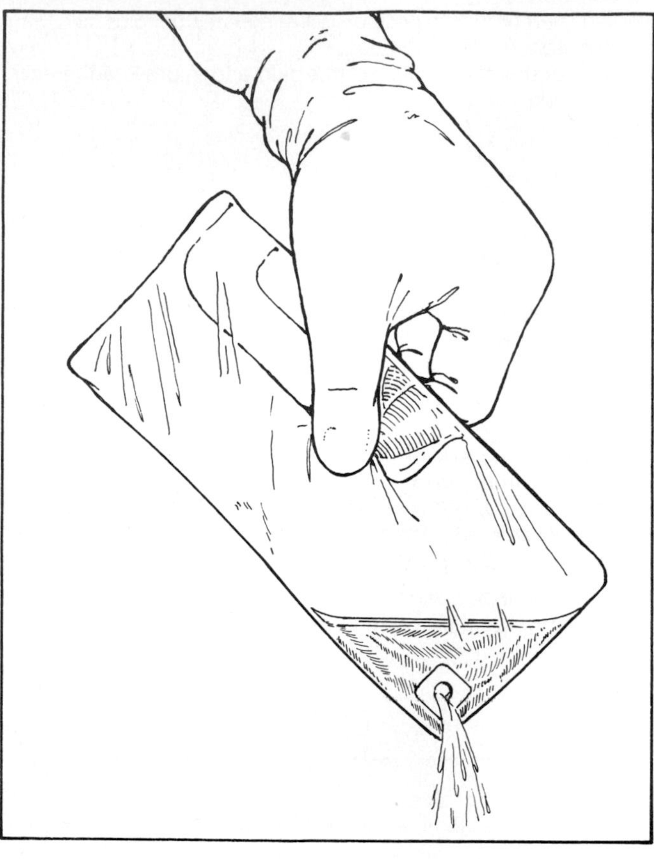

*FIG. 115-3* Emptying the urine bag.

11. Empty the urine from the bag through the opening at the base (i.e., pull tab) into a sterile specimen container (Fig. 115-3). Discard the urine bag.

***Special Considerations:*** *Do not attempt to pour the urine out from the perineal opening in the bag as it is difficult to control and may lead to contamination. If the child's intake and output is being monitored, note the amount of urine and document appropriately.*

12. Cleanse genital area and apply clean diaper.
13. Properly label the urine specimen and indicate the date and time of collection on the laboratory requisition. Deliver the specimen and requisition to the laboratory promptly.

For reliable counts, urine must be plated for culture within 2 hours of collection, or within 24 hours if refrigerated at 4° C or preserved in an evacuated urine culture tube (Goodman et al, 1985; and Lewis and Alexander, 1980).

***Special Considerations:*** *Consult policy/procedure manual of institution for any special handling instructions.*

## Evaluation Outcomes

1. An adequate urine specimen is collected.
2. Perineal skin irritation from the procedure is minimized.

## Observational Guidelines

Observe the urine for clarity, color, odor, and amount. Review laboratory results when available.

Observe child's perineum for irritation, comparing to initial assessment.

## Documentation

Record the collection of the specimen on the child's medical record, including the date, time of collection, clarity, color, odor, and amount of urine.

# SKILL 116 Assisting with Suprapubic Urine Aspiration

*Kelly Lannon Henderson*

It can be difficult to collect a urine specimen from infants that will yield interpretable results when cultured. A urine specimen may be obtained by using a urine bag (see Skill 115), by catheterization (see Skill 68), or by suprapubic aspiration (SPA). Catheterization or suprapubic aspiration are methods frequently used when rapid, accurate diagnosis is essential because of the child's clinical condition, since there is a high contamination rate with the urine bag method (see the box on p. 750 in Skill 115). In infants less than 1 year old (both male and female), SPA is a safe and aseptic method for obtaining a urine culture. SPA prevents the problem of urethral contamination and the trauma associated with catheterization. While the physician generally performs this procedure, the nurse often gathers the equipment and assists with holding the child.

## NURSING DIAGNOSES

Pain related to insertion of aspiration needle; Potential for injury related to complications from suprapubic needle puncture; Anxiety related to urine collection by suprapubic aspiration.

| Steps | Rationale |
|---|---|
| **Assessment** | |
| 1. Review physician's order for collection of urine specimen. Determine planned time for the procedure. | Verification of time and method of collection of urine specimen allows for gathering necessary equipment and assuring appropriate specimen collection. |
| 2. Assess for signs and symptoms of a urinary tract infection: fever; hematuria; flank pain; cloudy urine with sediment; itching; pain or burning with urination; frequent voiding; and/or a change in the color, amount, or odor of the urine. | Presence of any of these signs/symptoms may suggest the presence of bacteria in the urine. A urinary tract infection can be an inflammatory response to mechanical trauma, chemical irritation, or bacterial invasion, which may affect the urethra, bladder, and/or kidney.<br>***Special Considerations:*** *Signs and symptoms of a urinary tract infection vary depending on the location of the infection and on the causative agent. A suprapubic urine aspiration may also be done as part of a work-up for sepsis and/or an unknown source of infection.* |
| 3. Assess the family's understanding of the need to obtain the urine specimen, and the method that will be used. | Determining the family's present knowledge of the procedure provides a starting point for teaching and allows family to ask questions and express concerns.<br>***Special Considerations:*** *Refer to individual facility policy for information regarding need to obtain a signed consent form for the procedure.* |
| 4. Assess for any food or drug allergies. | Iodine is generally used to cleanse the skin before the suprapubic puncture. Knowledge of an allergy dictates the use of another agent.<br>***Special Considerations:*** *An allergy to shellfish could signify a possible reaction to iodine. If one or both of the parents are allergic to iodine/betadine, inform the physician before the procedure.* |
| 5. Determine whether child has been on any antibiotic therapy if the specimen is being sent for a culture. | If the child has been taking antibiotics it should be noted on the laboratory requisition for a urine culture to ensure accurate results. |
| 6. Assess for signs of dehydration. Gently palpate infant's bladder for fullness. Ask the family if they know when the child last voided. | To increase the chances of a successful aspiration, the bladder should be full enough to be palpated above the symphysis and the infant should not have voided in the last 30 to 60 minutes before the procedure. Perforation of the bowel is more likely in the dehydrated child (Morton and Lawande, 1982). |

| Steps | Rationale |
|---|---|
| | ***Special Considerations:*** *If infant has just recently voided or the bladder does not feel full enough by palpation then wait until the infant receives fluids, either oral or IV, to ensure hydration and establish urine in the bladder. Collaborate with the physician to reschedule the procedure. However, avoid a rapid fluid intake, which may result in a false low organism count (Whaley and Wong, 1991).* |
| 7. Assess for abdominal distension. | Distension of the bowel with gas increases the risk of perforation. |

## Planning and Goal Setting

| Steps | Rationale |
|---|---|
| 1. Gather equipment needed for the procedure:<br>a. Sterile gloves for the physician; nonsterile gloves for the nurse. | Gathering equipment ahead of time facilitates an efficient procedure.<br>***Special Considerations:*** *Consult with the physician to determine glove size and syringe and needle preferences (see step 1 c). An additional pair of sterile gloves should be available in case of contamination.* |
| b. Antiseptic solution—alcohol, betadine/iodine, or other appropriate solution. Prepackaged swabs are frequently used. | Cleansing the abdominal area at the insertion site will prevent contaminating the urine specimen with microorganisms that are present on the skin during penetration. |
| c. 22 or 23 gauge, 1 or 1½ inch needle, and at least a 10 ml syringe. Ask for the physician's preference.<br>d. Sterile gauze—2 x 2 in or 4 x 4 in. | The size and length of the needle used will depend on the infant's size, and on the physician's personal preference. |
| e. Sterile specimen container for culture or urinalysis. | A sterile container is used to transport the specimen.<br>***Special Considerations:*** *Facility policy as to acceptable container will vary, therefore check the policy to prevent unacceptable specimen handling.* |
| f. Completed laboratory requisition with the following: child's name, date, and time of specimen collection (fill in when specimen collected). Note on the requisition that the specimen was obtained by suprapubic aspiration.<br>g. Adhesive bandage. | Completion of requisition before obtaining the urine specimen prevents possible confusion with other specimens and allows more rapid transport to the laboratory. |
| 2. Recruit an assistant for restraining or assisting the physician if needed. | A second person may be needed to assist with holding the child and/or to hand the physician supplies to maintain a sterile field. |
| 3. Develop individualized nursing goals of care:<br>▪ To assist with obtaining an adequate, uncontaminated urine specimen.<br>▪ To minimize discomfort for the child during the procedure. | |

## Implementation

| Steps | Rationale |
|---|---|
| 1. Prepare the family for the procedure. Explain the method to be used (see also Skill 1). | This will help decrease anxiety in the family during the performance of the procedure. |
| 2. Put on nonsterile gloves. | Gloves should be worn if manually compressing the urethra, and should the infant void or have a stool during the procedure. |
| 3. Recheck diaper to be sure infant has not voided since assessment. | If the infant has voided within the last 30 minutes, the chances for a successful aspiration are decreased. |
| 4. Position the infant in a supine, frog leg position: place hands on the infant's knees, and forearms over the infant's arms to restrain them (Fig. 116-1). | Proper positioning of the child will allow good visualization of the abdominal area and the site for aspiration. The infant's hands and feet should be firmly restrained so that they will not contaminate the area for the aspiration. The infant needs to be still to prevent injury. A second person may need to assist with restraining. |
| 5. During the preparation period and before aspiration, urethral compression can be applied. In females, apply anterior rectal pressure, and in the male, apply pressure externally to the penile urethra (Kulberg, 1983). | Urethral compression prevents the infant from voiding, therefore ensuring a better chance for a successful SPA. |
| 6. The physician cleanses the suprapubic and abdominal area with the antiseptic solution. | Cleansing the abdominal area at the insertion site will prevent contaminating the urine specimen with microorganisms that are present on the skin. |
| 7. Continue securely restraining the infant. The physician puts on the sterile gloves and locates the symphysis pubis. | The ideal puncture site is just above the symphysis pubis, (0.5 to 1 cm) in the midline. |
| 8. Using the needle, puncture the skin at the selected site with a rapid, stabbing motion at a 10 to 20 degree angle to the perpendicular aiming slightly cephalad (Fig. 116-2). | |

| **Steps** | **Rationale** |
|---|---|

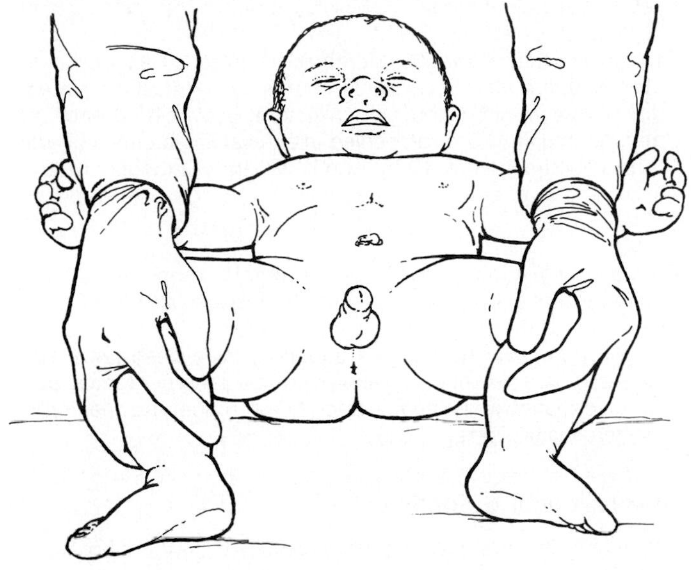

***FIG. 116-1*** Child is placed in a supine, frog-legged position.

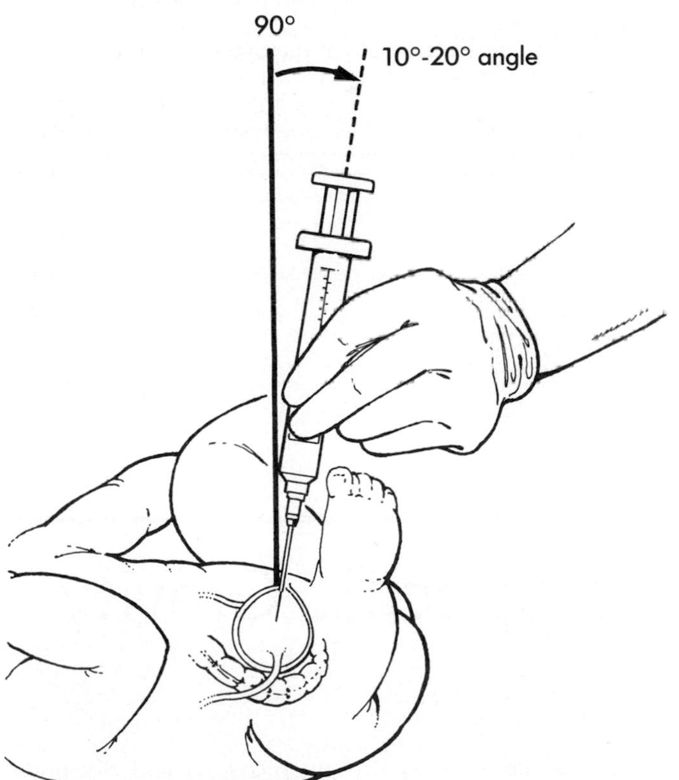


***FIG. 116-2*** Needle is inserted at a 10° to 20° angle.

9. While advancing the needle, light suction is exerted on the syringe. At a depth of about 1 inch, the bladder should be entered and urine will flow into the syringe.

***Special Considerations:*** *During this time continue to hold the infant as still as possible, providing verbal comfort and distraction.*

10. The physician aspirates the urine specimen, then withdraws the needle and applies pressure using sterile gauze at the puncture site.

Pressure is applied to provide hemostasis.

11. Transfer the urine specimen into the appropriate sterile specimen container for transport to the laboratory.
12. While maintaining pressure over the puncture site, clean the antiseptic solution off the infant's stomach.

| Steps | Rationale |
|---|---|
| 13. Check the gauze at the site to verify that bleeding/drainage has ceased. Cover the area with an adhesive bandage. | |
| 14. Attach proper identification label to the container and send the specimen to the laboratory promptly with the appropriate requisition. | If the specimen is incorrectly identified it can cause diagnostic or therapeutic errors. For reliable counts, urine must be plated for culture within 2 hours of collection, or within 24 hours if refrigerated at 4° C or preserved in an evacuated urine culture tube (Goodman et al, 1985; and Lewis and Alexander, 1980). |
| 15. Observe the aspiration site every hour for 4 hours after the procedure for signs of bleeding, drainage, redness, swelling, or bruising. Notify the physician if indicated. | |
| 16. Monitor urine output following procedure for presence and amount of hematuria. | Transient hematuria is the most common complication. The amount of blood in the urine should decrease with each successive void (Morton and Lawande, 1982). |
| 17. Monitor vital signs and temperature and assess abdomen for signs and symptoms of complications such as: elevated temperature, abdominal distension, decreased bowel sounds, a change in vital signs, or respiratory distress. | Complications, which occur infrequently, have been reported. These include bowel perforation with resulting peritonitis, abscess formation in the needle tract, hemorrhage, and anaerobic bacteremia (Kulberg, 1983). |

| Evaluation Outcomes | Observational Guidelines |
|---|---|
| 1. An adequate, uncontaminated urine specimen is obtained to confirm the presence or absence of bacteria. | Note that an adequate specimen was obtained; review laboratory results when available. |
| 2. Potential complications of SPA are prevented or minimized. | Note presence of hematuria, and gross bleeding. Assess vital signs and temperature, and assess abdomen. Note appearance of puncture site. |
| 3. The family is informed and prepared for the procedure. | Ask family to describe purpose of the procedure method used. Family expresses appropriate concern, expresses relief when procedure is completed, and does not exhibit signs of anger. |
| 4. The discomfort experienced by the child during the procedure is minimized. | The child fusses or cries minimally and responds quickly to comfort measures following the procedure. |

### Documentation

Record that the procedure was done and if urine was collected. Note the time, amount, and date of the collection, and the color and appearance of the urine. Record how the infant tolerated the procedure. Record ongoing aspiration site checks and observation for signs/symptoms of complications. If any of these are present or develop, document notification of the physician.

# *SKILL* 117 Measuring Specific Gravity

*Lydia Johnson*

Specific gravity is a simple method of examining urine in order to determine its concentration. Urine specific gravity is the ratio of the weight of solutes excreted by the kidney to a unit of water. Measuring urine specific gravity yields important information about the child's health state to the health care professional (Bowker et al, 1986).

The concentration of urine will depend on the body's state of hydration, renal function, and regulatory mechanism function. With dehydration the urine specific gravity will increase; with fluid volume excess the urine specific gravity will decrease. The measurement of urine specific gravity may be done by the nurse quickly and efficiently in any setting with the appropriate tools and technique.

## NURSING DIAGNOSES

Fluid volume deficit related to failure of regulatory mechanisms, fever, or infection; Fluid volume deficit related to diarrhea, vomiting, diaphoresis, excessive drainage, or dietary changes; Fluid volume excess related to compromised regulatory mechanisms or excessive fluid/sodium intake.

| **Steps** | **Rationale** |
|---|---|

## Assessment

1. Determine child's age and developmental level, including toilet training status.

These factors help determine how the specimen will need to be collected. The age and developmental level also provide comparison for assessing behaviors of dehydration/fluid volume excess.

2. Assess child's hydration status including (see Skill 64):
   a. Skin turgor.
   b. Edema.
   c. Color.
   d. Intake/output records.
   e. Behavior.

The child's hydration status should be compared to the specific gravity results.

***Special Considerations:*** *Conditions that can affect specific gravity are dehydration/fluid volume excess, diuretics, renal failure and diabetes insipidus.*

3. Review institution's policy regarding measurement of specific gravity and normal range of values. Specific gravity measurement between 1.010 and 1.025 is usually considered normal.

Institutional procedure will determine which materials and equipment will be needed for performing the specific gravity test.

***Special Considerations:*** *All staff should perform specific gravity testing in the same manner to provide continuity and reliability in test results.*

## Planning and Goal Setting

1. Determine urine collection method.
   a. Diaper sample.
   b. Potty hat.
   c. Foley.
   d. Urine collection bag.

A variety of methods can be used to collect urine. The urine does not need to be sterile but should be free from contaminants. The method should not affect the specific gravity result (Strobach and Kratina, 1982; Suri, 1988; and McConnell, 1982).

***Special Considerations:*** *Studies comparing diaper samples to collection bags have not included testing of diapers with absorbent gel material e.g., Ultra Pampers.*

2. Gather supplies.
   a. Syringe (1 ml to 10 ml).
   b. Needle (if collecting from a Foley).
   c. Specific gravity measurement tool: refractometer or Chemstrip 9 Multistick.
   d. Tissue.
   e. Gloves.

Having all supplies ready improves efficiency and yields increased contact time with the child/family.

***Special Considerations:*** *A calibrated hydrometer is seldom used in pediatrics since a large amount of urine (at least 20 ml) is needed for testing. For this procedure see Perry and Potter, 1990. Verify that strips are not expired because this will affect the accuracy of the results.*

3. Develop nursing goals of care:
   - To obtain an adequate urine specimen to test for specific gravity.
   - To accurately determine urine specific gravity.

## Implementation

1. Collect urine sample (may be sterile or nonsterile) from collection device using appropriate technique. Aspirate urine from:
   a. Diaper.
   b. Collection bag.
   c. Potty hat.
   d. Foley.

The urine specimen does not need to be sterile but free from contaminants.

***Special Considerations:*** *To collect urine from a diaper sample without absorbent gel material, aspirate urine from the wettest portion of the diaper (Fig. 117-1) or remove the wet absorbent substance from the diaper and place it into the barrel of a 5 ml syringe, then replace the plunger into the barrel and compress plunger to extract urine from the diaper sample (Suri, 1988; Waskerwitz, 1987). If using a diaper with absorbent gel material, place a 2 × 2 inch or 4 × 4 inch gauze sponge inside the diaper and, after the child has voided, aspirate urine from the gauze sponge. Stebor (1989) reported no significant change in specific gravities taken from diaper samples up to 4 hours after urination, provided the diaper was closed and taped to prevent evaporation and was not exposed to air, heat, or light.*

2. Draw urine specimen of .75 ml to 1.0 ml into syringe.

This is an ample specimen for specific gravity determination.

***Special Considerations:*** *Will need more than this amount if using a hydrometer to measure specific gravity.*

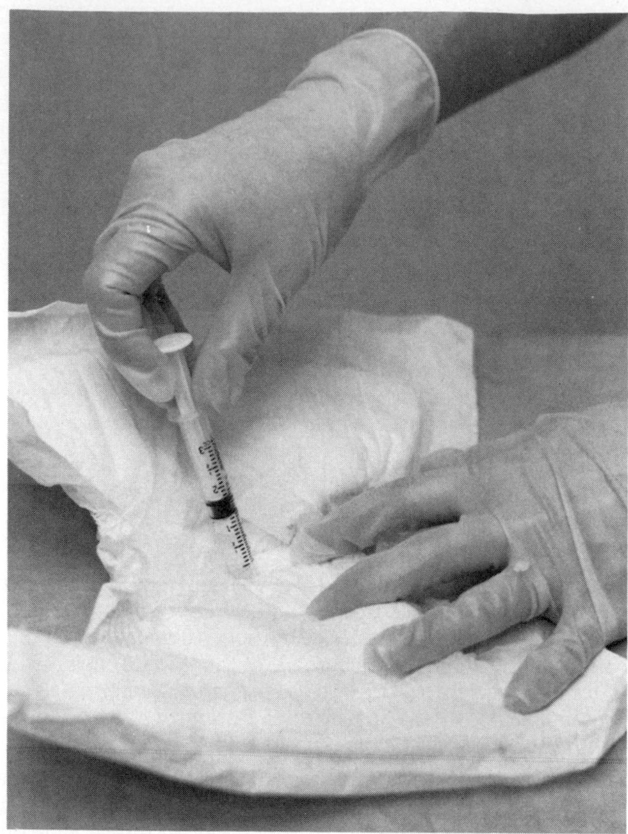

***FIG. 117-1*** Urine is aspirated from wettest portion of the diaper.

| **Steps** | **Rationale** |
|---|---|
| 3. Test urine sample on specific gravity measurement tool. | Refer to institution's policy/procedures to identify specific gravity measurement device to be used. |
| a. Refractometer—Lift cover slide off mirror lens. Turn refractometer on (light will come on). Place large drop of urine onto lens and lower cover slide. Look through eye piece and read specific gravity result. There will be numbers on the right hand side. The specific gravity result will be the number where the dark line ends. | ***Special Considerations:*** *The lens must be clean from dust or other particulate in order to obtain most accurate result.* |
| b. Chemstrip 9 Multistick—Remove strip from bottle and replace cap. Apply large drop of urine onto test strip pads. Immediately begin timing test as directed on bottle. After timing is completed, shake excess urine from test strip. Compare test strip color to color chart on side of bottle for specific gravity result. | |

## Evaluation Outcomes

1. An accurate specific gravity reading is obtained from a urine specimen.

## Observational Guidelines

Compare the specific gravity result to the initial assessment of the child, the intake/output record, and the appearance of the urine.

## Documentation

Record the specific gravity result, including the following data: name of child; time of day test done; test result; and any difficulty or unusual findings encountered doing the test.

# SKILL 118 Testing for Pinworm Infection

*Donna Phillips Smith*

Pinworms *(Enterobius vermicularis)* are the most common helminth infection in the United States (Benenson, 1985). These highly contagious nematodes flourish in crowded conditions such as schools and child care centers. Pinworms infect 33% to 80% of school-age children at some point (Henley and Sears, 1985). Estimates of prevalence in institutionalized children is as high as 90% (Patient Care, 1983). Diagnosis of pinworm infection is difficult, since it is seldom identified by traditional stool sampling. A more effective method of confirming diagnosis is the easily performed "tape test."

## NURSING DIAGNOSES

Pain (pruritus) related to pinworm infestation; Sleep pattern disturbance related to pruritus and/or incontinence; Potential for infection (family) related to insufficient knowledge to avoid exposure to parasite.

| Steps | Rationale |
|---|---|
| **Assessment** | |
| 1. Assess for primary symptom of intense perianal itching. Other common symptoms include irritability, poor quality of sleep, bedwetting, whining, and short attention span. | The adult female pinworm migrates out of the child's relaxed anal sphincter during sleep to lay eggs. This movement causes intense perianal itching. **Special Considerations:** *In young girls, the pinworms may migrate into the vagina and urethra causing vaginal and urinary tract infections and secondary enuresis. Infection may also be asymptomatic (Katzman, 1989).* |
| 2. Review facility policy on specimen collection. | Facility policy may vary as to acceptable specimen container or transport method. **Special Considerations:** *Pinworms are seldom identified in a stool specimen (Henley and Sears, 1985).* |
| **Planning and Goal Setting** | |
| 1. Time the test when the child first awakens and before arising, bathing, or toileting. | The eggs laid by the female pinworm during the night must be obtained before they are removed by scratching, wiping with toilet tissue, or bathing to avoid a negative test result. |
| 2. Assemble items:<br>a. Wooden tongue blade (depressor).<br>b. Transparent tape (not translucent or "frosted").<br>c. A commercially available paddle may be used instead of a wooden tongue blade depressor or transparent tape.<br>d. Gloves.<br>e. A glass laboratory slide, clean glass jar, or plastic bag. | Gathering items in advance facilitates specimen collection. **Special Considerations:** *The commercially available paddle with only one sticky surface is less efficient and more costly (Patient Care, 1983).* |
| 3. Develop an individualized nursing goal of care:<br>▪ Obtain an adequate specimen to test for the presence of pinworm ova. | |
| **Implementation** | |
| 1. Loop a 3 inch section of tape firmly around the end of the tongue blade, with the sticky side out, folding in the edges to adhere to the blade (Fig. 118-1). | Use of a wooden tongue blade provides a firm surface to facilitate adherence of the ova. Two sticky surfaces allow greater contact of the anal area, to increase the chance of ova collection. |
| 2. Remove the child's diaper or undergarments. | Removal of these items is necessary to provide access to the anal area. |
| 3. With a gloved hand, separate the child's buttocks to expose the perianal region. | Gloving of the hand touching the perianal region will prevent transmission of infection. |

| Steps | Rationale |
|---|---|

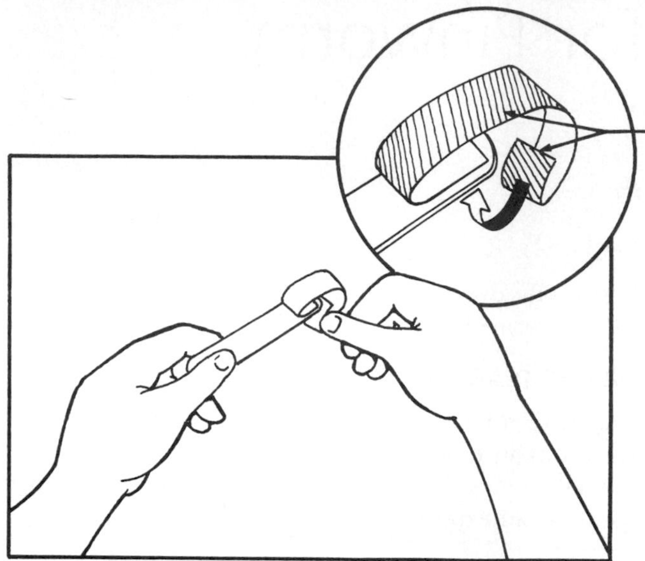

***FIG. 118-1*** Tape is looped around tongue blade to expose sticky surfaces.

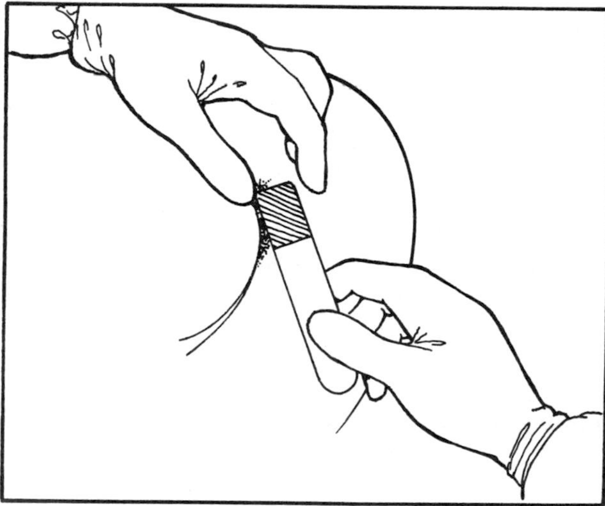

***FIG. 118-2*** The taped blade is pressed against the anal sphincter for specimen collection.

4. With the other hand, place the taped blade up to the anal sphincter pressing the blade to one side, then to the other, using the tape on both sides (Fig. 118-2).

The eggs and sometimes the adult pinworm will adhere to the tape and can be identified through the tape when viewed under a microscope.

5. Carefully remove the tape from the blade, and place sticky side down on a glass slide, or place the blade in a clean glass jar or plastic bag, according to facility policy. Label container with the child's name and time of collection and transport as necessary.
6. Rediaper or assist the child to redress.

Redressing permits the child to begin the morning routine.

7. Repeat the test three consecutive mornings if no pinworms or ova are identified.

False negatives are common. A negative finding is only accepted after 3 to 4 tests (Henley and Sears, 1985).

***Special Considerations:*** *Parents may be asked to collect tapes at home three consecutive mornings before bringing them for examination.*

## Evaluation Outcomes

1. Adequate specimens are collected to demonstrate the presence or absence of pinworms.

## Observational Guidelines

Check laboratory reports, or observe for ova or adult pinworms under a microscope.

### Documentation

Document on agency record each performance of the test and delivery of the tapes. If findings are positive, record medication administration and instructions to repeat dosage in two weeks. Also document child/family education concerning environmental measures to prevent reinfestation and infestation of others.

### Child and Family Teaching

1. *Treatment.* Physicians frequently treat the whole family based on positive findings in one member. Treatment is usually a single dose administration of medication, but must be repeated in two weeks to prevent reinfestation from developing larvae.
2. *Environmental measures.* Following medication treatment, all bedding and clothing should be washed in hot water. Bedrooms and bathrooms should be vacuumed or damp mopped. The toilet seat should be cleaned with a disinfectant, leaving it on several minutes, then wiping with paper towels (Sears, 1985). For the two to three week treatment period, the family should change undergarments and pajamas daily, washing these garments in hot water. They should also wear long, snug fitting pajamas. Showers are preferable to tub baths (Benenson, 1985). The child's fingernails should be cut short to prevent collecting eggs under the nails. Encourage the family to practice good handwashing, including scrubbing under the nails, before eating and after toileting.

### Home Care Modifications

A flashlight can be used to quickly inspect the anal area at night while the child is sleeping. If adult pinworms are seen, however, it may be very distressing to the parents. Lack of findings is not conclusive (Katzman, 1989). Having them perform the tape test at home, and placing the tapes in a container to bring in for inspection may be preferable (Patient Care, 1983).

# *SKILL* 119 Obtaining a Throat Culture

*Lisa K. Anderson*

A throat culture is an important diagnostic tool in the identification and differentiation of the causative agent in a pharyngeal or tonsillar infection. Between 80% and 90% of sore throats in children have a viral etiology (Whaley and Wong, 1991). The remaining 10% to 15% are caused by beta-hemolytic streptococci (Corbett, 1987). As in the collection of other cultures, correct technique is essential to avoid contamination of the culture and facilitate accurate medical diagnosis and treatment.

Other upper airway pathogens such as *Bordetella pertussis, Haemophilus influenza*, and respiratory syncytial virus (RSV) are sampled and cultured by using variations of the throat culture. These variations include the posterior nasopharyngeal (PNP) swab and nasal washings (see the box on the following page). For collection of a lower airway specimen (sputum), see Skills 87 and 92.

### NURSING DIAGNOSES

Anxiety related to unmet informational needs about purpose and procedure for throat culture; Potential for infection related to erythema, lesions, or exudate in the throat; Suffocation related to tracheal edema.

## *VARIATIONS IN THROAT CULTURE COLLECTION METHODS*

Respiratory syncytial virus (RSV) accounts for up to one half of all hospital admissions for respiratory disease in infants (Macdonald, 1985). Various methods of obtaining upper respiratory secretions for RSV culture have been used—throat swabs, nasopharyngeal swabs, and nasal washings. Comparison studies indicate that, although throat and nasopharyngeal specimens are easier to obtain, RSV is isolated more frequently and in less time from nasal washings (Hall and Douglas, 1975; Treuhaft, Soukup, and Sullivan, 1985; Masters et al, 1987; Nederhand et al, 1989).

Nasal washings are obtained by instilling 3 to 7 ml of phosphate buffered saline (PBS) into the child's nostril with a rubber bulb syringe and then collecting the nasal secretions and saline by immediate suction with the same bulb syringe. To facilitate the procedure, the child's head should be tipped back at a 70° angle. The bulb syringe should be inserted and collected in one squeeze-and-release motion (Hall and Douglas, 1975). The specimen may then be transferred from the syringe to a sterile specimen container, and either promptly transported to the laboratory, or inoculated into culture media at the bedside (Hall and Douglas, 1975). If the specimen is to be taken to the laboratory, it should be at room temperature and inoculated into culture media within 2 hours (Treuhaft, Soukup, and Sullivan, 1985) to facilitate maximum viral isolation.

Follow the basic technique for a throat culture outlined in this skill when obtaining a specimen for RSV using equipment specific to the collection of viral specimens (e.g., viral culturettes; algiswabs).

Nasopharyngeal swabs are frequently used to diagnose a *Bordetella pertussis* infection. Cough plates are no longer the recommended method of diagnosis (Behrman and Vaughan, 1987). NP swabs are also used to detect *Haemophilus influenzae* infection. A thin flexible wire with a small, tightly wrapped cotton tip is used for nasopharyngeal culture. The opposite end of the wire is usually looped for easier handling.

With the child adequately restrained (see Skill 51) and the head slightly tilted back, push the tip of the child's nose upward. Insert the swab through the nostril along the floor of the nose into the nasopharynx (see Fig. 119-1). Do not aim upward because the swab will not reach the posterior pharynx (Hughes and Buescher, 1980). If desired, slightly bending the wire 1 to 2 inches from the tip (depending on the size of the child) may facilitate insertion and location of the posterior pharynx. Leave in place a few seconds, then remove the wire and place in the appropriate media for prompt transport to the laboratory.

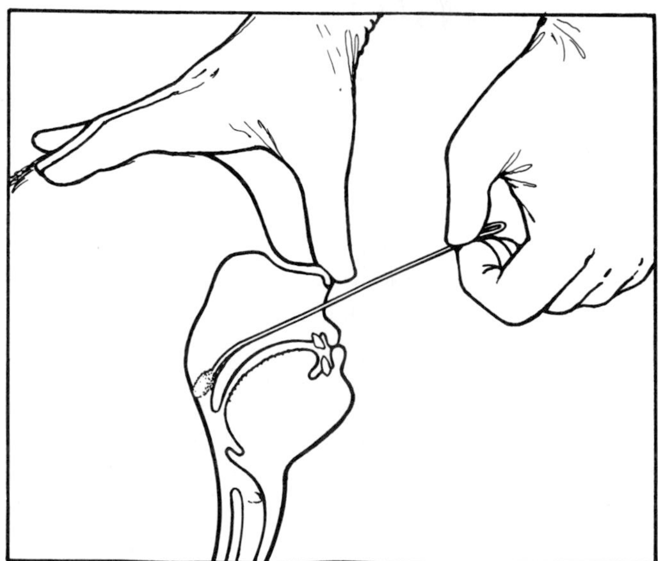

***FIG. 119-1*** The swab is inserted through the nostril, along the floor of the nose, into the nasopharynx.

## Assessment

| Steps | Rationale |
|---|---|
| 1. Review physician's order for specific test to be done on specimen, and lesions, exudate, or areas of the throat to be cultured. | Proper specimen collection will eliminate need for repetition and expedite the diagnostic process. |
| 2. Assess child's level of knowledge and understanding of the procedure, as well as previous experiences with the procedure. | Child's age, developmental level, and previous experience will help determine the level of cooperation to be expected. |
| 3. Assess child's ability to follow instructions and the need for assistance in collecting specimen. | If child is unable to cooperate or follow instructions, it will be necessary to solicit help for restraining the child during collection of specimen. |
| 4. Assess pharyngeal area. | Location of erythema, lesions, or exudate in the throat should be noted to facilitate the quick collection of an optimal amount of microorganisms. |
| 5. Review child's history and presenting symptoms for suspected epiglottitis: rapid onset; drooling; high fever; wet or absent cough; muffled voice; and sitting with open mouth, jaw thrust forward, and protruding tongue (Battaglia, 1986). | Throat culture should not be attempted if acute epiglottitis is suspected. The trauma induced by swabbing the pharynx or tonsils, however slight, could accelerate the rapid progression of the disease, increasing edema and totally occluding the airway (Battaglia, 1986; Thomas, 1984). |
| 6. Determine current antibiotic therapy. | Antibiotic therapy may alter culture results.<br>***Special Considerations:*** *Throat culture should be obtained before initiating antibiotic therapy, if possible.* |

## Planning and Goal Setting

| Steps | Rationale |
|---|---|
| 1. Gather equipment: | |
| a. Latex gloves. | Gloves serve as a physical barrier against secretions. |
| b. Tongue depressor. | |
| c. Sterile swab. | Cotton, dacron, or calcium alginate swabs should be used for throat culture (Traister, 1983). |
| d. Sterile culture tube. | Culture tube may contain a buffered gel media or may be part of a kit including swab and culture tube, e.g., Anaswab by Scott Laboratories, Sulphur, Louisiana.<br>***Special Considerations:*** *There are a number of diagnostic kits available for rapid identification of streptococcal infections; however, some authorities question the kits' sensitivity as a substitute for culture (Whaley and Wong, 1991).* |
| e. Flashlight or freestanding light source. | |
| f. Labels and laboratory requisition. | |
| 2. Explain procedure to child and family (see Skill 1). Demonstrate how to open mouth wide and say "ahh." Show the child all equipment, and allow child to handle it if desired. (Use sterile swab for collection.) Describe sensations child may feel during collection (e.g., "tickling," mild gagging). | Saying "ahh" relaxes the throat muscles and helps minimize contraction of the constrictor muscle of the pharynx, thereby decreasing the gag reflex (Kozier and Erb, 1987). |
| 3. Develop individualized goals of nursing care:<br>▪ Minimize child/family anxiety concerning the procedure.<br>▪ Obtain an adequate culture in a timely manner, uncontaminated by oral secretions.<br>▪ Minimize trauma to the pharyngeal/tonsillar area. | |

## Implementation

| Steps | Rationale |
|---|---|
| 1. Have older child or adolescent sit erect in bed or chair. Young child or infant should be placed on his or her back with head against the bed or pillow. Assistant should restrain arm and head of child, if necessary. | Collecting the specimen may produce minor, temporary discomfort or gagging, especially if mucosa is inflamed. Young children should be restrained to prevent mucosal damage caused by reflexive movement when the tonsils are touched by the swab.<br>***Special Considerations:*** *A family member should not be asked to restrain the child. Restraint by a family member may produce feelings of guilt in the family member and feelings of betrayal in the child.* |
| 2. Instruct child to open the mouth wide and say "ahh." Infants will open the mouth and pharynx optimally during crying. | ***Special Considerations:*** *Family member may be helpful in persuading the child to open the mouth.* |

| Steps | Rationale |
|---|---|
| 3. Position light source to illuminate the area to be cultured. | Proper visualization of area facilitates obtaining specimen from desired area of the throat. ***Special Considerations:*** *If a free-standing light source is not available, an assistant should hold the flashlight.* |
| 4. Insert tongue depressor gently into mouth with nondominant hand. Cover the anterior half of the tongue, and depress to hold tongue down, and visualize the pharyngeal area. | Placing the tongue depressor farther back on the tongue can cause gagging or discomfort. |
| 5. With a sweeping motion, quickly swab the tonsillar surface or tonsillar fossa, paying particular attention to areas of erythema or exudate (Traister, 1983) (Fig. 119-2). Do not touch the tongue, buccal mucosa, or palate with the swab at any time. Swab only one side for each culture taken (Smith and Duell, 1985). | Touching other areas of the mouth will contaminate the specimen with resident oral bacteria. ***Special Considerations:*** *Group A beta-hemolytic streptococcal cultures are best obtained by swabbing only the tonsillar surface or fossa (Wagner, 1986).* |

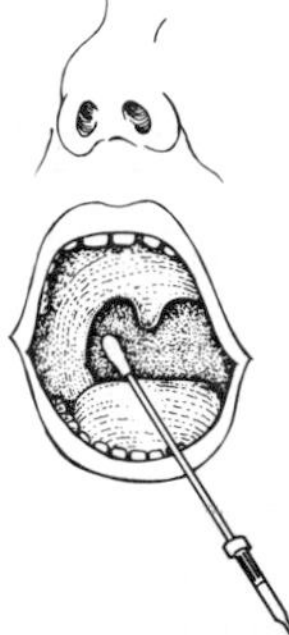

***FIG. 119-2*** The tonsillar surface is swabbed with a quick, sweeping motion.

From Perry AG and Potter PA: Clinical nursing skills and techniques, ed 2, St Louis, 1990, The CV Mosby Co.

| Steps | Rationale |
|---|---|
| 6. Withdraw the swab, and insert into the culture media. If swab stick extends above the top of the tube, cut or break off the stick. Secure the culture tube cover or lid. | Immediate placement of specimen into the culture media facilitates bacterial growth. ***Special Considerations:*** *Some culture kits require squeezing an ampule to release medium to preserve organisms.* |
| 7. Dispose of tongue depressor in waste receptacle. | Proper disposal prevents transmission of microorganisms. |
| 8. Label culture with child's identification, time and date of collection. | |
| 9. Promptly transport culture tube and completed requisition to laboratory. Record child's identification, date and time of collection, source of specimen, and current antibiotic therapy on the requisition. | Ideal bacterial growth conditions are provided in the laboratory. |
| 10. Provide comfort measures, and cool oral fluids if permitted. | Cool oral fluids will soothe pharyngeal irritation. Holding, stroking, comforting or praising, and enlisting a family member to support the child will decrease anxiety and ease coping. |

| Evaluation Outcomes | Observational Guidelines |
|---|---|
| 1. The child and family are adequately prepared for the throat culture collection. | Ask the family to summarize the reasons for throat culture. Note child's attempts at cooperation during the procedure. |
| 2. Throat culture is completed in a timely manner, and an adequate specimen is collected, uncontaminated by oral secretions. | Check laboratory reports for results. |
| 3. Trauma to the pharyngeal or tonsillar area is absent or minimal. | Assess by direct visualization of the pharyngeal area after specimen collection. Monitor respiratory status, and compare with baseline assessment. |
| 4. Specimen is properly handled and promptly delivered to laboratory to facilitate medical diagnosis and treatment. | Check laboratory reports for results. |

## Documentation

Record date and time of culture collection; record appearance of specimen; Note preprocedural and postprocedural teaching of child and family; document child's response to and tolerance of procedure.

# *SKILL* 120 Measuring Blood Glucose by Fingerstick

*Margaret P. Ireton*

The introduction of blood glucose monitoring (BGM) in the late 1970s has probably influenced diabetic control more than any other factor in the last 20 years (Travis, Brouhard, and Schreiner, 1987). The fingerstick method of measuring blood glucose levels is relatively painless and provides immediate results (Davidson, 1986). The use of capillary blood for glucose monitoring has been found to have an accuracy of approximately plus or minus 10% of the obtained blood serum results when the monitoring equipment is used according to instructions (Hilton, 1982).

Blood glucose monitoring can be easily taught to the school-age child and family members, is generally well tolerated by children, and may be performed in any setting. Blood glucose monitoring is a major factor in managing insulin-dependent diabetes mellitus (IDDM), but may be used any time frequent blood glucose assessment is indicated, e.g., total parenteral nutrition. Because of the variety of BGM systems available, it is not possible to provide specific guidelines for each device. Therefore this skill presents general guidelines applicable to all systems.

## NURSING DIAGNOSES

Altered health maintenance related to lack of information about purpose and procedure for capillary blood glucose measurement; Pain related to skin puncture by lancet; Potential for tissue injury related to child's/family's incorrect puncture procedure for fingerstick, movement of finger by child, or frequent use of same puncture site.

| Steps | Rationale |
|---|---|
| **Assessment** | |
| 1. Determine child's age, developmental level, current health status, and ability and willingness to cooperate. | Child's age, personality, cognitive and developmental abilities, self control, and motivation influence cooperation. The child's current health status affects ability to self-perform the blood glucose check.<br>***Special Considerations:*** *Most children can be involved at an age-appropriate level in the procedure:*<br>▪ *Preschoolers (3 to 6 years old): Start involvement with simple tasks such as pressing on/off button of meter or pressing release button on lancing device.*<br>▪ *School-age: Perform procedure with supervision.*<br>▪ *Adolescence: Perform procedure independently.* |
| 2. Determine whether child has been previously diagnosed with diabetes mellitus or is newly diagnosed. | Initial learning needs and teaching strategies used for the newly diagnosed child may differ from those relating to the child having management difficulties.<br>***Special Considerations:*** *See Child and Family Teaching for additional assessment guidelines for the child with management problems.* |
| 3. Review physician's order and institution's policy to determine time, frequency, or special conditions necessitating blood glucose monitoring. | Physician determines the routine glucose testing schedule based on the child's present health status and potential for fluctuation of the blood glucose level. Also, many institutions have a policy regarding frequency of blood glucose monitoring. |
| 4. Review child's medical history and current status for factors influencing the frequency and timing of blood glucose measurements and possible risk factors. | Assessing major influences on the fluctuation of the child's blood glucose level provides rationale for the frequency and timing of additional blood glucose measurements that may need to be performed. |
| a. Emotional stressors. | During emotional stress hormones are secreted that counteract the actions of insulin, allowing the blood sugar to increase (Travis, Brouhard, and Schreiner, 1987). |
| b. NPO status for surgery or tests. | Fasting may result in hypoglycemia and should be closely monitored.<br>***Special Considerations:*** *Type of IV fluids, medications, and present state of diabetic control influence the risk for hypoglycemia while NPO.* |

| Steps | Rationale |
|---|---|
| c. Strenuous exercise. | Blood glucose level may increase or decrease in response to strenuous exercise immediately or several hours later (Travis, Brouhard, and Schreiner, 1987). **Special Considerations:** *The most common response to exercise is a decrease in blood glucose over ½ to 2 hours.* |
| d. Meals, snacks, concentrated glucose preparations, glucagon, IV dextrose solutions during the past 24 to 36 hours. | The body's source of glucose is food. When ingested, all foods convert to glucose in some percentage (carbohydrate—100%, protein—58%, fats—10%). Food quantity is an important influence on post-prandial glucose level. Preparations and solutions containing dextrose also elevate glucose level. |
| e. Insulin administration. | Blood glucose level decreases in response to insulin administration. The pattern of response varies depending on type of insulin. |
| f. Physiologic stressors, e.g., infectious process, vomiting, surgery. | An increase in glucose level in response to physiologic stressors relates to an increase in counterregulatory hormones, e.g., epinephrine, adrenalin, glucagon, and cortisone (Travis, Brouhard, and Schreiner, 1987). |
| g. Hematocrit. | If the hematocrit is abnormal, an inaccurate blood glucose level may be obtained from a meter. A serum glucose is indicated for an accurate measure. |
| 5. Assess skin integrity of preferred sites for: | Visual inspection of the skin identifies potential sites and areas to avoid. |
| a. Signs of infection. | Puncture sites provide a portal of entry for microorganisms which may cause infection. |
| b. Bruises. | Puncture made through a bruised area may cause pain. |
| c. Extremely calloused area. | Frequent skin punctures may result in calluses at preferred sites. Thickly calloused areas lack the vascularity needed for obtaining a blood specimen. |

## Planning and Goal Setting

| Steps | Rationale |
|---|---|
| 1. Plan the procedure collaboratively with child/family based on assessment. | Collaborative planning enhances the child's cooperation with the procedure and motivation to learn. |
| 2. Select an environment that is comfortable, private, well-lit, free from distracting stimuli, and has access to a sink, faucet, and firm counter top. | Choosing a suitable environment enhances the child's ability to learn and perform the skill correctly. |
| 3. Gather and assemble equipment and supplies: | Accurate test results depend on the technique and the availability and condition of the equipment and supplies. |
| a. Alcohol swab (optional). | Either soap and water or an alcohol wipe are acceptable to cleanse the fingerstick site. |
| b. Cotton ball or clean tissue. | A cotton ball or tissue may be placed on the site after blood is obtained. |
| c. Lancet and automatic lancing device (optional), e.g., Soft touch, Penlet, Autolet. | These devices deliver a quick and consistent puncture at a given depth of penetration, thus ensuring adequate blood flow. **Special Considerations:** *An automatic device is recommended for children but child and family should learn both manual and mechanical methods in case of device failure (Whaley and Wong, 1991). Most lancing devices have pediatric platforms or endcaps that control penetration depth.* |
| d. Blotting material, e.g., tissue, or type required by specific system. | Excess blood from the reagent pad is blotted or wiped according to the product's instructions before the strip is placed in the meter. **Special Considerations:** *Use only recommended type of blotting material (Davidson, 1986). Several "no-wipe" systems are designed to decrease user error by eliminating need to remove excess blood from the reagent strip.* |
| e. Blood glucose reagent strip. Verify that strip is: compatible with meter or chart; not discolored; not past expiration date; and in original container, marked with date first opened. | Accurate results are dependent upon these criteria being met. **Special Considerations:** *If 4 months have elapsed since container was first opened, discard strips. Store reagent strips in original container, at room temperature and away from direct sunlight and high humidity.* |
| f. Blood glucose reflectance meter or specific color chart for measuring blood glucose levels. | Glucose reflectance meters provide a more sensitive measurement of blood glucose concentrations than color charts. |

**Steps** | **Rationale**

***Special Considerations:*** *For children or family members who are color blind or have difficulty distinguishing colors, a meter with a readout is the preferred method of measurement (Whaley and Wong, 1991).*

g. Any other supplies specified by procedure manual of meter; or instructions accompanying strips, or color chart (e.g., an accurate timing device, if a meter is not used).

Proper timing and correct techniques as outlined by the product's procedure manual enhance accuracy and reliability of test results.

4. Prepare equipment:

Preparing equipment in advance facilitates safe and efficient performance of the procedure with less anxiety for the child.

a. Adjust and set glucose reflectance meter:
   - Calibrate according to manufacturer's directions.

Meters require checking and adjustment before measuring glucose levels to provide accuracy. Calibration of meter varies according to brand.

   - Check batteries for viability.

Weak or dead batteries affect timeliness of measurement.

   - Check program code or number to match number on bottle or box of reagent strips, if applicable.

Program numbers must match on the meter and reagent strip bottle to enhance accuracy on certain meters.

b. Assemble automatic lancing device. Leave protective cap on sharp end of Autolet device until just before puncture.

Capillary blood is obtained by using an automatic lancing device in accordance with manufacturer's recommendations.

5. Develop individualized goals of nursing care:
   - To obtain an accurate blood glucose level.
   - To prevent tissue injury and infection at site of puncture.
   - To minimize child's anxiety and discomfort.
6. Develop individualized child and family goals:
   - Child/family will verbalize knowledge related to blood glucose measurement.
   - Child/family will be able to accurately perform blood glucose check.
   - Child/family will demonstrate proper care of equipment and supplies.

## Implementation

1. Explain to the child and family the principles and considerations for using supplies and equipment while demonstrating the procedure.

Explanations help to reduce fear and anxiety and to promote positive coping behaviors. Variance in procedure occurs with specific reagent strips and meters.

***Special Considerations:*** *Refer to package inserts and manufacturer's instructions for specific procedure.*

2. Remove reagent strip from container or individual foil wrap, replacing lid, if applicable. If container is being opened for first time, place date on label.

Exposure of the strips to moisture, air and light can result in chemical changes in the reagent pads, thereby invalidating test results.

3. Place clean reagent strip on dry paper towel or on a clean, dry, firm surface with reagent pad up, or place directly into the meter.

Reagent pads can become contaminated by touch or contact with damp surfaces.

***Special Considerations:*** *The test strip is placed in the meter before obtaining blood with some systems (e.g., One Touch meter by Lifescan, Inc.).*

4. Instruct or assist child in hand-washing using warm water and soap, rinsing and drying thoroughly.

Washing hands in warm, soapy water cleanses the skin and promotes blood flow to puncture site.

5. Position child comfortably in bed or in chair.

Good positioning enhances access to the puncture site and promotes the child's comfort and safety.

6. Select and prepare site, preferably using the sides of the fingertips (see Fig. 120-1).

The sides of the fingertips have a better capillary blood flow and are less sensitive to pain than the palmar surface.

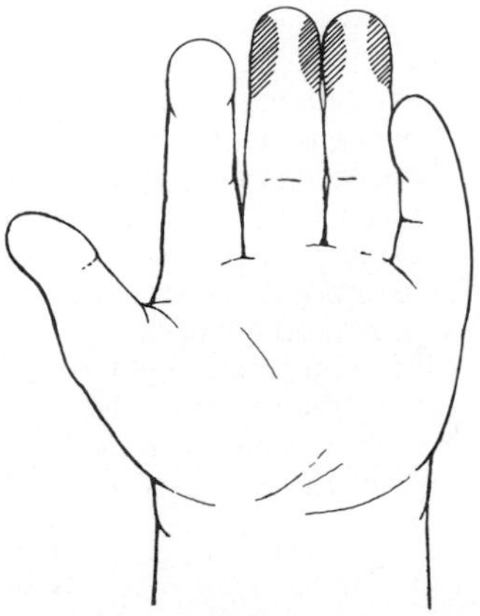

***FIG. 120-1*** Preferable sites for puncture.

| Steps | Rationale |
|---|---|
| a. Instruct child to dangle selected hand at side and "milk" selected finger. | Lowering hand below heart level and milking the finger facilitates blood flow to the site. |
| b. Wipe site with alcohol swab (optional). | ***Special Considerations:*** *The site must be dry before puncture to avoid diluting the blood sample. When alcohol is used to cleanse site, avoid skin contact with reagent test pad since the resulting chemical reaction may cause false readings.* |
| c. Position child's finger firmly in gloved nondominant hand (see Skill 121). | Positioning of site enhances the child's safety and facilitates adequate puncture. |
| 7. Using gloved dominant hand, remove protective cover from sharp end of lancet. If applicable, place automatic lancing device firmly against site. Activate device according to manufacturer's operating instructions. | ***Special Considerations:*** *If using manual method, use the technique described in Skill 121.* |
| 8. Turn puncture site toward floor. Apply moderate and even pressure around the puncture site then release, repeating until a large, hanging drop of blood at least 5 mm in diameter is obtained. | A large hanging droplet of blood ensures coverage of the reagent test pad, without smearing. "Milking" the finger in order to produce an adequate drop of blood does not adversely affect blood sugar results (Davidson, 1986).<br>***Special Considerations:*** *It is unnecessary to remove the first drop of blood for glucose measurement (Davidson 1986).* |
| 9. Holding the reagent strip level, quickly apply the hanging drop of blood to cover the pad of the test strip. | Holding the glucose strip level enhances the proper absorption of the blood by the total surface area of the reagent pad to provide the correct chemical reaction. Smearing an insufficient amount of blood to cover all of the reagent pad invalidates test results. |
| 10. Activate the timer on meters that require a timing process according to manufacturer's instructions. | Proper timing of blood exposure to the reagent pad chemicals is necessary to ensure accurate test results.<br>***Special Considerations:*** *The sequence of activating the timer and placing the hanging drop of blood on the pad varies with the specific meter. Refer to manufacturer's instructions.* |
| 11. If blotting is required for the product being used, place the blood covered reagent strip on a firm, flat, dry surface. | Keeping the reagent strip flat facilitates even dispersal of blood on the reagent pad. A moist surface may contaminate and dilute the blood-covered reagent strip, invalidating the test results. |
| 12. If needed, apply gentle pressure to puncture site with dry cotton ball or clean tissue. | Gentle pressure to bleeding site promotes hemostasis. Children may also become anxious at the sight of their own bleeding and covering the site may reduce their anxiety.<br>***Special Considerations:*** *Do not apply pressure with alcohol wipe because it may produce a stinging sensation.* |
| 13. After the appropriate time has elapsed (when applicable), remove the excess blood from the reagent pads gently and quickly (2 seconds) according to product manual. Repeat this step a second time using a clean area of the blotting material. | Inadequate pressure to blot reagent pads can produce falsely elevated test results and contaminate the meter. Excessive pressure or blotting for too long may produce a falsely low blood glucose reading.<br>***Special Considerations:*** *If blotting causes the reagent pad to split or separate, repeat the procedure with a new strip and a fresh drop of blood from a different site.* |
| 14. Insert and position the reagent strip in the reflectance meter (if applicable) according to manufacturer's directions. | Failure to insert the reagent strip correctly and in a timely manner affects light reflection and invalidates test results. |
| 15. Following completion of the timing cycle, read the blood glucose level on the digital display of the reflectance meter or, if using a color chart, follow directions on the reagent strip bottle for comparison of test pad(s) results with color chart. | The digital reading provides immediate feedback on the glucose level of the capillary blood. |
| 16. After result is noted: | |
| a. Remove the used reagent strip from the meter and discard. | Prompt removal of strip from the meter prevents contamination of the meter. |
| b. Turn off reflectance meter. | Some meters turn off automatically, after a programmed length of time but turning them off manually immediately after use extends the life of the battery. |
| c. Safely and properly discard used supplies. Dispose of lancets into a sharps container. | Safe disposal of used supplies prevents injury and possible spread of microorganisms. |
| d. Clean equipment according to manufacturer's directions. | Clean equipment enhances the accuracy of results and can prolong the life of the equipment. |
| e. Return equipment to its proper storage area. | Proper storage prevents damage and allows easy access for the next use. |

| Steps | Rationale |
|---|---|
| 17. Discuss meaning of test results with child and/or family; encourage their questions. | Responding to questions and sharing information with the child and family reinforces their cooperation, encourages their participation, increases their knowledge, and clarifies existing misconceptions regarding the procedure. |
| 18. Praise child for cooperation and participation. | Positive reinforcement increases the child's self-esteem and encourages future cooperation and participation. |
| 19. Report abnormal findings to physician and/or follow prescribed protocol for abnormal blood glucose levels. | Abnormal blood glucose levels may indicate a need to readjust aspects of the child's diabetic management, or may require immediate intervention (Travis, Brouhard, and Schreiner, 1987). |

| Evaluation Outcomes | Observational Guidelines |
|---|---|
| 1. Accurate blood glucose reading obtained. | Review recorded glucose measurements. Compare present results with child's laboratory glucose level, previously recorded results, present symptomatology, and criteria for acceptable glucose levels. |
| 2. Trauma and infection at the puncture site are prevented or minimized. | Note presence of redness, swelling, bleeding, bruising or tenderness at puncture sites on daily basis. |
| 3. Child's anxiety and discomfort related to procedure is minimal. | Observe child's response to procedure. Note any motor behavior, verbal responses or nonverbal behavior that indicate anxiety or discomfort. Note child's motivation and willingness to cooperate and participate in performing the procedure. |
| 4. Child/family accurately perform blood glucose measurement. | Note any hesitancies or inaccuracies. Observe child and/or family perform a blood glucose measurement. |
| 5. Child/family demonstrate proper care of equipment and supplies. | Observe how child/family handle and care for equipment and supplies. Ask child and/or family to verbalize correct care of equipment and supplies. |

## Documentation

Record date, time, blood glucose results, and any comments about pertinent behaviors influencing the results in child's personal blood glucose log and in the appropriate area of child's medical/nursing record. Record assessment of knowledge and skills regarding blood glucose measurement by fingerstick, type of reagent strip and glucose meter used, factors influencing technique, successes and errors in technique, usual pattern of testing, child's blood glucose level and response to each glucose check, any complications, any abnormal findings, and child/family teaching.

## Child and Family Teaching

1. For the child previously diagnosed with diabetes mellitus experiencing problems with control, an in-depth assessment of the child/family's knowledge and skill regarding blood glucose monitoring is indicated. This information individualizes teaching efforts and enhances effectiveness. Additional initial assessment information to obtain includes understanding of purposes and goals of blood glucose monitoring; level of motivation; factors that may hamper ability such as impaired vision or impaired manual dexterity; method of testing and recording results, testing schedule practices, and if testing is initiated in response to signs and symptoms of hypoglycemia/hyperglycemia; and demonstration of proper use and care of equipment and supplies.
2. Observe the child/family's technique in performing blood glucose monitoring. Observation allows further assessment and provides an opportune time for teaching. Note strengths and weaknesses in technique to allow an encouraging approach.
3. Discuss the child/family's protocol for responding to abnormal glucose levels, including criteria for repeating the glucose checks, criteria for contacting the physician; guidelines for adjusting insulin in response to exercise or illness; and nutritional management (Travis, Brouhard, and Schreiner, 1987). Emphasize that serious complications and hospitalization may be prevented or minimized if prompt action according to established guidelines is taken in response to abnormal glucose levels.

# SKILL 121 Obtaining Capillary Blood

*Dora Bradley*

Capillary blood collection is performed to obtain blood for a requested laboratory analysis. This method is preferred over venipuncture if the capillary blood is suitable for the desired test. It is considered less painful, traumatic, and invasive, and requires less blood than venipuncture.

## NURSING DIAGNOSES

Anxiety related to unmet informational needs about purpose and procedure for capillary blood collection; Pain related to skin puncture by lancet.

| Steps | Rationale |
|---|---|
| **Assessment** | |
| 1. Review physician's order and laboratory requirements before the procedure for: a. Type of test(s). b. Amount of blood needed. c. Specimen containers needed. d. Special timing requirements. e. Special measures to be taken, e.g., NPO, medication administration. | Reviewing orders ensures that the specimen meets requirements for obtaining accurate results. ***Special Considerations:*** *Amounts of blood needed for analysis may differ with age of child, actual test, and the kind of testing instrumentation used by the laboratory. For drug levels, start timing for IV drugs after the infusion is completed. Timing for peaks and troughs differs for each drug. If special timing is not requested, draw all required tests at the same time to decrease the number of punctures. In a neonate or infant, or any time that blood volume may be an issue, specimen collection may be done at intervals.* |
| 2. Assess for risk factors and contraindications: | Assessment of these factors assists collecting the specimen accurately with minimal trauma. |
| a. Physical status. | Capillary blood collection is contraindicated in the infant in shock or one with severe polycythemia. |
| b. Bleeding disorders, low platelet count, anticoagulant therapy. | Abnormal clotting mechanisms increase the child's risk for developing local ecchymosis and bleeding. |
| c. Allergy to iodine preparations. | Because iodine solutions are often used to cleanse the skin before puncture, identification of an allergy avoids a possible reaction. |
| 3. Determine potential puncture sites based on: a. Age. | Age determines potential puncture sites. ***Special Considerations:*** *The heel is usually used for infants. Fingertips or earlobes may be used in older children.* |
| b. Frequency of punctures. | If punctures are being performed frequently or on a regular basis, sites should be rotated. ***Special Considerations:*** *Assess previous sites for infection.* |
| c. Condition of potential sites. | Avoiding areas with compromised blood flow, local edema, local infection, ecchymosis, or open lesions prevents further trauma and promotes accurate results. |
| 4. Determine the child's and family's understanding of the procedure's method and purpose. Ask if the family desires to be present during procedures (see Skill 1). | Assessing the child's and family's understanding of the procedure is essential in maintaining communication and promoting cooperation. It also allows child and family an opportunity to ask questions. Family presence during procedures can be a support to the child. ***Special Considerations:*** *Be aware of the child's reaction to blood leaving the body and address these reactions according to the developmental level.* |
| **Planning and Goal Setting** | |
| 1. Assemble all equipment and supplies: | Assembling the appropriate equipment assists in performing the procedure efficiently, allowing more time to support the child. |
| a. Disposable lancets or microlancets: For infants, do not use lancets longer than 2.5 mm. Longer lancets may be used for older children. Visually examine lancet tip to make certain it is not dull or barbed. | Necrotizing osteochondritis from lancet penetration of the underlying calcaneus bone is the most serious complication of infant heel puncture and can be avoided by puncturing less than 2.4 mm and at the outer aspect of heel (Blumefeld, Turi, and Blanc, 1979). |

| Steps | Rationale |
|---|---|
| b. Alcohol or povidone-iodine swabs or other antibacterial solution at room temperature. | Antiseptic solutions reduce the introduction of microorganisms into the blood when the lancet punctures the skin. Cold solutions may cause vasoconstriction in the puncture site, making blood collection more difficult. **Special Considerations:** *Use preparations other than an iodophor solution to cleanse when an iodine allergy or sensitivity is suspected or known. Alcohol and povidone-iodine are used with caution, and the skin is rinsed after use in preterm infants (Kuller, Lund, and Tobin, 1983). These solutions may cause severe irritation in very low birth-weight infants.* |
| c. Appropriate specimen containers, including correct identification labels. | **Special Considerations:** *Heparinized capillary tubes are needed if capillary blood gases are being collected.* |
| d. Small specimen bag. | |
| e. Completed laboratory requisition. | |
| f. Sterile 2 × 2 inch gauze pads. | |
| g. Gloves. | |
| h. Chemical compress or warm cloth compress. | Compresses are used to dilate the blood vessels to the puncture site, most commonly for heel sticks. |
| i. Any other items necessary for specific laboratory tests, e.g., ice. | Chilling of the specimen is sometimes required to slow down the metabolic activity that may alter test results. Capillary blood gases are the most common example of this. |
| j. Linen protector. | |
| 2. Consider potential sites and select most suitable. | These sites are highly vascularized yet have fewer nerve endings and thus provide the best sites for capillary blood collection. |
| a. Plantar surface of heel, avoiding the anteromedial surface (Fig. 121-1). | The anteromedial surface of the heel is avoided because fibrosis and scarring in the area of calcaneus nerve can occur, causing pain when the child begins to walk (Whaley and Wong, 1991). **Special Considerations:** *The heel is the site of choice for infants, especially premature infants. Heel sticks should not be done once a child is walking since calluses on the heel make puncture more difficult and an infection may develop once the infant begins to walk on the punctured foot (Hazinski, 1984). Frequent heel punctures have also been linked with plantar wart development at a later age (Whaley and Wong, 1991).* |

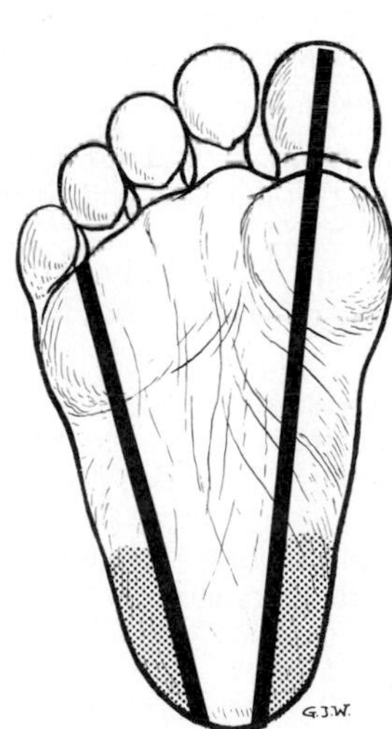

***FIG. 121-1*** Puncture sites on sole of infant's foot.

From Whaley LF and Wong DL: Nursing care of infants and children, ed 4, St Louis, 1991, The CV Mosby Co.

| Steps | Rationale |
|---|---|
| b. Finger; middle or ring finger preferred. | The index finger is used for more activities and avoiding a puncture to this finger can prevent future discomfort. **Special Considerations:** *Fingers are preferred sites for children over 2 years old.* |
| c. Inferior edge of the earlobe. | The ear lobe is less sensitive to pain and the skin is thin. **Special Considerations:** *It may be difficult to control bleeding from the earlobe, if the child has a hemorrhagic disease. Hemoglobin levels may be slightly higher from earlobe blood and leukocyte counts are less reliable (Hughes and Buescher, 1980).* |
| d. Great toe. | The medial aspect near the tip of the toe can be used for capillary blood collections (Hughes and Buescher, 1980; Nurse's Reference Library, 1981; Hazinski, 1984). **Special Considerations:** *The other toes are less suitable for capillary blood collection.* |

| Steps | Rationale |
|---|---|
| 3. Determine a suitable place to perform the procedure, preferably not the child's bed. | Maintaining the child's room as a safe place reduces anxiety and fear that may lead to sleeping difficulties. |
| 4. Recruit an assistant if necessary. | Stability of the site is necessary to control puncture depth, and facilitate collecting the blood in appropriate containers. |
| 5. Develop individualized goals of nursing care:<br>▪ Obtain an adequate specimen of capillary blood meeting requirements for accurate analysis.<br>▪ Minimize trauma, discomfort and complications at the puncture site.<br>▪ Minimize child's and family's anxiety. | |

## Implementation

| Steps | Rationale |
|---|---|
| 1. Prepare child for procedure (see Skill 1). | |
| 2. Apply warm compress to selected site.<br>a. Moist heat or special heel warming products (chemical compresses).<br>b. Temperature between 37° and 40° C.<br>c. 5 to 10 minutes duration (Whaley and Wong, 1991). | Warming of the puncture site produces vasodilatation and increases the blood flow to the site, making blood collection easier. It also causes greater mixing of arterial and venous blood, which makes the results more useful. Compress temperature greater than 40° C may cause burns, especially in neonates and premature infants because of fragile skin.<br>***Special Considerations:*** *Site will appear "flushed" when ready for capillary puncture. Do not use dry heat. Use warm tap water for cloth compresses. An infant with poor circulation may require the compress for a greater duration. If circulation is poor, the skin is also more susceptible to burn. Wrapping a clean disposable diaper around the compress helps to avoid rapid evaporation and cooling of the compress, which could cause vasoconstriction.* |
| 3. Protect linen from blood contamination. | Soiled linens are distressing to some children and require the additional work of a linen change. Linens with blood also increase the risk of blood-borne disease transmission.<br>***Special Considerations:*** *The disposable diaper used to hold the compress in place makes a suitable linen protector.* |
| 4. Cleanse the puncture site with antiseptic solution in a circular motion from the site outward. Allow skin to air dry or wipe dry with sterile gauze. | Cleansing the site reduces risk of infection. Puncturing through a wet film of antiseptic may produce hemolysis and prevent formation of a rounded "bead," making collection difficult.<br>***Special Considerations:*** *Avoid waving hand or blowing on site to enhance drying process because this may introduce airborne organisms.* |
| 5. Using nondominant hand, hold the extremity firmly and stabilize the puncture site, pulling the skin taut. | Firmly positioning the extremity helps ensure the safety of the child, and facilitates adequate puncture of the site and acquisition of the needed blood specimen. Taut skin provides a flat surface for puncture. |
| a. Foot (Fig. 121-2):<br>▪ Grasp heel of infant with the second and third fingers behind the ankle.<br>▪ Place thumb over the arch of the foot.<br>▪ Support the top of the foot with the fourth and fifth fingers (Alstrom et al, 1987).<br>b. Finger, small child (Fig. 121-3):<br>▪ Cup dorsal surface of child's hand in palm, curling child's fingers inward.<br>▪ Place own index finger over bent fingers.<br>▪ Separate selected finger, place it over index finger; secure by placing thumb on top and middle finger behind.<br>c. Finger, older child (Fig. 121-4):<br>▪ Select either the child's third or fourth finger turning child's hand palm side up.<br>▪ Place index and middle finger on the nail side of child's finger.<br>▪ Place thumb on child's finger above potential puncture site.<br>d. Earlobe:<br>▪ Hold earlobe securely between index finger and thumb. | Holding the foot properly facilitates an adequate puncture to the heel without injury to the underlying calcaneus. |

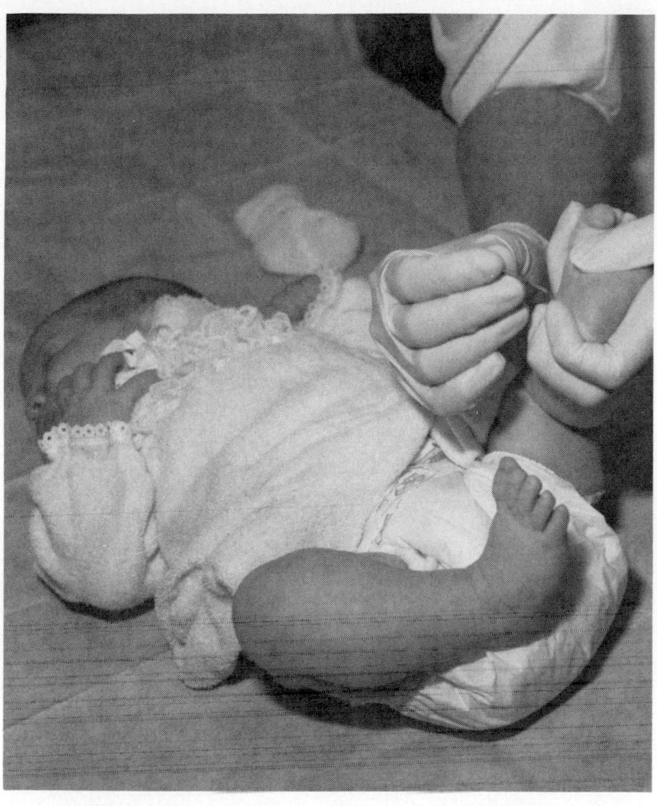

***FIG. 121-2*** Proper restraint of the foot facilitates adequate puncture.

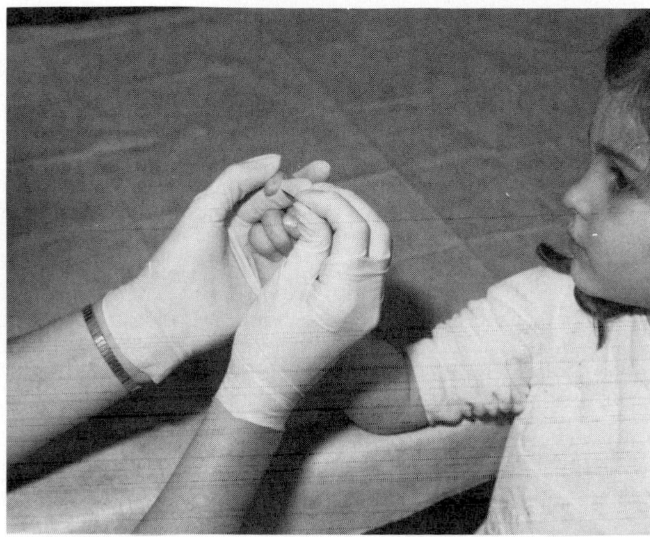

***FIG. 121-3*** Finger of small child is secured for collection of capillary blood.

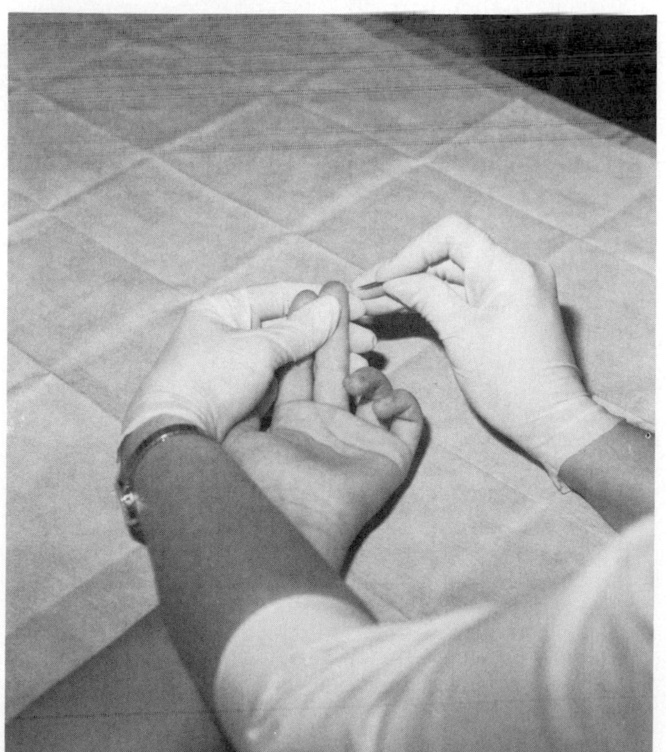

***FIG. 121-4*** For older child, hand is turned palm-side up.

| Steps | Rationale |
|---|---|
| e. Great toe:<br>▪ Use thumb and index finger to grasp toe at the distal toe joint. | |
| 6. Inform the child when the puncture is to occur, but avoid "planting" the idea of pain (Whaley and Wong, 1991) (see Skill 52). | Informing the child enhances his or her sense of control and allows preparation for discomfort. Avoiding planting the idea of pain allows for variation in sensory perception and also contributes to child's control in describing reactions (Whaley and Wong, 1991). |
| 7. Grasping lancet firmly with dominant hand, puncture skin with one continuous motion perpendicular to the skin. | A firm, continuous motion ensures an adequate puncture.<br>***Special Considerations:*** *Insufficient depth of the incision is a common source of error. Do not use round puncture instruments such as a hypodermic needle or autolet lancet as these will not produce a free flow of blood. Depth of incision may be more difficult to control if a scalpel blade is used.* |
| a. Heel:<br>▪ Puncture the skin at the outer aspects of the heel (see Fig. 121-1).<br>b. Finger, small child:<br>▪ Make puncture 3 mm from the nail bed.<br>▪ Apply pressure with the thumb and index finger.<br>▪ Bend fingers so puncture site is the lowest point of the finger (Alstrom, et al, 1987).<br>c. Finger, older child:<br>▪ Puncture approximately 3 mm from the nail bed (Alstrom et al, 1987) (see Fig. 121-4).<br>d. Earlobe:<br>▪ Puncture the edge approximately 10 to 15 mm from cheek.<br>▪ Apply slight pressure with the thumb and index finger.<br>e. Great toe:<br>▪ Puncture medial aspect near tip of toe.<br>▪ Make incision in a horizontal angle across the footprint pattern. | |
| 8. Wipe the first drop of blood away with sterile gauze pad. | First drop of blood may contain interstitial fluid, which can dilute specimen and cause false results. |
| 9. Apply moderate and even pressure around the puncture site then release, repeating until specimen is obtained. | Intermittent pressure assists with the capillary blood flow.<br>***Special Considerations:*** *Avoid massaging or "milking" the extremity because this causes venous congestion (Alstrom et al, 1987; Meites and Monte, 1979).* |
| 10. Reassure child about any concerns he or she may have while collecting specimen, e.g., being "drained" of blood. | Reassurance prevents the child from developing additional fears or anxieties.<br>***Special Considerations:*** *While collecting specimen, make simple comments, e.g., "You're really making lots of nice red blood" to reassure child that blood is continually being produced and replaced by the body (Whaley and Wong, 1991).* |
| 11. When an adequate volume of blood appears, fill the blood specimen container to the appropriate level and seal. | |
| a. Microtainer tube—hold tube at angle below horizontal, touching the tip to underside of drop. | This position allows blood to flow freely through top and down the tube wall. |
| b. Capillary tube—introduce tip of tube in the droplet. | Blood flows freely into tube as a result of capillary action.<br>***Special Considerations:*** *Avoid "scraping" blood sample off skin. This may bruise the child and cause hemolysis of the blood cells. If volume of blood is not adequate, it may be necessary to make another incision or select another site.* |
| 12. Gently agitate tubes with additives by rotating back and forth 8 to 10 times or gently inverting several times. *Do not* shake the tubes. Place in ice if appropriate (Perry and Potter, 1990; Nurse's Reference Library, 1981). | Rotating or inverting tubes ensures complete mixing of the additive with the blood and prevents coagulation. Shaking can result in hemolysis of red blood cells, thus altering accuracy of results. |
| 13. Upon completion, apply pressure at the puncture site with a dry sterile pad until the bleeding stops. | Applying pressure promotes hemostasis.<br>***Special Considerations:*** *The use of adhesive bandages has been discouraged for infants/toddlers because of a potential for aspiration. A dry sterile pad is preferred. If the older child requests an adhesive bandage, one may be used. If ecchymosis occurs, warm compresses increase circulation, aid removal of extravasated blood, and decrease pain (Whaley and Wong, 1991).* |

| Steps | Rationale |
|---|---|
| 14. Comfort the child, if necessary, and praise cooperation. | |
| 15. Label blood specimen with proper identifying information and transport to laboratory with correct requisition as soon as possible. | Proper identification prevents redraws, erroneous results, and/or diagnostic and therapeutic errors. Inaccurate results may occur if the blood is left in tubes for extended periods. |

| Evaluation Outcomes | Observational Guidelines |
|---|---|
| 1. An adequate amount of capillary blood is properly obtained. | Check tests results, particularly noting incomplete or hemolyzed results. |
| 2. Complications of puncture are prevented or minimized. | Observe puncture site for bleeding or ecchymosis following puncture. Reinspect puncture site at intervals for signs of infection: redness, warmth, swelling, drainage. |
| 3. Discomfort and anxiety for the child as a result of the procedure is prevented or minimized. | Observe child's behavioral and verbal responses during the procedure. Note the amount of effort required to comfort after the procedure. |

## Documentation

Record name of test drawn; date and time draw occurred; site used for puncture and observation of site post-procedure. Note the amount of blood collected and any special occurrences, e.g., multiple stick, traumatic puncture. Document child's reaction to the procedure and reporting of results to physician, especially "stat" or abnormal results.

# SKILL 122 Performing a Venipuncture

*Kelly McCampbell*

Venipuncture is performed to obtain blood for laboratory tests that reveal information about the child's condition or allow proper treatment. This procedure can be very traumatic for the child because the need for venipuncture is not fully understood by the child and the fear of pain is strong. Every effort should be made to decrease the number of venipunctures necessary.

## NURSING DIAGNOSES

Anxiety related to unmet informational needs about purpose and procedure for venipuncture blood collection; Pain related to insertion of venipuncture needle; Potential for injury related to hemorrhage at puncture site, nerve injury, infection or thrombosis.

| Steps | Rationale |
|---|---|
| **Assessment** | |
| 1. Review medical record and laboratory requirements to determine:<br>a. Type of test(s).<br>b. Amount of blood needed.<br>c. Prerequisite conditions or specific timing.<br>d. Diet and medical history. | The type of test to be performed determines the selection of collection tubes and supplies, e.g., ice. Certain diagnostic tests require preliminary conditions for obtaining accurate results. Numerous drugs and their metabolites affect test results by pharmacologic or chemical interference (Nurse's Reference Library, 1981). Blood loss from numerous samplings can significantly reduce total circulating blood volume. Therefore minimum amounts necessary to perform tests should be obtained.<br>***Special Considerations:*** *Blood loss should be replaced once it totals 5% to 7% of the child's circulatory volume (Hazinski, 1984). Fasting blood sugar and drug peak and trough are examples of tests requiring specific conditions and timing. An example of chemical interference may be seen when high dosages of ascorbic acid cause elevations in blood sugar.* |

| Steps | Rationale |
|---|---|
| 2. Assess factors that may influence site selection and planning: | Assessing these factors can assist in a positive outcome to the procedure. |
| a. Child's age and size. | Needle selection will depend on the size of the child. The child's age will influence his or her ability to cooperate with the procedure. |
| b. Visibility and palpability of vein (see Fig. 97-1): | Visible and palpable veins are easier to access. |
| ▪ Antecubital fossa and dorsum of hand veins are easily visualized and palpated in the older child. | The most common sites of venipuncture are the veins of the extremities, especially the arm and hand (Whaley and Wong, 1989). **Special Considerations:** *Use of the lateral cephalic vein is preferred in the antecubital fossa. Using the median cubital vein increases the risk of hematomas, creating an arteriovenous fistula, and injury to the median nerve (Dunn, 1987).* |
| ▪ Saphenous and marginal veins in the foot and leg, and scalp veins. | These veins can be used in infants as they may be easily located. However, foot and leg veins have a greater risk of infection or thrombosis (Millam, 1985). |
| ▪ Femoral and external jugular veins. | These large veins are used occasionally when unable to access other veins or large amounts of blood are needed. **Special Considerations:** *Venipuncture in these veins is sometimes restricted to physician/practitioner. Refer to institutional policy.* |
| c. Condition and location of veins: | |
| ▪ Extremity with an infusing IV. | Avoid using a vein near an IV infusion as the sample may be diluted or contain concentrations of IV fluids (Perry and Potter, 1990). **Special Considerations:** *If no alternative site is available, apply the tourniquet below the IV site and use a vein other than the one with the IV.* |
| ▪ Scar tissue. | Vein entry may be more difficult through extensive scar tissue. |
| ▪ Hematoma at potential site. | A hematoma indicates existing injury to a vessel's wall (Perry and Potter, 1990). This may alter the ability to obtain an accurate sample from the vessel. |
| d. Child's preference for site. | Allowing the older child the option of selecting the site enhances his or her sense of control and, thus cooperation. |
| e. Allergy to iodine preparations. | Iodine preparations that are often used to cleanse the skin may need to be avoided if allergy or sensitivity exists. |
| 3. Assess child for any possible risks for venipuncture: a. Bleeding disorders. b. Anticoagulant therapy. c. Decreased platelet count. | Presence of abnormal clotting abilities increases the risks of bleeding or hematoma formation. Minimizing number of venipunctures, using a phlebotomist with high level skill, and applying pressure at the site for longer periods become essential precautions. |
| 4. Determine the child/family's understanding of the procedure's method and purpose. Ask the family's preference for presence during procedure. | Assessment of this data influences the teaching preparation and emotional support needed. **Special Considerations:** *Past experiences with venipuncture may increase the child/family's anxiety. Children, even older ones and especially those whose condition warrants frequent blood draws, may fear the loss of their blood. Not understanding hemopoiesis, they mistakenly believe that withdrawing blood is life-threatening (Whaley and Wong, 1989). A family's response to the prospect of venipuncture may also be influenced by culturally determined health beliefs (see Skill 41).* |
| 5. Determine the child's ability to cooperate with procedure and the possible need for restraint and assistants. | Infants and small children who are unable to cooperate require proper positioning and restraining to minimize movement and ensure safety (Whaley and Wong, 1989). |

## Planning and Goal Setting

| Steps | Rationale |
|---|---|
| 1. Gather supplies: | Collecting supplies improves efficiency and minimizes the overall procedure time. |
| a. Tourniquet—select one of the following: ▪ Flexible rubber tubing. ▪ ⅜-inch penrose drain. ▪ Flat rubber velcro tourniquet. ▪ Small rubber band. ▪ Sphygmomanometer cuff. | The tourniquet impedes venous flow, resulting in venous distension without occluding arterial flow. **Special Considerations:** *When using a sphymomanometer cuff, inflate it to just above systolic blood pressure, maintain for 30 to 60 seconds, and then deflate the cuff to just above the diastolic blood pressure. To ensure that arterial flow is not interrupted, check for capillary blanching distal to the tourniquet.* |

| Steps | Rationale |
|---|---|
| b. Antibacterial cleansing solution at room temperature—select one of the following:<br>▪ Povidone-iodine.<br>▪ Tincture of iodine.<br>▪ Alcohol.<br>▪ Chlorhexidine gluconate (HIBICLENS). | Antibacterial cleansing prevents the introduction of bacteria into the blood when the needle pierces the skin. Cold solution may cause vasoconstriction.<br>***Special Considerations:*** *Select alternative antibacterial solution if the child is allergic to iodine preparations. Alcohol and povidone-iodine are used with caution, and the skin is rinsed after use in preterm infants (Kuller, Lund, and Tobin, 1983). These solutions may cause severe irritation in very low birth weight infants.* |
| c. Cotton ball or dry gauze. | These are used to apply pressure to the puncture site until the bleeding stops and prevent stinging caused by applying an antiseptic swab to a puncture site. |
| d. Adhesive bandage strips (optional). | The adhesive strip can be applied to the site after applying pressure.<br>***Special Considerations:*** *Adhesive strips reassure some children that their vital fluids will not leak out through the puncture site (Whaley and Wong, 1989). However, others are strongly opposed to the application of an adhesive strip. If possible, allow the child to choose. "Spot" Band-Aids pose an aspiration risk to young children (Pediatric Alert, 1987).* |
| e. Appropriate blood specimen containers, including correct identification labels. | Using the appropriate containers ensures proper testing of the specimen, thus enhancing accuracy of the results and reducing risk of redraw. |
| f. Completed laboratory requisition. | Completing the requisition facilitates delivery of the specimen to the laboratory. |
| g. Linen protector (towel, blue pad, etc.). | Protecting the linens facilitates clean-up. |
| h. Gloves. | Wearing gloves conforms with 1987 Centers for Disease Control guidelines if contact with blood is anticipated. |
| i. Any other test specific items, e.g., ice. | Chilling the specimen is sometimes required to slow metabolic activity that may alter test results.<br>***Special Considerations:*** *Proper chilling of a specimen requires the use of chipped ice or ice and water in a plastic bag or container. Large cubes of ice do not allow adequate contact between specimen and coolant to be effective.* |
| j. Syringe technique: | |
| ▪ Sterile needle, preferably butterfly or scalp-vein—23 to 25 gauge (infants and small children). | Smaller bore needles reduce trauma to vein wall (Perry and Potter, 1990). However, large bore needles reduce the risk of specimen hemolysis (National Committee for Clinical Standards, 1982). The lumen should be large enough to allow free flow of blood. The butterfly needle is often preferred because it is easier to manipulate than other catheters or needles.<br>***Special Considerations:*** *Check the patency of the needle by injecting air before the venipuncture. A wet needle or syringe may increase hemolysis of the specimen.* |
| ▪ Disposable syringes—3 ml greater than volume needed. Attach syringe to end of butterfly tubing. | The syringe is used to withdraw the specimen.<br>***Special Considerations:*** *Using smaller syringes affords better control and reduces likelihood of collapsing the vein from excessive negative pressure.* |
| ▪ Large bore transfer needles, e.g., 18 gauge. | The transfer needle is used to transfer the blood from the syringe to the collection tube. A large bore reduces hemolysis of the specimen. |
| k. Vacutainer technique:<br>▪ Evacuated (Vacutainer) tubes.<br>▪ Vacutainer needle holder. | |
| ▪ Vacutainer sterile, double-ended needles (23 to 25 gauge for infants and smaller children, 20 to 21 gauge for older children and adolescents). | Double-ended needles allow several tubes to be attached in quick succession. |
| 2. Determine a suitable location to perform the venipuncture with adequate lighting, preferably not in child's bed. | Maintaining the child's room as a safe place reduces anxiety and fear that may lead to sleeping difficulties. |
| 3. Find an assistant other than a family member if the child needs to be restrained. | Family should not be asked to help hold a child for a painful procedure because it may elicit guilt feelings and may interfere with the ability to maintain trust of the child. At least one other person is needed to help restrain the child. |

| Steps | Rationale |
|---|---|
| 4. Develop individualized goals of nursing care:<br>▪ Obtain an adequate blood specimen under required conditions for accurate analysis.<br>▪ Minimize discomfort, trauma and risk of infection at venipuncture site.<br>▪ Minimize the child's and family's anxiety. | |

## Implementation

| Steps | Rationale |
|---|---|
| 1. Prepare the child for the procedure (see Skill 1). | ***Special Considerations:*** *Explaining to the child that blood is continually being produced may reduce anxiety about blood loss being life threatening.* |
| 2. Position the child and restrain site as necessary (see Skill 51 and Fig. 51-1). | Improper restraints and positioning can result in unsuccessful or repeated attempts.<br>***Special Considerations:*** *A papoose board may be used for infants and younger children. A supine position is preferred, but the older, cooperative child may choose a comfortable position.* |
| 3. Place tourniquet or sphygmomanometer cuff approximately 2 to 4 inches above the selected site for a duration of no longer than 1 to 2 minutes. If veins appear to be large, distended, and highly visible, omit the use of the tourniquet. | The tourniquet or cuff impedes venous flow to the heart, causing veins to dilate. Prolonged application may alter test results, cause pain, and result in venous stasis (Perry and Potter, 1990). Using a tourniquet on large, distended veins increases the risk of hematoma.<br>***Special Considerations:*** *Serum potassium levels may be falsely elevated by prolonged tourniquet use. Avoid the use of a tourniquet when drawing a specimen for ammonia and lactic acid because tourniquet trauma can cause an elevation in these levels (Hughes and Buescher, 1980).* |
| 4. Base final site selection on assessment factors. Employ additional techniques to facilitate vein location, if necessary: | |
| a. Gravity. | Holding the limb dependent and below the horizontal level of the body induces vein distension. |
| b. Warm compresses for 10 to 15 minutes. | Applying warm compresses increases local vasodilation.<br>***Special Considerations:*** *Ensure that tourniquet is released during this time.* |
| c. Gentle rapping or "flicking" veins with fingertips. | Rapping or flicking promotes vasodilation.<br>***Special Considerations:*** *This technique is contraindicated with ammonia levels, lactic acid, or anticoagulation studies because it may alter the results (Hughes and Buescher, 1980).* |
| d. Alcohol swabbing. | The sheen from the wet alcohol may make the veins more visible. |
| 5. Palpate selected vein with index finger, noting firmness, elasticity, and absence of pulsation. Remove tourniquet when selection is complete. | Healthy and patent veins are elastic and rebound on palpation (Perry and Potter, 1990). Pulsation indicates arterial rather than venous flow.<br>***Special Considerations:*** *Arteries may be superficial in neonates, therefore careful palpation is necessary to avoid inadvertent arterial puncture.* |
| 6. Arrange linen protectors under selected site. | This lessens the chance of soiling the linens.<br>***Special Considerations:*** *Soiled linens are distressing and create a necessity for a linen change after the procedure. Also, soiled linens increase the risk of transmission of blood-borne diseases.* |
| 7. Cleanse the skin with antiseptic solution in a circular motion outward for approximately 5 cm (2 inches). Allow to air dry at least 2 minutes. | Allowing the skin to air dry increases the solution's bacteriocidal action and also decreases the "sting" when needle is inserted.<br>***Special Considerations:*** *Do not wave hand or blow over cleansed site because airborne organisms may be introduced. Avoid shaving a site on the scalp since microabrasions caused by shaving can be potential sites for infection.* |
| 8. Reapply tourniquet. | Release of tourniquet during cleansing allows normal venous flow. Reapplication to again produce venous distension is necessary for successful venipuncture. |
| 9. Hold needle in dominant hand with protective needle sheath removed. | Use of the dominant hand provides better control for the venipuncture. |

| Steps | Rationale |
|---|---|
| 10. Stabilize the vein. Place thumb of nondominant hand 1 inch below the site and draw skin taut or place thumb and first finger on opposite sides of vein and draw skin taut. | Stabilizing the vein prevents movement during venipuncture. |
| 11. Inform child when skin puncture will occur, but avoid "planting" idea of pain (Whaley and Wong, 1989) (see Skill 52). | Informing the child enhances the sense of control and allows child to prepare for discomfort. Avoiding planting the idea of pain allows variation in sensory perception and contributes to child's control in describing reactions (Whaley and Wong, 1989). |
| 12. Holding bevel up, insert needle about ½ inch below selected site at a 30° angle from the skin. | The lower angle reduces the risk of penetrating both walls of the vein. Bevel up position reduces vein trauma (Perry and Potter, 1990).<br>***Special Considerations:*** *If the vein is large, enter directly with one quick, steady motion. If the vein is small, enter skin lateral to the vein first.* |
| 13. Once the skin is penetrated, decrease the angle of the needle so that it is almost flush but not touching the skin. | Positioning the needle more parallel to the vein reduces the risk of puncturing the distal wall of the vein. Also, if the needle slides along the skin, organisms may be introduced. |
| 14. Gently advance the needle into the vein until a blood return is noted. | A blood return indicates presence in the vein.<br>***Special Considerations:*** *A "pop" may be felt as the needle enters the vein (Perry and Potter, 1990). No more than two unsuccessful attempts at venipuncture should be made by any one person (policy may vary according to the institution).* |
| 15. Withdraw appropriate amount of blood:<br>*Vacutainer technique:* | |
| a. Grasping the vacutainer firmly, advance the specimen tube stopper onto the needle without further advancing the needle in the vein. | By advancing the needle into the stopper, the tube's vacuum is broken, causing blood to flow rapidly into the tube. Further advancing the needle into the vein risks distal vein wall penetration.<br>***Special Considerations:*** *Vacutainer tubes have a premeasured amount of additive for a specific amount of blood. Allow the tube to fill only as much as the vacuum pulls in. To maintain the vacuum in the tube, do not advance it onto the vacutainer needle until the bevel of the needle is under the skin.* |
| b. Once tube is filled, firmly grasp the vacutainer, remove tube, and insert additional tubes as needed. | Adhering to the correct "order of draw" is necessary to avoid cross-contamination of specimens and invalidation of results (Table 122-1).<br>***Special Considerations:*** *Coagulation testing is never performed on the first tube of blood collected because tissue thromboplastin can contaminate the initial venipuncture and invalidate the results. When a citrate tube is the only test ordered, use the "two-tube technique" by filling a nonadditive tube first (Calam and Cooper, 1982).* |

***TABLE 122-1*** "Order of Draw" for Collecting Blood Specimens into Tubes

| Tube | Color-Top | Test Type | Additives | Function | Agitate |
|---|---|---|---|---|---|
| 1 | 2 bottles of solution | Blood culture | Nutrients | Promote growth of bacteria | Yes |
| 2 | Red | Serum studies (e.g., SMA, SMAC) | None | Not applicable | No |
| 3 | Blue | Coagulation studies (e.g., prothrombin time) | Trisodium citrate | Prevent clotting | Yes |
| 4 | Green | Plasma studies (e.g., chromosomal analysis) | Heparin (sodium, lithium, or ammonium) | Prevent clotting | Yes |
| 5 | Purple/ Lavender | Whole blood studies (e.g., Hct, Hgb, platelet count) | EDTA-K3 | Prevent clotting | Yes |
| 6 | Gray | Glucose determinations in serum or plasma (e.g., fasting blood sugar) | Glycolitic inhibitor (e.g., sodium fluoride, powdered oxalate) | Anti-glycolitic | No |

Adapted from Calam R and Cooper M: Recommended "order of draw" for collecting blood specimens in additive-containing tubes, Clin Chem 18(6):1399, 1982.

| Steps | Rationale |
|---|---|
| *Syringe technique:* | |
| a. Gently aspirate with the attached syringe to obtain the needed amount of blood. | Aspiration creates the vacuum needed to withdraw blood. Too forceful aspiration can cause vasospasm, vein collapse, attachment of vein wall to needle and/or hemolyze the specimen. ***Special Considerations:*** *If blood flow is slow or stops, release of pressure may allow flow to return.* |
| b. Keep needle stabilized while withdrawing blood. | Needle movement may cause dislodgement or discomfort. ***Special Considerations:*** *When drawing multiple samples, release the tourniquet 1 minute after beginning blood draw to prevent hemoconcentration of samples (Nurse's Reference Library, 1981).* |
| 16. Discontinue venipuncture. | |
| a. If using syringe technique, release suction on plunger. | Releasing the suction prevents sudden inflow of air into the syringe when the needle is removed. |
| b. Release tourniquet if still applied. | Releasing the tourniquet reduces vein engorgement and thus reduces bleeding at site when needle is removed. |
| c. Holding cottonballs or gauze gently at site, quickly withdraw needle from vein. | Applying pressure while the needle is still in place may produce discomfort. |
| d. Immediately apply firm pressure to site until bleeding has stopped. | Pressure stops the bleeding at the puncture site and reduces the risk of hematoma formation. ***Special Considerations:*** *When using the antecubital site, flexing the arm with the cotton ball in place has been shown to cause more bruising than direct pressure over the site (Dyson and Bogod, 1987).* |
| 17. Allow family member to comfort and hold child and/or praise child for efforts. | ***Special Considerations:*** *A simple comment such as, "You really make lots of nice red blood" reassures the child that blood is continually being produced by the body (Whaley and Wong, 1989).* |
| 18. If using syringe technique, immediately transfer blood to the appropriate specimen containers using large bore needles to pierce vacuum tubes or remove stoppers of tubes and gently expel blood down sides of tube. Do not force blood into tubes. Reapply stoppers. Adhere to the "order of draw" sequence (see Table 122-1). | Transferring the blood in this manner reduces the incidence of foaming and hemolysis of red blood cells. ***Special Considerations:*** *When using evacuated tubes, it is best to allow the vacuum in the tube to withdraw the correct amount of blood since injecting can result in under or overfilling, foaming, and possible hemolysis.* |
| 19. Gently agitate tubes with additives by rotating back and forth 8 to 10 times or gently inverting several times. *Do not* shake the tube (Perry and Potter, 1990; Nurse's Reference Library, 1981). | Rotating or inverting tubes ensures complete mixing of the additive with the blood and prevents coagulation. Shaking can result in hemolysis of red blood cells, thus altering accuracy of results. |
| 20. Inspect venipuncture site to ensure that all bleeding has stopped. | Prolonged bleeding may indicate a problem with the child's clotting ability. Additional pressure may be needed. |
| 21. Apply adhesive strip or tape over cotton ball. | Applying an adhesive strip or tape creates pressure on the puncture site, reducing blood oozing and preventing infection by keeping the site clean. ***Special Considerations:*** *Infants can take adhesive strips off and swallow or aspirate them. Care should be taken to prevent such an occurrence (Pediatric Alert, 1987).* |
| 22. Properly label and transport all specimens to laboratory as soon as possible with completed requisition. | Inaccurate results may occur if the blood is left in the tubes for an extended period of time. Improperly labeled specimens can result in a blood redraw, or diagnostic and therapeutic errors. |

| Evaluation Outcomes | Observational Guidelines |
|---|---|
| 1. An adequate amount of venous blood is properly obtained. | Review laboratory reports for results, especially noting incomplete or hemolyzed results. |
| 2. Complications of venipuncture are prevented or minimized. | Inspect venipuncture site for redness, swelling, drainage, warmth, bleeding, and/or hematoma formation. |
| 3. Discomfort and anxiety to the child as a result of the procedure is prevented or minimized. | Note child's behavior, verbalized comments during procedure, and amount of time and degree of difficulty in comforting the child afterward. |

### Documentation

Record type of specimen(s) collected, date and time of specimen(s) collection, and equipment used, e.g., type and size of needle. Note amount of blood collected, site used for venipuncture, and observation of site after procedure. Document difficulty of procedure, e.g., multiple sticks required, traumatic puncture resulting in hematoma, and indicate child's reaction to the procedure. Record name and credentials of persons doing procedure, and reporting of results to physician, especially "stat" or abnormal results.

# *SKILL* 123 Obtaining Blood Specimens from Venous Access Devices

*Lisa K. Anderson*

One of the advantages of central venous access device (VAD) placement in the seriously or chronically ill child is the ease of obtaining blood specimens from the device. In comparison to peripheral blood sampling, obtaining specimens from partially implanted devices (PIDs) and accessed totally implanted devices (TIDs) eliminates the pain of repeated needle sticks for the child (thus decreasing the child's and family's anxiety) and supports the medical plan of care by facilitating procurement of adequate samples in a timely fashion. Potential complications during specimen collection include introduction of air or microorganisms into the VAD, accidental dislodgement or displacement, or occlusion from inadequate flushing (Marcoux, Fisher, and Wong, 1990).

### NURSING DIAGNOSES

Potential for infection related to continual exposure of partially implanted devices to external environment or frequent interruption of skin integrity for venous access of totally implanted devices; Potential for injury related to hemorrhage at puncture site, air embolus, or inadequate restraint during venous collection; Anxiety related to unmet informational needs about the purpose and procedure for venous access device blood collection.

| Steps | Rationale |
|---|---|
| **Assessment** | |
| 1. Determine the type of VAD placed. For a totally implanted device (TID), assess if device is currently accessed. | The type of VAD influences both planning and implementation of the procedure. |
| 2. Review ordered laboratory tests requiring blood. Determine any prerequisite conditions (e.g., NPO), specific timing (e.g., drug levels), or special handling of the specimen. | The type of test ordered determines amount of blood needed for specimen, prerequisite conditions, and may influence collection time. Combining specimen collection when possible minimizes repeated entry into the central venous system and may decrease the risk of injury and/or infection. ***Special Considerations:*** *Pharmacologic and coagulation studies may require peripheral blood, rather than central venous catheter samples, to be more accurate (Moore, et al, 1986). Check agency or laboratory procedure manual.* |
| 3. Assess for current function of VAD and history of blood sampling from the device. | History and current use of VAD to obtain blood samples provides a baseline for assessing device function. |
| 4. Assess child/family's knowledge about the VAD and use for blood sampling. | An understanding of the function of the VAD may increase the level of cooperation from child and family. The child's perception of blood sampling must be assessed, since many children fear that removing blood from their bodies is life-threatening (especially children whose conditions require frequent sampling of blood) (Whaley and Wong, 1989). |

| Steps | Rationale |
|---|---|
| **Planning and Goal Setting** | |
| 1. Have family members at bedside to observe procedure, if possible. | Observation enhances family members' knowledge about VAD, and their presence may support the child emotionally. ***Special Considerations:*** *Parent/family teaching of blood withdrawal is usually not done, since this procedure occurs most often in the clinic or hospital setting.* |
| 2. Prepare child and family for the procedure (see Skill 1). | Preparation helps decrease the child's anxiety about the procedure. |
| 3. Obtain an assistant to help maintain the child's position and/or ensure aseptic technique. | Assistance may be necessary to prevent injury to the child or damage to the device and to ensure asepsis. |
| 4. Assemble equipment. | |
| a. Alcohol swabs. | |
| b. Two 10 ml Luer-Lok syringes filled with sterile normal saline. | Normal saline is used to flush the device before and after drawing blood samples. ***Special Considerations:*** *More than 10 ml of saline may be used to flush TIDs after blood sampling. One study demonstrated a 50% reduction in occlusion of TIDs when the amount of saline used to flush the catheter was increased from 10 ml to between 15 and 20 ml (Bagnall and Ruccione, 1987). Check agency's procedure.* |
| c. Empty 10 ml (minimum volume) sterile syringes (at least two syringes). | One syringe is used to aspirate and discard fluid; the others are used in collection of samples. Use of a syringe with a volume of less than 10 ml puts excessive pressure on TID ports and may cause the catheter to dislodge from the port internally (Wezel-Bolen, 1986). |
| d. Sterile Luer-Lok injection cap (if TID/PID not being used for continuous infusion). | |
| e. Sterile, capped needle (if PID/TID is being used for continuous infusion). | A sterile, capped needle may be used to maintain asepsis of the disconnected end of the continuous infusion tubing. |
| f. Blood collection tubes. | ***Special Considerations:*** *Consult the laboratory for the appropriate tubes to contain blood samples.* |
| g. Additional supplies for PID:<br>▪ 1-inch waterproof tape.<br>▪ Smooth cannula clamp (except for Groshong catheter). | A smooth clamp should be used to prevent damage to the catheter. Since Groshong catheters have a valve on the distal end to prevent reflux of blood, a clamp is not needed (Marcoux, Fisher, and Wong, 1990). |
| ▪ One 10 ml Luer-Lok syringe containing 3 to 10 ml of heparinized saline (10 units/ml) (Hickman or Broviac)<br>*OR*<br>▪ One 10 ml Luer-Lok syringe containing 5 to 10 ml normal saline (Groshong only). | ***Special Considerations:*** *Refer to Skill 110.* |
| h. Additional supplies for TID:<br>▪ Supplies to access TID (see Skill 110).<br>▪ Clamp (if not a part of Huber needle attachment).<br>▪ One 10 ml Luer-Lok syringe containing 3 to 5 ml of heparinized saline (100 units/ml) | TID must be flushed with heparinized saline if not being used for continuous infusion. |
| 5. Develop individualized goals of nursing care:<br>▪ Appropriate venous blood samples will be obtained in a timely manner.<br>▪ Venous access device will remain patent and functional for its designated use.<br>▪ Venous access device complications will be prevented or minimized.<br>▪ Child/family will experience minimal anxiety during the procedure. | |
| **Implementation**  | |
| 1. Wash hands for 1 minute with antibacterial soap. | Handwashing reduces surface bacteria to help prevent infection. |
| 2. To withdraw blood from a PID: | |
| a. Remove tape holding loop of catheter if present. | Untaping the catheter improves handling and avoids kinks in the tubing that can restrict fluid flow. |
| b. If continuous fluids are being infused, stop the infusion. | |

| **Steps** | **Rationale** |
|---|---|
| c. Clamp catheter (except Groshong) with the smooth cannula clamp (see Skill 110). | Hickman and Broviac catheters should be clamped before "opening the system" to prevent blood loss or air embolism. Groshong catheters have a valve on the distal end to prevent reflux and do not require clamping. |
| d. If PID is sealed by an injection cap, remove tape tab and clean outside of cap and catheter tip with alcohol swab. If PID is connected to IV tubing for continuous infusion, remove tape tab and clean junction with alcohol swab. | ***Special Considerations:*** *If the PID is multilumen, the larger lumen is usually used for obtaining blood samples (Perry and Potter, 1990).* |
| e. Remove injection cap and discard. If PID is connected to IV tubing, disconnect catheter from tubing. Place sterile capped needle on end of IV tubing. Maintain asepsis carefully. | Injection caps should never be reused because of the risk of introducing microorganisms. The capped needle maintains sterility of the IV tubing during the procedure. |
| f. Attach 10 ml Luer-Lok syringe filled with saline to catheter. Unclamp catheter if clamped. | |
| g. Rapidly flush catheter with saline, avoiding excessive pressure. Reclamp the catheter (except Groshong). | Flushing clears the catheter of infusion or heparin flush fluid and validates patency. |
| h. Attach empty sterile 10 ml syringe to catheter. Unclamp catheter. | |
| i. Aspirate 3 to 5 ml of blood. Reclamp catheter (except Groshong). Remove syringe and discard aspirate according to facility policy. | Aspirating blood to discard removes blood that may be diluted and could cause inaccurate test results.<br>***Special Considerations:*** *If blood cultures are ordered, the initial blood aspirated may be sent for culture, rather than discarded.* |
| j. Attach empty sterile 10 ml syringe to catheter. Unclamp catheter (if clamped) and aspirate appropriate volume of blood for sample. Reclamp catheter (except Groshong). | ***Special Considerations:*** *If more than 10 ml of blood is required for tests, repeat step, taking care to clamp/unclamp catheter when attaching and removing syringe.* |
| k. Remove syringe. Transfer blood specimen immediately to appropriate tubes. | Rapid transfer helps prevent clotting of the blood specimen to obtain accurate results. |
| l. Attach 10 ml Luer-Lok saline-filled syringe to catheter, unclamp (if clamped), and rapidly flush catheter with saline. Reclamp catheter (except Groshong). Apply new injection cap.<br>*OR*<br>For continuous infusion, remove sterile capped needle from tubing, and reattach tubing to catheter. | Rapid flushing clears the catheter of blood to help maintain patency. |
| m. Using 1-inch waterproof tape, apply tape around injection cap and catheter (or catheter/tubing junction), folding each end of tape over on itself. Unclamp catheter (if clamped). | Taping is a safety measure to prevent dislodgement of injection cap (or IV tubing) and catheter (Wezel-Bolen, 1986). |
| n. Rapidly flush the injection-capped catheter with heparinized saline but avoid excessive force (see Skill 110).<br>*OR*<br>Reestablish continuous infusion at appropriate rate. | Flushing ensures patency of the PID.<br>***Special Considerations:*** *Groshong catheters are flushed with normal saline.* |
| 3. To withdraw blood from a TID: | |
| a. Access TID (if needed) with Huber needle and attached extension tubing (see Skill 110). | |
| b. If continuous fluids are being infused, stop the infusion. | |
| c. Clamp the extension tubing. | |
| d. Follow step 2d through 2k above. | The procedure for drawing blood from TIDs is the same as for PIDs, with the extension tubing functioning as the catheter. |
| e. If Huber needle is to be removed after samples are obtained, attach 10 ml Luer-Lok syringe of heparinized saline to extension tubing.<br>*OR*<br>If Huber needle is to remain in place, apply sterile injection cap to tubing, scrub with alcohol swab for one minute; apply sterile needle to 10 ml Luer-Lok syringe of heparinized saline, and insert needle into injection cap. | |
| f. Unclamp tubing and rapidly inject heparinized saline into TID, avoiding excessive force (see Skill 110 for flushing procedure). | Flushing ensures patency of infusion port and catheter. |
| 4. Send all properly labeled blood samples to laboratory in a timely manner. | Prompt analysis of specimens facilitates medical plan of care. |
| 5. Dispose of all supplies and equipment appropriately. | |

| Steps | Rationale |
|---|---|
| **Evaluation Outcomes** | **Observational Guidelines** |
| 1. Blood sampling is completed in a timely manner and adequate uncontaminated specimens are collected. | Check laboratory reports for results. |
| 2. Venous access device remains patent and functional. | Device can be irrigated easily, and blood samples are easily aspirated. |
| 3. The child remains free of complications associated with accessing central venous devices. | Monitor for elevated temperature, chills; shortness of breath, chest pain; pain, numbness, or tingling of extremity on the same side of body as catheter; erythema or exudate at catheter insertion site (PID) or needle insertion site (TID); leaking of fluid, edema at insertion site. |
| 4. Child and family experience minimal anxiety during procedure. | Assess verbal and nonverbal behaviors (e.g., crying, pulling away, irritability). |

## Documentation

Document date and time of blood sampling; type of blood tests for which samples were drawn; patency of catheter and any difficulty with irrigation or aspiration of VAD; amount and concentration of heparinized saline flush used to irrigate catheter; and any complications or adverse conditions observed during procedure. If child is fluid restricted or is otherwise being closely monitored for fluid imbalance or blood loss, record amount of fluid injected or withdrawn from catheter.

# *SKILL* *124* Assisting with Lumbar Puncture

*Lisa K. Anderson*

A lumbar puncture is a medical procedure involving the insertion of a needle into the subarachnoid space of the lumbar spinal canal for diagnostic or therapeutic purposes. The needle is inserted betwen the L3 and L4 vertebrae to avoid damage to the spinal cord or major nerve roots. Once the spinal needle is in place: (1) cerebrospinal fluid (CSF) pressure may be measured by the attachment of a manometer onto the needle; (2) fluid may be withdrawn for analysis; (3) fluid may be withdrawn to reduce cerebrospinal pressure; and/or (4) medication may be injected intrathecally (into the subarachnoid space).

In the pediatric setting, lumbar puncture is most often used as a diagnostic tool in central nervous system infection or inflammation (Hazinski, 1984). CSF withdrawn during the puncture is sent to the laboratory for culture, Gram stain, cell count, and protein and glucose content. In addition, the color and character of the fluid must be noted. Normal CSF is colorless and clear. Blood in the first drops of CSF collected may indicate a traumatic tap secondary to entering a vein, or rarely, an intraventricular hemorrhage. Normal CSF results for a child above 6 months of age are listed below (Tucker et al, 1988).

Pressure: 70 to 200 mm of water
Color: colorless, clear
Glucose: greater than 40 mg/100 ml
Protein (total): less than 40 mg/100 ml
Red blood cells: none
White blood cells: 0 to 4
Microorganisms: none

Children diagnosed with certain types of cancer frequently have a lumbar puncture upon diagnosis and at intervals throughout their disease course. The procedure determines the presence or absence of leukemic cells and provides a means for intrathecal injection of antineoplastic chemotherapy as indicated in the treatment regimen.

### NURSING DIAGNOSES

Anxiety related to perceived threat to body integrity or unmet informational need about lumbar puncture procedure; Pain related to needle insertion and positioning for procedure; Potential for injury related to respiratory distress due to positioning, neurological impairment due to CSF leakage, or hemorrhagic shock due to excessive bleeding at the puncture site.

| Steps | Rationale |
|---|---|
| **Assessment** | |
| 1. Assess neurologic status of child:<br>a. Vital signs (pulse, respirations, blood pressure).<br>b. Level of consciousness.<br>c. Pupillary response.<br>d. Movement of extremities.<br>e. Sensation.<br>f. Fontanels (if open). | Initial assessment provides a baseline for postprocedure observation. Also, increased intracranial pressure is a contraindication in most cases.<br>***Special Considerations:*** *Lumbar puncture may be performed with caution on the infant with signs of increased intracranial pressure. If these signs are present in the older child with fused cranial sutures, the procedure should be postponed because of the possibility of herniation of the medulla through the foramen magnum with the sudden release of CSF during the puncture (Hazinski, 1984).* |
| 2. Assess age and size of child. | Positioning and needle size depend on age and size. |
| 3. Assess child's level of knowledge about the procedure and ability to understand and follow instructions. | Understanding of the procedure and the ability to follow instructions determines the level of cooperation.<br>***Special Considerations:*** *An assistant may be needed to help the child maintain positioning during the procedure to avoid injury and prolonging procedure.* |
| 4. Review physician order, medical record, and nursing assessment to determine purpose of lumbar puncture and to identify allergies to antiseptic solutions and local anesthetics. | An awareness of the purpose of the procedure determines equipment essential to complete procedure. If the child is allergic to iodine solution or local anesthetic agents, these agents should not be used during the procedure to avoid allergic reactions.<br>***Special Considerations:*** *Alternative cleansing solutions may be substituted, e.g., Hibiclens.* |
| **Planning and Goal Setting** | |
| 1. Review medical record for signed authorization for procedure. Obtain if not present, according to facility policy (see Skill 8). | Written authorization is required for most invasive procedures. |
| 2. Determine location for the procedure (treatment room, child's room, etc.) Consider factors such as lighting, ease of accessibility to child after positioned, and presence of roommate. | ***Special Considerations:*** *Use of the treatment room for a young child promotes the feeling of his or her room as a safe place.* |
| 3. Gather equipment:<br>a. Lumbar puncture tray, to include:<br>▪ Sterile gauze sponges (4 × 4 inch). | Sponges are used to clean and apply pressure to puncture site. |
| ▪ Sterile towel.<br>▪ Sterile drape. | Towel and drape maintain the sterile field. |
| ▪ 2 to 3 spinal needles (with obturators). | Size of needle must be appropriate for age and weight of child.<br>***Special Considerations:*** *Guidelines for needle selection:*<br>*Newborn—22 gauge 1½ inch.*<br>*Infant/child—22 gauge 1½ inch.*<br>*Adolescent—21 gauge 2½ inch.*<br>*Extra unopened needles should be readily available in case the puncture is repeated.* |
| ▪ Local anesthetic agent (Xylocaine 1%). | ***Special Considerations:*** *Physician personal preference may vary on the use of a local anesthetic. The wheal produced may obstruct landmarks in the newborn/small infant.* |
| ▪ Syringe with 25 gauge ⅝ inch needle attached. | Syringe and needle are used to inject local anesthetic at the site. |
| ▪ Three to four sterile fluid collection tubes numbered and with caps. | CSF is collected in the tubes.<br>***Special Considerations:*** *Consult physician to determine number of separate tubes needed for CSF collection.* |
| ▪ Adhesive bandage. | An adhesive bandage is generally the only dressing used to cover the puncture site following the procedure. |
| b. Antiseptic cleansing solution (povidone-iodine). | Topical cleansing of puncture site prevents infection by local flora. |
| c. Sterile gloves. Determine physician's size preference. | ***Special Considerations:*** *An extra pair should be available in case of contamination during procedure.* |
| d. Stool or chair for physician. | Lumbar puncture is best performed at eye level with the child's spine. |
| e. Strong light source. | Adequate illumination of the site facilitates successful completion of the procedure. |
| f. Manometer with 3-way stopcock (optional); may be included in the tray. | A manometer may be used to measure CSF pressure. |

| Steps | Rationale |
|---|---|
| g. Labels and laboratory requisitions. | ***Special Considerations:*** *Label the tubes by number, according to the sequence in which CSF is collected; e.g., Tube No. 1 is the first sample collected.* |
| h. Medication for intrathecal injection, if planned. | |
| 4. Explain the procedure to child and family (see Skill 1). | Anxiety is decreased and coping ability is increased by an honest, appropriate, thorough explanation of the procedure and assists the child in development of coping strategies. ***Special Considerations:*** *Describe the positioning necessary during the procedure and enlist child's participation in demonstration. Use diagrams of puncture site and "play trays" of equipment used during the lumbar puncture to facilitate explanation and permit child to adjust to the reality of the procedure and express feelings in a nonthreatening environment (Maul-Mellot and Adams, 1987).* |
| 5. Assist the child to void before the procedure, if developmentally appropriate. | Length of procedure and anxiety may cause the child to become incontinent. Voiding during the procedure may cause embarrassment for the older continent child. |
| 6. Develop individualized goals of nursing care: ▪ Minimize child's discomfort during procedure and postprocedure. ▪ Prevent postprocedure complications such as infection, injury, headache, and hemorrhage. ▪ Prevent positioning-related injury during the procedure. ▪ Minimize child/family's anxiety before, during, and after procedure. | |

## Implementation

| Steps | Rationale |
|---|---|
| 1. Prepare equipment. a. Open lumbar puncture tray (if desired by physician) using aseptic technique. | ***Special Considerations:*** *Do not open tray more than 15 minutes before procedure, in case there is a change in the child's status. This also minimizes the risk of contamination of equipment.* |
| b. Pour antiseptic cleansing solution into appropriate container on sterile field if solution is not supplied in the tray. | |
| c. Open glove outerwrap. | |
| d. Place extra spinal needles and gloves within close proximity, if packaged separately. | Extra needles and gloves should be available in the event of contamination or repeat puncture. |
| 2. Transport child to the treatment room or provide privacy if the procedure is to be done in the child's room. | |
| 3. Position the child for lumbar puncture: The child should be positioned nearest to the side of the table from which the physician will work. The child will be facing away from the physician and toward the person restraining him or her. | ***Special Considerations:*** *Physician may express preference for position of child.* |
| a. Newborn/small infant—Modified side-lying position with partial neck extension (Fig. 124-1): Place infant on his or her side with the back close to the edge of table. The spine is maintained in a flexed position by holding infant with one hand behind the neck and shoulders and the other hand behind the thighs. Maintain the neck in partial extension, not flexed toward the chest (Whaley and Wong, 1989). | This age group is prone to respiratory distress secondary to a soft, pliable trachea. Maintaining the neck in partial extension facilitates chest expansion and diaphragm excursion. |
| b. Infant—Sitting position (Fig. 124-2): Place infant with buttocks at the edge of table. Flex the neck so that the chin rests on the chest and immobilize the infant's arms and legs with hands (Whaley and Wong, 1989). Position diaper or absorbent pad under genital area to absorb urine or stool. | This position allows for adequate flexion of the lumbar spine in this age group. Presence of diaper or pad prevents contamination of the sterile field. ***Special Considerations:*** *Manometer readings of CSF pressure are inaccurate with the infant in the sitting position. Extreme flexion of the neck may be contraindicated for the infant with respiratory distress. Head support can be achieved by altering hand position or using the upper body to maintain the infant's head position. Prolonged positioning and the stress of needle insertion may cause the infant to void.* |

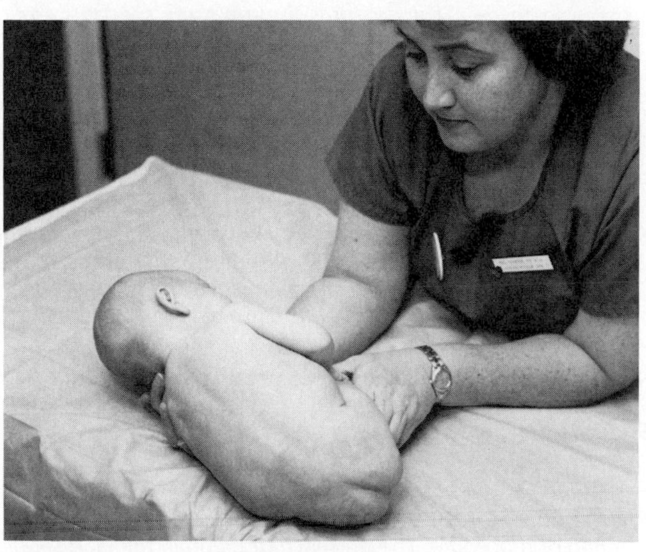

***FIG. 124-1*** Modified side-lying position for lumbar puncture.

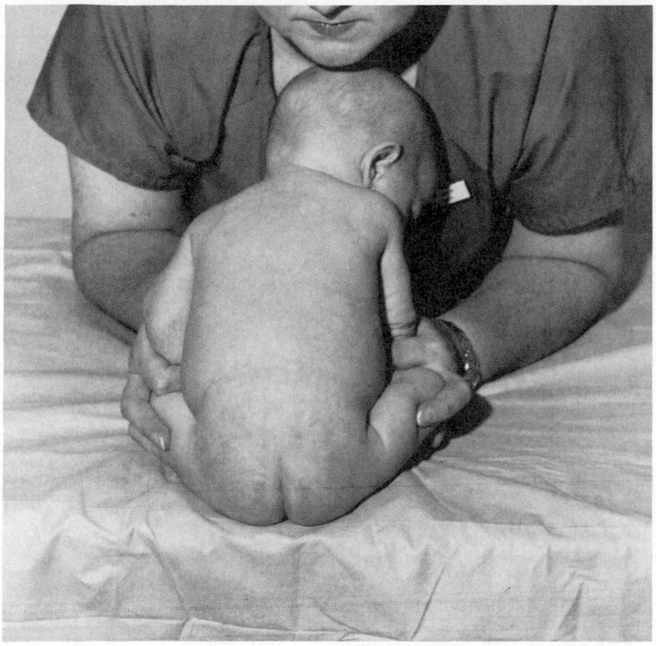

***FIG. 124-2*** Infant sitting position allows for flexion of lumbar spine.

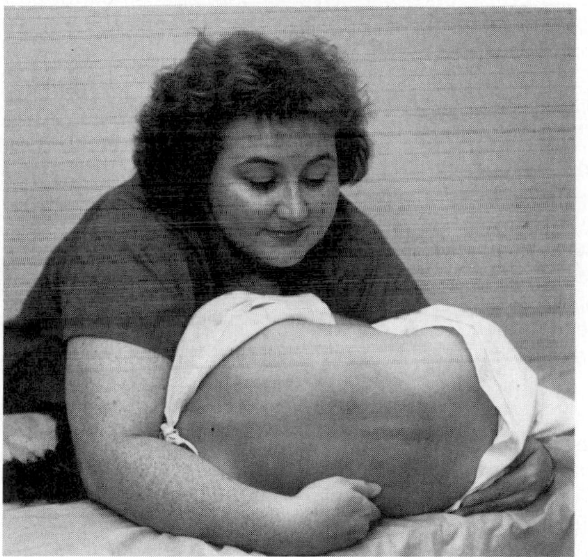

***FIG. 124-3*** Older child in side-lying position.

| Steps | Rationale |
|---|---|
| c. Older infant/child—Lateral decubitus position (Fig. 124-3): Place the child on side with the back close to edge of table. The spine is maintained in a flexed position by holding the child with one hand placed behind the neck and the other behind the thighs. The head and neck should be fully flexed. | Flexion of the lumbar spine facilitates separation of the vertebrae and insertion of the spinal needle into the subarachnoid space. ***Special Considerations:*** *Additional personnel may be necessary to assist child in maintaining this position.* |
| 4. Hold child securely in the correct position throughout the procedure. | Safety of the child and timely completion of the procedure is dependent upon maintenance of the optimal flexed-lumbar spine position. |
| 5. Talk to the child in a soothing, calm tone of voice throughout the procedure. | External anxiety perceived by the child reinforces his or her own anxiety. |
| a. Explain sensations that child is experiencing as they occur. | Explanation increases child's ability to develop an accurate perception of the situation. |

| Steps | Rationale |
|---|---|
| | ***Special Considerations:*** *Use age-appropriate language. For example:*<br>▪ *Young child—"The doctor is putting some special soap on your back now. Does that feel cold?"*<br>▪ *Older child—"The doctor is cleaning all the germs from your skin with a special soap. How does that feel?"* |
| b. Encourage the child to use coping mechanisms practiced before the procedure. | Using coping strategies helps the child gain mastery of anxiety he or she may be experiencing. |
| c. Identify and accept the child's behavior and feelings. | This facilitates establishment of a trusting relationship and validates the child's feelings.<br>***Special Considerations:*** *The infant may be reassured by soothing, cooing noises and physical closeness. Offer praise to the older child for any attempts at compliance and validate child's perceptions; e.g., say "It is hard to lie still, but I can tell you are trying very hard."* |
| 6. After spinal needle is in place, assist the physician in holding manometer (if using). Stabilize the manometer by holding it at the top. | Needle position is maintained and contamination of sterile field is prevented.<br>***Special Considerations:*** *Additional personnel may be necessary to assist the physician if the manometer is to be used, because the primary concern is the maintenance of the child's position.* |
| 7. Note the color and character of the CSF as it is collected by the physician. Note "opening" and "closing" pressures if a manometer is used. | ***Special Considerations:*** *Include this information in documentation of procedure. The presence of blood in the fluid should be verified with physician as to the cause.* |
| 8. After needle is withdrawn, apply direct pressure to the puncture site with a sterile gauze sponge until bleeding or leakage of CSF is stopped. | CSF loss and bleeding are minimized.<br>***Special Considerations:*** *Maintain lateral or sitting position of child during this time as much as possible to permit stabilization of CSF pressure.* |
| 9. Remove remaining cleansing solution (povidone-iodine) from skin with clean washcloth and warm water or alcohol and gauze sponges. Apply adhesive bandage to the site. | Povidone-iodine may cause skin irritation for some children after prolonged contact. Covering the site prevents infection. |
| 10. Provide comfort measures for the child. Maintain the child in a reclining position as much as possible during this time. | Comforting the child helps child to regain composure and communicates feelings of empathy and concern. The reclining position may help prevent post-tap headache, although this measure is unproven. |
| 11. Ensure that caps on all sterile collecting tubes are securely closed. | Closing tubes securely prevents loss or contamination of the specimens.<br>***Special Considerations:*** *An assistant may be needed to facilitate prompt handling, labeling, and transport of specimens.* |
| 12. Apply labels with complete patient information and send to laboratory with requisition for ordered tests, according to facility policy. | Proper labeling of specimens facilitates diagnosis and treatment of the child.<br>***Special Considerations:*** *Commonly ordered tests for diagnosis of meningitis include:*<br>*Tube 1: culture, Gram stain.*<br>*Tube 2: protein, glucose.*<br>*Tube 3: cell count.*<br>*Tube 4: viral culture.* |
| 13. Return the child to his or her room and family; allow family to provide further comfort measures. | The reunion of child and family allays fears and allows further soothing of the child. |
| 14. Instruct family and child in postprocedural expectations: | Involving the family and child in postprocedural education provides them with a sense of control. |
| a. Maintain reclining position for 1 to 6 hours. | A headache may occur post-tap, although the exact mechanism is unknown. A reclining position may be helpful. |
| b. Provide adequate fluid intake. | Fluids orally or intravenously aid in replacing CSF loss.<br>***Special Considerations:*** *Fluids may be restricted for some children and/or contraindicated orally.* |
| c. Provide analgesics (see Skill 52). | Procedural positioning and postprocedural headache may cause discomfort.<br>***Special Considerations:*** *Avoid analgesics that may interfere with accurate neurologic assessments.* |
| d. Monitor for effects of medication injected intrathecally (if appropriate). | |

| **Steps** | **Rationale** |
|---|---|
| 15. Reassess child's neurologic status every 15 to 30 minutes until stable:<br>a. Vital signs (pulse, respiration, blood pressure).<br>b. Level of consciousness.<br>c. Pupillary response.<br>d. Movement of extremities.<br>e. Sensation. | A decrease in CSF with increased intracranial pressure may cause herniation of the medulla. Signs and symptoms of herniation include:<br>▪ Decreased level of consciousness.<br>▪ Change in heart rate (tachycardia or bradycardia).<br>▪ Pupil dilation with sluggish response to light.<br>▪ Widening pulse pressure.<br>▪ Apnea.<br>▪ Abnormal posturing. |
| 16. Assess puncture site frequently. A small amount of blood or clear drainage is normal. | Complications of lumbar puncture include CSF leak, bleeding from the site, and infection at the site. |

| **Evaluation Outcomes** | **Observational Guidelines** |
|---|---|
| 1. The child and family are adequately prepared for procedure. | Ask the family to summarize the reason for lumbar puncture. Note child's attempts at cooperation during the procedure. |
| 2. The child is properly positioned during procedure and experiences minimal or no respiratory distress. | Adequate spacing between vertebrae in flexed spinal column permits needle insertion. Assess skin color, rate, depth, and quality of respirations. Child is not injured by breaking restraint and the sterile field is maintained. |
| 3. Neurologic status of child is monitored during procedure and returns to baseline after procedure. | Observe vital signs, pupillary response, level of consciousness, ability to move and feel all extremities; compare to baseline assessment. |
| 4. Complications of the procedure are prevented or minimized. | Observe the puncture site for excessive bleeding, CSF leak, or erythema and purulent drainage; assess for persisting discomfort at site or headache. Monitor vital signs and temperature. |
| 5. Discomfort to the child is minimized. | Observe for crying, resistance, inability to cooperate. Ask child to describe level of discomfort. Note how easily the child is comforted. |
| 6. Procedure is completed in a timely manner and adequate specimen is collected and properly handled to facilitate diagnosis and treatment. | Check laboratory reports for results. |
| 7. Postprocedure expectations are understood by child and family. | Ask the family to verbalize important postprocedure activities for the child; e.g., bedrest and fluid intake. |

## Documentation

Record date and time procedure performed and by whom (physician). Note nursing observations during and after procedure (vital signs, neurologic status, color, clarity, and pressure of CSF, assessment of puncture site). Document sending specimen to laboratory. Record child's tolerance of procedure (headache, neurologic status, anxiety) and document postprocedure teaching of expectations to child and family.

# SKILL 125 Assisting with Bone Marrow Biopsy

*Lisa K. Anderson*

Bone marrow aspiration or biopsy is the collection of hematopoietic marrow from thin flat bones for the purposes of examination of cellular components (erythrocytes, granulocytes, megakaryocytes), examination for presence of fibrotic tissue or neoplasm, and removal of marrow for treatment and readministration during bone marrow transplant (Perry and Potter, 1990). During bone marrow aspiration, the marrow is withdrawn through a needle by suction. Bone marrow biopsy requires the cutting of a small sliver of bone and marrow, utilizing a slightly different type of needle. This procedure is most often used in the diagnosis and treatment of cancers such as leukemia and lymphoma, and hematologic conditions such as thrombocytopenic purpura, aplastic anemia, and immunoglobulin disorders.

## NURSING DIAGNOSES

Pain related to needle insertion and bone marrow aspiration/biopsy; Potential for infection related to introduction of needle through skin into tissue and bone, immunosuppression; Potential for injury related to hemorrhagic shock due to altered coagulation and excessive bleeding at puncture site; Anxiety related to perceived threat to body integrity or unmet informational need about biopsy procedure.

| Steps | Rationale |
|---|---|
| **Assessment** | |
| 1. Assess child's vital signs and hematologic status:<br>a. Red cell count.<br>b. White cell count.<br>c. Platelet count.<br>d. Hemoglobin.<br>e. Hematocrit.<br>f. Vital signs (temperature, pulse, respirations, blood pressure). | An initial assessment of vital signs provides a baseline for postprocedure assessment. Abnormal cell counts and hemoglobin/hematocrit values predispose the child to complications after the procedure (e.g., bleeding, infection).<br>***Special Considerations:*** *The child undergoing bone marrow aspiration or biopsy may have abnormal laboratory values secondary to the disease process being evaluated by the procedure.* |
| 2. Assess child's age, developmental level, and level of knowledge about the procedure and ability to follow instructions (see Skill 25). | An understanding of the procedure and the ability to follow instructions determine the level of cooperation during the procedure. Excessive movement or active resistance during procedure may cause injury or prolong procedure. |
| 3. Review medical record and nursing assessment to identify allergies to medications and antiseptic solutions. | Use of antiseptic solutions or local anesthetic agents that the child is allergic to may cause a reaction. |
| 4. Review medical record to determine purpose of procedure. Determine laboratory tests (if any) to be performed. | Purpose determines whether biopsy or aspiration is indicated, which dictates the type of equipment to be used. |
| 5. Assess the need for sedation or prophylactic pain medication. If sedation is to be given via the intravenous route, assess the need for IV access (continuous or heparin lock). | Insertion of needle and aspiration or biopsy of marrow is a very painful and traumatic procedure for a child (Hamner and Miles, 1988).<br>***Special Considerations:*** *If preprocedure sedation is to be given, time administration for peak effect during the actual biopsy/aspiration (see Skill 52).* |
| 6. Assess child's usual coping strategies during painful procedures. | Children who experience painful procedures often develop personal coping strategies that can be encouraged and used in future encounters with pain.<br>***Special Considerations:*** *Maximum use of coping strategies is especially important if the child is awake during the procedure.* |

| Steps | Rationale |
|---|---|

## Planning and Goal Setting

1. Review medical record for signed authorization form for procedure. Obtain, if not present, according to facility policy (see Skill 8).

   Written authorization is required for most invasive procedures.

2. Determine location for procedure (surgical area, treatment room, child's room). Factors to consider include lighting, ease of accessibility to child for secure positioning and aspiration, and privacy.

   ***Special Considerations:*** *Use of the child's room for a painful procedure should be avoided, if at all possible, to maintain perception of the room as a safe place.*

3. Gather equipment.
   a. Bone marrow aspiration/biopsy tray, to include:
   - Antiseptic cleansing solution (povidone-iodine).

     Topical cleansing of puncture site prevents infection by local flora.
     ***Special Considerations:*** *An alternative solution (e.g., Hibiclens) may be substituted if the child has an allergy to iodine.*

   - Sterile gauze sponges (4 × 4 inches).

     Sponges are used to clean puncture site.

   - Sterile towels.
   - Sterile drape.

     Towels and drape maintain sterile field.

   - Local anesthetic agent for injection (lidocaine, Xylocaine).
   - Sterile syringes: two 3 ml, two 20 to 60 ml.
   - Sterile needles: two 25 gauge ⅝ inch.

     3 ml syringe and 25 gauge needle are used to inject local anesthetic. Large syringes are used for marrow aspiration.

   - Bone marrow needle: appropriate size for child.

     ***Special Considerations:*** *Consult physician, practitioner, or health facility manual to determine size of needle, based on size and/or age of child. Examples of needles available:*
     - *Aspiration—18 gauge Jamshidi needle with stylet; length 1$\frac{1}{16}$ to 1$\frac{7}{16}$ inches.*
     - *Biopsy—11 to 13 gauge Jamshidi needle with stylet and metal probe; length 4 inches*

   b. Sterile gloves—correct size for physician/practitioner.

   ***Special Considerations:*** *An extra pair of sterile gloves should be available in case of contamination during procedure.*

   c. Sterile gauze sponge (2 × 2 inches).
   d. Tape.
   e. Antiseptic ointment (povidone-iodine).

   Gauze, tape, and ointment are used to dress the puncture site to prevent infection.
   ***Special Considerations:*** *If the child is allergic to povidone-iodine, another antibiotic ointment may be used, e.g., Neosporin.*

   f. Pain medication or sedative, as ordered by physician.

   Bone marrow aspiration has been identified as a very painful and traumatic procedure for children (Hamner and Miles, 1988).
   ***Special Considerations:*** *A variety of pharmacologic interventions have been used to provide partial or complete analgesia, including local lidocaine infiltration, general anesthesia (Perin and Frase, 1985), Ketamine (Forlini, 1987), and fentanyl (Wong, 1989).*

   g. Masks for personnel (if indicated).

   ***Special Considerations:*** *Masks may be used, but their effectiveness in preventing transmission of microorganisms to the immunocompromised child is unproven.*

   h. Glass microscope slides with slide covers; specimen containers with preservative solution.

   ***Special Considerations:*** *Consult with physician/practitioner and/or facility manual to determine equipment necessary to transport marrow for examination.*

   i. Labels and laboratory or histology requisition.

4. Prepare child/family for procedure. Determine whether family wishes to be present during the procedure (see Skill 1). Information to include:
   a. Necessary positioning.
   b. Length of procedure (generally 20 to 30 minutes).
   c. What child will experience.
   d. Unless heavy sedation or general anesthesia is planned, expect pain when local anesthesia injected, when biopsy needle enters the periosteum, and for a few seconds when the marrow is aspirated.
   e. If parent is to be present, role is to provide emotional support by touch and talking to child.

   An honest, thorough, age-appropriate explanation of the reasons for and steps involved in the procedure decreases anxiety. The child's ability to cope may be increased by a discussion and rehearsal of coping strategies. Presence of a parent or family member may decrease the child's fear.
   ***Special Considerations:*** *A "play tray" of procedure equipment may be used to demonstrate and involve the child in therapeutic expression of feelings in a nonthreatening environment (Maul-Mellott and Adams, 1987). Although family attendance during procedure is controversial, most children want a parent present (Hamner and Miles, 1988).*

5. Develop individualized goals of nursing care:
   - Prevent positioning-related injury to the child during procedure.

| Steps | Rationale |
|---|---|
| ▪ Minimize child's discomfort during procedure and after the procedure. <br> ▪ Minimize child/family's anxiety concerning the procedure. | |

## Implementation

| Steps | Rationale |
|---|---|
| 1. Prepare equipment: <br> a. Open bone marrow aspiration/biopsy tray (if physician/practitioner preference) and set up sterile field. If tray is not available, organize individual equipment on a sterile field. | ***Special Considerations:*** *Do not open tray more than 15 minutes before procedure, to minimize risk of contamination of equipment.* |
| b. Pour antiseptic cleansing solution into appropriate container on sterile field if solution is not supplied in tray. | |
| c. Open glove outerwrap. | ***Special Considerations:*** *Extra gloves must be available in the event of contamination or second puncture.* |
| d. Place extra bone marrow needles within close proximity to sterile field. | |
| 2. Transport child/family to procedure location. | ***Special Considerations:*** *If family member is present during procedure, position them at the child's head, making it possible for them to offer physical and verbal support (Fochtman and Foley, 1982).* |
| 3. Assist child to assume position as indicated by physician/practitioner for procedure. | |
| a. Posterior iliac crest: child assumes prone position with pillow or blanket placed under hips to elevate the selected site (Whaley and Wong, 1989). | ***Special Considerations:*** *The posterior or anterior iliac crests are the sites of aspiration most often chosen in children. The tibia may be the chosen site for infants (Whaley and Wong, 1989; Fochtman and Foley, 1982). Modifications of position may be accomplished by using a pillow or folded blanket under or beside the hips or lower extremities.* |
| b. Anterior iliac crest: child assumes supine position with modifications made to facilitate visualization and accessibility of site. | |
| c. Tibia: infant is placed in supine position with modifications made to facilitate visualization and accessibility of site. | |
| 4. Restrain child securely in the correct position throughout the procedure. | Safety of the child and timely completion of procedure depend on maintenance of the correct position. <br> ***Special Considerations:*** *Few children are able to maintain position without restraint. The ideal situation requires two persons, one to immobilize the upper body and one to immobilize the lower body (Whaley and Wong, 1989).* |
| 5. Communicate with the child during the procedure. | Constant communication promotes relaxation and establishes trust. |
| a. Explain sensations that the child is experiencing as they occur. | Explanation enhances the development of accurate perceptions of the experience. |
| b. Remind the child to use coping strategies practiced before procedure. | By using coping skills, the child works toward mastery of anxiety. |
| c. Identify and accept the child's behavior and feelings. | Acceptance of negative or positive behavior and feelings facilitates the trust relationship. <br> ***Special Considerations:*** *Attempt to soothe the infant or young child with soft words of comfort. Praise and encourage older children for any attempt at compliance.* |
| 6. Assist physician/practitioner with equipment, as necessary (e.g., handing syringes, slide preparation). | ***Special Considerations:*** *Additional personnel may be required. Laboratory personnel may need to be present to receive and prepare specimens.* |
| 7. Note amount and appearance of bone marrow aspirate or biopsy. | Amount and appearance of aspirate/biopsy needs to be documented in the child's record. |
| 8. After the needle is removed, apply direct pressure to the site for 5 to 15 minutes with sterile gauze sponge, followed by the application of a pressure bandage or adhesive bandage (Duke University, 1983). | Pressure and bandage facilitate hemostasis. <br> ***Special Considerations:*** *If the child's platelet count is less than 50,000, a pressure bandage is required (Fochtman and Foley, 1982).* |
| 9. Assist physician/practitioner with preparation of specimens for transport to laboratory (as necessary), according to facility policy. Label all specimens correctly. | Proper labeling of specimens with child's identification, time of collection, and source of specimen facilitates diagnosis and/or treatment of the child. |

| Steps | Rationale |
|---|---|
| 10. Gently remove remaining povidone-iodine solution from skin with clean washcloth and warm water or alcohol and gauze sponges. | Povidone-iodine may cause skin irritation for some children after prolonged contact. |
| 11. Provide comfort measures for the child (see Skill 1). | Comforting the child helps maintain the trust relationship and decreases the child's anxiety level. |
| 12. Return child to his or her room; allow family to provide further comfort measures. If procedure is performed in child's room, remove all equipment as soon as possible. | Returning to a nonthreatening environment helps the child regain composure and distance self from the experience. |
| 13. Instruct child and family in postprocedure expectations. | Postprocedure education promotes feelings of control and enhances coping ability. |
| a. Child should rest or play quietly for 30 minutes to 1 hour (O'Rourke, 1986). | Active play or strenuous activity may hinder hemostasis at puncture site. |
| b. Vital signs will be monitored. | Assessment of vital signs verifies child's physiologic status in response to procedure (Perry and Potter, 1990). |
| c. Notify nurse if dressing at puncture site becomes blood-soaked; allow bandage to remain in place for at least 8 hours (Fochtman and Foley, 1982). | Potential complication of procedure is bleeding at the site of aspiration or biopsy. |
| 14. Monitor vital signs every 15 to 30 minutes until stable. | Pulse elevation or decreased blood pressure may signal hemorrhage. |
| 15. Assess bandage over puncture site frequently. | Assessment detects continued bleeding. |
| 16. After dressing is removed, assess the puncture site for signs of infection. | The most common complication of procedure is infection of the bone marrow. Pain, discoloration, drainage, or edema at the site is significant.<br>***Special Considerations:*** *If the child's absolute neutrophil count is less than 1000/mm$^3$, purulent drainage may not be present, even if the site is infected (Pikl, 1981).* |

## Evaluation Outcomes / Observational Guidelines

| Evaluation Outcomes | Observational Guidelines |
|---|---|
| 1. The child and family are adequately prepared for procedure. | Ask the family to summarize the reason for procedure. Note child's attempts at cooperation during and after procedure. |
| 2. The child is properly positioned during procedure. | Secure positioning and visualization of the site permits smooth needle insertion for aspiration or biopsy. Specimen is obtained. |
| 3. Discomfort to the child is minimized during procedure. | Observe for crying, resistance, inability to cooperate. Ask child to describe level of discomfort. Note how easily the child is comforted. |
| 4. Complications of the procedure are prevented or minimized. | Assess vital signs and compare to baseline. Observe site for absence of bleeding; assess for signs of infection (e.g., erythema, warmth, edema). |
| 5. Procedure is completed in a timely manner and adequate specimen is collected, properly handled, and transported to the laboratory. | Procedure is completed in 20 to 30 minutes. Check laboratory reports for results. |
| 6. Postprocedure expectations are understood by child and family. | Ask the child and family to verbalize important aspects of postprocedure care. |

## Documentation

Record date and time procedure performed and by whom; nursing observations during and after procedure (vital signs, amount and appearance of specimen, and assessment of site). Note specimens sent to laboratory. Record child's tolerance of procedure. Document preprocedure preparation and postprocedure teaching to child and family.

## UNIT XVIII

## PRODUCT REFERENCES AND TEACHING RESOURCES

### Books

Wong DL and Whaley LF: Clinical manual of pediatric nursing, ed 3, St Louis, 1990, The CV Mosby Co.
Includes home care instructions on obtaining a urine sample.

### Organizations

American Diabetes Association (ADA)
National Service Center
1660 Duke Street
Alexandria, VA 22314
(703) 549-1500

## REFERENCES


Adcock EW and Consolvo CA: Fluid and electrolyte management. In Merenstein G and Gardner S, editors: Handbook of neonatal intensive care, ed 2, St Louis, 1989, The CV Mosby Co.

Alstrom T et al: Recommendation for collection of skin puncture blood from children, with special reference to production of reference values, Scand J Clin Lab Invest 47:199-205, 1987.

Bagnall H and Ruccione K: Experience with a totally implanted venous access device in children with malignant disease, Oncology Nurs Forum 14(4):51-56, 1987.

Battaglia JD: Severe croup: the child with fever and upper airway obstruction, Pediatr Rev, 7(8):227-233, 1986.

Behrman RE and Vaughan VC III, editors: Nelson textbook of pediatrics, ed 13, Philadelphia, 1987, WB Saunders Co.

Benenson AS, editor: Control of communicable diseases in man, ed 14, Washington, DC, 1985, American Public Health Association.

Bergman M: Principles of diabetes management, New York, 1987, Elsevier Science.

Blumefeld TA, Turi GK, and Blanc WA: Recommended site and depth of newborn heel skin punctures based on anatomical measurements and histopathology, Lancet, 1(8110):230-233, 1979.

Bowker C et al: Focus on urinalysis, Nurs Times 82(17):1-6, 1986.

Calam R and Cooper M: Recommended "Order of Draw" for collecting blood specimens into additive-containing tubes, Clin Chem 18(6):1399, 1982.

Corbett JV: Laboratory tests and diagnostic procedures with nursing diagnoses, ed 2, Norwalk, Conn, 1987, Appleton and Lange.

Davidson M: Diabetes mellitus: diagnosis and treatment, ed 2, New York, 1986, John Wiley & Sons Inc.

Delameter A et al: Self-monitoring of blood glucose by adolescents with diabetes: technical skills and utilization of data. The Diabetes Educator 15(1):56-61, 1989.

Droeske SC and Francis SA: Pediatric diagnostic procedures, New York, 1981, John Wiley & Sons.

Duke University Hospital Nursing Services: Guidelines for nursing care: process and outcome, Philadelphia, 1983, JB Lippincott Co.

Dunn HP: Venipuncture hazards, NZ Med J 100(816):33, 1987.

Dyson A and Bogod D: Minimising bruising in the antecubital fossa after venepuncture, Br Med J 294(6588):1659, 1987.

Fischback F, editor: Manual of laboratory diagnostic tests, ed 2, Philadelphia, 1984, JB Lippincott Co.

Follansbee D: Assuming responsibility for diabetes management: what age? what price? The Diabetes Educator 15(4):347-352, 1989.

Fochtman D and Foley G, editors: Nursing care of the child with cancer, Boston, 1982, Little, Brown & Co.

Forlini J, Morin DM, and Treacy S: Painless pediatric procedures, Am J Nurs 87(3):321-323, 1987.

Garcia L: Special laboratory examinations for parasitic infections, Pediatr Clin North Am 32(4):1047-1061, 1985.

Goodman L et al: A urine preservative system to maintain bacterial counts, Clin Pediatr 24(7):383-386, 1985.

Guthrie D and Guthrie R: Nursing management of diabetes mellitus, ed 2, St Louis, 1982, The CV Mosby Co.

Hall C and Douglas R: Clinically useful method for the isolation of respiratory syncytial virus, J Infect Dis 131(1):1-4, 1975.

Hamner S and Miles M: Coping strategies in children with cancer undergoing bone marrow aspirations, J Assoc Pediatr Oncol Nurs 5(3): 11-15, 1988.

Hazinski MF: Nursing care of the critically ill child, St Louis, 1984, The CV Mosby Co.

Henley M and Sears J: Pinworms: a persistent pediatric problem, MCN 10(2):111-113, 1985.

Hilton BA: Does diabetic control really make a difference? Can Nurse 78:49-52, 1982.

Hughes W and Buescher E: Pediatric procedures, ed 2, Philadelphia, 1980, WB Saunders Co.

James W, White S, and Yanklowitz B: Allergic contact dermatitis to compound tincture of benzoin, J Am Acad Dermatol 11(5):847-850, 1984.

Katzman EM: What's the most common helminth infection in the US? MCN 14(3):193-195, 1989.

Kozier B and Erb G: Techniques in clinical nursing, a nursing process approach, ed 2, Menlo Park, Calif, 1987, Addison-Wesley Publishing Co.

Kulberg A: Urinalysis and urine culture, Top Emerg Med 5(1):47-59, 1983.

Kuller J, Lund C, and Tobin C: Improved skin care for premature infants, MCN 8:200-203, 1983.

Lewis JF and Alexander JJ: Overnight refrigeration of urine specimens for culture, So Med J 73(3):351-352, 1980.

Lohr J, Donowitz L, and Dudley S: Bacterial contamination rates in voided urine collections in girls, J Pediatr 114(1):91-93, 1989.

Macdonald NE: RSV update: time to alter your clinical approach? J Resp Dis 6(4):11-16, 1985.

Marcoux C, Fisher S, and Wong D: Central venous access devices in children, Pediatr Nurs 16(2):123-133, 1990.

Masters H et al: Comparison of nasopharyngeal washings and swab specimens for diagnosis of respiratory syncytial virus by EIA, FAT, and cell culture, Diagn Microbiol Infect Dis 8:101-105, 1987.

Maul-Mellot SK and Adams JN: Childhood cancer: a nursing overview, Boston, 1987, Jones & Bartlett Publishers Inc.

McConnell D: Urinalysis: a common test, but never routine, Nursing 12(2):108-111, 1982.

McDonald N et al: Efficacy of chlorhexidine cleansing in reducing contamination of bagged urine specimens, Can Med Assoc J 133:1211-1213, 1985.

Meites S and Monte JL: Skin-puncture and blood-collecting techniques for infants, Clin Chem 25(1):183-188, 1979.

Millam DA: How to get into hard-to-stick veins, RN 48(4):34-35, 1985.

Montana J: Glucose meters, J Pediatr Nurs: 4(2):132-136, 1989.

Moore C et al: Nursing care and management of venous access ports, Oncol Nurs Forum, 13(3):35-39, 1986.

Moore DS and Bauer CS: Effect of prepodyne as a perineal cleansing agent for clean catch specimens, Nurs Res 25(4):259-261, 1976.

Morton RE and Lawande R: The diagnosis of urinary tract infection: comparison of urine cultures from suprapubic aspiration and midstream collection in a children's out-patient department in Nigeria, Ann Trop Paediatr 2(3):109-112, 1982.

National Committee for Clinical Laboratory Standards, Publications H3-A2, H14-A, H18-T, H1-A2, Villanova, Penn: 1982, NCCLS.

Nederhand K et al: Respiratory syncytial virus: a nursing perspective, Pediatr Nurs 15(4):342-345, 1989.

Nurse's Reference Library: Diagnostics, Springhouse, Penn, 1981, Intermed Communications, Inc.

O'Rourke A: A bone marrow procedure guide, Oncol Nurs Forum 13(1):66-67, 1986.

Pediatric Alert: Fingersticks, Band-Aids and aspiration—a reader's caution, Pediatric Alert, p 72, Aug 1987.

Perin G and Frase D: Development of a program using general anesthesia for invasive procedures in a pediatric outpatient setting, J Assoc Pediatr Oncol Nurs 3(4):8-10, 1985.

Perry A and Potter P: Clinical nursing skills and techniques, ed 2, St Louis, 1990, The CV Mosby Co.

Pikl BH, editor: Massachusetts General Hospital manual of pediatric nursing practice, Boston, 1981, Little, Brown & Co.

Rademaker M and Kirby JD: Contact dermatitis to a skin adhesive, Contact Dermatitis 16(5):297-298, 1987.

Reams PK and Deane DM: Bagged versus diaper urine specimens and laboratory values. Neonatal Network 6(6):17-20, 1988.

Ross D and Ross S: Stress reduction procedures for the school-age hospitalized leukemic child, Pediatr Nurs 10(6):383-395, 1984.

Rowe PC: The Harriet Lane handbook, Chicago, 1987, Year Book Medical Publishers, Inc.

Saez-Llorens X et al: Bacterial contamination rates for non-clean catch and clean catch midstream urine collections in uncircumcised boys, J Pediatr 114(1): 93-95, 1989.

Sears JR: To prevent reinfestation (author's response), MCN 10(6):377, 1985.

Smith S and Duell D: Clinical nursing skills presented in the nursing process, Los Altos, Calif, 1985, National Nursing Review.

Stebor A: Posturination time and specific gravity in infants' diapers, Nurs Res 38(4):244-245, 1989.

Strobach M and Kratina S: Diaper versus bag specimens; a comparison of urine specific gravity values, MCN 7(3):198-201, 1982.

Suri S: Simplifying urine collection from infants and children without losing accuracy, MCN 13(6):438-441, 1988.

Thomas DO: Are you sure it's only croup? RN 47(12):40-43, 1984.

Traister M: Throat cultures, Topics in Emergency Medicine 5(1):40-46, 1983.

Travis L, Brouhard B, and Schreiner B: Diabetes mellitus in children and adolescents, Philadelphia, 1987, WB Saunders Co.

Treuhaft M, Soukup J, and Sullivan B: Practical recommendations for the detection of pediatric respiratory syncytial virus infections, J Clin Microbiol 2(2):270-273, 1985.

Tucker S et al: Patient care standards: nursing process, diagnosis, and outcomes, ed 4, St Louis, 1988, The CV Mosby Co.

Wagner D: To get a better strep culture, Emerg Med 18(5):152-154, 1986.

Waskerwitz M: Obtaining urine specimens from diapers, J Assoc Pediatr Oncol Nurs 4(1-2):50, 1987.

Wezel-Bolen GV: Technological advances in the care of children with chronic illnesses, Pediatrics: nursing update 1(11), Princeton, NJ, 1986, Continuing Professional Education Center, Inc.

Whaley LF and Wong DL: Essentials of pediatric nursing, ed 3, St Louis, 1989, The CV Mosby Co.

Whaley LF and Wong DL: Nursing care of infants and children, ed 4, St Louis, 1991, The CV Mosby Co.

When worms cause intestinal infection, Patient Care 17(14):257-281, 1983.

Wong D: Personal communication, April 5, 1989.

# UNIT XIX Emergency Measures

# SKILL 126 Performing Cardiopulmonary Resuscitation

*Patricia A. Jamerson*

In infants, children, and adolescents, cardiopulmonary arrest most often occurs following progressive deterioration of respiratory and cardiac function that is usually initiated by a respiratory arrest. Most resuscitations occur in children under 1 year of age with the majority being in infants less than 4 months old (Chameides, 1988). Sudden infant death syndrome (SIDS) is the primary cause of pediatric arrests; other events that may precede an arrest are respiratory illness, accidents, smoke inhalation, and suffocation by foreign objects (e.g., toys, plastic objects, food) (Chameides, 1988). Few children survive cardiopulmonary arrest (7% to 60%); about one third of the children that do survive have neurologic sequelae (Chameides, 1988; Eisenberg, Bergner, and Hallstrom, 1983; Lewis et al, 1983; Fiser and Wrape, 1987; Ludwig, Kittrick, and Parker, 1984; Torphy, Minter, and Thompson, 1984). Early recognition of the child at risk for respiratory arrest and effective management of arrests that do occur can improve the outcomes seen.

## NURSING DIAGNOSES

Ineffective airway clearance related to tracheobronchial obstruction; Altered tissue perfusion (cardiopulmonary, cerebral, renal, or peripheral) related to interruption of arterial/venous blood flow; Potential for injury related to skin and tissue trauma from excessive suctioning, chest compressions, and/or intravenous medication extravasation; Potential for aspiration related to gastric distension from excessive ventilation.

| Steps | Rationale |
|---|---|
| **Assessment (Pre-arrest)** | |
| 1. Assess patency of airway. | Special attention to airway patency is necessary because most arrests in infants and children are respiratory.<br>***Special Considerations:*** *Improper positioning of the head or aspirated objects may occlude the airway. As obligate nose breathers, infants may experience airway obstruction whenever the nose is blocked.* |
| 2. Assess respiratory status. | Noting subtle decompensatory changes in respiratory function enables early recognition and stabilization of a pre-arrest condition. |
| a. Respiratory rate. | ***Special Considerations:*** *Tachypnea is usually the first sign of respiratory distress and may not be accompanied by other signs. As the child fatigues, the rate may decrease within the normal range; this should* not *be misconstrued as a sign of improvement. An ominous sign in the child is bradypnea; whereas, the infant may have periods of apnea.* |

| Steps | Rationale |
|---|---|
| b. Breath sounds. | Abnormal breath sounds such as: stridor (a sign of upper airway obstruction), prolonged expiration accompanied by wheezing (sign of bronchial or bronchiolar obstruction), diminished or absent breath sounds, and grunting are indications of respiratory distress. |
| c. Work of breathing (respiratory effort of accessory muscle use). | Nasal flaring, suprasternal, intercostal, or substernal retractions, head bobbing, and see-saw respirations are all signs of increased respiratory effort. |
| d. Color. | Cyanosis of the mucous membranes may be seen in hypoxia. In older children, cyanotic nail beds may also indicate hypoxia. Cyanosis alone is not a reliable indicator of the degree of hypoxemia and is a late sign of respiratory distress (Hazinski, 1984). |
| 3. Assess cardiovascular status. | The primary responsibility of the cardiovascular system is perfusion of the tissues. When perfusion is inadequate, hypoxia and accumulation of acids within the tissues lead to cellular damage. Detecting early changes in cardiovascular status may prevent such damage. |
| a. Heart rate. | ***Special Considerations:*** *In the presence of hypoxemia, the infant generally responds with bradycardia, whereas the older child is initially tachycardic and becomes bradycardic with further decompensation.* |
| b. Blood pressure. | Hypotension is a late sign of cardiovascular collapse. |
| c. Peripheral pulses. | Thready, absent, or bounding pulses may indicate shock. |
| d. Skin perfusion:<br>▪ Color.<br>▪ Skin temperature.<br>▪ Capillary refill. | Pallor, mottling, peripheral cyanosis, decreased temperature, and prolonged capillary refill (>3 seconds) are early signs of decreased perfusion.<br>***Special Considerations:*** *In neonates, acrocyanosis is normal, but neonates will appear gray or ashen as perfusion diminishes.* |
| e. Level of consciousness. | As perfusion to the brain decreases, there is a progression of observable changes beginning with mood swings (e.g., agitation, confusion, lethargy) to decreased awareness of parents, decreased responsiveness to voice, decreased responsiveness to pain, and finally unresponsiveness. |
| f. Muscle tone. | Muscle tone decreases as perfusion decreases. |
| g. Reflex response. | Reflex response becomes depressed as perfusion diminishes. |
| h. Urine output. | Urine output decreases as tissue perfusion diminishes (<2 ml/kg/hr in the neonate; <1 ml/kg/hr in the child). |
| 4. Determine age of child. | Guidelines of resuscitation vary according to the child's age. The American Heart Association/American Academy of Pediatrics make the following distinctions:<br>▪ Newborn—birth to discharge from hospital.<br>▪ Infant—0-12 months.<br>▪ Child—1-8 years.<br>▪ Adult—8 years and older. |
| 5. In the neonate, review the maternal-fetal history for indicators of asphyxia. | Asphyxia is the major factor leading to a need for resuscitation of the neonate. |
| 6. Review medical history for factors that may influence resuscitative efforts:<br>a. Congenital anomalies.<br>b. Chronic condition (e.g., bronchopulmonary dysplasia).<br>c. Trauma. | Modifications may be necessary to meet special needs of the child. |

## Planning and Goal Setting

| Steps | Rationale |
|---|---|
| 1. Obtain appropriate equipment (Table 126-1) for age and size and keep in highly visible, easily accessible location. | Advance preparation and availability of proper equipment promote a more successful resuscitation because rapid intervention minimizes cellular damage.<br>***Special Considerations:*** *An emergency cart/box should be organized based on priority and accessibility of equipment. Avoid cluttering the cart with unnecessary supplies and equipment.* |

***TABLE 126-1*** **Cardiopulmonary Resuscitation Equipment**

| Equipment | Neonate | Infant | Child | Adolescent |
|---|---|---|---|---|
| Suctioning | Bulb syringe<br>#10 DeLee trap<br>#5-10 catheter | #8-10 catheter | #10-14 catheter | #12-14 catheter |
| Resuscitation Bags | <750 ml | <750 ml | 1000-1500 ml | 1500-2000 ml |
| Masks | Premature<br>Newborn | Infant<br>Child | Child | Small adult/adult |
| Oral airways | 00-0 | 1 | 2-4 | >5 |
| Endotracheal tubes | 2.5-4.0<br>Uncuffed | 3.5-4.0<br>Uncuffed | 4.0-5.5<br>Uncuffed | 6-8<br>Uncuffed/cuffed |
| Laryngoscope blades | 0-1<br>Straight | 1<br>Straight | 1-2<br>Straight/curved | 2-3<br>Straight/curved |
| Orogastric/nasogastric tube | 5-8 Fr. | 8-10 Fr. | 10-14 Fr. | 14-18 Fr. |
| Intravascular catheters | | | | |
| umbilical catheters | 3½, 5 Fr. | | | |
| butterfly | 23-25 gauge | 21-25 gauge | 16-20 | 16-20 |
| over-the-needle | 22-24 gauge | 20-24 gauge | 16-20 | 14-18 |
| Intracath | | 19 gauge | 16 | 14 |

Additional supplies:
Oxygen flowmeter, oxygen tubing, laryngoscope handles and blades, batteries, stylettes, scissors, gloves, syringes, needles, medications, cardiac monitor and electrodes, tape, and stethoscope.

Adapted from Bloom R and Cropley C: *Textbook of neonatal resuscitation,* Dallas, 1987, American Heart Association; and Chameides L: *Textbook of pediatric advanced life support,* Dallas, 1988, American Heart Association.

| Steps | Rationale |
|---|---|
| a. Resuscitation bag with manometer. | ***Special Considerations:*** *Self-inflating and anesthesia bags are available for infants and children. Self-inflating bags should have a reservoir for delivery of nearly 100% oxygen. It is preferable not to have a pop-off valve, but to be able to manually bypass the pressure limits in children with poorly compliant lungs (e.g., near drownings). An in-line manometer provides a means by which to monitor airway pressure (Chameides, 1988). Anesthesia bags require careful adjustment of gas flow and should only be used by individuals skilled in their use.* |
| b. Mask. | Appropriate mask size is critical to achieve an airtight seal. The mask should cover the chin, mouth, and nose without covering the eyes. |
| c. Endotracheal tubes. | Endotracheal tube selection should be based on the child's size. The tube size may be estimated in an emergency by selecting a tube that approximates the outside diameter of the child's little finger. Tubes 0.5 mm smaller and larger than the anticipated size should also be readily available (Chameides, 1988).<br>***Special Considerations:*** *Cuffed tubes are not necessary in children under 8 years as the cricoid cartilage serves as a functional cuff.* |
| d. Laryngoscope blades. | Blade selection is based on the age and size of the child. Straight blades are preferred for neonates and infants to better visualize the glottis, which is cephalad and anterior. |
| e. Oral airway. | Oral airways are available in a variety of sizes. The appropriate size may be estimated by approximating the length of the airway to the distance from the central incisors to the angle of the jaw. Incorrect placement or an airway that is too large displaces the tongue into the pharynx and obstructs the airway (Chameides, 1988). |
| f. Suction devices: catheters and tonsil tip. | Flexible suction catheters are useful for aspirating thin secretions from the endotracheal tube, nasopharynx, or mouth; whereas, tonsil suction is more useful in the removal of thick secretions and particulate matter from the pharynx (Chameides, 1988). |
| g. Intravascular catheters, spinal needle, or bone marrow needle. | Intravenous or intraosseous access is necessary to infuse fluids and certain emergency medications. |
| h. Orogastric tube. | Orogastric tubes are used to decompress air from the stomach and prevent aspiration of gastric contents. |

**TABLE 126-2** Drugs in Neonatal and Pediatric Cardiopulmonary Resuscitation

| Medication/Concentration | Indication | Dose/Route/Frequency | Considerations |
|---|---|---|---|
| Atropine sulfate<br>0.1 mg/ml | Bradycardia accompanied by poor perfusion. | 0.02 mg/kg (0.2 ml/kg)<br>IV, IT, IO<br>May repeat at 5 minute intervals to maximum dose. | Minimum dose is 0.1 mg.<br>Maximum dose is 1 mg in the infant/child and 2 mg in the adolescent.<br>Low doses lead to a paradoxical bradycardia. |
| Bretylium tosylate<br>50 mg/ml | Ventricular fibrillation or tachycardia not responsive to Lidocaine and defibrillation. | 5 mg/kg first dose<br>IV<br>Give over 8-10 minutes in the conscious child. May repeat in 20 minutes with 10 mg/kg. | May worsen dysrhythmias in digitalized child.<br>Nausea, vomiting, hypotension, or hypertension are side effects. |
| Calcium chloride<br>10% solution 100 mg/ml | Hypocalcemia, calcium channel blocker overdose, hyperkalemia, or hypermagnesemia. | 20 mg/kg (0.2 ml/kg)<br>IV<br>May repeat in 10 minutes. | Severe dysrhythmias may develop in digitalized children.<br>May cause significant bradycardia.<br>Flush well after administration to avoid precipitates.<br>Chemical burns may occur if infiltrates.<br>Other calcium salts should not be considered during resuscitation because hepatic metabolism is necessary to deliver ionized calcium. |
| Epinephrine<br>1:10,000 (0.1 mg/ml) | Bradycardia and to enhance response to defibrillation. | 0.01 mg/kg (0.1 ml/kg)<br>IV, IT, IO<br>May be repeated every 5 minutes. | Inactivated by sodium bicarbonate; depressed action in acidosis. |
| Glucose<br>D25W (250 mg/ml)<br>D10W (100 mg/ml) | Hypoglycemia. | 500-1000 mg/kg<br>IV | D25W is very hyperosmolar and may cause sclerosing of the veins or intraventricular hemorrhage in the neonate.<br>Monitor glucose and start infusion. |
| Lidocaine<br>10 mg/ml (1%)<br>20 mg/ml (2%) | Ventricular dysrhythmias. | 1 mg/kg bolus<br>IV, IT, IO<br>May repeat in 10 to 15 minutes. | A continuous infusion should be started if dose is repeated.<br>May cause CNS, myocardial, and circulatory depression. |
| Naloxone<br>0.4 mg/ml<br>1.0 mg/ml | Respiratory depression. | 0.1 mg/kg birth to 20 kg<br>2.0 mg/dose over 20 kg<br>IV, IM, SQ, IT<br>Repeat every 2 to 3 minutes as needed. | May precipitate withdrawal symptoms in the infant of a narcotic-addicted mother. Duration of action is shorter than narcotic action, necessitating readministration. |
| Sodium bicarbonate<br>1 mEq/ml (8.4%)<br>0.5 mEq/ml (4.2%) for neonates | Documented metabolic acidosis. | 1 to 2 mEq/kg or 0.3 × kg × base deficit<br>IV, IO<br>Infuse slowly over minimum of 2 minutes (1 mEq/kg/minute).<br>May repeat every 10 minutes.<br>Total dose for 24 hours not to exceed 8 mEq/kg. | Effective ventilations are necessary to avoid increased acidosis from metabolites of sodium bicarbonate.<br>Tissue necrosis may develop from infiltration into the skin.<br>Flush IV line after administration to avoid precipitate formation.<br>Excessive administration may lead to metabolic acidosis, hypernatremia, hyperosmolarity, and intraventricular hemorrhage. |
| Volume expanders<br>5% albumin<br>Whole blood<br>Blood products<br>Lactated Ringer's<br>Plasmanate<br>Normal saline | Hypovolemia or blood loss resulting in shock. | 10 ml/kg<br>IV, IO<br>Infuse over 5-10 minutes.<br>May be repeated. | Hyperosmolarity may lead to intraventricular hemorrhage or pulmonary edema.<br>Improved perfusion may also correct acidosis. |

Abbreviations: IV = intravenous, IT = intratracheal, IO = intraosseous, IM = intramuscular, SQ = subcutaneous
Adapted from: Bloom R and Cropley C: Textbook of neonatal resuscitation, Dallas, 1987, American Heart Association; Chameides L: Textbook of pediatric advanced life support, Dallas, 1988, American Heart Association; Standards and guidelines for cardiopulmonary (CPR) and emergency cardiac care (ECC), JAMA 255:2905-2984, 1986; Zaritsky A: Cardiopulmonary resuscitation in children, Clin Chest Med 8:561-571, 1987; Emergency drug doses for infants and children and Naloxone use in newborn = clarification, Pediatrics 83:803, 1989.

| Steps | Rationale |
|---|---|
| 2. Check supplies and test equipment for proper function. | A successful resuscitation is partially dependent on properly functioning equipment.<br>***Special Considerations:*** *Facility policy should establish the frequency of these checks.* |
| 3. Maintain familiarity with equipment utilization, location of supplies, and administration of emergency drugs. Maintain certification in resuscitation skills. | Familiarity with skills and equipment promotes better performance in the midst of crisis, resulting in a more successful resuscitation. |
| 4. Precalculate emergency drug doses based on child's weight and post at bedside (Table 126-2). Consider using preprinted information sheets. | Precalculating doses saves time and minimizes errors that may occur during the resuscitation crisis. |
| 5. Develop an individualized child goal:<br>▪ Child will achieve and maintain effective ventilation and adequate tissue perfusion. | |

## Implementation

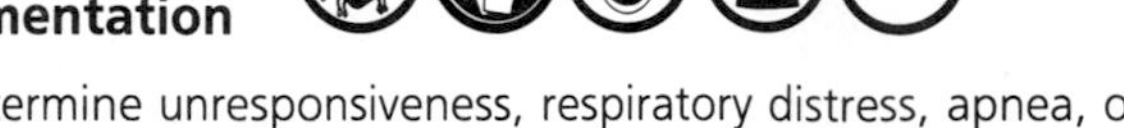

| Steps | Rationale |
|---|---|
| 1. Determine unresponsiveness, respiratory distress, apnea, or pulselessness. | Speed and skill in initiating resuscitative maneuvers helps maintain oxygenation to the brain and other vital organs (Chameides, 1988). |
| 2. Call for help. | A successful resuscitation depends on immediate intervention, preferably with more than one rescuer present. The child should not be left alone for the nurse to obtain equipment and supplies.<br>***Special Considerations:*** *If the family is present, direct a member of the nursing staff or clergy, if possible, to accompany the family to a nearby private location; keep them informed of events.* |
| 3. Position infant/child on back on a flat, firm surface. | The supine position provides accessibility for assessment and intervention.<br>***Special Considerations:*** *An alert child should not be forced to lie down. The child should be allowed to remain with the family and oxygen equipment introduced gradually (Chameides, 1988). The neonate should be placed in a preheated radiant warmer in slight Trendelenberg position. If newly delivered, dry well and remove wet towels to avoid cold stress, which increases oxygen requirements.* |
| 4. Open the airway by positioning the head in a slightly extended position using the head-tilt/chin-lift maneuver (Fig. 126-1). | Proper positioning may eliminate airway obstruction which caused the respiratory arrest.<br>***Special Considerations:*** *The less rigid trachea of the neonate or infant is prone to collapse and airway obstruction if the neck is hyperextended or under extended. In the presence of neck injury, a jaw-thrust maneuver should be used instead.* |
| 5. In the neonate, suction the mouth, then nose with a bulb syringe, DeLee trap, or suction catheter using pressures less than 100 mm/Hg (4 inches Hg) (see Skill 87). | Suctioning may eliminate airway obstruction. The mouth is suctioned first to avoid aspiration of any substances in the oropharynx if the infant would gasp upon suctioning the nose.<br>***Special Considerations:*** *Excessive suction pressures and/or deep suctioning may result in tissue trauma. Vigorous, deep suctioning may also cause vagal stimulation, which may lead to apnea and bradycardia (Bloom and Cropley, 1987).* |
| 6. Observe for respiratory effort.<br>a. Place ear close to child's mouth and nose.<br>b. Watch for rise and fall of chest and abdomen.<br>c. Listen for exhaled air.<br>d. Feel for exhaled air. | Positioning and or suctioning may eliminate airway obstruction that resulted in respiratory arrest. |
| 7. If no spontaneous respirations are noted, initiate positive pressure ventilations by mouth or with a resuscitation bag, watching for a rise and fall of the chest. | Ventilations are the most important resuscitation step and should be initiated as soon as possible to avoid cardiac arrest from prolonged hypoxemia.<br>***Special Considerations:*** *In the neonate try flicking or slapping the sole of the foot two or three times before initiating ventilations.* |

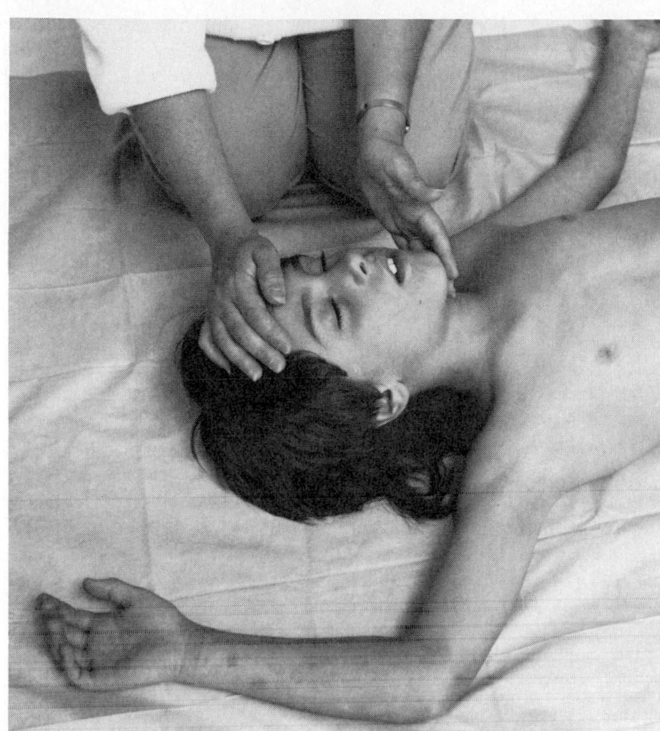

***FIG. 126-1*** The head-tilt/chin-lift maneuver.

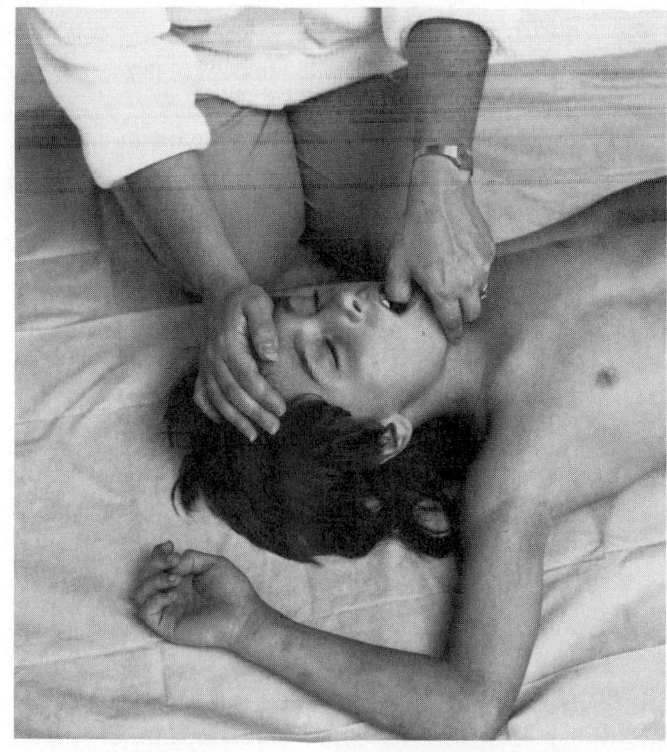

***FIG. 126-2*** The tongue-jaw lift.

| Steps | Rationale |
|---|---|
| a. Resuscitation bag: Using a bag and mask or bag and endotracheal tube, provide 90% to 100% oxygen by the following parameters. | ***Special Considerations:*** *A resuscitation bag needs to be readily accessible for the neonate at all times.* |
| *Neonate:* | |
| At a flow rate of 5 liters/minute (lpm) deliver 40 to 60 breaths per minute at the following pressures: | |
| ▪ First 2 to 3 breaths (in newly delivered): 30 to 40 cm $H_2O$. | Two to three times normal lung pressures are needed to initially expand the alveoli (Bloom and Cropley, 1987). |
| ▪ Normal lungs: 15 to 20 cm $H_2O$. | |
| ▪ Chronic lung disease: 20 to 40 cm $H_2O$. | |
| *Infant/child/adolescent:* | |
| At a flow rate of 10 to 15 lpm, deliver two slow breaths (1 to 1.5 seconds per breath). Deliver subsequent breaths at a rate of: ▪ Infant: 20 breaths per minute. ▪ Child: 15 breaths per minute. ▪ Adolescent: 12 breaths per minute. | Giving breaths slowly allows an adequate volume of air to be delivered at the lowest possible pressure, preventing gastric distension (Chameides, 1988). ***Special Considerations:*** *The flow rate varies with an anesthesia bag. Minimums required to prevent hypercarbia are 2 lpm in children less than 10 kg, 4 lpm in children between 10 and 50 kg, and 6 lpm in children over 50 kg (Chameides, 1988).* |
| b. Mouth: *Infant:* ▪ Form tight seal by placing mouth over infant's mouth and nose. ▪ Using just enough pressure to cause the chest to rise, give two slow (1 to 1.5 seconds per breath) ventilations, allowing the chest to deflate between breaths. ▪ Continue at a rate of 20 breaths per minute. *Child/adolescent:* ▪ Form tight seal by placing mouth over child's mouth and pinching the nose. ▪ Using just enough pressure to cause the chest to rise, give two slow (1 to 1.5 seconds per breath) ventilations, allowing the chest to deflate between breaths. ▪ Continue at the following rates: (1) Child—15 breaths per minute. (2) Adolescent—12 breaths per minute. | |
| 8. If resistance to air flow is met, troubleshoot and make appropriate corrections. Insert an oral airway if resistance persists. | Inadequate seal or airway obstruction caused by inappropriate head position, secretions, or foreign objects in the airway may create resistance to air flow. ***Special Considerations:*** *Soft tissues or congenital abnormalities (e.g., choanal atresia) may interfere with effective ventilations. Ineffective ventilations which persist may be an indication to use more pressure or a need for intubation; however, increased rates and pressures may lead to pneumothoraces.* |
| 9. If resistance persists, suspect foreign body airway obstruction. Take steps to relieve the obstruction. *Infant:* Deliver a series of four back blows and four chest thrusts. Repeat series following a breathing attempt (see Step 7). a. Straddle infant over the rescuer's arm or lay infant across the rescuer's lap with the head lower than the trunk and firmly supported. b. Use opposite hand to forcefully deliver 4 back flows (Fig. 126-3). c. Turn the infant as a unit on the rescuer's thigh, head still lower than trunk. d. Provide chest thrusts by performing slow chest compressions (see step 12). | ***Special Considerations:*** *Methods used to relieve foreign body obstruction are considered controversial. At this time, no interference is recommended if the child can cry, cough, or breathe. Blind finger sweeps are contraindicated as the foreign object may be pushed farther down the airway. However, visualized foreign objects may be removed using the tongue-jaw lift (Chameides, 1988) (Fig. 126-2). Assisted ventilations should not be used in the conscious child. If the first breath provided after attempts to relieve airway obstruction is successful, a second breath can be given before resuming resuscitative measures. If the breath is unsuccessful, the series of maneuvers should be repeated.* ***Special Considerations:*** *The Heimlich Maneuver is not used on infants because of the risk of intraabdominal trauma.* |
| *Child/adolescent:* Perform Heimlich maneuver. Repeat maneuver after a breathing attempt until obstruction is relieved (see step 7). | |
| a. Place heel of one hand on top of the other between the umbilicus and xiphoid process (Fig. 126-4). | ***Special Considerations:*** *Emesis may occur. Suction equipment should be readily available to prevent potential aspiration.* |
| b. Deliver 6 to 10 quick upward abdominal thrusts into the abdomen. | |

| **Steps** | **Rationale** |
|---|---|

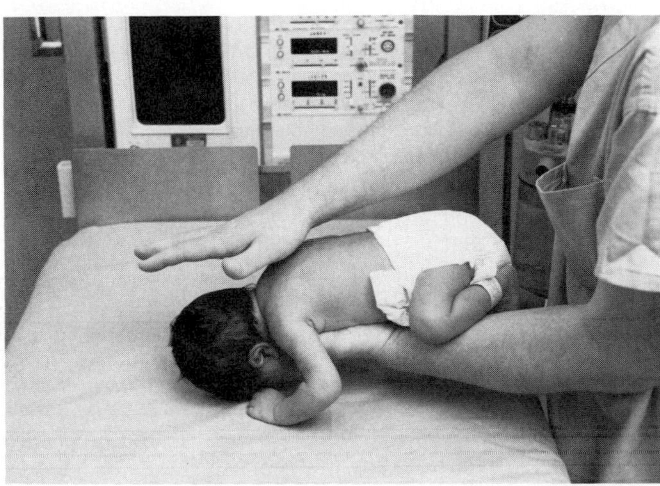

***FIG. 126-3*** Delivering back blows to infant.

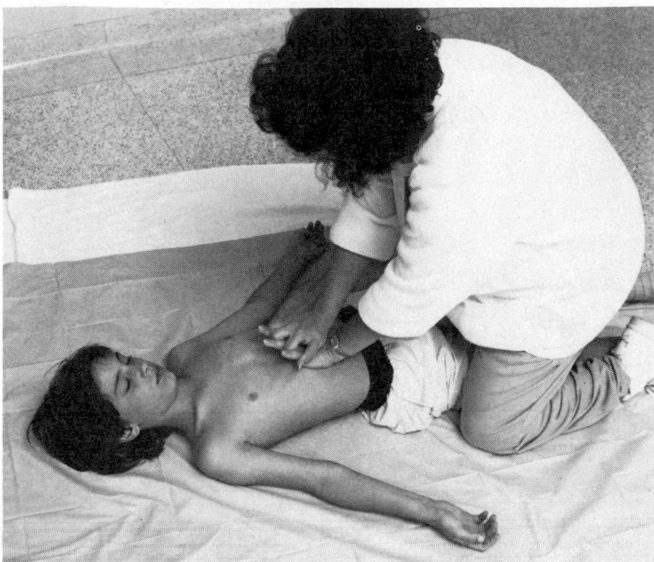

***FIG. 126-4*** Placement of hands for Heimlich maneuver.

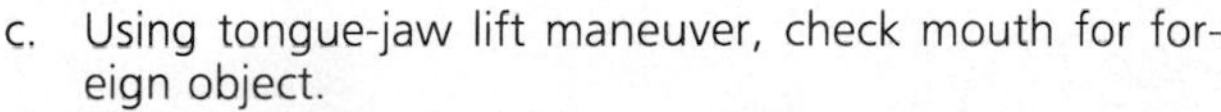

c. Using tongue-jaw lift maneuver, check mouth for foreign object.

d. If foreign object is visible, use finger sweep to remove.

10. Evaluate heart rate and pulses.

*Neonate:* Auscultate apically for 6 seconds after 15 to 30 seconds of effective ventilations.

The apical route provides an accurate method of determining the heart rate.

***Special Considerations:*** *Misinformation about the heart rate may be obtained by evaluating the umbilical cord or peripheral pulses. Peripheral pulses may be difficult to palpate and are easily obliterated in the neonate. Pulsations through the umbilical cord rarely persist past the first minute of life. Palpation of the carotid artery is contraindicated in neonates and infants because airway obstruction may occur.*

*Infant:* Palpate brachial pulse for presence of pulsations by lightly placing index finger just above the antecubital space on the side closest to the body (Fig. 126-5).

*Child/adolescent:* Gently palpate carotid artery for pulsations.

The carotid artery is the most accessible, and pulsations will persist when peripheral pulses are no longer palpable (American Medical Association, 1986).

***Special Considerations:*** *Because of vagal stimulation, slowing of the heart rate may occur by applying pressure to the carotid artery.*

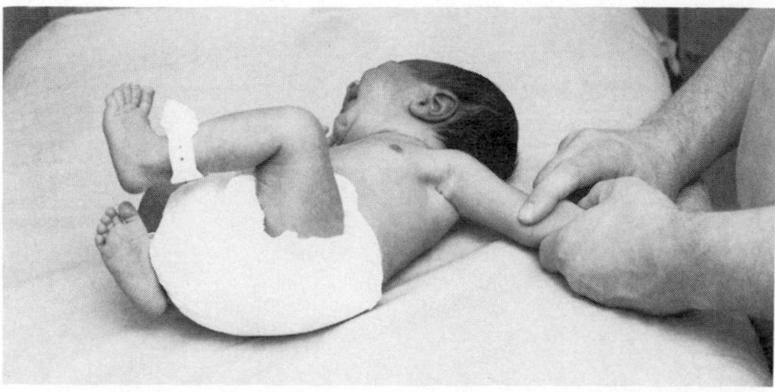

***FIG. 126-5*** Palpation of brachial pulse in infant.

**Steps** | 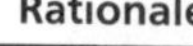 **Rationale**

11. Initiate chest compressions if the following criteria are noted:
*Neonate:* A heart rate below 60 bpm or between 60 to 80 bpm and not rising.
*Infant/child/adolescent:* Absence of pulsations.

Cardiac compressions mechanically generate cardiac output. Cardiac output is insufficient to maintain tissue perfusion when the neonate is bradycardic.

12. Use proper technique to provide chest compressions. Do not take digits or heel of hand off child's skin between compressions.

Improper technique may lead to pneumothoraces, fractured ribs, or laceration of the liver. Maintaining skin contact between compressions prevents loss of positioning on the sternum.

***Special Considerations:*** *Adult mechanical devices to depress the sternum should not be used on children (American Medical Association, 1986). Child-sized devices are not available.*

*Neonate:*

a. Place digits over sternum just below the nipple line.
b. Deliver at a rate of 120 bpm in a ratio of 3 compressions to 1 breath.
c. Depress to a depth of ½ to ¾ inch.

***Special Considerations:*** *There are two acceptable techniques to use in providing chest compressions in the neonate. (Bloom and Cropley, 1987).*

1. *Thaler (two-thumb method): The thumbs are placed side-by-side or directly on top of one another, while the fingers encircle the chest (Fig. 126-6).*
2. *Two-finger method: The tips of the middle and index or middle and ring fingers are used to compress the chest while the other hand provides back support. The fingers should be perpendicular to the sternum (Fig. 126-7).*

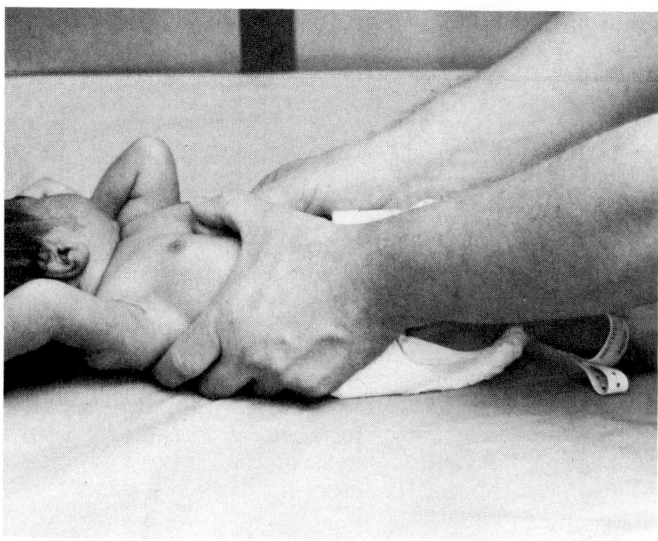

***FIG. 126-6*** Thumb placement for Thaler method.

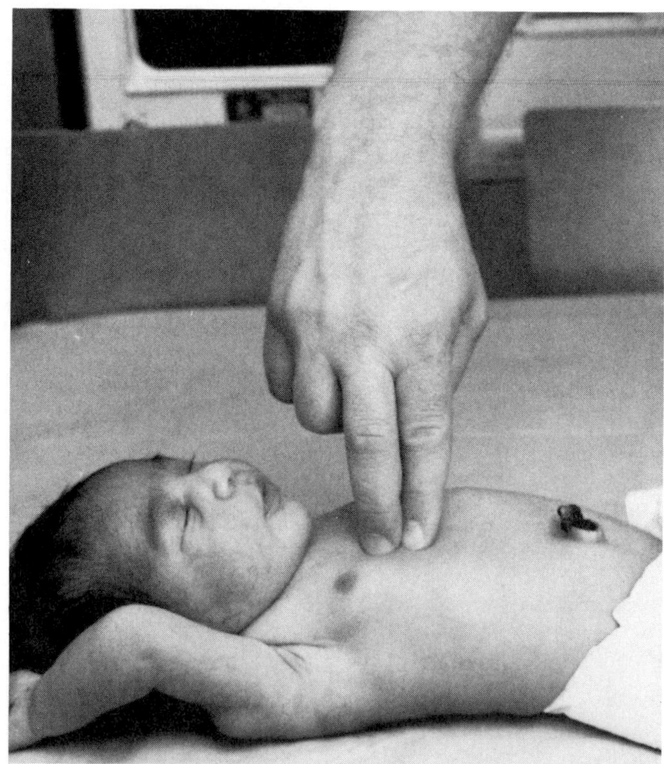

***FIG. 126-7*** Placement of the two-finger method of chest compression.

*Infant:*

a. Position fingers over sternum one finger width below nipple line.
b. Deliver at a rate of 100 bpm and a ratio of 5 compressions per breath.
c. Depress sternum ½ to 1 inch.

*Child/adolescent:* Locate placement by sliding middle finger along lower edge of ribcage to notch where ribs and sternum meet (Fig. 126-8).

| **Steps** | **Rationale** |
|---|---|

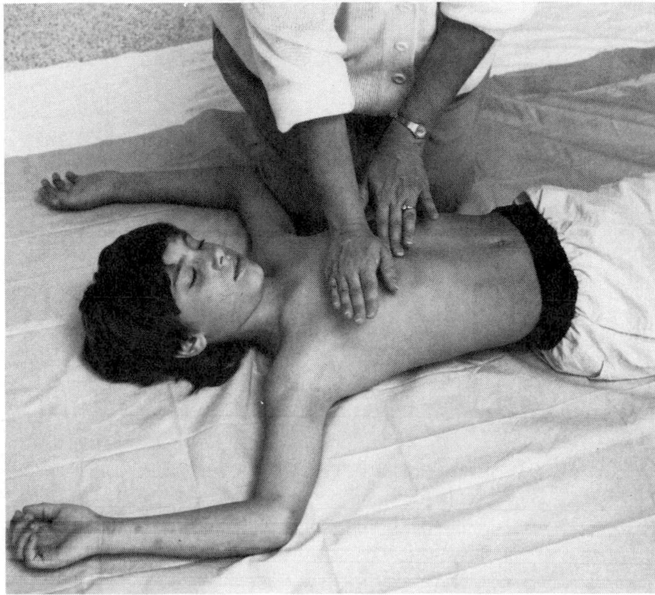

***FIG. 126-8*** Locating placement for chest compression in the older child/adolescent.

*Child:*
a. Place heel of hand next to index finger on sternum.
b. Deliver at a rate of 80 to 100 bpm in a ratio of 5 compressions per breath.
c. Depress sternum 1 to 1½ inches.

*Adolescent:*
a. Place heel of hand next to index finger on sternum. Place other hand on top, locking fingers to avoid touching the chest.
b. Deliver 80 to 100 compressions per minute in a ratio of 15 compressions to 2 breaths.
c. Depress sternum to a depth of 1½ to 2 inches.

13. Reevaluate heart rate and pulses throughout resuscitative effort:
    *Neonate:* Auscultate apical rate every 30 seconds.
    *Infant/child:* Palpate pulses after 10 cycles of compressions and breaths.
    *Adolescent:* Palpate pulses after 4 cycles of compressions and breaths.

Further indications for intervention are based on the heart rate.
***Special Considerations:*** *In the delivery room the Apgar score may be used to help evaluate resuscitation. The Apgar should be reevaluated every 5 minutes until a score of 8 or better is achieved or resuscitation measures are discontinued. Since resuscitative measures should be instituted before the 1 minute score is obtained, the Apgar cannot be used as a guide to resuscitation (Bloom and Cropley, 1987).*

14. Discontinue compressions when the following criteria are met or resuscitative efforts are aborted.
    *Neonate:* Heart rate is 80 beats per minute (bpm) or above.
    *Infant/child/adolescent:* Palpable pulses are present.
15. Continue positive pressure ventilations as described after ceasing chest compressions until the following criteria are met or resuscitative efforts are aborted.
    *Neonate:* Ventilate 40 times per minute until heart rate exceeds 100 bpm and spontaneous respirations are present.
    *Infant:* Ventilate 20 times per minute until spontaneous respirations are present.
    *Child:* Ventilate once every 4 seconds until spontaneous respirations are present.
    *Adolescent:* Ventilate once every 5 seconds until spontaneous respirations are present.

| Steps | Rationale |
|---|---|
| 16. Assist with intubation if ventilations are ineffective, the child is unable to protect airway (gag reflex absent), prolonged artificial ventilation is required, or direct suctioning of the trachea is necessary. | Endotracheal intubation provides direct airway access and a more effective means of ventilation.<br>***Special Considerations:*** *The endotracheal tube may be used as an alternate route for the administration of certain emergency medications (see Table 126-2). Intubation is also indicated if a diaphragmatic hernia exists to eliminate gastric distension. Direct suctioning of the trachea is necessary if the infant has not yet taken a breath or cried, and thick meconium is present.* |
| a. Before intubation assemble necessary equipment and check for function (see Table 126-1 for sizes):<br>▪ Laryngoscope handle.<br>▪ Laryngoscope blade.<br>▪ Suction catheter or tonsil suction.<br>▪ Resuscitation bag and mask.<br>▪ Oxygen source.<br>▪ Tape. | Preparation and evaluation of equipment minimizes unnecessary delays and additional trauma. |
| b. While preparing to intubate, continue artificial ventilations with a bag-valve-mask using 100% oxygen. | Oxygenation should be maintained to prevent additional hypoxemia. |
| c. Provide free-flow oxygen during intubation attempt. | An oxygen-enriched environment minimizes hypoxia that may occur during intubation procedure. |
| d. Limit intubation attempts to 20 seconds; provide bag-mask ventilation between attempts. | Prolonged attempts at intubation may result in profound hypoxemia since ventilation is interrupted. |
| e. Monitor heart rate continuously during attempt. Terminate intubation attempt and provide bag-mask ventilations with 100% oxygen if:<br>▪ Infant's heart rate drops below 80 bpm.<br>▪ Child's heart rate drops below 60 bpm. | Intubation may cause vagal stimulation resulting in bradycardia. |
| f. After intubation confirm placement by:<br>▪ Observing for chest expansion upon ventilation.<br>▪ Auscultating for equal, bilateral breath sounds.<br>▪ Observing for condensation of water vapor in endotracheal tube.<br>▪ Obtaining chest x-ray after tube has been secured with tape. | Proper placement is essential to avoid profound hypoxemia and gastric distension.<br>***Special Considerations:*** *In infants and neonates the stomach should also be auscultated to rule out intubation of the esophagus. The thin chest wall allows radiation of ventilated sounds from the stomach to the lung fields, providing misleading information.* |
| g. Note and record centimeter marking on endotracheal tube at gum line. | Notation of tube placement provides baseline information that can be used to periodically validate present position. |
| h. Avoid excessive motion of the head and neck (see Skill 94). | Neck flexion may move the endotracheal tube further into the airway while neck extension or rotation may lead to extubation. |
| 17. Obtain vascular access using the largest, most accessible vein that does not require interruption of resuscitation (see Skill 97). | Vascular access is necessary to administer fluid and certain medications and to obtain blood specimens.<br>***Special Considerations:*** *Vascular access may be difficult to obtain, particularly in children under 3 years old. An intraosseous route may be used in this age group for the administration of fluids and medications (Peck and Altieri, 1988).* |
| 18. Correctly administer emergency medications as determined by weight and route (see Table 126-2). The preferred routes in order of priority are: | Medications are used to stimulate the heart rate, improve perfusion, correct metabolic acidosis and correct dysrhythmias and electrolyte imbalance.<br>***Special Considerations:*** *Atropine is not recommended in the neonatal period, nor is calcium unless there is a documented hypocalcemia (Bloom and Cropley, 1987).* |
| a. Central venous (femoral, internal and external jugular, subclavian and umbilical veins). | A more rapid onset and higher peak concentration is obtained through central venous administration (Chameides, 1988). |
| b. Peripheral venous (scalp, cephalic, basilic, antecubital, saphenous, and dorsal arch of the hand or foot) (see Skill 97). | Peripheral veins provide numerous sites for the administration of fluids and medications.<br>***Special Considerations:*** *Vascular access may be difficult in the child that is perfusing poorly. Supradiaphragmatic vessels provide better delivery of medication into the system than vessels below the diaphragm (American Medical Association, 1986). Scalp vessels are impractical during resuscitative measures (Chameides, 1988).* |
| c. Intraosseous (tibia in infants and young children). | The intraosseous route is a relatively safe and effective route to administer fluids, epinephrine, whole blood, calcium, lidocaine, atropine, and sodium bicarbonate (Chameides, 1988). |

| Steps | Rationale |
|---|---|
| d. Endotracheal tube. | The endotracheal tube may be used for administration of certain medications (see Table 126-2) when vascular access is not available.<br>***Special Considerations:*** *Utilizing a feeding tube to instill the medication and diluting the drug with 1 to 2 ml of normal saline may aid delivery to the lower tracheobronchial tree.* |
| 19. Insert a nasogastric or orogastric tube if positive pressure ventilations are provided longer than 2 minutes. | During ventilation air enters the esophagus, causing gastric distension, upward displacement of the diaphragm, decreased lung capacity, and an increased risk of aspiration. Placement of a gastric tube decompresses the stomach and helps prevent aspiration (Bloom and Cropley, 1987).<br>***Special Considerations:*** *As obligate nose breathers, infants may develop respiratory distress from the use of a nasogastric tube.* |
| 20. Direct attention to correction of acidosis, hypoxemia, hypothermia, hypocalcemia, and/or hypoglycemia while continuing cardiopulmonary resuscitation and emergency drug therapy. | During the course of resuscitative efforts, other serious problems may develop that require intervention. |

| Evaluation Outcomes | Observational Guidelines |
|---|---|
| 1. Basic and advanced life support measures are provided promptly and without interruption. | Evaluate timing and sequence of events; review written record. |
| 2. Child is adequately oxygenated and ventilated; perfusion is maintained. | Assess respiratory rate, effort, and breath sounds. Monitor blood gases, pulse oximetry, and/or transcutaneous readings. Assess heart rate, rhythm, and pulse characteristics. Monitor blood pressure. Assess color and capillary refill. Assess level of consciousness, muscle tone, and reflex response. Monitor urine output, electrolyte levels, BUN, and creatinine. |
| 3. Child experiences minimal or no complications as a result of resuscitative measures. | Compare postarrest with prearrest neurologic status. Assess airway for signs of trauma. Note bruises and lacerations of chest. Monitor for signs/symptoms of pneumothorax, fractured ribs, and lacerated liver. Assess for abdominal distension. Assess IV site for patency, extravasation, and chemical burns. |

## Documentation

Document the events preceding the arrest, and the time and type of arrest. Note interventions performed, the personnel involved, and the child's response to interventions. Indicate the time and child's status when resuscitation efforts stopped.

UNIT XIX

### PRODUCT REFERENCES AND TEACHING RESOURCES

Wong DL and Whaley LF: Clinical manual of pediatric nursing, ed 3, St Louis, 1990, The CV Mosby Co.
Includes home care instructions for Infant CPR, Child CPR, Caring for the choking infant, and caring for the choking child.

### REFERENCES

American Medical Association: Standards and guidelines for cardiopulmonary (CPR) and emergency cardiac care (ECC), JAMA 255:2905-2984, 1986.

Bloom R and Cropley C: Textbook of neonatal resuscitation, Dallas, 1987, American Heart Association.

Chameides L: Textbook of pediatric advanced life support, Dallas, 1988, American Heart Association.

Eisenberg M, Bergner L, and Hallstrom A: Epidemiology of cardiac arrest and resuscitation in children, Ann Emerg Med 12:627-674, 1983.

Emergency drug doses for infants and children and Naloxone use in newborn = clarification, Pediatrics 83:803, 1989.

Fiser D and Wrape V: Outcome of cardiopulmonary resuscitation in children, Pediatr Emerg Care 3:235-238, 1987.

Hazinski MF: Nursing care of the critically ill child, St Louis, 1984, The CV Mosby Co.

Lewis J et al: Outcome of pediatric resuscitation, Ann Emerg Med 12:297-299, 1983.

Ludwig S, Kittrick R, and Parker M: Pediatric cardiopulmonary resuscitation, Clin Pediatr 23:71-75, 1984.

Peck KR and Altieri M: Intraosseous infusions: an old technique with modern applications, Pediatr Nurs 14(4):296-298, 1988.

Torphy D, Minter M, and Thompson B: Cardiopulmonary arrest and resuscitation of children, Am Dis Child 128:1099-1102, 1984.

Wong DL and Whaley LF: Clinical manual of pediatric nursing, ed 3, St Louis, 1990, The CV Mosby Co.

Zaritsky A: Cardiopulmonary resuscitation in children, Clin Chest Med 8:561-571, 1987.

# APPENDIX A Immunizations

Rosemary Liguori

Providing appropriate immunizations to prevent many of the serious childhood infectious diseases is a complex process that includes an awareness of the issues, controversies, and risks involved. Information must be provided in a sensitive, professional manner to achieve the primary goal of protecting the child's health.

Nursing responsibility for immunizations extends far beyond actual administration of the vaccine. The nurse must:

1. Possess a thorough knowledge of the current American Academy of Pediatrics' (1988) recommended immunization schedule (Table A-1). Familiarity with the alternative schedule for children not immunized in the first year of life (American Academy of Pediatrics, 1988) is also essential. Because recommendations are subject to change or vary because of research findings, the discovery of new vaccines, and increased levels of incidence or outbreaks of a disease, nurses must seek to acquire up-to-date information.
2. Cultivate an awareness of the issues and controversies present in immunization administration (see the box on p. 810). An assessment of the family's beliefs, values, and feelings is required to identify barriers to compliance with an immunization schedule. The family must be informed in a calm, professional, and accurate manner of the side effects and risks of immunization (see the box on p. 811), in addition to the risks of not being immunized.
3. Screen for possible contraindications or exceptions to specific vaccines. Minor, nonfebrile illnesses do *not* make the use of a vaccine inadvisable. Febrile illnesses are considered on an individual basis according to the vaccine and the likelihood that delaying immunization will result in the child not receiving the vaccine at the desired age. Careful assessment for contraindications or exceptions is instrumental in helping to prevent or minimize inherent immunization risks (see Table A-2).
4. Know the product type and recommended route of administration (see Table A-3 and the box on p. 813, Step 2). Concurrent with the responsibility to properly administer the vaccine is the nurse's obligation to minimize minor reactions that may accompany immunizations (see the box on p. 813). Review the side effects and risks for the specific vaccine with the family so that they will be prepared for the commonly occurring, mild, temporary reactions and will recognize signs of more severe reactions that warrant contacting a practitioner.

Following administration, document in the child's permanent record as required by the National Childhood Vaccine Injury Act of 1988 for childhood mandated vaccines (American Academy of Pediatrics, 1988): 1) type of vaccine; 2) date of administration; 3) manufacturer and lot number; and 4) name, address, and title of person administering vaccine. Additional documentation should include route of administration and site (if parenteral), expiration date of the vaccine, and all pertinent data concerning risks, benefits, side effects, and steps taken to minimize reactions. Reporting of significant adverse reactions is also required (American Academy of Pediatrics, 1988).

## INFORMATIONAL MATERIALS FOR PARENTS

Lederle Biologicals
A Division of American Cyanamid Company
Wayne, New Jersey 07470
Offers: Immunization and your child's health (363-7).

Hib Infection–Suite 1900
40 West 57th St.
New York, NY 10019
Offers: Your child and Hib infection. Send a self-addressed stamped envelope.

## UPDATES AND CONTROVERSIES REGARDING SPECIFIC VACCINES

### *HAEMOPHILUS INFLUENZAE* TYPE b (Hib)

Until 1985 little protection from the devastating effects of the Hib bacterium existed. In that year, a vaccine from the Hib capsular polysaccharide (polyribosylribitol phosphate [PRP]) was licensed for use with children ages 2 to 5 (Campion and Casto, 1988). Unfortunately, the highest risk age group for Hib is infants, and the vaccine failed to consistently elicit a protective response in younger children.

In 1987 an Hib conjugate vaccine (Hib polysaccharide covalently bound to diphtheria toxoid [PRP-D]) was licensed for use. This new conjugate induces a greater immune response at a younger age than the PRP, and the immune response is longer lasting. The PRP-D may be given simultaneously with the DTP at different sites. The safety of simultaneous administration with oral polio vaccine or measles-mumps-rubella vaccine has not been established.

In 1988 an alternate Hib vaccine was licensed—the HbOC (*Haemophilus* b conjugate vaccine [diphtheria $CRM_{197}$ protein conjugate]). The HbOC is considered equal to the PRP-D in safety, cost, and inferred efficacy, so administration of either vaccine is recommended for protection from Hib infection (American Academy of Pediatrics, 1989). No serious adverse reactions have been reported with either vaccine; only minor local swelling, tenderness, and fever have been reported (Campion and Casto, 1988; American Academy of Pediatrics, 1989). Previously, a single dose of the vaccine at 18 months was recommended; the recommended age has now been changed to 15 months (JAMA, 1990). Efficacy is being determined for children younger than 15 months. Children who have invasive Hib infection before 24 months of age should still be immunized because the immune response may not have been complete (Centers for Disease Control, 1988).

### MEASLES (Rubeola)

Far from being eradicated, widespread outbreaks of this potentially serious, even fatal, disease continue, especially in recent years. Cases are analyzed by the Centers for Disease Control to determine whether they were preventable (occurring in persons for whom the vaccine is currently recommended) or nonpreventable. The majority of nonpreventable cases (60% to 72%) occur in school and college-aged persons who have been immunized (American Academy of Pediatrics, 1989; Grimes and Woolbert, 1989), many at the age of 9 to 12 months, but it was later determined that maternal antibodies interfered with the immune response at this age. Therefore, in 1976 the recommended age for vaccination was changed to 15 months. In 1989 the American Academy of Pediatrics issued new immunization guidelines to further address potential gaps in coverage: 1) in addition to the routine dose now given at 15 months, give a second dose of MMR at entrance to middle or junior high school; 2) for high-risk areas, vaccinate children at 12 months of age, then again as above; 3) during outbreaks in high-risk areas, monovalent measles vaccine may be given to infants as young as 6 months, following the above recommendations for two routine doses later; and 4) revaccinate all children born after 1957 who have not received two doses after 12 months of age. More changes are likely in the future as research continues with this particularly resistant disease.

### PERTUSSIS

Pertussis vaccine (in the combined DTP) has incurred well-publicized controversy about adverse reactions. It may cause severe systemic reactions, especially transient or permanent central nervous system disorders. However, the sequelae of pertussis disease are similarly grave and pose a risk to a greater proportion of the population. Careful screening for contraindications and exceptions to administering the DTP minimizes the likelihood of serious adverse reactions.

Children who experience mild to moderate reactions to the pertussis vaccine (e.g., redness, edema, induration and tenderness at the site, fretfulness, vomiting, crying, and mild to moderate fever) should continue to receive it according to schedule, although the child will likely have the same reaction upon subsequent doses (American Academy of Pediatrics, 1988). Nurses should also be aware that many alleged serious vaccine reactions can be attributed to other coincidentally occurring factors (American Academy of Pediatrics, 1988). For example, Griffin et al (1990) reported that serious neurological events are rarely if ever caused by DTP immunizations in a child who was previously normal without a prior history of seizures. There is also no evidence of an increased risk of Sudden Infant Death Syndrome (SIDS) after receiving the vaccine (Griffin, 1988). New formulations are under investigation in the United States and other countries for a vaccine that will cause fewer reactions (Katz, 1987).

### POLIOMYELITIS

The introduction of the inactivated polio virus (IPV) vaccine by Salk in the mid-1950s and the Sabin oral attenuated polio virus (OPV) vaccine in the early 1960s has almost completely eliminated the threat of paralytic polio in the United States. Irregularities associated with the two vaccines, especially the OPV, require careful consideration for safe immunization. The IPV is reportedly very safe but less effective than the OPV both in conferring lifelong immunity and in preventing gastrointestinal tract replication of wild polio viruses encountered in nature. An enhanced potency IPV is currently available and efficacy studies are under way (American Academy of Pediatrics, 1988).

The OPV is linked to a rare risk (1 in 2.5 million doses) of vaccine-associated paralysis. This paralysis often affects the unimmunized, partially immunized, or immunodeficient family members of the recipient, who are exposed to the excreted vaccine. Vaccine-associated paralysis is far more likely to occur following the first OPV dose rather than subsequent doses.

Because of this risk, assessment of the child and close contacts is indicated before administering a polio vaccine. If the child or anyone in the household is immunodeficient, IPV is recommended. It is also recommended that unimmunized family members of the child scheduled for an OPV vaccine receive two doses of IPV before the child's dose (American Academy of Pediatrics, 1988). There is concern that the extra appointment needed may result in failure to comply with the child's immunization (Katz, 1987), however, it minimizes the vaccine-associated paralysis risk to the adult members. Although OPV is currently recommended for routine immunization, future recommendations may change based on enhanced potency IVP investigations.

## IMMUNIZATIONS WITH REPORTED REACTIONS

### DTP

**Mild (within 2 days)**

1. Temperature elevation (101° F to 103° F) for 24 to 48 hours.
2. Redness, edema, induration, tenderness at injection site.
3. Irritable, fretful behavior.
4. Anorexia, vomiting.
5. Change in sleep patterns (more or less than usual).
6. Transient urticarial rashes.

**Severe (within 2 days)**

1. Anaphylactic allergic reaction to vaccine—rare.
2. Temperature of 104.9° F or greater.
3. Persistent, unconsolable crying for 3 hours or more.
4. High-pitched, unusual crying.
5. Convulsion (with or without fever).
6. Collapse with a shocklike state (hypotonic-hyporesponsive).
7. Encephalopathy within 3 to 7 days (1:140,000 doses): severe alterations of consciousness and focal neurologic signs. Permanent neurologic deficits occur in approximately one-third of these cases (1:330,000) (American Academy of Pediatrics, 1988).

### OPV

**Rare**

1. Paralytic polio in recipients and close contacts (1:2.5 million doses) (Katz, 1987).

### MMR

**Mild (5 to 15 days)**

1. Fever of 103° F or higher.
2. Transient rash.
3. Lymphadenopathy.
4. Febrile seizures.
5. Aching and swelling of joints.
6. Pain, numbness, tingling sensation of feet and hands (rare).

**Severe**

1. CNS reaction, including encephalitis and encephalopathy (1:3 million doses).
2. Chronic arthritis (rare).
3. Nerve deafness; orchitis (rare).

### Hib VACCINE

**Mild**

1. Local site irritation (redness and swelling).
2. Temperature elevation of 101° F or higher, within 24 hours.

***TABLE A-1*** **Recommended Schedule for Active Immunization of Normal Infants and Children***

| Recommended Age | Immunization(s)† | Comments |
|---|---|---|
| 2 months | DTP, OPV | Can be initiated as early as age 2 weeks in areas of high endemicity or during epidemics |
| 4 months | DTP, OPV | 2-month interval desired for OPV to avoid interference from previous dose |
| 6 months | DTP | A third dose of OPV is not indicated in the United States but is desirable in geographic areas where polio is endemic |
| 15 months | Measles, mumps, rubella (MMR) | MMR preferred to individual vaccines; tuberculin testing may be done at the same visit |
| 18 months | DTP,‡§ OPV,‖ PRP-D | See footnotes |
| 4-6 years | DTP,¶ OPV | At or before school entry |
| 14-16 years | Td | Repeat every 10 years throughout life |

*For all products used, consult manufacturer's package insert for instructions for storage, handling, dosage, and administration. Biologics prepared by different manufacturers may vary, and package inserts of the same manufacturer may change from time to time. Therefore, the physician should be aware of the contents of the current package insert.

†DTP = diphtheria and tetanus toxoids with pertussis vaccine; OPV = oral poliovirus vaccine containing attenuated poliovirus types 1, 2, and 3; MMR = live measles, mumps, and rubella viruses in a combined vaccine; PRP-D = *Haemophilus* b diphtheria toxoid conjugate vaccine; Td = adult tetanus toxoid (full dose) and diphtheria toxoid (reduced dose) for adult use.

‡Should be given 6 to 12 months after the third dose.

§May be given simultaneously with MMR at age 15 months.

‖May be given simultaneously with MMR at 15 months of age or at any time between 12 and 24 months of age.

¶Up to the seventh birthday.

AUTHOR'S NOTE: Recent updates to these recommendations include: 1) use of either PRP-D or the newly licensed HbOC (*Haemophilus* b conjugate vaccine [diphtheria $CRM_{197}$ protein conjugate]) for immunization against *Haemophilus influenzae* type b at 15 months of age (American Academy of Pediatrics, Committee on Infectious Diseases: *Haemophilus influenzae* type b conjugate vaccines: update, Pediatrics 84(2):386-387, 1989; JAMA, 1990; and 2) a second dose of MMR at entrance to middle or junior high school (American Academy of Pediatrics, Committee on Infectious Diseases: Measles: reassessment of the current immunization policy, Pediatrics 84(6):1110-1113, 1989.

From Report of the Committee on Infectious Diseases, ed 21, 1988, Elk Grove Village, Ill, American Academy of Pediatrics.

**TABLE A-2** Contraindications to Routine Immunizations

| Contraindications (exceptions) | Rationale | Nursing considerations |
|---|---|---|
| **DIPHTHERIA, TETANUS, PERTUSSIS (DTP)** | | |
| Febrile illness (Minor, nonfebrile illness is not a contraindication) | Signs and symptoms associated with the illness may be erroneously attributed to the vaccine | Explain reason for postponement to family and reschedule immunization at earliest return visit |
| Immediate, severe, anaphylactic reaction to previous administration of one of these vaccines | Hypersensitivity to some component in the vaccine may result in a severe reaction during reimmunization | Take a history of reactions to previous vaccines or a vaccine component, e.g., thimerosal |
| **PERTUSSIS** | | |
| Neurologic disorder, e.g., infantile spasms, uncontrolled epilepsy, or progressive encephalopathy, characterized by progressive developmental delay or changing neurologic findings | Danger of serious reaction to pertussis vaccination is possibly increased if any of these conditions are present when receiving the vaccine and may result in confusion about causation of neurologic findings | Take a detailed neurologic history including past convulsions, fainting spells, tremors, and specific reactions to DTP; report any such findings to practitioner before administering the vaccine |
| Personal (not family) history of convulsions | | |
| Have or suspected of having neurologic conditions, e.g., tuberous sclerosis, certain inherited metabolic or degenerative diseases that predispose to seizures or neurologic deterioration | | |
| Any of the following reactions *after* receiving pertussis vaccine: Encephalopathy within 7 days; a convulsion, with or without fever, occurring within 3 days; persistent, inconsolable screaming or crying for 3 or more hours or an unusual high-pitched cry within 48 hours; collapse or shocklike state within 48 hours; temperature of 40.5° C (104.9° F) or greater, unexplained by another cause, within 48 hours; an immediate severe or anaphylactic reaction to vaccine (extremely rare) | | |
| **MEASLES, MUMPS, AND RUBELLA (MMR); LIVE POLIO VIRUS (OPV)** | | |
| Febrile illness (Minor, nonfebrile illness is not a contraindication) | Signs and symptoms associated with the illness may be erroneously attributed to the vaccine | Explain reason for postponement and reschedule immunization at earliest return visit |
| Anaphylactic reaction to neomycin (Minor, delayed reaction of an erythematous pruritic papule after MMR inoculation is not a contraindication to a second dose) | Severe neomycin sensitivity can result in systemic anaphylactic reactions in allergic person receiving vaccine containing trace amounts of neomycin | Take a careful history of allergic reactions to neomycin<br>Report positive findings to practitioner before administering vaccine |
| Pregnancy (Live oral poliovirus vaccine may be given if substantial risk of exposure is present. Inactivated polio virus [IPV] is preferred if immunization can be completed before anticipated exposure) | Theoretic risk to fetus | Take careful history of all women of childbearing age for possibility of pregnancy or conception within next three months |
| Congenital disorders of immune function<br>Immunosuppressive therapy (except investigational varicella vaccine); may immunize 3 months after immunosuppressive therapy is discontinued | Depressed immune functions prevent antibody response to vaccines; fatal vaccine-associated infections can occur | Emphasize to family need to avoid child's exposure to these viral infections; stress importance of regular immune globulin therapy to provide passive protection in selected children |
| Children on steroid therapy are evaluated for the risk of live virus vaccines | Duration and dosage of steroids affect immune system differently | Advise family that household contacts should not receive oral poliovirus vaccine because the virus can be transmitted to the immunocompromised child |
| Children with symptomatic or asymptomatic human immunodeficiency virus (HIV) infection should receive all routine vaccine except oral poliovirus vaccine (Inactivated polio virus [IPV] can be given although its effectiveness may be reduced) | Reports of severity of actual infection are thought to outweigh potential risks from vaccines | |
| **MEASLES AND MUMPS** | | |
| Anaphylactic egg hypersensitivity (Milder forms of allergy to egg or chicken feathers are not a contraindication) | Severe egg hypersensitivity may result in systemic anaphylactic reactions in allergic person receiving vaccine containing trace amounts of egg antigens | Take a careful history of allergic reactions to egg<br>Report positive findings to practitioner before administering vaccine |

From Wong D and Whaley L: Clinical manual of pediatric nursing, ed 3, St Louis, 1990, The CV Mosby Co.

**TABLE A-3** Vaccine Types and Routes of Administration

| Vaccine* | Type | Route |
|---|---|---|
| DTP | Toxoids and inactivated bacteria | Intramuscular |
| *Haemophilus* b | Polysaccharide | Subcutaneous, intramusuclar |
| | Polysaccharide-protein conjugate (PRP-D) | Intramuscular |
| | Diphtheria $CRM_{197}$ protein conjugate (HbOC) | Intramuscular |
| Measles | Live virus | Subcutaneous |
| MMR | Live viruses | Subcutaneous |
| Mumps | Live virus | Subcutaneous |
| Poliomyelitis: | | |
| OPV | Live virus | Oral |
| IPV | Inactivated virus | Subcutaneous |
| Rubella | Live virus | Subcutaneous |
| Tetanus and Td, DT | Toxoids | Intramuscular |

*DTP = diphtheria and tetanus toxoids and pertussis vaccine; PRP-D = *Haemophilus* b diphtheria toxoid conjugate; IPV = Inactivated poliovirus vaccine; MMR = measles, mumps and rubella vaccine; OPV = oral poliovirus vaccine; Td = tetanus and diphtheria toxoid for adult (≥7 years old) use; DT = diphtheria and tetanus toxoids.
Adapted from Report of the Committee on Infectious Diseases, ed 21, 1988, Elk Grove Village, Ill, American Academy of Pediatrics.

## TIPS TO MINIMIZE IMMUNIZATION REACTIONS

1. Take a careful history before administration to determine possible contraindications/exceptions to giving the vaccine, e.g., reactions to previous vaccines or to components in the vaccine (see Table A-2). Report significant findings to the practitioner.
2. For vaccines intended for the intramuscular route, select a needle of adequate length to appropriately reach the muscle mass. For DTP injections, a 1-inch needle injected at a 45 degree angle to the long axis of the leg in the vastus lateralis muscle is preferred (Hicks et al, 1989). Subcutaneous injection of vaccine intended for intramuscular injection may increase the risk of local reaction (American Academy of Pediatrics, 1988).
3. Prophylactically administer acetaminophen before injection of DTP vaccine (Lewis, 1988). Recommend an age-appropriate dose of acetaminophen to be given every 4 to 6 hours for 2 days.
4. Suggest using a cold compress (washcloth, covered ice bag) on a red or tender injection site for short periods of time (5 to 10 minutes every 30 minutes), for about the first 24 hours. Then apply warm or cold compresses as needed.
5. Assess family members at risk from OPV because of partial or nonimmunized status, or immune deficiency state. Appropriately immunize child and/or family members (see box on Updates and Controversies Regarding Specific Vaccines on p. 810).
6. Reassure the family that many children have mild reactions that are temporary.
7. Advise family to contact practitioner immediately if severe reactions occur.

## REFERENCES

American Academy of Pediatrics: Report of the committee on infectious diseases, ed 21, Elk Grove, Ill, 1988, The American Academy of Pediatrics.

American Academy of Pediatrics: Measles: reassessment of the current immunization policy, AAP News 5(7):6-7, 1989.

American Academy of Pediatrics: *Haemophilus influenzae* type b conjugate vaccines: update, Pediatrics 84(2):386-387, 1989.

Campion J and Casto D: *Haemophilus influenzae* type b conjugate vaccine, J Pediatr Health Care, 2(4):215-217, 1988.

Change in administration schedule for *Haemophilus* b conjugate vaccine, JAMA, 263(18):2429, 1990.

Griffin MR: Risk of sudden infant death after DTP vaccination, N Engl J Med 319(9):618-623, 1988.

Griffin MR et al: Risk of seizures and encephalopathy after immunization with diphtheria–tetanus–pertussis vaccine, JAMA 263(12): 1641-1645, 1990.

Grimes D and Woolbert LF: Measles outbreaks: who are at risk and why, J Pediatr Health Care 3(4):187-193, 1989.

Hicks JF et al: Optimum needle length for diptheria-tetanus-pertussis inoculation of infants, Pediatrics 84(1):136-137, 1989.

Katz S: Controversies in immunization, Pediatr Infect Dis J 6(6):607-613, 1987.

Lewis J: Prophylactic acetaminophen administration with DTP vaccination, Am J Dis Child 142:62-65, 1988.

U.S. Centers for Disease Control: Morbidity and mortality weekly report, pp 49-52; 57 Feb 3, 1989.

Wong D and Whaley L: Clinical manual of pediatric nursing, ed 3, St Louis, 1990, The CV Mosby Co.

# APPENDIX B Relaxation Techniques

Deborah Kay Brantly

## Distraction

Distraction is a method of coping and relaxation that involves focusing attention on something other than the stressor. It is best used during a stress-producing event. Distraction can simply involve directing a child to focus on an object or a person with the use of gentle touch to help maintain the child's focus. Having a child count during a procedure is a distraction technique. A more complex distraction exercise requires the child to make up a story to tell himself or herself during the stressful event or to concentrate on a future event, e.g., going to the playroom afterwards. Distraction is a simple technique that can be modified to fit all age groups. The younger child may do best by screaming or looking at someone as a distraction. A younger child may also need more guidance than the older child who is better able to independently focus on an object or future event.

### Example/sample script

*Focusing on an object:*

Have the child select an object in the room, e.g., a spot on the wall, a picture, a door handle, or button. Be sure the child's view of the object will not be obstructed at any time, especially if this technique is being used during a procedure. Direct the child to concentrate on the object.

*Concentrating on future events:*

Ask the child what he or she would like to do after the stressful procedure. (Make sure the event will occur.) Direct the child to think about the event in great detail—what he or she will do, what it will be like, etc. The child can say, "In a little while this will be over and then I will . . ." anytime he or she feels an increase in stress. Suggested events include being back in the child's room, playing in the playroom, coloring, painting, eating ice cream, going shopping with parent, going for a walk, or playing in the park.

## Rhythmic Breathing

Rhythmic breathing produces relaxation by concentrating on one's own breathing pattern. The child is asked to breathe in a slow, rhythmic manner. It aids the relaxation process to repeat the word "relax" as the child exhales. Rhythmic breathing should be continued for at least 2 to 4 minutes to produce relaxation. (See Figs. B-1 and B-2 for correct relaxation postures.) Rhythmic breathing is used for children 4 years and older. Younger children, particularly, may need to repeat the word "relax" as they exhale.

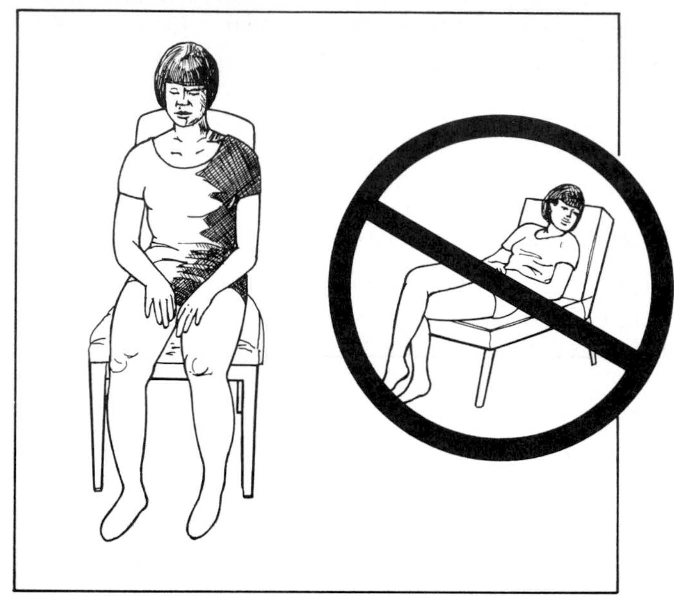

***FIG. B-1*** A balanced sitting position is conducive to relaxation.
Modified from DiMotto JW: Relax, Am J Nurs 84(6):754-758, 1984.

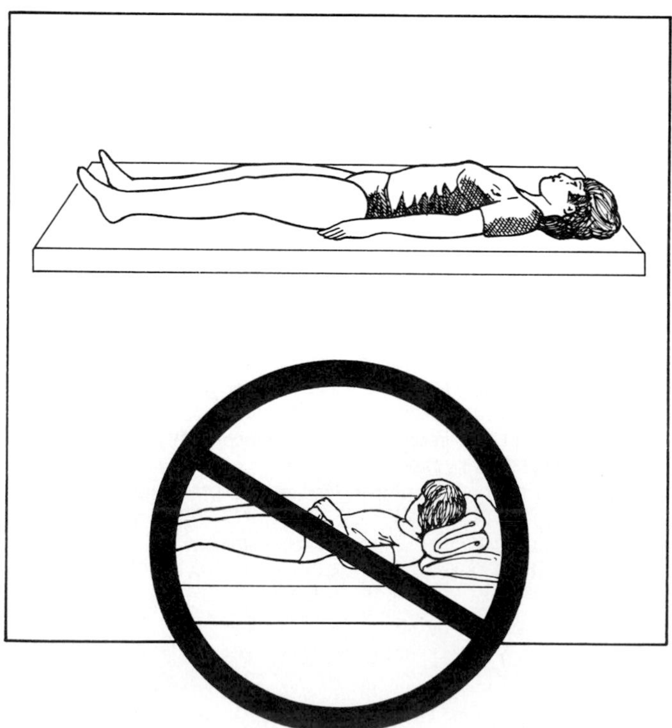

***FIG. B-2*** The child maintains alignment of head and spine when lying down to relax.
Modified from DiMotto JW: Relax, Am J Nurs 84(6):754-758, 1984.

***Example/sample script***

"Take one deep breath." (Pause) "As you lie there comfortably, pay attention to your breathing." (Pause 5 seconds) "Breathe normally and comfortably. Air goes in . . . air goes out." (Pause) "In 2, 3, and out 2, 3 . . ." Keep breathing like that. (Pause 5 seconds) "If you like, you can say the word 'relax' as you breathe out." (Pause 5 to 10 seconds) "Concentrate on your breathing." (Pause) "Breathe out the tension." (Pause) "Relax . . . Relax . . ." (Pause) "In 2, 3, and out 2, 3" (Pause) (Continue in this way until the child is virtually motionless except for breathing and seems relaxed.) "I'm going to count backwards from 3 and when I get to 1 you can open your eyes. Ready? 3-2-1."

## Progressive Muscle Relaxation

This method achieves relaxation through the focused concentration, then release, of tension in successive muscle groups. Adolescents are able to participate in more lengthy sessions and especially enjoy progressive muscle relaxation. However, shortened versions of the technique may be used with children as young as 5. Consider the child's attention span, tolerance of inactivity, and ability to follow commands when deciding on the appropriateness of this method. Many times progressive muscle relaxation is used in conjunction with other techniques. If the child wishes, background music or environmental sounds can be employed to enhance relaxation.

***Example/sample script***

"Lie back quietly." (Pause) "Take a deep breath and slowly let it out, releasing tension as you breathe out." (Pause 3 to 5 seconds) "Breathe normally and comfortably." (Pause 3 to 5 seconds) "Pay attention to your special feeling of relaxation." (Pause 5 seconds) "Clench your right fist." (Pause 3 to 5 seconds) "Now relax your right fist. Notice the difference between clenching and relaxing." (Pause 5 seconds) "Clench your right fist again, tight and hard." (Pause 3 to 5 seconds) "Now relax your right fist." (Pause 5 seconds) "Clench your left fist, as tight as you can." (Pause 3 to 5 seconds) "Now release your left fist and relax. Tense your left fist again." (Pause 3 to 5 seconds) "Now release your left fist." (Pause 5 seconds) "Now tense your right arm." (Pause 3 to 5 seconds) "Let go of the tension and relax." (Pause 5 seconds) "Tense your right arm again." (Pause 3 to 5 seconds) "Release your right arm and relax." (Pause 5 seconds) "Now your left arm. Tighten it hard." (Pause 3 to 5 seconds) "Release your left arm and relax. Tighten your left arm again." (Pause 5 seconds) "Release your left arm and relax." (Pause 5 seconds) "Now smile a big smile and wrinkle up your forehead." (Pause 3 to 5 seconds) "Relax your face." (Pause 5 seconds) "Smile again—as tight and big as you can." (Pause 3 to 5 seconds) "Now relax your smile and smooth out your forehead." (Pause 5 to 10 seconds) "Shrug up your shoulders, real hard." (Pause 5 seconds) "Now let go of the tension and relax your shoulders." (Pause 5 seconds) "Let the relaxation proceed as you feel your special feeling of relaxation." (Pause 5 seconds) "Shrug your shoulders again, up high." (Pause 5 seconds) "Now relax your shoulders and feel the difference relaxation can make." (Pause 10 seconds) "Take a deep breath now and hold it." (Pause 3 seconds) "Let it out and breathe normally." (Pause 5 seconds) "Again take a deep breath and hold it." (Pause 3 seconds) "Now slowly let it out. Again breathe normally and calmly." (Pause 5 seconds) "Relax your entire body as much as you can." (Pause 5 seconds) (Proceed in the same manner by directing the child to successively tense the abdomen, legs, and feet.) "You can become twice as relaxed as you are now. Notice any tension in your body and simply release it." (Pause 5 to 10 seconds) "Feel your special feeling of relaxation and concentrate on relaxing. You may feel heavy or you may feel light. Perhaps you feel limp, like a rag doll, or maybe even warm." (Pause 5 to 10 seconds) "Forehead smooth, jaw relaxed, neck and shoulders relaxed." (Pause 5 seconds) "Let the relaxation proceed." (Pause 5 to 10 seconds) "Right hand relaxed, right arm relaxed, left hand relaxed, left arm relaxed." (Pause 5 to 10 seconds) "Breathing is calm and easy, abdomen relaxed." (Pause 5 seconds) "Right leg relaxed and left leg relaxed." (Pause 5 to 10 seconds) "Deeper and deeper relaxation." (Pause 5 seconds) "When you are perfectly relaxed you are unwilling to move a single muscle." (Pause 5 to 10 seconds) "Relax." (Pause 10 seconds) "I am going to count backwards from 5. When I get to 1 you will open your eyes and feel relaxed and refreshed." (Pause 5 seconds) "5-4-3-2-1."

## Imagery and Visualization

Imagery and visualization involve focusing on mental images. It "is an extension of everyday thought processes like daydreaming. It is the use of one's imagination, rather than the focusing on existing stimuli (distraction)" (Hockenberry and Bologna-Vaughan, 1985). Imagery and visualization are used in many ways. Imagery usually involves the child imagining himself or herself in a different place or scene that is pleasant. It can also involve substituting an image for a sensation, e.g., pain. Imagery can be useful in many situations, e.g., it can offer the child with a chronic condition the opportunity to "experience" a prohibited activity. Imagery can transport the hospitalized child to a safer place where he or she is cared for by family and friends. For the child with cancer, it can serve to reduce stress and increase comfort, thus mobilizing immunologic support in fighting the disease (Hall, 1982-83). Visualization uses images that are more task-oriented, e.g., the child visualizes going through a painful procedure successfully or the person with a disability learns a new self-care technique (Coburn and Manderino, 1986). During the imaging procedure, it is acceptable for the child to relate what he or she is imaging and for the nurse to ask about the image and the child's feelings. Because the images are created by the child, it is important to respond spontaneously to the images and to explore their meaning. Often a child's fears and anxieties are revealed during imagery, and the imagery experience allows the child to mentally master a stressful situation.

Imagery is useful for all ages. It is a highly participative technique. In the younger child, it captivates his or her fantasy world and gives it structure. The younger child may tend to talk more than needed, giving details that seem to be unrelated. Continue to explore the image and the child's feelings. Frequently it serves as a metaphor for the child's experience.

#### *Example/sample script*

*Imagery:*

"Now just settle down comfortably and quietly. Imagine yourself somewhere you really enjoy." (Pause 3 seconds) "Now with that place in your mind, look around and see what's around you." (Pause 3 seconds) "What do you see?" (Pause while the child relates image) "Is there anything else in your view?" (Pause while child responds) "Just stay there enjoying it for a while." (Pause 5 to 10 seconds) "What does it feel like there?" (Pause while child relates feelings) "Anything else?" (Pause while child responds) "Is there anything else noticeable about your special place?" (Pause as child responds) "Enjoy your special place a little while longer before you leave." (Pause 10 to 15 seconds) "All right, now, it's time to leave. See yourself coming out. How are you leaving? Walking? Flying? Floating? (Pause as child responds) "When you're completely out, open your eyes."

*Visualization:*

Using a procedure similar to imagery, help the child to visualize mastering a difficult situation, e.g., going through a procedure successfully.

### Music and Environmental Sounds

Music or environmental sounds can be used alone or may be combined with other stress-reducing techniques to promote relaxation. Music should be played softly and deemed restful. Classical music "is most conducive to relaxation because its rhythms and harmonic structures are often perceived as soothing" (DiMotto, 1984). Instrumental music is most restful because it allows the mind to wander. Environmental sounds are usually tape recordings of sounds in nature, e.g., streams, ocean, rain, and wind. Music and environmental sounds can be used for children 4 years of age and older. When planning such sessions be sure to adjust the length of time to the child's developmental level. The younger child may need prompting from an adult, e.g., "What do you hear in the music? Close your eyes and concentrate."

### REFERENCES

Coburn J and Manderino M: Stress inoculation: an illustration of coping skills training, Rehab Nurs 11(1):14-17, 1986.

DiMotto JW: Relax, Am J Nurs 84(6):754-758, 1984.

Hall M: Using relaxation imagery with children with malignancies: a developmental perspective, Am J Clin Hypn 25(2-3):143-149, 1982-1983.

Hockenberry M and Bologna-Vaughan S: Preparation for intrusive procedures using noninvasive techniques in children with cancer: state of the art vs new trends. Can Nurs 8(2):97-102, 1985.

# APPENDIX C Calculating Safe Dosages for Children

*Kristie S. Nix*

The two most frequently used methods of calculating safe doses are based on weight or body surface area. These two methods should be used whenever possible as they are more reliable than other techniques, e.g., Clark's rule or Young's rule, which should be used only to verify doses when recommendations based on weight or body surface area are unavailable.

## Dose Based on Weight in Kilograms

***Steps***

1. If necessary, convert child's weight in pounds to kilograms.
2. Review medication reference to determine recommended safe range in milligrams/kilogram (mg/kg).
3. Multiply child's weight by the lower and upper limits of the dose range.
4. Compare physician's order with dose range to determine if medication dose is safe.
5. Doses outside recommended range should be verified with physician.

***Example***

Child weighs 22 pounds.
Conversion: 1 kg = 2.2 lb
22 ÷ 2.2 = 10 kg
Reference text states recommended dose range is 30 to 50 mg/kg/day in 4 divided doses.
10 kg × 30 = 300 mg/day
10 kg × 50 = 500 mg/day
Child's range = 300 to 500 mg/day
Order reads: Give 100 mg q6h.
100 mg given q6h = 100 × 4 = 400 mg/day
Conclusion: Dose falls in safe range.

## Dose Based on Body Surface Area (BSA)

***Steps***

1. Obtain child's height and weight measurements.
2. Use nomogram (Fig. C-1) to determine child's BSA ($m^2$):
   a. Find and mark child's height on left column, weight on right column.
   b. Place a ruler between the two measurements and connect with a line.
   c. Find BSA in the middle column.
3. Review medication reference to determine recommended child dose: multiply BSA by recommended $mg/m^2$
4. If child's recommended dose in $mg/m^2$ is not given, adult dose may be used for calculation:
   a. Divide child's BSA by 1.73 ("normal" adult BSA).
   b. Multiply result by recommended adult dose.
5. Prescribed dose which differs from calculation should be verified with physician.

***Example***

Child is 80 cm tall and weighs 12 kg.

Mark 80 cm on the left, 12 kg on the right: join with a straight edge (Fig. C-1).

BSA = 0.53 $m^2$
Reference states child dose = 50 $mg/m^2$
50 mg × 0.53 = 26.5 mg

Reference text recommends adult dose only:
500 mg daily
0.53 ÷ 1.73 = .31
500 mg × .31 = 155 mg daily for this child

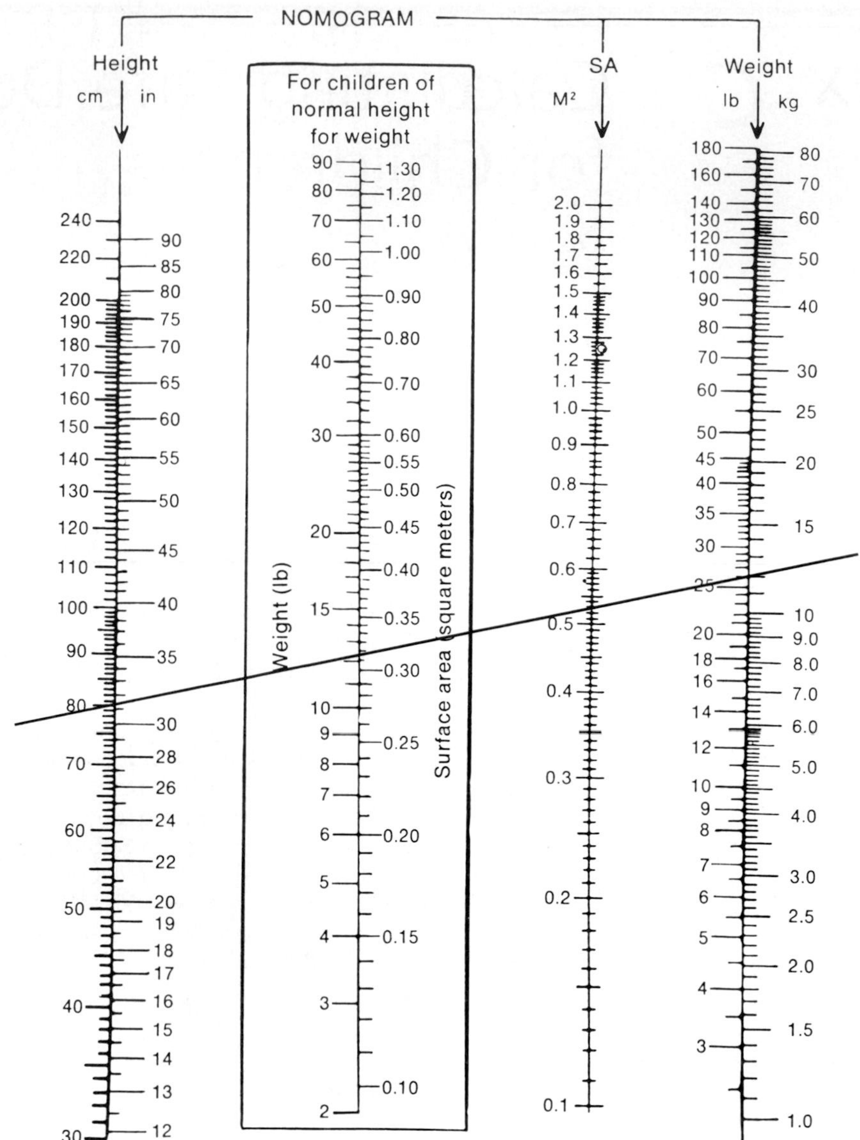


***FIG. C-1*** West nomogram (for estimation of surface areas). Surface area is indicated where straight line connecting height and weight intersects surface area (SA) column or, if patient is roughly of normal proportion, from weight alone (enclosed area).

Modified from data of Boyd E by West CD; from Behr RE and Vaughan VC, editors: Nelson textbook of pediatrics, ed 12, Philadelphia, 1983, WB Saunders Co.

# APPENDIX D Intravenous Infusion Solutions Commonly Used in Children

*Kristie S. Nix*

| Description | Approx. pH | mOs/L | Caloric value/L | mEq L Na | K | Ca | Cl | Other | Indications | Potential complications |
|---|---|---|---|---|---|---|---|---|---|---|
| **CARBOHYDRATES IN SODIUM CHLORIDE** | | | | | | | | | | |
| Dextrose 5% in NaCl 0.2% | 4.3 | 320 | 170 | 34 | | | 34 | | Daily maintenance of fluids, sodium, and chloride; Rehydration; Establish renal function; Maintenance carbohydrates | |
| Dextrose 5% in NaCl 0.3% | 4.3 | 365 | 170 | 56 | | | 56 | | | |
| Dextrose 5% in NaCl 0.45% | 4.3 | 405 | 170 | 77 | | | 77 | | | |
| Dextrose 5% in NaCl 0.2% with 20 mEq KCl/L | 4.2 | 360 | 170 | 34 | 20 | | 34 | | Potassium maintenance (with KCl additive) | Hyperkalemia |
| **SODIUM CHLORIDE SOLUTIONS** | | | | | | | | | | |
| NaCl 0.45% | 4.8 | 154 | | 77 | | | 77 | | Na and Cl replacement; Restore intravascular volume in shock; Metabolic alkalosis; Marked electrolyte imbalance; Initiate and terminate blood transfusion (0.9%) | Hypernatremia; Acidosis; Hypokalemia; Intravascular volume excess |
| NaCl 0.9% | 4.8 | 308 | | 154 | | | 154 | | | |
| **ELECTROLYTE SOLUTIONS** | | | | | | | | | | |
| Ringer's Lactate | 6.3 | 273 | 9 | 130 | 4 | 3 | 109 | Lact. 28 | Volume replacement, e.g., mild acidosis, burns, surgical losses; Multiple electrolyte replacement | Intravascular volume excess |
| Dextrose 5% in Ringer's Lactate | 5.0 | 525 | 170 | 130 | 4 | 3 | 109 | Lact. 28 | | |
| Ringer's | 6.0 | 309 | | 147 | 4 | 4 | 155 | | | |
| Normosol M in Dextrose 5% in water | 5.2 | 368 | 170 | 40 | 13 | | 40 | Mg. 3 Acet. 16 | Multiple electrolyte replacement; Rehydration | |
| Plasmalyte M in Dextrose 5% | 5.0 | 376 | 170 | 40 | 16 | 5 | 40 | Mg. 3 Acet. 12 Lact. 23 | | |
| **CARBOHYDRATES IN WATER** | | | | | | | | | | |
| Dextrose 5% in Water | 5.0 | 253 | 170 | | | | | | Vehicle for drug administration (D5W); Rehydration (rarely used with infants); Temporary replacement for hyperalimentation or medication incompatible with hyperalimentation; Hypernatremia | Water intoxication; Osmotic diuresis; Hyperinsulinism; Hypokalemia |
| Dextrose 10% in Water | 4.6 | 505 | 340 | | | | | | | |

Adapted from Trissel LA: ASHP handbook on injectable drugs, ed 5; Bethesda, MD, 1988, American Society of Hospital Pharmacists, Inc.
Slight manufacturer variations in composition from Table values.

# Index

## T

## U



## V



## W



## X



## Z